T0295055

VETERINARY HERBAL MEDICINE

VETERINARY
HERBAL MEDICINE

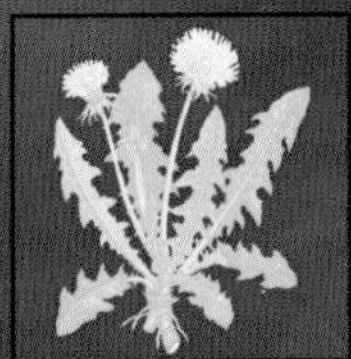

Susan G. Wynn, DVM, RH (AHG)
Bell's Ferry Veterinary Hospital
Acworth, Georgia
Adjunct Faculty, College of Veterinary Medicine
University of Georgia
Athens, Georgia

Barbara J. Fougère, BSc, BVMS(Hons),
MODT, BHSc(Comp Med), CVA(IVAS),
CVCP, CV Herb Med, MHSc(Herb Med) Enr
All Natural Vet Care
Sydney, Australia

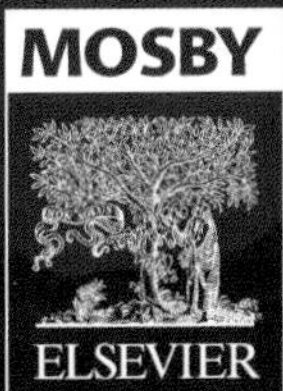

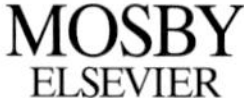

MOSBY
ELSEVIER

11830 Westline Industrial Drive
St. Louis, Missouri 63146

VETERINARY HERBAL MEDICINE

ISBN-13: 978-0323-02998-8
ISBN-10: 0-323-02998-1

Notice

Knowledge and best practice in this field are constantly changing. As new research and experience broaden our knowledge, changes in practice, treatment, and drug therapy may become necessary or appropriate. Readers are advised to check the most current information provided (i) on procedures featured or (ii) by the manufacturer of each product to be administered, to verify the recommended dose or formula, the method and duration of administration, and contraindications. It is the responsibility of practitioners, relying on their own experience and knowledge of the patient, to make diagnoses, to determine dosages and the best treatment for each individual patient, and to take all appropriate safety precautions. To the fullest extent of the law, neither the Publisher nor the Authors assumes any liability for any injury and/or damage to persons or property arising out of or related to any use of the material contained in this book.

The Publisher

Library of Congress Cataloging-in-Publication Data

Veterinary herbal medicine / [edited by] Susan G. Wynn, Barbara J. Fougère.
p. ; cm.
Includes bibliographical references and index.
ISBN-13: 978-0-323-02998-8
ISBN-10: 0-323-02998-1
1. Alternative veterinary medicine. 2. Herbs—Therapeutic use. I. Wynn, Susan G. II. Fougère, Barbara.
[DNLM: 1. Phytotherapy—veterinary. 2. Veterinary Medicine–methods. 3. Medicine, Herbal–methods. SF 745.5 V586 2007]
SF745.5.V4844 2007
636.089′5321—dc22

2006047201

Publishing Director: Linda Duncan
Publisher: Penny Rudolph
Developmental Editor: Shelly Stringer
Publishing Services Manager: Pat Joiner
Senior Project Manager: Karen M. Rehwinkel
Senior Designer: Jyotika Shroff

Printed in India

Last digit is the print number: 19 18 17 16 15 14 13

Contributors

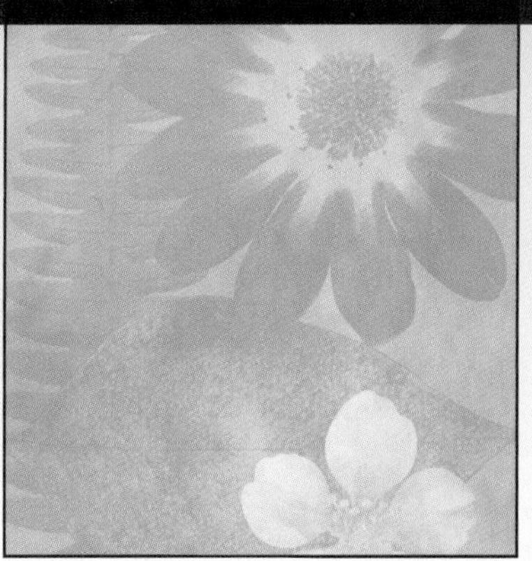

James Martin Affolter, PhD (Botany)
Professor
University of Georgia Department of Horticulture;
Director of Research
State Botanical Garden of Georgia
University of Georgia
Athens, Georgia

Chapter 17: Conserving Medicinal Plant Biodiversity

Kerry Martin Bone, BSc (Hons); Dip Phyt (Diploma in Phytotherapy)
Adjunct Associate Professor
School of Health
University of New England
Armidale, New South Wales, Australia;
Director of Research
Research & Development
MediHerb Pty Ltd
Warwick, Queensland, Australia

Chapter 7: Evaluating, Designing, and Accessing Herbal Medicine Research

William Bookout, BS, MBA
President, Genesis Limited;
President, National Animal Supplement Council
Valley Center, California

Chapter 8: Regulation and Quality Control

Marina Martin Curran, BSc (Hons), MSc
School of GeoSciences
University of Edinburgh
United Kingdom

Chapter 3: Ethnoveterinary Medicine: Potential Solutions for Large-Scale Problems?

Cindy Engel, PhD, MRSS
Lecturer, Open University
Clover Forge Farm
Suffolk, United Kingdom

Chapter 2: Zoopharmacognosy

Terrence S. Fox, BS (Hon), MS, PhD
Buck Mountain Botanicals
Miles City, Montana

Chapter 16: Commercial Production of Organic Herbs for Veterinary Medicine

Joyce C. Harman, DVM, MRCVS
Harmany Equine Clinic, Ltd
Washington, Virginia

Chapter 21: Herbal Medicine in Equine Practice

Hubert J. Karreman, VMD
Penn Dutch Cow Care
Quarryville, Pennsylvania

Chapter 22: Phytotherapy for Dairy Cows

Linda B. Khachatoorian, RVT
Product Manager
Genesis Limited
Valley Center, California

Chapter 8: Regulation and Quality Control

Tonya E. Khan, DVM, BSc
Veterinarian
Mosquito Creek Veterinary Hospital
North Vancouver, British Columbia, Canada

Chapter 3: Ethnoveterinary Medicine: Potential Solutions for Large-Scale Problems?

Robyn Klein, RH (AHG), MS, Medical Botanist
Adjunct Professor
Department of Plant Sciences
Montana State University
Bozeman, Montana

Chapter 10: Medical Botany

Cheryl Lans, MSc, PhD
Postdoctoral Scholar
Department of Sociology
University of Victoria
Victoria, British Columbia, Canada

Chapter 3: Ethnoveterinary Medicine: Potential Solutions for Large-Scale Problems?

Steven Paul Marsden, DVM, ND, MSOM, LAc, Dipl. Chinese Herbology, RH(AHG)
Instructor
International Veterinary Acupuncture Society
Fort Collins, Colorado;
Member, Board of Directors
National College of Naturopathic Medicine
Portland, Oregon;
Co-founder, Edmonton Holistic Veterinary Clinic
Edmonton, Alberta, Canada;
The Natural Path Clinic
Edmonton, Alberta, Canada

Chapter 5: Overview of Traditional Chinese Medicine: The Cooking Pot Analogy

Chapter 13: Herbal Energetics: A Key to Efficacy in Herbal Medicine

Constance M. McCorkle, PhD
Senior Research Scientist and President
CMC Consulting
Falls Church, Virginia;
Graduate Faculty Member
University of Fairfax
Vienna, Virginia

Chapter 3: Ethnoveterinary Medicine: Potential Solutions for Large-Scale Problems?

Andrew Pengelly, DBM, ND, BA, FNHAA
Program Convener and Lecturer in Herbal Therapies
School of Applied Sciences
University of Newcastle
New South Wales, Australia

Chapter 17: Conserving Medicinal Plant Biodiversity

Robert H. Poppenga, DVM, PhD, Diplomate, American Board of Veterinary Toxicology
Professor of Clinical and Diagnostic Veterinary Toxicology
California Animal Health and Food Safety Laboratory System
University of California School of Veterinary Medicine
Davis, California

Chapter 12: Herbal Medicine: Potential for Intoxication and Interactions With Conventional Drugs

David W. Ramey, DVM
Ramey Equine
Calabasas, California;
Adjunct Faculty
College of Veterinary Medicine and Biomedical Sciences
Colorado State University
Fort Collins, Colorado

Chapter 9: A Skeptical View of Herbal Medicine

Robert J. Silver, DVM, MS
Boulder's Natural Animal: An Integrative Wellness Center
Boulder, Colorado

Chapter 6: Ayurvedic Veterinary Medicine: Principles and Practices

Eric Yarnell, ND, RH(AHG)
President, Botanical Medicine Academy
Seattle, Washington;
Adjunct Faculty
Department of Botanical Medicine
Bastyr University;
Adjunct Faculty
Herbal Healing Program
Tai Sofia Institute;
Visiting Professor
Pochon CHA University
Seoul, Korea;
Chief Financial Officer,
Healing Mountain Publishing, Inc.;
Vice President, Heron Botanicals, Inc.
Seattle, Washington

Chapter 11: Plant Chemistry in Veterinary Medicine: Medicinal Constituents and Their Mechanisms of Action

Ellen Zimmerman, MA
Austin School of Herbal Studies
Austin, Texas

Chapter 15: Designing the Medicinal Herb Garden

Preface

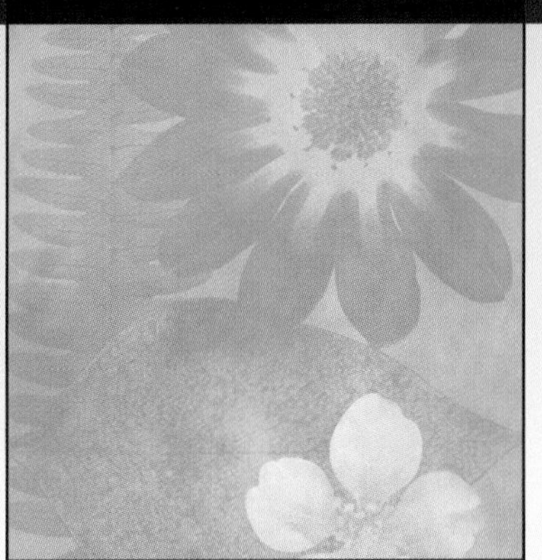

Consumers of medicine and veterinary medicine have shown that they desire a variety of medical approaches. Herbal medicine just can't seem to die, and has persisted no thanks to us veterinarians—our clients and nonveterinary herbalists have kept it alive. Skeptics have mourned the loss of medical independence, and have argued that medical research and practice should not be beholden to public opinion. In fact, the last hundred years of medical trajectory is the result of the Flexner report, which aimed to shut down sectarian medicine. Flexner's sponsor, the Carnegie Foundation, believed that medical education should not be independent and commercialized, but that it in fact should answer to public and charitable interests (Hiatt, 1999). People want herbal medicine. This is our attempt to help veterinarians explore and begin to offer it.

We recognize that challenges still exist. It may be some time until we clearly understand how herbs and drugs interact. Standardization is a contentious issue, recommended by researchers and resisted by herbalists. In our view, herbal medicine is unique among medical specialties in that we are guided by the past, whereas most of medicine is inspired by new and untested remedies. Still, we support research that clarifies these issues, and our hope is that researchers in this field will recognize the expertise and experience of herbalists already active in clinical investigations of their tools.

With this book, we hope that we can contribute to the re-emergence of the art of veterinary herbal medicine.

Acknowledgments

This book is the result of collaboration between extraordinary experts in a variety of fields. By bringing them together, we hope we have presented a new picture of herbal medicine to the veterinary profession. We could not have done it without our authors, and we have also relied upon reviewers to survey the information for errors. We thank Joni Freshman, Patricia Kyritsi Howell, Beth Lambert, Sherry Sanderson, Roy Upton, David Winston, and Eric Yarnell for previewing some of the chapters for accuracy. Any errors that remain belong to us and should not reflect on their work.

Of course, we stand on the shoulders of giants, and the resources of herbalists who come before us have been invaluable. We would like to especially thank Henriette Kress, Michael Moore, Paul Bergner, David Winston, Michael Tierra, James Duke, Daniel Moerman, Kerry Bone, Simon Mills, Berris Burgoyne, and many more who have shared their knowledge in books and on their websites, as well as the authors of the many ethnomedical, scientific herbals, and antiquarian veterinary texts, too many to be named, in our libraries.

We also acknowledge the tireless efforts of our editors, in particular Shelly Stringer and Karen Rehwinkel. Many thanks to our family and friends, who waited patiently for us to finish so that we could regain our free time.

Susan Wynn would particularly like to thank her parents, Jack and Linda Wynn, her students, her coworkers at Bell's Ferry Veterinary Hospital, and finally, Barbara Fougère, for their heartening reassurances about this project.

A special thanks from Barbara Fougère to Lyndy Scott and Karl Walls for your support and encouragement. And to Susan Wynn, its been a real pleasure—a challenging, stimulating, and very exciting journey working with you. Thank you.

Together we would also like to especially acknowledge the many animals who have given their lives for the sake of scientific research. If, in the evidence-based medicine scheme, their sacrifices are meaningless to our patients, we are the poorer for it.

Contents

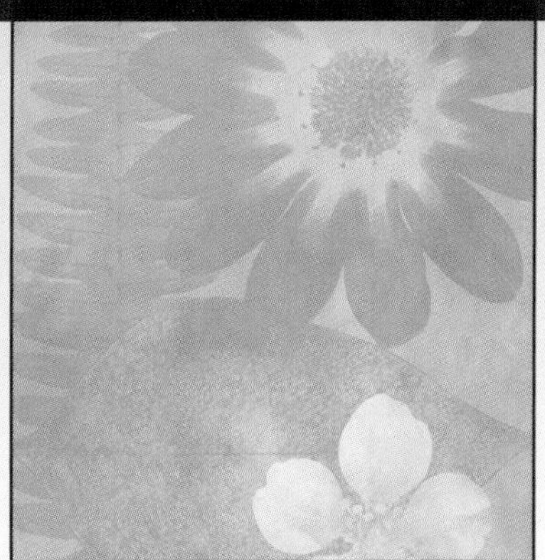

VETERINARY
HERBAL MEDICINE

Introduction: Why Use Herbs?

Susan G. Wynn and Barbara J. Fougère

CHAPTER 1

"Plants are nature's alchemists, expert at transforming water, soil, and sunlight into an array of precious substances, many of them beyond the ability of human beings to conceive, much less manufacture. While we were nailing down consciousness and learning to walk on two feet, they were, by the same process of natural selection, inventing photosynthesis (the astonishing trick of converting sunlight into food) and perfecting organic chemistry. As it turns out, many of the plants' discoveries in chemistry and physics have served us well. From plants come chemical compounds that nourish and heal and poison and delight the senses, others that rouse and put to sleep and intoxicate, and a few with the astounding power to alter consciousness—even to plant dreams in the brains of awake humans."

Botany of Desire, Michael Pollan

Herbal medicine represents a synthesis of many fields—botany, history, ethnomedicine, and pharmacology. Embarking on the study of this field means that veterinarians will be required to reframe the way they think about medicine. Many challenges await us. We are asked to consider plants we learned in toxicology as useful medicines. We are told, in the age of evidence-based medicine, that old authorities (some who lived as long as 2000 years ago) still have something to teach us. Our knowledge about these medicines comes from plant scientists, food scientists, pharmacologists, lay herbalists, and farmers—and we are asked to respect them as equal partners in herbal education and discovery. Even as we become comfortable and familiar with these plants, we are told that we won't be able to use them unless we become active in conservation efforts. Herbal medicine asks a lot but gives the practitioner more in return.

Why use an herb when we have available to us established, effective treatments for so many medical conditions? Most herbalists would answer this way: When conventional treatments are both safe and effective, they should be used. Unfortunately, that isn't the case for many serious chronic medical conditions—chronicity is virtually defined by the fact that medicine isn't working. Herbs represent an additional tool for the toolbox. For some, the fact that animals have been thought to treat themselves using herbs is reason enough to try them. For some herbalists, herbs also represent a different approach to the practice of medicine, that is, using the complex formulas "developed" by plants over millennia in relationship with the rest of the beings on the planet. These combinations of chemicals nourish, heal, and kill, but by using rational combinations in the practice of medicine, herbalists believe they attain longer lasting, more profound improvements (Box 1-1).

HERBS ARE NOT SIMPLY "UNREFINED DRUGS"

Complex Drugs With Complex Actions

Plants may contain many dozens of chemical constituents. Some of these have pharmacologically unique and powerful activity and have been tapped by the drug industry to develop new pharmaceuticals. However, the other ingredients in plants may have important activity as well. Consider, for example, the vitamins, minerals, flavonoids, carotenoids, sugars, and amino acids contained in a plant—do these assist effector cells in mounting the physiologic response initiated by the "drug"? And do constituents with lesser pharmaceutical activity than the one "recognized" active constituent play any role?

These complex drugs offer the sick patient a greater range of effects. Because there are many conditions for which the etiopathogenesis is unknown, providing the patient with a choice of biochemical solutions makes sense. Take, for example, Saint John's Wort for depression, as compared with paroxetine or sertraline.

The "active constituents" of Saint John's Wort and their studied actions include the following (Butterweck, 2003; Simmen, 2001):

- Amentoflavone: inhibits binding at serotonin (5-HT)(1D), 5-HT(2C), D(3) dopamine, delta opiate, and benzodiazepine receptors
- I3, II8-biapigenin: inhibits binding at estrogen–alpha receptor, benzodiazepine receptors
- Quercitrin, isoquercitrin, hyperoside, rutin, quercetin, amentoflavone, and kaempferol inhibit dopamine beta-hydroxylase
- Hypericin: binds D(3) and D(4) dopamine receptors, beta-adrenergic receptors, human corticotrophin-releasing factor (CRF1) receptor, sigma receptors, and

NPY Y1 receptors; inhibits activation of *N*-methyl-D-aspartate (NMDA) receptors

- Hyperforin: binds D(1) and, to a lesser extent, other dopamine receptors, 5-HT, opiate, benzodiazepine, and beta-adrenergic receptors; inhibits Na-dependent catecholamine uptake at nerve endings; inhibits high-affinity choline uptake; inhibits neuronal uptake of serotonin, norepinephrine, dopamine, gamma-aminobutyric acid (GABA), and L-glutamate through mechanisms different from synthetic selective serotonin reuptake inhibitors (SSRIs) (more reminiscent of tricyclic antidepressants [TCAs]); affects cell membrane fluidity; and enhances glutamate, aspartate, and GABA release
- Hyperin: decreases malondialdehyde and nitric oxide levels in injury model; decreases Ca influx in brain cells
- Pseudohypericin: inhibits activation of NMDA receptors

BOX 1-1

Reasons Whole Herbs Are Preferred to Isolated Active Constituents

- The whole herb or whole extract is already understood from history and clinical trials.
- The herb's constituents have complex actions that may benefit the patient through additive, antagonistic, or synergistic effects.
- Some constituents may not be stable when isolated.
- Most active constituents may be unknown.

Receptor Activity: Saint John's Wort Constituents

	5-HT	5-HT (1D)	5-HT (2C)	D(1) Dopamine	D(3) Dopamine	D(4) Dopamine	Delta Opiate	Benzodiazepine	Estrogen Alpha	Beta-adrenergic	Sigma	NPY Y1	NMDA	CRF1
Amentoflavone		✓	✓		✓		✓	✓						
12, II8-Biapigenin								✓	✓					
Hypericin					✓	✓				✓	✓	✓	✓	✓
Hyperforin	✓			✓	✓	✓	✓	✓		✓				
Pseudohypericin													✓	

5-HT, serotonin; NMDA, *N*-methyl-D-aspartate; CRF, corticotrophin-releasing factor.

Uptake Effects: Saint John's Wort Constituents

	Na-dependent Catecholamine Uptake	Inhibit High-affinity Choline Uptake	Inhibit Low-affinity Choline Uptake	Serotonin	Norepinephrine	Dopamine	GABA	L-glutamate
Hyperforin	✓	✓	✗	✓	✓	✓	✓	✓

GABA, gamma-aminobutyric acid.

Other Effects: Saint John's Wort Constituents

	Dopamine Beta-hydroxylase	Change Membrane Fluidity	GABA Release	Aspartate Release	Glutamate Release	Malondialdehyde Levels	Nitric Oxide Levels	Decrease Neuronal Calcium Influx
Quercitrin	✓							
Isoquercitrin	✓							
Rutin	✓							
Quercetin	✓							
Kaempferol	✓							
Hyperoside	✓							
Hyperforin		✓	✓	✓	✓			
Hyperin						✓	✓	✓

GABA, gamma-aminobutyric acid.

Paroxetine is a pure SSRI; sertraline is an SSRI that binds beta-adrenergic receptors. These are much more defined actions, as would be the action of many of the single constituents of Saint John's Wort. Treatment of patients with depression may require trial and error drug treatment, and the first drug prescribed is often ineffective. Offering a plant drug with multiple actions gives the body a multitude of possible solutions at one time.

As a whole, Saint John's Wort cannot be compared with any known drug. When asked which is the single active ingredient of any herb, the drumbeat of the herbalist will always be: **The Plant Is the Active Constituent!**

Synergy

The chemical compounds in plant medicines may have additive, antagonistic, or synergistic effects. For instance, foxglove is less toxic than its active ingredient digoxin because the digoxin is diluted out by other plant constituents, some of which may antagonize its action. Additive effects are fairly easily quantified when the individual chemicals are well defined. Synergistic effects are more difficult to quantify and are the subject of some investigation into the effects of plants.

Synergy between plant components may take pharmacodynamic forms or pharmacokinetic forms. In pharmacokinetic synergy, one component may enhance intestinal absorption or utilization of another component. Pharmacodynamic synergy occurs when two compounds interact with a single target or system. Not all of these interactions fit the strictest physicochemical definition of synergy, and Williamson (2000) has suggested that these should be called *polyvalent* actions of plant medicines.

Barberry *(Berberis aquifolium)* contains berberine, an alkaloid with documented antigiardial, antiviral, and antifungal properties. It is also an anti-inflammatory and has been shown to modulate prostaglandin levels in renal and cardiovascular disease. Herbalists have long used berberine-containing plants (which also include Goldthread *[Coptis* spp*]* and Goldenseal) for treating patients with infection. Use of the single drug berberine may lead to antibacterial resistance, although herbalists appear to use the whole plants repeatedly with no ill effects. One group asked the question, "Why don't bacteria easily develop resistance to berberine-containing plants?" Stermitz et al screened barberry plants for known multiple drug resistance inhibitors and found one—5-methoxyhydnocarpin (Stermitz, 2000). A seemingly unimportant constituent contained in barberry may synergistically enhance the effectiveness of the berberine it contains.

Other examples of purported synergism may be seen in plant medicines. Wormwood *(Artemisia annua)* is the source of the antimalarial compound, artemisinin. The flavonoids contained in the plant apparently enhance the antimalarial activity of this compound in vitro (Phillipson, 1999). Similar types of activity have been determined for compounds found in kava, valerian, dragon's blood *(Croton draconoides)*, and licorice (Williamson, 2000).

HERBAL PRESCRIPTIONS ARE INDIVIDUALIZED FOR EACH PATIENT

Herbal Simples and Specifics

In earlier times, a single herb that was appropriate for a particular condition was called a *simple*. For example, use of cranberry for a urinary tract infection is a simple prescription. Simple prescriptions allow new practitioners to learn about individual herbs thoroughly, one at a time, before taking the next step to formula design.

Some American eclectic practitioners (specifically, John M. Scudder, MD) taught that herbs have specific indications for use. According to this system of specific diagnosis and specific treatment, single herbs were recommended for a particular condition or diagnosis with associated symptoms. For example, quite a few herbs are appropriate for diarrhea (as there are drugs for diarrhea). Some herbs are considered astringents; others are demulcents. Some come with the accompanying features of soothing the respiratory tract or the skin as part of their therapeutic spectrum. A *specific* is chosen with the patient's overall health or disease picture in mind, when the herbalist possesses this depth of knowledge. Specific prescriptions reflect the growing popularity of homeopathy during the 19th century, and the herb symptom picture descriptions in John Scudder's specific medication are superficially similar to homeopathic symptom pictures (Table 1-1).

Herbal Formulas

In herbal medicine, polypharmacy is de rigueur; herbalists try to anticipate and treat associated problems and possible adverse effects of treatment in a proactive way. An herbal formula may provide the following for any individual patient:

1. One or more herbs that provide multiple mechanisms by which the major sign or complaint can be resolved
2. If these herbs do not fit the specific picture of the patient, the formula may provide herbs to reduce adverse effects or support other signs
3. Herbs that support other signs or systems in need

Formula design can be complicated or simple, and more information on this process can be found in Chapter 19, Approaches in Veterinary Herbal Medicine Prescribing.

HERBS OFFER A DIFFERENT APPROACH TO CHRONIC DISEASE

The diseases that dominate human medicine are different today from the ones described 100 or 1000 years ago. Animal health and disease have changed in sometimes similar ways; we currently have good treatment options for patients with bacterial and parasitic diseases, for instance, but we face challenges with cancer and allergic and degenerative diseases. For this, if for no other reason, the traditions of herbal medicine deserve another look.

Conventional pharmacology currently has no place for considering alteratives, tonics, and adaptogens—these represent just some of the activities that are possibly

TABLE 1-1

Specific Medication: Comparison of Cough Remedies

Herb	Action Against Cough	Other Indications for the Herb	Other Characteristics of the Herb
Licorice	Demulcent, antispasmodic, anti-inflammatory	Urinary tract inflammation, intestinal spasm	Suppresses cortisol breakdown; do not use in patients with hyperadrenocorticism
Elecampane	Aromatic stimulant and tonic	Digestive weakness	Very safe herb
Slippery elm	Demulcent	Chronic digestive disorders	Very safe herb
Lobelia	Nauseant, emetic, expectorant, relaxant, antispasmodic, diaphoretic, sialagogue, sedative; secondarily, occasionally cathartic, diuretic, and astringent	Formerly, for spasmodic problems from muscular tetany to seizures	Very strong herb—effective at low doses
Thyme	Tonic, carminative, emmenagogue, and antispasmodic	Flatulence, colic, headache	Safe herb in culinary doses

unique to plant medicines. Adaptogens, for instance, increase nonspecific responses to stress, usually without adverse effects and are often taken for long periods. Alteratives were formerly considered (among other things) blood cleansers, but today, we view alteratives as herbs that restore or correct absorptive and excretory functions.

The traditions of Traditional Chinese Medicine, Ayurveda, and other ethnomedical systems are even more unfamiliar for modern veterinarians trained in the scientific tradition. This is no excuse, however, for ignoring the possibilities when conventional medicine fails to serve our patients. These traditions offer hundreds to thousands of years of empirical experience, and the alternative perspective may open new avenues for scientific investigation. Veterinary herbalists do not graduate from these traditions—they learn from them.

SUMMARY

Herbal medicine is used in ways that differ from the ways conventional pharmacologic drugs are used. Because herbs have nutritional elements, and because pharmaceutical elements interact with one another polyvalently, the clinical effects may have greater depth and breadth than those seen in drug therapy. Patient prescriptions are based on both the pharmacology AND the traditional indications for the herbs.

For many of the reasons cited here, and for other reasons, veterinarians are using herbal medicine again. A recent survey of 2675 veterinarians in Austria, Germany, and Switzerland suggested that approximately three quarters of veterinarians in those countries are using herbal medicine, especially for chronic diseases and as adjunct therapy (Hahn, 2005).

Most veterinarians view their animal patients as kin, and veterinary herbalists may expand the family even further. Native Americans who depended on their domesticated animals (such as the Plains tribes and their horses) had greater knowledge of plant medicine than did other tribes (Stowe, 1976). Herbalists await scientific investigation of plant medicines but also learn from the plants themselves, acknowledging the ancient and evolving relationship between plants and mammals.

References

Butterweck V. Mechanism of action of St John's wort in depression: what is known? CNS Drugs 2003;17:539-562.

Hahn I, Zitterl-Eglseer K, Franz CH. Phytomedizin bei hund und katze: internetumfrage bei Tierärzten und Tierärztinnen in Österreich, Deutschland und der Schweiz. Schweiz Arch Tierheilk 2005;147:135-141.

Phillipson JD. New drugs from plants—it could be yew. Phytother Res 1999;13:1-7.

Simmen U, Higelin J, Berger-Buter K, et al. Neurochemical studies with St. John's wort in vitro. Pharmacopsychiatry 2001; 34(suppl 1):S137-S142.

Stermitz FR, Lorenz P, Tawara JN, Zenewicz LA, Lewis K. Synergy in a medicinal plant: antimicrobial action of berberine potentiated by 5′-methoxyhydnocarpin, a multidrug pump inhibitor. Proc Natl Acad Sci U S A. 2000 Feb 15;97(4):1433-1437.

Stowe CM. History of veterinary pharmacotherapeutics in the United States. JAVMA 1976;169:83-89.

Williamson EM. Chapter. In: Ernst E, ed. *Herbal Medicine: A Concise Overview for Professionals*. Oxford: Butterworth-Heinemann; 2000.

PART I

Historical Relationship Between Plants and Animals

Zoopharmacognosy

Cindy Engel

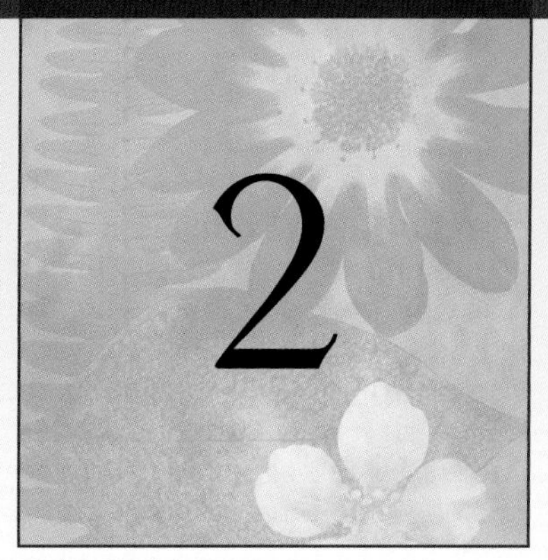

CHAPTER

Folklore asserts that animals instinctively know how to medicate their ills from the herbs they find growing wild. Traditional herbalist Juliette de Bairacli Levy writes that sick animals partake "only of water and the medicinal herbs which inherited intelligence teaches it instinctively to seek." Around the world, traditional herbalists use observations of sick wild animals to find new medicines. Benito Reyes of Venezuela, for example, claims to have discovered the antiparasitic benefits of the highly astringent seeds of the Cabalonga tree *(Nectandra pinchurim)* by observing emaciated animals scraping and chewing the fallen seeds.

As a result of such folklore, there is a common lay assumption that animals unerringly know which herbs to use for which ills. However, this overly romantic view of the wisdom of an all-knowing animal is clearly incorrect. Both wild and domestic animals are known to poison themselves by feeding on toxic substances, repeatedly return to feed on toxic but intoxicating plants, and sometimes quite clearly fail to successfully medicate their ills. Such failures could suggest that animals are in fact incapable of helping themselves when ill and have in the past kept the topic of animal self-medication off the research agenda.

However, a growing body of scientific evidence shows that animals—not only mammals but birds and insects—are self-medicating a variety of physical and psychological ills. Such behavioral strategies though, like all strategies, are fallible; however, it is the limits of efficacy that are of great interest to those working in the field of animal health. Because self-medication strategies have the potential to greatly enhance the health of animals in our care, we would be wise to explore them more closely.

SELF-REGULATION

Living systems are inherently self-regulatory. Behavior is one means by which animals regulate their physiologic and psychological states. For example, overheated animals move into the shade, where it is cooler; dehydrated, they search for water; anxious, they seek safety. However, behavioral self-regulation is far more refined than this. Deprived of only one amino acid, rats increase their consumption of novel foods until they find a diet that is rich in that missing amino acid. Furthermore, they learn an aversion to foodstuffs that are deficient in only one amino acid (Rogers, 1996; Fuerte, 2000). Lambs monitor the carbohydrate and protein content of their diet and adjust their feeding accordingly. If deprived of phosphorus, sheep not only identify a phosphorus-rich diet but also learn a preference for the foods that correct deficiency malaise (Villalba, 1999; Provenza, 1995).

Reviewers conclude that such nutritional wisdom is achieved via a combination of postingestive hedonic feedback and individual learning. They propose that "behavior is a function of its consequences" (Provenza, 1995, 1998). This is true of health maintenance in general, that is, the individual assesses via hedonic feedback—"Do I feel better or worse after doing that?"

The cost to an individual of not maintaining health can be high. Consequently, natural selection has honed a variety of behavioral health maintenance strategies reviewed most recently by Hart (1990, 1994) and Huffman (1997a). As Hart points out, behavior is often the *first line of defense* against attack by pathogens and parasites. As a result, animals use behavioral strategies for avoiding, preventing, and therapeutically addressing threats to survival.

NATURE'S LARDER—POWERFUL PHARMACOPOEIA

Animals must obtain the nutrients and energy they need from a larder that is constantly changing in composition and is often well defended. Moreover, nutrients and energy often come packaged with varying quantities of nonnutrients, many of which are bioactive. This bioactivity is not a fixed phenomenon either. These nonnutrients can be toxic, intoxicating, or medicinal, depending on dose, frequency of consumption, and combination with other foodstuffs, as well as on the changing internal conditions of individual animals.

Priority is given to finding sufficient nutrients and energy without consuming too many toxic defensive compounds. Adaptive taste preferences and biochemical detoxification processes help in this regard. The task requires not only adaptive physiologic characteristics but also continuous self-regulation at the behavioral level. A food that is safe on one occasion may be unsafe on another. The postingestive effects of each feeding bout must be monitored, so that survival is not threatened. Put simply, foods that create unpleasant sensations are avoided, those that create pleasant sensations or remove unpleasant sensations such as deficiency malaise are preferred.

As animals use hedonic feedback to find ways of remedying the unpleasant sensations of dietary deficiencies, and of avoiding the worst chemical defenses of plants and insects foods, so they can also find ways of removing the unpleasant sensations of disease and injury.

Early research on insects distinguished normal feeding from pharmacophagy (Boppre, 1984). Further refinement included a new term—zoopharmacognosy—that described the discoveries of animals who were apparently using medicinal herbs to treat illness (Rodriguez, 1993).

Huffman described a set of conditions that would help primatologists discriminate self-medication from normal feeding in wild primates. First, the animal should show signs of being ill (preferably with some quantifiable test as evidence of sickness). Second, it should seek out and consume a substance that is not part of its normal diet and that preferably should have no nutritional benefit. Its health should then improve (again, established quantifiably by tests) within a reasonable time, commensurate with the known pharmacology of the substance. Laboratory analysis of the plant or substance is then needed to establish that the amount consumed contains enough active ingredients to bring about the changes observed.

Although these criteria are helpful for identifying possible instances of self-medication in the field, they do not define self-medication. As we shall see, recent research on various animal species (both wild and domesticated) illustrates the broad spectrum of approaches that animals use to self-medicate.

Wild Medicine—Beneficial Diets

Everyday diets include beneficial nonnutritional components. A few of many possible examples are described here.

In the rain forests of Costa Rica, mantled howler monkeys are infested with different quantities of internal parasites, depending on where they live. Those living in La Pacifica have high levels of parasites, and those living in Santa Rosa have low levels. None of the heavily infested group has access to fig trees *(Ficus* spp), but the less infested group has many fig trees available. South Americans traditionally use fresh fig sap to cure themselves of worms because the sap decomposes worm proteins (Stuart, 1990; Strier, 1993; Glander 1994).

In the Fazenda Montes Claros Park in southeastern Brazil, endangered muriquis (or woolly spider monkeys) and brown howler monkeys are completely free of all intestinal parasites—a startling and unexpected discovery. In another location, both species are infested with at least three species of intestinal parasites. The main difference between monkeys in the two locations is that the worm-free monkeys have access to a greater selection of plants used as anthelmintics by local Amazonian people (Stuart, 1993).

The everyday diet of great apes contributes much to the sustainable control of parasites. Chimpanzees at Mahale Mountains National Park, for example, eat at least 26 plant species that are prescribed in traditional medicine for the treatment of internal parasites or the gastrointestinal upset that they cause (Huffman, 1998).

In Brazil, the gold and red maned wolf roams the forest at night hunting small prey but taking up to 51% of its diet from plants. By far, its favorite is the tomato-like fruit of Lobeira, or Wolf's fruit *(Solanum lycocarpum).* Although these fruits are more plentiful at certain times of year, the wolf works hard to eat a constant amount throughout the year, suggesting that this fruit is of some significant value. Researchers at Brazilia Zoo found that they could not help their captive wolves survive infestation with a lethal endemic giant kidney worm unless they fed Lobeira daily to their packs (daSilveira, 1969).

Correlations have been noted too in domestic diets and worm loads. When commercially raised deer in New Zealand were grazed on forage containing tannin-rich plants such as chicory, farmers needed to administer less chemical de-wormer (Hoskin, 1999). Furthermore, given a choice, parasitized deer and lambs select the bitter and astringent Puna chicory, thereby reducing their parasite load (Schreurs, 2002; Scales, 1994). Tannin-rich plants such as this are commonly selected in moderate amounts by free-ranging animals. Researchers in Australia and New Zealand have found that certain types of forage such as *Hedysarum coronarium, Lotus corniculatus,* and *L. pedunculatus,* which contain more useful condensed tannins, can increase lactation, wool growth, and live weight gain in sheep, apparently by reducing the detrimental effects of internal parasites (Aerts, 1999; Niezen, 1996). Tannin-rich pastures may also provide opportunities for ungulates to regulate bloat (McMahon, 2000).

Occasionally, even extra large doses of astringent tannins may be consumed. Janzen described how the Asiatic two-horned rhinoceros occasionally eats so much of the tannin-rich bark of the mangrove *Ceriops candolleana* that its urine turns dark orange. He postulated that the rhinoceros may be self-medicating against endemic dysentery, pointing out that the common antidysentery medicine—clioquinol (Enterovioform)—consists of about 50% tannin (Janzen, 1978).

Adaptive Taste Preferences

Evidence suggests that animals seek out particular tastes because of the adaptive consequences. Tannins usually deter mammals from eating plants because their astringency puckers and dries the tongue and impairs digestion by binding proteins. However, as we have seen, tannins are not avoided entirely. Given a choice, deer avoid selecting food with the lowest tannin levels and instead select those containing moderate amounts, suggesting that a certain amount of tannin is attractive to them (VerheydenTixier, 2000). It appears such taste preferences may be adaptive because of the impact of tannins on intestinal parasites. When domesticated goats were fed polyethylene glycol (PEG), which deactivates tannins, numbers of intestinal parasites increased (Kabasa, 2000). Sheep, goats, and cattle increase tannin consumption when fed the deactivating PEG. Alternatively, when fed high-tannin diets, lambs increase PEG intake (Provenza, 2000). These results indicate an attempt to self-regulate tannin consumption to an optimal level.

As we shall see in the next section, other so-called feeding deterrents are sought out when their potent bioactive effects outweigh taste aversions.

Bioactive Botanicals—Toxin or Medicine?

Chimpanzees have similar taste preferences to humans. They prefer sweet over bitter foods. In the Mahale Mountains of Tanzania is a small shrub, *Vernonia amygdalina,* known as bitter leaf. Its extreme bitterness successfully keeps most indigenous animals away, although introduced domesticated goats appear unable to identify the risks; consequently, another common name for this plant is "goat killer." When local chimpanzees are sick, they seek out this bitter, toxic plant, carefully strip off the outer layers of shoots, and chew and suck the juicy bitter pith.

The plant is considered a very strong medicine by local people who use it to treat malarial fever, stomachache, schistosomiasis, amoebic dysentery, and other intestinal parasites (Huffman, 1989). Pig farmers in Uganda supply their animals with branches of this plant, in limited quantities, to treat intestinal parasites.

Bitter pith chewing is rare, but chimpanzees with diarrhea, malaise, and nematode infection recover within 24 hours (similar to the recovery time of local Tongwe people who use this medicine). The behavior clearly influences nodular worm infestation. In one example, fecal egg count dropped from 130 to 15 nodular worm eggs within 20 hours of chewing bitter pith. Bitter pith chewing is more common at the start of the rainy season, when nodular worms increase (Huffman, 1997b) (Figure 2-1). Furthermore, scientists have noticed that chimpanzees with higher worm loads, or those that appear to be more ill, tend to chew *more* bitter pith than those with lower infestation levels.

Vernonia amygdalina from Mahale contains seven steroid glucosides, as well as four sesquiterpene lactones, capable of killing parasites that cause schistosomiasis, malaria, and leishmaniasis. The sesquiterpene lactones (previously known to chemists as "bitter principles") are not only anthelmintic but also antiamoebic, antitumor, and antimicrobial. The outer layers of the shoots and leaves of the shrub, which chimpanzees so carefully discard, contain high levels of vernonioside B1 that would be extremely toxic to a chimpanzee. Not only can chimpanzees find a suitable plant to alleviate their symptoms, they can also find the right *part* of the plant to be effective without harm (Ohigashi, 1991, 1994).

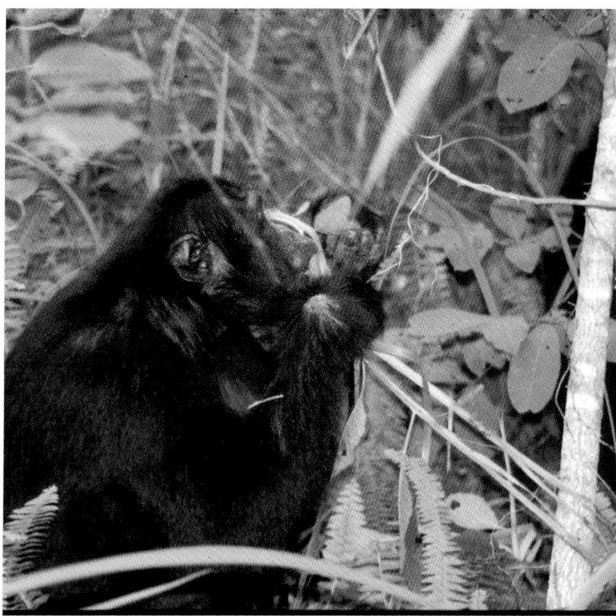

Figure 2-1 Chimpanzee sucks on the bitter pith of *Vernonia amygdalina* (bitter leaf) in Tanzania. *(Courtesy Michael Huffman.)*

It is possible that bitterness in plants may be an effective indicator of medicinal properties: it generally indicates toxicity, but it is this very toxicity that is so effective against parasites. This plant is not just bitter, it is the most bitter plant the chimpanzees can find in the forest. One slurp of its juice will make an adult human wince. Chimpanzees and other animals normally avoid it, but appetitive or tolerance changes may take place during sickness. Sick human patients will apparently tolerate more bitter herbal prescriptions, but as health improves, their tolerance of bitters declines. The mechanism that brings about these changes is not yet known, but experimental evidence supports the idea of an adaptive taste preference for bitters.

Laboratory mice were used to explore the link between illness and consumption of bitters. Experimental mice were given a choice between two water bottles—one contained only water, and the other, a bitter-tasting chloroquine solution that would combat malarial infection. Control mice were given only water. Those mice infected with malarial parasites and given access to chloroquine experienced significantly less infection and mortality than did infected mice with no access to chloroquine. Malarial infection was reduced because mice took approximately 20% of their water from the bottle containing the bitter chloroquine solution. However, consumption of chloroquine was not related to malarial infection. Given a choice, both sick and nonsick mice took small doses of the bitter solution, supporting the idea of an adaptive taste preference for moderate consumption of bitters (Vitazkova, 2001).

It is not only primates, or even vertebrates, that use herbal medicines to control parasites. Even insects do it.

It has long been known that certain butterflies harvest and store the toxic cardiac glycosides from milkweed plants, and that this stash protects them against some predatory birds. However, these glycosides also protect butterfly larvae from internal parasites. It is not clear whether these benefits are merely incidental to feeding, yet the dietary choice is distinctly beneficial.

Scientists who study insect parasitoids (lethal parasites) have found convincing evidence that insects do self-medicate. Woolly bear caterpillars of the tiger moth can be injected with the eggs of parasitic tachinid flies. Fly larvae develop inside the caterpillars, feeding off their fat reserves and finally bursting out of the abdominal wall. Under laboratory conditions, infected caterpillars usually die from this experience. However, when Richard Karban and his colleagues at University of California Davis started rearing their caterpillars in outdoor enclosures, they noticed that the survival rate of parasitized caterpillars was much higher. Outside, the caterpillars had access to plant species not provided in the laboratory. Given a choice, healthy caterpillars chose to feed on lupine *(Lupinus arboreus),* and parasitized caterpillars preferred to feed on hemlock *(Conium maculatum).* Having parasites affected dietary choices, and the change in diet improved chances for survival. Although hemlock, which is known to contain at least eight alkaloids, does not kill the parasites, it helps caterpillars survive infection (Karban, 1997).

Geophagy

Geophagy—the consumption of soil, ground-up rock, termite mound earth, clay, and dirt—is extremely common in mammals, birds, reptiles, and invertebrates. The habit is still found among many contemporary indigenous peoples, including the Aboriginal people of Australia and the traditional peoples of East Africa and China (Abrahams, 1996).

Geophagy is far more common in animals that rely predominantly on plant food and is more common in the tropics. Historically, the explanation for geophagy was that animals ate earth for the purpose of gaining minerals, such as salt (sodium chloride), lime (calcium carbonate), copper, iron, or zinc. Certainly, wild animals do seek minerals from natural deposits, but a need for minerals is by no means a universal explanation for geophagy. There are many cases in which the soils eaten are not rich in minerals; they sometimes even have *lower* levels of minerals than the surrounding topsoil. Recent geophagy research indicates that the small particle clay profile of soil is often the prime reason for geophagy.

In the body, clays can bind mycotoxins (fungal toxins), endotoxins (internal toxins), manmade toxic chemicals, and bacteria, and they can protect the gut lining from corrosion, acting as an antacid and curbing diarrhea. In short, clay is an extremely useful medicine.

The benefits of clay to animal health have been known for some time. Addition of bentonite clay improves food intake, feed conversion efficiency, and absorption patterns in domestic cattle by 10% to 20%. Clay-fed cattle also experience less diarrhea and fewer gastrointestinal ailments (Kruelen, 1985). In addition, veterinarians find clay an effective antacid. Free-ranging cattle help themselves to clay by digging out and licking at subsoils.

High in the Virunga Mountains of Rwanda, mountain gorillas mine yellow volcanic rock from the slopes of Mount Visoke. After loosening small pieces of rock with their teeth, they take small lumps in their powerful leathery hands and grind them to a fine powder before eating (Schaller, 1964). Gorillas are more likely to mine rock in the dry season, when they are forced to change their diet to plants such as bamboo, *Lobelia,* and *Senecio,* which contain more toxic plant secondary compounds than are found in their usual diet. Along with this change in diet comes diarrhea (a natural response to rid the body of toxins); this extra loss of fluid during the dry season could be a serious health problem for the gorilla (Fossey, 1983). Halloysite, the type of clay found in the subsoil eaten by mountain gorillas, is similar to kaolinite, the principal ingredient in Kaopectate, the pharmaceutical commonly used to soothe human gastric ailments. Kaolinite helps reduce the symptoms of diarrhea by absorbing fluids within the intestine (Mahaney, 1995).

Wild chimpanzees take regular mouthfuls of termite mound soil and scrape subsoils from exposed cliff faces or river banks. When scientists spent 123 hours looking specifically at the health of chimpanzees eating termite mound soil, they found that all were unwell, with obvious diarrhea and other signs of gastrointestinal upset (Mahaney, 1996). Analyses of termite mound soils show them to be low in calcium and sodium but high in clay (up to 30%), more specifically, in the same sort of clay used by mountain gorillas and sold by human chemists to treat gastrointestinal upsets in the West. Termite mound soils are used not only by chimpanzees but also by many other species, such as giraffes, elephants, monkeys, and rhinoceroses.

In the rain forests of the Central African Republic, forest elephants and other mammals have created large treeless licks on outcrops of ancient subsoils (Figure 2-2). Most are high in minerals, but almost a third of the licks have lower levels of minerals than surrounding soils. The one thing *all* the sites have in common is a clay content of over 35%. These elephants feed primarily on leaves all year round, except for 1 month—September—when ripening fruit is so abundant that they change to eating mainly fruits. Leaves generally contain defensive secondary compounds to deter herbivores; ripe fruits do not. A change from eating leaves to fruits would therefore dramatically reduce the consumption of toxic secondary compounds—a natural experiment to see whether toxin consumption equates with clay consumption. The only month in which elephants reduce their visits to the clay licks is during that fruit-eating month—September (Klaus, 1998)!

In the tropical forests of South America, too, clay consumption is particularly common in parrots, macaws, monkeys, tapirs, peccaries, deer, guans, curassows, and chachalacas. After studying geophagy in the Amazon forest of Peru for many years, Charles Munn concluded that nearly *all* vertebrates that feed on fruits, seeds, and leaves also eat clay. On an average day, he has observed

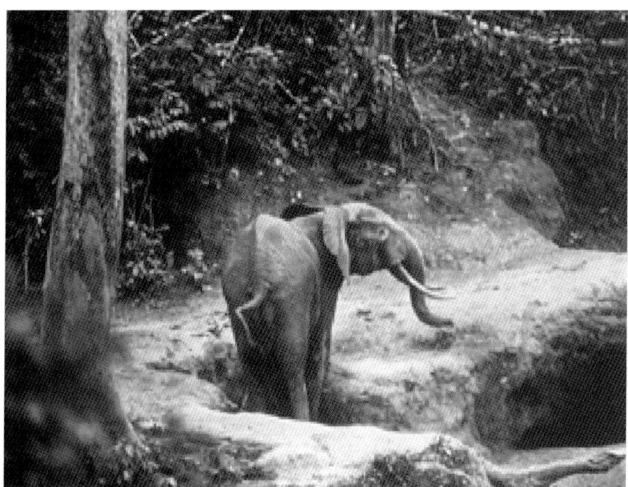

Figure 2-2 Elephants dig down to find clay deposits in Central Africa. *(Courtesy Martin Gruber.)*

up to 900 parrots from 21 species and 100 large macaws gathering to feed on the eroding riverbanks, biting off and swallowing thumb-sized chunks of orange clay (Mayer, 1999).

In 1999, the hypothesis that animals eat clay for the purpose of inactivating plant toxins was tested experimentally with macaws by James Gilardi and a team of scientists at the Davis California campus. First, they established that seeds eaten by macaws contain toxic plant alkaloids. Then, they fed one group of macaws a mixture of a harmless plant alkaloid (quinidine) plus clay. A second group of macaws were fed just the quinidine, without any clay. Several hours later, the macaws that ate the quinidine *with* clay had 60% less alkaloid in their blood than did the control group, demonstrating that clay can indeed prevent the movement of plant alkaloids into the blood. What surprised the scientists though was that the clay remained in the macaws' gut for longer than 12 hours, meaning that a single bout of geophagy could protect the birds for quite some time. It is suspected that clay not only prevents plant toxins from getting into the blood, but it also lines the gut and protects it from the caustic chemical erosion of seed toxins (Gilardi, 1999). Because macaws do not have a diarrheal response to toxins, the consumption of clay may be an essential part of their diet, allowing them to successfully use foods that other animals are unable to tolerate.

It is evident that clay is sought by many animals with gastrointestinal malaise—often caused by plant toxins but also by internal pathogens. In fact, eating clay is used as an *indicator* of gastrointestinal upset in rats (Takeda, 1993). Rats are unable to vomit, and when they are experimentally poisoned with lithium chloride, they eat clay; this "illness response behavior" is dose dependent, that is, the more sick they feel, the more clay they eat. If they are then given saccharin (a sweet taste) with the poison, they learn to associate the sweet taste with the feeling of nausea. They will then eat clay even when given saccharin alone (Sapolsky, 1998).

Scientists who research geophagy agree that, as a strategy, it has many benefits. The Director of the Geophagy Research Unit in Utah, William Mahaney, concludes, "All geophagy is a form of self-medication." Archaeological nutritionist Timothy Johns proposes that geophagy may be the earliest form of medicine and concludes that, although some soils can be a source of nutrients (minerals and/or trace elements), the primary benefit of clay consumption is its effect of countering dietary toxins and, secondarily, the effects of parasites. This explains why plant eaters need to eat earth, and why this practice is more common in the tropics, where plants are more heavily defended by toxic secondary compounds.

Mechanical Scours

Great apes (i.e., chimpanzees, bonobos, and gorillas) do something peculiar with hairy leaves. They assess a potential leaf with their hands, mouth, and tongue while it is still attached to the plant; then, if it is desirable, they pick it, fold it in concertina fashion, and swallow it whole without chewing (Figure 2-3). In each bout, apes swallow from one to one hundred leaves, which are later excreted undigested. Across Africa, they use leaves from at least 34 different species of herbs, trees, vines, and shrubs. Some contain bioactive phytochemicals, others do not; however, *all* are rough in surface texture with hooklike microstructures called *trichomes* (Wrangham, 1977; Huffman, 1997, 2003).

Leaf swallowing, as it is known, is more common at the beginning of the rainy season, when nodular worm infestation starts to increase; many of the apes seen doing this are clearly suffering from symptoms of nodular worm infestation, including diarrhea, malaise, and abdominal pain (Huffman, 1997). After decades of research, scientists discovered that the rough texture of leaves acts as a mechanical scour, scraping loose intestinal worms out through the gut. Rough leaves also stimulate diarrhea and speed up gut motility, helping the animal to shed worms and their toxins from the body. This is likely to provide rapid relief from feelings of gastrointestinal malaise (Huffman, 2001).

It seems that leaf swallowing is particularly effective against nodular worms because they move around freely in the large intestine looking for food and mates. Other worms (such as threadworms and whipworms) burrow into the mucosa of the small intestine and thereby probably escape the scraping effects of rough leaves. However, leaf swallowing has also helped chimpanzees at Kibale National Park, Uganda, to rid themselves of a particularly heavy outbreak of tapeworms *(Bertiella studeri)* (Wrangham, 1995).

It is thought that the unpleasant sensations of abdominal pain, diarrhea, and bowel irritation of nodular worm and tapeworm infestations could be the triggers for leaf swallowing or the chewing of bitter pith (Huffman, 1997).

Primates are not the only species to seek out mechanical scours. Biologists have long known that bears somehow rid themselves of internal parasites before hibernation. Alaskan brown bears in Katmai National

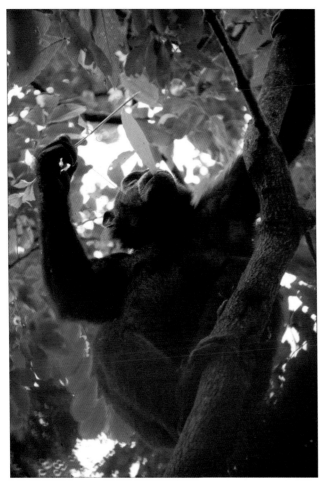

Figure 2-3 Chimpanzee selects hairy Aspilia leaf in Tanzania. *(Courtesy Michael Huffman.)*

Park change their diet before hibernation. Highly fibrous, sharp-edged, coarse sedge *(Carex* spp [Cyperaceae]*)* appears in large dung masses almost completely composed of long tapeworms. The coarse plant material scrapes out the worms in a similar way to the rough leaves swallowed by chimpanzees (Huffman, 1997). Physical expulsion also seems to be used by Canadian snow geese. Just before migration, they deposit large boluses of undigested grass and tapeworms in their dung. When they reach their migration destination, they are clear of tapeworms. In both brown bears and snow geese, worms are being shed at a time of critical nutritional stress—a time when carrying these parasites would greatly reduce the animal's chances of survival.

Wolves eat grass, and wolf scats have been found that contain both grass and roundworms (Murie, 1944). Tigers are reported to eat grass "when hungry," although if heavily infested with worms, they may appear emaciated. Samples of the droppings of wild Indian tigers consist almost entirely of grass blades, and in at least one case, a tapeworm was found inside (Schaller, 1967). Both domestic dogs and cats occasionally chew grass—possibly a residual self-medication strategy of their wild ancestors.

Traditional herbalists use physical scours as a method of worm control. With chemical de-wormers (herbal or nonherbal), there is a delicate balance between a dose toxic enough to harm the parasites yet not the host. These nontoxic physical remedies used by wild animals may be a particularly useful addition to parasite control in modern farming, where parasites are increasingly resistant to drugs (Huffman, 2003).

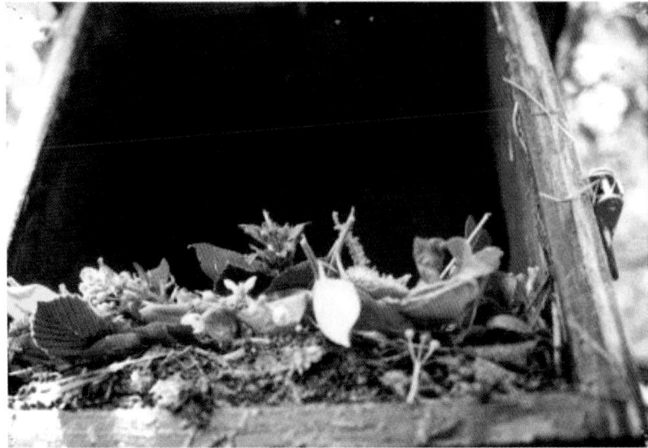

Figure 2-4 European starlings fill nest box with pungent herbs at hatching time. *(Courtesy Helga Gwinner.)*

Topical Applications

Birds and mammals also use nature's pharmacy externally on their skin and in their immediate environment. In these examples, they are exploiting the volatile components of plant and insect secretions.

During nesting time, male European starlings collect a selection of aromatic herbs to bring back to the nest (Figure 2-4). In North America, they preferentially select wild carrot *(Daucus carota),* yarrow *(Achillea millefolium),* agrimony *(Agrimonia parviflora),* elm-leaved and rough goldenrod *(Solidago* spp*),* and fleabane *(Erigeron* spp*),* even when they are not the most common plants nearby. These herbs are all highly aromatic. Furthermore, they contain more volatile oils, in greater concentrations, than are found in aromatic plants close at hand that are not selected.

Back at the nest, the fresh herbs are woven into the nest matrix and topped up all the while the chicks are hatching. The benefits of these herbs to the chicks are evident. Chicks in herb nests have a significantly greater chance of surviving into the next season than do chicks in nests from which the herbs have been removed (Clark, 1988).

Chicks do not eat or actively rub against these pungent herbs, yet when herbs are removed from nests, chicks become infested with more mites. More specifically, chicks in nests that contain wild carrot have higher hemoglobin levels than do those without, again suggesting that they are losing less blood to blood-sucking mites.

Preferred plants contain monoterpenes and sesquiterpenes (such as myrcene, pinene, and limonene) that are harmful to bacteria, mites, and lice in the laboratory. These herbs are particularly effective against the harmful bacteria *Streptococcus aureus, Staphylococcus epidermidis,* and *Pseudomonas aeruginosa*. Lining the nest with pungent herbs is adaptive in that it has a number of different beneficial effects on chicks (Clark, 1985).

In Panama, white-nosed coatis, relatives of raccoons, rub their coats with resin from the *Trattinickia aspera* tree that has a camphor- or menthol-like smell. This resin is used by local Guaymi Indians to repel biting flies. Chemists at Cornell University have identified sesquiterpene lactones in the resin that are repellent to fleas, lice, ticks, and mosquitoes.

In the mosquito-ridden llanos of central Venezuela, wedge-capped capuchin monkeys rub the secretions of large millipedes into their skin. The active ingredients are benzoquinones, which are potentially carcinogenic but antimicrobial and repellent to insects such as the bothersome mosquitoes (Valderrama, 2000).

LABORATORY EXPLORATIONS OF SELF-MEDICATION

Although biologists were initially surprised by examples of self-medication observed in the field, the ability of animals to self-medicate has been used in laboratory experiments for many years. Self-selection of drugs is commonly used in pain, addiction, and mental health research.

Laboratory experiments show that mice actively self-medicate feelings of anxiety. In one example, one group of mice received electric shocks to the feet ("acute physical stress"), and the other group was forced to witness *another* mouse getting a foot shock ("acute emotional stress"). Both groups of mice had free access to morphine, but only the mice exposed to emotional stress self-administered the morphine (Kuzmin, 1996). A similar effect is seen with cocaine self-administration in emotionally stressed rats (Ramsey, 1993).

Scientists in the Ukraine found that stressed rats learned to self-administer strobe lighting at certain frequencies that changed electrical activity in the brain, thereby calming heart rhythm and lowering blood pressure. The rats thereby ingeniously calmed themselves down (Shlyahova, 1999). A feeling of anxiety is clearly unpleasant, and it is surely the animal's desire to *feel* better that drives this kind of behavioral self-regulation.

The welfare of animals in intensive farming is a contentious issue, and any objective measure of their suffering is useful in the debate. A team of veterinary scientists at Bristol University in the United Kingdom have used chickens' ability to self-medicate as proof that they suffer pain. Broiler chickens have been artificially selected to grow extremely quickly, turning food into meat at the expense of bone growth. Their legs therefore are often not strong enough to support their weight, and they frequently suffer broken leg bones. Lame birds go off their food and remain still, unwilling to walk—even to the water trough. However, 1-month-old birds can rapidly learn to select feed that contains the painkilling analgesic carprofen; in addition, the amount of painkiller the birds eat increases with the severity of lameness. Carprofen tastes slightly peppery and can cause gastrointestinal upset. Sound birds tend to avoid the drugged feed, suggesting that they find it unpleasant (Danbury, 2000).

Broiler chickens can also self-medicate stress. It has long been known that supplementing chicken feed with vitamin C (ascorbic acid) helps chickens cope better with heat stress, but producers have difficulty knowing when, and by how much, to supplement the feed. Mike Forbes and his colleagues at Leeds University in the United Kingdom solved this problem by allowing individual birds to self-medicate. To do this though, birds need some way of *detecting* the tasteless, colorless, and odorless vitamin C. Birds have acute color vision and readily learn color associations. By coloring feed that contains vitamin C, researchers revealed that birds could learn the positive effects of colored feed within 3 days and could self-medicate as and when necessary.

Kutlu and Forbes (1993) suggest that vitamin C works by reducing production of the stress hormone corticosterone, thereby reducing other symptoms of chronic stress. They point out that self-medication with vitamin C could be applied to other forms of stress such as parasite infection, high humidity, and high production rates.

MECHANISMS OF ANIMAL SELF-MEDICATION

It is clear that the behavioral repertoires of mammals and birds include many remedial strategies other than those involving the consumption of bioactive phytochemicals. The physical scraping actions of fibrous scours, the topical and local use of volatile oils, and the absorptive properties of clays illustrate the wider landscape of self-medication.

It seems we need to consider at least three nonexclusive mechanisms of self-medication:

1. Adaptive dietary/behavioral preferences—for example, adult mice have taste preferences for moderate levels of bitters that protect them from disease; deer have taste preferences for tannins that affect parasite levels. Both bitters and tannins are normally considered feeding deterrents.
2. Adaptive illness response behaviors—for example, rats seek clay when nauseous.
3. Exploratory hedonic feedback—for example, chicks rapidly learn the beneficial analgesic effects of distasteful drugged food.

APPLICATIONS OF SELF-MEDICATION

Understanding how animals attempt to self-medicate is essential if we are to provide optimal conditions for self-regulation.

Much of the self-medication we see can be explained by hedonic feedback. This ensures that animals only rarely attempt to consume highly toxic substances and prefer to consume those that confer rapid positive feedback. When it comes to finding relief from discomfort, hedonic feedback ensures that animals use safer, less potent "medicines" and resort to the stronger, often more toxic medicines only on rare occasions. This means that continuous moderate self-regulation will be more common than dramatic curative strategies using strong medicines. In other words, much self-medication is unseen.

The limits of hedonic feedback are also worth considering. Because individuals use substances that provide a "feel good factor," they are vulnerable to intoxication and even addiction. Although not described here, both intoxication and addiction occur in wild and domestic species. Just because an animal readily consumes a certain substance does not mean that the substance is safe for consumption in unlimited quantities.

Self-medication via hedonic feedback is a fairly blunt instrument; the animal feels discomfort and tries a range of things until the discomfort is eased. This form of self-medication is aimed at relieving symptoms—not at the pathogen per se. This means that self-medication may or may not affect the pathogen. In some cases, such as when apes scour intestinal parasites, the action that removes the discomfort also removes the pathogen, but this is not always the case. Although Karban's caterpillars survived infestation with normally lethal parasitoids by self-medicating on potent alkaloids, the parasites themselves were unharmed.

It is also important to consider the role that learning plays in the refinement of self-medication strategies. Even those strategies that are apparently innate are usually refined through experience. Young male starlings, for example, have a selective preference for collecting a wide range of pungent plants at hatching time; however, the profile of those choices is refined with experience, so that older males show similar localized preferences. Chimpanzees too seem to need experience on the benefits of leaf swallowing to refine their self-medicating skills.

It is clear that birds and mammals are able to rapidly find remedies in unfamiliar compounds. Laboratory studies on pain relief and stress reduction demonstrate the readiness of rodents and birds to try novel strategies. This has management implications. In their attempt to remove feelings of unease, disease, and discomfort using what is available locally, inexperienced and poorly provisioned animals may try to self-medicate with unsuitable, even unsafe materials. It is therefore essential that safe choices be provided to them for use as potential medicines.

Health maintenance strategies are flexible but are not infallible. The ability to successfully self-medicate requires a complex mix of innate behavioral strategies and refinement attained via learning (experience). It is not appropriate to leave sick animals to fend for themselves —even free-ranging animals—in the hope that they will find some way of self-medicating, especially naïve or domesticated animals. The more opportunities animals have to learn the consequences of their actions, the better.

Domestication has not selected individuals for their ability to self-regulate, and the domestic environment often provides little opportunity for trial and error, experience with potentially toxic bioactive materials, or learning from the observations of others. Even so, given the paucity of research in this area, it is apparent from the examples presented here that domestic animals retain a surprising array of self-medicating abilities.

Incorporating our embryonic understanding of self-medication into animal health management requires that we acknowledge the individual's ability to self-regulate. This means providing individual animals with access to as many potential natural medicines as possible ad libitum. For example, although clay can provide numerous health benefits for ungulates, it is not necessarily best practice to administer clay in standardized form, say via feed, to the whole herd. This is not allowing for self-regulation. It is far better to provide clay licks for individuals to use as and when required.

The essential provision of plant biodiversity for all animals (not only herbivores) cannot be overemphasized. Exposure to diverse flora is especially important during early years when the banes and benefits of certain tastes are being developed by the individual.

Another area that veterinarians might consider is self-administration of certain drugs (herbal or non-herbal). Self-selection of appropriate levels of veterinary medication looks promising, especially for analgesia and carminatives, as long as there is no danger that hedonic feedback may lead to overindulgence.

Although more research is urgently needed, it is clear that there exists an exciting opportunity for encouraging—even exploiting—an individual's ability to self-regulate health status.

References

Abrahams PW, Parsons JA. Geophagy in the tropics: a literature review. The Geographical Journal 1996;162:63–73.

Aerts RJ, Barry TN, McNabb WC. Polyphenols and agriculture: beneficial effects of proanthocyanidins in forages. Agric Ecosyst Environ 1999;75:1–12.

Boppré M. Redefining pharmacophagy. J Chem Ecol 1984;10: 1151–1154.

Clark L, Mason JR. Effect of biologically active plants used as nest material and the derived benefit to starling nestlings. Oecologia 1988;77:174–180.

Clark L, Mason JR. Use of nest material as insecticidal and anti-pathogenic agents by the European starling. Oecologia (Berlin) 1985;67:169–176.

Danbury TC, Weeks CA, Chambers JP, Waterman-Pearson AE, Kestin SC. Self-selection of the analgesic drug carprofen by lame broiler chickens. Veterinary Record, March 11, 2000.

daSilveira EKP. O.lobo-guara *(Chyrsocyon brachyrus)*. Possival acao inhibidoria de certas solancas sobre o nematoide renal. Vellozia 1969;1:58–60.

Fossey D. *Gorillas in the Mist*. London: Hodder & Stoughton; 1983.

Fuerte S, Nicoladis S, Berridge, KC. Conditioned taste aversion in rats for a threonine-deficient diet: demonstration by the taste reactivity test. Physiol Behav 2000;68:423–429.

Gilardi JD, Duffey SS, Munn CA, Tell LA. Biochemical functions of geophagy in parrots: detoxification of dietary toxins and cytoprotective effects. J Chem Ecol 1999;25:897–919.

Glander KE. Nonhuman primate self-medication with wild plant foods. In: Etkin N, ed. *Eating on the Wild Side: The Pharmacologic, Ecologic, and Social Implications of Using Non-cultigens*. Tucson, Ariz: University of Arizona Press; 1994:227–239.

Hart BL. Behavioral adaptations to pathogens and parasites: five strategies. Neurosci Biobehav Rev 1990;14:223–294.

Hart BL. Behavioural defence against parasites: interaction with parasite invasiveness. Parasitology 1994;109:S139–S151.

Hoskin SO, Barry TN, Wilson PR, Charleston WAG, Hodgson J. Effects of reducing anthelmintic input upon growth and faecal egg and larval counts in young farmed deer grazing chicory *(Cichorium intybus)* and perennial ryegrass *(Lolium perenne)* white clover *(Trifolium repens)* pasture. J Agric Sci 1999;132: 335–345.

Huffman MA. Animal self-medication and ethno-medicine: exploration and exploitation of the medicinal properties of plants. Proc Nutr Soc 2003;62:371–381.

Huffman MA. Current evidence for self-medication in primates: a multidisciplinary perspective. Yearbook Phys Anthropol 1997a;40:171–200.

Huffman MA, Caton JM. Self-induced gut motility and the control of parasite infections in wild chimpanzees. Int J Primatol 2001;22:329–346.

Huffman MA, Gotoh S, Turner LA, Hamai M, Yoshida K. Seasonal trends in intestinal nematode infection and medicinal plant use among chimpanzees in the Mahale Mountains, Tanzania. Primates 1997b;38:111–125.

Huffman MA, Ohigashi H, Kawanaka M, et al. African Great Ape self-medication: a new paradigm for treating parasite disease with natural medicines? In: Ageta H, Ami N, Ebizuka Y, Fujita T, Honda G, eds. *Towards Natural Medicine Research in the 21st Century*. Amsterdam: Elsevier Science; 1998.

Huffman MA, Seifu M. Observations on the illness and consumption of a possibly medicinal plant *Vernonia amygdalina* by a wild chimpanzee in the Mahale Mountains National Park, Tanzania. Primates 1989;30:51–63.

Janzen DH. Complications in interpreting the chemical defences of trees against tropical arboreal plant-eating vertebrates. In: Montgomery GG, ed. *The Ecology of Arboreal Folivores*. Washington: Smithsonian Institute Press; 1978:73–84.

Kabasa JD, OpudaAsibo J, terMeulen U. The effect of oral administration of polyethylene glycol on faecal helminth egg counts in pregnant goats grazed on browse containing condensed tannins. Trop Anim Health Prod 2000;32:73–86.

Karban R, English-Loeb G. Tachinid parasitoids affect host plant choice by caterpillars to increase caterpillar survival. Ecology 1997;78:603–611.

Klaus G, Klaus-Hugi C, Schmid B. Geophagy by large mammals at natural licks in the rain forest of the Dzanga National Park, Central African Republic. J. Trop. Ecol 1998;14:829–839.

Kruelen DA. Lick use by large herbivores: a review of benefits and banes of soil consumption. Mam Rev 1985;15:107–123.

Kutlu HR, Forbes JM. Self-selection of ascorbic acid in coloured foods by heat-stressed broiler chickens. Physiol Behav 1993;53:103–110.

Kuzmin A, Semenova S, Zvartau EE, Van Ree JM. Enhancement of morphine self-administration in drug naïve, inbred strains of mice by acute emotional stress. Eur Neuropsychopharmocol 1996;6:63–68.

Mahaney WC, Aufreiter S, Hancock RGV. Mountain gorilla geophagy: a possible seasonal behavior for dealing with the effects of dietary changes. Int J Primatol 1995;16:475–488.

Mahaney WC, Hancock RGV, Aufreiter S, Huffman MA. Geochemistry and clay mineralogy of termite mound soils and the role of geophagy in chimpanzees of Mahale Mountains, Tanzania. Primates 1996;37:121–134.

Mayer W. Feat of clay. Wildlife Conservation Magazine, June 1999.

McMahon LR, McAllister TA, Berg BP, et al. A review of the effects of forage condensed tannins on ruminal fermentation and bloat in grazing cattle. Can J Plant Sci 2000;80: 469–485.

Murie A. *The Wolves of Mount McKinley*. Washington DC, US Department of the Interior. Fauna Series 1944;5:59.

Niezen JH, Charleston WAG, Hodgson J, Mackay AD, Leathwick DM. Controlling internal parasites in grazing ruminants without recourse to anthelmintics: approaches, experiences and prospects. Int J Parasitol 1996;26:983–992.

Ohigashi H, Huffman MA, Izutsu D, et al. Toward the chemical ecology of medicinal plant use in chimpanzees: the case of *Vernonia amygdalina* Del. A plant used by wild chimpanzees possible for parasite-related diseases. J Chem Ecol 1994;20: 246–252.

Provenza FD. Post-ingestive feedback as an elementary determinant of food preference and intake in ruminants. J Range Manage 1995;48:2–17.

Provenza FD, Buritt EA. Self-regulation of polyethylene glycol by sheep fed diets of varying tannin concentrations. J Anim Sci 2000;78:1206–1212.

Provenza FD, Villalba JJ, Cheney CD, Werner SJ. Self-organisation of foraging behaviour: from simplicity to complexity without goals. Nutr Res Rev 1998;11:199–222.

Ramsey NF, Van Ree JM. Emotional but not physical stress enhances intravenous cocaine self-administration in drug-naïve rats. Brain Res 1993;608:216–222.

Rodriguez E, Wrangham RW. Zoopharmacognosy: the use of medicinal plants by animals. In: Downum KR, Romeo JT, Stafford H, eds. *Recent Advances in Phytochemistry 27: Phytochemical Potential of Tropical Plants*. New York: Plenum Press; 1993:89–105.

Rogers W, Rozin P. Novel food preferences in thiamine-deficient rats. J Compar Physiol Psychol 1996;61:1–4.

Sapolsky RM. Junk food monkeys. London Headline 1998:156.

Scales GH, Knight TL, Saville DJ. Effect of herbage species and feeding level on internal parasites and production performance of grazing lambs. N Z J Agric Res 1994;38:237–247.

Schaller G. *The Deer and the Tiger: A Study of Wildlife in India*. Chicago, Ill: University of Chicago Press; 1967.

Schaller G. *The Year of the Gorilla*. Chicago, Ill: University of Chicago Press; 1964.

Schreurs NM, Lopez-Villalobos N, Barry TN, Molan AL, McNabb WC. Effects of grazing undrenched weaner deer on chicory or perennial ryegrass/white clover on the viability of gastrointestinal nematodes and lungworms. Vet Rec 2002;151: 348–353.

Shlyahova AV, Vorobyova TM. Control of emotional behaviour based on biological feedback. Neurophysiology 1999;31:38–40.

Strier KB. Menu for a monkey. Natural History, 1993.

Stuart MD, Greenspan LL, Glander KE, Clarke M. A coprological survey of parasites of wild mantled howler monkeys. J Wildlife Dis 1990;26:547–549.

Stuart MD, Strier KB, Pierberg SM. A coprological survey of wild muriquis *Brachyteles arachnoids* and brown howling monkeys *Aloutta fusca*. J Helminth Soc, 1993.

Takeda N, Hasegawa S, Morita M, Matsunaga T. Pica in rats is analogous to emesis: an animal model in emesis research. Pharmacol Biochem Behav 1993;45:817–821.

Valderrama X, Robinson JG. Seasonal anointment with millipedes in a wild primate: a chemical defense against insects? J Chem Ecol 2000;26:2781–2790.

VerheydenTixier H, Duncan P. Selection for small amounts of hydrolysable tannins by a concentrate selecting mammalian herbivore. J Chem Ecol 2000;26:351–358.

Villalba JJ, Provenza FD. Nutrient-specific preferences by lambs conditioned with intraluminal infusions of starch, casein, and water. J Anim Sci 1999;77:378–387.

Vitazkova S, Long E, Glendinning J. Mice suppress malaria infection by sampling a "bitter" chemotherapy agent. Anim Behav 2001;61:887–894.

Wrangham RW. Feeding behaviour of chimpanzees in Gombe National Park, Tanzania, In: Clutton-Brock TH, ed. *Primate Ecology*. New York: Academic Press; 1977:504–538.

Wrangham RW. Leaf swallowing by chimpanzees, and its relation to a tapeworm infection. Am J Primatol 1994;37:297–303.

Ethnoveterinary Medicine: Potential Solutions for Large-Scale Problems?

3

CHAPTER

*Cheryl Lans, Tonya E. Khan, Marina Martin Curran, and Constance M. McCorkle**

WHAT IS EVM?

Also sometimes called veterinary anthropology (McCorkle, 1989),[†] ethnoveterinary medicine or EVM can be broadly defined in this way:

> The holistic, interdisciplinary study of local knowledge and its associated skills, practices, beliefs, practitioners, and social structures pertaining to the healthcare and healthful husbandry of food, work, and other income-producing animals, always with an eye to practical development applications within livestock production and livelihood systems and with the ultimate goal of increasing human well-being via increased benefits from stockraising (McCorkle, 1998a).

This definition suggests the myriad scientific disciplines that are implicated in the research and development (R&D) and application of EVM. It also signals attention to all aspects of a people's knowledge and practices in animal healthcare, productivity, and performance, that is, their diagnostic (including ethologic) understandings; preventive, promotive, and therapeutic skills and treatments; and a wide range of health-related management techniques.

These aspects in turn embrace local *Materia medica,* which include minerals and animal products or parts, as well as plants and human-made and natural materials; modes of preparation and administration of ethnoveterinary medicaments; basic surgery; various types of immunization; hydro, physical, mechanical, and environmental treatments and controls; herding, feeding, sheltering, and watering strategies; handling techniques; shoeing, shearing, marking, and numerous other husbandry chores such as ethnodentistry; management of genetics and reproduction; medicoreligious acts; slaughter, as one medical option; and all the various socio-organizational structures and professions that discover, devise, transmit, and implement this knowledge and expertise. These human elements span not only traditional healers of animals (Mathias, 2003) but also families, clans, castes, tribes, communities, cooperatives, dairy associations, other kinds of grassroots development organizations, and more.

Impelled in large part by livestock development projects around the world, EVM has evolved to embrace other topics, such as zoopharmacognosy (animals' self-medication) as a possible source of EVM ideas; participatory epidemiology; gendered knowledge, tasks, and skills in EVM (Davis, 1995; Lans, 2004); safety in handling and processing food and other products from animals; product marketing and associated agri-business skills; conservation of biodiversity in terms of natural resources, including animal genetic resources (Köhler-Rollefson, 2004); health- and husbandry-related interactions between domestic and wild animals; ecosystem health (i.e., how animals, humans, and their environment can interact to protect or improve the health of all three); EVM-related primary education curricula in rural areas and in training programs for veterinary professionals and paraprofessionals; and policy, institutional, and economic analyses in most of the foregoing realms.

For fuller discussions of all the previously listed topics and themes in EVM, see related studies in Reference Section (Mathias, 2004; McCorkle, 1995, 1998b; McCorkle, 2001). It is important to mention, however, that by far the most-studied element of EVM is veterinary ethnopharmacopoeia, especially the use of botanicals.

*The authors would like to acknowledge important inputs to this chapter by Dr. Med. Vet. Evelyn Mathias. She contributed data on the history of EVM, of which she was one of the leading pioneers. She also shared recent information on avian influenza, as per a study of this subject that she was preparing in Spring 2006.

†Because they are so voluminous yet also often recondite, references to the history of EVM and to specific examples of knowledge and techniques from one or another culture are not cited one-by-one in this introduction. Rather, such references are mentioned only if they cannot be found in one or more of the sources by Martin, Mathias/Mathias-Mundy, McCorkle, and their co-authors that are cited in the text. These all represent formal publications released as books or as articles in peer-reviewed disciplinary outlets spanning agriculture, anthropology, international development, and veterinary medicine. These items are more readily accessible to interested readers.

WHERE DID EVM COME FROM?

All over the world and down through the ages, people who keep livestock have developed their own ideas and techniques for meeting the health and husbandry needs of their food, farm, and work animals. Their knowledge and skills may be hundreds or even thousands of years old. Classic cases include Ayurveda in India and acupuncture and herbal medicine in China, all of which were (and are) practiced for animals as well as for humans. These and a few other traditions of EVM have long-standing written records, like scrolls of the Talmud and the Bible's Old Testament, which occasionally advise on Jewish pastoralism; Sri Lankans' 400-year-old palm leaf manuscripts on cattle and elephant health and husbandry; early military manuals from numerous peoples on the health care, conditioning, and training of warhorses and draught animals; and, probably most ancient of all, hieroglyphic papyri on Egyptians' care of sacred bulls.

In preliterate or still-nonliterate societies, EVM was and is perforce passed down verbally across the generations. With the 14th century Renaissance in Europe, however, literacy and publishing opportunities expanded and nascent scientific disciplines emerged, some of which occasionally mentioned EVM—most notably, agriculture, botany, medicine (both human and veterinary), folklore studies, and anthropology. In the so-called developing world, European colonialism from the 16th to the 20th century stimulated the production of government reports, personal memoirs, enterprise records, and so forth, by civil servants and technical staff, missionaries, large landowners and ranchers, and others who worked or traveled in the colonies. Some of these authors chronicled their observations and impressions of native veterinary knowledge and practices—albeit often in very ethnocentric and unflattering terms. But even today, much of EVM is transmitted orally. To take just one example, this is still the case for local acumen about the care and training of hunting dogs and mules in parts of rural United States (personal communication, from C. M. McCorkle, for her native state of Missouri).

However, not until the 1970s did a noticeable number of peer-reviewed scientific articles, book chapters, special journal issues *(Ethnozootechnie),* and report series (as from the UN's Food and Agriculture Organization [FAO]) emerge that were devoted to "traditional," "indigenous," or later, "local" or "community-based" animal healthcare and husbandry. From the 1970s onward, an ever-growing number of graduate theses and dissertations in anthropology and, especially, veterinary medicine also addressed EVM. These initially spanned a few universities in Africa, India, and West Germany, plus at least four in France. Later they were joined by Dutch and UK (notably Edinburgh) universities, along with several prestigious schools in the United States (e.g., Cornell, Harvard, Stanford, Tufts).

HOW HAS EVM EVOLVED?

On the basis of a review of emerging literature along with firsthand research in 1980 among Quechua stockraisers in the high Andes of South America, EVM was finally codified in 1986 as a legitimate field of scientific R&D (McCorkle, 1986). An annotated bibliography on EVM and related subjects followed soon thereafter (Mathias-Mundy, 1989). Published by a US agricultural university program of indigenous knowledge studies within a series on technology and social change, this item was available only as "grey literature." Nevertheless, it was in high demand. Only in 1996 did the first formally published anthology of scientific studies dedicated solely to EVM reach print (McCorkle, 1996).

Between 1986 and 1996, however, the field of EVM literally exploded. This explosion was ignited and thereafter fanned by various fuels.

One major stimulus was the World Health Organization's project to incorporate valid human-ethnomedical techniques and—on the model of barefoot doctors in China—local medical practitioners into real-world strategies for achieving WHO's goal of "basic healthcare for all." EVM seeks to do likewise for livestock; e.g., via the creation of cadres of community-based veterinary paraprofessionals (ILD Group 2003) that ideally deliver both conventional and ethno-options. EVM embraces a cost-effective return to the "one medicine" concept, in which such healthcare services are delivered jointly to both animals and humans—especially in poor and/or remote areas (Green, 1998; McCorkle, 1998b; others in the special section on human and animal medicine in this issue of *Agriculture and Human Values*), along with the creation of cadres of community-based veterinary paraprofessionals (IDL Group, 2003) that, ideally, deliver both conventional and ethnomedical options.

Another stimulus was the developed world's burgeoning, billions-of-dollars clamor for more healthful and organic food products (including those for livestock), as well as safer, more natural medical options with fewer adverse effects for both humans and (especially companion) animals.

Probably most important, however, was the growing realization among international livestock developers and even some early policymakers that conventional, formal sector, "high-tech" (thus also high-cost) healthcare and husbandry interventions transferred from the developed world could not sustainably meet the basic stockraising needs of most rural people in the developing world, where every rural community keeps animals, as do many urban inhabitants as well. This realization grew out of the on-farm experiences of agricultural, animal, and social scientists and veterinarians in governmental and nongovernmental overseas field projects.

An early public-sector leader in this regard was the US Small Ruminant Collaborative Research Support Project. Begun in 1979 in Peru, but growing and continuing until 1997, it involved some 15 US agricultural universities and research centers that worked in cooperation with literally hundreds of governmental and nongovernmental organizations (NGOs) in Bolivia, Brazil, Indonesia, Kenya, Morocco, and Peru.

Pioneering international NGOs in EVM included: in the US, Heifer Project International (HPI), notably in Cameroon and the Philippines; the Philippines-based

International Institute for Rural Reconstruction (IIRR); and the UK Intermediate Technology Development Group (ITDG), which worked particularly in East Africa. Later NGO leaders included India's ANTHRA group, which focuses on livestock development among women in that country; also in India, the Bharatiya Agro Industries Foundation (BAIF); Germany's League for Pastoral Peoples (LPP), especially with its work on camels; the US Christian Veterinary Mission; and Vétérinaires Sans Frontières (VSF/Switzerland, 1998).

A related factor in the EVM explosion appears to have been the growing volume of articles or papers published in well-known and respected journals or presented at established disciplinary conferences in Europe and the United States. Initially most such items were written about the developing world by developed-world scientists and field practitioners. However, these groups' serious engagement of the topic seems in turn to have empowered and motivated their counterparts in the developing world to document and report on their own emic (i.e., native) knowledge and field-based observations in EVM. Had these counterparts done so previously, they would have risked ridicule by their national peers who would have perceived them as nonscientific, ignorant, backward, or even superstitious. Indeed, this same fate was suffered by many developed-world explorers of EVM in the 1970s and 1980s.

It was also helpful that between 1986 and 1996, new outlets and technologies came into being for more rapid, informal, and globally inclusive exchanges of EVM observations and information across a much wider range of national and disciplinary groups. A pioneering outlet in this regard was the *Indigenous Knowledge and Development Monitor.* Based first in the United States and later in the Netherlands, this development magazine was published from 1993 to 2001 and was distributed *gratis* to developing world subscribers. In 1999, it was followed by a global electronic mailing list devoted solely to EVM. Recently, this list was expanded topically and renamed the Endogenous Livestock Development List (http://groups.yahoo.com/group/ELDev/). Although initiated and funded in the developed world, all these efforts relied on hands-on management by and content input from a panel of editors who represented nearly all continents of the globe.*

In hindsight, perhaps it is not surprising that this period also saw an increase in grants for R&D and conferences on EVM. Funding came from agencies such as Sweden's Foundation for Science, the Swiss Agency for Development and Cooperation, the World Bank, FAO, and national federations of local grower or dairier groups. Furthermore, most of these funds were earmarked for livestock projects, researchers, or organizations associated with the developing world, albeit often with *pro bono* input from colleagues in the developed world. This carried forward the sincere spirit of peer-based North/South collaboration established by earlier public-sector (whether bilateral or multilateral) and NGO efforts, as mentioned previously.

A notable example is the first-ever international conference, *Ethnoveterinary Medicine: Alternatives for Livestock Development.* Held in India in 1997, it was supported by the World Bank and many other donors, plus pharmaceutical companies. This event was hosted by India's BAIF based on a proposal written by Indian, German, UK, and US scientists. Together they thereafter produced two volumes of formal abstracts and proceedings (Mathias, 1999). The conference boasted 33 formal papers and nearly as many poster papers on EVM. Disciplines represented ran from A (anthropology) to Z (zoology) and included all the animal and veterinary sciences in between, along with traditional veterinary praxis as represented by local healers from India.

At this point, a patent need arose to update, expand, and more tightly focus the 1989 bibliography referenced earlier. This was done, and the bibliography was released through a major publishing house in international development, with financial support provided by the UK Department for International Development. The new bibliography (Martin, 2001) boasted 1240 annotations spanning 118 countries, 160 ethnic groups, and 200 health problems of 25 livestock breeds and species. It covered publications dated through December of 1998.

Since 1998, EVM has rocketed ahead. Publications are increasing exponentially, now with a greater number of developed-world authors researching or writing about EVM in their own cultures and native lands. Recent examples of publications and conferences in this vein come from Canada (TAHCC, 2004), Italy (Guarrera, 1999, 2005; Manganelli, 2001; Pieroni, 2004), the Netherlands (van Asseldonk, 2005), and Scandinavia (Waller, 2001).

This trend is due in part to the fact that established scientific outlets in numerous disciplines—like the *Revue Scientifique de l'Office Internationale des Epizooties* (OIE, 1994)—are now more open than ever to papers on EVM. Also, new outlets are coming into being. For instance, the *Journal of Evidence-Based Complementary and Alternative Medicine* plans to mount a series of articles on EVM beginning in 2006. Even more important is the fact that the literature is beginning to demonstrate a salubrious move up from mere description of EVM knowledge and practices to more critico-analytic and applied studies. The two cases presented in this chapter are indicative.

Scientific meetings on EVM have likewise burgeoned—whether in the form of sessions set aside for EVM at long-standing events like the University of Utrecht (Netherlands) Symposium on Tropical Animal Health and Production, or entire conferences devoted only to EVM. The range of topics presented has also broadened such that workshops and conferences have been created to accommodate specialized interests in a particular region, species, or type of EVM. Moreover, such events are increasingly mounted and funded by developing-world organizations and governments. Consider the following history.

In 1994, 1996, and 1998, the NGOs IIRR, ITDG, and VSF held workshops on EVM in Southeast Asia, Eastern Africa, and Sudan, respectively. Meanwhile, in 1997, LLP convened a workshop on both EVM and conventional practices for camel health and husbandry (Köhler-

*See the Resources section at the end of this chapter for additional resources.

Rollefson, 2000). In 1999, a conference was held in Italy on "Herbs, Humans and Animals—Ethnobotany & Traditional Ethnoveterinary Practices in Europe" (Pieroni, 2000). In 2000, an international conference on EVM was mounted in Africa and hosted by Nigeria's Ahmadu Bello University (Gefu, 2000).

Later, a participatory workshop on EVM was held in the Canadian province of British Columbia, funded by the Social Sciences and Humanities Research Council of the government of Canada (see http://bcics.uvic.ca/bcethnovet/rationale.htm). The year 2005 witnessed the first Pan-American conference on EVM in Latin America, which was organized and hosted by a Guatemalan university, with financial support provided by the Guatemalan government. Also in 2005, various Mexican universities, research centers, and government agencies hosted an international conference on animal genetics and the invaluable animal germplasms, including disease-resistant ones that local peoples have developed and husbanded down through time.

Upcoming in 2006 is a key conference on the same issue, which has been organized by LPP and is being funded and hosted by the Rockefeller Foundation at its prestigious Bellagio Centre in Italy. Also in 2006, the British Society of Animal Science is organizing a special conference/workshop on veterinary ethnobotany targeted to both plant and animal researchers and emphasizing, "the role of plants and their derived products as a means of preventing or treating diseases of animals and improving health" in an environmentally sustainable way.

Even more impressive is the number of universities and associated research centers that now include curricula on EVM. Besides the Netherlands, Nigerian, and UK universities already mentioned, some others include Ethiopia's Addis Ababa University, Mexico's Universidad Autónoma de Chiapas, Rwanda's University Centre for Research on Traditional Pharmacology and Medicine, and the University of the West Indies. In addition, particularly in Africa, technical units or components of traditional medicine have been incorporated into a number of government livestock, veterinary, or medical agencies.

WHY THE INTEREST IN EVM?

The appeal of EVM can be summarized as bulleted below. Most of these considerations apply to both developing and developed nations.

- Particularly among poor or remote stockraisers who can neither afford nor may access expensive or distant conventional healthcare options, validated EVM techniques may be the most realistic choice.
- This may also be true for wealthier and better-situated stockraisers insofar as the conventional services on offer may not respond to these producers' particular veterinary needs.
- Whether for poor or rich stockraisers, depending on their production systems and market conditions, the value of the animals in question may not warrant the cost of professional veterinary care and inputs.
- Especially if they are imported, the desired commercial drugs may not be available; if they are available, supplies may be expired, insufficient, or even adulterated.
- Other problems with commercial medicines are that veterinary professionals to advise on them may be absent. Stockraisers (especially those illiterate in the language on the drugs' labels and instructions) may be uncertain about their indications, dosages, and even modes of administration. Dangers here include not only the obvious ones for patients but also the problem of escalating chemoresistance.
- As a rule, people are more comfortable receiving healthcare services from known, trusted, local, and co-ethnic practitioners, such as traditional healers or respected livestock extensionists who are from the same community, speak the same tongue, and are themselves stockraisers.
- In emergencies or fast-spreading epidemics, there simply may not be time for anything other than local practitioners and treatments. To the extent that such help and treatment are cheaper, they make for better returns to stockraising and thus are more sustainable.
- Again, particularly among poor and remote rural populations, opportunities are available for cheaper and more sustainable services via the joint extension of human and veterinary traditional and modern medicine to both people and livestock.
- People in many cultures are concerned about adverse effects from food or environmental pollution associated with powerful modern drugs and biocides. Ethnomedical alternatives may prove more benign.
- Indeed, long-time savvy about the local ecology, livestock and wildlife ethology, natural resources, and so forth may result in management interventions that are even more effective in preventing disease in the first place—thus avoiding the dangers or costs of therapy of any sort, whether conventional or ethno-medical.
- Studies of EVM treatments and practices in different cultures and between different biosocial groups within them (e.g., women vs men, high vs low castes) may bring to light useful new *Materia medica* or techniques for promoting, protecting, or restoring the health and well-being not only of animals but also of people.

WHERE IS EVM HEADED NEXT?

Along with others, all the benefits outlined previously have been attested to in the larger literature on EVM. Doubtless, readers will think of others. But beyond providing more culturally comfortable, practical, and economical alternatives or complements to conventional medical approaches, R&D in EVM may conceivably help solve problems left in the wake of, or new to, conventional medicine. An example of the former is ailments that have become resistant to overprescribed or misused commercial drugs like antibiotics and commercial parasiticides. Viral diseases exemplify the latter, in that antigenic shifts may render conventional vaccination responses unrealistic (Atawodi, 2002). Such shifts come about when two varieties of a virus concurrently infect the same host, allowing genomes to recombine into a novel subtype.

Of course, various limitations to EVM have been noted in the literature. Among others are the following claims (after Fielding, 2000).

- For ethnoveterinary botanicals, the required type and amount of (especially) plant materials may not be available when needed, particularly if the plants in question are seasonal or nonlocal, or if herds or flocks are very large.
- Even when the materials are available, the mode of administration may not be practical for large herds or flocks.
- EVM treatments are too site-specific to justify R&D investments designed to modify them for more universal application.
- EVM has little or nothing to offer against acute viral disease.

The first and second concerns above are certainly valid. But the literature suggests that they apply equally to conventional treatments because of import, supply, or price problems with commercial drugs—whether in the developing or the developed world. A case in point involves experiences in modern-day France regarding the relative availability and efficacy of conventional and EVM treatments for sudden outbreaks of sheep disease, some of which are viral (Brisebarre, 1996).

In response to the third bullet above, this omnibus claim has been largely debunked. Time and again, historically and contemporaneously, and across different continents and cultures, the same or similar plant or other materials and management techniques have been reported for the same or similar livestock and human health problems. Indeed, many so-called modern pharmaceuticals for both animals and people derive from plants and other materials (or their molecular models) used in traditional medicine. In 1990, it was estimated that world sales of medicines derived from plants discovered by indigenous peoples amounted to US $43 billion.

With increased bioprospecting (Clapp, 2002), this trend has intensified and become even more profitable (Lans, 2003). In the developing and the developed world, companies that process or merely package and then retail or wholesale "natural," "organic," or "ancient" alternatives based on ethnomedicine for livestock and humans have expanded, proliferated, and specialized. In the past decade alone, a number of companies have sprung up in Europe and on the East and West coasts of the United States to distribute EVM-based herbal preparations, many of which are imported from India. Some of these enterprises even specialize in preparations for a single animal species such as horses (Stephen Ashdown, DVM, personal communication).

More intriguing is the fourth bullet's claim that EVM has little or nothing to offer against viral diseases. To date, this statement has gone largely uncontested in the EVM literature. Meanwhile, the effectiveness of a wide variety of EVM treatments for parasitic and bacterial ills, wounds and fractures, fertility and obstetric problems, and numerous husbandry needs has been clearly documented.

The primary conventional response to viral epidemics is mass vaccination. However, this approach can have drawbacks that go even beyond those implied for conventional veterinary medicine discussed earlier. These concerns are listed here:

- Viruses may mutate so rapidly that research, development, production, and administration of an appropriate vaccine cannot keep pace.
- Depending on the disease that is diagnosed, it is not always possible to distinguish infected from already vaccinated animals. In the absence of strict immunization records, this makes it difficult to tightly target the populations to be vaccinated. Thus, the costs of vaccine purchase and administration will mount insofar as some animals are treated two or three times over.
- As noted earlier, the cost of treatment may outstrip the value of the animals in question. This is particularly true for small stock like poultry.
- Even after animals have been immunized with an effective vaccine, they may continue to shed the virus. This risks further mutation or reinfection.
- Mass vaccination also risks eliminating the 1% or 2% of a population that has some natural immunity to the virus. Yet such animals could serve as prime breed stock in the future (Köhler-Rollefson, 1998).

In light of the foregoing considerations and in response to the question of "Where is EVM headed next?" the following sections offer two literature-based cases that illustrate EVM potentials for prevention and control of viral disease, whether in livestock or people.

EVM AND VIRAL DISEASES: TWO CASES FROM POULTRY PRODUCTION

The cases presented here focus on major viral disease in family poultry enterprises in the developing world. There, more than 80% of poultry are raised in such enterprises. These "backyard birds" provide up to 30% of household protein intake in the form of eggs and meat. Trade in these poultry products and (depending on the culture) in fertilized eggs, chicks, and live birds also contributes significantly to household nutrition and income. Often, this income is used to step up the family farming enterprise through the purchase of larger stock, like pigs, sheep, goats, or even cattle and buffalo (Ibrahim, 1996).

Family poultry enterprises normally consist of small to medium-sized flocks of free-ranging birds. They are typically owned and cared for by household women and children. Generally, producers endeavor to supply their flocks with local or purchased feed supplements; various types of protection from predators and the elements; assistance in incubation and chick fostering; and more. However, rarely do they employ costly commercial veterinary inputs.

Arguably, viruses are responsible for the most massive and pervasive economic losses from disease of poultry worldwide—especially in family enterprises, but also in agro-industrial poultry production. Newcastle's disease (ND) is perhaps the best known of these banes. However, much in the news of late is avian influenza (AI), which constitutes a new strain of the centuries-old "fowl plague"—today, generally called simply "bird flu."

Developed-world producers can ward against such threats with modern immunizations, albeit with the drawbacks already noted. However, many family poultry enterprises in the developing world simply cannot afford commercial vaccines—even where these are available and reliable (i.e., unexpired, unadulterated, or unfalsified), with trained personnel to administer them (such as community-based paraprofessionals). Although some ethnoveterinary vaccines of variable efficacy do exist for viral diseases of poultry,* poor or remote people in the developing world rely primarily on plant-based prophylactic measures to stave off such ills in their birds.

The question is: Do any such measures really make any difference? To begin to answer this, Cases 1 and 2 below respectively address: Africans' phytomedical treatments for ills identified as ND; and Africans' and other peoples' botanicals for responding to unspecified respiratory signs in poultry, which are here taken as suggestive of AI. Unless otherwise indicated, for Case 1, production data on ND in Africa are drawn from Guèye 1997, 1999, and 2002. For both cases, technical background on the etiological agents and clinical signs of both ND and AI is based mainly on Alexander 2000 and 2004 plus Tollis 2002. Both OIE and WHO offer a periodically updated technical and other information on AI at their websites (www.oie.int. and http.www/who.org).

Finally, it should be noted that for both cases, the references to and discussion of EVM treatments for ND and probable incidences of AI are only illustrative. They derive from a convenience sample of English-language publications available to the first two authors, rather than from an exhaustive review of pertinent EVM or human ethnomedical literature globally.

*Although this chapter deals only with plant-based treatment, note that native peoples of Africa, Asia, and later Europe also elaborated indirect and direct methods of inoculating against viral ills.—notably, foot-and-mouth disease, rinderpest (cattle plague), and poxes (camel, cow, fowl, and in humans, smallpox). Indirect methods consist mainly of controlled exposure. Direct methods entail administering various preparations derived from tissue, blood, scabs, mucous, or saliva from infected animals to healthy stock. Some of these techniques are still in use today, including for poultry. All were based in (and indeed, gave rise to) what is now considered sound medical science. For historical and efficacy details, consult Schillhorn van Veen 1996 plus items in Martin 2001.

CASE 1: NEWCASTLE'S DISEASE

ND is especially devastating to free-ranging flocks in developing countries, where it kills 70% to 80% of unvaccinated birds every year. ND was first identified in 1926 in Newcastle-upon-Tyne, England, and simultaneously in Java, Indonesia. However, almost certainly, these were not the first outbreaks.

ND is caused by an enveloped RNA virus of the Paramyxoviridae family. It can infect at least 241 species of birds. Chickens are particularly susceptible, whereas waterfowl are often asymptomatic. Today, ND is described in terms of multiple pathotypes. The velogenic strain is the most virulent and occurs as two subtypes—viscerotropic and neurotrophic. The former is characterized by diarrhea, facial edema, nasal discharge, and, often, sudden death. The latter manifests as respiratory and subsequently neurologic signs, along with high mortality without gastrointestinal lesions.

Although a thermostable vaccine against ND exists, family flocks in Africa are rarely immunized due to the reasons discussed previously. Family-level producers instead rely on their own local/indigenous knowledge and resources. Indeed, Africans' choice of EVM to treat poultry diseases in general reportedly ranges from 55% of family producers in Mozambique to 79% in Botswana. Across Africa, people use many botanicals to control ND. Usually, the *Materia medica* are crushed and then mixed into birds' drinking water.

Table 3-1 lists a sampling of the plants involved in such preparations, labeled by the names given in the original scientific paper about them. As discussed in the following paragraphs, a number of these plants have proved promising for combating ND.

Aloe secundiflora

Aloe species are used extensively for a variety of poultry diseases across Africa, including *Aloe excelsa* for fowlpox—another viral disease. In a controlled experiment, an extract of *Aloe secundiflora* was prepared in much the same way as villagers prepare it. It was composed of the inner gel, containing antiviral polysaccharides such as acemannan, and the outer sap, containing anthraquinone glycosides. The extract was administered to or withheld from treatment or control groups of chickens purposely infected with ND at the same time. Administered at the time of infection, this traditional medicine decreased mortality by 21.6%. Pretreatment with the extract for 2 weeks before infection decreased mortality by 31.6% (Waihenya, 2002).

Because most farmers are aware of the seasonality of ND, pretreatment is feasible. The anthraquinone components in *Aloe* species (aloenin and aloin) are at least partially responsible for the anti–ND virus activity (Waihenya, in press). Indeed, enveloped viruses seem to be particularly sensitive to anthraquinones. These biochemicals have been demonstrated to impair the influenza, pseudorabies, and varicella-zoster viruses, as well as herpes simplex virus (HSV) types 1 and 2 (Andersen, 1991; Sydiskis, 1991).

Azadirachta indica

This plant acts against both ND (Babbar, 1970; Kumar, 1997) and foot-and-mouth disease viruses (Wachsman, 1998). However, its usefulness against ND is likely better explained by its anti-inflammatory and immune-stimulating properties (Boeke, 2004; Sadekar, 1998a).

CASE 1: NEWCASTLE'S DISEASE—cont'd

Capsicum spp

These are widely used worldwide to treat patients with a variety of diseases, particularly in polyprescriptions with other plant materials. The key constituent is capsaicin, which may improve disease resistance in poultry (Guèye, 1999). For controlling ND, African families use *Capsicum* (especially *Capsicum frutescens*) in combination with other species such as *Aloe secundiflora, Amaranthus hybridicus, Iboza multiflora, Khaya senegalensis,* and *Lagenaria breviflora* (Guèye, 1999, 2002; ITDG, 1996). Although one clinical trial found that a combination with *Citrus limon* and *Opuntia vulgaris* was not effective in controlling ND (Mtambo, 1999), further study of *Capsicum* seems justified.

Cassia tora

Similar to aloes, this plant contains significant quantities of anthraquinones (Koyama, 2003), which explains its demonstrated activity against ND (Mathew, 2001). Related species with anti–ND virus activity include *Cassia auriculata* (Dhar, 1968) and *Cassia fistula* (Babbar, 1970; Mathew, 2001).

Euphorbia ingens

In a small clinical trial (Guèye, 2002), branches of this plant were crushed and soaked in chickens' drinking water overnight. When this water was administered at the same time that the birds were infected with ND, mortality decreased by 38.4% in comparison with controls. With pretreatment, mortality fell by 100%. Many other *Euphorbia* species or their chemical constituents possess significant antiviral activity. Examples include *Euphorbia compositum* against respiratory syncytial virus and influenza (Glatthaar-Saalmüller, 2001a), *Euphorbia thymifolia* and *Euphorbia tirucalli* against HSV (respectively, Lin, 2002; Betancur-Galvis, 2002), *Euphorbia australis* against human cytomegalovirus (HCMV; Semple, 1998), and *Euphorbia grantii* and *Euphorbia hirta* against polio and coxsackie viruses (Vlietinck, 1995).

Beyond the five species just discussed, also promising are five other EVM plants listed in Table 3-1, because they possess scientifically demonstrated antiviral activity for various human diseases. These plants and the corresponding human diseases and research references are displayed in Table 3-2.

Although the antiviral properties of EVM treatments for ND are important, other EVM responses to ND may provide symptomatic relief or immune system support. These effects should not be overlooked. This is especially true for family poultry, which are almost invariably infected with velogenic ND. In this regard and in relation to Table 3-2, it should be noted that Africans use *Adansonia digitata* (Tal-Dia, 1997), *Mangifera indica* (Sairam, 2003), *Strychnos potatorum* (Biswas, 2002), and *Ziziphus abyssinica* (Adzu, 2003) to assuage diarrhea in livestock and humans. They also employ bronchorelaxants based on *Adansonia digitata* (Karandikar, 1965) and *Cassia didymobotrya* (Kasonia, 1997).

Finally, all the following plants used in African EVM have been shown to have immune-enhancing properties: *Allium sativum* (Kyo, 2001), *Aloe vera* (Tan, 2004), *Azadirachta indica* (Sadekar, 1998a), *Mangifera indica* (Garcia, 2003; Makare, 2001), *Piper nigrum* (Chun, 2002), *Tephrosia purpurea* (Damre, 2003), and *Trigonella foenum-graecum* (Bin-Hafeez, 2003).

TABLE 3-1

Plants Used in African Ethnoveterinary Medicine for Newcastle's Disease

Ethnoveterinary Medicine Plants	Family	Part(s) Used	Reference(s)
Adansonia digitata	Bombacaceae	Fruit	Guèye, 1997
Agave americana + pepper fruit and soot	Agavaceae	Leaf	ITDG, 1996
Agave sisalana	Agavaceae	Leaf, stalk	Guèye, 2002
Agave sisalana + *Aloe secundiflora,* pepper fruit, and "oswawandhe" root	Agavaceae	Leaf/leaf/fruit/root	ITDG, 1996
Allium sativum	Liliaceae	Bulb	Alders, 2000
Aloe spp	Liliaceae	Leaf	Guèye, 2002 ITDG, 1996
Aloe nuttii	Liliaceae	Unspecified	Kambewa, 1999
Aloe nuttii + *Kigelia aethiopica, Sesamum angolense,* and soil	Liliaceae	Unspecified	Kambewa, 1999

Continued

TABLE 3-1

Plants Used in African Ethnoveterinary Medicine for Newcastle's Disease—cont'd

Ethnoveterinary Medicine Plants	Family	Part(s) Used	Reference(s)
Aloe secundiflora	Liliaceae	Leaf	Minja, 1999
Aloe secundiflora + *Agave sisalana*, pepper fruit, and "oswawandhe" root	Liliaceae	Leaf/leaf	ITDG, 1996
Aloe secundiflora + *Capsicum* spp and *Amaranthus hybridus*	Liliaceae	Leaf/fruit/leaf	ITDG, 1996
Amaranthus hybridus + *Capsicum* spp and *Aloe secundiflora*	Amaranthaceae	Leaf, flower/ fruit/leaf	ITDG, 1996
Anacardium spp	Anacardiaceae	Unspecified	Guèye, 2002
Anogeissus leiocarpus	Combretaceae	Root	PRELUDE, nd
Apodytes dimidiata	Icacinaceae	Leaf, stalk	Guèye, 2002
Azadirachta indica	Miliaceae	Bark, leaf	Guèye, 2002
Butyrospermum paradise + *Combretum micranthum* and *Ficus gnaphalocarpa*	Sapotaceae	Barks	Guèye, 2002
Capsicum spp	Solanaceae	Seed	ITDG, 1996
Capsicum annuum	Solanaceae	Seed	ITDG, 1996
Capsicum annuum + *Iboza multiflora*	Solanaceae	Fruit/leaf	Guèye, 2002
Capsicum frutescens + *Lagenaria breviflora*	Solanaceae	Seed/fruit	Guèye, 2002
Capsicum spp + *Amaranthus hybridus* and *Aloe secundiflora*	Solanaceae	Seed, fruit/leaf, flower/unspecified	ITDG, 1996
Capsicum spp + *Khaya senegalensis*	Solanaceae	Seed/bark	Guèye, 1999
Cassia didymobotrya	Caesalpiniaceae	Leaf	Guèye, 2002
Cassia sieberiana	Caesalpiniaceae	Bark	Guèye, 2002
Cassia tora	Caesalpiniaceae	Leaf, stalk	Guèye, 2002
Cissus quadrangularis	Vitaceae	Leaf, stalk	Guèye, 2002
Citrus limon + *Capsicum frutescens* and *Opuntia vulgaris*	Rutaceae	Fruit/fruit/stem	Mtambo, 1999
Combretum micranthum + *Butyrospermum paradoxum* and *Ficus gnaphalocarpa*	Combretaceae	Barks	Guèye, 2002
Diplorhynchus condylocarpon	Apocynaceae	Leaf, stalk	Guèye, 2002
Euphorbia ingens	Euphorbiaceae	Branch	Guèye, 2002
Euphorbia metabelensis	Euphorbiaceae	Latex	Guèye, 2002
Euphorbia tirucalli	Euphorbiaceae	Leaf, stalk	Guèye, 2002
Ficus spp	Moraceae	Leaf, stalk	Guèye, 2002
Ficus gnaaphalocarpa + *Combretum micranthum* and *Butyrospermum paradoxum*	Moraceae	Bark	Guèye, 2002
Guibourtia coleosperma	Caesalpiniaceae	Leaf, stalk	Guèye, 2002
Iboza multiflora + *Capsicum annuum* or *Euphorbia ingens*	Lamiaceae	Leaf/fruit/stem	Guèye, 2002
Inula glomerata	Asteraceae	Leaf, stalk	Guèye, 2002
Khaya senegalensis + *Capsicum* spp	Meliaceae	Bark/unspecified	Guèye, 1999
Kigelia aethiopica + *Aloe nuttii*, *Sesamum angolense*, and soil	Bignoniaceae	Unspecified	Kambewa, 1999
Kigelia africana	Bignoniaceae	Leaf, stalk	Guèye, 2002
Lagenaria breviflora + *Capsicum frutescens*	Cucurbitaceae	Fruit	Guèye, 2002
Lamnea acida	Unspecified	Bark	Guèye, 2002
Mangifera indica	Anacardiaceae	Bark, leaf	Alders, 2000 Guèye, 2002
Mucuna spp	Fabaceae	Leaf	ITDG, 1996
Ochna pulchra	Ochnaceae	Leaf, stalk	PRELUDE, nd
Parkia filicoidea	Fabaceae	Bark	Guèye, 1997, 2002
Physostigma mesoponticum	Fabaceae	Unspecified	Kambewa, 1999
Piper nigrum	Unspecified	Fruit	Guèye, 2002
Sesamum angolense + *Aloe nuttii* and *Kigelia aethiopica*	Pedaliaceae	Unspecified	Kambewa, 1999
Strychnos potatorum	Loganiaceae	Leaf, stalk	Guèye, 2002
Swartzia madagascariensis	Caesalpiniaceae	Bark	Guèye, 2002
Synadenium volkensii	Euphorbiaceae	Bark	PRELUDE, nd
Tephrosia vogelii	Fabaceae	Unspecified	Kambewa, 1999
Tylostemon spp	Lauraceae	Unspecified	Kambewa, 1999
Ziziphus abyssinica	Rhamnaceae	Leaf, stalk	PRELUDE, nd

TABLE 3-2

Plants Used in African Ethnoveterinary Medicine for Newcastle's Disease That Act Against Viruses in Humans

EMV Plants	Active Against	References
Adansonia digitata	HSV1/2, poliovirus, SINV	Ananil, 2000; Hudson, 2000
Allium sativum	HSV1/2, HRV2, parainfluenza 3, *Vaccinia* virus, VSV, HCMV, murine CMV, influenza B	Guo, 1993; Liu, 2004; Nagai, 1973; Weber, 1992
Cassia didymobotrya	VSV	Cos, 2002
Combretum micranthum	HSV1/2	Ferrea, 1993
Mangifera indica	HSV1/2	Yoosook, 2000; Zheng, 1990; Zhu, 1993

CMV, Cytomegalovirus; *HCMV,* human cytomegalovirus; *HRV2,* human rhinovirus type 2; *HSV1/2,* herpes simplex virus type 1 or 2; *SINV,* Sindbis virus; *VSV,* vesicular stomatitis virus.

CASE 2: AVIAN INFLUENZA

Similar to ND, AI is caused by an enveloped RNA virus, but from the Orthomyxoviridae family. It is a type A influenza that is further categorized according to membrane proteins into 15 hemagglutinin (H1 to H15) and 9 neuraminidase (N1 to N9) subtypes. This virus replicates in the respiratory and gastrointestinal systems, with the corresponding clinical signs and modes of shedding. Wild waterfowl are the natural hosts, but other birds and even mammals can become infected. First documented in 1878, AI is clinically classified as having low or high pathogenicity (LPAI or HPAI). LPAI is usually asymptomatic in wild waterfowl but causes mild or even severe disease in domestic poultry. Untreated HPAI in domestic birds approaches 100% mortality.

The last three major antigenic shifts in type A influenza led to the human pandemics of Spanish, Asian, and Hong Kong flu in 1918, 1957, and 1968. Spanish flu was the most devastating of these. It infected 20% to 40% of the world's population, and it took more than 20 million human lives (Hien, 2004).

In 1997, a new strain of HPAI (H5N1) was detected in humans in Hong Kong. Formerly found only in birds in Asia, this strain has lately been reported in wild or domestic fowl in Africa, Eastern and Western Europe, and the Middle East. As of the time of this writing (late February 2006), 91 zoonotic deaths from H5NI have reportedly occurred. Virtually all of these have involved poultry workers who were in direct contact with the nasal, respiratory, or fecal discharges of infected animals. So far, no human-to-human transmission has been definitively confirmed. However, this new, virulent strain has an estimated mortality rate of anywhere between 50% and 72% in directly infected humans. Although this figure is obviously in flux, by comparison, mortality from the Spanish flu was only 2.5%.

Given the possible threat to human health from this new strain of AI, and given that respiratory signs are the more distinctive ones for differential diagnosis of AI, a review of EVM botanicals for preventing or controlling the clinical signs of unspecified respiratory disease in poultry hardly seems amiss. To this end, Table 3-3 documents a wide variety of plants used in EVM in these regards. As with ND, the plant materials are usually administered in the drinking water of flocks.

Three species stand out here in terms of their documentation in both EVM and human (see Table 3-4) medical literature for their promise in combating viral disease.

Allium sativum **(Garlic)**

Clinically, the constituents of garlic are antiviral to influenza (Yakovlev, 1950) and possibly also beneficial when administered before infection (Nagai, 1973). Fresh garlic is virucidal against herpes simplex virus types 1 and 2 (HSV1 and HSV2), human rhinovirus type 2, parainfluenza 3, *Vaccinia* virus, and vesicular stomatitis virus (Weber, 1992).

Andrographis paniculata

Families in India boil this whole plant in 2 L of water until half the water evaporates. Then, they add 2 handfuls of uncooked, milled rice and leave the mixture to stand overnight. The next morning, it is fed with the flocks' regular food. In vitro and clinical studies indicate that either alone (Thamlikitkul, 1991) or in combination with *Eleutherococcus senticosis* (Melchior, 2000; Spasov, 2004), *A. paniculata* reduces the severity of symptoms associated with respiratory infections in humans—including colds, sinusitis, and influenza (Cáceres, 1999; Glatthaar-Saalmüller, 2001b). Moreover, this plant or its constituents possess activity against hepatitis B (Mehrotra, 1990), human immunodeficiency virus, i.e., HIV (Chang, 1991), and respiratory syncytial virus (Ma, 2002). Also, it has potent antiinflammatory (Panossian, 2002) and immune-stimulating (Kumar, 2004) properties. These may

Continued

CASE 2: AVIAN INFLUENZA—cont'd

account for the amelioration of respiratory signs observed in chickens. It is interesting to note that the plant's isolated andrographolide constituents are not as immune stimulating as is the crude extract employed in family poultry enterprises in India (Melchior, 2000).

Nicotiana glauca

Both in vitro and clinical studies show that the aqueous extract of this tobacco plant increased survival of chick embryos infected with influenza virus. Moreover, studies indicate that unlike ostrich and other birds or many mammals, chickens can eat the leaf without experiencing any obvious adverse effects (Watt, 1962).

Turning from these three plants to others listed in Table 3-3, *Heliotropium indicum* has powerful anti-inflammatory properties (Srinivas, 2000), as do *Eryngium foetidum* (Garcia, 1999), *Pimenta racemosa* (Garcia, 2004), and *Zingiber officinale* (Penna, 2003). *Momordica charantia* (Spreafico, 1983), *Trigonella foenum-graecum* (Bin-Hafeez, 2003), and *Zingiber officinale* (Tan, 2004) all exhibit immune-enhancing properties.

The fourth and last table in this chapter (Table 3-4) lists EVM plants from Tables 1-1 and 1-3 that are used for apparent viral diseases of poultry and that share the same genus, or are even the same species, as plants demonstrated to have anti-influenza or antiviral activity in humans.

Among the items in Table 3-4, it should be noted that *Citrus* species contain relatively large quantities of flavonoids such as hesperitin from *Citrus junos*, which significantly inhibits influenza A virus in vitro (Kim, 2001). Hesperidin is also anti-inflammatory (Emim, 1994). *Euphorbia compositum* and *Mahonia aquifolium* both show anti-influenza activity. The latter is also immunomodulatory (Kostalova, 2001), although it has demonstrated no activity against AI in vitro (Sauter, 1989).

Other EVM plants of interest have known antiviral properties, although their anti-influenza activity may remain unknown. For instance, *Curcuma longa* is anti-inflammatory (Joe, 2004); as a feed additive, it improves broiler performance (Al-Sulton, 2003). *Ocimum sanctum* wards against inflammation and, specifically for poultry, the immunosuppressive effects of infectious bursal disease (Godhwani, 1987; Sadekar, 1998b). *O. sanctum* also has other immunomodulatory effects (Mediratta, 2002). *Ocimum gratissimum* is active against HIV (Ayisi, 2004). Various species of *Plantago,* a popular Chinese medicine for infectious diseases, are antiviral or immune stimulating for HSV2, adenovirus, and human respiratory syncytial virus (Chiang, 2002, 2003; Gomez-Flores, 2000; Li, 2004). *Plantago palmata* combats coxsackievirus (Vlietinck, 1995).

Finally, plants reported as having anti-influenza effects for humans merit mention. Even though they may not be referenced in the EVM literature, they may be suggestive for future R&D or application in EVM. A few examples are *Crataegus crus-galli, Euonymus europaeus, Fragaria vesca, Ribes rubrum, Ribes uva-crispa, Sambucus nigra, Solanum nigrum,* and *Viburnum opulus* (Sauter, 1989).

TABLE 3-3

Plants Used in Ethnoveterinary Medicine Worldwide for Respiratory Signs in Poultry

EVM Plants	Part(s) Used	Location	Reference(s)
Allium cepa	Bulb	India	IIRR, 1994
Allium sativum	Bulb	India, West Indies	IIRR, 1994; Lans, 2001
Capsicum annuum	Fruit	Africa	Guèye, 1999
Citrus aurantifolia	Fruit juice, peel	West Indies	Lans, 2001
Citrus aurantium	Fruit juice, peel	West Indies	Lans, 2001
Citrus limetta	Fruit juice, peel	West Indies	Lans, 2001
Coffea arabica	Beans	West Indies	Lans, 2001
Coffea robusta	Beans	West Indies	Lans, 2001
Colocasia esculata	Tuber	Africa	ITDG, 1996
Curcuma longa	Rhizome	India	IIRR, 1994
Eryngium foetidum	Leaf	West Indies	Lans, 2001
Eriobotrya japonica	Unspecified	Italy	Viegi, 2003
Euphorbia metabelensis	Latex	Africa	Guèye, 1999
Heliotropium indicum	Mature leaf	Philippines	IIRR, 1994
Mahonia aquifolium	Root	Canada	TAHCC, 2004

TABLE 3-3

Plants Used in Ethnoveterinary Medicine Worldwide for Respiratory Signs in Poultry—cont'd

EVM Plants	Part(s) Used	Location	Reference(s)
Momordica charantia	Stem, leaf	West Indies	Lans, 2001
Nicotiana tabacum	Leaf	Africa	Guèye, 1999
Nicotiana glauca	Leaf	Africa	Watt, 1962
Ocimum micranthum	Unspecified	Honduras	Ketzis, 2002
Ocimum sanctum	Leaf	India	IIRR, 1994; Kumar, 1997
Pimenta racemosa	Leaf	West Indies	Lans, 2001
Piper guineense	Fruit	Africa	Guèye, 1999
Plantago major	Unspecified	Italy	Viegi, 2003
Ricinus communis	Leaf	West Indies	Lans, 2001
Spondias pinnata	Young leaf	Philippines	IIRR, 1994
Trigonella foenum-graecum	Seed	India	IIRR, 1994
Zingiber officinale	Rhizome	India	IIRR, 1994

TABLE 3-4

Plants (or Closely Related Ones) Used in Ethnoveterinary Medicine for Viral Diseases or Respiratory Signs in Poultry That Act Against Viruses in Humans

Ethnoveterinary Medicine Plants	Same or Closely Related Plants	Active Against	Reference(s)
Cassia didymobotrya, Cassia sieberiana, Cassia tora	*Cassia mimosoides*	HSV1	Sindambiwe, 1999
Citrus aurantifolia, Citrus aurantium, Citrus limetta, Citrus limon	*Citrus junos*	Influenza type A	Kim, 2001
Combretum micranthum	*Combretum hartmanni*	HIV	Ali, 2002
Curcuma longa	Same	HIV	Barthelemy, 1998; Mazumder, 1995
Euphorbia metabelensis	*Euphorbia compositum*	Influenza	Glatthaar-Saalmüller, 2001a
Eriobotrya japonica	Same	Rhinovirus	DeTommasi, 1992
Ficus spp	*Ficus ovata*	HSV, poliovirus	Ananil, 2000
Ficus gnaphalocarpa	*Ficus polita*	HIV	Ayisi, 2003
Mahonia aquifolium	*Mahonia bealei*	Influenza	Zeng, 2003 OK
Momordica charantia	Same	HIV, HSV1, poliovirus, HSV1, SINV, HSV	Bourinbaiar, 1995; Jiratchariyakul, 2001; Lee-Huang, 1990; Schreiber, 1999 Foà-Tomasi, 1982; Beloin, 2005; Bourinbaiar, 1996
Nicotiana glauca, Nicotiana tabacum	*N. glauca*	Influenza	Watt, 1962
Plantago major	Same	HSV2	Chiang, 2002
Ricinus communis	Same	HSV, SINV	Mouhajir, 2001
Tephrosia vogelii	*Tephrosia madrensis, Tephrosia viridiflora, Tephrosia crassifolia*	Dengue virus	Sánchez, 2000
Zingiber officinale	Same	Rhinovirus	Denyer, 1994

HIV, Human immunodeficiency virus; *HSV1/2,* herpes simplex virus type 1 or 2; *SINV,* Sindbis virus.

POTENTIAL SOLUTIONS FOR LARGE-SCALE PROBLEMS?

This chapter began with a brief overview of the evolution of EVM. From roots doubtless dating back to the dawn of human domestication of animals, EVM has today become a globally recognized and multidisciplinary field of study and application. Beyond that, however, this chapter has endeavored to suggest how—whether bench, field, or literature based—R&D in EVM is not just an historical or academic pursuit. Rather, it is a living, breathing field that holds promise for addressing many animal and also human concerns regarding health, safety, and the environment in both the developing and developed worlds, especially as these two worlds become ever more entwined in the process of globalization. Moreover, EVM may hold greater potential than was heretofore suspected for one of the most recalcitrant categories of disease—viral infection.

This last point is illustrated by a sampling of the literature on plant-based treatments used in EVM to prevent or control two major viral diseases of livestock (here, poultry) worldwide—Newcastle's disease and avian influenza (the latter based presumptively on respiratory signs). Both strike wild as well as domesticated birds, and typically cause respiratory (as well as gastrointestinal) distress. However, AI poses a particular danger to humans. Thus EVM botanicals for ND and AI are compared with literature on the use of the same or closely related species with known activity against viral disease in humans. The four tables presented in this chapter reveal 25 overlapping items. Two plants in particular stand out for their frequent occurrence: *Cassia didymobotrya* and *Combretum micranthum.* Along with other *Cassia* species, also noteworthy are species of *Citrus, Euphorbia,* and *Nicotiana.*

Taken together, these preliminary, literature-based findings suggest that EVM may hold greater promise for preventing, controlling, or at least alleviating the clinical signs of viral disease than was previously thought—especially when conventional treatments are unavailable, unaffordable, or unreliable. Also, EVM could conceivably play a supporting or a multitiered role in the control of viral disease.

Illustrating for AI and depending on the immune-enhancing or anti-influenza properties of the plants administered, EVM could possibly increase birds' resistance to the disease; if LPAI is present, decrease the chances of its mutating into HPAI; during an outbreak of HPAI, help prevent or slow the spread of HPAI to otherwise healthy animals; and generally, reduce environmental contamination with the influenza virus. Also, it may be that pretreatment could be effective with AI as it has been with ND, but this remains to be investigated.

More broadly, analyses of the sort presented in this chapter can point out which EVM treatments merit further study and evaluation for their value against one or another disease in one or more species of livestock, or even humans. Again illustrating for AI, to the extent that EVM can help decrease viral contamination of the environment, then to that extent, too, it can decrease humans' exposure to AI. That would in turn reduce the chances of an antigenic shift that might provoke a new pandemic of human influenza.

None of this is to say, however, that conventional techniques should be replaced across-the-board by semi- or even fully-validated EVM treatments—whether the latter consist of phytomedicines, indigenous inoculations, ethnosurgical or more mechanical or husbandry interventions. Particularly for viral diseases, EVM treatments await further research outside the lab or the literature. Like conventional techniques, EVM treatments must also be verified using the actual livestock species in question under controlled on-station and then on-farm conditions.

Nor do EVM treatments obviate the need for sound husbandry and biosecurity measures, whether for viral or other contagious diseases. However, this is to say that the effectiveness of conventional measures can almost certainly be augmented by EVM measures. It is also to say that—faced with pandemic threats such as that posed by AI, and echoing the wisdom of WHO as much as 30 years ago—it would be foolish not to investigate all promising preventive, control, or mitigation options that might derive from EVM savvy for enhancing the health and well-being of animals, humans, or both.

References

Adzu B, Amos S, Amizan MB, Gamaniel K. Evaluation of the antidiarrhoeal effects of *Ziziphus spina-christi* stem bark in rats. Acta Trop 2003;87:245-250.

Alders RG. Sustainable control of Newcastle disease in rural areas. In: Alders RG, Spradbrow PB, eds. SADC Planning Workshop on Newcastle Disease Control in Village Chickens. Proceedings of an International Workshop. ACIAR Proceedings No. 103; March 6-9, 2000; Maputo, Mozambique.

Alexander DJ. A review of AI in different bird species. Vet Microbiol 2000;74:3-13.

Alexander DJ, Bell JG, Alders RG. Technology review: Newcastle disease with special emphasis on its effect on village chickens. International Conference of the Food and Agriculture Organization; February 12-13, 2004; Rome, Italy.

Ali H, König GM, Khalid SA, Wright AD, Kaminsky R. Evaluation of selected Sudanese medicinal plants for their in vitro activity against hemoflagellates, selected bacteria, HIV-1-RT and tyrosine kinase inhibitory, and for cytotoxicity. J Ethnopharmacol 2002;83:219-228.

Al-Sulton SI. The effect of *Curcuma longa* (turmeric) on overall performance of broiler chickens. Int J Poultry Sci 2003;2:351-353.

Ananil K, Hudson JB, de Souzal C, et al. Investigation of medicinal plants of Togo for antiviral and antimicrobial activities. Pharm Biol 2000;38:40-45.

Andersen DO, Weber ND, Wood SG, Hughes BG, Murray BK, North JA. *In vitro* virucidal activity of selected anthrquinones and anthraquinone derivatives. Antiviral Res 1991;16:185-196.

Atawodi SE, Ameh DA, Ibrahim S, et al. Indigenous knowledge system for treatment of trypanosomiasis in Kaduna state of Nigeria. J Ethnopharmacol 2002;79:279-282.

Ayisi NK, Nyadedzor C. Comparative in vitro effects of AZT and extracts of *Ocimum gratissimum, Ficus polita, Clausena anisata, Alchornea cordifolia,* and *Elaeophorbia drupifera* against HIV-! And HIV-2 infections. Antiviral Res 2003;58:25-33.

Babbar OP, Chowdhury BL, Singh MP, Khan SK, Bajpai S. Nature of antiviral activity detected in some plant extracts screened in cell cultures infected with Vaccinia and Ranikhet disease viruses. Indian J Exp Biol 1970;6:304-312.

Barthelemy S, Vergnes L, Moynier M, Guyot D, Labidalle S, Bahraoui E. Curcumin and curcumin derivatives inhibit Tat-mediated transactivation of type 1 human immunodeficiency virus long terminal repeat. Res Vir 1998;149:43-52.

Beloin N, Gbeassor M, Akpagana K, et al. Ethnomedicinal uses of Momordica charantia (Cucurbitaceae) in Togo and relation to its phytochemistry and biological activity. J Ethnopharmacol 2005;96:49-55.

Betancur-Galvis LA, Morales GE, Forero JE, Roldan J. Cytotoxic and antiviral activities of Columbian medicinal plant extracts of the *Euphorbia* genus. Mem Inst Oswaldo Crus 2002;97:541-546.

Bin-Hafeez B, Haque R, Parvez S, Pandey S, Sayeed I, Raisuddin S. Immunomodulatory effects of fenugreek *(Trigonella foenum graecum* L.*)* extract in mice. Int Immunopharmacol 2003;3:257-265.

Biswas S, Morugesan T, Sinha S, et al. Antidiarrhoeal activity of *Strychnos potatorum* seed extract in rats. Fitoterapia 2002;73:43-47.

Bourinbaiar AS, Lee-Huang S. The activity of plant-derived antiretroviral proteins MAP30 and GAP31 against herpes simplex virus infection in vitro. Biochem Biophys Res Commun 1996;219:923-929.

Bourinbaiar AS, Lee-Huang S. Potentiation of anti-HIV activity of anti-inflammatory drugs, dexamethasone and indomethacin, by MAP30, the antiviral agent from bitter melon. Biochem Biophys Res Commun 1995:208:779-784.

Brisebarre AM. Tradition and modernity: French shepherds' use of medicinal bouquets. In: McCorkle CM, Mathias E, Schillhorn van Veen TW, eds. *Ethnoveterinary Research & Development.* London, UK: Intermediate Technology Publications; 1996: 76-90.

Cáceres DD, Hancke JL, Burgos RA, Sandberg F, Wikman GK. Use of visual analogue scale measurements (VAS) to assess the effectiveness of standardized *Andrographis paniculata* extract SHA-10 in reducing the symptoms of common cold. A randomized double-blind placebo study. Phytomedicine 1999;6: 217-223.

Chang RS, Ding L, Chen GQ, Pan QC, Zhao ZL, Smith KM. Dehydroandrographolide succinic acid monoester as an inhibitor against the human immunodeficiency virus. Proc Soc Exp Biol Med 1991;197:59-66.

Chiang LC, Chiang W, Chang MY, Ng LT, Lin CC. Antiviral activity of *Plantago major* extracts and related compounds *in vitro.* Antiviral Res 2002;55:53-62.

Chiang LC, Chiang W, Chang MY, Ng LT, Lin CC. *In vitro* cytotoxic, antiviral and immunomodulatory effects of *Plantago major* and *Plantago asiatica.* Am J Chin Med 2003;31:225-234.

Chun H, Shin DH, Hong BS, Cho WD, Cho HY, Yang HC. Biochemical properties of polysaccharides from black pepper. Biol Pharm Bull 2002;25:1203-1208.

Clapp R, Crook C. Drowning in the magic well: Shaman Pharmaceuticals and the elusive value of traditional knowledge. J Environ Devel 2002;11:79-102.

Cos P, Hermans N, DeBruyne T, et al. Further evaluation of Rwandan medicinal plant extracts for their antimicrobial and antiviral activities. J Ethnopharmacol 2002;79:155-163.

Damre AS, Gokhale AB, Phadke AS, Kulkarni KR, Saraf MN. Studies on the immunomodulatory activity of flavonoidal fraction of *Tephrosia purpurea.* Fitoterapia 2003;74:257-261.

Davis D. Gender-based differences in the ethnoveterinary knowledge of Afghan nomadic pastoralists. Indigenous Knowledge and Development Monitor 1995;3:3-5.

Denyer CV, Jackson P, Loakes DM. Isolation of antirhinoviral sesquiterpenes from ginger (*Zingiber officinale*). J Nat Prod 1994;57:658-662.

DeTommasi N, DeSimone F, Pizza C, et al. Constituents of *Eriobotrya japonica.* A study of their antiviral properties. J Nat Prod 1992;55:1067-1073.

Dhar ML, Dhar MM, Mehrothra BN, Dhawanan BN, Ray C. Screening of Indian plants for biological activity. Ind J Exp Biol 1968;6:232-247.

Emim JA, Oliveira AB, Lapa AJ. Pharmacological evaluation of the anti-inflammatory activity of a citrus bioflavonoid, hesperidin, and the isoflavonoids, duartin and claussequinone, in rats and mice. J Pharm Pharmacol 1994;46:118-122.

Ferrea G, Canessa A, Sampietro F, Cruciani M, Romussi G, Bassetti D. In vitro activity of a *Combretum micranthum* extract against herpes simplex virus types 1 and 2. Antiviral Res 1993;21:317-325.

Fielding D. Ethnoveterinary medicine in the tropics—key issues and the way forward? Available at: http://taa.org.uk/Fieldingdone.htm. Accessed 13th March 2006.

Foà-Tomasi L, Campadelli-Fiume G, Barbieri L, Stripe F. Effect of ribosome-inactivating proteins on virus-infected cells. Inhibition of virus multiplication and of protein synthesis. Arch Virol 1982;71:323-332.

García D, Leiro J, Delgado R, Sanmartin L, Ubeira FM. *Mangifera indica* L. extract (Vimang) and mangiferin modulate mouse humoral immune responses. Phytother Res 2003;17:1182-1187.

García MD, Fernandez MA, Alvarez A, Saenz MT. Antinociceptive and anti-inflammatory effect of the aqueous extract from leaves of *Pimenta racemosa* var. ozua (Mirtaceae). J Ethnopharmacol 2004;91:69-73.

García MD, Sáenz MT, Gómez A, Fernández MA. Topical anti-inflammatory activity of phytosterols isolated from *Eryngium foetidum* on chronic and acute inflammation models. Phytother Res 1999;13:78-80.

Glatthaar-Saalmüller B, Fallier-Becker P. Antiviral action of *Euphorbium compositum* and its components. Forsch Komplementarmed Klass Naturheilkd 2001a;8:207-212.

Glatthaar-Saalmüller B, Sacher F, Esperester A. Antiviral activity of an extract derived from roots of *Eleutherococcus senticosus.* Antiviral Res 2001b;50:223-238.

Godhwani S, Godhwani JL, Vyas DS. *Ocimum sanctum:* an experimental study evaluating its anti-inflammatory, analgesic and antipyretic activity in animals. J Ethnopharmacol 1987;21: 153-163.

Gomez-Flores R, Calderon CL, Scheibel LW, et al. Immunoenhancing properties of *Plantago major* leaf extract. Phytother Res 2000;14:617-622.

Green EC. Etiology in human and animal medicine. Agr Human Values 1998;15:127-131.

Guarrera PM. Traditional antihelmintic, antiparasitic and repellent uses of plants in Central Italy. J Ethnopharmacol 1999;68: 183-192.

Guarrera PM, Forti G, Marignoli S. Ethnobotanical and ethnomedicinal uses of plants in the district of Acquapendente (Latium, Central Italy). J Ethnopharmacol 2005;96:429-444.

Guèye EF. Diseases in village chickens: control through ethnoveterinary medicine. ILEILA Newsletter 1997;13:20.

Guèye EF. Ethnoveterinary medicine against poultry diseases in African villages. World Poultry Sci J 1999;55:187-198.

Guèye EF. Newcastle disease in family poultry: prospects for its control through ethnoveterinary medicine. Paper presented at: 27th World Veterinary Congress; September 25-29, 2002; Tunis, Tunisia. Available at: http://www.cipav.org.co/lrrd/lrrd14/5/guey145a.htm Accessed 13th March 2006.

Guo NL, Lu DP, Woods GL, et al. Demonstration of the anti-viral activity of garlic extract against human cytomegalovirus in vitro. Chin Med J (Engl) 1993;106:93-96.

Hien TT, deJong M, Farrar J. AI—a challenge to global health care structures. N Engl J Med 2004;351:2363-2365.

Hudson JB, Anani K, Lee MK, DeSouza C, Arnason JT, Gbeassor M. Further investigations on the antiviral activities of medicinal plants of Togo. Pharm Biol 2000;38:46-50.

Ibrahim MA, Abdu PA. Ethno-agroveterinary perspectives on poultry production in rural Nigeria. In: McCorkle CM, Mathias E, Schillhorn van Veen TW, eds. *Ethnoveterinary Research & Development.* London, UK: Intermediate Technology Publications; 1996:103-115.

IDL Group. *Community-Based Animal Health Workers: Threat or Opportunity?* Crewkerne, UK: The IDL Group; 2003.

IIRR. Ethnoveterinary Medicine in Asia: An Information Kit on Traditional Animal Health Care Practices, vol 4. Silang, Cavite, Philippines: IIRR; 1994.

ITDG, IIRR. *Ethnoveterinary Medicine in Kenya: A Field Manual of Traditional Animal Health Care Practices.* Nairobi, Kenya: IIRR; 1996:136-137.

Jiratchariyakul W, Wiwat C, Vongsakul M, et al. HIV inhibitor from Thai bitter gourd. Planta Med 2001;67:350-353.

Joe B, Vijaykumar M, Lokesh BR. Biological properties of curcumin-cellular and molecular mechanisms of action. Crit Rev Food Sci Nutr 2004;44:97-111.

Kambewa BMD, Mfitilodze MW, Hüttner K, Wollny CBA, Phoya RKD. The use of indigenous veterinary remedies in Malawi. In: Mathias E, Rangnekar DV, McCorkle CM, eds. Ethnoveterinary Medicine: Alternatives for Livestock Development: Proceedings of an International Conference; November 4-6, 1997; Pune, India. Part 2. Validation of Ethnoveterinary Medicine. Pune, India: BAIF Development Research Foundation; 1999. Available at: http://www.vetwork.org.uk/pune10.htm. Accessed 13th March 2006.

Karandikar SM, Joglekar GV, Balwani JH. Beneficial effect of *Adansonia digitata* (gorakha chinch) in bronchial asthma and allergic skin disorders. Indian Med J 1965;59:69-70.

Kasonia K, Ansay M. A recognition of rural knowledge: medicinal plants and traditional veterinary medicine of central Africa (testing the traditional veterinary pharmacopoeia). In: Mathias E, Rangnekar DV, McCorkle CM, eds. *Ethnoveterinary Medicine: Alternatives for Livestock Development. Proceedings of an International Conference;* November 4-6, 1997; Pune, India.

Ketzis K, Brown D. Medicinal plants used to treat livestock ailments in Honduras. Journal of Herbs, Spices and Medicinal Plants 2002;10:55-64.

Kim HK, Jeon WK, Ko BS. Flavanone glycosides from *Citrus junos* and their anti-influenza virus activity. Planta Med 2001;67: 548-549.

Köhler-Rollefson I, Bräunig J. Anthropological veterinary medicine: the need for indigenizing the curriculum. Paper presented at: 9th AITVM Conference; September 14-18, 1998; Harare, Zimbabwe.

Köhler-Rollefson I, McCorkle CM. Domestic animal diversity, local knowledge, and stockraiser rights. In Bicker A, et al, eds. *Development and Local Knowledge: New Approaches to Issues in Natural Resource Management, Conservation and Agriculture.* New York, NY: Routledge, Taylor & Francis Group; 2004:164-173.

Köhler-Rollefson I, Mundy P, Mathias E. A Field Manual of Camel Diseases: Traditional and Modern Veterinary Care for the Dromedary. London: ITDG Publishing and the League for Pastoral People; 2000.

Kostalova D, Bukosvky M, Koscova H, Kardosova A. Anticomplement activity of *Mahonia aquifoium* bisbenzylisoquinoline alkaloids and berberine extract. Ceska Slov Farm 2001;50:286-289.

Koyama J, Morita I, Kawanishi K, Tagahara K, Kobayashi N. Capillary electrophoresis for simultaneous determination of emodin, chrysophanol, and their 8-beta-D-glucosides. Chem Pharm Bull 2003;51:418-420.

Kudi AC, Myint SH. Antiviral activity of some Nigerian medicinal plant extracts. J Ethnopharmacol 1999;68:289-294.

Kumar R, Singh DP, Chaturvedi VK, Pathak RC. A note on antiviral property of Neem *(Melia azadirachta)* and Tulsi *(Ocimum sanctum)* against Newcastle disease virus. Indian J Comp Microbiol Immunol Infect Dis 1997;18:192-193.

Kumar R, Sridevi K, Kumar N, Nandur S, Rajagopal S. Anticancer and immunostimulatory compounds from *Andrographis paniculata.* J Ethnopharmacol 2004;92:291-295.

Kyo E, Uda N, Kasuga S, Itakura Y. Immunomodulatory effects of aged garlic extract. J Nutr 2001;131:1075s-1079s.

Lans C. Creole remedies: case studies of ethnoveterinary medicine in Trinidad and Tobago. Wageningen University dissertation no. 2992; 2001.

Lans C. Struggling over the direction of Caribbean medicinal plant research. Futures 2003;35:473-491.

Lans C, Brown G, Borde G, Offiah VN. Knowledge of traditional medicines and veterinary practices used for reproductive health problems in human and animal health. J Ethnobiol 2004;23:187-208.

Lee-Huang S, Huang PL, Nara PL, et al. MAP30: a new inhibitor of HIV-1 infection and replication. FEBS Lett 1990;272:12-18.

Li Y, Ooi LSM, Wang H, But PPH, Ooi VEC. Antiviral activities of medicinal herbs traditionally used in southern mainland China. Phytother Res 2004;18:718-722.

Lin CC, Cheng HY, Yang CM, Lin TC. Antioxidant and antiviral activities of *Euphorbia thymifolia* L. J Biomed Sci 2002;9:656-664.

Liu ZF, Fang F, Dong YS, Li G, Zhen H. Experimental study on the prevention and treatment of murine cytomegalovirus hepatitis by using allitridin. Antiviral Res 2004;61:125-128.

Ma S-C, Du J, But PP-H, et al. Antiviral Chinese medicinal herbs against respiratory syncytial virus. J Ethnopharmacol 2002;79: 205-211.

Makare N, Bodhankar S, Rangari V. Immuno-modulatory activity of the alcoholic extract of *Mangifera indica* L. in mice. J Ethnopharmacol 2001;78:133-137.

Manganelli RE, Camangi F, Tomei PE. Curing animals with plants: traditional usage in Tuscany (Italy). J Ethnopharmacol 2001;78:171-191.

Martin M, Mathias E, McCorkle CM. *Ethnoveterinary Medicine: An Annotated Bibliography of Community Animal Healthcare.* London: ITDG Publishing; 2001.

Mathew T, Mathew Z, Taji SA, Zachariah S. A review of viricidal Ayurvedic herbs of India for poultry diseases. J Am Holistic Vet Med Assoc 2001;20:17-21.

Mathias E. Ethnoveterinary medicine: harnessing its potential. Vet Bull 2004;74:27N-37N.

Mathias E, McCorkle CM. Traditional livestock healers. Rev Sci Tech de l'Office International des Epizooties 2003;23:277-284.

Mathias E, Rangnekar DV, McCorkle CM, Martin M, eds. *Ethnoveterinary Medicine: Alternatives for Livestock Development. Proceedings of an International Conference;* November 4-6, 1997; Pune, India. Vol 1 and 2. Pune, India: BAIF Development Research Foundation; 1999. Available at: http://www.vetwork.org.uk/pune10.htm. Accessed 13th March 2006.

Mathias-Mundy E, McCorkle CM. *Ethnoveterinary medicine: An annotated bibliography.* From Bibliographies in Technology and Social Change, No. 6. Ames: Iowa State University, Technology and Social Change Program; 1989.

Mazumder A, Raghavan K, Weinstein J, Kohn K, Pommier Y. Inhibition of human immunodeficiency virus type-1 integrase by curcumin. Biochem Pharmacol 1995;49:1165-1170.

McCorkle CM. Back to the future: lessons from ethnoveterinary RD&E for studying and applying local knowledge. Agric Human Values 1995;12:52-80.

McCorkle CM. Ethnoveterinary medicine. In: Schoen AM, Wynn SG, eds. *Complementary and Alternative Veterinary Medicine.* St. Louis, MO: Mosby; 1998a:713-741.

McCorkle CM. An introduction to ethnoveterinary research and development. J Ethnobiol 1986;6:129-149.

McCorkle CM. Veterinary anthropology. Human Organization 1989:48(2):156-162.

McCorkle CM, Martin M. Parallels and potentials in animal and human ethnomedical technique. Agriculture and Human Values 1998b:15:139-144.

McCorkle CM, Mathias E, Martin M. Introduction. In: *Ethnoveterinary Medicine: An Annotated Bibliography of Community Animal Healthcare.* London: ITDG Publishing; 2001:1-33.

McCorkle CM, Mathias E, Schillhorn van Veen TW, eds. *Ethnoveterinary Research & Development.* London, UK: Intermediate Technology Publications; 1996.

Mediratta PK, Sharma KK, Singh S. Evaluation of immunomodulatory potential of Ocimum sanctum seed oil and its possible mechanism of action. J Ethnopharmacol 2002;80:15-20.

Mehrotra R, Rawat S, Kulshreshtha DK, Patnaik GK, Dhawan BN. *In vitro* studies on the effect of certain natural products against hepatitis B virus. Indian J Med Res 1990;92:133-138.

Melchior J, Spasov AA, Ostrovskiu OV, Bulanov AE, Wikman G. Double-blind, placebo-controlled pilot and Phase III study of activity of standardized *Andrographis paniculata* Herba Nees extract fixed combination (Kan Jang) in the treatment of uncomplicated upper-respiratory tract infection. Phytomedicine 2000;7:341-350.

Minja MMJ. The Maasai wonder plants. Paper presented at: People and Plants Training Workshop, Tropical Pesticides Research Institute; March 15-18, 1999; Arusha, Tanzania.

Mouhajir F, Hudson JB, Rejdali M, Towers GHN. Multiple antiviral activities of endemic medicinal plants used by Berber people of Morocco. Pharm Biol 2001;39:364-374.

Mtambo MMA, Mushi EJ, Kinabo LDB, et al. Evaluation of the efficacy of the crude extracts of *Capsicum frutescens, Citrus limon* and *Opuntia vulgaris* against Newcastle disease in domestic fowl in Tanzania. J Ethnopharmacol 1999;68:55-61.

Nagai K. Experimental studies on the preventive effect of garlic extract against infection with influenza virus. Jpn J Infect Dis 1973;47:321.

OIE (Office International des Epizooties). Early Methods of Animal Disease Control. Revue Scientifique et Technique de l'Office International des Epizooties 1994;13.

Panossian A, Davtyan T, Gukassyan N, et al. Effect of andrographolide and Kan Jang—fixed combination of extract SHA-10 and extract SHE-3—on proliferation of human lymphocytes, production of cytokines and immune activation markers in the whole blood cells culture. Phytomedicine 2002;9:598-605.

Penna SC, Medeiros MV, Aimbire FS, Faria-Neto HC, Sertie JA, Lopes-Martins RA. Anti-inflammatory effect of the hydralcoholic extract of *Zingiber officinale* rhizomes on rat paw and skin edema. Phytomedicine 2003;19:381-385.

Pieroni A, ed. *Herbs, Humans and Animals/Erbe, Uomini e Bestie.* [Engl/Ital] Startseite, Germany: Verlag Köln; 2000.

Pieroni A, Howard P, Volpato G, Santoro RF. Natural remedies and nutraceuticals used in ethnoveterinary practices in inland southern Italy. Vet Res Commun 2004;28:55-80.

PRELUDE Medicinal Plants Database, Specialized in Central Africa, Metafro Infosys. Belgium: Royal Museum for Central Africa. Available at: http://www.metafro.be/prelude. Accessed 13th March 2006.

Sadekar RD, Kolte AY, Barmase BS, Desai VF. Immunopotentiating effects of *Azadirachta indica* (Neem) dry leaves powder in broilers, naturally infected with IBD virus. Indian J Exp Biol 1998a;36:1151-1153.

Sadekar RD, Pimprikar NM, Bhandarkar AG, Barmase BS. Immunopotentiating effect of *Ocimum sanctum* Linn dry leaf powder on cell mediated immune (CMI) response in poultry, naturally infected with IBD virus. Indian Vet J 1998b;75:168-169.

Sairam K, Hemalatha S, Kumar A, et al. Evaluation of anti-diarrheal activity in seed extracts of *Mangifera indica.* J Ethnopharmacol 2003;84:11-15.

Sánchez I, Gomez-Garíbay F, Taboada J, Ruíz BH. Antiviral effect of flavonoids on the dengue virus. Phytother Res 2000;14:89-92.

Sauter C, Wolfensberger C. Anticancer activities as well as antiviral and virus-enhancing properties of aqueous fruit extracts from fifty-six European plant species. Eur J Cancer Clin Oncol 1989;25:987-990.

Schreiber CA, Wan L, Sun Y, Lu L, Krey LC, Lee-Huang S. The antiviral agents, MAP30 and GAP31, are not toxic to human spermatozoa and may be useful in preventing the sexual transmission of human immunodeficiency virus type 1. Fertil Steril 1999;72:686-690.

Semple SJ, Reynolds GD, O'Leary MC, Flower RLP. Screening of Australian medicinal plants for antiviral activity. J Ethnopharmacol 1998;60:163-172.

Sindambiwe JB, Calomme M, Cos P, et al. Screening of seven selected Rwandan medicinal plants for antimicrobial and antiviral activities. J Ethnopharmacol 1999;65:71-77.

Spasov AA, Ostrovskij OV, Chernikov V, Wikman G. Comparative controlled study of *Andrographis paniculata* fixed combination, Kan Jang® and an Echinacea preparation as adjuvant, in the treatment of uncomplicated respiratory disease in children. Phytother Res 2004;18:47-53.

Spreafico F, Malfiore C, Moras ML, et al. The immunomodulatory activity of the plant proteins *Momordica charantia* inhibitor and pokeweed antiviral protein. Int J Immunopharmacol 1983;5:335-343.

Srinivas K, Rao MEB, Rao SS. Anti-inflammatory activity of *Heliotropium indicum* Linn. and *Leucas aspera* Spreng. in albino rats. Indian J Pharmacol 2000;32:37-38.

Sydiskis RJ, Owen DG, Lohr JL, Rosler KHA, Blomster RN. Inactivation of enveloped viruses by anthraquinones extracted from plants. Antimicrob Agents Chemother 1991;35:2463-2466.

TAHCC. Alternative Animal Health Care in British Columbia: A Manual of Traditional Practices Used by Herbalists, Veterinarians, Farmers and Animal Caretakers. Victoria, British Columbia, Canada: The Traditional Animal Health Care Collaborative; 2004.

Tal-Dia A, Toure K, Sarr O, et al. A baobob solution for the prevention and treatment of acute dehydration in infantile diarrhea. Dakar Med 1997;42:68-73.

Tan BK, Vanitha J. Immunomodulatory and antimicrobial effects of some traditional Chinese medicinal herbs: a review. Curr Med Chem 2004;11:1423-1430.

Thamlikitkul V, Dechatiwongse T, Theerapong S, et al. Efficacy of *Andrographis paniculata*, Nees for pharyngotonsillitis in adults. J Med Assoc Thai 1991;74:437-442.

Tollis M, DiTrani L. Recent developments in AI research: epidemiology and immunoprophylaxis. Vet J 2002;164:202-215.

Van Asseldonk AGM, Beijer H. *Herbal Folk Remedies for Animal Health in the Netherlands.* The Netherlands: Institute for Ethnobotany and Zoopharmacognosy; 2005.

Viegi L, Pieroni A, Guarrera PM, Vangelisti R. A review of plants used in folk veterinary medicine in Italy as basis for a databank. J Ethnopharmacol 2003;89:221-244.

Vlietinck AJ, Van Hoof L, Totte J, et al. Screening of hundred Rwandese medicinal plants for antimicrobial and antiviral properties. J Ethnopharmacol 1995;46:31-47.

VSF/Switzerland. Ethnoveterinary Workshop—Malual Kon, Sudan; November 9-12, 1998; Nairobi, Kenya (unpublished paper).

Wachsman MB, Castilla V, Coto CE. Inhibition of foot and mouth disease virus (FMDV) uncoating by a plant-derived peptide isolated from *Melia azedarach* L leaves. Arch Virol 1998;143:581-590.

Waihenya RK, Mtamba MMA, Nkwengulila G. Evaluation of the efficacy of the crude extract of *Aloe secundiflora* in chickens experimentally infected with Newcastle disease virus. J Ethnopharmacol 2002;79:299-304.

Waihenya RK, Mtambo MMA, Nkwengulila G, Kayser O, Hafez HM. Antiviral activity of the crude extract and fractions obtained using high performance liquid chromatography of Aloe secundiflora against Newcastle disease virus. Fitoterapia. Journal of Tropical Microbiology and Biotechnology, 2005 (1), 2005, 10-13

Waller PJ, Bernes G, Thamsborg S, et al. Plants as de-worming agents of livestock in the Nordic countries: historical perspective, popular beliefs and prospects for the future. Acta Vet Scand 2001;42:31-44.

Watt JM, Breyer-Brandwijk MG. *The Medicinal and Poisonous Plants of Southern and Eastern Africa*. London: E&S Livingstone Ltd; 1962:987.

Weber N, Andersen DO, North A, Murray BK, Lawson LD, Hughes BG. In vitro virucidal effects of *Allium sativum* (garlic) extract and compounds. Planta Med 1992;58:417-423.

Yakovlev AI, Zviagin SG. Influence of phytocides on virus influenza A. I. Action of the volatile components from garlic and onion on influenza A. Bull Biol Med 1950;29:284-387.

Yoosook C, Bunyapraphatsara N, Boonyakiat Y, Kantasuk C. Anti–herpes simplex virus activities of crude water extracts of Thai medicinal plants. Phytomedicine 2000;6:411-419.

Zeng X, Lao B, Dong X, et al. Study on anti-influenza effect of alkaloids from roots of Mahonia bealei in vitro [Chinese]. Zhong Yao Cai 2003;26:29-30.

Zheng MS. Antiviral effect of mangiferin and isomangiferin on herpes simplex virus. Chin Med J 1990;103:160-165.

Zhu XM, Song JX, Huang ZZ, Wu YM, Yu MJ. Antiviral activity of mangiferin against herpes simplex virus type 2 in vitro. Acta Pharmacol Sin 1993;14:452-454.

Resources

Other internet resources that readers interested in EVM may consult include those listed in McCorkle 2001 plus later additions such as the following:

www. ethnopharmacology.org of the International Society for Ethnopharmacology

www.ethnovetweb.com, Dr. Med. Vet. Evelyn Mathias' Ethnoveterinary Medicine website

www.ik-pages.net on indigenous knowledge generally

www.metafro.be/preludehttp://www.metafro.be/prelude, for an ethnobotanical database for Africa; for plants used in human or, more rarely, animal ethnomedicine, Phytomedica@ egroups.com

www.unesco.org/most/bpikreg.htm and **http://www. vetwork.org.uk/pune10.htm** for the 1997 India conference mentioned in the text; http://www.asa2000.anthropology.ac. uk/kohler/kohler.html

Examples of scientific journals other than purely veterinary ones that occasionally include articles on EVM can be appreciated in the Martin et al. 2001 bibliography.

The Roots of Veterinary Botanical Medicine

Susan G. Wynn and Barbara J. Fougère

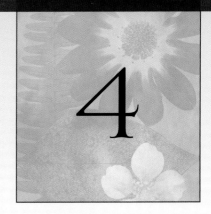

CHAPTER

Today, veterinarians frequently study the names and properties of herbs, yet they may have little or no personal experience of the nature of the plant, its environment, its taste, and its properties. Theoretical knowledge is sterile compared with traditional herbalists' approach of tasting each herb, experiencing its unique qualities, and discerning its properties. Herbalists like Shen Nong Dioscorides and many others learned from their direct experience; this is invaluable even today. Observing herbs and tasting them directly or by infusion, decoction, pills, or formulas is of great benefit, as is taking the herbs for a course of therapy to experience the effects. Herbalists who follow this path will know at a deep experiential level what it is they are prescribing.

Herbal medicine is one of the oldest forms of treatment known and used by all races and all peoples. The World Health Organization (WHO) estimates that botanical medicines are used by 70% of the world's population (Eisenberg, 1998), and it is no surprise that people have used the same plant medicines for the animals in their care as long as animals have been associated with human life. Thus, the history of veterinary botanical medicine, the oldest form of veterinary medicine, has followed a parallel route alongside the evolution of human medicine for much of history. Indeed, herbal medicine itself has undergone a number of philosophical shifts over time, but from antiquity until now, it has remained fundamentally unchanged in tone. Herbal medicine is empiricist, holistic, and vitalist in orientation, and some herbalists argue that it should remain so, even as modern medicine tries to incorporate the use of herbs as "drugs" seeking the "active constituent." This "scientism," perhaps bordering on reductionism, is simply a new philosophy in the larger picture of herbal medicine.

The earliest indications for the use of plants as treatments date back to prehistoric times, with herbs found in graves older than 60,000 years. How did people begin to use plants as medicines? Two main theories are suggested. One is trial and error with final development of a system of thought (such as Traditional Chinese Medicine, one of the best developed systems) and passage of this empiric knowledge from person to person, shaman to shaman, healer to healer. The other is, to our Western mind, a mystical communication between healer and plant, wherein the herbalist directly discovers the plant's medicinal qualities. In many indigenous cultures, the process whereby the plant informs the healer is indeed a spiritual phenomenon that is treated with reverence. Is biochemical screening for biological activity more or less efficient than communing with a plant? Only time will tell. What we do know is that herbs have been used and recorded throughout antiquity in both human and animal medicine.

ANTIQUITY

Evidence suggests that Ayurveda, developed in India, is perhaps the earliest medical system. The Rig veda, the oldest document of human knowledge, written between 4500 and 1600 BCE, mentions the use of medicinal plants in the treatment of humans and animals. The "Nakul Samhita," written during the same period, was perhaps the first treatise on the treatment of animals with herbs. Chapters dealing with animal husbandry like "Management and Feeding" appear in ancient books like *Skandh Puran, Devi Puran, Harit*, and others. Palkapya (1000 BC) and Shalihotra (2350 BC) were famous veterinarians who specialized in the treatment of elephants and horses (Unknown, 2004). King Asoka (274-236 BC) engaged people to grow herbs for use in the treatment of sick and aged animals (Haas, 1992). Medicines that are mentioned in early Ayuvedic texts (200 BC-AD 200) of Charaka Samhita include ricinus, pepper, lily, and valerian.

Vasant Lad describes the basis for Ayurveda ("life science") in a way that is reflected in the Tao of Chinese medicine and echoes the humors of Greek medicine:

> "According to Ayurveda, every human being is a creation of the cosmos, the pure cosmic consciousness, as two energies: male energy, called *Purusha* and female energy, *Prakruti*. *Purusha* is choiceless passive awareness, while *Prakruti* is choiceful active consciousness. *Prakruti* is the divine creative will. . . . The structural aspect of the body is made up of five

elements, but the functional aspect of the body is governed by three biological humors [or doshas]. Ether and air together constitute *vata;* fire and water, *pitta;* and water and earth, *kapha. Vata, pitta,* and *kapha* are the three biological humors that are the three biological components of the organism. They govern psycho-biological changes in the body and physio-pathological changes too. *Vata-pitta-kapha* are present in every cell, tissue, and organ. In every person, they differ in permutations and combinations. [The balance in the doshas can be effected by] hereditary, congenital, internal, external trauma, seasonal, natural tendencies or habits, and supernatural factors." (Lad, 1996)

In China, one of the oldest known and longest preserved *Materia Medica* was compiled in 3700 BC by a Chinese emperor named Shen Nong. Shen Nong (the Divine Farmer) is the legendary originator of Chinese herbal medicine. He is credited with tasting hundreds of herbs, selecting those that were suitable as remedies, and describing their properties. As a result of his efforts, numerous herbs became routinely used for healthcare, and knowledge was handed down by oral tradition for centuries. His book of medicinal herbs listed herbal *Materia Medica* for both humans and animals. It is interesting to note that it discussed the antifever properties of *Artemesia annua* (Chinese wormwood), which has now been shown to be extremely effective against malaria.

When these herbs were described in a formal manner, the book was named after Shen Nong, known today as the *Shen Nong Ben Cao Jing (Herbal Classic of Shen Nong).* The earliest mention of a text called *Shen Nong Jing (Classic of Shen Nong)* came from authors who lived during the period immediately following the fall of the Han Dynasty (220 AD), suggesting that it might have been compiled during the latter part of the Han Dynasty. It is thought that Shen Nong lived from 2737 BC to 2697 BC—nearly 5000 years ago; this is why it is common to hear that Chinese medicine has a history of 5000 years. However, we are able to access little information about how herbal medicines were used before the compilation of the Shen Nong herbal—about 1800 years ago.

The *Shen Nong Ben Cao Jing* describes for the first time the flavors (sour, salty, sweet, bitter, acrid/pungent), natures (cold, hot, warm, cool), functions, and indications for the herbs. Herbs were classified according to their efficacy and toxicity, and the terms *sovereign* (or king), *minister, assistant,* and *envoy* were described to define the function of an herb within a formula. According to the *Ben Cao,* "Medicinals should coordinate [with each other] in terms of yin and yang, like mother and child, or brothers. . . . to treat cold, one should use hot medicinals. To treat heat, one should use cold medicinals." Shen Nong clearly tasted the herbs and fit their characteristics into the Tao, the philosophy that guided people's understanding of their world. Herbs were tools that interacted with people to shift and balance their bodies back to health. An English language translation of the ancient *Shen Nong Ben Cao Jing* has been published (Yang, 1997).

The earliest Chinese medical practitioners treated both people and animals until the Zhou dynasty (1122-770 BC), when veterinary medicine became a separate branch

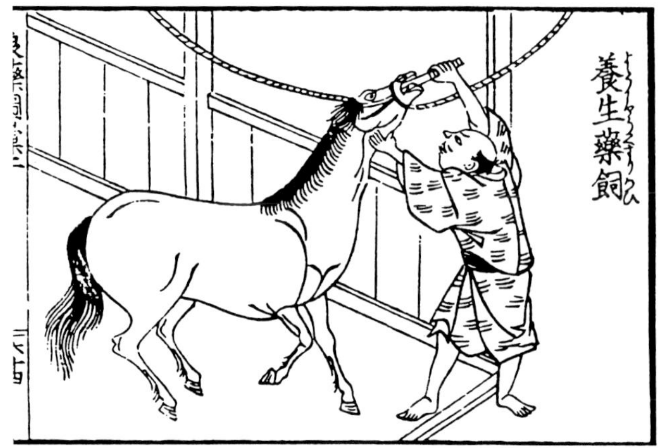

Figure 4-1 Administering liquid medicine with a bamboo bottle is an aspect of the old Chinese-Japanese art of horse healing, *Ryoyaku-ba-ryn-benkai*, as portrayed in *Zisanshi* (first edition, Kyoto [1759]; second edition, Yedo [1859]). *(From Dunlop RH, Williams DJ. Veterinary Medicine: An Illustrated History. St. Louis, Mo: Mosby; 1996.)*

of traditional Chinese medicine (Schoen, 1994), and in China, the first mention of diseases and treatments of horses appeared in writings of the Shang Dynasty (1766-1027 BC). One of the first texts in Chinese veterinary medicine was *Bai Le's Canon of Veterinary Medicine*, written by Sun Yang in approximately 650 AD (Figure 4-1).

In Mesopotamia, the Sumerians used cuneiform written language from about 3500 BC. The earliest extant clay tablet from Sumeria dates from about 2100 BC; it contains 15 medical prescriptions and mentions 120 mineral drugs and 250 plant-derived medicines. These included asafetida, calamus, crocus, cannabis, castor, galbanum, glycyrrhiza, hellebore, mandragon, menthe, myrrh, opium, turpentine, styrax, and thyme. The largest surviving medical treatise is from about 1600 BC; it is entitled "Treatise of Medical Diagnoses and Prognoses." Although the names of the medicines used then do not translate well, it is probable that milk, snakeskin, turtleshell, cassia, thyme, willow, fir, myrtle, and dates were also used (Janick, 2002). The Code of Hammurabi (circa 1780 BC), another famous document arising from Babylonian society, discussed treatments of animals, costs of treatments, and penalties for mistreatment and errors (Swabe, 1999).

The Edwin Smith Papyrus (found in Egypt and preserved at the New York Academy of Medicine) dates from 1700 BCE. These scrolls include a surprisingly accurate description of the circulatory system, noting the central role of the heart and the existence of blood vessels throughout the body. They describe the use of herbs such as senna, honey, thyme, juniper, pomegranate root, henbane, flax, oakgall, pinetar, bayberry, ammi, alkanet, aloe, cedar, caraway, coriander, cyperus, elderberry, fennel, garlic, wild lettuce, myrrh, nasturtium, onion, peppermint, papyrus, poppy, saffron, watermelon, and wheat. The Ebers Papyrus (now in University Library at

Leipzig) dates from about 1500 BC and contains more than 800 prescriptions. Some of these are very complicated, containing such ingredients as opium, hellebore, salts of lead and copper, and blood, excreta, and viscera of animals (Haas, 1999). Many more of the ancient scrolls were housed in the Library of Alexandria, which was destroyed by fire in 47 BCE. However, early evidence of veterinary herbal medicine is found in ancient Egyptian parchments such as the Kahun Veterinary Papyrus (dating around 1900 BC) (Karasszon, 1998), on which cattle feature prominently.

Ancient Greek and Roman societies began developments in veterinary medicine in similar, yet slightly different directions compared with the Egyptians. The "Hippiatrika" is one of the first documents we see that relates to Roman practitioners and their study of horses (Walker, 1991). "Hippiatros" was a term used in Greece around 500 BC to refer to horse doctors (Swabe, 1999). The horse was central in Greek and Roman society because members of society depended on it for military and trade functions. Earlier on (between 383 BC and 322 BC), Aristotle, sometimes called "the Father of Veterinary Medicine," became very influential in Greek society. Physiology, comparative anatomy, and pathology were a few of the specialized areas that Aristotle discussed in his writings. He compared animal and human anatomy and physiology and disease in writings such as *Historia Animalium, De Partibus Animalium, De Generatione Animalium,* and *Problematicum* (Karasszon, 1998). Another important influence on both veterinary and herbal medicine was Hippocrates (460-377 BC). He wrote *Corpus Hippocraticum,* in which he described more than 200 plants, and he is credited with the development of the humoral theory (Figure 4-2).

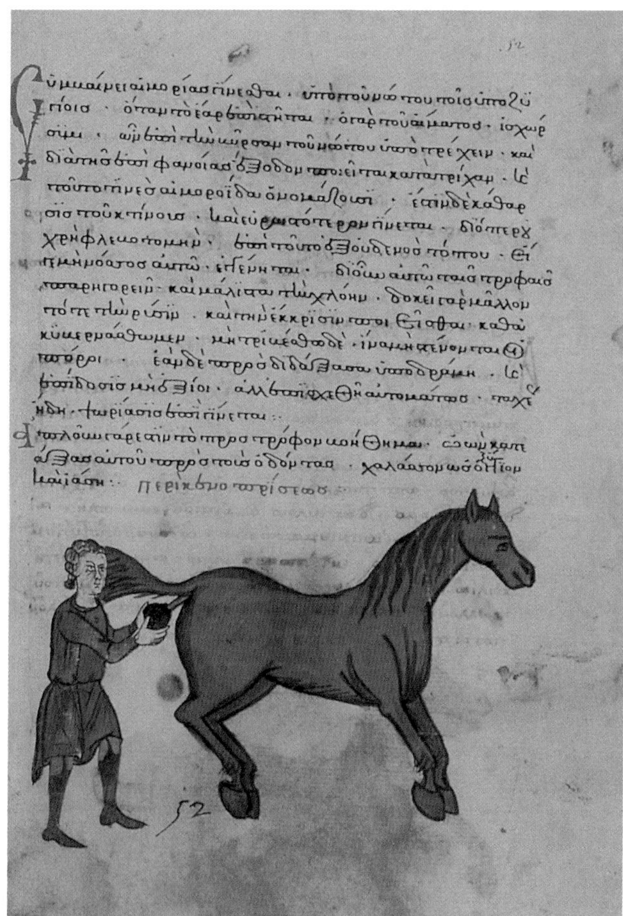

Figure 4-2 An illustration from the 14th century *Hippiatrika* manuscript showing treatment of distention in a horse. Much of the information on horse care found in the *Hippiatrika* came from the Greeks, and the use of oil and wine for medicinal purposes is frequently prescribed. Here, a clyster of wine, oil, soda salt, and sap from wild cucumber roots is being administered to relieve the distention. *(Cod. G. 2233. Bibliothèque Nationale, Paris) (From Dunlop RH, Williams DJ. Veterinary Medicine: An Illustrated History. St. Louis, Mo: Mosby; 1996.)*

HUMORAL THEORY

The idea of the Four Humors became popular in Ancient Greece from about 400 BC. It probably originated in Indian Ayurvedic medicine, where it was picked up by travelers and taken to the Greek empire (which included the present-day countries of Greece, Egypt, Turkey, and Italy). However, it is attributed to Hippocrates. At this time, thinkers were beginning to explain events in the world around them in terms of natural phenomena rather than blaming the gods and spirits. They established that all things were made up of the four elements air, water, fire, and earth. These elements were also linked to the four seasons and to body fluids or "humors"—blood, phlegm, black bile, and yellow bile. Illness was thought to result when these humors lost their natural balance, and health could be restored by rebalancing the humors. This theory was very important because it encouraged doctors to look for natural causes of disease and to provide physical, rather than spiritual treatments.

The rise of rationalism meant that doctors were now observing patients and reasoning toward a logical cure, just as the Chinese had done. Hippocrates reasoned that medicine could be applied without ritual because disease was a natural phenomenon and not a supernatural event. He argued that some acute diseases were self-limiting and should not necessarily be treated, and that diet and exercise were vital in preventing and treating conditions of the human body. The humoral theory remained very influential for more than a thousand years and was not seriously challenged until the 15th century. It is interesting to note that it is related in many ways to the philosophical basis of Traditional Chinese Medicine and of many other traditional medical practices (Table 4-1).

MEANWHILE IN JAPAN

Kampo (also written *Kanpo*) is based on Traditional Chinese Medicine and literally means "the Han Method," referring to the herbal system of China that developed during the Han Dynasty. Cultural contact between China and Japan has occurred since ancient times. There is a story about a Chinese Emperor (reign: 221-210 BC) who is said to have sent emissaries by ship on the Eastern Sea

TABLE 4-1

Humor	Associated Element	Energetic Qualities
Blood	Air	Hot, moist
Phlegm	Water	Cold, moist
Black bile	Earth	Cold, dry
Yellow bile	Fire	Hot, dry

to find the herb of immortality; it is suggested that they returned from Japan at the end of their mission with ganoderma (lingzhi; Japanese: *reishi*). Some Chinese medical works were introduced to Japan as early as the 4th or 5th Century AD, coming first by way of Korea, which had adopted Chinese medicine by that time. Historical records indicate that a Korean physician named Te Lai came to Japan in 459 AD, and that a Chinese Buddhist named Zhi Cong brought medical texts with him to Japan via Korea in 562 AD. It was during this period that the Chinese written language was adopted in Japan, which enabled people to learn from China about Buddhism, Confucianism, governmental organization, and the divination arts and opened the way for study of Chinese medicine. Kampo encompasses acupuncture and other components of Traditional Chinese Medicine but relies primarily on prescription of herb formulas. It differs today from the practice of Chinese herbal medicine in mainland China primarily in its reliance on a different basic collection of important herb formulas and a somewhat different group of primary herbs. Kampo medicine is widely practiced in Japan today (Dharmananda, 2004).

THE RISE OF ROME

A first century Roman (Lucius Junius Moderatus Columella) wrote 12 volumes of *On Agriculture*. Volume VI dealt with cattle, horses, and mules; volume VII with sheep, goats, pigs, and dogs; and volume VIII with poultry and fowl. In volume VI, we find reference to the use of garlic in cattle:

> "It will be no use to give cattle a satisfying diet, unless every care is taken that they are healthy in body and that they keep up their strength. Both these objects are secured by administering, on three consecutive days, a generous dose of medicine compounded of equal weights of the crushed leaves of lupine and of cypress, which is mixed with water and left out of doors for a night. This should be done four times a year-at the end of spring, of summer, of autumn, and of winter. Lassitude and nausea also can often be dispelled if you force the whole raw hen's egg down the animal's throat when it has eaten nothing; then, on the following day, you should crush spikes of 'Cyprian' or ordinary garlic in wine and pour it into the nostrils."

He also recommended for bloat in cattle a drench of wild myrtle and wine mixed with hot water. For ulceration of the lungs, he recommended administration of cabbage leaves baked in oil. He also recommended a seton (a foreign body, more recently of cloth, introduced into tissue to elicit drainage or form an open tract for drainage of a wound) of white hellebore through the ear and a daily mixture of leek juice, olive oil, and wine to "avert death of cattle" (Smithcors, 1957).

The decline of Ancient Greece corresponded with the rise of the Roman Empire, and many Greek scholars moved to Rome. Two Greek scholars working in Rome had an influence on herbal medicine. Dioscorides of Anazarbus (Pedianos Dioskurides) was a careful observer and naturalist, botanist, and skilled physician and is known today for the famous work *De Materia Medica*, published in the year 65 AD. This book listed more than 500 plants and was translated into many languages, including Persian, Hebrew, and Anglo-Saxon. The organization of Dioscorides' work followed the pattern of one plant, one chapter. Following the description of the plants, some indications for use were described.

Origins of the Name "Veterinarian"

The origins of the term "veterinarian" are not clear, but classical Roman derivation seems likely. Animal caretakers were named *souvetaurinarii,* and pack animals were called *veterina*. The *veterinarium* was the compound in Roman military encampments where pack animals were kept. Columnella wrote a famous text on agriculture that included information on animal husbandry, and he used the term *veterinarius* for those who cared for livestock other than horses. Men who cared for horses were called *mulomedicus*.

(Dunlop, 1996)

Dioscorides classified plant medicines according to the state of the plants themselves (with seasonal variations) and their effects on people—this was a drug affinity system (Riddle, 1985) that had little to do with mystical powers or cosmic relationships that would later characterize the alchemical herbology of Culpepper. It became the foremost classical source of modern botanical terminology and the leading pharmacologic text for the next 1600 years. An illuminated copy prepared in the year 512 is now housed in the Österreichische Nationalbibliothek.

The second Greek physician who had a lasting impact was Claudios Galenos (131-201 AD), who is generally referred to as Galen. He learned much about anatomy through his work treating professional gladiators. He developed an interest in anatomy and skills as a surgeon, and he dissected pigs, goats, and apes and applied what he found to the human body. He was strongly influenced by Hippocrates' Four Humors and his theory was built on Hippocrates' idea that the body was made up of four liquids—blood, phlegm, yellow bile, and black bile—and that imbalances in one of these humors might be treated with a substance that opposed that tendency. For instance, psoriasis is considered a hot and dry condition, so Galen would suggest that the patient drink cool liquids, eat cold foods, and use a cool, wet herb such as plantain. He wrote more than 500 books on medicine and developed a system of pharmacology and therapeutics. Galen's humoral theory and Alexandrian Greek medicine shaped Islamic and European medicine for the next 1400 years. His books were used at medical schools until the Renaissance.

Other early Roman writers of note on the topic of veterinary medicine include Vegetius, author of *Mulomedicina,* a comprehensive equine veterinary text compiled from works of the previous authors Pelagonius, Chiron, and Apsyrtus (Mezzabotta, 1998).

THE DARK AGES

When Rome fell in 476 AD, Greek medicine was temporarily lost to Europe. Civilization as it was during the reign of Rome ceased to exist, and it took centuries for the level of Roman societal achievements in living standards, culture, architecture, and medical practice to be regained. When Galen's ideas were rediscovered after Crusaders and Byzantine scholars returned to Europe, his system again became medical dogma for hundreds of years.

But first, Europe had to endure the Dark Ages, when medicine was characterized in two ways—the storage and adaptation of Greek knowledge by Christian monasteries, and folk medicine.

During the Dark Ages, Christian monasteries played a crucial role in preserving the knowledge of the ancients. Monks painstakingly copied classical texts, which were traded or passed on to other eminent individuals or institutions. Monks also cared for the sick and injured because there were very few physicians. So, monks not only preserved but also developed skills in the use of herbs and natural medicine. Each monastery maintained its own herbal garden and kept others up-to-date with advances in medical treatments.

The writings of the Dark Ages in Europe are largely lost to us, but some books from those times remain. Anglo-Saxon herbals were published from the 7th to the 11th centuries (Table 4-2). The medicine of this age incorporated many charms, in addition to the plants; Christian prayers probably replaced older pagan charms over time. The herbs that appeared most commonly included betony, vervain, peony, yarrow, mugwort, and waybroad

TABLE 4-2

Examples of Anglo-Saxon Veterinary Medicine

Diagnosis	Treatment	Source
Sick cattle	"Take the wort, put it upon gledes and fennel and hassuck and "cotton" and incense. Burn all together on the side on which the wind is. Make it reek upon the cattle. Make five crosses of hassuck grass, et them on four sides of the cattle and one in the middle. Sing about the cattle the Benedicite and some litanies and the Pater Noster. Sprinkle holy water upon them, burn upon them incense and give the tenth penny in the Church for God, after that leave them to amend; do this thrice."	*Lacnunga*
To prevent sudden death in swine	"Sing over them four masses, drive the swine to the fold, hang the worts upon the four sides and upon the door, also burn them, adding incense and make the reek stream over the swine." *or* "Take the worts of lupin, bishopwort, hassuck grass, tufty thorn, vipers bugloss, drive the swine to the fold, hang the worts upon the four sides and upon the door."	*Lacnunga*
Elf-shot horse	"If a horse be elf-shot, then take the knife of which the haft is the horn of a fallow ox and on which are three brass nails, then write upon the horse's forehead Christ's mark and on each of the limbs which thou mayest feel at; then take the left ear, prick a hole in it in silence, then strike the horse on the back, then it will be healed. And write upon the handle of the knife these words—'Benedicite omnia opera Domini dominum.' Be the elf what it may, this is mighty for him to amend." *or* "If a horse or other neat be elf-shot take sorrel-seed or Scotch wax, let a man sing twelve Masses over it and put holy water on the horse or on whatsoever neat it be; have the worts always with thee. For the same take the eye of a broken needle, give the horse a prick with it, no harm shall come."	*Leech Book of Bald*
"If a beast drinks an insect"	Sing this: "Gonomil, orgomil, marbumil, marbsai, tofeth."	*Leech Book of Bald*
Drowned bees	Place them in warm ashes of pennyroyal and then, "they shall recover their lyfe after a little tyme as by ye space dissertation."	*The Boke of Secretes of Albartus Magnus of the Virtues of Herbes, Stones, and Certaine Beastes*

(plantain). There are four known texts from the 10th century; these are now held by the British Museum and include *Leech Book of Bald, Lacnunga, Herbarium of Apuleius* (a translation from the 5th century), and a translation from Petronius' *Practica Petrocelli Salernitani* entitled περί Διδαξέως (which means "about learning/instruction").

One of the most interesting Middle European monastic personalities was German abbess Hildegard von Bingen (1098-1179). Remnants of Greek medicine were evident in her writings, which retained some of the old herb characteristics but introduced a new spiritualism that reflected her love of God and her Old Testament belief that everything in creation was made to serve man (Hozeski, 2001):

> "Every herb, however, is either warm or cold. They spring up this way. The warmth of herbs signifies the soul and the cold of herbs signifies the body."

And:

> ". . . for the earth has many useful herbs that reach out to people's spiritual needs, and yet they are distinct from people. In addition, the earth has useless herbs that reflect the useless and diabolical ways of humans."

Hildegard wrote *Causeae et Curae* and *Physica*, in which she described causes of diseases and their cures. She compiled the beginnings of a Germanic herbal knowledge and wrote widely on devotion, mysticism, and healing. She used the four-element and four-humor system, and her approach integrated body, mind, and spirit with specific prescriptions for herbs, diet, and gems. She also wrote *Liber Simplicis Medicinae*, in which she prescribed different herbs for cattle, goats, horses, pigs, and sheep (Haas, 2000). Currently, the writings of Hildegard are undergoing a revival in the German-speaking world.

Outside the monasteries, the wise women and traveling herbalists were using medicinal plants in ritual and magic. It was mainly these wise women who felt the brunt of the Inquisition, and many were burned as witches; because they relied on an oral tradition, their knowledge was widely lost. While Europe's Dark Ages trundled on under the influence of Christianity, Spain became a center of botanical research. Among other bright lights, Arab culture and society in the Near East advanced medicine to new heights.

Energetics of Herbs—The European Perspective
Coles' Art of Simpling (echoing Paracelsus and others of the time)

Temperate Plants and Fruits
Maidenhair, Asparagus, Licorice, Pine Nuts, Figs, Raisins, Dates, Woodruff, Bugle, Goat's Rue, Flaxweed, Cinquefoil.

Hot in the First Degree
Wormwood, Marshmallows, Borage, Bugloss, Oxeye, Beets, Cabbage, Chamomile, Agrimony, Fumitory, Wildflax, Melilot, Comfrey, Avens, Eyebright, Selfheal, Chervil, Basil, etc. Sweet Almonds, Chestnuts, Cypress Nuts, Green Walnuts, Ripe Grapes, Ripe Mulberries, Seeds of Coriander, Flax, Gromwell, etc.

Hot in the Second Degree
Brooklime, Green Anise, Angelica, Parsley, Mugwort, Betony, Groundpine, Fenugreek, Saint John's Wort, Ivy, Hops, Balm, Horehound, Rosemary, Savory, Sage, Maudlin, Ladies Mantle, Dill, Smallage, Marigolds, *Carduus benedictus*, Scurvygrass, Alehoose, Alexander, Archangel, Devilsbit, Sanicle, Capers, Nutmegs, Dry Figs, Dry Nuts, The Seeds of Dill, Parsley, Rocket, Basil, Nettle, The Roots of Parsley, Fennel, Lovage, Mercury, Butterburr, Hog's Fennel, etc.

Hot in the Third Degree
Asarabacca, Agnus, Arum, Dry Anixe, Germander, Bastard, Saffron, Centaury, Celandine, Calamint, Fleabane, Elecampane, Hyssop, Bays, Marjoram, Pennyroyal, Rue, Savine, Bryony, Pilewort, Bankcresses, Clary, Lavender, Feverfew, Mint, Watercresses, Hellebore, etc.

Hot in the Fourth Degree
Selatica, Cress, Spurge, Pepper, Mustardseed, Garlic, Leeks, Onions, Stonecrop, Dittander or Pepperwort, Garden Cresses, Crowfoot, Ros Solis, and the Root of Pellitory of Spain.

Cold in the First Degree
Orage, Mallows, Myrtle, Pellitory of the Wall, Sorrel, Woodsorrel, Burdock, Shepherd's Purse, Hawkweed, Burnet, Coltsfoot, Quinces, Pears, Roses, Violets.

Cold in the Second Degree
Blites, Lettuce, Duckmeat, Endive, Hyacinth, Plantain, Fleawort, Nightshade, Cucumbers, Chickweed, Dandelion, Fumitory, Wild tansy, Knotgrass, etc. Oranges, Peaches, Damsons, etc.

Cold in the Third Degree
Purslane, Houseleek, Everlasting, Orpine, etc. Seeds of Henbane, Hemlock, Poppy.

Cold in the Fourth Degree
Henbane, Hemlock, Poppies, Mandrake, etc.

Moist in the First Degree
Bugloss, Borage, Mallows, their flowers and roots; Pellitory, Marigolds, Basil and the roots of Satyrion, etc.

Moist in the Second Degree
Violets, Waterlily, Orage, Blites, Lettuce, Ducksmeat, Purslane, Peaches, Damsons, Grapes, Chickweed, etc.

Dry in the First Degree
Agrimony, Chamomile, Eyebright, Selfheal, Fennel, Myrtle, Melilot, Chestnuts, Beans, Barley, etc.

Dry in the Second Degree
Pimpernel, Shepherd's Purse, Wormwood, Vervain, Mugwort, Betony, Horsetail, Mint, Scabious, Bugle, *Carduus benedictus.*

Dry in the Third Degree
Southernwood, Ferns, Yarrow, Cinquefoil, Angelica, Pilewort, Marjoram, Rue, Savory, Tansy, Thyme, Hellebore.

Dry in the Fourth Degree
Garden Cresses, Wild Rue, Leeks, Onions, Garlic, Crowfoot.

ARABIC MEDICINE

Rational approaches to medicine were developed to the highest level in the Middle East, where Avicenna lived from 980 to 1037 AD. He is the most famous and influential of the philosopher scientists of Islam and was born in Persia (now Iran). Abdullah Ibn Ahmad Ibn al-Baytar, as he was known in his land, was a botanist (he described more than 1400 medical herbs, comparing them with the descriptions of ancient authors) and pharmacist. He further codified Galen's theory of using opposites to correct disease processes. His *Canon of Medicine* is one of the most influential medical books of all time. The *Canon* described the primary constituents of the human body as the elements—earth, air, fire, and water—that possess two qualities each. Earth is dry and cold, water is wet and cold, air is hot and moist, and fire is hot and dry. The humors are described as the primary body fluids that affect physiologic processes; they are themselves influenced by states of motion and rest. These humors include sanguineous (blood), serous (phlegm), bilious (choler or yellow bile), and atrabilious (melancholy, or black bile), which correspond with air, water, fire, and earth, respectively. Avicenna is credited with introducing astrology into medicine. Each humor possessed certain normal qualities and was associated with certain signs of the zodiac. Avicenna's *Canon* was widely read by Europeans after it was translated into Latin in the 12th century. From 1500 to 1674, more than 60 editions were published in Europe. It was the standard text for university medical training until the 18th century.

In the 12th century, Ibn al-Wwam wrote "Kitab Al-Falaha," a treatise on agriculture with a section on veterinary medicine. The 33rd chapter discusses diseases of the horse. Redness in the eye was said to be cured with rose water, blepharitis and conjunctivitis with centaury or saffron, mange in the ears or on the nose with saffron and sulphur, stomatitis with powder of pomegranate shells, headache with a linseed cataplasm, leeches in the mouth, nose, or throat with olive oil, and red urine with white pepper (Erk, 1960).

THE RENAISSANCE

The Renaissance represented a flourishing of new ideas and discoveries in all areas of human endeavor. Great herbals from all over Europe began to appear in the 16th century, with the advent of the printing press. These included *Herbarum Vivae Eicones* (1530) by Otto Brunfels; *Kreuter Buch* (1542) by Jerome Boch; *De Historias Stirpium* (1542) by Loenhart Fuchs; *New Herball* (1551) by William Turner; *Commentary on Dioscorides* (1544) by Pier Andrea Mattioli; *Croydeboeck* (1554) by Rembert Dodoens, and *Herball* (1597) by John Gerard. Fuchs' herbal is particularly distinguished as providing a new standard for plant illustrations. Leaves from copies of the herbal printed in the 16th century are regularly offered for sale on Ebay!

One of the greatest challenges to the traditional Galenic humoral practice of medicine came from Phillipus Theophrastus Bombastus von Hohenheim (1493-1541), also known as Paracelsus. He was the son of a doctor and became an alchemist who contributed greatly to the discovery of medicinal effects of metals. Paracelsus was from a time when the discovery of the New World by Columbus called into question every construct developed by modern thought of the time. He rejected the theoretical dogma of Hippocrates and Galen for experimental medicine. He was particularly interested in the intrinsic property of a remedy—plant or mineral—and not necessarily the relationships and properties attributed to it by the ancients (Wood, 2000). Paracelsus said that the size of the dose determined whether the substance was a poison or a medicine.

He believed that humans functioned chemically and that illness should be treated chemically, and he introduced the use of chemical drugs in place of herbal remedies. He opened the way for exploration of new remedies, including opium and the inestimable calomel—mercury. He was a firm believer in the Doctrine of Signatures, which linked the physical properties and habitat of a plant with its possible actions and indications. It is recorded that Paracelsus used Saint John's Wort topically for gangrene in horses (Mulder, 1994).

DOCTRINE OF SIGNATURES

The Doctrine of Signatures is an ancient theory that reemerged in Europe through the efforts of Paracelsus, and again in the 16th century with Jakob Böhme (1575-1624), a shoemaker in Görlitz, Germany, who wrote "Signatura Rerum; The Signature of All Things." This doctrine espoused the philosophy that God stamped his "signature" on a plant to show how it might be used for medicine. As an example, two very different plants that resemble lung tissue are named "lungwort." *Pulmonaria officinalis* has broadly lanceolate leaves that are mottled to look like lung parenchyma; the other plant, *Sticta pulmonaria*, is a lichen in which the structure resembles the pulmonary tree. The doctrine of signatures is not unique to Europe. Ancient medical practices, including Chinese medicine, contain elements of it, and Israeli folk medicine practices reflect some of this thought (Dafni, 2002). Certain of the precepts inherited from Europe were found in the early 1900s in isolated Appalachian communities of the United States.

People looked at plant shape, color, and taste for clues as to their medical uses. The form of the leaf, flower, or root might recall a certain organ. Ginseng root, for instance, is shaped like a human, and in Traditional Chinese Medicine, some vines, worms, and snakes are long and thin and are thought to easily enter the *jing-luo* (or meridians). Orchids often have bulbs or flowers shaped like testicles, hence their common name derived from the Greek word for testicle—"orchis." In addition, it was thought that some plants were usually found growing in association with others that complemented or remedied their actions. For instance, poison ivy can very often be found growing near jewelweed *(Impatiens capensis)*, which is thought to stop the itching when applied topically. Plant color is important as well. For instance, plants with yellow parts are often associated with the liver (recalling the yellow color of bile). Plants with red parts (like the root of bloodroot) might be associated with treatment of blood disorders. Blue plant parts might cool fevers, and purple parts are thought to manage blood infections.

The philosophy reflected the belief, "As above, so below." Taken to a greater extreme, one could fit all plants into the alchemical cosmology that grew in influence in the 16th and 17th centuries. The plant might, because of its taste sensation or color, be associated with one of the Elements (Spirit [Ether], Fire, Air, Earth, and Water) and may therefore be more closely aligned with certain types of diseases. This sympathetic magic was formalized in the great book by Nicholas Culpeper, *The English Physitian* [sic], which was written in 1652 and is still in print. Here is the description of dandelion found in an undated early 20th century edition of the book:

> "It is under the dominion of Jupiter. It is of an opening and cleansing quality, and therefore very effectual for the obstructions of the liver, gall, and spleen, and the diseases that arise from them, as the jaundice and hypochondriac [sic]; it opens the passages of the urine both in young and old; powerfully cleanses imposthumes and inward ulcers in the urinary passage, and by its drying and temperate quality, doth afterwards heal them . . . The distilled water is effectual to drink in pestilential fevers, and to wash the sores."

George Turberville wrote an influential book on the treatment of dogs in 1576, titled *The Noble Art of Venerie or Hunting*. His treatment recommendations reflected the beliefs of the day. To prevent "madness," or to obtain mostly male hunting dog offspring, for instance, he recommended that care in husbandry be paid to the phases of the moon and the signs of Gemini and Aquarius (Dunlop, 1996).

William Coles, author of *The Art of Simpling* (1656), knew of Culpeper, and although he apparently thought Culpeper went too far, he still believed in the Doctrine. He lists, for instance, Adder's tongue as an herb that should be used for curing the bite of an adder because of its shape. On the other hand, viper's bugloss *(Echium vulgare)* has speckled stalks (like a snake's skin), and this also makes it good for snake bites and for "poison" from scorpions and other venomous beasts. In addition,

> "Walnuts bear the whole Signature of the Head, the outward most green bark answerable to the thick skin wherewith the head is covered, and a Salt made of it is singularly good for wounds in that part, as the kernel is good for the brains which it resembles, being environed with a Shell, which imitates the Skull, and then it is wrapped up again in a silken covering somewhat representing the Pia Mater."

Coles provided a good example of how extreme this system could become under the cover of official doctrine:

> "And I know not why Sagittaria, or Arrowhead, should not be good for wounds made with the head of an Arrow, and Kidney beans for diseases of the Kidneys, though I confess I have not read to that purpose in any Author."

Yet he acknowledges that, although the doctrine is useful, not all plants are marked (Figure 4-3):

> "But because all Plants have not their Signatures, we are not rashly to conclude that they are therefore unfit for Medicinal uses, there being no necessity that all should be thus signed, though some be, for then the rarity of it, which is the delight, would be taken away by too much harping upon one thing.

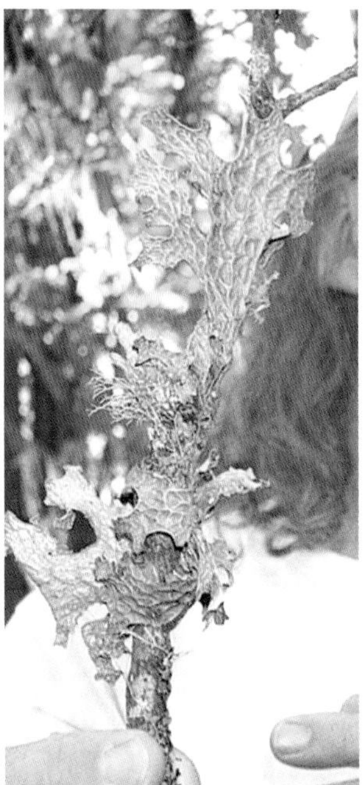

Figure 4-3 Lungwort has anatomic characteristics resembling lung parenchyma—a good example of naming a plant according to the doctrine of signatures.

In England, the Renaissance period produced several great botanists and herbalists. The first printed herbal in England was *Bancke's Herbal,* author unknown, from 1524. This work is probably a compilation from medieval manuscripts, and it has gone through many editions. The first illustrated herbal in England was *Grete Herball*, which is a translation of other herbals. Turner's *Herball* was an influential text, but the most famous English herbal was John Gerard's *The Herball or Generall Historie of Plantes*. This work was probably the result of the labor of another man, a Dr Priest, but Gerard's *Herball* is still known as the most beautiful of the English herbals because of the illustrations and its Elizabethan style. His work reflected the theory that herbs treat not only physical diseases but also those of the mind and spirit. Interestingly, Gerard describes methods of aromatherapy that involve the inhalation of volatile oils and the absorption of these through the skin into the circulatory system. The last great English herbalist of this period was John Parkinson, who wrote *Paradisus* in 1629 and the *Theatrum Botanicum* in 1640. The *Theatrum Botanicum* described more than 3800 plants and was the most complete and aesthetically beautiful English treatise on plants of the day. Rohde (1922) claims that the only herbal to devote an entire chapter to animals is Coles' *Art of Simpling* (1656) (see the box on p. 38).

Throughout the 16th century, the division between university-trained doctors and other practitioners such as midwives, herbalists, and bone crackers grew. The era of "homemade" practitioners had its roots in the tradition of the village healer, along with the increased numbers of publications made possible by the spread of the printing press. Written knowledge of medicine and herbs became available to masses. During the reign of Henry VIII, practitioners of contemporary alchemy and practitioners of traditional herbal medicine clashed. Untrained practitioners also referred to as "quacks" were common. To stop this flood of lay practitioners and the associated competition with trained physicians, starting in 1512, the English Parliament passed a series of Acts of Parliament to regulate the practice of medicine in England. However, to the dismay of the surgeons who tried to use one of the new acts to stop local healing women from practicing their home remedies, this resulted in the passing of what is known as "The Quacks' Charter." This new act allowed, "it shall be lawful to every person . . . having knowledge and experience of the nature of Herbs, Roots, and Waters . . . to practice, use, and minister . . . without suit, vexation, trouble, penalty, or loss of their goods." Modern herbalists refer to this Act as "The Herbalists' Charter." The practice of folk medicine and the use of herbs were distinguished and protected from the emerging medical paradigm.

This may be where herbal medicine diverged and began to develop a separate theory and practice from what would become the practice of medicine. It is under the protection of this Herbalists' Charter Act that natural therapists in England are still able to practice to this day.

CHEMICAL MEDICINE

Chemical medicine embodied in the tradition of alchemy attempted to distill different waters from herbs, minerals, and parts of animals, as opposed to Galenical preparations made from whole plant parts. It was a trend encouraged by Paracelsus, who was one of the first to realize that it was the "active constituents" or chemicals present in plants that interacted with the body and stimulated healing. A schism between herbal medicine and embryonic scientific medicine began.

This gap widened when medical science developed the concept of experiment as a way to gain knowledge. Renaissance thinkers like William Harvey (1578-1657) and Francis Bacon (1561-1626) were early authors of scientific medicine, now called "biomedicine," and the herbalists remained empiricists at heart and in practice for the next few hundred years. Paracelsus' discovery of chemical medicine, using metals and other new substances, a weakening of the church's grip on how disease was understood, systematic compilations and distribution of pharmacopeias with the introduction of the printing press, the anatomic research by Vesalius and experimental physiology of Harvey—all of these contributed to changing attitudes, or a "modernization" that left gentle herbal cures behind in the minds of the public. By the end of the 16th century, the followers of Paracelsus were actively promoting their new medicines, many of which (e.g., mercury) were extremely toxic. Paracelsus would have been appalled by the often violent reactions in patients that resulted in great suffering—quite the opposite of what he was attempting to achieve.

The 17th century was characterized by a number of developments. First, the discovery of the Americas led to the introduction of new and exotic medicines such as Peruvian bark (from South American species of *Cinchona).* It also saw an increasing number of books on the subject of self-treatment using herbs and simple cures. Nicholas Culpeper (1616-1654) was one of the most fervent critics of the imported exotic medicines. He initially studied to be a doctor and later, as an apothecary, trained at Cambridge. At that time, to restrict access to medical information, the language of choice for physicians was Latin. In Culpeper's opinion, this was an elitist ploy to keep the knowledge of herbs and healing from the masses. He translated the London pharmacopoeia into vernacular English and simplified the recipes, so that exotic foreign (and very expensive) ingredients were replaced with locally grown plants. In 1652, he published his classic, *The English Physician or an Astrologo-physical Discourse of the Vulgar Herbs of this Nation, Being a Compleat Method of Physick Whereby a Man may Preserve his Body in Health, or Cure himself being Sick, for threepence charge, with such Things as onlie Grow in England, they being Most Fit for English Bodies*. In it, he tied Galenical herbalism to astrology, as Avicenna had done, claiming that this was a predictable, consistent, and reliable system, but he also relied on a wealth of practical experience. Culpeper's permanent contribution was to make practical herbal medicine available to everyone. This book has had more than 40 editions, was the first medical book published in America, and still has a healthy spot in the used book trade today.

Early in the 18th century, Carl von Linne (Linnaeus) developed binomial nomenclature to denote every species of plant. In the preceding centuries, medicinal plants were identified by a single name, but that name might be given to several plants, or a plant could have multiple names. Plants could now be catalogued based on morphology, without any context in which to judge whether these plants were or had been useful in medicine. Some think that this is the precursor for random chemical screening of plants for the purpose of finding an active chemical—a process that is still used today but that has generally been found inefficient. Drug companies and researchers alike are now back to studying plants on the basis of their traditional uses, but thanks to Linnaeus, we can identify these plants with certainty.

THE FRENCH CONNECTION

Tracking forward in time now to the 17th century, the link between Western herbal medicine and veterinary medicine grew stronger as did the importance of animal husbandry and agriculture to support the rising human population in Europe. As domestic animals became increasingly valuable, so did the need to study them in greater depth. Claude Bourgelat in Lyons, France, opened the first veterinary medicine school on February 13, 1762.

The school was founded by Louis XV and was designed mainly for the study of the diseases and treatments of livestock. In 1764, the school was transferred to Paris, and in 1766, the Royal Veterinary School of Alfort was opened, as was the Jardin des Plantes. Veterinary students grew medicinal plants, collected, dried, and prepared extracts, and distilled them to produce drugs. Activities at the renamed Alfort Imperial Veterinary School of 1803 included the systematic study of plants, toxic plants, and spices and medicinal plants.

THE AMERICAS

Little is known of herbal practice by natives in North, Central, or South America because they left no written record. What we do know survives in the practice of remaining indigenous peoples and the pioneers who colonized the United States and in a very few descriptive herbals compiled by explorers. Europeans learned some aspects of Native American healing and exported many of these remedies to Europe. Land grant colleges were started very early, and herbariums and study of plant material were part of university study.

One of the early Central American herbals is *Codex de la Cruz-Badiano* (Badianus manuscript) of 1552, originally known as *Libellus de Medicinalibus Indorum Herbis*. The book was written in Nahuatl (an Aztec language) by Martin de la Cruz, an Aztec physician of the 25-year-old Spanish colony called *New Spain* (now Mexico) and translated by Juan Badiano. The illuminated text contains such familiar herbs as thistle, clover, oak, cypress, beans, senna, wormwood, artichoke, cress, tobacco, nettles, and jimson weed. North American native practices have been preserved by word of mouth and revived by modern ethnobotanists in a number of books (Moerman, 1998; Weslager, 1973; Densmore, 1974; Hutchens, 1991).

In the United States, herbal practice evolved from colonial times to the early 20th century. Initially, the Puritans brought herbs and herb seeds from Europe, in addition to their copies of Culpeper's *English Physician*. William Byrd II (1674-1744) reported that Virginia gardens of his time usually contained the following herbs: angelica, anise, borage, burnet, chives, coriander, dill, fennel, garlic, marjoram, parsley, rosemary, savory, sorrel, and yarrow.

The first description of herbs that would grow in North America was *New England's Rarities Discovered*, written by "John Josselyn Gentleman" in 1672. Josselyn described native herbs and explains in detail how the Native Americans used them. He also described plants that were brought from England and forever changed the American plant landscape with their invasiveness, such as couch grass, shepherd's purse, dandelion, stinging nettle, plantain, chickweed, and comfrey.

In the 18th and early 19th centuries, the *Materia Medica* enlarged and changed to include American herbs, primarily those of Eastern forests. Pioneers learned these herbs from natives. At the same time, botanists were hard at work discovering and describing unique American plants and their use by American Indians. One such famous botanist was Constantine Rafinesque (1784-1841), who spent time with natives to write his masterpiece, *New Flora of North America* (1836).

As European doctors immigrated and the United States opened its own medical schools, the bloodletting, salivation from calomel administration, and other horrific practices soon became "regular medicine."

HEROIC MEDICINE

The 17th and 18th centuries saw the increasing use of chemical medicine, as well as the introduction and practice of heroic medicine. As European doctors immigrated and the United States opened its own medical schools, the heroic practices of the time included materials such as animal feces and burnt animal matter in medicines; the use of debilitating procedures such as bloodletting; and the administration of chemicals such as mercury, arsenic, and antimony, mainly for the purpose of inducing purging, which was considered cleansing to remove possible toxins. Heroic medicine no doubt caused enormous suffering among patients. The public and the medical profession were becoming polarized, and medical reform was imminent.

Herbal medicine's great revival occurred in the early 1800s in rebellion against heroic medical practices, but was also a reflection of the Jacksonian political climate of the times. Nineteenth century capitalism promoted economic self-sufficiency and nationalistic confidence. Applied science was freed from philosophy and became an instrument of the culture. Lay reformers and practitioners promoted new theories that the public found easy to accept. Medical schools were privatized, and licensure was eventually eliminated because it was considered elitist. This situation laid the foundation for medical sects, which developed and flourished in America throughout the 19th century.

No wonder healers with a different approach were able to make an extraordinary impact on medical practice. Samuel Thomson (1769-1843) was one of those who changed the course of medicine in the United States. Thomson, a self-taught herbalist, birthed *Botanic Medicine* and taught about the power of the body to heal itself. He learned some of the arts of herbal medicine from a local woman, the Widow Benton, and went on to develop a system that was to spark a revolution against the dominant "heroic" model of medicine. Thomson's initial model emphasized "sweating out" the disease influence and restoring "animal warmth" with herbs and a sweat bath; some herbalists believe that this model is borrowed directly from certain Native American practices. His herbal pharmacopoeia consisted of cayenne pepper to produce sweating, and lobelia and buckthorn to produce vomiting and purging, with rests in between, which earned him and his followers the appellation "steam and puke doctors." Although it was still considered heroic, his treatment was aimed at stimulating self-healing—a rediscovered Hippocratic doctrine.

His system became known as the Thomsonian System of Practice, which he patented in 1813 and which was practiced throughout the United States as a franchise known as the "Improved System of Botanic Practice of Medicine." He licensed agents to be educated and receive his products, and by 1939, more than 3,000,000 members made up his Friendly Botanic Society. Many doctors and herbalists began referring to themselves as Thomsonians to distinguish themselves from the "regular" physicians of 19th century America.

The interest in herbal medicine was rekindled, but its success and appeal to the masses would bloom only after a group of medical doctors took it on. Soon came the Neo-Thomsonians, who despite their teacher's complaints, greatly expanded the *Materia Medica*, probably on the basis of Native American uses of these herbs, as well as experimentation and empiric observations. The Physiomedical movement was a direct outgrowth of the Thomsonian movement, and its philosophy was to use only healing plants—toxins were not allowed, even if they were toxic plants and even in homeopathic doses. The Physiomedicals were vitalists who believed that the remedy only corrected abnormal tissue states, and that the vital force did the rest of the work of healing the patient. Eclectic medicine arose from these roots as a philosophy that subscribed to no particular dogma; it suggested that scientific and empiric methods would provide evidence for selection of the best methods of practice.

Wooster Beach, a student of Thomson's, opened two Eclectic hospitals in the northeastern United States, where the science of the time was combined with herbal treatments. Beach called this discipline "Eclectic" medicine. Alva Curtis and William Cook were two reformers who led the Physiomedical movement to open multiple schools in the East and Midwest. Later, Eclectics and Physiomedicalists built this combined scientific herbalism into a high medical art, and the publications of John Scudder, John King, Finley Ellingwood, Harvey Wickes Felter, William Cook, and John Uri Lloyd serve as valuable references for today's practicing herbalists.

Battlefield Medicine of the 19th Century

An interesting peek into the pharmacy of the Confederacy during the Civil War is given in Denney's work (1994). According to Denney, *The Confederate States Medical and Surgical Journal*, July 1864 issue, detailed a "standard supply table of indigenous remedies for field service and sick in general hospital." Herbs listed as stimulants were calamus, lavender, partridgeberry, sassafras, Seneca snakeroot, tulip tree, and Virginia snakeroot. Astringents were derived from white oak bark and leaves, bearberry bush, marsh rosemary, and sumac. Tonics recommended were American century, American Colombo, American gentian, blackberry or dewberry, dogwood, Georgia bark, hops, persimmon, sage, white willow, and wild cherry.

No major changes or movements occurred in European herbal medicine until American herbal practitioners came to the continent in the early 1800s with a new message. Albert Coffin, a charismatic medical doctor, modified the Thomsonian system somewhat and took it to England. The "nature cure" system became popular in Germany, where Father Sebastian Kneipp championed his famous "water cure." Benedict Lust brought this system to the United States, where he opened the first health food store in 1896, calling it the Kneipp Store. He founded the American School of Naturopathy, which granted degrees.

Some writers claim that, although the populist, self-help tone of the Eclectics and the Physiomedicalists brought them to their full power in the United States, their downfall lay in their failure to grant any validity to the germ theory. While regular medicine was building hospital-based academic practices and developing laboratory procedures that would revolutionize diagnostics and treatment, reform movements continued to insist on using part-time faculty and holding to a fully empiric view of the patient. Failure to adopt Council on Education guidelines and unwillingness to embrace new developments caused a wane in their popularity, and some of the schools fell to selling diplomas and graduating unqualified doctors. The last Eclectic college was closed in 1939, and not until the 1960s was significant interest in herbal medicine to rise again. The knowledge of herbal medicine built by the Eclectics and the Physiomedicalists was kept alive in the Naturopathic schools that began to open in the United States. Two Naturopathic books that sparked the renaissance in herbal medicine in the United States were Edward Shook's *Treatises in Herbology*, and John Christopher's *School of Natural Healing*, both of which were published in the 1960s.

Many of those who are interested in alternative modalities are familiar with the Flexner report, which is said to have been the death knell for herbal and homeopathic medicine in the early years of the 20th century. This report, entitled "Medical Education in the United States and Canada," was published in 1910, was funded by the Carnegie and Rockefeller Foundations, and was backed by the American Medical Association (AMA). Readers have found ample connections between the Rockefellers, pharmaceutical and industrial monopolies, and an ingrained opposition to the public's use of any medicine not dependent on the drug industry.

The report described American medicine as rife with sectarianism, disagreement about best treatments for patients, and, in some cases, frighteningly dirty and substandard facilities among the sectarian schools. Reformers did themselves in by not recognizing or instituting the changes recommended by Flexner—that schools should have up-to-date laboratory facilities, that faculty should be full-time teachers and researchers with hospital affiliations for bedside teaching, and that licensing should be reinstituted to ensure adequately educated doctors.

In their place, scientific medicine and chemical drugs with the backing of the increasingly powerful AMA and drug companies began to dominate the health industry. Botanical medicine, it was claimed, was no longer needed because all chemicals could be synthesized by extracting active constituents from plants. Most drugs currently in use originate from plants or are based on plant chemicals. Some of the most important examples include digitoxin from foxglove, aspirin from willow bark, morphine from poppy, vincristine from the Madagascan periwinkle. Not only do these plants provide the basis for synthesized drugs; to this date, they are still the raw material used in the synthesizing process. The reader can peruse the US Pharmacopoeia and, for that matter, the veterinary *Materia Medica*, to track this history of declining plant use as drug therapy grew in prominence during the 20th century.

From the 1920s to the 1950s, orthodox medicine in America and worldwide made significant leaps forward. Pharmaceutical companies began to mass produce drugs such as antibiotics, surgical techniques continued to advance, and new vaccines were developed. However, despite these developments, herbal medicine has undergone a resurrection since the 1960s and is increasingly being rediscovered as a source of treatments that can potentially prevent costly adverse effects of standard drug treatments and offer a different approach and opportunity for treatment when other treatments have failed (one of the most striking examples is Chinese Artemisia for malaria) (Abdin, 2002).

Presently, herbal medicine is used by herbalists as a complete system of healing, and by medical professionals as complementary therapy. However herbs fit into the practice of medicine, some guiding philosophy for their prescription is usually at work. Modern herbalists tend to claim that there are three main philosophies that undergird herbal use:

1. Scientific herbal medicine, or Phytotherapy—this is usually reductionistic, studying herbs and diseases in isolation to understand them as molecular interactions that are more easily measured than whole systems. Phytotherapists tend to use evidence-based treatments.
2. Heroic—In this philosophy, illness is seen primarily as an accumulation of toxins, worsening as people age. Treatment centers on detoxification and controlling one's exposure to toxins. Herbs used in this tradition are strong, generally starting with laxatives, diuretics, and diaphoretics.
3. Traditional medicine—This is the most holistic of the traditions. Traditional medicine, such as the Wise Woman tradition, Native American medicine, Chinese medicine, and other cultural medical systems, tends to view the organism as a whole, using simple herbs, physical activity, food, and emotional support to restore health.

Modern practitioners of herbal medicine tend to combine evidence-based practice with the knowledge of traditional uses of the herbs.

VETERINARY BOTANICAL MEDICINE

> If you find yourself with some spare time, visit a veterinary school library and access some of the older veterinary textbooks. Besides fascinating reading that describes techniques and conditions that seem old-fashioned now, the contrast is obvious in one field—therapeutics. Herbs form the very basis of veterinary medicines and, up until the 1960s, are found in most veterinary pharmacopoeias and textbooks.

The use of herbal treatments within veterinary medicine is not new, as we have seen. Herbs have been integral to all folk and cultural traditions, and study of these traditions is making a comeback (see Chapter 3, Ethnoveterinary Medicine: Potential Solutions for Large-Scale Problems). Even before academic researchers began to study traditional uses of herbs, lay authors were reviving the traditions. Juliette de Bairacli Levy was one of the first. She was born in England and apparently attended veterinary school for a short while before dropping out. She continued to learn natural medicine on her own and from gypsies, who became her friends. She is the author of five herbals that make very interesting reading indeed.

As the profession of veterinary medicine grew in the 17th and 18th centuries, advances in regular and herbal medicine continued to develop alongside those in human regular and herbal medicine. What is interesting to observe is how recently many herbs were considered orthodox within the veterinary profession (to at least the 1960s). It is also interesting to observe what some would consider alternative terms in the herbal literature, such as *alterative* and *carminative* as mainstream descriptors of plant actions in veterinary textbooks. During the 18th and 19th centuries, herbal medicine was entrenched in the veterinary profession. However, orthodox veterinary use of herbs did not follow the true tradition of herbal medicine, and typically, treatments called for combinations of herbs and inorganic substances.

Veterinarians became medical professionals following the establishment of veterinary schools. After the first school in Lyon was established, veterinary colleges were founded in Turin, Göttingen, Copenhagen, London, Edinboro, and other European cities. Horse doctors, farriers, and some lay animal experts were now considered quacks. Education centered on horses, but William Youatt, a British veterinarian, elevated the knowledge of canine medicine in his books that are still fairly easily found in the antiquarian trade.

In North America, the first established veterinary schools were located in Mexico and Canada. The first veterinary school in the United States was established at Cornell in 1894. Previous to this, veterinarians had formed professional organizations (such as the US Veterinary Medical Association [USVMA] in 1863 and regional associations), but these veterinarians may have had medical or other training. The Eclectics had their share of "veterinary reformers," two of whom were Nelson N. Titus and G. H. Dadd. Dadd's book, *The American Cattle Doctor* (published in 1858), explains the Reformed Practice. His "Creed of the Reformers" details Eclectic veterinary practice as follows:

> "We believe that a perfect system of medical science is that which never allows disease to exist at all; which prevents disease, instead of curing it, by means of a perfect hygienic system, proper modes of life, attention to diet, ventilation and exercise.
>
> "We believe that the next best system is that which, after disease has made its appearance, promptly meets its development by the use of such agencies as are perfectly in harmony with the laws of life and health, and physiological in their action; such, for example, as water, air, heat and cold, friction, food, drink, and medicines that are not usually regarded as poisons, and are known to prove congenial to the animal constitution.
>
> "We have no attachment to any remedy which experience shows unsafe; but on the contrary, we rejoice in the success of every attempt to sanative for disease-creating agents, and believe that a number of the articles which are still

occasionally used in the old school, will in time become obsolete, as medical science progresses.

"We hold that our opposition to any course of medical treatment should be in proportion to the mischief it produces, entirely irrespective of medical theories. Hence our hostility to the lancet.

"We do not profess to know more about anatomy, physiology, surgery, etc, than our allopathic brethren; but the superiority which our system claims over others is, in the main, to be found in our therapeutic agents, all of which are harmless, safe, and efficient. While they arouse the energies of nature to resist the ravages of disease, they act harmoniously with the vital principle, in the restoration of the system from a pathological to the physiological state."

It may be instructive to compare the treatments presented in various texts over the course of the 19th century. In the following paragraphs, three common conditions and suggested treatments for each of them are presented. The early authors (Varlo, Youatt, Hinds, and Lambert) were chosen to represent typical practices of the time, and Dadd and Titus are the quintessential Eclectic veterinary practitioners who reintroduced to the American veterinary profession plant medicine in the treatment of animals.

Diarrhea in Cattle

Varlo, 1785: "Take half a pint of verjuice [sour juice of crabapples or other unripe fruit], and mix in it an ounce of bole armoniac reduced to powder; or, for want of this, bruise to powder a large handful of kennel coal, and give it in a quart of new milk three mornings together."

Lambert (from Richardson, 1828): Calf scours: "You must take a pint of verjuice and clay that is burnt till it be red, or very well-burnt tobacco pipes, pound them to a powder and sift them very finely; put to it a little powder of charcoal, then blend them together and give it to the calf, and he will mend in a night's time for certain."

Dadd, 1858: "In the early stages of this disease, it is not always to be checked. It is often a salutary operation of nature to rid the system of morbific materials, and all that we can do with safety, is to sheathe and lubricate the mucous surfaces, in order to protect them from the acrid and stimulation properties of the agents to be removed from the alimentary canal. When the disease, of which diarrhea is only a symptom, proceeds from exposure, apply warmth, moisture, friction, and stimulants to the external surface, aided by the following lubricant—powdered slippery elm 1 ounce; powdered charcoal 1 tablespoon, boiling water 2 quarts. When the fecal charges appear more natural and less frequent, a tea of raspberry leaves or bayberry bark will complete the cure. When the disease assumes a chronic form, and the animal loses flesh, the following tonic, stimulating, astringent drink is recommended: Infusion of chamomile 1 quart, powdered caraway seeds 1 ounce, powdered bayberry $^1/_2$ ounce. For "scouring rot," the recipe is powdered charcoal 1 teacup full, common salt 2 ounces; Pyroligeneous acid half a wine glass (vinegar obtained from wood), warm water, 2 quarts.

Titus, 1865: Diarrhea: "This disease is better known than the method of cure. It is more difficult to cure this disease in horned cattle than in man, or any other animal. But I have never failed to effect a cure with the following treatment, if given in time: tincture of opium 2 ounces, tincture of kino 3 ounces, tincture of camphor 1 ounce, essence of peppermint 1 ounce, Paregoric 4 ounces. Mix, and given an ounce in 6 hours, until the disease abates; in bad cases, give injections of: slippery elm flower 2 ounces, morphine 20 grams, warm water 1 quart. The animal should have no water to drink; but should have a liberal allowance of linseed tea or some other mucilaginous drink. A tea made of the Indian arrow-root has been very effectual in curing the disease. The animal should be kept on dry food, and kept in a warm, comfortable place."

Canine "Itch" or Mange

Lambert (from Richardson, 1828): "Get brimstone, beat it into fine powder and sift it, then take an ounce of elecampane root, waterlily roots dried, and beat to a powder, of each one ounce, a little handful of bay salt dried and powdered; make an ointment with half a pint of oil of turpentine, and two ounces of hogs lard, and having rubbed the dog with a wool card (or some such thing) till the blood comes in some places, anoint him with this warm, and it will cure him."

Youatt, 1857: "Bleeding, aperient, and cooling medicines are indicated, and also applications of the subacetate of lead, or spermaceti ointment. A weak infusion of tobacco may be resorted to when other things fail, but it must be used with much caution. The same may be said of all mercurial preparations. The tanner's pit has little efficacy, except in slight cases. Slight bleedings may be serviceable, and especially in full habits; setons may be resorted to in obstinate cases. A change in the mode of feeding will often be beneficial, and also mercurial alteratives, as Aethiop's mineral with cream of tartar and nitre. The external applications require considerable caution. If mercury is used, care must be taken that the dog does not lick it. . . . Unguents are useful, but considerable care must be taken . . . Lotions of corrosive sublimate, decoction of bark, infusion of digitalis or tobacco effected some little good; but the persevering use of the iodine of potassium, purgatives, and the abstraction of blood very generally succeeded."

Dadd, 1858: "Powdered charcoal half a tablespoon full, powdered sulphur 1 ounce, soft soap sufficient to form an ointment. Apply externally for 3 successive days, at the end of which time, the animal is to be washed with castile soap and warm water, and afterwards wiped dry. The internal remedies consist of equal parts sulphur and cream of tartar, half a teaspoonful of which may be given daily, in honey. When the disease becomes obstinate and large, scabby eruptions appear on various parts of the body, take pyroligneous acid 2 ounces, water 1 pint, and wash parts daily, and keep animal on a light diet."

Equine Founder

Lambert (in Richardson, 1828): "If the founder is settled in the feet and legs, you may take from the horse one pint of blood, once in 3 days, put him in running water and let him stand 2 hours, morning and night, give him 1 day, four ounces of Glauber's salts, and the next day, one ounce of saltpeter, and in this manner, repeat these doses until the horse is well. The medicine may be given to the horse in moistened oats or meal, but he must not have much provender, until he gets well. Wash his legs down well with hot pot-liquor, or dishwater. The horse must be bled in the foot between the hair and the hoof."

Hinds, 1830: ". . . take off the shoe . . . Apply a bran poultice warm to the whole foot daily, but do not add to it any greasy or oily substances as is too often practiced . . . a number of contrivances for affording coolness and natural pressure to the sole and frog, besides the foregoing, have been resorted to, and among these the admixture of vinegar, alegar, verjuice, or solution of nitre with the clay, with the stopping, etc are well calculated to answer the purposes intended. Rubbing the knees with turpentine is also serviceable. Physic . . . either of the three evacuations being suppressed or imperfectly performed must be restored, and a purgative, a urine-ball, or a diaphoretic powder must be administered as occasion requires, and opportunity presents itself; of course, neither of those will be given while the animal is out of doors."

Youatt, 1857: "Bleeding is indispensable, and that to its fullest extent. If the disease be confined to the forefeet, 4 quarts of blood should be taken as soon as possible from the toe of each . . . poultices of linseed meal, made very soft, should cover the whole of the foot and pastern and be frequently renewed, which will promote evaporation from the neighboring parts, and possibly through the pores of the hoof, and, by softening and suppling the hoof, will relieve the painful pressure on the swelled and tender parts underneath . . . shoe should be removed . . . the sole pared . . . There is doubt as to the propriety of administering physic. The horse may find it difficult or impossible to rise, in which case much inconvenience will ensue from the operation of physic; or there may be danger, from the intense character of the fever in the feet often assumes, of producing a change in inflammation to the bowels or lungs, in which case the irritation of physic would probably be fatal. Sedative and cooling medicines should be diligently administered, consisting of digitalis, nitre, and emetic tartar . . . If no amendment be observed, three quarts of blood should be taken from each foot on the following day, and in extreme cases, a third bleeding of two quarts may be justifiable, and, instead of the poultice, cloths kept wet with water in which nitre has been dissolved immediately before, and in the proportion of an ounce of nitre to a pound of water, and wrapped round the feet. About the third day, a blister may be tried, taking in the whole of the pastern and coronet . . . The horse should be kept on a mash diet, unless green meat can be procured for him; and even that should not be given too liberally . . ."

Titus, 1865: The foot, like every other part, is liable to inflammation from various causes and particularly from violence, long continued action, and more especially, letting the horse drink cold water, when very warm from exercise.

As soon as the horse is discovered to be foundered, he should be placed in a vat of water about summer temperature; this is better than to place the horse in running water as this chills the horse and obstructs the circulation. When it gets too warm for the heat of the feet, it should be changed; it should be kept 2 or 3 degrees below the temperature of the body, and the horse should be kept constantly in it until all fever and inflammation have abated. If the horse cannot be kept on his feet, they should be kept constantly wet by means of cloths or a sponge. This treatment is an infallible cure, and will be found more effectual than all the medicines in the whole *Materia Medica.* It requires no medicine, excepting a dose of physic occasionally.

[One recipe for physic balls: Powdered aloes, 1 oz; powdered mandrake, $^1/_4$ oz; powdered ginger, $^1/_4$ oz {variations included the addition of blood root and peppermint}—balls are formed by adding honey]."

In 1878, Finlay Dun published the ninth edition of his popular textbook, *Veterinary Medicines, Their Actions and Uses.* He was a respected lecturer at the Edinburgh Veterinary College and an examiner in chemistry at the Royal College of Veterinary Surgeons. He details the use of remedies such as gentian as a bitter tonic—"useful in treating atonic digestion"—and dissolved Linseed tea or ale together with nitre and Epsom salts for treating "simple catarrh in the horse." Juniper is described as a topical irritant, a mild stimulant, a carminative, and a diuretic "of use in treating indigestion and flatulence, diminishing the evil effects of bad fodder and marshy pastures."

Herbs were still prominent in the veterinary literature into the 1900s. In Leeney (1929), *Home Doctoring for Animals,* fennel, aniseed, gentian, fenugreek, ginger, opium, cassia bark, cinnamon, caraway, peppermint, cumin, aloes, thymol, male fern, digitalis leaves, elm bark, camphor, capsicum, belladonna, Peruvian bark, linseed, quassia, oak bark, licorice, cinchona, and other herbs are featured in standard powders, ball, and drench recipes.

In Banham and Young's *Veterinary Posology* (1935), aloes, belladonna, buchu, caffeine, camphor, cannabis, capsicum, cinchona, cinnamon, crocus, turmeric, digitalis, eucalyptus, fenugreek, galangal, gentian, ginger jalap, juniper, lavender, lobelia, peppermint, myrrh, olive oil, senna, tamarind, thymol, uva ursi, and ginger took a prominent place beside the increasing numbers of chemical drugs that were proliferating at the time such as strychnine, arsenic, ammonium, apomorphine, atropine, iodine, zinc, lead salts, and many others.

Even into the 1960s, in Daykin's *Veterinary Applied Pharmacology and Therpauetics,* a textbook used in veterinary schools throughout the United Kingdom, Australia, and the United States, male fern, acacia, podophyllum, camphor, buchu, cascara, senna, peppermint, betel nut, calabar, kamala, licorice, aniseed, belladonna, ginger, and nux vomica, among others, still feature highly as contemporary medicines, along with vaccines, antibiotics, corticosteroids, and hormone treatments now available.

As the demise of herbal medicine occurred concomitantly with the rise of scientific medicine, veterinary medicine followed suit. Many of the patented herbal medicines used in veterinary medicine had become associated with the use of inorganic substances like mercury and arsenic. It is therefore not surprising that the use of such remedies came into some disrepute with the advent of "modern" pharmaceuticals. Perhaps paralleling the contemporary story of Western herbal medicine (Griggs, 1981), as pharmaceutical research changed the modern standard of medicine (including veterinary), within a decade, the study of herbs all but disappeared from the curriculum of veterinary schools. Instead, plants as treatments were replaced with the toxicology of weeds and "poisonous plants." As a result, few herbal remedies survive today in conventional veterinary practice.

VETERINARY BOTANICAL MEDICINE RENAISSANCE

Since perhaps the late 1970s, holistic veterinarians have created a renaissance of interest in and study of medicinal plants, plant-derived drugs, and phytotherapy. At the same time, organic agriculture has become more important, and the need to find nondrug treatments for food animals has pushed this rebirth in veterinary herbal medicine as well. "Clearly, a new opportunity had surfaced to improve the quality of practicing veterinary medicine by using herbal plants and their extracts to improve health, increase energy, facilitate healing, modify symptoms, help the immune system function, and improve quality and longevity of patients' lives" (Basko, 2002).

The first international veterinary herbal organization, the Veterinary Botanical Medicine Association, was formed in 2000 to develop responsible herbal practice by encouraging research and education, strengthening industry relations, keeping herbal tradition alive as a valid information source, and increasing professional acceptance of herbal medicine for animals. Currently, Ayurvedic medicine, Western medicine, Traditional Chinese herbs as well as Kampo and other systems of herbal medicine are employed by veterinary and animal herbalists throughout the world. Growth in interest is expected to continue as we reflect on the various traditions and scientific applications of herbal medicines and find their place within the context of veterinary medicine. Research must continue into the safety, efficacy, and appropriate applications of herbal medicines, along with their comparative costs and benefits in veterinary medicine.

Yet, although reductionism and experimental science have their place in veterinary medicine, they are simply a piece of the whole. Medicine and science are not the same. Although medicine has benefited greatly from the scientific approach, medical history always brings the pendulum back when dogma sets in, and it affirms the value of empiric observation. Evidence-based medicine is becoming part of veterinary practice. Even with perfect knowledge of the genetics, environment, psychology, and chaos potential of an individual patient, science may never allow us to predict his or her interaction with an herb or herbal practitioner—the individual practitioner reigns supreme in this decision making.

Western veterinary botanical medicine is still in its infancy, but the value of herbal medicine and of herbal medicine's approach to chronic disease (in particular) should not be underestimated. As we collectively learn more about herbal medicine and its applications to animals, we are sure to find herbs playing a far more extensive role in the care and health of our animals as a society. It is an exciting time to be on the bridge that spans the past and the future of veterinary herbal medicine.

Further Information on Herbal History

Griggs B. Green Pharmacy, Healing Arts Press, Rochester, Vt (1981, 1991, 1997)

Anderson FJ. *An Illustrated History of the Herbals*. New York: Columbia University Press; 1977

Berman A, Flannery MA. *America's Botanico-Medical Movements. Vox Populi*. New York: Pharmaceutical Products Press; 2001

Hammurabi. "Code of Hammurabi." April 29, 2004. http://www.yale.edu/lawweb/avalon/hamframe.htm

Columella http://www.gmu.edu/departments/fld/CLASSICS/columella.rr.html

Culpeper's *The English Physitian* of 1652: http://info.med.yale.edu/library/historical/culpeper/culpeper.htm

Grieves M. 1973. *A Modern Herbal*. This is a classic book originally published in 1931. It compliles information on herbs that is not easily accessible elsewhere. www.botanical.com/botanical/mgmh/comindx.html

Fuchs DeHistoria Stirpium: http://info.med.yale.edu/library/historical/fuchs/

The Academic Medical Library of Paris has an online version of Galen's works at: http://www.bium.univ-paris5.fr/histmed/medica/galien_va.htm

History of Maisons-Alfort Veterinary School Botanic Garden http://uiabotanique.free.fr/navigu/ist6eng.htm

World Association for the History of Veterinary Medicine. Available at: http://wahvm.vet.uu.nl. Contains bibliographic listings of source manuscripts and books, links to veterinary libraries, and searchable databases.

***

A surviving chapter on herbal medicine to treat animals (1656).
William Coles, 1656. The Art of Simpling.

Chapter XXXI: Of such Plants as have operation upon the bodies of Bruit Beasts.

Though the Bodies of Men be more tender than any other Creatures, fuller of Diseases, and easier to be wrought upon, and so the greatest number of Plants is applicable to them, yet Bruit Beasts also have some share in the Physical use of Plants as well as they. For a Toad being over-charged with the poison of the Spider, as is ordinarily believed, hath recourse to the Plantain leaf which cures him. The Weasel when she is to encounter the Serpents, arms herself with eating of Rue. The Dog when he is sick at the Stomach knows the Grass that will cure him, eats of it, falls to his Vomit and is well. When the Cat is sick, she goes to Nepal or Catmint, of which there is this old Rhyme:

If you set it, the Cats will eat it.
If you sow it, the Cats won't know it.

If the Ass be oppressed with melancholy, he eats of the herb asplenium, or miltwaste, and so eases himself of the swelling of the Spleen. (Vitruvius saith, that the Swine in Candy, feeding thereon, were found to be without Spleens.) So, the wild Goats being shot with Darts, or Arrows, cure themselves with Dittany, which Herb hath that power to work them out of the Body, and to heal up the wound. The Swallow makes use of Celandine, which is therefore called Chelidonium, the Linnet and Goldfinch of Eyebright, for the repairing of their own, and their young ones' sight. And here, though I am no Leech, yet I shall set down such Plants as I have seen and read, are used by Leeches, and the manner of applying them to Cattle, and such unusual Accidents as happened to them by their operation. The Leaves of black Bryony bruised with Wine and laid upon the forenecks of Oxen that are galled with the yoke, helpeth them. When a Cow hath newly Calved, they give her unthreshed Rye out of the Barn to make her clean, as they call it. If the Calf be dead in the Cow's Belly, they give her Savine to make her cast it. When a Cow is troubled with the Tail Evil, they make an Incision toward the lower end of the Tail, where the Evil is, and put therein Rue, Pepper, and Salt, which will cure them. And if Hogs or other Cattle be subject to the Murrain, it is usual with them, and almost with every Husbandman, to cut an hole in the ear or Dewlap, and put therein a piece of the root of Bear's-foot, which some call Pegging, some Settering, and therefore, the plant is by some called Setterwort. Hay sodden

Continued

in Water till it be tender, and applied hot to the Chaps of Beasts, which are Chapfallen, through too much abstinence, either by long standing in the Pound or Stable without meat, is a present remedy. Ground Ivy stamped and mixed with a little Aloe and Honey, and strained, taketh away the Pin and Web, or any grief out of the eyes of Horses or Cows, or other Beast, being squirted into the same with a Syringe. It is reported that if one cast Lysimachia, or loosestrife between two Oxen when they are fighting, they will part presently, and being tied about their necks, it will keep them from fightling. Cocks having eaten Garlic are most stout to fight, and so are Horses. A Serpent doth so hate the Ash tree, that she will not come nigh the shadow of it, but she delights in Fennel very much, which she rates to clear her eyesight. If you are troubled with Moles in your Gardens or other Grounds, put Garlic, Leeks, or Onions in their passages, and they will leap out of the ground presently. Adder's tongue wrapped in Virgin's wax, and put into the left ear of any Horse, will make him fall down as if he were dead, and when it is taken out again, he becomes more lively than he was before. If Asses chance to feed much upon Hemlock, they will fall so fast asleep, that they will seem to be dead, insomuch that some thinking them to be dead indeed, have flayed off their skins, yet after the Hemlock done operating, they have stirred and wakened out of their sleep, to the grief and amazement of the owners, and to the laughter of others. If a Horse cannot piss without pain, take an Elder bough full of Leaves, and strike him gently therewith, and cover his Head, Neck, and Body with the same Leaves, and it will help him much. Wood Nightshade, or Bittersweet, being hung about the neck of Cattle that have the Staggers helpeth them. The roots of Gentian, or the juice of them, or in the decoction of the Herb or Root, being given to Cattle to drink, freeth them from the Botts and Worms, and many other Diseases, as also when they begin to swell being poisoned by venomous Worm or Tick, which often lick up with the Grass; as also when such sorms, or other hurtful vermin, have bitten Kine by the Udders, or other tender places, which presently thereupon swell and put them in so great pain, that it makes them forsake their meat, do but take the Leaves of Gentian and stroke the bitten place with the juice of them, and they by two or three times are helped and cured. He that desires further information in cures of this nature, let him read the works of Gervase Markham, who had one very well upon this subject (1668).

References

Abdin MZ. Artemesinin, a novel antimalarial drug: biochemical and molecular approaches for enhanced production. Planta Med 2002;69:289-299.

Banham GA, Young WJ. Veterinary Posology: Table of Veterinary Posology. London: Bailliere Tindall & Cox; 1935.

Basko I. Introduction to Veterinary Western herbology. Proceedings of the 17th Annual Conference of the American Holistic Veterinary Medical Association; September 28-October 1, 2002; Eugene, Ore.

Coles W. *The Art of Simpling: An Introduction to the Knowledge and Gathering of Plants.* St Catharine's, Ontario: Kessinger Publishing; 1968.

Culpeper N. *The English Physitian.* Reprint, No date.

Dadd GH. *The American Cattle Doctor,* A.O. Moore, Agricultural Book Publisher. New York. 1858.

Dafni A, Lev E. The doctrine of signatures in present-day Israel. Economic Botany 2002;56:328-334.

Daykin PW. *Veterinary Applied Pharmacology and Therapeutics.* London: Bailliere Tindall & Cox Ltd; 1964.

Denney RE. *Civil War Medicine: Care and Comfort of the Wounded.* New York: Sterling Publishing Corp, Inc; 1994:11.

Densmore F. *How Indians Use Wild Plants for Food, Medicine and Crafts.* New York: Dover Publications; 1974.

Dharmananda S. Kampo medicine. The practice of Chinese herbal medicine in Japan. Portland, Ore: Institute for Traditional Medicine. Available at: http://www.itmonline.org/arts/kampo.htm 25 March 2004.

Dun F. *Veterinary Medicines: Their Actions and Uses.* 5th ed. David Douglas, Edinburgh 1878:580.

Dunlop RH, Williams DJ. *Veterinary Medicine: An Illustrated History.* St. Louis: Mosby; 1996.

Eisenberg D, Davis R, Ettner S, et al. Trends in alternative medicine use in the United States 1990-1997; results of a follow up survey. JAMA 1998;280:1569-1575.

Erk N. A study of the veterinary section of Ibn Al-Awwam's Kitab Al Falala. MSU Vet 1960;21:42-44.

Focus on: Farmers' reliance on ethnoveterinary practices to cope with common cattle ailments. Richardson Josiah, compiler. The New-England Farrier and Family Physician, 1828.

Gresswell G; Gresswell C, Gresswell A. 1887. The Veterinary; pharmacopoeia, materia medica, and therapeutics . . . 1886. London: Bailliere, Tindall.

Griggs B. *Green Pharmacy: A History of Herbal Medicine.* New York: Viking Press; 1981.

Haas KB. Animal therapy over the ages. Early Botanical Medicine Veterinary Heritage 2000;23:6-8.

Haas KB. The father of wildlife rehabilitation. Wildlife Rehabil Today (Spring) 1992;3:52.

Haas LF. Papyrus of Ebers and Smith. J Neurol Neurosurg Psychiatry 1999;67:578.

Hinds J, Smith TM. *The Veterinary Surgeon,* 1830.

Hozeski BW. (Transl) Hildegard's Healing Plants: from her medieval classic *Physica* Boston, MA: Beacon Press 2001.

Hutchens AR. *Indian Herbalogy of North America.* Boston, Mass: Shambala Publications; 1991.

Janick J. 2002. Herbals: the connection between horticulture and medicine. History of Horticulture Lecture Series, Purdue University. Available at: http://www.hort.purdue.edu/newcrop/history/lecture23/lec23l.html. Accessed September 22, 2004.

Karasszon D. *A Concise History of Veterinary Medicine.* Budapest: Akademiai Kiado; 1998.

Lad V. An introduction to Ayurvedic medicine. Health World Online. Available at: http://www.healthy.net/asp/templates/article.asp?PageType=Article&ID=373. Accessed September 22, 2004.

Leeney H. *MRCVS Home Doctoring for Animals.* London: Macdonald & Martin; 1929.

Markham G. *Markham's Farewell to Husbandry,* 9th edition, 1668.

Mezzabotta MR. 1998. Aspects of multiculturalism In: *The Mulomedicina of Vegetius.* Available at: http://academic.sun.ac.za/as/journals/akro/Akro45/mezzabot.pdf. Accessed September 20, 2004.

Moerman DE. Native American Ethnobotany. Timber Press, Portland OR. 1998.

Mulder JB. A historical review of wound treatments in animals. Vet Heritage 1994;17:17-27.

Riddle JM. Dioscorides on pharmacy and medicine. Austin, Texas: University of Texas Press, 1985.

Rohde ES. *The Old English Herbals.* London: Constable and Company; 1922. (reprinted in 1971 by. Dover Publications, Inc.)

Schoen A. Veterinary Acupuncture: Ancient Art to Modern Medicine. Sydney, Australia: Mosby; 1994.

Smithcors JF. *Evolution of Veterinary Art.* Kansas City, Mo: Veterinary Medical Publishing Company; 1957.

Swabe J. *Animals, Disease, and Human Society: Human-Animal Relations and the Rise of Veterinary Medicine*. New York: Routledge; 1999.

Titus NN. *The American Eclectic Practice of Medicine, As Applied to the Diseases of Domestic Animals*, 1865.

Unknown. History of herbal traditions. Available at: http://www.indianherbsltd.com. Accessed January 15, 2004.

Varlo C. *A New System of Husbandry*, vol I and II, 1785.

Walker RE. *Ars Veterinaria: The Veterinary Art From Antiquity to the End of the XIXth Century: Historical Essay*. Kenilworth, NJ: Schering-Plough Animal Health; 1991:17.

Weslager CA. *Magic Medicines of the Indians*. Somerset, NJ: The Middle Atlantic Press; 1973.

Wood M. *Vitalism: The History of Herbalism, Homeopathy, and Flower Essences*. Berkeley, Calif: North Atlantic Books; 2000.

Yang S (translator). *The Divine Farmer's Materia Medica*. Boulder, Colo: Blue Poppy Press; 1997.

Youatt W. *The Dog*, 1857.

Overview of Traditional Chinese Medicine: The Cooking Pot Analogy

CHAPTER 5

Steven Paul Marsden

In *Nei Jing Su Wen,* the 2000-year-old seminal classic that gave rise to all of Chinese medicine, it is stated that to be a master physician, one must master the use of metaphors as they apply to medicine and the body. Perhaps the best metaphor for the inner workings of the body as understood by Chinese medicine is that of a cooking pot suspended over a fire (Figure 5-1).

THE BODY AS A COOKING POT

Mastering the simple implications of this analogy eliminates much of the confusion surrounding Chinese medical physiology and pathophysiology, and provides a solid foundation for understanding the use of herbs in Chinese medicine.

The Kidneys and Essence

The best place to begin a discussion of the cooking pot analogy is with the fire underneath the pot. In Chinese medicine, this fire and the fuel that supplies it are the contributions of the Kidneys. Just as the fire is located underneath the pot, the Kidneys are located in the lower third, or *jiao*, of the body. In animals, this is equivalent to the caudal abdomen.

The "fuel" component of the Kidneys is Essence, or *Jing*. Essence is a sticky glutinous substance, tantamount to a sort of primordial ooze, which harbors the basic life force of the body. Tangible manifestations of this life-giving fluid stored in the Kidneys include semen, breast milk, and blood. It is not surprising then that Kidney failure was recognized early on in Chinese medicine as an important cause of anemia.

Essence is of two types—prenatal and postnatal—and is classified according to origin. Postnatal Essence is continually produced by the body through digestion. Foods that contain the raw materials that can be converted into Essence often are rich in animal protein. Cases of Kidney Essence deficiency, such as chronic renal failure in cats, are sometimes treated with the use of diets that are high in animal protein, calling into question the standard recommendation of most veterinary practitioners for low-phosphorus diets.

Prenatal Essence, which cannot be generated by the body, includes all hormones crucial to normal physical and sexual development, such as growth hormone, estrogen, testosterone, erythropoietin, and progesterone. Until the advent of synthetic versions by modern medicine, these hormones were irreplaceable once they were no longer produced by the body. Animals that lack prenatal Essence are thus prone to developmental abnormalities.

Although Essence has functions in the body in its own right, it can also be converted into just about anything else the body requires. In a sense, Essence was considered to function similarly to a stem cell in the bone marrow, with an inherent pleuripotentiality. Indeed, Chinese medicine recognized that the soft gelatinous material inside the cavities of bones was a major component of the body's Essence pool.

Chinese medicine extended the definition of marrow to also include the soft gelatinous tissues of the central nervous system housed within the cavities of the cranium and the spinal column. The relationship of these tissues to Essence seemed obvious in that their function routinely declined as organisms slowly ran out of life-giving Essence and approached death. Declines in hearing, cognitive function, and memory are examples of symptoms of Kidney Essence deficiency.

Because marrow is a key component of both bone and Essence, bone integrity likewise came to be associated with Kidney Essence. Loss of bone strength that manifests as osteoporosis in humans and as lower limb and back weakness in many companion animals is an additional key symptom of Kidney Essence deficiency.

The ability of Essence to be converted into a number of different substances in the body makes it similar in concept to cash in a savings account. Similar to cash, Essence can be spent in a number of ways, but all expenditures can roughly be classified as having a Yin or a Yang nature. Yang is roughly equivalent to energy, and Essence may be mobilized to create Yang energy that can then

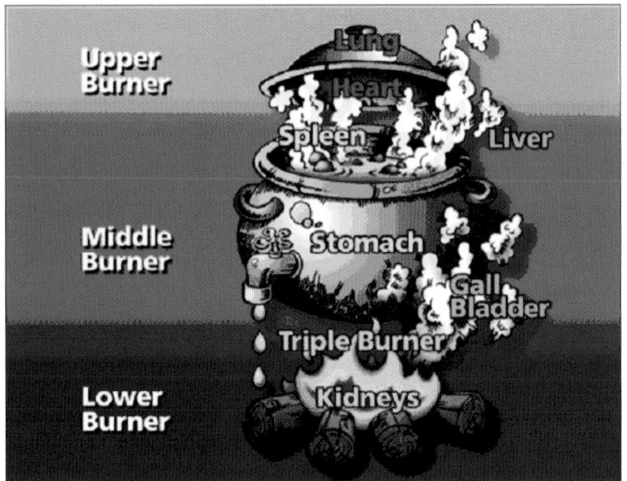

Figure 5-1 The body as a cooking pot.

warm or generally animate the body. Yin, or substance, may be produced from Essence to combat certain wasting conditions, or to keep the body moist during extremes of heat. Although it allows the organism to meet the temporarily high demands for Yin and Yang produced by disease or climate extremes, the penalty associated with Essence consumption is a potential shortening of the life span of the organism.

A third class of material produced by Essence is known as Qi (pronounced "chee"). Essence mobilization into Yin and Yang is the first step in this process, after which Yin and Yang interact to "ignite" each other. This process was envisioned to be somewhat similar to the powering of an oil lamp, wherein Yang energy is the spark, Yin is the oil, and the interaction of the two produces a flame known as Qi. Qi is the specific type of power consumed and stored by most of the internal organs. When an organ is lacking in power and is functioning poorly, it is thus often said to be Qi deficient. In the cooking pot metaphor for Chinese medical physiology, Qi is the flame that allows the cooking pot to function; the logs are the ultimate fuel source and represent Essence.

The Bladder

The Kidney's main function in Chinese medicine is as a storage depot of Essence; in conventional medicine, a main function is the management of body water stores through alterations in urine concentration. In Chinese medicine, urine concentration is believed to be performed by the Bladder, which is thereby considered an absorptive organ. Specifically, the Bladder is believed to accumulate water absorbed from the digestive tract by the Small Intestine; it then sorts the water into *pure* and *turbid* components. Only pure substances and fluids are considered appropriate for storage within the internal organs of the body. Turbid materials are duly excreted. The Bladder's function in storage and absorption is powered directly by the Kidney. Even in Chinese medicine, then, Kidney failure is considered the ultimate cause of a failure to concentrate urine, together with the common sequela of urinary incontinence.

BOX 5-1

Common Signs of Kidney Deficiency in Small Animals

- Profuse clear urine
- Urinary incontinence
- Anemia
- Lower limb and back weakness
- Deafness
- Vaginal discharge
- Cognitive dysfunction

Box 5-1 summarizes common symptoms of Kidney deficiency in small animals, as discussed earlier. Almost all symptoms are derived from a decline in body Essence, or *Jing*, over the life of the animal. It is not surprising, then, that these symptoms are also the most common signs of advancing age in both humans and animals.

The Spleen and the Stomach

The cooking pot hung over the fire of the Kidneys represents the digestive organs of Chinese medicine, particularly, the Spleen and the Stomach. The Spleen and the Stomach nourish the body by transforming raw materials in food into pure, useful substances such as Yang, Yin, Qi, Blood, and Essence. Apart from prenatal Essence, if a substance exists in the body, the Spleen and the Stomach are considered to have manufactured it. Their central location in the middle of the body matches this central role in manufacturing every one of its tissues.

The Stomach is the vessel in which the mechanical processes of digestion take place, including the secretion of digestive juices and peristalsis. When Stomach Qi does not promote peristaltic movement "downward" in an aboral direction but instead "rebels upward," the result is emesis. Food may also simply linger in the Stomach, producing halitosis through the direct connection between the Stomach and the mouth.

The Spleen is considered to facilitate assimilation following digestion through the microvilli and the pancreas. Absorption of amino acids, glucose, and fats by mediated cell transporters within both the gastrointestinal lumen and even the body as a whole results from the presence of sufficient Spleen power, or Qi. If Spleen function is inadequate, the products of the Stomach's efforts simply descend to be voided as watery, painless diarrhea, resulting in tissue atrophy and loss of weight. In Chinese medical parlance, then, the Spleen "raises the clear," such that only the turbid, or impure, descends to the Small and Large Intestines.

Given its complete lack of any digestive function in conventional medical physiology, the labeling of the Spleen as a digestive organ is a source of discomfiture for many veterinarians who attempt to study Chinese medicine. The initial conjecture that the Spleen was a digestive organ was reasonable, however, given its obvious prominence in the human body in the exact location where digestion was quite literally felt to take place. The Spleen's function was later determined as being filled by the pancreas; however, in humans, the pancreas is largely retroperitoneal and is almost indistinguishable from the adipose of the omentum, making it forgivable that the early Chinese did not identify it.

Once the error was made, it was difficult to undo. Because texts written even 1500 years ago are in daily use by Chinese medical practitioners, editing of all relevant Chinese medical literature would have been an onerous task, and it would have been unnecessary because Chinese medicine was not engaged in surgery or any physical manipulation of the organ itself. In the final analysis, it seemed less confusing and more harmless to simply acknowledge that, in light of present knowledge, a splenectomy could never cause digestive weakness, and that the practice of arbitrarily labeling the Spleen the organ of digestion can be continued for the purposes of discussion.

The products of digestion are numerous and include Blood, postnatal Essence, Yang, Yin, all fluids, and Qi. The stronger the function of the Spleen and the Stomach, the less often the organism must dip into its reservoir of Kidney Essence to meet the demands for these substances imposed by daily living. In the cooking pot diagram, we can see Essence dripping as a liquid fuel down to the woodpile and clouds of Qi wafting up to where these gather inside the lid of the cooking pot, or the Lung. Likewise, all other substances produced by the Spleen and the Stomach are stored only briefly before they are sent to the internal organ, where they are stored, or out into the circulation. The Liver is considered the main storage organ for Blood, and *Ying Qi* and Blood are the substances sent into the circulation. Ying Qi, which equates roughly to plasma, was correctly considered to carry the heavier or corpuscular elements of Blood. In keeping with the Spleen's general role of uptake and assimilation, when the Spleen's production of Ying Qi was deficient, Blood was not able to be held in the vessels, and it passively oozed out in a process known today as *diapedesis*.

The Spleen is the source of not only healthful fluids but pathologic ones as well. When the Spleen and the Stomach lack the power to adequately transform food and water into useful substances, the material that is produced instead is known as Dampness or Phlegm. Dampness and Phlegm behave as normal fluids do to some extent, going where normal fluids go, such as into the joints, the mouth, and the bloodstream; then, they simply accumulate as a useless detritus that provides the foundation for some of the most serious and common small animal disorders. Sometimes, the pathologic fluid accretes into masses; at other times, it simply serves as a source of friction with circulating energy, which it releases uselessly as heat. In the mouth, Dampness and Phlegm can be directly visualized as tenacious saliva or, especially in humans, as a thick, greasy coating on the tongue surface. Manufacture of Dampness and Phlegm is prevented when the fire under the cooking pot is adequate, and when the pot itself is not overfilled (Boxes 5-2 and 5-3).

BOX 5-2

Common Signs of Spleen and Stomach Pathology

COMMON SIGNS OF SPLEEN DEFICIENCY	COMMON SIGNS OF STOMACH PATHOLOGY/DISEASE
Muscle wasting and weakness	Vomiting and regurgitation
Watery painless diarrhea	Halitosis
Anemia	Excessive appetite
Hemorrhage	Thirst
Inappetance	Epigastric pain or distention
Lassitude	Dyspepsia
Dyspnea	
Pallor	

BOX 5-3

Common Signs of Dampness and Phlegm

- Masses
- Joint swelling
- Heat symptoms—increased appetite or thirst, restlessness, hyperexcitability, panting, insomnia, heat and exercise intolerance
- Polyuria
- Weight gains
- Exudates and discharges from the ears, skin, and eyes
- Slimy fluid and mucous in the stool and vomit
- Productive cough
- Tenesmus (organ wall swelling)

The Lungs and the Large Intestine

The major action of the Lungs and the Large Intestine is to gather, carry downward, and distribute Qi. In a sense, the Lungs are the quartermaster of the body, and early Chinese medical writings depicted them as the Minister placed in charge of guarding the Imperial granaries. Essentially, the Lungs gather Qi the way the lid of a cooking pot gathers steam. The Qi is then carefully distributed to certain centers of the body. The steam metaphor is appropriate, given that Qi is essentially considered to be a vapor. The cooking pot diagram depicts Qi as wafting up from the cooking pot and thus being solely produced by the Spleen. Qi is also inhaled, however, and it is a mix of Qi from air and from food that is distributed around the body.

One form of Qi produced by the Spleen and gathered by the Lungs is *Wei Qi.* Like Ying Qi, Wei Qi circulates within the bloodstream. From the blood, Wei Qi is envisioned to move out to the periphery, where it acts as a defensive barrier to pathogenic Qi, or *Xie Qi.* This early concept of the front line of the body's defenses being carried to the periphery via the circulation, where they confront pathogens, is a succinct summary of some of the intricacies that would be discovered almost 2 millennia later by immunologists and microbiologists.

Besides the circulation, Qi is also distributed by the Lungs to the fire in the woodpile beneath the cooking pot. Qi from the Lungs stored by the Kidneys helps ensure that the body's Essence stores are not mobilized to generate Qi but can instead be conserved to lengthen life. The storage of Lung Qi by the Kidneys is not a passive act, however. The Kidneys must have enough strength to reach up and actively grasp the descending Lung Qi. Dyspnea, asthma, and coughing result from the inability of Lung Qi to descend, whether because of Kidney weakness or because of physical obstructions such as mucus and Phlegm (Table 5-1).

TABLE 5-1

Types of Qi in the Body

Types of Qi	Translation	Function
Zhong Qi	Central Qi	Energy of digestion
Gu Qi	Food Qi	Energy derived from food
Da Qi; Tian Qi	Great or Heavenly Qi	Inhaled air (for this reason the Lungs are said to open to the nose and connect with the throat)
Zong Qi	Ancestral Qi	The aggregate of all Qi that has accumulated in the chest before departing to serve various functions; includes Gu Qi and Da Qi
Xie Qi	Pathogen	Exogenous cause of disease
Wei Qi	Defensive Qi	Resists pathogen invasion
Ying Qi	Plasma	Circulates with Blood and source perspiration
Zheng Qi	Righteous Qi	Sum complement of healthy Qi
Jing-Luo Qi	Channel and Vessel Qi	Circulating Qi; both Ying and Wei Qi circulate
Yuan Qi	Source Qi	Power supplied by the Kidney
Zang-Fu Qi	Organ Qi	Power possessed by each organ

The Large Intestine is considered loosely related to the Lungs in that it too functions to carry its contents downward. As in conventional medicine, the Large Intestine in Chinese medicine is believed to absorb a small amount of water, with most water being absorbed upstream in the Small Intestine.

Another similarity between the Lung and the Large Intestine is their dependence on a carefully controlled temperature. Qi, similar to all vapors, is extremely vulnerable to temperature fluctuations. If the Lungs become too cold, the moist Qi vapor may congeal into water; if the Lungs become too hot, the vapor evaporates and disappears. Within the Large Intestine, too much heat dries up the small amount of moisture that is present, creating stool dryness and constipation; too much moisture leads to diarrhea (Box 5-4).

The Heart and the Small Intestine (upper Jiao)

The Heart houses consciousness, or Shen. The immediate survival of an organism hinges, above all else, upon its ability to engage in an appropriate manner with its environment. The fact that the Heart is responsible for this power of discernment has earned it the title in Chinese medicine of Emperor of the body. As the Emperor, the Heart speaks for the rest of the body, accounting in part for the association in Chinese medicine of the tongue with the Heart. The Heart is nestled within the clear air, or Qi, of the Lungs, giving it the clarity of vision it needs to wisely rule the rest of the body. Consciousness is disturbed and even lost when this clarity is lost. In such a case, the Orifices of the Heart are said to be obstructed. A common condition in which this occurs is a grand mal seizure.

Because of the tendency for heat to rise, the Heart, in its lofty position under the lid of the cooking pot, has a tendency to accumulate fiery Yang energy. As such, it is an important source of Yang energy (or spark) for use by the Kidneys in the ignition of Yin to create Qi, or power. In turn, some of the Kidney Yin is steamed up by the resultant fire in the woodpile to cool the innately Yang Heart, serving to establish a mutually reciprocating and controlling relationship between the two organs.

Without the connection between the Heart and the Kidney, the lower body would become too cold and the

BOX 5-4

Common Signs of Lung and Large Intestine Disease

SIGNS OF LUNG PATHOLOGY/DISEASE	SIGNS OF LARGE INTESTINE PATHOLOGY/DISEASE
Dyspnea	Constipation
Cough	Diarrhea
Frequent colds in humans	
Neck and back pain	

upper body would become too hot. A common clinical syndrome in which this occurs is chronic renal failure in cats, wherein the heat in the upper burner, or Heart, creates uncontrollable thirst; coldness and weakness of the lower burner or Kidneys, on the other hand, result in poor urine concentration.

The Heart governs consciousness and receives extensive support from the Pericardium. The Pericardium is necessary to ensure that the Heart has an adequate blood supply; it serves as the interface between the Emperor and the rest of the kingdom. This caretaker role is emphasized in the *Nei Jing*, which details the pathways of the Heart channel but recommends only Pericardium points for the treatment of Heart disorders. Additionally, the *Nei Jing* describes pathogenic attacks on the Heart or Emperor as always ending in death, in that its Pericardium protector must have already been vanquished.

The function of the Small Intestine is considered loosely allied with that of the Heart; both organs are involved in prudent engagement with the environment. Although the Heart exhibits this prudence by governing the external interactions of the organism, the Small Intestine exhibits it by discerning the "clear" from the "turbid" in the chyme received from the Stomach. The pure water it extracts from the lumen is sent directly to the Bladder for final processing, and the turbid water is sent on for a final brief filtering by the Large Intestine (Box 5-5).

The Liver

The major action of the Liver is to facilitate movement, particularly of the circulation. Once the Heart has initiated the movement of Blood, the Liver becomes responsible for ensuring smooth laminar flow. The main requirement for smooth laminar flow is, in turn, an adequate blood supply. When the smooth flow of blood is disrupted, pain that is improved by movement results. If blood is particularly stagnant, bruising, hemorrhage, vascular engorgement, and tumors may result.

A by-product of adequate Qi and Blood circulation to the farthest reaches of the body by the Liver is the maintenance of healthy skin, hair, and nails. When circulation of Qi and Blood to the periphery is adequate, pathogenic Qi can invade with little resistance from the *Wei Qi*, producing skin rashes. In addition, inadequate Blood circulation can lead to desiccation of the Tendons, resulting in cramping pain and thinning and falling out of hair, which does not regrow; menstrual bleeding is painful, scanty, or erratic, resulting in dysmenorrhea, metrorrhagia, or amenorrhea; the fetus may fail to receive adequate nourishment, resulting in miscarriage; the cornea dries and desiccates, manifesting as keratoconjunctivitis sicca; a sense of inadequacy sets in that results in an enhanced sense of covetousness and fear; and vivid dreams disturb sleep.

The Spleen is the source of all fluids, including Blood; adequate Blood production by the Spleen ensures that the Liver has sufficient Blood with which to nourish the extremities. Unfortunately, when the Liver has an inadequate supply of Blood, a disharmony is created between the Liver, the Spleen, and the Stomach. The pressure brought to bear on the Spleen and the Stomach by the Liver overwhelms the two neighboring organs, further compromising Blood supply. Common clinical syndromes arising from the vicious cycle that ensues include hyperlipidemia, chronic active hepatitis, pancreatitis, ascites, gastric ulceration, and liver failure. All are amenable to treatments that restore harmony between the Liver and the Spleen.

The Gallbladder as a bile storage organ is considered relatively unimportant in Chinese veterinary medicine, as it is in conventional medicine. There is far more interest, however, in the Gallbladder acupuncture channel because it traverses the joints, most commonly causing lameness in the dog. The Gallbladder channel is discussed more fully in the next section (Table 5-2).

The Triple Burner and the Gallbladder

The major action of the Triple Burner and its cousin, the Gallbladder, is to facilitate the activity of all other organs. The Triple Burner has no Western organ equivalent but is

BOX 5-5

Signs of Heart Disease in Chinese Medicine

- Incontinence
- Seizures
- Agitation, confusion
- Cystitis
- Circulatory failure, or blood stasis

TABLE 5-2

Symptoms of Blood Deficiency and Its Sequelae*

Liver Blood Deficiency	Liver Qi Stagnation	Blood Stasis
Pale tongue	Lavender tongue	Purple tongue
Alopecia, hair dryness		
Thin pulses	Wiry pulses	Erratic pulses
Cramping pain	Distention; shooting pain	Stabbing localized pain
Recurrent skin rashes		
Fearfulness, territoriality	Irritability	
Vivid dreams		
	Colic	Masses
		Hemorrhage (dark clotted blood)

*Often all three syndromes may be present in the same animal, usually dogs.

perceived to be a sort of internal axis that provides a conduit for the movement of Qi and fluids up and down the body. In the cooking pot diagram, it is essentially the space between the fire and the pot, and the lid and the pot. Within the Triple Burner, Lung Qi descends to the Kidneys, taking with it water and fluids obtained from the Spleen and the digestive tract. Meanwhile, the Source Qi, depicted by Fire, moves up from the Kidneys to supply the various organs of the body. The Triple Burner is thus the intermediary between the rest of the body and the Source Qi of the Kidneys. It thus plays a similar role to the Pericardium, which acts as an intermediary with the Heart. Without the Triple Burner, no organs could access the fires of the Kidney. Because both the Pericardium and the Triple Burner are gatekeepers, they are considered related in Chinese medicine.

Similar to the Pericardium, the Gallbladder is closely related in function to the Triple Burner. Whereas the Triple Burner conducts energy internally, the Gallbladder channel is believed to deliver energy from the interior of the body to its surface. Once on the surface, the energy of the Gallbladder channel galvanizes the structures it passes through, such as the knee and hip joints. Congenital hip dysplasia, hind limb paralysis, and crucial ligament tears are just a few of the small animal conditions commonly treated via the Gallbladder and its channel (Table 5-3).

CONCLUSIONS

Chinese medicine is often dismissed by conventional medical practitioners as arcane and as having little relevance to modern medicine. It is clear, however, that the poetic and circular logic of Chinese medicine allowed it to speculate on the existence of dozens of physiologic processes and phenomena that would not be described by

TABLE 5-3

External Pathogens and Their Treatment

Pathogen	Definition	Treatment Goal	Indicated Flavor	Examples
Wind-Cold	Outer body layers and appendages most often affected. As the pathogen invades from the outside, the patient commonly experiences chills (even though body temperature may be high); aching of the neck, back, and head; and a superficially palpable pulse	Disperse Wind	Warm, pungent herbs are required. The expansive power of the pungent flavor helps push the cold pathogen out of the body. The warmth of the herb counters the coldness of the pathogen. In essence, spicy warm herbs (e.g., garlic) are called for, which often induce perspiration and have strong antimicrobial properties; this association between antimicrobial power and diaphoresis led most cultures to believe that resolution of colds and flu required the induction of perspiration	Cinnamon twigs, garlic, ephedra
Wind-Heat	Superficial (epithelial) body layers are involved, but symptoms are more overtly inflammatory. Symptoms may range from pharyngitis to skin wheals and pustules. Even some cases of acute diarrhea were classified in Chinese medicine as a special (Damp) form of Wind-Heat invasion, known as "summerheat"	Disperse Wind, clear Heat. In the case of summerheat, the orderly movement of Qi internally is obstructed by the invading pathogen, resulting in vomiting, diarrhea, and coughing	Pungent, cool herbs are needed to provide an effective outward push to pathogens of the skin and throat. Bitter and pungent herbs are used internally for summerheat invasion. The bitter taste has a vigorous descending effect, harnessing the explosive power of the pungent flavor and driving it downward. The net effect is an opening, dilating effect on smooth muscle, which relieves cramps and dilates bronchioles	Pungent, cool, superficially acting herbs consist of Mint leaves and many flowers, including Dandelion and Honeysuckle. Bitter, pungent herbs that carry Qi downward include Citrus peel, Apricot kernel, Coltsfoot herb, and Chamomile flowers

TABLE 5-3

External Pathogens and Their Treatment—cont'd

Pathogen	Definition	Treatment Goal	Indicated Flavor	Examples
Wind-Damp	Appendages and the back are particularly affected. Symptoms are worse from exposure to Damp weather and most often include aching joints. Fluid accumulations, such as edema and joint swelling, may be noted, along with moist, tacky skin eruptions. Wind-Damp invasion requires an internal predisposition to dampness. Damp is elaborated internally because of digestive weakness	Disperse Wind, drain Damp	Bland-tasting herbs "leech" out dampness, while also supporting the digestive power of the patient. This dual draining and supporting function is much like the sand of a beach on which a person's weight is supported but water is drained rapidly away. Wind-expelling herbs are pungent	Bland herbs include Coix seed, various fungi such as *Poria*, and the stigmata and silk of Corn. Pungent herbs that expel Wind-Damp include *Angelica pubescens* (Du Huo) and *Ledebouriella* (Fang Feng)
Cold	Cold invasion creates a sense of chilliness. Cold internally slows circulation and movement, resulting in stiffness and sometimes severe abdominal pain. Limb pain may also be observed—the application of warmth may bring pain relief	Warm Yang, expel Cold pathogens	Hot, pungent, spicy herbs warm the Yang. Pairing these with a bitter cathartic (e.g., Rhubarb root and rhizome) was believed to expel the pathogen. Bitter, warm, pungent herbs are notorious for their analgesic properties	Aconite, corydalis, fennel, and cinnamon bark are common examples
Heat	Heat invasion produces heat intolerance, perspiration, plethora, increased heart rate, thirst, dehydration, yellow exudation, and severe inflammation. Unrelenting or deeply entrenched heat leads to fluid loss, desiccation of the Blood, and circulatory failure	Clear Heat, Nourish Yin and move Blood in later stages	Heat-clearing herbs are always bitter. Herbs that replenish (i.e., rehydrate) Yin usually taste sweet and may have a glutinous texture. Blood-moving herbs may be bitter or bitter and pungent	Bitter herbs include natural sources of antimicrobials such as Peruvian bark, Oregon grape, and Goldenseal. Glutinous sweetish herbs include *Panax ginseng* and Slippery elm. Bitter or bitter, pungent Blood movers include *Angelica sinensis* (Dang Gui) and Peach kernel
Damp	Damp internally manifests as weight gain, oily discharge, abundant bland exudates, and tenesmus	Drain Damp	Bland herbs, as discussed earlier, are the mainstay of treatment	Other examples include *Polyporus* fungus and *Alisma*
Phlegm	Phlegm manifests as tangible tissue accumulations or tenacious catarrhal discharges	Transform Phlegm, soften nodules	Very hard lumps may require (mineral-laden) salty herbs, which are believed to be taken up by the lesions, which then imbibe moisture. Sweet, pungent herbs may also be used, with the sweet taste emolliating the lesion and the pungent taste breaking it up	Examples of mineral-laden herbs that are useful for breaking up indurations include Horsetail for bladder scar tissue and various seaweeds for thyroid goiter. Sweet, pungent herbs used in treating mass lesions and mucus include Poke root and Echinacea, respectively

conventional medical physiology for more than a thousand years. These processes include a notion of humoral immunity; a basic understanding of body water management, and the roles of the kidney, small intestine, and colon in that process; and the dependence of normal development on liquid substances (later called *hormones*), which, if lacking at birth, could not be replaced. Given their predictive value millennia ago, many conventional medical practitioners are revisiting the Chinese medical classics. Their goal is to determine whether these classics have new insights to offer, as veterinary medicine evolves out of its outdated belief in single "magic bullet" cures for chronic diseases and begins instead to recognize them as arising from complex interrelationships between organs and organ systems, much as Chinese medicine postulated centuries ago.

Ayurvedic Veterinary Medicine: Principles and Practices

CHAPTER

Robert J. Silver

INTRODUCTION TO AYURVEDIC VETERINARY MEDICINE

In recent years, there has been increased interest by the pharmaceutical industry in discovering medicines derived from other cultures. The hope is that these unique medical remedies can address disease conditions that do not respond well enough with conventional medicines. This upsurge of interest in medicines from other cultures, or *ethnomedicine*, is shared by the general populace as well.

More people than ever are studying and practicing Traditional Chinese Medicine, the ethnomedical system of China. The ethnomedical system of the subcontinent of India—Ayurveda—has attracted the interest of many people and practitioners in recent years. Today, in India, Ayurveda is still practiced side by side with conventional Western medicine. To become an Ayurvedic physician in India now, one must complete a Western medical degree followed by 8 years of training in Ayurvedic medicine.

Ayurveda has had a profound influence on the way medicine is practiced in every culture throughout the world. Ayurveda provides the historical foundation for the practice of the following:

- Traditional Chinese Medicine
- Western "Galenic" medicine
- Middle Eastern "Unani" ethnomedicine

Ayurvedic medical texts dating thousands of years BC document the treatment of livestock, horses, camels, and elephants with surgery and with herbal therapies. One such text is the *Mahabharata*, which dates back to circa 3000 BC (Mahabarat, 1958). The practice of ethnoveterinary medicine is as old as the domestication of livestock.

According to the World Health Organization (WHO), ethnomedical, or "traditional" medical practices are still used by 85% of people in developing countries as their first line of medical "defense" (WHO, 1988). The Food and Agricultural Organization (FAO) advocates the use of traditional medical practices for animal treatment in developing countries (Anjaria, 1984).

To use Ayurvedic therapies effectively, one does not need to have an understanding of the philosophy that underlies Ayurveda. Modern veterinarians can use Ayurvedic herbal therapies on the basis of the scientifically determined pharmacologic actions of the botanical compounds contained in these formulas. A large volume of basic and clinical research has been undertaken on the herbs of Ayurveda. Thus, in the World scientific literature, documentation is available that enables the veterinary practitioner to evaluate herb safety, efficacy, and dosing.

Ayurveda means, literally, "the Science of Life." Ayurveda is an ancient healing system that has its roots in India. Ayurveda is more than simply a compendium of procedures and therapies: Ayurveda is a way of life that relates an individual's existence to universal principles.

As a holistic healing system, Ayurveda encompasses not just the treatment of disease, but also the creation and maintenance of individual health and optimal wellness. It is a detailed and complete system that puts its emphasis on living in harmony with the laws of Nature and the Universe. Health in Ayurveda results from this harmonious integration of individual constitution with Nature and Universe.

The actual practice of Ayurvedic medicine involves the combined use of herbs, diet, massage, exercise, detoxification, and meditation. These therapies are prescribed to the patient as a result of the patient's Ayurvedic diagnosis.

Ayurvedic diagnosis is made after three sources of patient information are considered:

1. The practitioner's observations of the patient during the examination
2. A thorough medical, familial, and environmental history
3. A description of the medical problem in depth with details

It is important to stress again that a veterinarian need not adopt any or all of the principles and practices of Ayurvedic medicine to benefit from its use. Many Ayurvedic herbs are unique, coming from the very diverse panoply of ecosystems found in India. Many herbs from the Indian subcontinent contain phytochemicals that are not found in the herbs of the Western tradition. This is due, in part, to the more tropical climate and richly volcanic soil specific to the Himalayans and other mountain ranges in India. One such herb that is indigenous to India is the tree named *Boswellia serrata*, from which the oleo-resin boswellia is extracted. Another unique herbal from India is shilajeet, which is an organic exudate derived from a specific geologic formation that incorporates layers of organic sediment.

Ayurvedic herbs have a long and ancient history of use; thus, their effects and adverse effects have been evaluated empirically in great detail. This allows the practitioner a large degree of confidence in using these herbs safely and effectively in veterinary medical prescriptions.

This chapter provides some background information to assist the veterinary practitioner in understanding the basics of Ayurvedic thought; also provided are examples of which Ayurvedic medicines are prescribed in a modern veterinary practice and how this is done. A guide to some of the more commonly used Ayurvedic herbs and their clinical applications can be found at the end of this chapter.

HISTORY OF AYURVEDA

India possesses one of the oldest organized systems of medicine. Its roots can be traced back to the remote and distant past of human prehistory. Elements of Ayurvedic medicine can be found at the roots of nearly all traditional and modern systems of medicine in the world. Early written accounts describing the medicinal use of plants are found in the ancient Vedic texts. These writings originated in the period circa 3147 BC (Anjaria, 2002).

The Indian mythologic epic poem, "The Ramayana" (Ramayana, 1958), described Vaid Sushena from Sri Lanka treating the unconsciousness of Laxmanji with the use of a specific herb (not mentioned). Herbal treatments for animals are also emphasized in this text, dating back to circa 4000 BC (Anjaria, 2002). The Mahabharata (~3000 BC), another Indian classic (Mahabarat, 1958), includes a story of an animal trainer and a caretaker. Elsewhere in this ancient text are descriptions of "noted animal physicians." This book contains one of the earliest written records documenting the practice of veterinary medicine in ancient history. Somavanshi has reviewed the ethnoveterinary resources of ancient India. This review reports the availability and sources of ancient Indian literature from different libraries and documentation centers in India (Somavanshi, 1998).

Chapters that discuss animal husbandry practices appear in *Skanda Purana*, *Devi Purana*, and other lesser known texts. The horse played an important role in the lives of ancient people; because of this, equine ethnoveterinary medicine attained a glorified status in ancient India. Famous veterinarians were described: Palkapya, around 1000 BC, and Shalihotra, around 2350 BC, specialized in the treatment of horses and elephants. Elephants were also very important because of their role in ancient Indian culture as beasts of burden. The science of elephant medicine is detailed in many early Indian texts (Anjaria, 2002).

Shalihotra was the first to describe in writing detailed accounts of surgical and medical therapies (Shalihotra, no date). Shalihotra compiled an Indian *Materia Medica*, which provided step-by-step descriptions of methods of administration of herbs, including instructions on preparing medicines for injection.

Shalihotra is reported to have written the first book on veterinary treatments in Sanskrit. This text was called *The Shalihotra* and is considered to be the first book ever written to describe specific techniques in veterinary medicine, including the use of indigenous herbs in the treatment of working animals. Another text attributed to Shalihotra is *Ashva-Ayurveda*, which discussed treatment of the horse. Shalihotra is considered to be historically the first true veterinarian because of his contributions to the science of veterinary medicine (Anjaria, 2002).

A number of other ancient Indian texts not as well known as the texts previously discussed also contain chapters on veterinary medicine. Prescriptions for the treatment of animals have been detailed in these texts as well (Anjaria, 2002). Charak and Sushruta, 1220 BC and 1356 BC, respectively, compiled their observations on indigenous and herbal therapy as the *Charak Samhita* (medicine) and the *Sushruta Samhita* (surgery) (Charak Samhita, 1941). *Mrig Ayurveda* is another ancient text that describes the medical treatment of animals; it is sometimes loosely translated as *Animal Ayurveda*. A synonym of Mrig is *Pashu*, which often follows *Mrig* in parentheses. *Mrig (Pashu) Ayurveda* is considered to be a special branch of Ayurveda. This ancient text is stored in the Library of Gujarat Ayurveda University in Jamnagar, India. *Hasti Ayurveda* is a comprehensive text that contains material devoted to medicine for elephants (Anand, 1894).

The first veterinary hospital was built by King Ashoka (300 BC). He also developed operational protocols for veterinary hospitals regarding the use of botanical medicinals (Anjaria, 2002). Historically, Ayurvedic medicine expanded its influence into Asia, contributing to the development of Traditional Chinese Medicine. Buddhist monks practiced Ayurveda and planted Ayurvedic herb gardens along their peripatetic routes while spreading Buddhist thought and political influence throughout all the far corners of Asia. In this way, Ayurveda spread to Sri Lanka, Nepal, Tibet, Mongolia, Russia, China, Korea, Japan, and other parts of Southeast Asia.

The influences of Ayurvedic medicine reached as far as the empires of Egypt, Greece, and Rome. During the reign of Alexander the Great, Hindu physicians were used to treat snakebites and other ailments among the soldiers of the Grecian camp.

Some authorities believe that many Greek and post-classical philosophers like Paracelsus, Hippocrates, and Pythagoras may have actually visited India and the East and learned from Ayurvedic and other Eastern teachings; they then brought the medicines they found there back to Greece. The great Hellenic physician Dioscorides mentions many Indian plants in his work, including the use of datura for asthma, and nux vomica for paralysis and dyspepsia. The Roman Empire also relied heavily upon Indian medicines. Imports of ginger and other spices from India were so large that the famous Roman herbalist, Pliny, complained about the heavy drain of Roman gold for the purchase of Indian herbal medicines and spices and the effects of this on the Roman economy (Kapoor, 1990).

Ayurvedic medicine, with its ancient roots, also has a broad base of followers in our modern era. Ayurveda is actively practiced in India, and Ayurvedic practitioners can be found in increasing numbers in many countries of the modern world. In the United States, Deepak Chopra, MD, and the Transcendental Meditation movement of the Maharishi Mahesh Yogi, along with many others, have been instrumental in the establishment and promulgation of the concept and practice of Ayurvedic healing modalities.

PHILOSOPHIES UNDERLYING AYURVEDA

Considering that Ayurvedic thought historically preceded Traditional Chinese Medicine (TCM) and served as a basis (in part) for the development of TCM, it should be no surprise that many similarities can be noted between TCM and the basic structure and philosophy of Ayurvedic medicine. Contemporary veterinarians interested in systems of ethnomedicine have been studying the principles and practices of TCM by learning to practice veterinary acupuncture. These TCM-trained veterinarians will be able to more readily understand Ayurvedic medical principles and practices.

As an example, the concept that *Yin* and *Yang* are the fundamental underlying substances of the Universe in TCM finds a parallel in Ayurveda. *Purusha*, which is male in energy, is considered to be the Great Spirit. *Prakruti*, or Great Nature, is the representation of matter. The union of these two primal forces produces all things. Similar to *Yin* and *Yang*, *Purusha* and *Prakruti* are opposite yet complementary concepts.

Purusha and *Prakruti* as two complementary forces constitute together a single cohesive dynamic, called *Mahat*. They are continuously being created and destroyed in the same way that *Yin* becomes *Yang* and *Yang* becomes *Yin*. The joining of these two forces creates *Mahat*, or Cosmic Consciousness. In a similar fashion, in Taoist philosophy (which underlies the principles of TCM), the *Tao* contains the two forces of *Yin* and *Yang*.

The word *Prakruti* has two meanings according to the context in which it is used. In the context just described, *Prakruti* refers to Universal Nature. Most commonly though, *Prakruti* refers to Individual Nature, or individual constitution. Ayurveda is directed toward creating Life in harmony with *Mahat*. Disease is not natural—it is artificial and results from lack of balance with *Mahat*.

Ayurveda considers the Universe, as well as the physical bodies of humans, animals, and plants, to consist of five basic elements: Earth, Air, Fire, Water, and Ether. Ayurvedic thought also attributes five states that matter can embody: Solid, Liquid, Radiant, Gaseous, and Ethereal. The five elements in Ayurvedic thought are responsible for the physical nature of all visible and invisible matter in the universe.

Ayurveda teaches that a subtle energy called *Prana* is the "Life Force," or the *Qi* (of TCM) of the body. It binds body, mind, and spirit and orchestrates their smooth interaction. Similar to *Qi*, *Prana* is not air. Oxygen, however, is considered to be one of the agents of *Prana*.

Seven types of vital tissues *(Dhatus)* in the bodies of humans and animals are derived from food. These tissues include Plasma, Blood, Muscle, Fat, Bone, Bone Marrow and Nervous Tissue, and Reproductive Tissue. Plants have tissue types that correspond to these animal tissues. Each plant tissue nourishes its corresponding animal tissue. It is thought that each tissue nourishes the next tissue on the list (Table 6-1). Thus, the juice of the leaf nourishes the flowers and fruit; the flowers and fruit nourish the softwood, and so forth. Plant parts also relate to the five elements. These relationships are also outlined in Table 6-1.

THE TRIDOSHA

Critical to an understanding of Ayurvedic principles is the concept of the three *Doshas* (the group is known as the *Tridosha*) (Table 6-2), which describe the three basic characteristics found in all livings things from both Animal

TABLE 6-1

Ayurvedic Elements Associated With Mammalian and Plant Tissues

Plant Tissue or Part	Correspondence to Mammalian Tissue	Element Correspondence
Juice of leaf	Plasma	None
Flowers/Fruit	Blood	Fire/Ether
Softwood	Muscle	None
Gum, hard sap	Fat	None
Bark	Bone	None
Leaf	Bone marrow and nervous tissue	Air
Resin, sap	Reproductive tissues	None
Root	None	Earth
Stem and branches	None	Water
Seed	None	All five elements

TABLE 6-2

Comparison of the *Tridosha*

Dosha	Qualities	Anatomy and Physiology	Characteristics
Vata	Dry, light, cold, subtle, unstable, rough, clear and transparent; strongest of the *Doshas;* powerful and mobile in nature	Sensory organs, nervous system, respiratory system, digestion—separating the nutrients from the waste	Restless mind, weak memory; avoid confrontation; active and sensitive nature; express themselves through sport and creative pursuits, sometimes by overindulgence in pleasures, often sexual in nature.
Pitta	Heat, sharpness, liquidity, slight oiliness; blue and yellow colors; fleshy and unpleasant smell; pungent and sour tastes; fluidity	Eyes get red in the summer and after bathing; provides color shine and heat to the body; bodies tend to be hot and sweaty; enzymes and digestive function, hormones, acid, bile, stomach, small intestines	Intelligent, aware; vision, hunger, thirst, taste; precise, irritable, articulate, learned, proud; have an aggressive nature; are sharp and knifelike in anger
Kapha	Heavy, cool, soft, viscous, sweet, stable, slimy; sturdiness, plumpness, enthusiasm, wisdom, virility	Maintains oiliness of the body and organs; maintains general stability of the body; provides strength, patience, and virility; promotes smooth working of the joints; primary agent of all cellular development and reproductive activity	Courageous, tolerant, and generous; slow talkers; can be lethargic; phlegmatic, even lazy if not motivated by others; stable patient personality; honorable; not easily provoked, but difficult to calm down if provoked

and Plant Kingdoms. In Sanskrit, *Dosha* means, literally, "fault or error, a thing which can go wrong" (Svoboda, 1995). The three *Doshas* are described by the elements and energies inherent in each tendency. These qualities include factors like temperature, moisture, weight, and texture. The *Tridosha* represents three primal metabolic tendencies in the living organism. Each individual, whether human, plant, or animal, embodies one or a combination of two of the *Doshas.*

This embodiment is considered to be an organism's individual constitution. Balance among the members of the *Tridosha* results in health and homeostasis. Disease results from an imbalance among the three *Doshas.* Individual constitution also represents the type of disease to which an individual is most prone. Disease conditions that differ in nature from the individual are usually easy to treat. When the disease is the same *Dosha* as the individual, it is more difficult to treat because the constitution of the individual reinforces the disease pattern (Frawley, 1988).

The first *Dosha* is named *Vata,* which means "wind." *Vata* is dry and cold. It is the principle of kinetic energy and corresponds most closely to the TCM concept of *Qi* (Svoboda, 1995). *Vata* is associated with the mental phenomena of enthusiasm and concentration. It is concerned with processes that are activating and dynamic in nature. It is derived from the elements Ether and Air. *Vata* is the most powerful of the *Doshas* and is considered to be the "Life Force."

Vata governs all movement in the body, such as respiration, circulation, excretion, and voluntary action. It is located in the body below the navel in the bladder, large intestines, nervous system, pelvic region, thighs, bone marrow, and legs. Its principal organ is the large intestine. When *Vata* is out of balance, the primary symptoms are gas, colic, low back pain, arthritis, pruritus, and paralysis. Individuals with a *Vata* constitution are more susceptible to these symptoms. *Vata* symptoms include cold extremities, cold aversion, and aversion to cold food. Clinical manifestations of *Vata* pathology can also include hypertension and cardiac arrhythmias. Muscle spasms, back aches, dry eyes, dry skin, and a dull and rough hair coat are all symptoms of *Vata* pathology. In a veterinary context, breeds that have a *Vata* constitution are the ectomorphic ones, such as the Borzoi, the Greyhound, and the Afghan.

The second *Dosha, Pitta,* or bile, is derived from Fire and an aspect of Water. It is the principle of biotransformation and balance and is the cause of all metabolic processes in the body. It rules all of the enzymes and hormones in the body. It is most closely associated with the TCM concept of *Yang. Pitta* is associated with the mental processes of intellect and clear and focused concentration. *Pitta* governs the activities of the endocrine organs. It governs body heat, temperature (thermogenesis, thermal homeostasis), and all chemical reactions (Svoboda, 1995).

Pitta maintains digestive and glandular secretions, including digestive enzymes and bile. It is responsible for digestion, metabolism, pigmentation, hunger, thirst, sight, courage, and mental activity. Its location in the body is between the navel and the chest in the stomach, small intestines, liver, spleen, skin, and blood. Its primary location in the body though is the small intestines and, to a lesser extent, the stomach. When *Pitta* is out of balance, its primary manifestation is acid and bile, leading to inflammation. Humans with *Pitta* pathology complain of a burning sensation in the stomach or liver. Animals with a *Pitta* constitution have a mesomorphic constitution and a tendency toward "hot" behavior, such as might be found in a Rottweiler, Chow Chow, or Pit Bull terrier (Sodhi, 2003).

The third *Dosha*, *Kapha*, is derived from Water and Earth. It is the principle of cohesion and stability. It regulates *Vata* and *Pitta*. *Kapha* functions by way of the bodily fluids and is most closely associated with the TCM concept of *Yin*. When there is *Kapha* pathology, it corresponds to the TCM pathogenic factors of Damp and Phlegm. *Kapha* promotes properties that are conserving and stabilizing in nature, along with anabolic functions. It is responsible for keeping the body lubricated and is essential for maintenance of its solid nature, its tissues, its strength, and its sexuality. *Kapha* maintains substance, weight, structure, solidity, and body build and is associated with the mental properties of courage and patience.

Kapha integrates the structural elements of the body into stable form. It forms connective and musculoskeletal tissue. Its normal locations in the body are the upper part of the body and the thorax, head, neck, upper portion of the stomach, pleural cavity, fat tissues, and areas between joints. *Kapha*'s principal organ is the lungs. When out of balance, it manifests disease symptoms associated with being heavy and slow, leading to obesity. Humans with *Kapha* pathology complain of feeling heavy after eating, and they report a feeling of depression. *Kapha* people have slow speech and slow movements. Discharges may or may not be present in a *Kapha* imbalance. Veterinary patients with a *Kapha* constitution include the English bulldog, the Newfoundland, and the Great Pyrenees breeds, as well as the obese, sluggish Golden retriever.

For a living being to exist, it must employ characteristics of all three of the *Doshas*. This means it must have the following:

1. Tissue structure or anabolism in its *Kapha* quality.
2. Chemical processes or metabolism in its *Pitta* quality. *and*
3. Movement and elimination or catabolism in its *Vata* qualities.

Without any one of these qualities, life cannot exist. Seven combinations of the three *Doshas* in turn become the seven possible constitutions (Boxes 6-1 and 6-2).

The origins and pathogenesis of disease in Ayurvedic medical theory are considered to be the following:

- The buildup of waste products or toxins such as *Mala* and *Ama*
- The blockage of the *Srotas* (or nourishing vessels), most commonly by a buildup of waste products or toxins (*Mala* and *Ama*)
- The lack of appropriate nourishment to the vital tissues, often secondary to the blocked Srotas

BOX 6-1

The Seven Constitutions From the *Tridosha*

Vata	Anxious, fearful, light and "airy"; ectomorphic; prone to *Vata* diseases
Pitta	Aggressive and impatient, "fiery" and hot headed; mesomorphic; prone to *Pitta* diseases
Kapha	Stable and entrenched, heavy, wet and "earthy;" endomorphic; prone to *Kapha* diseases
Vata-Pitta	Blend of *Vata/Pitta* traits
Pitta-Kapha	Blend of *Pitta/Kapha* traits
Vata-Kapha	Blend of *Vata/Kapha* traits
Sama	Balanced *Vata/Kapha/Pitta* (rare)

Malas are the waste products of digested food and drink. The four categories of *malas*, or waste products, are as follows:

- Urine, feces, and sweat
- Fatty secretions from the skin and intestines, along with earwax
- Mucus of the nose, saliva, and tears
- Hair and nails

In Ayurvedic thought, digestion is the most important function of the body. Problems with digestion are considered to be the principal cause of disease. Ayurveda defines 13 different types of *Agnis*, or enzymes.

Agnis are enzymes that assist in the digestion and assimilation of food. *Agnis* (enzymes) are found in the mouth, stomach, and gastrointestinal tract *(jatharagnis)*, the liver *(bhutagnis)*, and in the tissues *(dhatvagnis)*.

Ama is considered to be the chief cause of disease. It is formed when there is a decrease in enzyme activity, or when food and drink are digested improperly. *Ama* takes the form of a liquid sludge and travels through the blood channels, as does the nourishing "chyle" from digestion. Because of its heavy nature, *Ama* lodges in different parts of the body, obstructing the channels and causing disease. Internal disease begins with *Ama*, and external diseases create *Ama*. In TCM, *Ama* corresponds to the pathogenic factor called *Phlegm*.

The diagnosis of *Ama* is made on the basis of the following signs:

- Thick, greasy coating on the tongue
- Feces and turbid urine with a foul odor
- Feces that contain undigested food
- Feces accompanied by abundant bad-smelling flatulence

Just as there are channels, meridians, or vessels in TCM, Ayurveda has the *Srotas*. These are the subtle body channels through which certain types of energy move through the organism. *Srotas* are the energetic equivalents of physical structures such as nerves and blood vessels. This makes them responsible for the transportation of

BOX 6-2

Seasons and Times According to *Tridosha*

Vata

Season: Fall (September—November) Avoid *Vata*-promoting foods during *Vata* months

Time: 2 PM until sunset (6 PM); 2 AM until sunrise (6 AM)

Life cycle: Old age

Digestive cycle: After

Key word: Dry

Promoting foods: Dried fruit, apples, melon, potato, tomato, eggplant, ice cream, beef, peas and green salad, high-protein foods

Inhibiting foods: Sweet fruits, coconut, brown rice, red cabbage, bananas, grapes, cherries, oranges

Pitta

Season: Summer (June-August) Avoid *Pitta*-promoting foods during *Pitta* months

Time: 10 AM-2 PM; 10 PM-2 AM

Life cycle: Adulthood

Digestive cycle: During

Key word: Hot

Promoting foods: Spicy and pungent food, peanut butter, sour fruit, banana, papaya, tomato, garlic *(Allium sativum)*

Inhibiting foods: Mangoes, oranges, pears, plums, sprouts, green salad, sunflower seeds, asparagus, mushrooms

Kapha

Season: Winter (December-February) Avoid *Kapha*-promoting foods during *Kapha* months

Time: 6 AM (sunrise) until 10 AM; 6 PM (sunset) to 10 PM

Life cycle: Childhood

Digestive cycle: Before

Key word: Heavy

Promotional foods: Bananas, melons, coconuts, dates, papayas, pineapples, dairy products

Inhibiting foods: Pomegranate *(Punica granatum)*, cranberry, basmati rice, sprouts, chicken

Note: Early spring months (March–April) produce *Kapha* aggravation; thus, *Kapha*-promoting foods need to be avoided then. The later spring months (April–May) create *Pitta* aggravation.

energies through the entire body; thus, they serve an important nourishing function.

Large *Srotas* are considered to correspond to the physical form of the large and small intestines, uterus, arteries, and veins. Small *Srotas* correspond to the capillaries. Healthy bodies have open and free-flowing channels. Disease commonly occurs when overly abundant waste materials, such as the *Ama* and the *Mala* (discussed previously), clog up the *Srotas*, which are the conducting tubules or channels through which the body's energy comes and goes, thus contributing to a regional deficiency in nourishment that leads to symptoms and disease.

In addition to the physical structures associated with the *Srotas*, Ayurveda recognizes that underlying the physical body are nonphysical "subtle bodies" that are derived from higher planes of consciousness. These subtle bodies provide the energetic warp and woof that allows matter to be organized on the physical plane. The *Srotas* provide channels for the movement of energy and fluid through the Physical Body. In the Vital Body, *Prana* moves through subtle channels and nodes called *Nadis* and *Chakras*, respectively. The *Pranic* body affects the physical body by influencing the *Srotas*, which flow synchronously with the *Nadis*.

The *Chakras* are located along the most important *Nadis*—the *Sushumna*, or Central Conduit. The Central Conduit is located in the same physical location as the central sulcus of the spinal cord. Because the spinal cord and the *Sushumna* exist on different planes, they can occupy the same physical space simultaneously.

According to Ayurvedic thought, the three categories of disease include the following (Zysk, 1996):

- Diseases that originate within the body (hereditary, congenital, and *Dosha*-related or constitutional)
- Diseases that originate outside the body (trauma and external pathogens such as bacteria and viruses)
- Diseases that originate from "supernatural" sources (seasons, planetary influences, curses, and acts of God)

AYURVEDIC DIAGNOSTIC PRACTICES

Ayurveda has a well-established system of diagnosis, similar in some respects to TCM. An initial examination is made using visual observation, palpation, and questioning. The detailed examination determines the patient's physical constitution type and mental status. The diagnostician tries to discover any indications of imbalances or abnormalities in the patient. Susruta (cited in Frawley, 1988) writes as follows:

> ". . . the physician should interrogate the patient about his complaints in detail. He should use the five senses of sight, touch, hearing, smell, and taste, in addition to his verbal inquiry."

Some Ayurvedic physical diagnostic tests are not common to Western medical practice. Tongue diagnosis and pulse diagnosis are two unique diagnostic tools that a Western practitioner can readily learn and use clinically to add new perspectives that can enhance the patient's understanding of his or her condition.

Ayurvedic tongue diagnosis is based on observation of the geographic location on the tongue of superficial color and surface coatings. The different locations, colors, and surface coatings have specific diagnostic interpretations. The tongue that shows *Vata* aggravation is dry, rough, and cracked. *Pitta* aggravation shows up as red and hot and is associated with a burning sensation in the mouth. *Kapha* aggravation tongues are wet, slimy, and coated.

Pulses are considered to provide important information to assist the clinician in his or her quest to understand the patient and gain control over disease. Pulse taking makes use of the physical interaction of physician and patient. For the veterinarian, whose patient does not speak of the condition, pulse taking can provide another dimension for gaining insight into the animal and its condition.

Pulse diagnosis is used by most Ayurvedic practitioners. It was introduced as an Ayurvedic diagnostic around the 9th century AD. For the Ayurvedic pulse, the hands are positioned similarly to TCM positioning. In dogs and cats, the femoral artery is palpated. The radial artery of the right hand is palpated for human males, and the left hand is palpated for females. In Ayurvedic tradition, palpation of a pulse wave at the index finger that feels like a snake indicates *Vata*. If the pulse feels like a frog at the middle finger, this indicates *Pitta*. If the pulse wave at the ring finger feels like the movement of a swan or a peacock, then the predominant dosha is *Kapha*. In other words, pulse quality variation can help the clinician to determine constitution. In a similar way, femoral pulse variation in animals can be useful to a skilled Ayurvedic practitioner for determining constitutional pathology (Table 6-3).

Additional diagnostic parameters are gathered by the practitioner through detailed observations of the patient and examination of the urine. Observations of the patient's demeanor in the examination room helps with the practitioner's diagnosis. Consideration is given to patient body type, ambulation—both in and out of the examination room—and the appearance of patient skin, haircoat, pads, nails, and hooves. Also of importance to a thorough diagnosis is the nature, quantity, and quality of vocalizations. Urine examination involves the free-catch collection of the first urine mid stream in a clear glass jar. After sunrise, the urine is examined for color and degree of transparency (Box 6-3).

After visual inspection, a few drops of sesame oil are placed in the urine and examined in the sunlight. Shape, movement, and diffusion of the oil in the urine are prognosticators. The drops will form different shapes, giving an indication of which *Doshas* are involved. Visual examination of various parts of the body aid the Ayurvedic veterinarian in diagnosis. Tongue, skin, nails, and other physical features point out which *Doshas* are most involved in the patient's diagnosis. The physical condition of the body can be related to the *Tridosha* (Box 6-4).

Three types of prognoses are recognized in Ayurvedic medicine:

1. Easily curable
2. Palliative
3. Incurable/Difficult to cure

If the disease-type and patient constitution are different, it is easy to cure the disease, but if the disease type and patient constitution are the same, the disease is difficult to cure.

The ability to cure a patient is also dependent on the season in which he or she is being treated. Thus, if the disease, constitution, and season correspond to the same *Dosha*, then the disease is nearly impossible to cure (Zysk, 1996). Treatment in Ayurveda is dependent on the *Tridosha* of the patient. The patient's constitution is taken into account, and therapy is directed toward balancing the excesses (reducing excess first, then supporting deficiency). This balance is achieved through a combination of dietary therapy, lifestyle alterations, detoxification, and herbal therapies.

BOX 6-3

Urine Diagnosis According to the *Tridosha*

DOSHAS	COLOR	TRANSPARENCY	SHAPES
Vata	Pale-yellow	Oily	Snakelike
Pitta	Intense yellow, reddish, or blue		Umbrella
Kapha	White	Foamy and muddy	Pearl shaped

BOX 6-4

***Tridosha* Diagnosis Based on Physical Characteristics**

TRIDOSHA	PHYSICAL CONDITION OF THE BODY
Vata	Coldness, dryness, roughness, and cracking
Pitta	Hotness and redness
Kapha	Wetness, whiteness, and coldness

TABLE 6-3

Guide To Ayurvedic Pulses

Dosha	Pulse Description	Pulse Sensation	Tongue
Vata	@ index finger, feels like a snake	Motion is irregular or zigzagging	Dry, rough, and cracked
Pitta	@ middle finger, feels like a frog	Has a jumping motion	Red and hot, associated with a burning sensation in the mouth
Kapha	@ ring finger, feels like a swan or peacock	Movement is slow	Wet, slimy, and coated

PRINCIPLES OF AYURVEDIC HERBAL THERAPY

Ayurveda is a "holographic" and "holistic" system (Svoboda, 1995). It is stated in the *Charaka Samhita* that

> "Everything that exists in the vast external universe also appears in the internal cosmos of the body, the microcosm, in altered form."

One example of this correspondence of macrocosm to microcosm is the relationship between the Five Elements of Ayurveda and the five parts of a plant. The root is equal to the element, Earth; the stem and branches correspond to the element, Water; the plant's flowers are considered to contain the Fire element; the leaves correspond to the element of Air; the fruit is the element of Ether; and the seed contains all five elements.

This macrocosm/microcosm relationship can also be seen in the way that plants are categorized in Ayurveda according to the seven bodily tissues *(Dhatus)*. A correspondence is noted between the tissues of the Plant Kingdom and the tissues of the Animal Kingdom. In Box 6-5, the plant tissue is listed to the right of the animal tissue it is associated with. The tissues of plants have activity on the tissues of the mammalian body to which they correspond. Of all plants, the tree is considered to be the ultimate expression of the Plant Kingdom, in the same way that the human being is considered to be the ultimate expression of the Animal Kingdom (Frawley, 1988).

Each part of the plant is chosen for its medicinal appropriateness, taking into account its characteristics with respect to the following four qualities:

1. Five Elements
2. Taste
3. Temperature
4. *Tridosha*

Ayurvedic Plant Properties

Plant properties are defined by Ayurveda according to their energetics. These energetics are determined by the herb's taste, heating or cooling nature, postdigestion effects, and special potency effect on target organs. From these selection criteria, the individualized herbal remedy is chosen to match or balance the Ayurvedic diagnosis that reflects the characteristics specific to the Ayurvedic patient (Sodhi, 2003).

Taste (rasa)

Six primary tastes have been described: Sweet, Sour, Salty, Pungent (AKA Acrid), Bitter, and Astringent. The taste of an herb directly affects the nervous system; this begins the first process of digestion performed by the salivary glands.

Energy (virya)

Energy defines the heating or cooling nature of an herb. Hot herbs create thirst, fatigue, sweating, a burning sensation, and dizziness. Cool herbs refresh, calm, and promote tissue balance.

Postdigestion effect (vipaka)

Following digestion, the six herbal tastes are transformed into three postdigestion tastes: Sweet, Sour, and Pungent. Sweet remains sweet. Salty becomes sour. Sour remains sour. Pungent, bitter, and astringent become pungent following digestion. The Sweet taste is associated with the mouth and stomach. The Stomach is also associated with the taste sour, as is the small intestine. The large intestine is associated with the taste, pungent.

Special potency (prabhava)

Herbs have unique, subtle, and more specific qualities.

BOX 6-5

Animal–Plant Tissue Correspondence

ANIMAL TISSUE	PLANT TISSUE
Plasma	Juice of leaf
Blood	Resin, sap
Muscle	Softwood
Fat	Gum, hard sap
Bone	Bark
Marrow and nerve tissue	Leaf
Reproductive tissue	Flowers and fruit

Ayurvedic Herbs Grouped by Therapeutic Category

The herbs of Ayurveda are organized in a number of ways. Categorizing the herbs according to their taste, temperature, and other energetic qualities, including the herb's relationship to the *Tridosha*, has been discussed previously. Perhaps the most useful way to categorize herbs is to do so according to their therapeutic impact on the patient. Grouping herbs in this fashion allows the practitioner to choose herbs that are most pertinent when he or she is addressing a patient's medical condition.

The following therapeutic categories are common to all ethnomedical systems of herbal medicine. Examples of Ayurvedic herbs are provided in each category (Sodhi, 2003).

Alterative

Herbal detoxifiers and blood "cleansers," with anti-infective properties. Antipyretic in nature, these herbs cool the blood and reduce *Pitta*. Diseases addressed by this group of herbs include fever, sore throat, otitis, acne, dermatitis, and, in some cases, cancer. *Aloe vera (Aloe barbadensis)*, neem *(Azadirachta indica)*, and sandalwood *(Santalum album)* are examples.

Anthelmintic

Pungent or bitter-tasting herbs help to eliminate parasites, bacteria, fungus, virus, and yeast.

Ajwain *(Trachyspermum ammi)*, cloves *(Syzygium caryophyllata)*, garlic *(Allium sativum)*, pomegranate *(Punica granatum)*, pumpkin seeds are examples.

Astringent
Tissue-firming, condensing, compacting action on the body. Arrests excessive discharge and secretions. Uses include alleviating diarrhea and bleeding.

Nutmeg *(Myristica fragrans)*, saffron, turmeric *(Curcuma longa)*, ginger *(Zingiber officinale)*, haritaki *(Terminalia chebula)*, amla *(Phyllanthus emblica)* and Bibhitaki (AKA Bahera, *Terminalia belerica*) are examples.

Bitter tonic and antipyretic
Prescribed in moderation, the bitter nature of these herbs can suppress digestion and reduce the assimilation of digesta. Bitter herbs are used in purification, sedation, and heat-dispelling and heat-reducing therapies.

Chirata *(Swertia chirata)*, kutki *(Picrorrhiza kurroa)*, neem *(Azadirachta indica)*, *Aloe vera (Aloe barbadensis)*, and gentian *(Gentiana kuroo)* are examples.

Carminative
Dispel flatulence, pain, and bloating, promoting normal gastrointestinal peristaltic function. Aromatic herbs such as spices belong to this category.

Ajwain *(Trachyspermum ammi)*, asafetida *(Ferula foetida)*, basil *(Ocimum sanctum)*, bay leaves, cardamom *(Elettaria cardamomum)*, cinnamon *(Cinnamomum zeylanicum)*, cloves *(Syzygium caryophyllata)*, garlic *(Allium sativum)*, nutmeg *(Myristica fragrans)*, turmeric *(Curcuma longa)*, coriander *(Coriandrum sativum)*, cumin *(Cuminum cyminum)*, and fennel *(Foeniculum vulgare)* are examples.

Diaphoretic
Stimulate perspiration, improve circulation, and dispel fevers and chills as part of their function in removing toxins.

Cool herbs include coriander *(Coriandrum sativum)*, spearmint, peppermint, and chamomile

Hot herbs include basil *(Ocimum sanctum)*, camphor, cardamom *(Elettaria cardamomum)*, cinnamon *(Cinnamomum zeylanicum)*, cloves *(Syzygium caryophyllata)*, ginger *(Zingiber officinalis)*, and eucalyptus *(Eucalyptus globulus)*.

Diuretic
Increase urine production through direct effects on the kidney and urinary bladder.

Barley, buchu, coriander *(Coriandrum sativum)*, fennel *(Foeniculum vulgare)*, Gokshura *(Tribulus terrestris)*, punarva *(Boerhaavia diffusa)*, uva ursi, and Ajwain *(Trachyspermum ammi)* are examples.

Emmenagogue
Promote and regulate menstruation in women.

Aloe vera *(Aloe barbadensis)*, cotton root and seed *(Gossypium herbaceum)*, licorice *(Glycyrrhiza glabra)*, Shatavari *(Asparagus racemosus)*, and saffron are examples.

Expectorant and demulcent
Promote the elimination of phlegm and mucus from the body. Indirectly, clear lungs and nasal passages and soothe the gastrointestinal tract.

Ginger *(Zingiber officinale)*, licorice *(Glycyrrhiza glabra)*, calamus *(Acorus calamus)*, cardamom *(Elettaria cardamomum)*, cinnamon *(Cinnamomum zeylanicum)*, cloves *(Syzygium caryophyllata)*, pipali *(Piper longum)*, and eucalyptus *(Eucalyptus globulus)* are examples.

Laxative and purgative
Relieve constipation and promote bowel movements, thus eliminating *Mala* or waste products and promoting health.

Castor seed oil *(Ricinus communis)*, bran, senna *(Cassia italica)*, *Aloe vera (Aloe barbadensis)*, flaxseed *(Linum usitatissimum)*, ghee (clarified butter), licorice *(Glycyrrhiza glabra)*, prunes, psyllium seed *(Plantago ovata)*, warm milk, Trifal, Haritaki *(Terminalia chebula)*, Bahera (AKA Bibhitaki; *Terminalia bellerica*), and Ambla *(Emblica officinalis;* AKA amla *[Phyllanthus emblica])* are examples.

Nervine and antispasmodic
Promote improved nervous system function by sedation or by stimulation.

Ashwagandha *(Withania somnifera)*, licorice *(Glycyrrhiza glabra)*, Gotu Kola *(Centella asiatica)*, Guggul *(Commiphora mukul)*, valerian *(Valeriana officinale)*, and sandalwood (*Santalum album*) are examples.

Stimulent and digestive
Promote energy, activity, and digestive process. Hot in energy, pungent in taste.

Spices, ginger *(Zingiber officinale)*, garlic *(Allium sativum)*, Ajwain *(Trachyspermum ammi)*, asafetida *(Ferula foetida)*, black pepper *(Piper nigrum)*, cloves *(Syzygium caryophyllata)*, and onion *(Allium cepa)* are examples.

Nutritive tonics
Nourish the tissues of the body and increase weight and bone density.

Almonds, Amla *(Emblica officinalis;* AKA *Phyllanthus emblica)*, coconut, dates, honey, licorice *(Glycyrrhiza glabra)*, milk, sesame seeds *(Sesamum indicum)*, and Shatavari *(Asparagus racemosus)* are examples.

Rejuvenating tonics (single herbs)
Rejuvenate mind and body and reverse aging process (Box 6-6).

BOX 6-6

Tonic Herbs for the *Tridosha*

Vata tonic:	Ashwagandha *(Withania somnifera)*, garlic *(Allium sativum)*, Guggul *(Commiphora mukul)*, and Haritaki *(Terminalia chebula)*
Pitta tonic:	Amla *(Emblica officinalis)*, Gotu Kola *(Centella asiatica)*, saffron, and Shatavari *(Asparagus racemosus)*
Kapha tonic:	Bibhitaki, AKA Bahera *(Terminalia bellerica)*, Guggul *(Commiphora mukul)*, and Pipali *(Piper longum)*

Rejuvenating rasayanic tonics (special combination formulas)

Special combinations of herbs that have been used for hundreds of years for the purposes of rejuvenation and improved vitality. Ayurvedic practitioners recommend that after 40 years of age in humans, and the corresponding age of entry into the years of "middle age" for animals, that some or all of these formulas be taken on a regular basis to improve overall health and well-being. Rasayana tonics, for best results, must be ingested over long periods. Rasayana herbal therapy is considered to be very safe, both at elevated dosages and for very long periods of time.

Ashwagandha *(Withania somnifera)*, although a single herb, is considered a powerful Rasayana therapy. Most Rasayana herbal therapies consist of special combinations of herbs.

Trifala is considered to be a Rasayanic tonic herb combination for Rasayanic therapy. Trifala is made up of three herbs: *Emblica officinalis* (AKA *Phyllanthus emblica* [Amla]), *Terminalia ballerica* (Bahera; AKA Bibhitaki), and *Terminalia chebula* (Haritaki).

Shilajeet, another Rasayana herbal therapy, is derived from organic, bituminous exudates found under rock formations that are located in the northwestern Himalayas. It is specifically applied to genitourinary infections, diabetes, bronchial asthma, and stomach problems.

Chavanprash is a complex herbal paste that consists of clarified butter (ghee), honey, and approximately 40 different herbs, including Amla; it is processed specially to produce this paste, which is used as a condiment or spread on bread or other foods.

Aphrodisiac

These herbs rejuvenate both male and female reproductive organs, in terms of sexual or reproductive function.

PRINCIPLES UNDERLYING AYURVEDIC HERBAL MEDICINALS

It is uncommon for a practitioner of Ayurvedic medicine to use a single, individual herb as the herbal therapy for a patient. These are called "singulars" or singles. More commonly, the practitioner will formulate a complex medicinal that will include a variety of herbs, minerals, and trace metals, in specific proportions and processed in specific ways so as to create a "whole" that is greater than its parts—more potent, more biologically active, and less likely to produce adverse effects than any of the individual herbs involved.

Each formulation has a unique character, whose activity may be quite different than the activity of its ingredients. A few formulations have been in use for thousands of years that serve as examples of this. For instance, Triphala (AKA Trifala, Trifal) is one of these ancient combination formulas that has taken on a life of its own. It consists of three fruits that in combination have properties far different than each of its constituents.

These fruits include *Terminalia chebula* (Haritaki), *Terminalia bellerica* (Bahera), and *Phyllanthus emblica* (AKA *Emblica officinalis* [Amla]). This formula is an alterative, adaptogenic rejuvenating compound. It has digestive benefits and provides some laxative and diuretic activity. This herb also has found uses as a topical solution for wound care and burns. Trifala can be used to treat patients with clinical conditions such as indigestion, carbohydrate intolerance, anemia, diabetes, chronic lung conditions, hypertension, hypercholesterolemia, skin disorders, conditions of the eye, and yeast infections.

The three herbs have effects on each other, thus increasing each of their individual potencies by virtue of their unique interaction. Herb-to-herb interactions make up the foundation of Ayurvedic herbal prescriptions. *Synergism* is one such interaction. *Opposition* occurs when ingredients in the formulation have opposite effects on each other. Often, this principle is used to create increased balance in a formula or to reduce potential adverse effects. Laxative or diuretic herbs can be added in small amounts to a formula so as to reduce the possibility of toxin buildup. This is called *protection*.

Circulatory-stimulating herbs, added in small amounts to a formulation, can improve that formulation's absorption and bioavailability. Ginger, for instance, in addition to improving a formula's absorption, speeds up the circulation so as to distribute that formula's ingredients to the body that much more quickly. Ginger also serves as a digestive aid, protecting the stomach from irritation. In this capacity, ginger provides the formulation with *enhancement* (Sodhi, 2003).

AYURVEDIC HERBS COMMON TO WESTERN CULTURES

Ayurveda, as a 5000-year-old system of healing, has influenced the development of many other systems of healing. As was discussed earlier in this chapter, the Egyptians, Greeks, and Romans all traveled to India to bring back indigenous medicinal and herbal therapies. Over thousands of years, many of these herbs have inserted themselves into common usage in both our Western culture and the Traditional Medicine of China and East Asia. Many of these herbs can now be found in the kitchen and on the spice rack, as well as in our herbal pharmacies (Table 6-4).

THE PRACTICE OF AYURVEDIC VETERINARY MEDICINE

Adapting the principles of Ayurveda to a conventional veterinary practice begins with understanding the following four Ayurvedic axioms:

1. The natural state of the individual is to be healthy.
2. Disease can be prevented at its premanifestation stage by maintaining and modifying the balance of the *Tridosha* in a seemingly healthy individual.
3. The root cause of disease is a lowering of the internal fire *(Agni)* of digestion, which is considered to be a deficiency of the enzyme systems that drive a healthy digestive process.
4. The body possesses an innate ability to heal itself (Barnett, 1996).

Thus, the Ayurvedic veterinary practitioner regards the diet and digestive system as central to the healing

TABLE 6-4

Some Effective Ayurvedic Herbs That Are Commonly Found in Our Kitchens (Williamson, 2002)

Common Name	Botanical Name	Ayurvedic Name	Common Clinical Applications
Garlic	*Allium sativum*	*Lasan*	General tonic, addresses conditions of the digestive, respiratory, nervous, reproductive, and circulatory systems.
Turmeric	*Curcuma longa*	*Haldi*	General tonic and blood purifier, anti-inflammatory agent, analgesia in arthritis and rheumatism and for the common cold. It finds a particular use in diseases of the liver such as jaundice, and as a cholegogue; it has also been used as an anodyne, antimalarial, antiepileptic, aperitif, carminative, diuretic, and vermifuge. Topical use for insect bites and wounds as an antiseptic.
Sweet Basil	*Ocimimum sanctum*	*Tulsi*	Demulcent, diaphoretic, expectorant for bronchitis, insecticide, anthelmintic, laxative, stimulant, anti-inflammatory cardiotonic, and blood purifier
Black Pepper	*Piper nigrum*	*Golmirch, kalmirch*	Stomach and digestive complaints, colds, bronchitis. Other uses include for neuralgia, and scabies. Topical use as an anodyne for pain due to cold and neuralgia, for hemorrhoids and dermatologic disorders.
Pomegranate	*Punica granatum*	*Anar, Dadim*	Bark, root, and fruit are put to ethnoveterinary use for intestinal worms in poultry and ruminants. Fruit and leaves are used to treat eye diseases in swine and ruminants. Leaves and stem are used for diarrhea in swine.
Fenugreek	*Trigonella foenum-graecum*	*Methi*	Topically, as a poultice, relieves swelling, treats burns, and on hair follicles, prevents premature graying of the hair. Internally, the seeds increase lactation, the leaves are good for indigestion and disorders of the gallbladder. A decoction of the herb is used for leukorrhea and addresses hyperglycemia; thus finds its way into formulas for diabetes.
Ginger Root	*Zingiber officinale*	*Adrak* (fresh), *Sonth* (dried)	Rheumatism, inflammation; diuretic, carminative, aphrodisiac.

process for patients with disease, and as essential for those patients in whom the establishment of "Wellness" is a priority.

The Ayurvedic veterinary practitioner establishes an Ayurvedic diagnosis, generally through observation and history, and thus defines the nature of the disease problem. Then, the practitioner recommends specific dietary therapies, perhaps with the addition of digestive enzymes or raw foods, along with the inclusion of active, beneficial, probiotic bacterial cultures in the patient's diet.

Herbal therapies are used that address the biomedical definition of the patient's disease(s) and that help to balance the animal's *Tridosha*.

Ayurvedic veterinary medicine is not as complex as Ayurvedic human medicine because of of our more limited understanding of domestic animal disease, compared to human medical conditions. Thus, some elements of Ayurvedic medicine that address spirituality, higher thought, and meditation, as well as some of the Panchakarma therapies of purgation, are not as readily applied or used in the practice of Ayurvedic medicine with veterinary patients.

It is not uncommon for Ayurvedic herbal therapies to be used in a simple fashion with domestic animals. Use of an herb for its historically or scientifically derived application in a specific, biomedically defined medical condition is common to the practice of Ayurvedic veterinary medicine.

In this sense then, the non-Ayurvedic practitioner of veterinary medicine can use these herbs as therapeutic modalities without being specifically cognizant of the principles and practices of Ayurvedic medicine or the specific Ayurvedic techniques of diagnosis and therapy.

AYURVEDIC THERAPEUTIC PROTOCOLS FOR VETERINARY PRACTICE*

*Protocols and Dosages, courtesy Dr T. Sodhi (a founder of Ayush Herbs, Redmond, WA), are for dried, powdered herbs. See Chapter 24, under individual herb monographs, for alternative dosing recommendations.

Anemia

(Sodhi, 2003)

Causes: Chronic renal failure, feline leukemia, myelofibrosis.

Therapy: Withania somnifera (Ashwagandha). 100 mg/kg BID (can administer up to 4-6 times the recommended dosage for greater effectiveness without toxicity).

Immune-mediated hemolytic anemia (IMHA)
Therapy: Trifala and Ashwagandha (can administer up to 4-6 times the recommended dosage [100 mg/kg BID] of each or combined 50:50).*

*Traditional herbal digestive combination consisting of *Terminalia chebula*, *Terminalia bellerica*, and *Emblica officinalis*.

Allergic Bronchitis and Feline Asthma

(Sodhi, 2003)
Therapy: Tylophora (Tylophora indica), Trifala, and Ashwagandha (*Withania somnifera*).
Dosage: 100 mg/kg BID of a 33:33:33.combination formula.

Autoimmune Conditions

(Sodhi, 2003)
Therapy: Ashwagandha *(Withania somnifera)*, Trifala, a proprietary liver formula:* (*Andrographis paniculata, Berberis aristata, Boerhaavia diffusa, Calotropis gigantea, Eclipta alba, Picrorrhiza kurroa, Solanum nigrum, Swertia chirata, Tephrosia purpurea, Raphanus sativa, Terminalia arjuna, Belleric myrobalan, Terminalia chebula, Emblicus officinalis*), cease vaccinations; home-cooked diet, digestive enzymes, and stress reduction. Immunocompromised animals may need to receive Ashwagandha, liver support, and digestive enzymes for their entire lives.

*Livit-2™, Ayush Herbs.

Herbs for Healthy Immune Function

(Anjaria, 2002)
Allium sativum
Curcuma longa
Ocimum sanctum
Phyllanthus emblica
Solanum nigrum
Terminalia chebula
Tinospora cordifolia
Tribulus terrestris
Withania somnifera

Cognitive Dysfunction and Geriatrics

(Sodhi, 2003)
Therapy: Ashwagandha *(Withania somnifera)* and *Bacopa monniera*.

Dermatologic Conditions

(Sodhi, 2003)
Therapy: Neem *(Azadirachta indica)* leaf tea topical soaks, neem oil topically to ears, neem orally. For inflammatory skin lesions, I use a proprietary *Boswellia* formulation* (Boswellia, ginger, Ashwagandha, turmeric, glucosamine sulfate, chrondroitin sulfate); for chronic mite infestations or dermatophytosis, use Ashwagandha and Trifala, in addition to neem, internally, combined with supportive herbs in a proprietary formula.† These supportive herbs are *Phyllanthus emblica, Terminalia bellerica, Terminalia chebula, Tinospora cordifolia*, and *Rubia cordifolia*. Neem can also be used topically, and traditionally, this use was more common than internal use. Dietary changes, including the addition of omega-3 and omega-6 fatty acids to meals, home-made hypoallergenic diets, and oatmeal baths, are used for resistant atopic individuals.

*Boswellia Plus™, Ayush Herbs.
†Neem Plus™, Ayush Herbs.

Herbs for Skin and Hair

(Anjaria, 2002)
Allium sativum
Azadirachta indica
Boerhaavia diffusa
Cedrus deodara
Commiphora mukul
Curcuma longa
Ferula foetida
Phyllanthus emblica
Piper nigrum
Withania somnifera

Epilepsy

(Sodhi, 2003)
Therapy: Support liver with Livit-2™ (described under Autoimmune Conditions) and administer Ashwagandha *(Withania somnifera)* in a proprietary formula that also contains *Mucuna pruriens*, Ashwagandha, Gotu Kola, and *Valeriana officinalis**. Monitor phenobarbital and bromide levels if patient is on anticonvulsant therapy, as dosages may need to be adjusted. The dose of Livit-2™ may be adjusted as much as 2 times higher than maintenance dose, if liver enzymes are elevated.

*Mucuna Plus™, Ayush Herbs.

Giardiasis

(Sodhi, 2003)
Therapy: A proprietary digestive tonic* that contains the following herbs: *Azardirachita indica* (neem), *Embelia ribes* (vidanga), *Piper longum* (pipali), *Aegel marmelos* (bilwa), *Momordica charantia* (Karela), *Ocimum basilicum* (tulsi), *Holarrhena antidysenterica* (kutaja), and *Berberis aristata* (daruharidra); add additional *Aegle marmelos* (bilwa powder) and kutki, also known as *Picrorrhiza kurora*, to increase the formula potency against this protozoal parasite. Therapy may need to be long term, occasionally up to 6 months, depending on the condition of the animal and reexposure to pathogens.

*AP-Mag™, Ayush Herbs.

Hepatic Conditions

(Sodhi, 2003)

Therapy: Phyllanthus amarus and Livit-2™ (described previously). If ascites is present, a proprietary diuretic formula*, containing standardized extracts of *Didymocarpus pedicellata* (patharphori), *Saxifraga ligulata* (pashanbhed), *Rubia cordifolia* (manjistha), *Achyranthes aspera* (apa marga), *Tribulus terrestris* (gokhru), *Ocimum basilicum* (Tulsi), *Crataeva religiosa* (Varun), *Mimosa pudica* (lajwanti), *Dolichos biflorus* (kulthi), *Cyperus rotundus* (nagarmotha), and Shilajeet, can assist the kidneys in promoting diuresis.

*Rentone™, Ayush Herbs.

Herbs for the Liver

(Anjaria, 2002)

Allium sativum
Andrographis paniculata
Boerhaavia diffusa
Curcuma longa
Eclipta alba
Phyllanthus amarus
Solanum nigrum
Terminalia chebula
Tinospora cordifolia

Inflammatory Bowel Disease and Colitis

(Sodhi, 2003)

Therapy: Restricted diet: avoid wheat, corn, soy, and potentially allergenic proteins. Livit-2*, Boswellia Plus (both described previously) for inflammation.[†] Herbs for regulating digestive function are also used. Feeding omega-3 and omega-6 fatty acids, and adding digestive enzymes of plant origin. Trifala[‡] and deglycyrrhized licorice root *(Glycyrrhiza glabra,* AKA DGL*)* are used in patients with more severe symptoms. Rotating the diet every 3 to 4 months can also be helpful.

*Livit-2™, Ayush Herbs.
[†]Boswellia Plus™, Ayush Herbs.
[‡]Traditional digestive tonic consisting of *Terminalia chebula, Terminalia bellerica,* and *Emblica officinalis.*

Herbs for Gastrointestinal Conditions

(Anjaria, 2002)

Acacia catechu
Aegle marmelos
Andrographis paniculata
Asparagus racemosus
Holarrhena antidysenterica
Plantago ovata
Trigonella foenum-graecum
Azadirachta indica
Commiphora mukul
Ferula foetida
Ocimum sanctum
Piper nigrum
Punica granatum
Tribulus terrestris

Lower Urinary Tract Problems

(Sodhi, 2003)

Therapy: Diet modification, avoidance of stress, Ashwagandha *(Withania somnifera)* for its adaptogenic properties, and herbs such as shilajeet and *Tribulus* and others* for their direct benefit to the organs of the urinary system. Concurrent use of cranberry extract and vitamin C may improve patient response to therapy.

*Rentone™, Ayush Herbs.

Osteoarthritis

(Sodhi, 2003)

Therapy: Ashwagandha *(Withania somnifera)* combined with *Boswellia serrata* has enhanced anti-inflammatory properties to improve patient comfort. Ashwagandha also contains an anabolic plant steroid, lactone, which may help to build muscle mass secondary to disuse atrophy. Ashwagandha possesses calming properties as well, which also improve patient comfort levels. Arthritic animals sleep better, giving them a chance to reduce their stiffness and soreness. *Boswellia* has been studied, and in a variety of clinical trials, it has proved to be a potent anti-inflammatory agent.

Herbs for Musculoskeletal Conditions

(Anjaria, 2002)

Allium sativum
Asparagus racemosus
Azadirachta indica
Boswellia serrata
Commiphora mukul
Curcuma longa
Piper nigrum
Plantago ovata
Trigonella foenum-graecum
Withania somnifera
Zingiber officinale

Hypothyroid Conditions in Dogs

(Sodhi, 2003)

Therapy: Guggul, liver support* and *Phyllanthus amarus* may help patients with frankly reduced serum T_4 values. Home cooking and elimination of vaccinations are also recommended by this author. Dogs will respond over 3 to 6 months with improved haircoat and weight loss. Patients who have borderline values can benefit from this program alone. Patients with abnormal values will have an improved response when this program is used concurrently with exogenous thyroid hormone supplementation.

*Livit-2™, Ayush Herbs.

Herbs to Improve Milk Production

(Anjaria, 2002)
Leptadenia reticulata
Asparagus racemosus
Trigonella foenum-graecum

Renal Tonic Herbs

(Anjaria, 2002)
Boerhaavia diffusa
Crataeva nurvala
Tribulus terrestris

CURRENT STATUS OF AYURVEDIC VETERINARY MEDICINE

The subcontinent of India has one of the most ancient cultures in the world. In contrast, modern-day India has achieved a very high level of advanced scientific progress. As a result of the scientific technological transformation of Indian culture, the ancient healing art of Ayurveda has undergone its own transformation, guided by scientific studies and technology. In India today, there is a new type of Ayurvedic physician or veterinarian who still uses the ancient wisdom inherent in Ayurveda but integrates that wisdom into contemporary scientific understanding of the human body, and of the actions of drugs and herbal formulations.

Modern pharmaceutical companies in India now produce Ayurvedic herbal formulations that are not "*Dosha* specific" but that apply to all body types. The roots of these broad-spectrum formulations can be found described in the ancient classic texts of Ayurveda. Indian pharmaceutical research has focused on gaining an understanding the action of the herbs of Ayurveda. This research ranges from the basic pharmacognosy of the Ayurvedic herbs to publication of hospital-based, standardized clinical trials to establish scientifically the effects and effectiveness of a number of herbs and combination herbal formulations.

VETERINARY CLINICAL TRIALS AND CONTROLLED STUDIES

> "Research on traditional medicinal plants is an important facet of biomedical research. A considerable amount of literature on veterinary herbal drug research, clinical trials, pharmacology, and basic research has been generated with a view to scientifically systematize the ethnoveterinary medicinal practices and folklore claims on herbal treatments. Research efforts by the National Laboratories and Veterinary, Medical, Pharmacy, and Science Colleges in India have established detailed data regarding herbs—their effects and effectiveness and safety."
>
> (Anjaria, 2002)

Two works of the Indian Council of Medical Research have been published. One text, *Medicinal Plants of India*, volume 1, presents work on more than 310 plants; volume 2 provides data collected on another 550 species of plants. The other text, Iyengar's *Bibliography of Investigated Medicinal Plants*, covers more than 2500 medicinal plants investigated over a period of 25 years (1950-1975) and cites nearly 400 references (Anjaria, 2002).

Unfortunately, of the studies analyzed in the Iyengar text, it was found that only 1.36% ended in actual clinical trials. However, 1.95% of the research reviewed did involve animal model experimental studies (Anjaria, 2002).

One such study on the effects of nutmeg *(Myristica fragrans)*, also a common culinary spice, evaluated its effects on blood pressure, diarrhea, and pain (Grover, 2002). Nutmeg extracts were able to correct diarrhea in guinea pigs without any adverse impact on blood pressure. Another study that was a cooperative project between the University of Sydney and the Department of Pharmaceutical Studies at Andhra University, India, evaluated the impact on blood pressure of an Ayurvedic herb known for centuries for its benefit for patients with cardiac disease and hypertension. *Terminalia arjuna* is the main herb in a number of formulas directed toward improving cardiovascular function (Nammi, 2003). In this study, an alcohol extract of *Terminalia arjuna* was administered to anesthetized dogs, and hemodynamic parameters were collected. It was concluded that a peripheral mechanism of vasodilation likely aids in the reduction of blood pressure, thus confirming the traditional application for this herb in patients with cardiac disease and hypertension.

Quite a few studies have been performed to investigate the impact that a variety of Ayurvedic herbs have on patients with type 2 diabetes mellitus. One study in experimentally induced diabetic rats determined that *Embelia ribes* possesses statistically significant antihyperglycemic effects on the rats in this study when compared with nontreated controls. The authors conclude, "The results of test drug were comparable [with] glipazide (25 mg/kg, orally), a standard oral antihyperglycemic agent." This is the first pilot study to provide biochemical evidence of the potential of *E. ribes* in the treatment of patients with diabetic dyslipidemia (Bhandari, 2002).

Momordica charantia, or bitter melon—an edible vegetable—has a long history of use in the treatment of humans with diabetes in India. In this placebo-controlled study, the fresh juice of *M. charantia* was administered orally to streptozotocin (STZ)-induced diabetic rats. It was found that the juice partially reversed all diabetes-induced effects measured in this study. Treatment of STZ-induced diabetic rats with *M. charantia* juice normalized the structural abnormalities of peripheral nerves. The results of this study indicate that *M. charantia* can exert marked beneficial effects in diabetic rats; moreover, it can regulate glucose uptake into jejunal brush border vesicles and stimulate glucose uptake into skeletal muscle cells similar to the response obtained with insulin (Ahmed, 2004).

Many of the culinary spices commonly found in our kitchens have been the subject of intense investigation into their biomedically defined actions. Many spices came into usage not just for their taste, but also for their activity as antioxidants and antimicrobial agents. These spices served to preserve foods long before the advent of refrigeration. Turmeric and ginger, common spices of Asia, have been found to possess potent anti-inflammatory and antioxidant properties (Chainani-Wu, 2003).

Ayurvedic herbs are being studied for their ability to augment immune function. Asparagus *(Asparagus racemosus)*, Ashwagandha *(Withania somnifera)*, and Guduchi *(Tinospora cordifolia)* were evaluated for their ability to improve immune function in mice subjected to cyclophosphamide chemotherapy for sarcoma-producing ascites. Investigators found that treatment of ascitic sarcoma-bearing mice with a formulation of total extracts of *Withania somnifera* and *Tinospora cordifolia* (80:20) and an alkaloid-free polar fraction of *Withania somnifera* resulted in protection toward cyclophosphamide-induced bone marrow effects, and immunoprotection, as indicated by a significant increase in white cell counts and specific antibody titers (Tables 6-5 and 6-6) (Diwanay, 2004).

TABLE 6-5

Twenty-six of the Most Investigated Ayurvedic Herbs

Botanical Name and Part Used	Selected Constituents	Principle Actions and Uses
Abrus precatorius; seeds and roots	Steroidal fraction (oil)	Antifertility
Acorus calamus; rhizomes	A and B-arasone	Tranquilizing, antitubercular
Allium sativum; bulbs	Allin essential oil	Cholesterol lowering; antibacterial; antidiabetic; anti-inflammatory
Azadirachta indica: stem, bark, leaves	Sodium nimbidinate; nimbidin; nimbidol; azadirachtin	Antibacterial; antitubercular; antiviral; antifungal; antihelmintic; insecticidal; diuretic
Boerhaavia diffusa; roots	Punarnavine	Anti-inflammatory
Boswellia serrata; gum, resin	Boswellic acids, beta sitosterol	Anti-inflammatory; spares gastrointestinal system; synergistic with glucosamine; indicated for inflammatory bowel disease and colitis, as well as pruritic skin disease and asthma
Centella asiatica; whole plant	Brahmosides, glycosides (asiaticoside), alkaloids (hydrocotyline), valerine, beta-sitosterol, ascorbic acid	Tranquilizing; anabolic; promotes wound healing
Plectranthus barbatus, formerly Coleus forskohlii	Forskolin (diterpenoid compound)	Addresses cardiac output; reduces intraocular pressure; asthma, antihistaminic properties; increases thyroid hormone production; atopic dermatitis; K9 dose = 100 mg BID
Commiphora mukul; gum resin	An unidentified crystalline steroidal compound	Anti-inflammatory; antirheumatic
Curcuma longa; rhizome	Curcumin sodium; curcuminate	Anti-inflammatory; antiarthritic
Emblica officinalis; Phyllanthus emblica; seeds	Phyllembin; ascorbic acid	Anabolic; antibacterial; resistance building
Glycyrrhiza glabra; peeled root	Glycyrrhizin; glycyrrhetic acid	Anti-inflammatory; antiarthritic; antipyretic
Gymnema sylvestris	Gymnemic acid	Antidiabetic
Holarrhena antidysenterica; seeds, bark	Alkaloids: conamine, conkurchine; conessimine, conessine, etc.	Antidiarrheal; antidysenteric; antiamebic; antibacterial
Momordica charantia; fruits	Charantin	Antidiabetic
Nardostachys jatamansi; roots	Valeranone (jatamansone)	Tranquilizing; antihypertensive; antiarrhythmic
Picrorrhiza kurroa; roots	Picrorrhizin; kutkin	Choleretic; antihepatotoxic; antibacterial; cure for jaundice
Psoralea carylifolia; seeds	Psoralen; isopsoralen	Useful in leukoderma; antibacterial; antihelmintic
Pterocarpus marsupium; heartwood	Pterostilbene	Antidiabetic
Syzygium cumini; Eugenia jambolana; seeds	Jamboline	Antidiabetic
Tribulus terrestris; fruits	Tribuloside potassium	Diuretic
Tylophora asthmatica; Tylphora indica; stem	Tylophorine; tylophorinine	Antiasthma; anticancer

Continued

TABLE 6-5

Twenty-six of the Most Investigated Ayurvedic Herbs—cont'd

Botanical Name and Part Used	Selected Constituents	Principle Actions and Uses
Vinca rosa; whole plant	Vinblastine; reserpine	Anticancer; antihypertensive; antibacterial; antidiabetic
Withania ashwagandha; *Withania somnifera*; roots	Withaferin-A, etc.	Tranquilizing; cardiotonic; antibacterial; antifungal; anticancer; antiarthritic
Zingiber officinale	Gingerols, shogaols zingerone, zingiberone, etc.	Antiemetic; anti-inflammatory; hepatoprotective; inhibits platelet-activating factor (PAF); antipyretic; antioxidant; immunomodulatory; thermogenic; antiviral; nematodicidal; insect repellent; molluscicidal activity

(Anjaria, 2002)

TABLE 6-6

Quick Guide to the Most Commonly Used Ayurvedic Herbs in Veterinary Practice

Botanical and Common Names	Ayurvedic Name	Actions and Applications
Achyranthes aspera Chaff-flower	Apamarg	Young leaves steamed and eaten like spinach. Potassium rich. Traditional uses include diuretic, lithotriptic
Aegle marmelos Bael or Bael fruit	Bilva	Clinically proven to address amebic dysentery and chronic diarrhea, and to improve digestive activity and appetite
Allium sativum Garlic	Lahsan	One of the most studied herbs in the world, garlic has many benefits: It improves digestive, respiratory, nervous, cardiovascular, and reproduction function. Indications include colds, coughs, asthma, heart disease and hypertension, arrhythmias, dermatitis, and rheumatism
Aloe barbadensis *Aloe vera*	Kumari	Gel and thickened leaves are used. Tonic to renew female nature Indicated for fever, constipation, obesity, inflammatory skin conditions, swollen glands, conjunctivitis, bursitis, jaundice, hepatitis, splenomegaly, hepatomegaly, and intestinal helminthiasis
Andrographis paniculata Green chiretta; Creat	Kalmegh	Liver tonic, heart tonic. Positive cardiac ionotrope, alterative, anthelmintic, febrifuge, anti-inflammatory. Antineoplastic benefits have been documented
Asparagus racemosus Asparagus (wild); Sparrow-grass	Shatavari	Roots promote lactation and are used for their demulcent, diuretic, aphrodisiac, tonic, alterative, antiseptic, and antidiarrheal properties. Used to treat debility, infertility, impotence, and reduced libido in women, menopause, stomach ulcers, hyperacidity, dehydration, lung abscesses, hematemesis, cough, herpes, leucorrhea, and chronic fevers
Azadirachta indica Chinaberry; Neem tree; Margosa	Neem or Nimba	An evergreen tree, Neem is considered to be one of the most important herbal detoxicants in Ayurvedic medicine. Most of the tree is used: leaf, root, seed, root bark, gum, fruits, flowers, stems, and oil. Ethnoveterinary uses vary, depending on which part of the tree is used. *Bark:* Vomiting, burning sensation near the heart, fatigue, fever, thirst, bad taste in the mouth, cough, ulcers, inflammations, leprosy, blood disorders, urinary discharges; can also cause loss of appetite. In poultry, the bark is used to address wounds, diarrhea, ticks, and lice, and as an insect repellent. *Leaf:* Eye disorders, biliousness, skin diseases, inflammation, earache, rheumatism, boils, blood impurities. Also used to treat abscesses and commonly applied after castration. Leaves have also been found to be useful for bleeding, udder infections, fever, foot rot, and lice in ruminants. Also serve as an insect repellent. Neem leaves are commonly placed in bags of grain to ward off insect infestations. *Decoction of leaf:* As a gargle in stomatitis and for gingival and periodontal disease

TABLE 6-6

Quick Guide to the Most Commonly Used Ayurvedic Herbs in Veterinary Practice—cont'd

Botanical and Common Names	Ayurvedic Name	Actions and Applications
Azadirachta indica, Continued	Neem, *Continued*	*Tender young leaves:* Eye and skin diseases, leprosy *Old leaves:* Help cure ulcers rapidly *Young branches:* Cough, asthma, hemorrhoids, tumors, urinary discharges *Ripe and unripe fruits:* Urinary discharges, skin diseases, tumors, hemorrhoids, toothache *Seeds:* In ruminants, used for ticks and as an insect repellent in all species *Oil of the seed:* Used to treat skin disorders topically *All of the plant parts share the following applications:* Helminthiasis, oral wounds, glossitis, *Escherichia coli* bacillosis, hepatomegaly, jaundice, hemorrhagic dysentery, and intestinal wounds; constipation, indigestion, respiratory and throat disorders; asthma, pleuropneumonia, and swelling of the mucous membranes in the lungs and respiratory tract. Common skin disorders such as dermatophytosis, alopecia, eczema, urticaria, and scabies are also addressed by all the parts of the tree. Miscellaneous indications for Neem include metritis, tetanus, stranguria, swelling of the kidney, mastitis, otitis, ear abscesses, rinderpest, and rheumatism. ***Therapeutic Actions of Neem*** *Medicinal and Pharmacologic Activities, General Attributes* • Antifungal • Antibacterial • Antiviral • Antidiabetic • Antimalarial • Antipyretic • Antiulcer • Anxiolytic • Hepatoprotective • Hypoglycemic activity • Anti-inflammatory • Immunomodulatory • Antitumor • Antiifertility • Insecticidal activity: This is the main attribute for which Neem is known. Seed extracts have been found to disrupt the growth and development of tobacco caterpillar larvae and of *Spodoptera litura*. The leaf was measured to have the second highest activity after seed extracts. Other insecticidal effects include alteration of insect ovarian function and blockage of insect ecdysis and maturation. ***Specific Attributes of Plant Parts*** *Bark:* Tonic; Refrigerant, Anthelmintic *Leaf:* Carminative, Expectorant, Anthelmintic, Insecticidal *Young branches:* Anthelmintic *Flowers:* Stimulant, Stomachic, Bitter, Anthelmintic *Ripe and Unripe Fruits:* Oily, Bitter, Hot, Purgative, Anthelmintic *Seeds:* Oil, bitter, anthelmintic. Neem is considered to be quite safe; it possesses a wide margin of safety. Moderate use is not associated with any signs of toxicity. The dose that kills 50% of the population (LD_{50}) of a 50% ethanolic extract of the stem bark was >1 g/kg body weight when given intraperitoneally in rats. Excessive dosages are associated with liver and kidney changes of laboratory animals. There are no cases on record of adverse reactions or toxicity to this herb in humans. ***Dosage*** Infusion (tea) 1-10 mL TID Powder 0.5-1 g TID Oil (most common use is topical, this dosage is for internal use): 0.05 mL-0.5 mL TID

Continued

TABLE 6-6

Quick Guide to the Most Commonly Used Ayurvedic Herbs in Veterinary Practice—cont'd

Botanical and Common Names	Ayurvedic Name	Actions and Applications
Bacopa monniera Thyme-leaved gratiola	*Brahmi*	Small, creeping herb; grows easily in damp areas. Considered a brain tonic; improves intellect, asthma, hoarseness, insanity, and, of most frequent use, epilepsy in dogs and cats. Anticonvulsant, antiviral, immunostimulant, antipyretic, antineoplastic, cardiotonic, hypotensive.
Berberis aristata or English barberry	*Daruhaldi* or *Daruharidra*	Used for febrile conditions, hepatomegaly, splenomegaly, conjunctivitis, chronic dysentery, jaundice, hepatitis, and diabetes. Hepatitis, cholecystitis, giardiasis, amebiasis, gastric ulcers.
Boerhaavia diffusa Pigweed, spreading pigweed	*Punavarna*	Beneficial effect on kidney and liver function, diuretic. Commonly used to address ascites secondary to liver disease.
Boswellia serrata Indian olibanum tree	*Salai*	Extract of resin collected from the sap of this tree has been used for centuries to address pain and inflammation. Traditional uses include rheumatism, dysentery and diarrhea, and inflammatory skin disease. Has anti-inflammatory, expectorant, and diuretic properties. Very safe; studies indicate that *Boswellia* produces none of the adverse effects commonly associated with anti-inflammatory pharmaceuticals, such as ulcers, gastritis, and adverse cardiovascular effects. Recent studies confirm its value for rheumatoid arthritis and osteoarthritis, musculoskeletal pain in general, and ulcerative colitis and Crohn's disease. Also effective for inflammatory skin diseases such as psoriasis and for bronchial asthma. Inhibits both cyclooxygenase and lipoxygenase enzyme systems, thus reducing inflammation by reducing production of proinflammatory mediators of pain. *Dosage of Powdered Herb:* *Dogs:* 10-20 mg/kg BID *Cats:* 5-10 mg/kg BID (liquid forms are available)
Calotropis gigantea Swallow wart	*Akanda*	Analgesic, anti-inflammatory, antiviral. Traditional uses include asthma, rheumatoid arthritis, leprosy, and viral hepatitis.
Centella asiatica Gotu kola; Indian pennywort	*Kula kudi* or *Mandukparni brahmi*	Improves circulation, especially in nervous tissue. Traditional uses include topically for wound healing and internally as a nervine and brain tonic; improves memory. Benefits the heart, possesses anti-inflammatory and diuretic properties as well. Other plants have also been called Brahmi *(Bacopa monnieri).*
Cinnamomum cassia or *zeylanicum;* Cinnamon	*Dalchini*	Bark of the plant improves circulation, digestive function, and respiratory function. Traditionally used for colds, sinus congestion, bronchitis, and dyspepsia.
Plectranthus barbatus, formerly Coleus forskohli		A member of the mint family, this plant is found commonly at altitudes >1000 ft and <8000 feet, growing on dry, sunny slopes. The roots and leaves are the parts most commonly used. Active principle is forskolin, which is a diterpene volatile oil. Forskolin activates cyclic adenosine monophosphate (cAMP), which regulates involuntary smooth muscle activity, inhibits platelet aggregation and mast cell degranulation, has a positive ionotropic effect on cardiac muscle, and normalizes blood pressure. One indication for *Coleus forskohlii* use is conditions of the cardiovascular system. Forskolin has been studied extensively for its ability to lower intraocular pressure in glaucoma patients. It also has antihistaminic activity and can be effective in atopic and asthmatic patients. Its platelet aggregation-inhibiting properties make it useful for patients to help prevent strokes and occlusive coronary artery disease. Studies have also shown that this herb has the ability to promote thyroid hormone production. *Dosage:* *Dogs:* 5-10 mg/kg BID *Cats:* 2.5-5 mg/kg BID

TABLE 6-6

Quick Guide to the Most Commonly Used Ayurvedic Herbs in Veterinary Practice—cont'd

Botanical and Common Names	Ayurvedic Name	Actions and Applications
Commiphora mukul; Indian bedellium Guggul; gum-guggul	*Guggul*	A resinous gum derived from the sap of a tree. Guggul addresses lipid metabolism, thyroid metabolism, and benefits digestive function. Traditional applications include rheumatoid arthritis, obesity, dermatologic conditions, and lower urinary tract disorders. Topically, guggul has been used as a gargle for gingivitis, periodontal disease, and chronic tonsillitis. Guggul has been extensively studied with respect to its hypolipidemic, cholesterol-lowering and antiatherosclerotic activities. These studies have determined that guggal's impact on lipid metabolism results from the thyroid-stimulating activity of a ketosteroid—guggulsterone—found in this resinous extract.
Coriandrum sativum Coriander	*Dhanya*	Also known as cilantro or Chinese parsley. Indications include urinary tract infection, vomiting, indigestion, sore throat, dermatitis, hay fever, and allergies. It has diuretic and carminative (relieves gastrointestinal gas) activities.
Curcuma longa Turmeric	*Haldi* or *Hardira*	This rhizome is one of the most common culinary spices in Indian cooking. A member of the ginger family of herbs, it is used both fresh and dried for medicinal and culinary purposes. Indications include as a first line of defense following trauma. It has a global effect on all tissues in the body. It may be used as an anti-inflammatory agent. Studies have shown a comparable anti-inflammatory benefit to the nonsteroidal anti-inflammatory drug phenylbutazone, with inhibitory activity of both the cyclooxygenase and lipoxygenase proinflammatory enzyme systems. It provides hepatoprotective activity and functions as a choleretic and cholegogue. Turmeric's antioxidant properties have been extensively studied, and it has been shown to reduce the adverse effects of chemotherapy. Its early use as a culinary herb stems from this herb's antimicrobial activity, which aided in food preservation during a period of history that did not possess refrigeration. *Dosage of dried herb:* *Dogs:* $^1/_2$-1 tsp BID *Cats:* $^1/_4$ tsp BID *Curcuminoids (nutraceutical derivative of turmeric):* *Dogs:* 5-10 mg/kg BID *Cats:* 2.5-5 mg/kg BID
Cyperus rotundus Cyperus	*Motha* or *Mustaka*	The dried tuberous root is fragrant, and the essential oil derived from it is used in perfumes. The roots possess diuretic, diaphoretic, and astringent properties. Medicinally, it is used for gastrointestinal complaints.
Didymocarpus pedicellata	*Pathar phori*	(Means in Sanskrit: "that which breaks the stones"). Indications include upper and lower urinary tract disease, splenomegaly, hepatomegaly and cardiovascular disease.
Dolichos biflorus Horse gramplant	*Kulatha*	A culinary edible bean that is cooked or fried before use, with both astringent and diuretic properties. Indicated for urinary tract disorders.
Eclipta alba Trailing eclipta, False daisy	*Bhangra*	This herb is indicated for splenomegaly and hepatomegaly. It also has a reputation for stimulating hair growth. It is a cholegogue.
Elettaria cardamomum Cardamom		Colds, cough, bronchitis, asthma; improves intestinal absorption. Antiemetic, antieructation effect when combined with fennel. Excellent, safe digestive stimulants. Improves spleen function, scours phlegm from lungs and gastrointestinal tract, addresses *Kapha* pathology.
Emblica officinalis, AKA *Phyllanthus emblica* Indian gooseberry	*Amla*	(Also known as *Amlaki.*) Rich source of bioflavonoids and vitamin C. A plum-sized fruit containing up to 700 mg vitamin C per fruit. Rasayana, adaptogenic herb; indicated for anemia, asthma, bleeding gums, diabetes, colds, chronic lung disease, hyperlipidemia, hypertension, yeast infections, scurvy, and neoplastic conditions. *Dosage of dried herb:* *Dogs:* 10-20 mg/kg mg BID *Cats:* 5-10 mg BID

Continued

TABLE 6-6

Quick Guide to the Most Commonly Used Ayurvedic Herbs in Veterinary Practice—cont'd

Botanical and Common Names	Ayurvedic Name	Actions and Applications
Equisetum arvense Horsetail		A mineral-rich herb that provides substantial amounts of silica and other minerals extracted from the soil and converted to a colloidal, water-soluble form. It has diuretic properties and is used in the treatment of patients with arthritis and pulmonary tuberculosis.
Foeniculum vulgare Fennel seeds	*Saumph*	Commonly used for abdominal discomfort, dyspepsia, bloating, and colic. As a galactagogue, fennel stimulates milk production in lactating females, and as an emmenagogue, fennel promotes menstruation. Fennel has also been used for cystitis, to relieve the burning sensation during urination.
Ferula foetida Asafetida	*Hingu*	Plant resin. Used for indigestion, flatulence, abdominal distention, colic, constipation, arthritis, and epilepsy. Potent herbal, given orally, is effective for colic; can also be used topically for abdominal discomfort. Expels roundworms and flatulence. Improves appetite.
Glycyrrhiza glabra Licorice root	*Mulethi* or *Yashtimadhu*	Traditionally used for cough, cold, bronchitis, sore throat, laryngitis, stomach ulcers, gastric hyperacidity, and painful urination.
Gymnema sylvestris Gymnema	*Gurmar*	Traditionally used for dyspepsia, as a diuretic, and for snakebites (both internally and topically); most valuable application is for diabetes. Research has determined that the triterpene saponins contained in the leaves of *Gymnema* provide its hypoglycemic activity. These studies have also shown that *Gymnema* has an effect only on the blood sugar levels of patients with diabetes; normoglycemic patients are unaffected by it.
Indian coral powder		Derived from the marine invertebrate calcific skeleton of coral, this mineral herb is a rich source of calcium and magnesium. This mineral herbal product has traditional uses for cardiac disease, as a laxative, as a calmative agent, and for its diuretic properties.
Mucuna pruriens Cowhage or cowitch	*Kavach apikachlu*	A member of the legume family, this climbing tropical plant is consumed as a vegetable in India. The active medicinal principle is found in the seeds, which contain four alkaloids (macunine, macunidine, prurienine, and prurieninine) and several other bioactive phytocompounds such as dopamine, lecithin, and glycosides. Traditionally, the seeds are used as a tonic, stimulant, diuretic, purgative, emmenagogue, and aphrodisiac. The roots of this plant have been shown to produce uterine contractions. Indications for use include neurologic disease, renal infection, and dropsy. The hairs covering the seed coat of this plant are used as a vermifuge. Human patients with Parkinson's disease have benefited from this botanical medicine because of its dopamine content.
Mimosa pudica Sensitive plant	*Lajja* or *Lajwanti*	An oil extract of the seeds of this plant has been used traditionally for conditions of the urinary tract. The aqueous extract of the leaf is used topically in dressings for sinus conditions, sores, and hemorrhoids.
Mentha spp Mint		Addresses respiratory, digestive, nervous, and cardiovascular conditions. Indications include colds, fever, sore throat, laryngitis, headache, dyspepsia, nervousness, and agitation.
Momordica charantia Bitter melon	*Karela*	Treats worms, digestive disorders, and skin diseases. Studies have demonstrated a human immunodeficiency virus (HIV)-inhibiting effect. Major herb for lowering blood glucose in diabetic individuals.
Myristica fragrans Nutmeg	*Jaiphala*	Applications include abdominal discomfort, diarrhea, and intestinal gas. Also used for insomnia and anxiety. Improves intestinal absorption of nutrients. Considered to be beneficial for patients with inflammatory bowel disease.
Ocimum bacillicum Sweet basil; holy basil	*Tuls*	Antitussive, sinus congestion, headache, arthritis, rheumatism, fever, and abdominal distention. Possesses rejuvenative and stimulating properties, as well as antiviral, antibacterial, antifungal, and anthelmintic activity. Additionally, basil leaves have been found to be anti-inflammatory, antipyretic, diuretic, carminative (reduces gastrointestinal gas), demulcent, diaphoretic, expectorant, and cardiotonic in action. In addition to the leaves, the seeds of sweet basil are demulcent, diaphoretic, diuretic, and stimulating. Commonly used for chronic constipation and hemorrhoids, and topically as a poultice for skin sores or sinus congestion.

TABLE 6-6

Quick Guide to the Most Commonly Used Ayurvedic Herbs in Veterinary Practice—cont'd

Botanical and Common Names	Ayurvedic Name	Actions and Applications
Phyllanthus niruri or *Phyllanthus amarus* Stone breaker, shatter stone	*Bhuivali*	Actions include astringent, stomachic, and diuretic. Therapeutically, this plant addresses conditions of the liver, including jaundice and viral hepatitis B. Proven to possess antibacterial properties contained in the alkaloid fractions of the leaves, *Phyllanthus* can also be used for chronic diarrhea and infections of the genitourinary tract. *Dosage:* *Dogs:* 10 mg/kg TID *Cats:* 5-10 mg/kg TID
Picrorrhiza kurroa Yellow gentiana	*Kutkin* or *Kutki*	A small, hairy perennial herb. The rhizome contains the active principles kutkin, picroside-1, and kutkoside-1. Actions include hepatoprotection, mild laxative, cholegogue, anthelmintic, and antifungal. Has been shown to lower serum cholesterol in humans. Has been used in hyperbilirubinemic and epileptic patients. Other indications include amebiasis, giardiasis, and hepatitis.
Piper longum Long pepper	*Pippili*	Antiparasitic, expectorant. Benefits the liver, spleen, and lymphatics and is considered to be a blood "cleanser." Studies have demonstrated this herb's ability to increase secretory immunoglobulin A (IgA). Improves circulation, digestion, and immune function. Active ingredients of this herb include piperine, piplartine, sesamin, piplasterol, pipelonguminin, steroids, and glycosides. The roots and fruits of this plant are used traditionally for diseases of the respiratory tract and as an analgesic and counterirritant for musculoskeletal pain and inflammation. It is used as a snuff for coma or drowsiness. It is also used as a cholegogue for gallbladder disease.
Piper nigrum Black pepper	*Marichi*	Improves digestion and circulation. Helps to remove toxins via the colon; addresses obesity, sinus congestion. Hemostatic and anthelmintic agent. Use caution and lower doses in patients with inflammatory conditions—may aggravate.
Plantago ovata Blond psyllium Sponghel psyllium	*Isapghul*	In ethnoveterinary usage, Psyllium seeds are mixed with guar gum and used as cattlefeed. The dried seeds and husk are used for their demulcent, emollient, and laxative properties. Conditions commonly addressed by this herb include chronic constipation, amebic and bacillary diarrhea secondary to irritant conditions in the gastrointestinal tact, colds and coughs, bronchitis, rheumatism, kidney disorders, and urethritis.
Punica granatum Pomegranate	*Dadima*	The fruit, fruit rind, bark, and root of this plant contain the active medicinal principles. The fruit is used for sore throat, ulcers, colitis, conjunctivitis, and anemia. The bark has been found to have anthelmintic properties and activity against pinworms, roundworms, and tapeworms.
Raphanus sativa Black radish seed	*Muli*	The extract is used for liver disease and hemorrhoids, flatulence, amenorrhea, dyspepsia, strangury, cough, and paralysis.
Rauwolfia serpentina Serpentine root	*Chota card*	Traditional uses cover a variety of ailments from snakebite to mental illness. This herb is the source of the pharmaceutical drug reserpine, and it contains other alkaloids such as rescinnamine and desperindine. *Rauwolfia* is used in the management of hypertension. *Rauwolfia* exerts its effects via regulation of neurotransmitter metabolism at nerve endings. With more than 50 bioactive alkaloids in *Rauwolfia*, its biological activity is more complex than that of reserpine alone. Human hypertensive patients describe a general sense of euphoria, as well as a slowing of the pulse following ingestion of *Rauwolfia*. It has also been found that *Rauwolfia* exerts a calming effect on anxiety states. Because of the effect of *Rauwolfia* on blood pressure, it should be used at lower doses initially, while the patient is adapting to this powerful herb.
Rosa damascene		Derived from rose petals, this herb exerts a cardiotonic effect. It is also known for its actions as a calmative and digestive tonic.

Continued

TABLE 6-6

Quick Guide to the Most Commonly Used Ayurvedic Herbs in Veterinary Practice—cont'd

Botanical and Common Names	Ayurvedic Name	Actions and Applications
Rubia cordifolia Indian madder, dyers madder	*Manjit*	A vine found in the western Himalayas. Its leaves have tonic, antiseptic, and antidiarrheal activities. A tea made from both the leaves and the stem is effective in addressing dermatitis and as a vermifuge.
Santalum album Sandalwood	*Chandana*	Traditional uses include ophthalmic conditions, conditions of the genitourinary tract such as cystitis, urethritis, and vaginitis, and acute dermatitis, herpes virus infections, bronchitis, palpitations, and heatstroke.
Saxifraga ligulata	*Pakhanbhed*	Known as "the plant which breaks rocks in order to grow." The rhizomes contain the active principles, including tannins, which are astringent, diuretic, laxative, and lithotropic (which is from where it derives its name). Clinical indications for its use include kidney and urinary bladder stones, diarrhea, splenomegaly, and renal and pulmonary disease.
Sesamum indicum Sesame seeds	*Til*	Useful for chronic cough, weak pulmonary system, chronic constipation, gingivitis, and hair loss.
Shilajit or Sheelajeet		A thick organic mineral solution containing low-molecular-weight organic compounds. This "exudate" is found oozing out from the base of steep rock formations. It is considered to be a Rasayana herb, with far-reaching health benefits as a rejuvenative tonic. In clinical applications, shilajit addresses infections of the genitourinary tract, bronchial asthma, and conditions of the upper gastrointestinal tract and stomach.
Solanum nigrum Garden or black nightshade	*Makoi*	Possesses antiseptic, analgesic, and antiprotozoal activities in its use for hepatitis and rheumatoid arthritis. Hepatoprotective, antiulcer activity, anti-inflammatory.
Swertia chirata Chiretta Nepalese neem	*Kirat*	Traditionally used for liver disease and as a "blood purifier." This herb lowers fevers, benefits the stomach, and has anthelmintic properties.
Syzygium caryophyllata; Lavang caryophyllus aromaticus; Eugenia caryophyllata (all synonyms) Cloves		Dried flower buds contain the active principles. Stimulant, expectorant, carminative, analgesic, and aphrodisiac. Indicated for colds, coughs, asthma, indigestion, toothache, vomiting, hiccough, laryngitis, pharyngitis, hypotension, and impotence. Note: Cloves have been found to possess a toxic principle that affects cats, but not dogs.
Tephrosia purpura Wild indigo	*Dhamasia*	Used in cirrhosis of the liver, lymphatic blockage, and edema.
Terminalia arjuna Arjun, Terminalin	*Arjun*	Traditionally, this herb has been used in the treatment of patients with cardiovascular disease.
Terminalia belerica Belleric myrobalan	*Bahera* or *Bibhitaki*	Tall tree widely distributed throughout India and the foothills of the Himalayas. The fruit, which is rich in tannins, is used. Studies have demonstrated a beneficial impact on patients with asthma and chronic sinusitis. Its actions are antihistaminic, antitussive, antibacterial, antifungal, and antiyeast. Astringent, hemostatic agent, expectorant, and laxative. Commonly used in dysentery, bronchitis, and hepatitis This herb is used to balance *Kapha* body types.
Terminalia chebula Myrobalan	*Haritaki*	Derived from a large tree, the fruit, which is used medicinally, is rich in tannins and a plant sterol, beta-sitosterol. Studies indicate antiviral, antiyeast, antihistaminic, anti-inflammatory, laxative, and antibacterial activities for this herb. Antibacterial activity includes effectiveness against *E. coli, Salmonella typhosa, Salmonella paratyphosa* A, B, and C, *Cholera, Shigella, Klebsiella,* and *Pseudomonas*. This herb balances the *Dosha, Vata.*
Tinospora cordifolia, Gulancha tinospora	*Guruchi*	Whole plant used in scabies in swine. The vine is used to improve appetite, for dyspepsia, and to address internal parasites in ruminants and poultry. The stem, root, and whole plant are used in sprains, abscesses, tumors, wounds, broken horns, cracked tail, and anthrax; as a galactagogue; and in the treatment of patients with pneumonia, asthma, cough, swelling of the lungs, colic, constipation, tetanus, pox, and compound fracture. Anti-inflammatory, antispasmodic, and antipyretic properties.

TABLE 6-6

Quick Guide to the Most Commonly Used Ayurvedic Herbs in Veterinary Practice—cont'd

Botanical and Common Names	Ayurvedic Name	Actions and Applications
Trachyspermum ammi, AKA *Carum copticum* Wild celery	*Ajwain*	Ajwain wild celery seeds. Digestive and respiratory effects. Useful for colds, laryngitis, asthma, cough, colic, indigestion, and arthritis. Addresses *Vata*-type diseases.
Tribulus terrestris Caltrops	*Gokhrshur*	The spiny fruit of this herb contains sapogenins, diosgenin, gioenin, chlorogenin, and ruscogenin, among others. The calcium-rich leaves are used in cooking as a calcium supplement. The fruits of this plant are both tonifying and diuretic. Its traditional uses include urinary tract infections and stomach pain, and as a lithotriptic. The roots are known to improve appetite.
Trigonella foenum-graecum Fenugreek	*Methi*	This herb benefits the diabetic patient; improves lipid metabolism and digestive function. It is also used for bronchitis and chronic cough, colds and flu, allergies, and arthritis.
Triphala		Not a single herb, but a combination of three herbs that synergistically produce a unique effect in combination that is different from each herb's individual activity. It consists of a combination of the fruits of *Terminalia chebula*, *Terminalia bellerica*, and *Phyllanthus emblica*, AKA *Emblica officinale* (Amla). Although this herb has many applications, Triphala is most commonly used in its capacity as a rejuvenating or Rasayana formula and for its digestive benefits. This herb is covered in greater detail earlier in this chapter.
Tylophora indica Emetic swallow wort	*Anantamul*	Traditional uses for this herb include respiratory conditions such as asthma, bronchitis, whooping cough *(Bordetella bronchiseptica)*, dysentery, and diarrhea. It has also been recommended for rheumatism and gout. *Tylophora*, when used at higher dosages, has emetic and purgative effects.
Valeriana officinalis	*Tagar*	The root contains the active principles, which are most frequently used for conditions of anxiety. Valerian has sedative, anxiolytic, and muscle spasm–relieving properties.
Withania somnifera Winter cherry	*Ashwagandha Rasayana herb*	Similar to ginseng, has rejuvenating qualities; adaptogen, promotes health and longevity. Indications: Immune system enhancement, anemia, inflammation, bacterial infection, and diarrhea. Soothing to the nervous system, can benefit epilepsy patients.
Zingiber officinale Ginger	*Adarak* = fresh rhizome; *Sunthi* = dried rhizome	This commonly used culinary spice has stimulating, diaphoretic, expectorant, carminative, antiemetic, analgesic, and anti-inflammatory activities. Similar to its cousin turmeric, ginger reduces inflammation by inhibiting enzymes of both the lipoxygenase and cyclooxygenase pathways. Indications include colds, fever, nausea (is safe enough to be used by pregnant woman for morning sickness), motion sickness, vomiting, eructation, abdominal discomfort, headaches, heart disease, laryngitis, and arthritis. As do most culinary herbs, ginger possesses antimicrobial activity. Comparison studies have found ginger's antiemetic effect to be comparable with that of metoclopramide. Ginger is considered the "Universal medicine," because it balances all three *Doshas*: *Vata*, *Pitta*, and *Kapha*.

Sodhi, 2003.

SAFETY OF AYURVEDIC HERBS

The Centers for Disease Control and Prevention (CDC) published a *Morbidity and Mortality (MMWR) Weekly Report* on July 9, 2004, entitled "Lead Poisoning Associated With Ayurvedic Medications—5 States, 2000-2003" (MMWR, 2004). In this study, 12 cases of lead poisoning among adults in five states were associated with the ingestion of Ayurvedic formulations. The report goes on to state the following:

> "In this report, the majority of persons affected were of Asian Indian or East Indian descent. Several of the Ayurvedic medications analyzed did not contain lead. However other Ayurvedic preparations have been analyzed to contain from 0.4 to 261,200 ppm lead."

Certain branches of Ayurvedic medicine, as it is practiced in Asia, consider heavy metals to be therapeutic and encourage their use in the treatment of patients with certain ailments. All subjects in this study received their Ayurvedic medications in India or Nepal.

Although this is not a very large cross section of the total population at risk who are taking Ayurvedic medications, it is important to note that these formulations all had their origins in India. Most Ayurvedic preparations that are sold in the United States and Canada have been manufactured specifically for the Western consumer. It is important that the consumer query the company very closely when locating a supplier for Ayurvedic herbal products; he or she should demand to see certificates of analysis that guarantee product purity.

INTERNATIONAL BIAS AGAINST AYURVEDIC MEDICINE

Singh, in his article published in India in 2000 in the *Bulletin of the Indian Institute for the History of Medicine* describes the systematic bias against India that characterizes Western literature on the history of medicine. The author notes that many writers have "ignored the contributions of India in the development of medicine entirely," and other writers have "relegated India's role much behind other civilizations." He goes on to state: "Unnecessary and deliberate controversies on the dating and origins of Ayurveda have been elaborated by Western authors to emphasize the primacy of Greek versus Hindu medicine" (Singh, 2000).

In another Indian publication, an Indian physician writes,

> "It has been very difficult to get a contemporary view of Ayurveda because Indian doctors trained in allopathic medicine have become Westernized in their approach to medicine, so that they have lost touch with the deeper meaning of Ayurveda. On the other hand, most contemporary commentaries on ancient Ayurvedic texts have been written by Ayurvedic physicians (with a few notable exceptions), which naturally have the disadvantage of being written by people closely involved in the subject, thus lacking a detached view."
>
> (Dahanukar, 1989)

INFORMATIONAL RESOURCES

This chapter on Ayurveda has been carefully revised from its first publication (Schoen, 1998). Dr. C. Viswanathan, an Indian physician and orthopedic surgeon, reviewed that first chapter on the Web site of the Task Force for Veterinary Science. In his review, Dr. Viswanathan found a number of errors in the text directly related to the details of Ayurvedic history and philosophy.

In an honest attempt to correct these errors and avoid any further errors, this chapter has been reviewed for accuracy of content by the editors of the text *Ethnovet Heritage: Indian Ethnoveterinary Medicine: An Overview* (Anjaria, personal communications, 2004; Anjaria, 2000): Professor Jayvir Anjaria, who has completed 12 years of clinical veterinary field work treating animals with Western and Ayurvedic medicine; 20 years in research, teaching, and administration; and 14 years of consultancy with the pharmaceutical industry; Professor Shailendra Dwivedi, an Indian veterinarian with 23 years of experience as a teacher and extension scientist at the Indian Veterinary Research Institute (IVRI) Izatnagar; and Dr. Minoo Parabia, who has a Doctor of Philosophy degree in Ethnobotany and Taxonomy, has earned an honorary Ayurveda diploma, and treats about 100 patients free of cost (including daily medicine provisions) as his service to society.

References

Ahmed I, Adeghate E, Cummings E, Sharma AK, Singh J. Beneficial effects and mechanism of action of *Momordica charantia* juice in the treatment of streptozotocin-induced diabetes mellitus in rat. Mol Cell Biochem 2004;261:63-70.

Anand Ashram Series, Hasti-Ayurveda Treatise on Elephant Medicine, 1894.

Anjaria J. *Traditional System Vet Med for Small Farmers in India RAPA 80*. Rome, Italy: Food and Agriculture Organization; 1984.

Anjaria J; Parabia M; Dwivedi S, eds. *Ethnovet Heritage: Indian Ethnoveterinary Medicine: An Overview*. Ahmedabad, India: Pathik Enterprises Publishers; 2002.

Anonymous. Shalihotra (Ancient Script) (Sanskrit). Stored at Gujarat Ayurveda University Library, Jamnagar, India.

Barnett R, Barone J. *Ayurvedic Medicine: Ancient Roots, Modern Branches*. New Delhi, India: Concorp Management, Publishers; 1996.

Bhandari U, Kanojia R, Pillai KK. Effect of an ethanolic extract of Embelia ribes on dyslipidemia in diabetic rats. Int J Exp Diabetes Res. 2002;3:159-162.

Chainani-Wu N. Safety and anti-inflammatory activity of curcumin: a component of tumeric *(Curcuma longa)*. J Altern Complement Med 2003;9:161-168.

Charak S. In: *Sanskrit Charakacharya*. 3rd ed. Bombay, India: Vaid Jadavji Trikamji Pub. Sathyabhamabai Padurang, Nirnay Sagar Press; 1941.

Dahanukar S, Urmila T. *Ayurveda Revisited*. Bombay, India: Popular Prakashan; 1989.

Diwanay S, Chitre D, Patwardhan B. Immunoprotection by botanical drugs in cancer chemotherapy. J Ethnopharmacol 2004;90:49-55.

Frawley D, Lad V. *The Yoga of Herbs*. Twin Lakes, Wis: Lotus Press; 1988.

Grover JK, Khandkar S, Vats V, Dhunnoo Y, Das D. Pharmacological studies on *Myristica fragrans*—antidiarrheal, hypnotic, analgesic and hemodynamic parameters. Methods Find Exp Clin Pharmacol 2002;24:675-680.

Kapoor LD. *CRC Handbook of Ayurvedic Medicinal Plants*. Boca Raton, Fla: CRC Press, Inc; 1990.

Mahabarat. 1958 Ved Vyas Printed at Kalyan Karyala Geeta Press, Gorakhpur, India for Mahadev Ramchandra Jagushte, Surat, India.

MMWR Morb Mortal Wkly Rep. 2004;53:582-584.

Nammi S; Gudavalli R, Babu BS, et al. Possible mechanisms of hypotension produced 70% alcoholic extract of *Terminalia arjuna* (L.) in anaesthetized dogs. BMC Complementary and Alternative Medicine 2003;3:5.

Schoen A, Wynn S. Complementary and Alternative Veterinary Medicine. Mosby, St Louis, 1998.

Singh A. The bias against India in Western literature on history of medicine: with special emphasis on public health. Bull Indian Inst Hist Med Hyderabad 2000;30:41-58.

Sodhi T. Ayurveda in Veterinary Medicine. Proceedings of the AHVMA Annual Conference; September 20-23, 2003; Durham, NC.

Somavanshi R. 1998. Ethnobotanical approach in evaluation of ethnoveterinary practices. ICAR Summer Short Course on Techniques for Scientific Validation and Evaluation of Ethnoveterinary Practices. Izatnagar, India: Division of Medicine, IVRI; 1998:7-13.

Svoboda R, Lade A. *Tao and Dharma, Chinese Medicine and Ayurveda*. Detroit, Mich: Lotus Press; 1995.

Valmiki, Tulsikrut. Ramayana. 1958. Surat, India: Mahadev Ramchandra Jaguste; 1958.

Virdi J, Sivakami S, Shahani S, Suthar AC, Banavalikar MM, Biyani MK. Anti-hyperglycemic effects of three extracts from *Momordica charantia*. Ethnopharmacology 2003;88:107-111.

Williamson E, ed. *Major Herbs of Ayurveda*. London: Churchill Livingstone; 2002.

World Health Organization. Promotion and development of traditional medicine. WHO Technical Report ser. 622 (1988).

Zysk KG. In: Micozzi MD, ed. *Traditional Ayurveda, Fundamentals of Complementary and Alternative Medicine*. London: Churchill Livingstone; 1996.

PART II

Herbal Medicine Controversies

Evaluating, Designing, and Accessing Herbal Medicine Research

CHAPTER 7

Kerry Martin Bone

An ongoing debate among herbalists and natural therapists involves what role, if any, science must play in the future of herbal medicine. Some feel that the traditional basis of herbal medicine provides a completely adequate therapy and that the scientific investigation of herbs or herbal therapy has little to offer. They caution that the wholesale incorporation of scientific methods into the practice of herbal medicine will result in adverse changes—changes that will make herbal medicine less than what it is today. They fear that herbal medicine will lose its traditional basis, its insight, and its soul. Perhaps it will become a sick hybrid that is neither scientifically sound nor valid as a therapy; possibly, herbal medicine will become totally reductionist, with herbs, similar to many modern drugs, used only for superficial symptom control. Among some herbalists, science is seen as a technique for information gathering that is inferior to the knowledge derived from insight, inspiration, and intuition.

The more eloquent among herbalists argue that herbal medicine does not involve just complex medicines but rather requires a complex therapeutic approach that can be difficult to capture in clinical trials for the following reasons:

- Treatments are individualized, which makes difficult the design of meaningful clinical trials. One attempt that has been made in this direction is a clinical trial that included patients with irritable bowel syndrome in which individualized treatments were compared against a standard formulation and a placebo under double-blind conditions (Bensoussan, 1998).
- The patient–practitioner relationship counts. In other words, herbalists often reject the claim that the inability to eliminate observer bias in uncontrolled trials makes findings invalid in all cases, and that the relationship itself is therapeutic.
- Treatments may be provided for chronic diseases with waxing and waning signs. How can this be adequately addressed in trial design? Treatment effects may not be as simple as the disappearance of a single objective symptom. How can measures of well-being be incorporated into research design?

Although many of these considerations have bases in truth, it is not necessarily valid to reject scientific methods completely. First,the differentiation should be made between science and what can be called "scientism."

Science is a method for gathering and organizing information obtained from the natural environment. It is a very useful tool for gaining new information. Science is used to find truth, but this truth is never absolute. It is always relative to the particular conditions imposed by the information gathering. Moreover, science is always about theory. Hence, a good scientist accepts that a large body of information and knowledge is unknown to current science. This unknown knowledge can and will affect the scientific truths of today. In other words, much of what is accepted as obvious and true today will prove to be untrue in the future—this is the process of science. For example, in the 19th century, it was obvious and true to all scientists that light traveled in straight lines. However, Einstein later proved this to be untrue. This condition of scientific inquiry can be expressed in another statement that is relevant to the debate about the validity of natural medicine: Absence of evidence is not the same as evidence of absence. That is, if a phenomenon has not yet been measured in a scientific experiment, this does not necessarily mean that it is non-existent.

By contrast, scientism can be defined as a philosophical approach that accepts only that *current* scientific theories define the truth. For example, the human body functions only as a biochemical machine because this is current scientific theory. According to scientism, the existence of an organizing life force is not possible because it has not been established in a way that is acceptable to modern scientific methods. Not all scientists subscribe to scientism, and it is scientism that natural therapists should have concerns about—not open-minded scientific inquiry.

Used properly and in context, good science has much to offer. But what is the proper context for herbal medicine? Phytotherapy has been defined as the positive incorporation of science and tradition. In particular, scientific investigation is useful for providing the solid, factual, background information that any therapist needs. For example, science can tell us that *Ginkgo biloba* is good for circulation, or that *Hypericum perforatum* is a valid treatment for depression. However, traditional considerations will often be more relevant in guiding the phytotherapist regarding when to apply this information in a clinical situation. In this context, science is just one tool to be used in the consulting room. During a consultation, a good practitioner will assess the patient, whether human or animal, as an individual, using insight, logic, and common sense and supported by the appropriate use of scientific information. The treatment of the patient as an individual can never be outweighed by results of double-blind clinical trials.

At the other extreme, phytotherapists or natural therapists who embrace scientific information should be on guard against pseudoscience. The risk is serious that poor science or pseudoscience will render natural medicine an ineffective therapy. Characteristics of pseudoscience that allow its recognition include the following:

- Hypotheses presented as undisputed facts. The claim that Echinacea should not be used in autoimmune disease is one current example
- Hypotheses that can be neither proved nor disproved, that is, circular arguments
- Conclusions based on insufficient evidence
- Extrapolating excessively from a narrow context of results, for example, extrapolating from in vitro data to clinical situations without consideration of factors such as dose, metabolism, absorption, and distribution of active compounds
- Quoting obscure or old studies, or studies not published in peer review journals (a peer review journal is one for which accepted experts review papers for scientific quality before the time of their publication)
- Use of theories that are no longer accepted, for example, outdated theories about the nature of cancer
- Claim of scientific persecution (this does occur, of course, but is often used as an excuse for poor science)
- Development of theories that bear no relationship to experimental findings
- Use of scientific methods that are inappropriate for the purpose of proving or disproving a hypothesis

Science can develop and is developing phytotherapy by providing new information. However, many complex issues remain to be resolved, particularly in the field of pharmacologic research on herbs and its implications for quality, safety, and efficacy. If we do not get the science right by adapting experimental protocols to the particular requirements of doing good phytopharmacologic research, results will be at best useless and at worst downright misleading.

DESIGNING RELEVANT HERBAL MEDICINE RESEARCH

Ideally, pharmacologic research on herbs can provide evidence of activity (proof of efficacy), an understanding of how they work, information about quality and safety, leads for new applications, and supporting evidence for the use of whole extracts in preference to isolated chemicals.

Modern Drug Discovery

In modern drug discovery, the sequence of events usually occurs as follows. Desirable pharmacologic properties for treatment of patients with a particular disease are speculated. The search begins for chemical agents that have these properties in the right potency. They must lack other properties that cause undesirable adverse effects. Compounds may be natural, nature derived, or synthetic. Test tube and animal research precede any testing in humans, and most compounds do not make it! (Only one herbal product has been developed in this way: *Ginkgo biloba*.) Resultant drug medicines are often prepared around a one-dimensional, receptor-based, reductionist, mechanistic approach to disease, for example, suppress a particular aspect of the immune or inflammatory response, raise levels of a neurotransmitter, and so forth. In other words, it is often anticipated how the drug will work with consideration of the active mechanism.

Phytopharmacologic Discovery

The term *phytopharmacology* as used here applies to research on herbs as medicines. This is distinct from the copious research aimed at discovering new chemical entities (drugs) in plants, which are often exotic or toxic and unknown to the main herbal traditions.

Essential differences between modern drug discovery and the way research is conducted on medicinal plants relate more to cultural, socioeconomic, and regulatory issues than to inherent differences between the subject materials. In phytopharmacologic discovery, we usually start with human use. Only then might scientists become interested in understanding *how* the herb works. It is therefore possible that an herb might act through a pharmacologic mechanism that has not yet been discovered.

So, with phytopharmacology, generally, some evidence of clinical efficacy is found *before* a mechanism of action is proposed. However, some differences relate to the subject material, particularly the chemical complexity and the fact that the plant is a living thing. Mechanisms may be complex and numerous because of chemical complexity. True mechanisms may be unknown and multidimensional. Activity may be based on the relationship between patient and plant physiology (the medicine was once alive).

Why should phytochemicals have biological activity in humans? Baker suggests an evolutionary kinship (Baker, 1995). Enzymes in animals can share a common ancestry with enzymes or proteins in plants. Phytochemicals that are substrates of a plant enzyme may also be capable of being substrates of the corresponding human enzyme. In Baker's examples, phytochemicals interact with enzymes that metabolize animal hormones, leading to hormone-like effects. One of the best examples of this is glycyrrhetinic acid from licorice, which exerts a potent mineralocorticoid effect without ever interacting with mineralocorticoid receptors.

Herbs are complex. It was difficult enough to understand exactly how a drug like aspirin, a single chemical in use for more than 100 years, worked in the human body. The scientist who did so shared the Nobel Prize. In the case of a chemically complex herbal extract, the task is that much more difficult, perhaps even impossible with today's technology and today's one-dimensional approach to researching pharmacology and therapeutics.

Research techniques in phytopharmacology

It is worthwhile to examine the relative appropriateness of the research techniques used in phytopharmacology. On the face of it, these research techniques are the same as those used in conventional research:

- Molecular level: analyzing effects on enzymes, nucleic acids, proteins, etc.
- Subcellular level: analyzing effects on membranes and organelles
- Cells: analyzing effects on whole cells such as hepatocytes, lymphocytes, etc.
- Organs: analyzing effects on whole isolated organs such as heart, liver, etc.
- Animals: analyzing the whole animal response to an intervention in laboratory animals such as rats and mice
- Clinical: analyzing clinical effects on human or animal patients in a controlled setting such as the randomized controlled trial

These first four categories are studied as in vitro models. Given the chemical complexity of herbs, the uncertain pharmacokinetics of many phytochemicals, and the fact that most herbs are already used in humans, it is suggested that the best model for phytopharmacologic research is the 6-foot rat (i.e., the human volunteer) or other *clinical* patients such as dogs, cats, cows, and horses, using the appropriate species as a model.

Limitations of the In Vitro Test in the Context of Phytopharmacology: During an in vitro test, an herbal extract comes into direct contact with test cells, as shown in the diagram (Figure 7-1). Often, levels of exposure are unrealistic. But the reality, after an herb is orally administered, is very different, as is represented in the next diagram (Figure 7-2).

In other words, the cells of the body experience a modified version of the herbal extract and are often exposed to metabolites of the original compounds. Bowel flora play a special role here. In particular, some phytochemicals that are active in in vitro tests are not even absorbed. For this reason, extrapolation of in vitro research to whole body systems must be done with *great caution.* For more information on herbal pharmacokinetics and bowel flora metabolism of phytochemicals, the reader is referred elsewhere (Mills and Bone, 2000).

Examples of Phytopharmacologic Research on Humans and Domestic Animals: So, in the face of this uncertainty, the best research model for herbs is the one that most closely resembles the clinical patient. Listed here are some examples of pharmacologic research that has been done on humans, but the same types of research could be conducted in a veterinary context.

A number of opportunities exist in which one can creatively devise herbal research using human volunteers. Many uncertainties are dealt with using this type of research, including extrapolation to the patient, bioavailability, and dosage.

Examples include the following:

- Pharmacokinetics and bioavailability studies
- Ex vivo research on isolated cells. In this example, the volunteer is administered the herb; then, cells such as blood cells are removed from the person and are studied to ascertain whether any of their features differ from those before treatment; blood cells from someone who did not take the herb (i.e., a control) are also analyzed
- Use of noninvasive techniques (e.g., electroencephalography [EEG], electrocardiography [ECG], ultrasound, positron emission tomography [PET] scans, polysomnography)
- Change in physiologic function: hormone levels, urine output and quality, hepatic biotransformation, immune function, gastric acid output, etc.
- Performance: memory, cognitive function, intelligence quotient (IQ), endurance, recovery

Research Linking Quality and Efficacy

The issue of being able to relate the phytochemical content of an herb or herbal extract to its clinical efficacy is one of the potentially most fruitful areas of

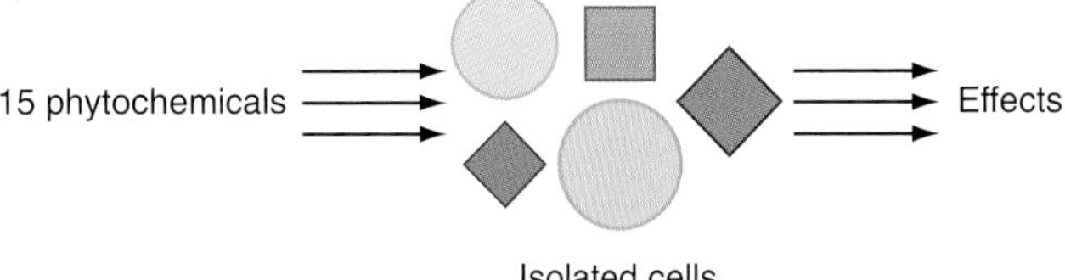

Figure 7-1 A diagrammatic representation of the *in vitro* test for an herbal extract.

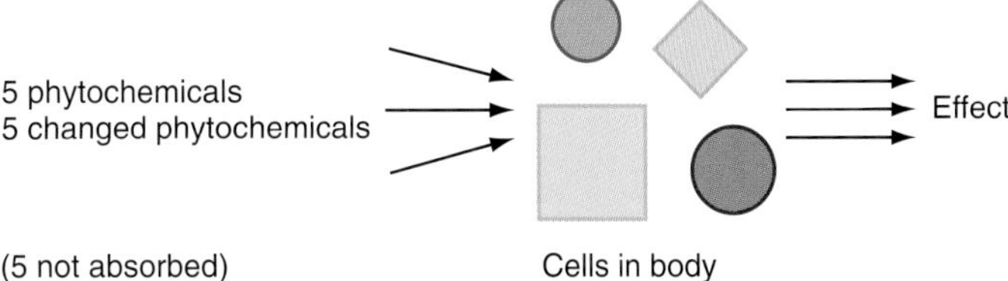

Figure 7-2 A diagrammatic representation of cellular exposure after oral ingestion of an herbal extract.

phytopharmacologic research but also one of the most complex, controversial, and difficult. Efficacy cannot occur without quality, but which phytochemicals in a plant define its quality from a therapeutic perspective?

The patient is a black box when it comes to many herbs; we do not know what is happening in terms of relating the clinical outcomes to the phytochemical input (Figure 7-3). But as represented in Figure 7-4, we can break the "black box" up into two components, whereby the digestive tract acts as a filtering process and often an agent of change (as discussed previously). If a plant compound is not absorbed (or its metabolites are not absorbed), we can probably discount its relevance from the quality perspective.

So, first, we need to determine the bioavailable constituents and then decide which bioavailable constituents are active. If a phytochemical is bioavailable (or its metabolites are bioavailable), this does not necessarily imply that it is important for activity.

Valerian—The hunt for the "active constituent"

The complex issue of relating the phytochemicals in a plant to its pharmacologic activity is well illustrated by research on valerian *(Valeriana officinalis)*. Research is often too focused on hunting for the active constituent. The example of valerian shows that the research emphasis over the years has shifted from one phytochemical class to another (Schumacher, 2002). The question, still not conclusively answered in the case of valerian, is whether one class is more important than another (Mills and Bone, 2000) (Box 7-1).

How to preserve or enhance quality in studies of therapeutic efficacy

What can we conclude about quality in the face of this complexity and uncertainty? In the absence of conclusive evidence linking phytochemical components to human therapeutic activity, several pragmatic research approaches can be used to preserve or enhance quality and establish credible evidence for particular phytochemicals as markers of quality:

1. Preserve as much as possible—qualitatively and quantitatively—the phytochemicals found in the fresh plant. For example, with the globe artichoke, losses of phytochemicals occur very quickly on poor drying owing to plant enzymatic activity.
2. Using pharmacologic models, determine which bioavailable phytochemicals contribute to activity, and ensure that levels of these components are optimized. There might be many compounds—not just one or one class of compounds. In the case of *Hypericum,* in vivo or human research has demonstrated that the following phytochemicals (or groups) have antidepressant activity following oral doses: hypericin and pseudohypericin solubilized by the oligomeric proanthocyanidins (OPCs); hyperforin; and flavonoids, in particular, hyperoside and isoquercitrin (Butterweck, 2003a).
3. Prove a particular product works clinically, and then ensure that all future products reflect the same phytochemical profile. The best example of this is *Ginkgo biloba.*

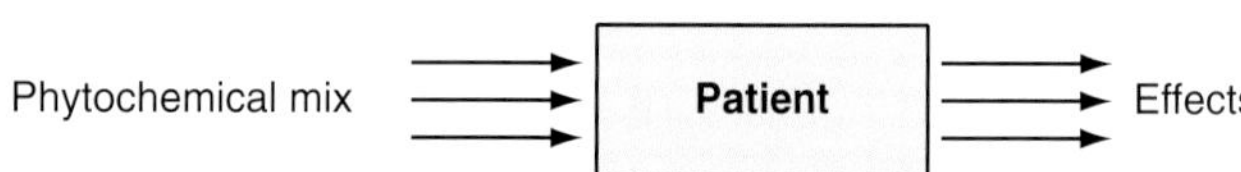

Figure 7-3 A representation of the patient as a black box in terms of clinical effects from an herbal extract. Which phytochemicals are important?

Referring to the first approach of preserving what is in the fresh plant as much as possible, does that mean there should be a preference for fresh plant tinctures? At the risk of being controversial, the postulated advantages of fresh plant tinctures are not supported by phytochemical fact. There is too much water in a fresh plant for the direct manufacture of a sufficiently concentrated preparation. However, there is another important concern. The high water content and the unquenched enzymatic activity mean that phytochemicals are being decomposed as the tincture is being made. Cichoric acid in *Echinacea purpurea* is now a well-known example of this (Bauer, 1989).

Enzymatic activity can still degrade important phytochemicals when the dried herb comes into contact with gastric juices. So, placing dried herbs in capsules can mean that enzymatic degradation starts again when the herb enters the stomach.

The experiment represented in Figure 7-5 was carried out in a simulated stomach and mimics what happens when equivalent quantities of *Echinacea* tops are ingested either as just the dried herb in a capsule or as an extract in a capsule (Lehmann, 2002).Cichoric acid levels degrade to almost zero for the dried herb, indicating that enzymatic activity is still present.

If an extract of the dried herb is often the best form to use because it avoids the problem of enzymatic activity, some important considerations should be observed:

- If compounds are known or suspected to be important for activity, it must be ensured that they are

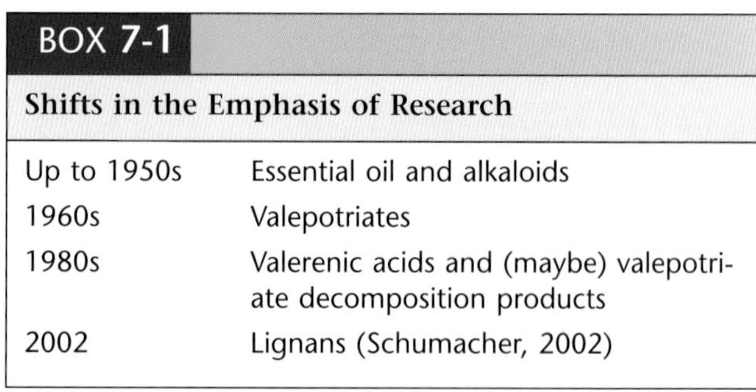

BOX 7-1

Shifts in the Emphasis of Research

Up to 1950s	Essential oil and alkaloids
1960s	Valepotriates
1980s	Valerenic acids and (maybe) valepotriate decomposition products
2002	Lignans (Schumacher, 2002)

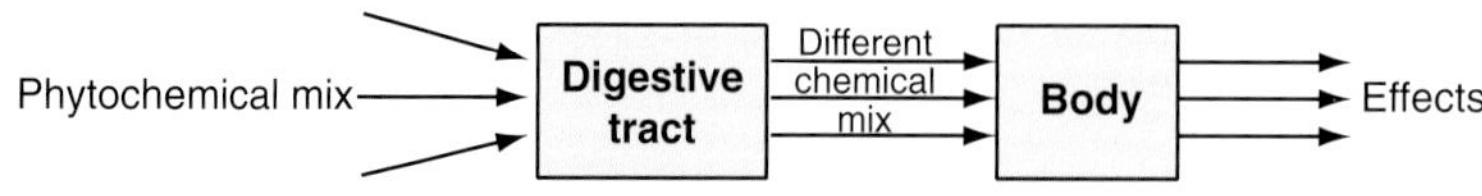

Figure 7-4 A two-component representation of the patient as a black box.

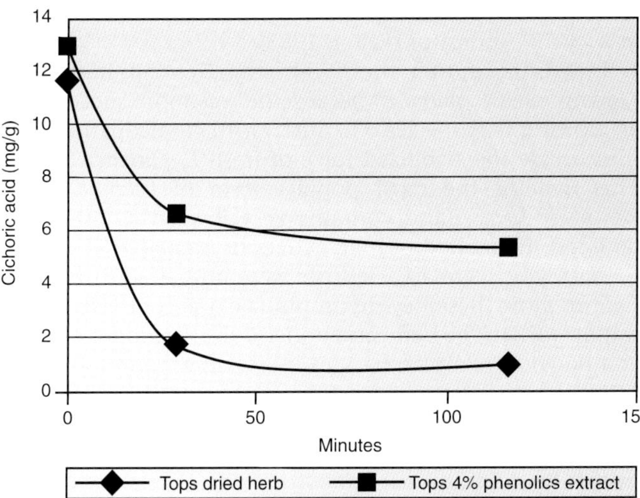

Figure 7-5 Cichoric acid degradation: dried herb versus extract.

optimized by extraction, but not at the undue expense of others.

- Water is a poor solvent—yet it has been used traditionally. What do we make of this? For example, that the astragalosides in *Astragalus* are not water soluble?
- The extraction should be optimized to the known phytochemistry of the plant. For example, if it is resinous or contains essential oil, use a high ethanol content.

Synergy, Addition, or Antagonism: Important Issues in Phytopharmacologic Research

A concept that is often invoked by herbalists is that of synergy. However, all the concepts listed here, namely, synergy, addition, and sometimes antagonism, are important in terms of understanding how an herb might act as a whole.

With synergy, the combined effect of two or more components is greater than that expected from their arithmetic combination. The opposite is antagonism. Additive effects, whereby several components are important for activity, are likely to be more common. For a more extensive discussion of these issues as they relate to plant medicine, the reader is referred elsewhere (Williamson, 2001).

It is important to note that synergy is not essential for justifying the use of the plant as a whole extract; demonstration of additive effects from several different phytochemicals is sufficient to justify this. Even in the absence of additive effects, the complex action of a variety of chemicals is a special characteristic of complex medicines. Which phytochemical do you isolate as the drug if they all contribute to the effect? An example of synergy can be seen in Table 7-1 (Kisa, 1981).

In this study, the potentiating effect of the laxative anthraquinone sennoside C on the purgative activity of sennoside A was assessed in vivo. A lower ED_{50} (the amount of material required to produce a specified effect in 50% of an animal population) means greater activity.

TABLE 7-1

Potentiating Effect of Sennoside C on the Purgative Activity of Sennoside A

Sennoside A : C Ratio	ED_{50} mg/kg
10 : 0	11.1
9 : 1	8.1
8 : 2	7.2
7 : 3	6.2
5 : 5	6.9
0 : 10	11.2

ED_{50}, the amount of material required to produce a specified effect in 50% of an animal population.

The ratio of sennoside A to sennoside C that gives the highest activity is similar to that which occurs naturally in senna, and a synergistic effect between the two compounds is demonstrated at this ratio. (If there was no synergy, the ED_{50} for any mixture of sennosides A and C would be in the range from 11.1 to 11.2 mg/kg.)

Enhanced bioavailability as a key aspect of synergy

The enhanced bioavailability of active phytochemicals from whole plant extracts is one of the most compelling arguments for using plant extracts, rather than isolated chemicals. Although several examples are now available in the literature, additional evidence of this phenomenon is needed. The most likely (and readily studied) example of synergy is that wherein an inactive component enhances the bioavailability of an active phytochemical.

Established examples with which the bioavailability from a complex extract is greater than that for the isolated phytochemical include the following:

- Kava lactones from *Piper methysticum* are more bioavailable than isolated lactones (Mills and Bone, 2000)
- Hypericin and pseudohypericin are made more bioavailable by the OPCs from *Hypericum* (Butterweck, 2003b)
- Daidzin from *Pueraria lobata* is more bioavailable than is isolated daidzin (Mills and Bone, 2000)

The Gaps in Our Knowledge

A highly important current challenge in phytopharmacology is recognizing and addressing the gaps in our knowledge of commonly used herbs. Despite their common use, and in some cases good clinical trial support for their activity, we still do not conclusively know the following:

- How *Echinacea* acts on the immune system, and which compounds are important
- How saw palmetto acts in benign prostatic hyperplasia
- How valerian acts on the nervous system
- The bioavailable compounds to be derived from hawthorn
- The pharmacologic basis of chaste tree activity

Clearly, if we wish to get the science right and make it relevant to commonly used herbs, there is a need to focus on answering these important questions. Recent advances have been made with *Echinacea* (see later) and chaste tree (Wuttke, 2003).

ECHINACEA: WHAT IS IMPORTANT?

It is relevant to discuss a new perspective on the complex issue of *Echinacea* and what makes it work. The following example serves to illustrate many of the issues outlined previously in terms of linking quality to efficacy. In Professor Bauer's review of the literature, he proposed that the following compounds have established immunologic activity in pharmacologic models (Bauer, 1991):

- Alkylamides
- Cichoric acid
- Polysaccharides
- Glycoproteins

Support for glycoproteins and polysaccharides derives only from in vitro research and human studies using intravenous doses (Bauer, 1991). Support for lipophilic components (cichoric acid and alkylamides) derives from in vitro, in vivo, and human studies (Bauer, 1991).

Why should polysaccharides be regarded as quality markers for *Echinacea* when

- No analytic methods are available to properly measure them
- Research was conducted with the use of intravenous treatments
- Poor bioavailability and absorption issues with oral treatments create great uncertainty?

Historical Context

Before new research developments for *Echinacea* are discussed, its use as an immune herb must be understood in its historical context. Information about the therapeutic value of *Echinacea* first came from American Indian tribes. Their use of *Echinacea* was then adopted by the Eclectics, a group of doctors who were prominent in the United States around the late 19th and early 20th centuries. By 1921, *Echinacea* (specifically the root of *E. angustifolia)* was by far the most popular treatment prescribed by Eclectic physicians (Wagner, 1996). The Eclectics used *Echinacea* for about 50 years, which is a relatively short time in the context of traditional use. However, given that the Eclectic use of *Echinacea* was based on tribal knowledge, and that they accumulated extensive clinical experience in its use, their traditionally used data are of high quality. The best sources of such data are King's American Dispensatory (Felter, 1983) and Ellingwood (1993).

What is also important to note is that the reputation of Echinacea as an immune herb came from solid traditional data generated by the Eclectics on only one form of *Echinacea*—a fluid extract of the dried root of *Echinacea angustifolia* extracted with the use of a high percentage of alcohol. We can call this a "traditional *Echinacea* extract," and because it is extracted in a high percentage of alcohol, the term *lipophilic extract* (fat loving) is also relevant. In particular, the Eclectics defined good quality *Echinacea* root "as imparting a persistent tingling sensation," which is a clear reference to alkylamide levels as a quality indicator (Felter, 1983).

In Europe during the 1930s, the German herbalist Madaus used *E. purpurea* because he was more successful at growing this species. His interest in homeopathy led him to use the stabilized juice of fresh *E. purpurea* tops. This remains the most popular form of *Echinacea* in Germany today (and contains very low levels of alkylamides). It is a hydrophilic extract of *Echinacea.*

Naturally, German scientists were interested in investigating how these new hydrophilic extracts of *Echinacea* might work in the body and undertook a search for active components. Polysaccharides possessing immunologic activity were isolated from the aerial parts of *E. purpurea* (Bauer, 1991). Some clinicians and scientists then mistakenly applied this research to the very different lipophilic or traditional *Echinacea* preparations and came to the conclusion that they were therapeutically inferior because of their low or absent content of polysaccharides. (The low levels of polysaccharides in traditional *Echinacea* extracts are due to the low starting levels in the root and the fact that high levels of alcohol do not effectively extract these water-loving molecules.)

However, many phytotherapists remained unconvinced. A key aspect of modern phytotherapy is a respect for traditionally generated knowledge; this suggests that a lipophilic extract of *E. angustifolia* root was the preferred form. Some believed that the concept of polysaccharides failed to explain what was unique about *Echinacea* and expressed concerns about the low oral bioavailability of such large polar compounds (Melchart, 2002). Because of their important role in primary metabolism, all plants contain polysaccharides. Moreover, the levels found in *Echinacea* preparations are not high when compared with mushrooms and other accumulators of polysaccharides such as *Althaea officinalis* and *Aloe* species. It is possible that *Echinacea* polysaccharides exert some unique and potent pharmacologic actions on the immune system, but this argument is not helped by research showing that many polysaccharides have immunologic activity (Egert, 1992).

So, what was clearly needed was a different understanding of *Echinacea,* especially of the phytochemicals important for the activity of traditional *Echinacea* products and their mode of action on the immune system.

New Insight Into Echinacea

These answers may have come in 2004, with the release of a number of developments at the International Congress on Natural Products Research, which was held in Phoenix, Arizona. At this conference, several papers were presented (as posters and oral presentations) that, when combined, provide new insight into the possible mechanism of action of traditional lipophilic extracts of *Echinacea.* As was mentioned earlier, such extracts are particularly rich in the phytochemicals known as *alkylamides* (or alkamides), but they also contain caffeic acid derivatives. (Caffeic acid derivatives include echinacoside and cichoric acid, depending on the species of *Echinacea.*)

An oral presentation by Dr Reg Lehmann from Australia presented important findings indicating that only the alkylamides (and not the caffeic acid derivatives) were found to be bioavailable with both an in vitro model and observations from a placebo-controlled pharmacokinetic trial in healthy volunteers (Matthias, 2004). In particular, only alkylamides could be detected in the blood plasma samples from volunteers taking an *Echinacea* root extract in tablet form. No other phytochemicals known to occur in *Echinacea* root were found in the plasma, despite their being present in the tablets. (If *Echinacea* is to have systemic effects on the immune system, then it is likely that the phytochemicals responsible for this must be systemically absorbed.)

These results were supported by an oral presentation by Professor Rudi Bauer of Karl Franzens University in Austria, whose team investigated the bioavailability of a 60% ethanolic extract of *Echinacea angustifolia* root in 12 healthy volunteers (Woelkart, 2004a). The alkylamides were shown to be rapidly absorbed after oral ingestion of the liquid.

Another significant discovery presented at the Congress was the observation by two separate research teams that the immune effects of *Echinacea* may be mediated by the interaction of *Echinacea* alkylamides with cannabinoid receptors. A Swiss research team found that an in vitro immune-modulating effect of a lipophilic *Echinacea* extract (and individual alkylamides) on monocytes/macrophages could be neutralized by the presence of agents that block CB2 cannabinoid receptors (Gertsch, 2004a,b). Bauer, in collaboration with US scientists, found that alkylamides from *Echinacea* were bound to both CB1 and CB2 cannabinoid receptors (Woelkart, 2004b). In particular, certain alkylamides exhibited selectivity for CB2 receptors.

Taken together, these developments presented at the Phoenix conference suggest the hypothesis that the alkylamides are largely responsible for the systemic immune effects of *Echinacea* lipophilic extracts, and that this immune-modulating activity is (at least in part) due to the interaction of alkylamides with cannabinoid receptors, specifically, CB2.

Cannabinoid research has undergone a tremendous transformation in the past 10 to 15 years. This progress was made possible by the discovery of the cannabinoid receptors (Berdyshev, 2000). Two cannabinoid receptors, CB1 and CB2, were originally found because they were activated by the major psychoactive component of marijuana *(Cannabis sativa)*—delta-9-tetrahydrocannabinol (Grotenhermen, 2004). CB1 receptors are highly localized in the central nervous system (CNS) and are believed to primarily modulate behavior; CB2 receptors predominate in immune tissues outside the CNS, especially the spleen, and are believed to modulate immune function (Ralevic, 2003).

When the cannabinoid receptors were first discovered, they were classified as orphan receptors because no endogenous molecules were known to stimulate their function. However, shortly thereafter, two major endogenous cannabinoids (endocannabinoids) were isolated (Grotenhermen, 2004). These are the arachidonic acid derivatives anandamide and 2-arachidonylglycerol (Grotenhermen, 2004). In fact, the structure of anandamide is strikingly similar to that of some *Echinacea* alkylamides.

Cannabinoid receptors are remarkably preserved across the animal kingdom, which suggests that they play an important developmental and physiologic role (Salzet, 2000; Fride, 2004). Much of the immune activity of the cannabinoid system appears to be mediated by the cytokine network. Cytokines include the interleukins (e.g., IL-3, IL-6), tumor necrosis factor-alpha (TNF-α), and the interferons (IFNs). Specific effects identified thus far for anandamide include the following (Klein, 2000):

- Decreased proliferation in a breast cancer cell line
- Increased IL-3– and IL-6–dependent immune cell line proliferation
- Increased IL-6 production in Theilervirus–infected astrocytes
- Decreased interleukins, IFN-γ and TNF-α in human peripheral blood mononuclear cells

These effects are similar to some of those found with *Echinacea* alkylamides or with lipophilic *Echinacea* extracts.

The research of the Swiss team was particularly insightful into one aspect of the mode of action of *Echinacea* alkylamides (Gertsch, 2004a). A lipophilic extract of *Echinacea purpurea* strongly stimulated TNF-α mRNA synthesis in peripheral monocytes—but not TNF-α production. In other words, *Echinacea*-induced new TNF-α transcripts (mRNA) were not translated into TNF-α itself. When monocytes were treated with lipopolysaccharide (LPS) or endotoxin, a powerful stimulator of the immune system, TNF-α protein production is substantially increased. However, coincubation of monocytes with LPS and *Echinacea* extract resulted in a strong inhibition of this effect of LPS.

Studies over a longer time span revealed additional insights. TNF-α mRNA was upregulated (around eightfold) by the *Echinacea* extract over a time span of 24 hours, whereas the constituent protein level of TNF-α was not changed. However, LPS-stimulated TNF-α protein expression was potently modulated by *Echinacea,* resulting in significant inhibition (~40%) during the first 20 hours and a subsequent prolongation of TNF-α production. The authors were able to show that all these effects of *Echinacea* extract on monocytes were produced by the interaction of *Echinacea* alkylamides with the CB2 receptors on these cells.

The results of this study suggest that *Echinacea* works as a modulator or facilitator of the immune response, rather than as an immune stimulant. In resting monocytes, it prepares them for a quicker immune response by inducing TNF-α mRNA. However, in overstimulated monocytes (as in the case of LPS), it first reduces and then extends their response in terms of TNF-α production. In particular, these key findings challenge the mythology that traditional *Echinacea* extracts will "overstimulate and wear out" the immune system, if taken continuously. On the contrary, we now have evidence (also confirmed by the Australian team) that *Echinacea* does not stimulate resting immune cells and moderates the excessive and probably detrimental responses of overstimulated cells, thereby prolonging their effective activity.

The importance of liver metabolism

The Australian research team also discovered some interesting factors that appear to govern the human bioavailability of *Echinacea* alkylamides. As was stated previously, only alkylamides were found in human plasma after ingestion of *Echinacea* tablets, but the levels were extremely variable, and first-pass liver metabolism was suspected as influencing this observation. The 2,4-diene alkylamides (predominant in *E. purpurea)* were found to be rapidly degraded by human liver microsomes; in contrast, the 2-ene alkylamides (predominant in *E. angustifolia)* were much more slowly degraded. More interesting was the discovery that the 2-ene alkylamide, undeca-2E-ene-8,10-diynoic acid isobutylamide, actually slowed down the rate of 2,4-diene alkylamide degradation. The protective effect of this major alkylamide is a highly novel finding, and it was deduced that only relatively small proportions of this compound will result in a product with enhanced bioavailability. This is the first work that supports the traditional use of *E. angustifolia* root preparations in that the 2-ene alkylamides are not found in *E. purpurea.* It also shows the value, from a pharmacokinetic perspective, of combining the root of *E. purpurea* with *E. angustifolia.* In other words, the alkylamides from *E. angustifolia* enhance the bioavailability of those in *E. purpurea.*

Whole root extracts are still valid

Several other research groups are now of the opinion that the alkylamides are the most important compounds for the pharmacologic activity of traditional *Echinacea* extracts. In addition to the teams discussed previously, a Canadian group found that alkylamides at very low oral doses significantly increase the phagocytic activity, as well as the phagocytic index, of alveolar macrophages in normal rats (Goel, 2002). Thus, a previously known immune function of *Echinacea* (increased phagocytic activity) can also be attributed to alkylamides.

Drugs that interact with CB2 receptors are under investigation at several research centers, and the temptation will no doubt be there to isolate the *Echinacea* alkylamides as a class of new immune-modulating drugs. However, the other components of an *Echinacea* extract probably serve a role in stabilizing the alkylamides, which are particularly prone to oxidation, and possibly have other functions as well. Hence, the use of whole root extracts is still preferable. On the other hand, growing, harvesting, drying, and extraction techniques should be tested and modified if necessary to ensure that good levels of alkylamides are maintained in traditional *Echinacea* products. In addition, the inclusion of alkylamide levels (per dose or per milliliter) on the label provides valuable and clinically relevant quality information.

ACCESSING RESEARCH INFORMATION ON HERBS

A number of databases and Internet sites can provide useful access to research studies on herbal medicine. By far, the most useful free site is PubMed, which is run by the National Library of Congress in the United States (Box 7-2). Pubmed has now made available MedlinePlus <http://medlineplus.gov/> . In addition to information on prescription and over-the-counter medicines, MedlinePlus includes over 100 herbal and supplement monographs from Natural Standard, an evidence-based, peer-reviewed collection of information on alternative treatments.

Note that most databases list titles and abstracts only. Full papers can be obtained through medical libraries or other services such as Infotrieve (Web site address: www4.infotrieve.com). Alternatively, a polite email to the author(s) often yields a prompt response. Most authors are only too pleased to provide a portable document format (PDF) copy of their article to interested readers.

Many Internet sites contain interesting herbal research and other medical data. A few of these are listed below:

- http://www.sciencedirect.com/
  This is an Elsevier Web site that features the *Journal of Ethnopharmacology.* The table of contents with abstracts can be viewed for issues back to 1982. Abstracts can also be retrieved by using the Author and Keyword Indexes, although these are lists rather than search engines.
- http://www.herbalgram.org/herbalgram/index.html
  This is part of the American Botanical Council's Web site; it provides information about its publication HerbalGram—how to order it and so forth. Several articles from HerbalGram are listed for download. Further information about other ABC publications (such as the Herb Reference Guide), education, and services is also listed.

BOX 7-2

Useful Internet Databases on Herbs

PubMed: US National Library of Medicine Article Citation Database
http://www.pubmed.org

Agricola: US National Agricultural Library Article Citation Database
http://agricola.nal.usda.gov/

APT Online (wildlife and zoo abstracts)
http://apt.allenpress.com/aptonline/?request=search-simple

STN is a service that provides pay for access to several relevant databases, including EMBASE, NAPRALERT, and CHEMABS. The Website address is
http://stneasy.cas.org.

APT, Allenpress Titles; STN, Databases in Science and Technology; EMBASE, Excerpta Medica pharmacologic and biomedical database; NAPRALERT, Natural Products Alert; CHEMABS, Chemical Abstracts database.

- http://www.botany.net/IDB/botany.html
  This is a directory of sites with subject groupings of crops, ethnobotany, herbal medicine, plant pathology, poisons, and weeds. Against most of the Web addresses is a one- or two-line explanation of the site.
- http://www.herb.umd.umich.edu/cgi-bin/herb/
  This is the site of the Native American Ethnobotany database; it provides very well-summarized information but is referenced.
- http://www.rrreading.com/
  This site contains information about how to subscribe to Robyn's Recommended Reading—a publication that reviews herbal medicine literature. The site also contains lists of recommended reading (books, journals, and articles) and links to other sites.
- http://www.escop.com/epjcontents.htm
  The European Phytojournal—the Official Newsletter of the European Scientific Cooperative On Phytotherapy (ESCOP)—free on the Web. Contents include the following:
  - Scientific papers from ESCOP international symposia
  - Regulatory reviews of the status of phytomedicines and phytotherapy in Europe
  - Regular updates of research and clinical literature
  - Links to relevant information resources and sites
  - News of ESCOP national association, members, and professional, educational, and other related activities
- http://www.bl.uk/collections/health/amed.html
  The British Library's Allied and Complementary Medicine Database (AMED). Comprises a selection of journals in complementary medicines, physiotherapy, occupational therapy, rehabilitation, podiatry, palliative care, and other professions allied to medicine. Includes abstracts for many records for articles published from 1995 onward. Covers relevant references to articles from more than 400 journals, many not indexed by other biomedical sources.
- http://www.ods.od.nih.gov/
  The National Institutes of Health (NIH) in the United States are the biggest source of health research and information in the world. The Office of Dietary Supplements in the NIH has put together this site to collect all the research carried out on supplements, such as vitamins, minerals, herbal products, and so forth, that has been reported in both orthodox and natural medicines. Although it is still being built, the site offers access to articles dating back about 10 years and is about the best of its kind for accessing nonbiased information about some over-the-counter herbals.

EVIDENCE-BASED MEDICINE

The final theme for this chapter, which is not directly related to phytopharmacology but is vitally related to the issue of biomedical research in phytotherapy, is that of evidence-based medicine (EBM).

Historically, evidence in medicine (and herbal medicine) has been based on case studies and practitioner observation. EBM was pioneered by researchers at McMaster University, Canada. They defined EBM as the conscientious, explicit, and judicious use of current best evidence in decision making about the care of *individual* patients. Decision making with the use of EBM is not limited to randomized controlled clinical trials, although it holds such studies in highest regard.

Evaluation criteria in EBM include the following:

- Are the results valid? Any bias in the design or confounding factors?
- What are the results? This is heavily influenced by the statistical methods employed.
- Will the results help my patient? Is it safe?

When we backtrack slightly to how a new drug is developed and approved, as well as to information on the clinical trials necessary to achieve this, it is evident that this is a highly artificial situation. Usually, trials include carefully selected groups of patients, typically middle-aged white men. Exclusion criteria aim to reduce the impact of confounding factors. However, this does not necessarily provide a true picture of the effect on other groups such as women, children, and the sick or elderly.

Do common medical practices reflect EBM? The following are common practices not supported by EBM. A meta-analysis of eight clinical trials found that the use of antibiotics in otherwise healthy people with acute bronchitis was not justified (Chandran, 2001). Antipyretic therapy has yet to prove effective in preventing febrile seizures (El-Radhi, 2003).

The Cochrane Reviews, which reflect the EBM approach, have the following to say about some common prescribing habits. Evidence for use of motility-enhancing drugs in nonulcer dyspepsia is inconclusive (Moayyedi, 2004). No evidence justifies the use of minocycline as front-line treatment in moderate acne (Garner, 2004). Evidence is inconclusive to support the use of spironolactone in acne (Farquhar, 2004). No convincing evidence indicates that tacrine is a useful long-term treatment for patients with symptoms of Alzheimer's disease (Qizilbash, 1998). The value of antibiotics in acute otitis media in children is modest, and their use is probably not justified against potential risks (Glasziou, 2004). Yet, these drugs are being used in these situations on a daily basis. If we put this into an economic perspective, the global dollar value of non-EBM use of drugs far exceeds the total global value of the whole herbal medicine market.

EBM and Phytotherapy

Attempts to generate evidence for phytotherapeutic practice must be consistent with the inherent properties of the medicines and the way they are used. Factors to be considered in the design of clinical trials on phytotherapy include individual variation in response to treatment; n of 1 or single patient trials could be an option here. Individual prescribing, the testing of combinations, and the use of appropriate clinical outcomes are all issues that need to be addressed. Despite these issues, a growing clinical evidence base supports the use of a number of key herbs. A German team recently summarized 58 systematic reviews of clinical trials involving specific herbal treatments (Linde, 2001).

TABLE 7-2

Levels of Evidence in Human Medical Decision Making

Levels of Evidence	
Level 1:	Evidence obtained from a systematic review of all relevant randomized controlled trials
Level 2:	Evidence obtained from at least one properly designed randomized controlled trial
Level 3:	Evidence obtained from well-designed controlled trials without randomization
	Evidence obtained from well-designed cohort or case control analytic studies, preferably from more than one center or research group
	Evidence obtained from multiple time series with or without the intervention. Dramatic results in uncontrolled experiments* could also be regarded as this type of evidence
Level 4:	Opinions of respected authorities, based on clinical experience, descriptive studies, or reports of expert committees
Traditional evidence	Does traditional use fit in here? Yes, according to the Australian Therapeutic Goods Administration—but at a lower level. There is a need to develop ways of defining this knowledge better, so that its acceptability and utility as evidence are strengthened. New techniques are available for analyzing generated data (e.g., Bayesian statistics). The correlation of the phytochemical content of a plant with its traditional use can also serve to strengthen the evidence base

*Such as the results of the introduction of penicillin treatment in the 1940s.

Although randomized, controlled clinical trials are considered to be the gold standard of evidence, other levels of evidence are outlined in Table 7-2.

Does Traditional Knowledge Constitute an Evidence Base?

Thomas Bayes was a Presbyterian minister in the mid-18th century. He developed an approach that is now used in statistics that incorporates previous knowledge to determine the probability that a hypothesis is true. Put another way, with Bayesian methods, probability is not treated as an intrinsic property of a system, but rather as a statement about an observer's state of knowledge of the system. An example is the sun rising and predicting whether it will rise the next day.

Bayesian methods might be particularly suited to attaching a level of evidence (or certainty) to the data generated from previous traditional use and current traditional practice. For more information on the issue of the role of traditional knowledge as an evidence base for modern herbal practice, see an excellent review by Simon Mills (Mills, 2002).

CONCLUSIONS

For scientific research to be valuable for modern herbal practice, scientists must do the following:

- Develop more meaningful models to relate phytochemical content to pharmacologic and clinical outcomes. Only then can quality, safety, and efficacy be meaningfully optimized
- Investigate further the concept that plants act as a whole and demonstrate synergy—a fact often talked about by herbalists, but for which there is relatively little pharmacologic evidence to date
- Better understand how commonly used herbs work
- Develop clinical models that better incorporate the way phytotherapy is practiced in a holistic context

Evidence-based phytotherapy should not necessarily adopt the same models as conventional medicine. There is a need to do the following:

- Develop clinical models that better reflect what is known about phytotherapy and how it is practiced
- Better establish traditional knowledge as an integral part of an evidence-based approach to phytotherapy

A Phytotherapist's Perspective

I would like to conclude by offering a personal perspective on phytopharmacologic research.

The philosopher and teacher Rudolf Steiner once said that, for every human illness, somewhere in the world, there exists a plant that is the cure. I believe that there is a healing potential locked inside plants that is integral to their evolution, just as it is part of human evolution to learn to tap this wonderful gift of Nature.

This is the passion of the herbalist as a scientist: to unlock the healing potential of plants by combining the time-honored wisdom of traditional knowledge with sound clinical experience and the rigor of scientific research. This quest can be achieved only by means of a total commitment to understanding the complex issues of quality and continuous improvement as they apply to medicinal plants.

ACKNOWLEDGMENTS

Thanks to Michelle Morgan, Berris Burgoyne, and Michael Thomsen for assistance with the section on accessing research information.

References

Baker ME. Endocrine activity of plant-derived compounds: an evolutionary perspective. Proc Soc Exp Biol Med 1995;208:131-138.

Bauer R, Remiger P, Jurcic K, et al. Influence of Echinacea extracts on phagocytotic activity. Z Phytother 1989;10:43-48.

Bauer R, Wagner H. Echinacea Species as Potential Immunostimulatory Drugs In: Wagner H, Farnsworth NR, eds. *Economic and Medicinal Plant Research,* vol 5. London: Academic Press; 1991:303-305.

Bauer R, Wagner H. Echinacea Species as Potential Immunostimulatory Drugs In: Wagner H, Farnsworth NR, eds. *Economic and Medicinal Plant Research,* vol 5. London: Academic Press; 1991:280-283.

Bensoussan A, Talley NJ, Hing M, et al. Treatment of irritable bowel syndrome with Chinese herbal medicine: a randomized controlled trial. JAMA 1998;280:1585-1589

Berdyshev EV. Cannabinoid receptors and the regulation of immune response. Chem Phys Lipids 2000;108:169-190.

Butterweck V, Christoffel V, Nahrstedt A, et al. Step by step removal of hyperforin and hypericin: activity profile of different *Hypericum* preparations in behavioral models. Life Sci 2003;73:627-639.

Butterweck V, Lieflander-Wulf U, Winterhoff H, et al. Plasma levels of hypericin in presence of procyanidin B2 and hyperoside: a pharmacokinetic study in rats. Planta Med 2003;69: 189-192.

Chandran R. Should we prescribe antibiotics for acute bronchitis? Am Fam Physician 2001;64:135-138.

Egert D, Beuschner N. Studies on antigen specificity of immunoreactive arabinogalactan proteins extracted from *Baptisia tinctoria* and *Echinacea purpurea.* Planta Med 1992;58: 163-165.

Ellingwood F. *American Materia Medica, Therapeutics and Pharmacognosy.* Portland, Ore: Eclectic Medical Publications; 1993.

El-Radhi AS, Barry W. Do antipyretics prevent febrile convulsions? Arch Dis Child 2003;88:641-642.

Farquhar C, Lee O, Toomath R, et al. Spironolactone versus placebo or in combination with steroids for hirsutism and/or acne (Cochrane Review). Chichester, UK: John Wiley & Sons, Ltd.; 2004.

Felter HW, Lloyd JU. *King's American Dispensatory.* 18th ed, 3rd rev. First published 1905, reprinted. Portland, Ore: Eclectic Medical Publications; 1983.

Fride E. The endocannabinoid-CB receptor system: importance for development and in pediatric disease. Neuro Endocrinol Lett 2004;25:24-30.

Garner SE, Eady EA, Popescu C, et al. *Minocycline for Acne Vulgaris Vulgaris:Efficacy and Safety* (Cochrane Review). Chichester, UK: John Wiley & Sons, Ltd.; 2004.

Gertsch J, Schoop R, Kuenzle U, et al. Alkylamides from *Echinacea purpurea* potently modulate TNF-alpha gene expression: possible role of cannabinoid receptor CB2, NF-κB, P38, MAPK and JNK pathways. Presented at: International Congress on Natural Products Research; July 31-August 4, 2004; Phoenix, Ariz. Lecture O:9.

Gertsch J, Schoop R, Kuenzle U, et al. Echinacea alkylamides modulate TNF-α gene expression via cannabinoid receptor CB2 and multiple signal transduction pathways. FEBS Lett 2004;577:563-569.

Glasziou PP, Del Mar CB, Sanders SL, et al. Antibiotics for acute otitis media in children (Cochrane Review). Chichester, UK: John Wiley & Sons, Ltd.; 2004.

Goel V, Chang C, Slama JV, et al. Alkylamides of *Echinacea purpurea* stimulate alveolar macrophage function in normal rats. Int Immunopharmacol 2002;2:381-387.

Grotenhermen F. Pharmacology of cannabinoids. Neuro Endocrinol Lett 2004;25:14-23.

Kisa K, Sasaki K, Yamauchi K, et al. Potentiating effect of sennoside C on the purgative activity of sennoside A. Planta Med 1981;42:302-303.

Klein TW, Lane B, Newton C, et al. The cannabinoid system and cytokine network. Proc Soc Exp Biol Med 2000;225:1-8.

Lehmann R, Penman K. Personal communication 2002.

Linde K, ter Riet G, Hondras M, et al. Systematic reviews of complementary therapies—an annotated bibliography. Part 2: Herbal medicine, BMC Complementary and Alternative Medicine, 2001. Available at: http://www.biomedcentral.com/1472-6882/1/5. Accessed February 24, 2004.

Matthias A, Penman KG, Bone KM, et al. Echinacea—what constituents are therapeutically important? Presented at: International Congress on Natural Products Research; July 31-August 4, 2004; Phoenix, Ariz. Lecture O:8.

Melchart D, Clemm C, Weber B, et al. Polysaccharides isolated from *Echinacea purpurea herba* cell cultures to counteract undesired effects of chemotherapy—a pilot study. Phytother Res 2002;16:138-142.

Mills S. Herbal medicine. In: Lewit G, Jonas WB, Walach H, eds. *Clinical Research in Complementary Therapies: Principles, Problems and Solutions.* Edinburgh: Churchill Livingstone; 2002:211-227.

Mills S, Bone K. Principles of Herbal Pharmacology, in *Principles and Practice of Phytotherapy: Modern Herbal Medicine.* Edinburgh: Churchill Livingstone; 2000:22-79.

Mills S, Bone K. Valerian, in *Principles and Practice of Phytotherapy: Modern Herbal Medicine.* Edinburgh: Churchill Livingstone; 2000:581-589.

Mills S, Bone K. Principles of Herbal Pharmacology, in *Principles and Practice of Phytotherapy: Modern Herbal Medicine.* Edinburgh: Churchill Livingstone; 2000:71.

Moayyedi P, Soo S, Deeks J, et al. Pharmacological interventions for non-ulcer dyspepsia (Cochrane Review).Chichester, UK: John Wiley & Sons, Ltd.; 2004.

Qizilbash N, Whitehead A, Higgins J, et al. Cholinesterase inhibition for Alzheimer disease: a meta-analysis of the tacrine trials. Dementia Trialists' Collaboration. JAMA 1998;280: 1777-1782.

Ralevic V. Cannabinoid modulation of peripheral autonomic and sensory neurotransmission. Eur J Pharmacol 2003;472:1-21.

Salzet M, Breton C, Bisogno T, et al. Comparative biology of the endocannabinoid system possible role in the immune response. Eur J Biochem 2000;267:4917-4927.

Schumacher B, Scholle S, Holzl J, et al. Lignans isolated from valerian: identification and characterization of a new olivil derivative with partial agonistic activity at A(1) adenosine receptors. J Nat Prod 2002;65:1479-1485.

Wagner H. Herbal immunostimulants. Z Phytother 1996;17: 79-95.

Williamson EM. Synergy and other interactions in phytomedicines. Phytomedicine 2001;8:401-409.

Woelkart K, Koidl C, Grisold A, et al. Pharmacokinetics and bioavailability of alkamides from the roots of *Echinacea angustifolia* in humans after oral application. Presented at: International Congress on Natural Products Research; July 31-August 4, 2004; Phoenix, Ariz. Lecture O:10.

Woelkart K, Xu W, Makriyannis A, et al. The endocannabinoid system as a target for alkamides from Echinacea roots. Presented at: International Congress on Natural Products Research; July 31-August 4, 2004; Phoenix, Ariz. Poster P:342.

Wuttke W, Jarry H, Christoffel V, et al. Chaste tree *(Vitex agnus-castus)* pharmacology and clinical indications. Phytomedicine 2003;10:348-357.

Regulation and Quality Control

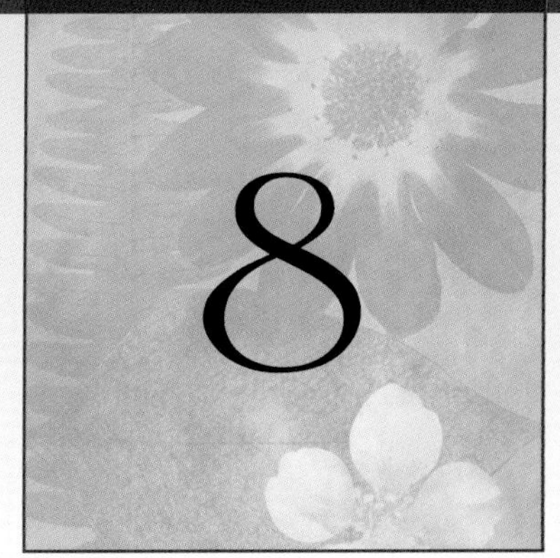

CHAPTER

William Bookout and Linda B. Khachatoorian

REGULATORY STATUS OF HERBAL MEDICINE WORLDWIDE

The regulatory status and quality control of herbs worldwide are as diverse as the countries they come from. The sophistication of herbal remedies often correlates with the technological advances of the countries that produce and use herbs or herbal products. Products range from teas to traditional crude pills to standardized herbal medicines (phytomedicines) produced in pharmaceutical facilities.

Sophisticated regulations control phytomedicines in some countries; in others, they are regarded as food or supplements, and therapeutic claims are prohibited. In countries where traditional or folk medicine is practiced extensively, no statutes may be in place to establish herbal medicines within a regulatory framework; however, many of these countries are developing regulations and guidelines with the help of the World Health Organization (WHO). In the international herbal trade market, economic incentive for many of these countries is increasing, and the potential for export of native herbal ingredients to countries that have implemented regulations has resulted in a higher standard for manufacturing practices.

In human herbal medicine, regulatory approaches for products range from a mandate of the same regulatory requirements as for drugs to exemption from all regulatory requirements. With regard to veterinary herbal medicines, the regulatory status is overall even less developed but is often considered to be equal to that for human herbal medicines. When veterinary herbal products are neither regulated nor registered, a responsible, fair system is needed to attest to proof of quality, to ensure safe and proper use, and to oblige companies to report adverse events.

Europe

The European Union has developed the "Directive on Food Supplements," which has been adopted by the European Parliament and took effect in August of 2005. The 25 countries that make up the European Union implemented the directive, which contains a "positive list" of vitamin and mineral ingredients that are allowed in food supplements.

The Codex Alimentarius Commission, a joint project of the Food and Agricultural Organization of the United Nations and the WHO, also adopted international guidelines on vitamin and mineral food supplements in the Summer of 2005. The Draft Guidelines for Vitamin and Mineral Food Supplements include "other ingredients," which may include herbs when included in a supplement. Food supplements that include herbal ingredients "should also be in conformity with the specific rules on vitamins and minerals." In addition, the World Trade Organization has developed an international Agreement on the Application of Sanitary and Phytosanitary Measures, which defines standards for food safety, veterinary drug and pesticide residues, contaminants, methods of analysis and sampling, and codes and guidelines for hygienic practice (American Herbal Products Association, 2005).

The European Agency for the Evaluation of Medicinal Products has developed guidance documents for Human and Veterinary Medicinal Product Quality (European Agency for the Evaluation of Medicinal Products, 2001). Guidance includes qualitative and quantitative measures of active substances; description of preparation methods, material controls, intermediate and finished testing procedures, and final stability tests.

The same agency has also developed guidelines on specifications, test procedures, and acceptance criteria for herbal medicinal products, herbal drugs, and herbal drug preparations (European Agency for the Evaluation of Medicinal Products, 2001). The document provides a uniform set of specifications for herbal products.

To further the standardization effort and to increase European scientific support, the phytotherapy societies of Austria, Denmark, Belgium, France, Germany, Ireland, Italy, Netherlands, Norway, Spain, Sweden, Switzerland, Turkey, and the United Kingdom founded the European

Societies' Cooperative on Phytotherapy (ESCOP). ESCOP objectives include: developing a coordinated framework to scientifically assess herbal medicines for humans, promoting their acceptance within general medical practices, and supporting phytotherapy research and the production of reference monographs.

China

Traditional Chinese Medicine production has been undergoing modernization, standardization, and internationalization efforts for the past 10 years. The "Five P's" that have formed the basis for these changes are: Good Agricultural Practice (GAP), Good Manufacturing Practice (GMP), Good Laboratory Practice, Good Clinical Practice, and Good Selling Practice. The focus on certification and registration of herbal/TCM manufacturers has been strong. Good Manufacturing Practices are fundamental requirements for registration. China has more than 1500 herbal material manufacturers that have completed GMP certification. The GAP outlines environmental conditions; seeds and propagation materials; cultivation practices; harvesting and primary processing; packaging, transportation, and storage; quality control; personnel and equipment; and documentation requirements. Good Agricultural Practices are being implemented, with farmers and raw ingredient suppliers reaching full compliance by 2007 (Starling, 2003).

Japan

Japan has also developed Good Agricultural and Collection Practices for Medicinal Plants (GACP) 2003. The GACP provides technical guidance for the production of medicinal plant materials for crude drugs, finished crude drugs, and Kampo medicines. Areas covered include cultivation and collection of medicinal plants, postharvest processing, and quality control of plant materials. Reference standards for the GACP include the Japanese Pharmacopoeia and Japanese Standards for Herbal Medicines. The regulation of herbal products in Japan is similar to that for chemical drugs.

Africa

African nations have a wealth of natural resources and have developed a renewal program for their plant genetic resources (International Environmental Law Research Centre, 2002-2003). The focus of the program will be on agriculture, health and nutrition, environment, poverty alleviation, and scientific/technical research. Herbal medicine for human and animal health is strong in local cultures and traditions, where the ratio of traditional herbalists to villagers is 1:200. Up to 80% of rural populations depend on traditional medicine to meet their primary healthcare needs. Realizing the potential of scientific, health, and economic impact, the Plant Genetic Resources program simultaneously focuses on strengthening environmental conservation through the development of national and regional programs.

Australia

The Australian Register of Therapeutic Goods (ARTG) was established under the Therapeutic Goods Act (TGA) of 1989. The ARTG database contains two basic lists—medicines and medical devices. A search of the ARTG database reveals more than 1000 "herbal" products that have been registered. Australia has adopted the guidelines produced by the European Agency for the Evaluation of Medicinal Products. The guidance documents for Human and Veterinary Medicinal Product Quality (European Agency for the Evaluation of Medicinal Products, 2001) include qualitative and quantitative measures of active substances, description of preparation methods, material controls, intermediate and finished testing procedures, and final stability tests.

Australia has also adopted the same agency's guidelines on specifications, test procedures and acceptance criteria for herbal medicinal products, herbal drugs, and herbal drug preparations (European Agency for the Evaluation of Medicinal Products, 2001). The document provides a uniform set of specifications for herbal products.

New Zealand

The regulation of herbal substances in New Zealand is the same as in Australia. This came about through the formation of a joint agency in December of 2003—the Trans-Tasman Therapeutic Products Agency—with full implementation in July of 2005. Core issues of the joint effort are identified in a consultation paper; these include definition of "herbal substance," naming of herbally derived substances that do not meet the definition, regulation of complex and nontraditional herbal extracts, expression of dry/fresh weight equivalence, extracts, and the standardization of herbal ingredients. Key objectives of the Trans-Tasman Therapeutic Products Agency were to develop a regulatory scheme for products to safeguard public health and safety in both Australia and New Zealand and to facilitate trade and closer economic relations between these countries. Therefore, New Zealand uses the same guidance documents for Human and Veterinary Medicinal Product Quality as those produced by the European Agency for the Evaluation of Medicinal Products.

Canada

In January of 2004, the Natural Health Products (NHP) regulations came into effect. These regulations establish NHPs as a subset of drugs, and allow a 6-year transition period. Canadian regulatory oversight will include the following: (1) premarketing review and approval; (2) GMP; (3) a manufacturing site license; (4) clinical trial processes; and (5) a postmarketing surveillance program for adverse reactions.

United States of America

The regulatory status and quality control processes applied to herbal supplements for use in animals are topics that are confusing and involve issues that most people do not clearly understand. Further complicating these issues is the fact the regulatory situation is changing rapidly as discussions between industry participants and regulatory agencies continue; therefore, what is true today may not be true tomorrow.

REGULATION OF SUPPLEMENTS FOR ANIMALS

The goals of this section are as follows:

- To provide the reader with enough information to enhance understanding of the current situation and to dispel some misconceptions or misunderstandings regarding the regulatory status of herbal supplements for animals in the United States
- To allow the reader to make more informed decisions when selecting a product by elevating level of knowledge and understanding regarding herbal products
- To clearly communicate how the reader can become personally involved in ensuring that these products will remain available and in elevating industry standards

Definitions

- **AAFCO (American Association of Feed Control Officials)**—a not-for-profit association with purpose to "establish and maintain an Association through which officials of any State, Province, Dominion, District, Territory, Republic, Commonwealth, or Federal or other governmental agency . . . may unite to explore the problems encountered in administering such (feed) laws, to develop just and equitable standards, definitions, and policies to be followed . . . to promote uniformity in laws, regulations, and enforcement policies, and to cooperate with members of industry . . ." (AAFCO, 2004). AAFCO is a nonregulatory association that recommends regulatory policy; however, it has no regulatory power in and of itself
- **Companion Animals**—a dog, cat, horse, or other animal not intended for human consumption. (In certain examples, such as for tax purposes, horses are considered livestock. However, in most cases, horses are not intended for human consumption in the United States and therefore are considered companion animals for purposes of administering supplements.)
- **DSHEA** (The Dietary Supplement Health and Education Act of 1994)—act that was passed by Congress and signed into law in October of 1994. (The DSHEA bill created formal categorical recognition for dietary supplements for humans. Language was not included for companion animals. Although supplements are available for animals that are similar to products marketed for people, the FDA has determined that DSHEA does not apply to animals.)
- **FFDCA**—Federal Food and Drug Cosmetic Act of 1934
- **FDA/CVM**—US Food and Drug Administration/Center for Veterinary Medicine
- **GRAS (Generally Recognized As Safe)**—substances considered to be food additives that are generally recognized as safe for their intended use within the meaning of section 409 of the FFDCA
- **National Animal Supplement Council (NASC)**—a not-for-profit industry trade association founded in 2001 that represents industry participants and other stakeholders involved in providing or using supplements for nonhuman food chain animals
- **NHFC (Nonhuman Food Chain)**—an animal (i.e., dog, cat, or horse) that is not considered to be part of the human food chain
- **Novel ingredient**—an ingredient that is unapproved or unrecognized as a feed ingredient
- **Supplements (FDA/CVM)**—The US Food and Drug Administration/Center for Veterinary Medicine describes supplements as follows: "The Center for Veterinary Medicine is often asked to comment on the status under the Act of products intended for the nutritional supplementation of foods for animals. Such products would include vitamins, minerals, protein supplements, and fatty acid sources. The diets of livestock, poultry, and fur-bearing animals are usually planned by nutritionists or other experts, and the nutritional ingredients are sold through industrial channels. On the other hand, nutritional supplements for companion animals such as cats, dogs, and horses not intended for food, as well as other pets, are mostly sold over the counter direct to lay customers and are generally intended merely for the dietary supplementation of the particular species for which they are intended." (FDA/CVM CPG 7126.04)
- **Supplements (NASC)**—The National Animal Supplement Council submitted a new definition to the FDA/CVM for consideration, which defined supplements for animals as follows: "The Federal Food, Drug, and Cosmetic Act (the Act), Sec. 201 (f), defines the term 'food' as an article used for food or drink for man or other animals including components of such articles. Furthermore, Sec. 201(ff) of the Act defines the term dietary supplement' as a product intended to supplement the diet that bears or contains one or more of the following dietary ingredients: vitamin; mineral; herb, or other botanical; amino acid; a concentrate, metabolite, constituent, extract, or combination of any ingredients described. Sec. 201(g)(1) defines the term 'drug' as (C) articles (other than food) intended to affect the structure or any function of the body of man or other animals (NASC, 2003)"

Background

Although supplements are commonly available for animals, similar to products available for human use, most people do not understand that there is no specific regulatory category for dietary supplements (herbal products) for animals. The timeline examines events that specifically created categorical recognition for human products now referred to as "dietary supplements," and it explains why the human category does not apply to supplements for companion animals (Box 8-1).

BOX 8-1

Evolution and Timeline

1900—No federal law exists to regulate food and drugs

1906—Pure Food and Drug Act established

1938—Federal Food Drug and Cosmetic Act established

1951—Durham-Humphrey Amendment—FDA classifies drugs as OTC or prescription only

1993—FDA publishes Advanced Notice of Rulemaking for Dietary Supplements

October 25, 1994—Dietary Supplement Health Education Act (DSHEA) becomes law

April 1996—FDA/CVM publishes notice in the Federal Register stating the reasons why DSHEA did not apply to animals. This opinion means that supplements for animals are considered either animal feed or unapproved drugs

February 1999—US Court of Appeals for the Third Circuit—the Court stated that it appears that the DSHEA does not apply to dietary supplements intended for veterinary use

1999 to 2001:

- Products increasing in demand and availability
- Novel Ingredients Task Force formed by American Association of Feed Control Officials (AAFCO)—unsuccessful
- Botanicals & Herbs Committee formed by AAFCO—unsuccessful

August 2001—Enforcement strategy for marketed ingredients announced by AAFCO. Perception on removing products from the marketplace is eminent

November 2001—National Animal Supplement Council (NASC) formed

April 2002—Initial meeting of industry resulted in submission of Compliance Plus proposal for industry self-regulation to AAFCO and FDA/CVM. Primary objectives:

- Establishing a nationwide adverse event reporting system
- Establishing research and risk management initiatives
- Establishing consistent labeling guidelines for nonfeed products
- Establishing quality systems requirements similar to Current Good Manufacturing Practices (cGMP) guidelines for human supplement products

July 2002—NASC submits ingredient definition for glucosamine for approval as a feed ingredient

August 2002—AAFCO-ESMI Committee recommends Comfrey as a target ingredient to be removed from animal feed because of safety concerns

January 2003—NASC submits ingredient definition for methylsulfonyl methane (MSM) for approval as a feed ingredient

January 2003—FDA/CVM declines to approve glucosamine as feed ingredient

February 2003—NASC focuses on completing ingredient risk assessment for all ingredients contained in members products and forms Scientific Advisory Committee (SAC)

July 2003—NASC submits ingredient risk recommendations for 631 ingredients following review of recognized panel of experts

August 2003—NASC completes adverse event reporting system for members; trains CVM personnel

August 2003—AAFCO–ESMI Committee recommends kava kava as a target ingredient to be removed from animal feed because of safety concerns

September 2003—State of Iowa announces intention to remove all products that contain unapproved ingredients on the basis of safety concerns. The announcement specifically includes glucosamine products

October–November 2003—NASC takes aggressive grass roots action resulting in compromise position that is acceptable to state officials and industry members

January 2004—FDA/CVM declines to approve MSM as feed ingredient

March 2004—NASC submits labeling guidelines for nonfeed products, based on intended use. Resulting communications, direction, and numerous discussions render feed ingredient pathway closed

April 2004—NASC submits quality systems requirements (QSR) documents for production of animal supplements

April 2004—NASC finalizes ingredient risk assessment profiles for all ingredients currently in the marketplace. Reports display quantitative data for use/risk by primary species

April—May 2004—NASC conducts training programs for all member companies for labeling, adverse event reporting requirements, use/range database, research initiatives, and quality system guidelines/requirements

July–August 2004—NASC conducts presentations at CVM and AAFCO with demonstrated accomplishments and provides access to data under confidentiality agreement

August 2004—AAFCO-ESMI Committee recommends pennyroyal oil as a target ingredient to be removed from animal feed because of safety concerns

Before President Clinton signed the Dietary Supplement Health Education Act, dietary supplements for humans were considered food or drugs. DSHEA created a specific category for dietary supplements and made allowances for these products to be legally marketed under certain provisions defined in the language of the bill. One of the primary items addressed the use of labeling claims. Overt drug claims that referred to a product involving the diagnosis, prevention, treatment, or ability to cure a disease were prohibited; however, claims involving a product's ability to effect the "structure or function" of the body were allowed.

Although it was widely assumed, most people do not realize that DSHEA did not mention the use of these products for animals. Examination of the Congressional record suggests that the issue of products being useful for companion animals was simply not considered when language for the Bill was discussed. Nonetheless, because the benefit of these products for humans has been recognized, the animal supplement industry continues to grow, and the availability of various products for animals increases.

In today's regulatory environment, in the absence of a specific category, supplements labeled for animals are considered animal feeds that contain unapproved ingredients or unapproved drugs, depending on intended use. In point of fact, neither category provides an appropriate or realistic pathway; however, the FDA/CVM further elaborated:

> "Thus, substances marketed as dietary supplements for humans still fall under the pre-DSHEA regulatory scheme when marketed for animals; that is, they are considered food, food additives, new animal drugs, or GRAS, depending on the intended use. Most of these types of products on the market would be considered unapproved and unsafe food additives or new animal drugs based on current intended uses. While these products are technically in violation of the law, they are of low enforcement priority except for when public or animal health concerns arise. CVM's concerns about certain dietary supplements focus on three main areas:
>
> 1. Human food safety—ingredients that are used in food animals, including horses that are used for food, must be shown to be safe for people who consume products from these animals. Without these data, there is no assurance that animal-derived food is safe.
> 2. Animal safety—ingredients must be shown to be safe for animals. CVM and AAFCO have not received data indicating that these products have actually been tested on animals to show that a particular level is appropriate or safe for the animals.
> 3. Manufacturing quality—supplements must be shown to be manufactured to a consistent standard (e.g., shown to contain a given amount of the ingredient).
>
> In addition, some of these products are being used and/or marketed to treat or prevent disease. This moves them from the supplement category into the drug category. CVM is concerned that these products have not been shown to be safe and effective. And some owners may be using these products in lieu of obtaining appropriate veterinary treatment for their animals (FDA Veterinarian, 2002)."

Many herbal ingredients have been given GRAS status by the FDA and the AAFCO and are categorized as feed additives, with their intended use defined as "spices and other natural seasonings and flavorings," or "essential oils, oleoresins, and natural extractives" (AAFCO, 2004). The quantity of the ingredient added to animal food should not exceed the amount reasonably required to accomplish its intended physical, nutritional, or other technical effect in the food (FDA 21 CFR Sec 582.1). When GRAS ingredients with the intended uses listed previously are incorporated into an animal supplement with the purpose being to "effect the structure or any function of the body," they are then considered by regulatory agencies to be unapproved ingredients, thereby causing the product to be "adulterated." Intended use is designated by claims made by the manufacturer in labeling and advertising statements (US Dept of Health and Human Services, 2004). Although current regulations do not contain a category for these GRAS ingredients intended for use as "animal supplements affecting the animal's body structure or function," an appendix list has been included.

Many industry members have tried to label these products as animal feed, in following the recommendations of the AAFCO. This regulatory pathway is inappropriate; however, in the absence of a specific alternative, the animal feed category was viewed as the only viable choice and came with its own set of challenges. There is no consistency among State Feed Control Officials in regulating these products or ingredients. Companies that attempt to provide supplement products and comply with feed guidelines are faced with inconsistency among the states. In other words, one state may allow the products to be sold or may require specific labeling on a formula that may not be acceptable to another state. It is quite clear that providers cannot develop and sell different labeled product for each different state. Some states have taken a hard line stand in issuing "stop sale" orders to companies when products are found in distribution. In an extreme example, the State of Iowa issued the following directive on September 18, 2003:

> "The attachment with this letter is a listing of the most commonly used drug claims, inappropriate claims for feed products, and unapproved ingredients. Those companies who will be registering feed products for the year 2004 are asked to review this list (antioxidants, probiotics, glucosamine and chondroitin, and unapproved feed additives were specifically mentioned). If you find that any of your company's product contain these label discrepancies or unapproved feed additives, please do not attempt to register these products. Please remove from your registration those products that are adulterated and are already in distribution. Your company will be allowed until December 1, 2003, the appointed date for the mailing of your small package pet food renewal, to remove these products from distribution or re-label the products so that they are within compliance of Iowa law. Adulterated products that are found in distribution will be placed on stop sale and removed from distribution (Iowa Department of Agriculture and Land Stewardship, 2003)."

Therefore, all products that contain unapproved feed ingredients labeled as animal feed would be removed from the marketplace. This crisis was averted because of a significant Grass Roots effort by the National Animal Supplement Council (www.nasc.cc) that focused on the State of Iowa.

What Exists Today?

More than 62% of American households own a nonhuman food chain (NHFC) animal (dog, cat, or horse) (American Pet Product Manufacturers, 2001), and 90% of veterinarians use supplements in their practice. Numerous studies indicate that about a third of these NHFC animals receive a daily dietary supplement (AVMA, 2002; Yankelovich Consultants, 2000; Healthy Pets 21

Consortium, 2001). Thus the rights of more than 20% of American households to give their horses, dogs, or cats supplements are affected by this issue.

Supplements used in NHFC animals closely resemble human dietary supplements, with ingredients such as glucosamine, methylsulfonyl methane (MSM), herbs, vitamins, and minerals. They are used by animal owners and veterinarians to assist with normal physiologic functions, enhance wellness, affect the structure/function of body tissues/systems, and—in the case of some products—avoid or forestall the need to euthanize their dog, cat, or horse.

In 1994, recognizing that an unpredictable, inconsistent, inappropriate regulatory pathway for dietary supplements was restricting access to products that had the potential to enhance wellness, Congress passed the Dietary Supplement Health Education Act (DSHEA). In 1996, while acknowledging that "the definition of dietary supplement in DSHEA does not explicitly state whether it includes or excludes animals other than man (Federal Register, 1996)," the FDA took the position that DSHEA should not apply to animals, citing arguments that relied largely on protection of the human food chain.

Because of the FDA's interpretation, which made no distinction between "production" and NHFC animals, no viable regulatory framework or approval pathway exists for NHFC animal supplements. Depending on their intended use, NHFC animal supplements are sometimes regulated as animal feeds with unapproved ingredients (subject to enforcement under potentially 50 different feed laws) and in some cases are regulated by the FDA Center for Veterinary Medicine as unapproved animal drugs.

With regard to human supplements, the FDA has stated the following:

> "Dietary supplements can be considered as falling somewhere along the continuum between conventional foods on the one hand and drugs on the other (Federal Register, 2003)."

However, with regard to NHFC animal supplements, the CVM claims to be prevented from taking a similar approach because "DSHEA does not apply to animal products." This inconsistency is a legislative oversight that finds no basis in logic.

A rational federal framework must be established to supersede the current ad hoc, patchwork regulatory policy applied to dietary supplements for NHFC animals, primarily dogs, cats, and horses. The present environment of high regulatory uncertainty—including "stop sale" orders from numerous state feed control officials—restricts consumer and possibly professional access to products and interferes with interstate commerce. Potentially imminent restrictions on animal owner access to products that are readily available for humans threaten to become an emotional issue affecting more than 20% of American households, but this can be avoided by a reasonable solution that accomplishes the objectives of all stakeholders.

Requirements of the Animal Medicinal Drug Use Clarification Act (AMDUCA)

Herbs are not specifically addressed by the US Food and Drug Administration (FDA) or the American Association of Feed Control Officials (AAFCO) and are not (as of this writing) considered drugs. Herbs are therefore not covered by the AMDUCA, which provides guidelines for extralabel use of drugs. Still, the record keeping and labeling guidelines are sensible in the absence of other regulatory guidelines and are listed below.

Record Requirements

- Animals identified, either as individuals or a group
- Animal species treated
- Numbers of animals treated
- Condition being treated
- Established names of the drug and active ingredients *(Editor's note: For herbs, the accepted common name and the taxonomic designation should be listed)*
- Dosage prescribed or used
- Duration of treatment
- Specified withdrawal, withholding, or discard time(s), if applicable, for meat, milk, eggs, or animal-derived food
- Records kept for 2 years (FDA may need access to these records to estimate risk to public health)

Label Requirements

- Name and address of the prescribing veterinarian
- Established name of the drug *(See note on herb names, above)*
- Any specified directions for use, including the class/species or identification of the animal or herd, flock, pen, lot, or other group; the dosage frequency and route of administration; and the duration of therapy
- Any cautionary statements
- Your specified withdrawal, withholding, or discard time(s) for meat, milk, eggs, or any other food

Industry Efforts

Through the NASC, industry members have attempted to work within the existing framework to obtain "feed ingredient definitions" for both glucosamine and MSM—two substances with a significant history of safe use in both NHFC animals and humans. The FDA rejected both applications, indicating, "We do not believe it is in the public interest to regulate glucosamine as food or a food additive under the FFDCA (FDA, 2002)," and responded with similar language for MSM.

The new animal drug approval (NADA) process is currently industry's only alternative and can cost many millions of dollars. Given the smaller market size, the rules against patenting natural ingredients, and the potential for substitution with similar human products that do not face such requirements, the business-limiting factors for animal supplement providers render the NADA process unrealistic.

In an attempt to address these issues, the National Animal Supplement Council, a nonprofit industry association representing approximately 70% of the industry, put forward a comprehensive program of industry self-regulation titled *Compliance Plus*, which was submitted in April of 2002 to both the FDA Center for Veterinary Medicine and AAFCO. *Compliance Plus* consists of four major initiatives:

1. A comprehensive adverse event reporting system (NAERS), which would ultimately be available to the public
2. A Scientific Advisory Committee to pursue new ingredient approvals and effectively manage risk
3. Truthful, nationally consistent labeling and elimination of overt drug claims
4. Quality systems requirements similar to proposed DSHEA GMPs

NASC has promptly delivered on each of the commitments made in the *Compliance Plus* program. The FDA/CVM has attempted to respond to the cooperation from the NHFC supplement industry by regulating NHFC animal supplements with an intended use other than feed as "unapproved drugs of low regulatory priority." However, this is not a viable long-term solution for several reasons:

- It leaves industry in the position of selling "unapproved products"
- Any product that provides comprehensive nutritional support (i.e., contains a multivitamin) would continue to be regulated under state feed laws, subject to stop sale orders by states if they contain "unapproved" feed ingredients
- Most troubling under this arrangement, the FDA may require that any product that contains any herbal ingredient (in even a minute amount) must be sold on a prescription basis. This would create significant turmoil, and many pet owners may decide to use human products, which are not developed for animals. Moreover, under *Durham-Humphrey*, NASC believes such a requirement should be imposed only for "drugs unsafe for self-medication (FDA 1998)." The FDA has not presented data to support the position that these products present high risk in NHFC animals, and NASC believes that NAERS data argue against such a sweeping characterization

Possible Solutions

Existing law is ill suited to regulate supplements for NHFC animals. Industry has attempted self-regulation and extensive cooperation with the AAFCO and the FDA/CVM but may not appear to be able to achieve an acceptable solution under existing law. In fact, depending on enforcement actions by the FDA and state feed control officials, a potential crisis looms. One option may be that Congress has the opportunity to avert an emotional constituent issue affecting 20% of households by supporting an amendment to explicitly include NHFC animals in DSHEA. Alternatively, the FDA could amend its 1996 opinion on the applicability of DSHEA for animals not in the human food chain. Yet another option would be to introduce a stand-alone bill that is specifically drafted to apply to supplements marketed for non-human food chain animals. In the near term, the CVM could issue guidance to industry, essentially creating a responsible solution that is jointly developed by industry leaders and regulatory agencies. Although it is most desirable, it remains to be seen whether or not this will be possible.

The Role of Veterinary Herbalists

One should stay informed and knowledgeable regarding the status of establishing a reasonable approach; this ensures that products will continue to be available from responsible providers. Routine updates are provided on the Internet at www.nasc.cc.

Veterinary herbalists should get involved if and when necessary. If a legislative solution is required, it will take a coordinated effort by all stakeholders to emphasize to elected officials the importance of the issue. Veterinarian and client involvement will be keys to success.

Industry participants who are working diligently to achieve an optimal outcome that will be in everyone's best interest should be supported. Some companies are making the investment to create optimal outcomes for all stakeholders.

QUALITY CONTROL

From a global standpoint, quality control issues regarding herbal ingredient production are rapidly improving because of the implementation of national regulations. Many production steps and manufacturers stand between the grower and the animal that is being given a finished product. At each production step, quality control measures should be implemented to guarantee the finished product. Examples of the many quality measures that manufacturers implement according to their role in the process include GAP, Good Wild Crafting Practice (GWP), Good Laboratory Practice (GLP), GMP, and Best Manufacturing Practice (BMP).

Quality control of an herbal product is necessary for quality veterinary medicine. Unfortunately, herbal products are often considered inferior to conventional medicine, in part because there is a paucity of scientific verification and, perhaps more importantly, because of the historically wide variation in the quality of herbal products. Veterinary herbal manufacturers must change this and produce herbal products that are of consistent quality and utility. This can be accomplished by ensuring that each quality step of production has been performed in compliance with the guidelines listed in the previous paragraph. Manufacturers that produce high-quality products will certify the processes.

The issues of quality in veterinary herbal medicine include the following:

1. Quality of the raw materials (GAP/GWP). Raw materials must be of the right species, grown under optimum conditions for that plant, and harvested properly. They

must be dried appropriately and must not be contaminated with extraneous materials, other plants, herbicides, and other items.

2. Laboratory characterization of raw materials (GLP). Consistent analytic procedures performed to test each batch of herbs for macroscopic identification, microscopic identification, phytochemical characterization, potential impurities/contaminants/degradation products (heavy metals, pesticides, fumigants), moisture, and foreign matter, along with microbiological testing, chemical testing, and verification via various laboratory techniques. A certificate of analysis is provided to the manufacturer which outlines laboratory testing and results (Box 8-2).
3. Good Manufacturing Practice/Best Manufacturing Practice (GMP/BMP) (US Food and Drug Administration, 1999). Written procedures and records for production include the following:
   - Master and batch production specifications, including weight or measure of each raw material used and specifications of the finished product, developed and used in the manufacturing process; any deviation from lot acceptance criteria; written, approved specifications; standards; extraction procedures; assay procedures; or other laboratory control mechanisms
   - Equipment use and cleaning and sanitation records, including dates of use and product and lot number of each batch processed
   - Written procedures and records that demonstrate that automatic equipment is installed, maintained, checked, and recalibrated as necessary to ensure that it is capable of performing the intended functions
   - Written procedures and records for reprocessing of a product, including receipt, storage and handling, sampling, and examination of original packaging material
   - Written procedures and records to ensure that correct labels and labeling and safe packaging materials are used
   - Samples of each batch of dietary supplement product that are retained and stored under conditions consistent with the product labeling
   - Records retained for 1 year after expiration of the shelf-life of a lot of the animal supplement product or 3 years from the date of manufacture, whichever is greater
   - Written procedures and records for distribution that are developed and used and include the following:
     - Procedures and records for tracing distribution of product
     - Procedures and records for recalling a product
     - Written procedures and records for handling complaints, which include
       - Procedures developed and used for handling all written and oral complaints regarding a product, including provisions for appropriate review and evaluation by the person or unit responsible for quality control
       - Records concerning the handling of complaints, including any investigation, investigational findings, and follow-up action taken
       - Records retained for 1 year after expiration of the shelf-life of a lot of the dietary supplement product or 3 years from the date of manufacture, whichever is greater
     - Observations: review of records to ensure that
       - Procedures established to ensure good manufacturing practices are applied in day-to-day operations
       - Product that does not meet manufacturing specifications for purity, quality, strength, and composition is not distributed
4. Quantitative analysis/assay of pharmacologic activity. Quantitative analysis provides a validated method for identifying a compound that is most commonly associated with the pharmacologic activity of an herbal ingredient. This may include qualitative markers identified by pharmacologic literature. Methods for analysis are published in official pharmacopoeias such as the *United States Pharmacopoeia and Natural Formulary*, the *British Herbal Pharmacopoeia*, or the *Pharmacopoeia of the People's Republic of China*. Guidelines for the validation of analytic procedures for veterinary medical products have been published by the FDA/CVM (FDA/CVM, 1999) and are part of the Veterinary International Cooperation on Harmonization (VICH) that was launched in 1996 in a program with the European Union and Japan. Although test method guidelines are written specifically for drugs and not for animal supplements, comparative testing for herbal products may use some of these methods, such as standard precision, linearity, replicate sampling, selectivity, retention times, and limits of detection.

Quality control of supplements for NHFC animals is probably as misunderstood as the regulatory environment. For the most part, people have the "reasonable expectation" that the products they purchase are produced to some quality standards. The following section summarizes the situation that exists today in the United States.

BOX 8-2

Documentation Requirements of Chinese Herbal Production Techniques and Processes (WHO, 2002)

- Origin of propagation material
- Planting time/quantity and area
- Seedling growth, transplantation
- Fertilization—time, amount, and method
- Pesticide use—(including insecticides, fungicides, and herbicides); amount, time, and method of use
- Collection—amount, fresh weight, processing, drying, reduced weight after drying, transportation, and storage
- Meteorological data and micro-climatic records
- Quality evaluation—records of plant properties and inspection results of materials
- Record keeping—all records kept at least 5 years

No mandatory nationally published quality or current Good Manufacturing Practice Standards that manufacturers are required to follow are in place for animal supplements. The NASC has published quality systems requirements (QSRs) that members are required to implement.

Finished product quality is a function of control of the processes involved in producing a product. Testing a finished product may be an indicator of product quality; for a single production run, however, it does not guarantee that these results will be repeatable for different batches produced. Even the strictest quality control procedures are not foolproof. Continued vigilance in monitoring adverse events is a critical component of a comprehensive quality control system.

This is not to say that there are no quality products on the market, or that one should be suspicious of every manufacturer of supplements for animals. It does mean that the consumer should be aware of the situation and informed enough to ask the right questions when making decisions about products to purchase or recommend.

Definitions

(National Animal Supplement Council, 2004)

- **Acceptance Criteria**—product specifications and acceptance/rejection criteria, such as acceptable quality level and unacceptable quality level, with an associated sampling plan that is necessary for decision making on whether to accept or reject a lot or a batch (or any other convenient subgroups of manufactured units)
- **Adequate**—that which is needed to accomplish the intended purpose in keeping with good public health practice
- **AER**—Adverse event report
- **Adverse event report**—a complaint about a supplement for a nonhuman food chain animal that is linked to any negative physical effect or health problem that may be connected to or associated with use of the product
- **BMPs**—Best Manufacturing Practice Standards
- **Batch or Lot**—one or more components or finished supplements for nonhuman food chain animals that consist of a single type, model, class, size, or composition produced under essentially the same conditions and intended to have uniform characteristics and quality within specified limits
- **cGMP or GMPs**—Current Good Manufacturing Practice Standards
- **Certificate of Analysis (COA)**—a technical report that adequately defines product composition for a batch of product (specific lot number) and whose results are based on manufacturing and test data that can be used to determine whether product or ingredient meets the written specifications and requirements previously set
- **Complaint**—any written, electronic, or oral communication that alleges deficiencies related to the identity, quality, durability, reliability, safety, effectiveness, or performance of a supplement for nonhuman food chain animals after it has been released for distribution
- **Component**—any raw material, substance, piece, part, software, firmware, labeling, or assembly intended to be included as part of the finished, packaged, and labeled supplement for nonhuman food chain animals
- **Composition**—as appropriate:
  - (1) the identity of an ingredient or supplement.
  - (2) the concentration of an ingredient (e.g., weight or other unit of use/weight or volume) or the potency or activity of one or more ingredients, as indicated by appropriate procedures and testing specifications.
- **Control Number**—any unique distinctive symbol, such as a distinctive combination of letters or numbers, or both, from which the history of the manufacturing, packaging, labeling, and distribution of the unit, lot, or batch of supplements for nonhuman food chain animals can be determined
- **Finished Product**—any supplement for nonhuman food chain animals that is suitable for use
- **NAERS**—he National Animal Supplement Council Adverse Event Reporting System
- **NASC Best Manufacturing Practice (BMP) Standards**—defined guidelines and criteria with which a member of the National Animal Supplement Council must comply to meet the minimum quality controls for the manufacture of high-quality products with known composition and purity. (The NASC Best Manufacturing Practice Standards provide the means by which one can understand, analyze, control, and document the manufacturing process used in the production of nonhuman food chain animal supplements through the implementation of standard operating procedures (SOPs) that define how the company will meet BMP Standards.)
- **Nonconformity**—not meeting a specified requirement
- **Quality Assurance**—the sum total of the organized arrangements made with the objective of ensuring that the final products are of the quality required for their intended use
- **Quality Audit**—a systematic, independent (not necessarily by a third party) examination of a company's quality system that is performed at defined intervals and at sufficient frequency to determine whether quality system procedures are being followed, that these procedures are implemented effectively, and that these procedures are suitable for achieving quality system objectives
- **Quality Control Procedure(s)**—a planned and systematic procedure for taking all actions necessary to prevent a product from becoming adulterated
- **Quality System Requirements (QSRs)**—the standards related to organizational structure, responsibilities, procedures, processes, and resources needed for implementing a quality management system
- **Raw Material**—any ingredient or component intended for use in the manufacture of a supplement
- **SOP**—the written standard operating procedures that are required to define, describe, and inform how a particular process is to be conducted or carried out. When followed, SOPs optimize product quality; reduce

potential contamination, mix-up, and errors; and improve efficiency of processes, procedures, record keeping, and productivity

Production and Process Controls

- **Master Production and Control Records**—To assure uniformity from batch to batch, a master production and control record shall be prepared for the manufacture of each ingredient and supplement, and shall be reviewed and approved by the quality control unit.
- **Batch Production and Control Records**
  - Individual batch production and control records shall be prepared and followed for each batch of product produced and shall include complete information related to the production and control of each batch. These records shall be an accurate reproduction of the appropriate master production and control record and shall include documentation that each significant step in the manufacture, processing, packing, or holding of the batch was accomplished.
  - Any deviation from written, approved specifications, standards, test procedures, or other laboratory control mechanisms shall be recorded and justified.

Understanding Product Quality

Anytime a supplement is purchased, it is natural for the purchaser to assume that the product has been produced according to some standards for quality and integrity. The expectation of quality is certainly reasonable; however, the assumption of quality may be dangerous. In my opinion, industry participants can be categorized in three ways:

1. Industry participants who are members of the National Animal Supplement Council. NASC provides member companies with components needed to develop, establish, implement, and follow quality processes for their particular business. Additionally, the association requires independent facility audits for evaluation of the key components, which helps ensure process control and continued vigilance.
2. Responsible supplement providers who are not members of NASC. Although NASC strategic objectives also involve regulatory issues, NASC membership is not required for a company to be considered a quality provider.
3. Opportunists—industry participants who do not live up to the standards that all consumers have the right to expect when purchasing a supplement for animals.

How can you determine which companies and products fit into which category? The answers require an understanding of the basics involved in producing a product and knowing the right questions to ask your supplier.

Quality really begins with the mindset and philosophy of the executive management team within the company. If the president of the organization is quality focused, this philosophy has a very good chance of permeating throughout the organization. How can someone determine whether the leadership of an organization is quality focused? One should not be afraid to call the company and ask questions regarding their quality procedures. At minimum, any supplier of supplements for animals should have a comprehensive quality manual in place for its organization. Every employee of the company should be familiar with the contents of the quality manual, as this document defines the SOPs that cover the entire scope of operations within the organization.

EUROPAM, the European Herb Growers Association, has produced Guidelines for Good Agricultural Practice (GAP) of Medicinal and Aromatic Plants, along with Good Wildcrafting Practices (EUROPAM, 2001). The WHO has also published guidelines on Good Agricultural and Collection Practices (GACP) for Medicinal Plants (WHO, 2003). Included in the WHO document are the GACP for Japan, the European Agency for Evaluation of Medicinal Products, and GAP for Traditional Chinese Medicinal Materials. Because many herbs used in the manufacture of animal supplements are produced internationally, the implementation of these various guidelines can help growers and manufacturers provide quality ingredients. Manufacturers who purchase raw materials from growers should have quality standards in the production process to ensure that each individual ingredient used in a particular formula meets defined standards and defined SOPs. These standards and acceptance criteria must be defined in writing.

Some companies that provide products have the formulas "tableted" or produced close to "final" form by contracted manufacturers. In this case, each company should have a quality manual that defines and documents the specific procedures that are applicable to its scope of operation.

Suppliers that label product and ship under their specific brand name must still have written SOPs that completely and thoroughly define the processes under their control. Essential components of SOPs that will ensure that quality products are consistently produced include the following:

- Acceptance criteria for the product
- How products are tracked to the first point of distribution
- An adverse event reporting system to alert the company of potential problems
- Explanation of which personnel have specific responsibility for quality

An example of quality control for a common herb—garlic (Allium sativum)

A high-quality herbal ingredient must begin with the grower. The seeding material must be identified botanically, with plant variety, cultivar, chemotype, and origin being noted on the medicinal plant record. Cultivation practices for quality medicinal and aromatic plants must begin with soil that has not been contaminated by sludge that contains heavy metals or chemicals. Fertilization should be performed with thoroughly composted manures that are free of human feces and appropriate for the plant species. Irrigation water should comply with quality standards and must be free of contaminants such as heavy metals, pesticides, herbicides, and hazardous substances.

Harvesting should be performed when the plant is at the best quality for the intended utilization and under the best possible conditions. All harvest equipment and containers should be clean, which reduces contamination of the plant. Harvested material should be promptly processed, taking into consideration the plant's active substances. According to the University of California, Davis, China produces about three quarters of the world garlic market (University of California, 2004). Manufacturers in China follow Good Agricultural Practices for Traditional Chinese Medicinal Materials set by the General Committee of the State Administration of Pharmaceutical Supervision. Although guidelines vary from one country to another, some, such as the Australia Therapeutic Goods Administration, are subject to the same standards as pharmaceuticals. Manufacturers must be certified to export products to countries that have these types of standards.

The US pharmacopoeial grade of garlic may be fresh or dried bulbs of *Allium sativum*, containing not less than 0.5% alliin (determined by liquid chromatography and calculated by dry weight) (Blumenthal, 1998). Garlic may be used fresh or carefully dried. Monographs published in different countries may not have the same quantitative requirements for the alliin content of garlic. Macroscopic and microscopic examination and high-performance liquid chromatography (Lawson, 1991; Han,1995) are common testing procedures.

Testing Final Products Versus Process Control

Testing is a valuable tool used after production has been completed to assess whether a product meets defined specifications. What it does not ensure is that consistency is achieved for all production lots or batches. Repeatability and consistency can be achieved only through control of the processes by which products are produced.

The American Herbal Pharmacopoeia (AHP) has developed herbal monographs, botanical and chemical references, analytical testing services, and quality control texts. High-performance thin-layer chromatography (HPTLC) has been identified as a quality assessment tool for the evaluation of herbal products. The Institute for Nutraceutical Advancement (INA) also recommends high-performance liquid chromatography for the assessment of alliin in garlic. The INA supports the production of high-quality botanical products through its Methods Validation Program, which provides analytic methods through which the need for global consistency in testing can be fulfilled. Many testing laboratories offer validation certification of herbal products; however, because the number of herbs and botanical products is great, many monographs and references have yet to be developed. When available, ingredient validation and analysis certification should be requested by manufacturers for the production of quality products (Figure 8-1).

One should think of testing and process control as one would the production of a diagnostic radiograph. Each processed film represents a production batch or lot of supplements. The individual who takes the radiograph (veterinarian or technician) may be able to produce a diagnostic film once, but other films may not qualify as diagnostic. In reviewing the example for radiographs, one should think of each step taken to produce a final film as specifications for an animal supplement.

- Test results for one production lot = One film
- Product specifications = Each step taken to produce the film
- Process control = Ensuring all steps taken to produce the film are correct

If the goal (acceptable specification) is to produce a diagnostic film, these variables must be controlled. Anatomic target, restraint devices, positioning, film size and speed, maintenance of the x-ray machine, technique chart, and film processing are a few of the variables that must be considered and controlled. All steps in the process must be controlled and evaluated so that repeatable results are achieved. The production of animal supplements is no different.

The FDA has advised consumers to consider four factors when making purchasing decisions about nutritional supplements (US Food & Drug Administration, 2002). It suggests that the manufacturer or distributor be contacted for answers to the following questions:

- Can label claims be substantiated through analytic testing?
- Is information available on the safety and efficacy of ingredients in the formulation?
- Is a quality control system in place to ensure that the product actually contains what is stated on the label and that the product is free of contaminants?
- Has the manufacturer received any adverse event reports from consumers who have used the product?

It is important for the reader to understand that consistent testing methods have not been published for all dietary supplement ingredients used for humans or animals, including herbal ingredients. This means that the only way that one product can be effectively compared with another is through assurance that ingredients are tested for purity before they are blended with other ingredients in the final product formulation.

US Pharmacopoeia (USP) Testing specifications should be followed, when available. If USP standards are not defined for a particular ingredient, testing should follow the highest standards generally agreed upon by the industry and should use qualified analytic laboratories. Other resources for testing methods include international pharmacopoeias and published monographs (US Food and Drug Administration, 1999).

When finished products are compared, outcomes should be compared with the use of identical testing methods. Typically, different grades of ingredients are available to suppliers, and cost varies widely depending on their purity, testing, and source. Because of the lack of consistently applied testing standards for ingredients, a supplier may meet label claims using one testing method and have significantly different results when using a different assay method.

Providers who use high-quality ingredients, who follow current Good Manufacturing Practice standards,

MAYWAY CORP.

Chinese Herbs & Herbal Products since 1969.

CERTIFICATE OF ANALYSIS

PRODUCT NAME:	DA SUAN, EXTRACT POWDER
BOTANICAL NAME:	ALLIUM SATIVUM
PART USED:	STEM
COUNTRY OF ORIGIN:	SHANGHAI, CHINA
ITEM NO.:	5018C / 5018CB
MW LOT NO:	SH03015
BATCH NO.:	03AM0304*04020310
BATCH SIZE:	25 KGS.
PACK SIZE:	25 KG/DRUM
REPORT DATE:	4/11/2003

ITEM	RESULTS
FORM	POWDER
IDENTIFICATION METHOD	TLC
PARTICLE SIZE	100 MESH
LOSS ON DRYING	3.2%
TASTE	CHARACTERISTIC
COLOR	PALE YELLOW
TAP DENSITY	0.49 G/ML
STANDARD	5:1 HERB TO EXTRACT
HEAVY METALS	<4 PPM
SO2	N/A
PESTICIDES	UNDETECTABLE
TOTAL PLATE COUNT	800/G
YEAST & MOLD	80/G
E .COLI	NEGATIVE
SALMONELLA	NEGATIVE
STAPHYLOCOCCUS AUREUS	NEGATIVE

*N.D.=none detected at 0.01 PPM

Mayway Corporation

Yvonne Lau
President
1/7/2005

1338 MANDELA PARKWAY, OAKLAND, CA 94607-2055 · tel: 1-510-208-3113 · fax: 1-510-208-3069 · www.mayway.com

Figure 8-1 Certificate of Analysis. (*Permission to use granted by Mayway Corp.*)

and who apply appropriate standardized analytic tests for label validation help ensure consistent product quality.

The National Animal Supplement Council

The National Animal Supplement Council is an industry group dedicated to protecting and enhancing the health of companion animals and horses throughout the United States. Founded in 2001, NASC is a not-for-profit all-industry association that consists of stakeholders concerned with the issues surrounding the supply of supplements for nonhuman food chain animals. Members include manufacturers, suppliers, veterinarians, distributors, dealers, retailers, and animal friends. NASC members include manufacturers of animal supplements who are committed to the highest current standards of quality and safety in the industry.

The NASC mission: "To promote the health and well-being of nonhuman food chain animals that are given supplements by establishing regulations which are Fair, Reasonable, Responsible, and Nationally Consistent."

The cornerstone of NASC members' pledge is the Compliance Plus[SM] quality program. This program provides a framework of best manufacturing practices for quality assurance and product safety, along with a commitment to ongoing research and development that stands alone in the industry.

NASC Member companies are required to

- Have a quality manual in place that meets the standards for the industry
- Follow proper labeling guidelines for both animal feed and nonfeed products
- Have an adverse event reporting and complaint system in place
- Follow the guidance of the organization's Scientific Advisory Committee for risk classification of ingredients (229 of the 653 ingredients reviewed were herbals)

NASC members who supply products may use the NASC seal on their product labels and can use the logo on advertising, provided they meet specific criteria that ensure that they are "in compliance" with strict policies and standards. This seal is awarded only after a member company successfully completes an independent facilities audit, which evaluates the criteria defined for NASC member companies. These requirements are mandatory for NASC members who supply supplements. The seal is a way for consumers to know that when they buy a product, they buy from a reputable manufacturer. Buying from NASC members is the best way that veterinarians and consumers can support efforts to improve the quality of animal supplements and preserve the availability of these supplements to US and international markets (NASC Mission Statement, www.nasc.cc).

The "Plus" in *Compliance Plus* refers to adverse event reporting, which was not provided under DSHEA, but which has been strongly encouraged by the FDA. The NASC Adverse Event Reporting System (NAERS) has been operational since 2003, during which time all NASC member companies have been required to monitor, evaluate, and act upon occurrences by filing monthly adverse event reports in a Web-enabled national reporting system. The NAERS captures critical information for each adverse event, including incident description, veterinarian involvement, contact information, investigation details, and risk assessment. The FDA/CVM has had full visibility on every adverse event in the system since training was provided in July of 2003; reporting tools allow the FDA to monitor adverse events by company, product, ingredient, species, and other categories.

Adverse Event Reporting

Even the best process controls are not infallible. Unexpected events can arise, or unknown "gaps" in even the most thorough quality systems can happen. Quality-focused companies strive to continually improve their processes under controlled circumstances. If all processes were perfect, there would never be any recalls; however, because no process is perfect, it is important for companies to remain vigilant in identifying potential issues early on and determining whether corrective action is necessary.

Potential problems may occur anywhere in the production process, with AERs usually resulting from ingredients or combinations of ingredients. Although process controls help establish specific control mechanisms, a documented adverse event reporting system such as the NASC NAERS is an essential component for responsible providers of animal supplements.

The NAERS also captures the total usage of NHFC animal supplements sold by industry members, enabling calculation of the incidence of adverse events relative to product usage, and helping in the establishment of fact-based, empiric estimates of true risk to animal health. In 2005, for example, more than 200 million NHFC supplement *administrations* resulted in 179 adverse events, or just less than 1 adverse event for every 1.5 million NHFC supplement administrations. These data strongly support continued access to NHFC supplements by animal owners. At the time of this writing, none of the adverse events reported in NAERS has been classified as serious or life threatening.

An example of an NAERS report for garlic use data is seen in Figure 8-2 (used with the permission of the NASC). Figure 8-3 demonstrates a consolidation of data on the ingredient Garlic for the years from 1999 through 2004.

Furthermore, the NAERS is designed to enable analysis of adverse event and usage data on an ingredient-by-ingredient basis for each primary species, giving FDA an unprecedented capability for efficiently maintaining surveillance of ingredient use and risk assessment going forward. This systematic, data-driven approach is an example of how industry and regulators, working together, can develop risk-based tools that allow continued access by NHFC animal owners to useful products, while at the same time providing vigilant protection of public and animal health. This can be extremely important when regulatory agencies have concerns with regard to ingredient risk because often these concerns are generated by reports of an adverse event occurring in another

National Animal Supplement Council
PO Box 2568
Valley Center, CA 92082
T: 760-751-3360

☐ Confidential

NASC INGREDIENT RISK REPORT

The following information is the proprietary property of the National Animal Supplement Council (NASC). Any use or dissemination of this information requires written permission from NASC.

Please Select An Ingredient Name:

INGREDIENT INFORMATION

Ingredient Name:	Garlic
No of NASC Registered Products with this ingredient:	46
Years Ingredient on the Market:	16 Year(s)

USAGE INFORMATION

In Dogs:

Minimum Usage:	0.24 mg/kg
Maximum Usage:	15.01 mg/kg
Straight Mean Usage:	11.24 mg/kg
Weighted Mean:	N/A

In Horses:

Minimum Usage:	0.00 mg/kg
Maximum Usage:	107.09 mg/kg
Straight Mean Usage:	11.03 mg/kg
Weighted Mean:	N/A

In Cats:

Minimum Usage:	0.96 mg/kg
Maximum Usage:	9.43 mg/kg
Straight Mean Usage:	6.60 mg/kg
Weighted Mean:	N/A

Figure 8-2 NASC NAERS ingredient risk report—garlic use data. (*Used with permission of the NASC.*)

NASC INGREDIENT RISK REPORT

Confidential

National Animal Supplement Council
PO Box 2568, Valley Center, CA 92082
T: 760-751-3360

The following information is the proprietary property of the National Animal Supplement Council (NASC). Any use or dissemination of this information requires written permission from NASC.

Please Note: The requirement for NASC members to enter AE reports began Q3 of 2003. Some companies were recording AEs prior to that time, and that data is displayed. NASC did not require reporting the number of administrations sold until Q3 2003, so data prior to that time is likely understated. Since we cannot be sure that the data prior to Q3 2003 are complete, we do not report AE Incidence prior to that time. Please direct questions about the NAERS system and the methodology to: Bill Bookout at NASC, 760-751-3360 or Paal Gisholt at SmartPak Equine at 774-773-1107.

AES AND ADMINISTRATIONS

In Dogs:

Year	Adverse Events Reported	Incidence Of AEs %	Serious Adverse Events Reported	Incidence Of Serious AEs %	Administrations Reported
2002 Total	0	0	0	0	14,810,764
2003 Total	0	0	0	0	24,766,232
2004 Total	0	0	0	0	12,120,749
Grand Total	0	0	0	0	51,697,745

In Horses:

Year	Adverse Events Reported	Incidence Of AEs %	Serious Adverse Events Reported	Incidence Of Serious AEs %	Administrations Reported
1999 Total	0	0	0	0	64,000
2000 Total	0	0	0	0	442,240
2001 Total	0	0	0	0	500,679
2002 Total	0	0	0	0	530,471
2003 Total	0	0	0	0	522,398
2004 Total	0	0	0	0	326,440
Grand Total	0	0	0	0	2,386,228

In Cats;

Year	Adverse Events Reported	Incidence Of AEs %	Serious Adverse Events Reported	Incidence Of Serious AEs %	Administrations Reported
2000 Total	0	0	0	0	140,700
2001	0	0	0	0	144,600
2002 Total	0	0	0	0	607,242
2003 Total	0	0	0	0	715,884
2004 Total	0	0	0	0	749,560
Grand Total	0	0	0	0	2,357,986

Adverse Event: "An Adverse Event is a type of Complaint where a patient has suffered any negative physical effect or health problem that MAY be connected to or associate with use of the product."

Serious Adverse Event: "An Adverse Event with a transient incapacitating effect (i.e. rendering the animal unable to function normally for even a short period of time, such as with a seizure) or nontransient (i.e. permanent) health effect. Transient vomiting or diarrhea do not constitute Serious Adverse Events. A purported Serious Adverse Event requires follow-up with a veterinarian. A layperson diagnosis does not constitute a Serious Adverse Event."

Figure 8-3 NASC NAERS ingredient risk report—garlic adverse events and administration history. (Used with permission of the NASC.)

species or caused by excessive exposure to or use of a single ingredient and not a blended formulation.

Quality Questions for Product Selection

- Do not be afraid to pick up the telephone, identify yourself as a customer, and ask to speak with the President of the company
- Ask the President to give you an overview of the company's quality control and quality assurance procedures
- Ask your sales representative to provide quality *documentation* for the ingredients used in the formulation and testing information for the finished product. At a minimum, the company should be able to provide Certificates of Analysis for the primary active ingredients used in the formulation. Be aware that standardized testing methods may not be established for every ingredient that may be contained in the formula. If these standards are published, look for testing and analytic methods that follow USP standards. If USP standards are not available, published monographs and pharmacopoeias provide information on testing methods
- Look for lot numbers on products
- Ask whether the production facility has been independently audited and certified by an independent auditing organization. If it has been, the company should be able to provide a certificate or letter that indicates the results of the audit
- If you do have an adverse event, call the company to report the occurrence. Evaluate how the report is handled and review any follow-up report from the company
- Ask technical questions and consider the answers. Decide whether you are comfortable with the technical support you receive

SUMMARY

From a global standpoint, the regulatory environment is one of inconsistency; however, progress is being made in adoption of a uniform approach to regulating herbal products. In the United States, much progress has been made toward achieving an acceptable compromise while not restricting reputable companies from providing beneficial products for animals.

Although quality begins with evaluation and testing of ingredients, many steps may affect product quality. For any company to produce a quality product, a comprehensive written system of process control is a mandatory requirement. This being said, even the most comprehensive quality systems are not infallible, which suggests that continued vigilance also must be a key quality requirement.

In our opinion, an optimal outcome can best be achieved when responsible members of industry, regulatory agencies or guiding bodies, clinicians, academia, and the scientific community work cooperatively to establish and implement a system that is fair, reasonable, responsible, and globally consistent. Through these efforts, herbal modalities may come to be recognized as viable options for animal and human healthcare.

ADDITIONAL SOURCES OF INFORMATION

- www.nasc.cc—National Animal Supplement Council; provides updates and recommended action regarding supplements for companion animals in the United States
- www.vm.cfsan.fda.gov/~dms/dietsupp.html—US Food and Drug Administration Center for Food Safety and Applied Nutrition (December 1, 1995), discussion of Dietary Supplement Health Education Act of 1994
- www.fda.gov/ola/2003/dietarysupplements1028.html—statement of John M. Taylor, Associate Commissioner for Regulatory Affairs, FDAFDA, before the Committee on Commerce, US Senate, October 28, 2003
- www.usp.org—US Pharmacopoeia (see Dietary Supplements)
- www.ahpa.org—American Herbal Products Association
- www.herbal-ahp.org/—American Herbal Pharmacopoeia

APPENDIX OF GRAS INGREDIENTS

- GRAS ingredients—US FDA 21 CFR (#225 ingredients)
- Sec. 582.1 Substances that are generally recognized as safe
  (1) The quantity of a substance added to animal food does not exceed the amount reasonably required to accomplish its intended physical, nutritional, or other technical effect in food; and
  (2) The quantity of a substance that becomes a component of animal food as a result of its use in the manufacturing, processing, or packaging of food, and which is not intended to accomplish any physical or other technical effect in the food itself, shall be reduced to the extent reasonably possible.
- Sec. 582.10 Spices and other natural seasonings and flavorings
- Sec. 582.20 Essential oils, oleoresins (solvent-free), and natural extractives (including distillates)
- Sec. 582.30 Natural substances used in conjunction with spices and other natural seasonings and flavorings
- Sec. 582.40 Natural extractives (solvent-free) used in conjunction with spices, seasonings, and flavorings
- Sec. 582.50 Certain other spices, seasonings, essential oils, oleoresins, and natural extracts

Common Name	Botanical Name of Plant Source
Alfalfa	*Medicago sativa L.*
Alfalfa herb and seed	*Medicago sativa L.*
Algae, brown	*Laminaria* spp and *Nereocystis* spp
Algae, brown (kelp)	*Laminaria* spp and *Nereocystis* spp
Algae, red	*Porphyra* spp and *Rhodymenia palmata (L.) Grev*
Allspice	*Pimenta officinalis Lindl*
Almond, bitter (free from prussic acid)	*Prunus amygdalus Batsch, Prunus armeniaca L.*, or *Prunus persica (L.) Batsch*
Ambergris	*Physeter macrocephalus L.*
Ambrette (seed)	*Hibiscus moschatus Moench*
Ambrette seed	*Hibiscus abelmoschus L.*
Angelica	*Angelica archangelica L.* or other spp of *Angelica*
Angelica root, seed and stem	*Angelica archangelica L.*
Angostura (cusparia bark)	*Galipea officinalis Hancock*
Angostura (cusparia bark)	*Galipea officinalis Hancock*
Anise	*Pimpinella anisum L.*
Anise, star	*Illicium verum Hook f.*
Apricot kernel (persic oil)	*Prunus armeniaca L.*
Asafetida	*Ferula assa-foetida L.* and related spp of *Ferula*
Balm (lemon balm)	*Melissa officinalis L.*
Balsam of Peru	*Myroxylon pereirae Klotzsch*
Basil	*Ocimum basilicum L.*
Basil, bush	*Ocimum minimum L.*
Basil, sweet	*Ocimum basilicum L.*
Bay	*Laurus nobilis L.*
Bay (myrcia oil)	*Pimenta racemosa (Mill.) JW Moore*
Bay leaves	*Laurus nobilis L.*
Bergamot (bergamot orange)	*Citrus aurantium L.* subsp *bergamia Wright et Arn.*
Bitter almond (free from prussic acid)	*Prunus amygdalus Batsch, Prunus armeniaca L.*, or *Prunus persica (L.) Batsch*
Bois de rose	*Aniba rosaeodora Ducke*
Cacao	*Theobroma cacao L.*
Calendula	*Calendula officinalis L.*
Camomile (chamomile) flowers, Hungarian	*Matricaria chamomilla L.*
Camomile (chamomile) flowers, Roman or English	*Anthemis nobilis L*
Camomile (chamomile), English or Roman	*Anthemis nobilis L.*
Camomile (chamomile), German or Hungarian	*Matricaria chamomilla L.*
Cananga	*Cananga odorata Hook f. and Thoms.*
Capers	*Capparis spinosa L.*
Capsicum	*Capsicum frutescens L.* or *Capsicum annuum L.*
Caraway	*Carum carvi L.*
Caraway, black (black cumin)	*Nigella sativa L.*
Cardamom (cardamon)	*Elettaria cardamomum Maton.*
Cardamom seed (cardamon)	*Elettaria cardamomum Maton.*
Carob bean	*Ceratonia siliqua L.*
Carrot	*Daucus carota L.*
Cascarilla bark	*Croton eluteria Benn.*
Cassia bark, Chinese	*Cinnamomum cassia Blume.*
Cassia bark, Padang or Batavia	*Cinnamomum burmanni Blume.*
Cassia bark, Saigon	*Cinnamomum loureirii Nees.*
Cassia, Chinese	*Cinnamomum cassia Blume.*
Cassia, Padang or Batavia	*Cinnamomum burmanni Blume.*
Cassia, Saigon	*Cinnamomum loureirii Nees.*
Castoreum	*Castor fiber L.* and *C. canadensis Kuhl.*
Cayenne pepper	*Capsicum frutescens L.* or *Capsicum annuum L.*
Celery seed	*Apium graveolens L.*
Cherry, wild, bark	*Prunus serotina Ehrh.*
Chervil	*Anthriscus cerefolium (L.) Hoffm.*
Chicory	*Cichorium intybus L.*
Chives	*Allium schoenoprasum L.*

Common Name	Botanical Name of Plant Source
Cinnamon bark, Ceylon	*Cinnamomum zeylanicum Nees.*
Cinnamon bark, Chinese	*Cinnamomum cassia Blume.*
Cinnamon bark, Saigon	*Cinnamomum loureirii Nees.*
Cinnamon leaf, Ceylon	*Cinnamomum zeylanicum Nees.*
Cinnamon leaf, Chinese	*Cinnamomum cassia Blume.*
Cinnamon leaf, Saigon	*Cinnamomum loureirii Nees.*
Cinnamon, Ceylon	*Cinnamomum zeylanicum Nees.*
Cinnamon, Chinese	*Cinnamomum cassia Blume.*
Cinnamon, Saigon	*Cinnamomum loureirii Nees.*
Citronella	*Cymbopogon nardus (L.) Rendle.*
Citrus peels	*Citrus* spp
Civet (zibeth, zibet, zibetum)	*Civet cats, Viverra civetta Schreber and Viverra zibethaSchreber.*
Clary (clary sage)	*Salvia sclarea L.*
Clove bud, leaf or stem	*Eugenia caryophyllata Thunb.*
Clover	*Trifolium* spp
Cloves	*Eugenia caryophyllata Thunb.*
Coca (decocainized)	*Erythroxylum coca Lam.* and other spp of *Erythroxylum*
Coffee	*Coffea* spp
Cognac oil, white and green	Ethyl oenanthate, so-called
Cola nut	*Cola acuminata Schott* and *Endl.*, and other spp of *Cola*
Coriander	*Coriandrum sativum L.*
Corn silk	*Zea mays L.*
Cumin (cummin)	*Cuminum cyminum L.*
Cumin, black (black caraway)	*Nigella sativa L.*
Curacao	Orange peel (orange, bitter *Citrus aurantium L.* peel)
Cusparia bark	*Galipea officinalis Hancock.*
Dandelion leaf and root	*Taraxacum officinale Weber* and *T. laevigatum DC.*
Dill	*Anethum graveolens L.*
Dog grass (quackgrass, triticum)	*Agropyron repens (L.) Beauv.*
Dulse	*Rhodymenia palmata (L.)*
Elder flowers	*Sambucus canadensis L.* and *S. nigra L.*
Estragole (esdragol, esdragon, tarragon))	*Artemisia dracunculus L.* (tarragon)
Fennel, common	*Foeniculum vulgare Mill.*
Fennel, sweet	*Finocchio (Florence Foeniculum vulgare Mill. var.) Fennel duice (DC.) Alex.*
Fennel, sweet	*Foeniculum vulgare Mill.*
Fenugreek	*Trigonella foenum-graecum L.*
Galanga (galangal)	*Alpina officinarum Hance.*
Garlic	*Allium sativum L.*
Geranium	*Pelargonium* spp
Geranium, East Indian	*Cymbopogon martini Stapf.*
Geranium, rose	*Pelargonium graveolens*
Ginger	*Zingiber officinale Rosc.*
Glycyrrhiza	*Glycyrrhiza glabra L.* and other spp of *Glycyrrhiza*
Glycyrrhizin, ammoniated	*Glycyrrhiza glabra L.* and other spp of *Glycyrrhiza*
Grains of paradise	*Amomum melegueta Rosc.*
Grapefruit	*Citrus paradisi Macf.*
Guava	*Psidium* spp
Hickory bark	*Carya* spp
Hops	*Humulus lupulus L.*
Horehound (hoarhound)	*Marrubium vulgare L.*
Horsemint	*Monarda punctata L.*
Horseradish	*Armoracia lapathifolia Gilib.*
Hyssop	*Hyssopus officinalis L.*
Immortelle	*Helichrysum angustifolium DC.*
Jasmine	*Jaminum officinale L.* and other spp of *Jasminum*
Juniper (berries)	*Juniperus communis L.*
Kelp	See algae, brown
Kola nut	*Cola acuminata Schott and Endl.*, and other spp of *Cola*
Laurel berries	*Laurus nobilis L.*
Laurel leaves	*Laurus* spp

Common Name	Botanical Name of Plant Source
Lavandin hybrids between	*Lavandula officinalis Chaix.* and *Lavandula latifolin Vill.*
Lavender	*Lavandula officinalis Chaix.*
Lavender, spike	*Lavandula latifolia Vill.*
Lemon	*Citrus limon (L.) Burm. f.*
Lemon balm	See balm
Lemon grass	*Cymbopogon citratus DC.* and *Cymbopogon flexuosus Stapf.*
Lemon peel	*Citrus limon (L.) Burm. f.*
Licorice	*Glycyrrhiza glabra L.* and other spp. of *Glycyrrhiza*
Lime	*Citrus aurantifolia Swingle.*
Linden flowers	*Tilia* spp
Locust bean	*Ceratonia siliqua L.*
Lupulin	*Humulus lupulus L.*
Mace	*Myristica fragrans Houtt.*
Malt (extract)	*Hordeum vulgare L.* or other grains
Mandarin	*Citrus reticulata Blanco.*
Marigold, pot	*Calendula officinalis L.*
Marjoram, pot	*Majorana onites (L.) Benth.*
Marjoram, sweet	*Majorana hortensis Moench.*
Mate 1	*Ilex paraguariensis St. Hil.*
Melissa	See balm
Menthol	*Mentha* spp
Molasses (extract)	*Saccharum officinarum L.*
Musk (Tonquin musk)	Musk deer, *Moschus moschiferus*
Mustard	*Brassica* spp
Mustard, black or brown	*Brassica nigra (L.) Koch.*
Mustard, brown	*Brassica juncea (L.) Coss.*
Mustard, white or yellow	*Brassica hirta Moench.*
Naringin	*Citrus paradisi Macf.*
Neroli, bigarade	*Citrus aurantium L.*
Nutmeg	*Myristica fragrans Houtt.*
Onion	*Allium cepa L.*
Orange leaf	*Citrus sinensis (L.) Osbeck.*
Orange, bitter, sweet, flowers, peel	*Citrus aurantium L.*
Oregano oreganum (Mexican oregano, Mexican sage, origan)	*Oreganum Lippia* spp
Origanum	*Origanum* spp
Palmarosa	*Cymbopogon martini Stapf.*
Paprika	*Capsicum annuum L.*
Parsley	*Petroselinum crispum (Mill.) Mansf.*
Peach kernel (persic oil)	*Prunus persica Sieb. et Zucc.*
Peanut stearine	*Arachis hypogaea L.*
Pepper, black	*Piper nigrum L.*
Pepper, cayenne, red	*Capsicum frutescens L.* or *Capsicum annuum L.*
Pepper, white	*Piper nigrum L.*
Peppermint	*Mentha piperita L.*
Persic oil	See apricot kernel and peach kernel
Peruvian balsam	*Myroxylon pereirae Klotzsch.*
Petitgrain	*Citrus aurantium L.*
Petitgrain lemon	*Citrus limon (L.) Burm. f.*
Petitgrain mandarin or tangerine	*Citrus reticulata Blanco.*
Pimenta	*Pimenta officinalis Lindl.*
Pimenta leaf	*Pimenta officinalis Lindl.*
Pipsissewa leaves	*Chimaphila umbellata Nutt.*
Pomegranate	*Punica granatum L.*
Poppy seed	*Papaver somniferum L.*
Pot marigold	*Calendula officinalis L.*
Pot marjoram	*Majorana onites (L.) Benth.*
Prickly ash bark	*Xanthoxylum* (or *Zanthoxylum*) *Americanum Mill.* or *Xanthoxylum clava-herculis L.*
Quince seed	*Cydonia oblonga Miller.*

Common Name	Botanical Name of Plant Source
Rose absolute, buds, flowers, fruit (hips)	*Rosa alba L., Rosa centifolia L., Rosa damascena Mill., Rosa gallica L.,* and vars. of these spp
Rose geranium	*Pelargonium graveolens*
Rose leaves	*Rosa* spp
Rosemary	*Rosmarinus officinalis L.*
Rue	*Ruta graveolens L.*
Saffron	*Crocus sativus L.*
Sage	*Salvia officinalis L.*
Sage, Greek	*Salvia triloba L.*
Sage, Spanish	*Salvia lavandulaefolia Vahl.*
Savory, summer	*Satureia hortensis L. (Satureja).*
Savory, winter	*Satureia montana L. (Satureja).*
Schinus molle	*Schinus molle L.*
Sesame	*Sesamum indicum L.*
Sloe berries (blackthorn berries)	*Prunus spinosa L.*
Spearmint	*Mentha spicata L.*
Spike lavender	*Lavandula latifolia Vill.*
St. John's bread	*Ceratonia siliqua L.*
Star anise	*Illicium verum Hook. f.*
Tamarind	*Tamarindus indica L.*
Tangerine	*Citrus reticulata Blanco.*
Tannic acid	Nutgalls of *Quercus infectoria Oliver* and related spp of *Quercus*. Also in many other plants
Tarragon	*Artemisia dracunculus L.*
Tea	*Thea sinensis L.*
Thyme, also white	*Thymus vulgaris L.* and *Thymus zygis var. gracilis Boiss.*
Thyme, wild or creeping	*Thymus serpyllum L.*
Triticum	See dog grass
Tuberose	*Polianthes tuberosa L.*
Turmeric	*Curcuma longa L.*
Vanilla	*Vanilla planifolia Andr.* or *Vanilla tahitensis JW Moore*
Violet flowers, leaves	*Viola odorata L.*
Wild cherry bark	*Prunus serotina Ehrh.*
Ylang-ylang	*Cananga odorata Hook. f.* and *Thoms.*
Zedoary	*Curcuma zedoaria Rosc.*

References

AAFCO Official Publication, Association of American Feed Control Officals, Oxford, IN, USA, 2004, p 69, 388.

American Herbal Products Association, "Codex Alimentarius and dietary supplements", Silver Spring, MD, USA, April 2005.

American Pet Product Manufacturers Association, Pet Owner Survey and Lifestyles and Media Study, Greenwich, CT, USA 2001.

AVMA Pet Owner Survey, Schaumberg, IL, USA 2002.

Blumenthal M, Busse WR, Goldberg A, Gruenwald J, Hall T, Riggings C, Rister R. The Complete German Commission E Monographs-Therapeutic Guide to Herbal Medicines, American Botanical Council, Austin, TX 1998.

EUROPAM, the European Herb Growers Association, GAP/GWP —Subcommittee, Brussels, Belgium, November, 2001.

European Agency for the Evaluation of Medicinal Products, Evaluation of Medicines for Human Use, Committee for Veterinary Medicinal Products (CVMP) EMEA/DVMP/815/00, London England, July 2001.

European Agency for the Evaluation of Medicinal Products, Evaluation of Medicines for Human Use, Committee for Veterinary Medicinal Products (CVMP) EMEA/DVMP/814/00, London, England, July 2001.

FDA, Code of Federal Regulations, Title 21, Vol 6, Sec 582.1, 2005.

FDA/CVM, Guidance for Industry, Validation of Analytical Procedures: Methodology #64, Rockville, MD, USA, July 1999.

European Agency for the Evaluation of Medicinal Products, Evaluation of Medicines for Human Use, Committee for Veterinary Medicinal Products (CVMP) EMEA/DVMP/814/00, July 2001.

European Agency for the Evaluation of Medicinal Products, Evaluation of Medicines for Human Use, Committee for Veterinary Medicinal Products (CVMP) EMEA/DVMP/815/00, July 2001.

FDA/CVM, Guidance for Industry, Validation of Analytical Procedures: Methodology #64, July 1999.

FDA/CVM, Personal Correspondence to NASC, Rockville, MD, USA, July 30, 2002. DAF 02327

FDA Veterinarian, Center for Veterinary Medicine, vol XVII, #III, May/June 2002.

FDA, The Evolution of US Drug Law, Rockville, MD, 1998.

FDA/CVM, Compliance Policy Guidance (CPG 7126.04), Sec. 690.100 Nutritional Supplements for Companion Animals, Rockville, MD, USA Available at: http://www.fda.gov/ora/compliance_ref/cpg/cpgvet/cpg690-100.html.

Federal Register, Department of Health & Human Services, Food and drug Administration, Rockville, MD, USA, Docket No. 95N-0308, April 22, 1996.

Federal Register, Department of Health & Human Services, Food and drug Administration, Rockville, MD, USA, Docket No. 96N-0417, March 13, 2003.

Han J, Lawson L, Hand G, and Han P. A Spectrophotometric Method for Quantitative Determination of Allicin and Total Garlic Thiosulfinates. Anal Biochem 1995;225:157-160.

Healthy Pets 21 Consortium *State of the American Pet Survey*, Ralston Purina, St. Louis, MO, October 2002.

International Environmental Law Research Centre, IELRC Working Paper, Plant Genetic Resources in Africa's Renewal, Geneva, Switzerland, 2002-2003.

Iowa Department of Agriculture and Land Stewardship, Des Moines, IA, September 18, 2003, personal correspondence.

Lawson LD, Wood SG, Hughes B. HPLC analysis of allicin and other thiosulfinates in garlic clove homogenates. Planta Medica 1991;57:263-270.

NASC Mission Statement, National Animal Supplement Council, Valley Center, CA, USA, 2001. Available at: www.nasc.cc

NASC Revised Language submitted to CVM, Valley Center, CA, USA, February 25, 2003.

National Animal Supplement Council, QSR Guidelines, Valley Center, CA, USA, April 2004.

Starling S, Functional Foods & Nutraceuticals, "China Rises to Global Challenge", Boulder, CO, USA April 2003.

University of California, Davis, CA, ASE 110, Crop Management Systems for Vegetable Production, Commercial Onion & Garlic Production, Fall 2004.

US Dept of Health and Human Services, FDA, Center for Drug Evaluation and Research, Rockville, MD, USA, Guidance for Industry—Botanical Drug Products, p.2, June 2004, p 2.

US Food and Drug Administration, Center for Food Safety and Applied Nutrition. "Tips for the Savvy Supplement User: Making Informed Decisions and Evaluating Information," Dietary Supplements, College Park, MD, USA, January 2002. Available at: http://www.cfsan.fda.gov/~dms/ds-savvy.html

US Food and Drug Administration, Center for Food Safety and Applied Nutrition, Food Advisory Committee Dietary Supplement Working Group on Ingredient Identity Testing Records and Retention, College Park, MD, USA, June 1999.

www.nasc.cc—Supplement Issues—State Issues—Iowa, National Animal Supplement Council, September 2003.

WHO Guidelines on Good Agricultural and Collection Practices (GACP) for Medicinal Plants, Annex 1-3, Geneva, 2003.

WHO Guidelines on Good Agricultural and Collection Practices for Medicinal Plants, Annex 1: People's Republic of China, State Administration of Pharmaceutical Supervision, Decree No.32, Good Agricultural Practice for Traditional Chinese Medicinal Materials, Geneva, Switzerland, April 2002.

Yankelovich Consultants Study. The State of the American Pet: A Study Among Pet Owners; prepared for Ralston Purina, 2000, Yankelovich Marketing, Chapel Hill, NC.

A Skeptical View of Herbal Medicine

David W. Ramey

CHAPTER

Of the various approaches to veterinary medicine that may be labeled "alternative" or "complementary" (among other labels), herbal and botanical medicine—defined here as preparations derived from plants, plant products, or fungi (including leaves, stems, flowers, roots, and seeds, used as crude products or in forms resulting from solvent extraction or decoction) that are used to prevent and treat diseases—may be simultaneously the most promising and the most frustrating.

Herbal medicine may be considered promising for several reasons. It is inarguable that some plants may contain pharmacologically active substances. Without question, a significant percentage of currently available pharmaceutical products derive from plant sources. Furthermore, it cannot be asserted that humans have now examined every available plant for every conceivable biologically active compound; that is, it is possible—even likely—that some therapeutic substances available in plants have yet to be discovered. Thus, it is hardly implausible to think that as yet undiscovered or unrecognized plants that contain pharmacologically active compounds may hold promise for the treatment of animals (and humans) with certain medical conditions.

However, with this unrealized promise come numerous frustrations. Articles and books on herbal and botanical medicine are replete with inaccurate information, unsupported suggestions, and inappropriate speculation. For all the promise offered by herbal medicines, of those relatively few that have been examined, most have been found wanting. The promise of pharmacologically active substances derived from plant sources is often obscured by nonsense, hype, and inaccuracy. Thus, for crude plant preparations to again enter the mainstream of medicine, many obstacles must be overcome. In particular, the truth must overcome the hype, which, unfortunately, is often a daunting task for the truth. A skeptical view of herbal therapies looks at some of the facts versus the many fallacies that permeate the field.

THE HISTORICAL USE OF PLANTS AS MEDICINE

It is certainly true that humans have employed various medicinal plants, often in association with magic or religious tenets, to treat their ailments and presumably those of their animals. Therefore, one argument used in favor of the use of herbal and botanical medicine is an appeal to the longevity of the therapy. Otherwise stated, herbal medicines are said to have withstood the "test of time" and should therefore be employed. Both practitioners and owners may believe that such remedies are safe and effective, even though they have not seriously questioned whether this is true (Ernst, 1995a).

It should be immediately noted that the "test of time" standard is inadequate when it comes to assessing the reliability of any human endeavor, including those involving the practice of medicine (Ernst, 1998a). Some notoriously unreliable enterprises have been associated with humankind for many thousands of years. For example, people have used astrology—the attempt to foretell one's future by looking at the stars—for thousands of years, although there is no credible evidence for its usefulness and ample evidence to refute it. Similarly, therapeutic phlebotomy (bleeding) is one of the oldest known medical interventions; it has generally been abandoned only in the last century or so (except for its use in a very few conditions) and is still used in some societies. Curiously, and in keeping with the general response of some modern herbalists to scientific criticisms of their remedies, even when bleeding was finally shown to be ineffective, it was not bleeding itself, but the new type of controlled trial, that was doubted (Lilienfeld, 1982). Finally, even medications that *were* used for thousands of years have subsequently been shown to have serious adverse effects. For example, a traditional Oriental formula, *Sho-saiko-to,* was said to have been used for 2000 years in China without adverse effects, but it came to be associated with serious liver damage in Japan in a case report of 4 patients (Itoh, 1995). Thus, the "test of time" is not a reliable indicator of safety or efficacy.

Nevertheless, some evidence for the use of herbal and botanical medicines dates back to the Neanderthal period (Kleiner, 1995). Once historical records began, prescriptions for the use of various plants became part of the medical tradition of virtually every society. Even today, herbal medicines are an important component of traditional medicine in virtually every culture (Vickers, 1999). Once traditions of plant medicine were established, they eventually became more developed. So, for example, the 16th century saw European medical schools creating botanical gardens to grow medicinal plants (Akerele, 1993). When the European expansion occurred, beginning in the late 15th century, European explorers encountered medicinal plants from other cultures and began to send them back to Europe. These plants, originating from Central and South America, profoundly influenced European treatments of the 16th and 17th centuries (Duran-Reynals, 1946). As America became colonized, housewives of the colonial period would gather plants and wild herbs, such as sarsaparilla, horehound, and dandelion, and hang them to dry for future use (Blanton, 1930). Indeed, until the 20th century, most medicinal remedies were botanicals, and, through trial and error, a few were considered to be helpful.

Over time, more formal programs involving the use of herbal and botanical remedies arose. For example, in the United States between 1836 and 1911, 13 physiomedical colleges, which substituted botanical medicines for pharmaceutical drugs and promoted beliefs in a "vital force" that permeated the body and to which healing powers were attributed, opened and then closed their doors (Haller, 1997). In the United States and to a lesser extent in Europe, the Thomsonian movement of the mid-1800s became popular by endorsing herbal remedies for health and medicine (in addition to advocating steaming the body to overcome the "power" of cold). However, contrary to assertions that herbal remedies are time honored, the influence of herbalists and their remedies, as well as the power of the other medical sects, waned over time. This likely occurred because these practitioners could no longer match the advances of science and accompanying improvements in medicine, which removed them from the public trust that developed as those advances continued.

The history of veterinary applications of herbals and botanicals is perhaps as long as, but somewhat less well documented than, that of similar applications in human medicine (Haas, 2000). For example, black and white hellebore treatments *(Helleborus niger* and *Veratrum album*, respectively*)* were used by Pliny in the first century AD. as a seton (drain) through the ears of horses or sheep; in the early 20th century, they were used as purgatives, emetics, anthelmintics, and parasiticides (although they caused death in many animals). Historical prescriptions for herbal use—such as pounded apricot kernels combined with pig fat for the treatment of animals with hoof ailments, or guang barley combined with food chewed by a child for the treatment of animals with hoof wounds—can be found in 6th century Chinese *Qimin yaoshu* (Ramey, 2001). The medicinal practices of native North Americans are a rich source of veterinary herbal prescriptions (Vogel, 1970). Botanical "horse medicines" were provided for the treatment of horses during the American Civil War (Merillat, 1935). Even as late as 1957, popular books continued to list such substances as aconite, belladonna, cinchona, ipecac, nux vomica (strychnine), and tobacco for veterinary use (Hiscox, 1957). However, such titles became scarcely evident until the latest revival of interest in the use of herbal and botanical veterinary remedies.

Chinese Herbal Medicine

A vast, somewhat haphazard tradition of herbal and botanical medicine has existed in China for centuries (Unschuld, 1986); variants of this tradition have apparently held fascination for some practitioners of veterinary medicine. In addition to plants and herbs, the historical practice of Chinese medicine used materials of animal and mineral origin—both individual substances and prescriptions composed of several substances. The first recipes date from the Han dynasty (roughly 200 BC–200 AD); the oldest find to date is the *Wushier bingfang*, dating from 167 BC. Early Chinese medicinals were described primarily by their flavors, as well as by their heating and cooling properties (similar to the humoral theories of the Greeks). Later, specialized Materia Medica texts (bencao) were compiled. In late Ming times, the most important of the Chinese herbal texts, *Bencao Gangmu* ("General Outline of Materia Medica") by Li Shizhen, was published in 1596 (after the author's death). It contains many recipes designed for the treatment of patients with specific illnesses, as was typical of the practice of Chinese herbal medicine throughout history.

Some modern practitioners of Chinese herbal medicine have attempted to assimilate some theoretical aspects of various historical practices of Chinese medicine into their own approach to medicine (Wynn, 2003). This has resulted in practice approaches that are quite different from those of historical China. In fact, modern "Chinese" herbalism has little relationship to the traditional practice of herbal medicine that began in China—in fact, it diverges widely from it.

In China, the approach to the practice of medicine has never followed a single, unified approach. Rather, two systems of medicine developed over time. One was based on the theories of "systematic correspondence" (yin-yang, five phases, etc.); the other, using herbal and other medicines, prescribed various concoctions for the treatment of patients with disease symptoms, without recourse to those theories. The theories associated with more esoteric approaches preserved their validity only in areas that lay beyond empirical examination. However, for a brief period, primarily in the 13th to 15th centuries, attempts were made to incorporate herbal medicine into more theoretical approaches. Ultimately, such attempts failed.

Failure to assimilate arcane theories into Chinese herbal medicine occurred perhaps in part because such theories failed to explain real pathologic processes that *were* noted by Chinese physicians (e.g., leprosy). Instead of relying on concepts such as *yin* and *yang*, Chinese physicians attempted to treat patients with leprosy and other real diseases through a purely pragmatic approach without the need for theoretical underpinnings. Unfortunately, such approaches were largely unsuccessful. The life expectancy in 19th century China has been estimated at around 25 years (Caldwell, 1999) and there is certainly no indication that any such remedies provide a cure for real pathologic processes; none are in evidence today. In addition, Chinese physicians recognized that certain substances or combinations of substances had the same effects on different patients with the same problem. Thus, for real disease symptoms, even in the absence of underlying knowledge of the pathology of disease, the herbal prescriptions of historical China were propounded in essentially the same way as those in other parts of the world—without consideration for sex, age, constitution, or even preference of the individual (Unschuld, 1988).

For decades, pharmaceutical companies have conducted screening programs to investigate Chinese medical preparations; despite this, in the search for new compounds, only a few Chinese drugs have found their way into modern medicine. As of 1987, it was noted that about 7000 species of plants were used in China as herbal remedies but that only 230 of the most commonly used ones had been subjected to in-depth pharmacologic, analytic, and clinical studies (Chang, 1987). The most important of those Chinese medicines to come into common use, *ma huang*, contains ephedrine, a substance that has recently been banned by the US Food and Drug Administration (US FDA Web site, 2004a). However, so far, traditional Chinese medicines have not led to an enrichment of the international pharmacopoeia; investigations—for example, of artemisinin *(Qinghaosu)* and its derivatives for the treatment of patients with malaria (Balint, 2001)—are ongoing.

HISTORICAL REALITY CHECK

The fact that herbal and botanical products have been used throughout history may suggest, to some, that such products are effective medicines; however, a critical look reveals that such an assertion is not correct. In my opinion, an approach to medical therapy that relies on crude botanicals and botanical preparations is not likely to be, and has not been, useful for the treatment of patients with disease or the maintenance of health.

When the historical efficacy of herbal medications is discussed, the salient question is, "Effective compared with what?" In fact, during the heyday of herbal and botanical medicine, other medical treatments, such as bleeding or prescribing large doses of mercury salts (calomel), were largely ineffective—even toxic. Thus, the use of a plant product that was not acutely toxic would have been expected to be of less obvious harm to the patient compared with other interventions and, therefore, more desirable. Furthermore, the fact that herbal medications were widely used may simply reflect that plants were readily available for use by all, and that outside health care was simply not affordable or available for many humans or animals.

Throughout history, it cannot be asserted that herbal and botanical medicines were responsible for any measurable improvement in human or animal health. Mortality curves remained surprisingly similar over thousands of years and under diverse cultural conditions (Cairns, 1986). For example, examination of skeletons from a 40,000-year-old Paleolithic society in Morocco shows that 50% of the population had died before age 38. Before the advent of modern pharmacology in the 20th century, life was "poor, nasty, brutish, and short" (Thomas Hobbs, 1588–1679). When compared with the mortality curves of preagrarian societies, those of 19th century cities were largely identical, although death rates spiked during years of infectious epidemics. In 1900, Western life expectancy was 45 years.

By 1996, this expectancy had increased to 76.1 years. The high rates of morbidity and short life spans that are consistent throughout history and across cultures were due, at least in part, to the inability to prevent or effectively treat infectious diseases (Huxtable, 1999). The dramatic changes in life expectancy that occurred in the 20th century were largely due to clean water, vaccination, and the ability to control infection via effective pharmaceuticals.

In addition, historical assessments of herbal therapies must be made in light of vast differences between historical and current use of the products. In the past, the emphasis for the use of herbal medications was on treatment of symptoms, rather than underlying disease conditions (which had yet to be identified). Ironically, and particularly so in light of the holistic claims that may be made currently for herbal preparations, elimination of the symptom, rather than elimination of the underlying problem, was the criterion used for treatment "success." For example, if a fever abated because the patient ingested willow bark, the treatment would have "worked," although the disease process that caused the fever might have been unaffected. In addition, herbal and botanical remedies were generally applied for vague, all-encompassing conditions (e.g., liver malfunction), rather than for specific indications.

Again, the vague nature of such historical prescriptions should not be surprising in light of the fact that these remedies were prescribed in an era when the causes of disease were uncertain, when different diseases with the same symptoms could not be differentiated, and when the treating doctor had few tools at his or her disposal. In addition, the long-standing use of plants as medicine did not lead to an overall increase in knowledge about their use, nor was such use codified in any meaningful way. Throughout most of history, whether in China, India, or European societies, no effective way of conveying useful information had been developed. As a result, historical herbalists copied extensively from one another over millennia and mixed accurate (by modern standards) information with nonsense, misconceptions, and inaccuracies.

In fact, the true usefulness of historical texts as guides for modern practice is extremely limited. In historical texts, true plant identities are doubtful, in regard to both genus and species. Furthermore, if such treatments failed when they were applied, this was not likely to be noted—the societal acceptability of risk in the treatment of patients with disease was higher (Huxtable, 1999). In fact, the only way to separate the beneficial from the useless or hazardous was through anecdotes relayed mainly by word of mouth (Angell, 1998). Nor would the appearance of such information necessarily have been useful; even when they became available, most people lacked the means, the literacy, and the mobility to obtain or read textbooks.

Given those limitations, the history of botanical preparations does not provide a good template for modern medical prescription. The nature of the historical claims made for efficacy of various plants and the vague nature of the conditions treated makes it exceedingly difficult to objectively evaluate the true utility of the remedies employed today. Furthermore, the historical "successes" attributed to botanicals carried a cost. As noted, the indications for using a given botanical were poorly defined. Dosages were unavoidably arbitrary and ill defined because concentrations of active ingredients were unknown. Any number of contaminants may have been present. It is most important to note that, as with many other tools used in the historical practice of medicine, many of the remedies simply did not work; some were harmful or even deadly. Accordingly, although historical records of the use of medicinal plants may make for interesting reading, such records cannot be used as accurate guides for many currently advocated uses of herbal and botanical products.

THE HISTORICAL USE OF PLANTS AS DRUGS

Limitations of the historical use of plants aside, it is inarguable that the active ingredients of some currently used pharmaceuticals are identical to, or derived from, plants that were used historically as historical folk remedies. Herbal and botanical sources may be the origin of as many as 30% of all modern pharmaceuticals (Kleiner, 1995). For example, aspirin (acetylsalicylic acid) is derived from salicylic acid, which, as salicin (salicyl alcohol plus a sugar molecule), occurs in the flower buds of the meadowsweet *(Filipendula,* formerly *Spirea)* and in the bark and leaves of several poplars and willows, notably the white willow *(Salix alba).* Historically, it was noted that white willow bark extracts had some effectiveness as a pain remedy; indeed, the seminal Greek physician Hippocrates reportedly prescribed willow bark and leaves for fever and the pain of childbirth. Other cultures have soaked willow leaves and applied them topically for use as a painkiller. Digoxin, another pharmacologically active compound, is derived from the foxglove plant, *Digitalis* spp. (at least 12 varieties of the plant are known). Historically, foxglove was found to be helpful for "dropsy" (ascites or edema). Quinine, first isolated from the bark of the cinchona tree *(Cinchona calisaya)* in 1820, was an important antipyretic. As the cost declined and as it became more readily available, quinine was used for the treatment of fever of virtually any origin ("fever" being a common reason for the prescription of plant preparations throughout history). Indeed, the use of quinine as an antipyretic became so widespread in the days after the Civil War that the American Medical Association (AMA) tried unsuccessfully to convince the federal government to grow the cinchona tree in the United States (Ackernecht, 1943).

However, simple facts about the historical use of plants as medicine may not reveal other important considerations that may have led to their decline. After all, it is highly unlikely that people would abandon safe, effective, readily available, and inexpensive medications for no reason. As such, although salicin (the parent of salicylate drugs) was first isolated in the 19th century and was used in crude form as willow bark long before that, to ingest 1 g of salicin from willow bark, a person must ingest at least 14 g of the bark. In addition, the tannins in willow bark (as well as salicin itself) are very irritating to the stomach lining; however, this consideration may not have been important in the historical use of plant preparations because adverse effects were an accepted part of historical medical therapy (Huxtable, 1998). Furthermore, as with many plant preparations when compared with the pharmaceutical products derived from them, salicin is only about half as potent as aspirin.

The use of digitalis preparations for the treatment of patients with heart disease carried its own set of problems. According to detailed descriptions from historical texts, each of the 12 varieties of digitalis plants had active compounds, although the quality of those compounds varied. Seeds of the plant have at least six different biologically active chemical variations, with cardiac and other effects. The potency of digitalis preparations deteriorated rather quickly over a few months, even when the preparations were kept hermetically sealed. Additional difficulties arose because various digitalis compounds had different rates of absorption from the gastrointestinal tract. Finally, variations from batch to batch depended on growing conditions (Osol, 1955).

The use of quinine declined simply because newer and better products were developed. In the 1880s, research with coal tars led to the development of synthetic antipyretics. These products quickly took the place of quinine. Over time, this trend has continued, and plant preparations have essentially disappeared from the mainstream therapeutic armamentarium because newer synthetic drugs gave greater consistency and more targeted efficacy.

THE MYTH OF "NATURAL"

Historical usage notwithstanding, popular modern herbalism has achieved much of its popularity through bombastic claims, such as that its therapies are safer, holistic, or more "natural." Many promoters of natural herbal products promote the myth that they are somehow superior to the same products produced synthetically in a laboratory. No scientific basis exists for such claims. A chemical is a chemical. For example, no difference has been discerned in the vitamin C that is obtained from natural biosynthetic processes in rose hips and that which is made in the laboratory of a chemical manufacturer. The word "natural" implies only the source and does not indicate that the product is, in fact, superior. Rather, it appears to be used mostly as a marketing term.

Nor does "natural" imply that herbal medications are safe. Many people think that herbal medicines, because they are natural, are harmless (Ernst, 1995b). This is wrong. Nothing about herbs automatically makes them nontoxic simply because they are natural. Natural toxins have the same mechanisms of toxicity as synthetic toxins. For example, cabbage and broccoli contain a chemical whose breakdown products act in the same manner as those of dioxin—one of the most feared industrial contaminants. Dioxin is carcinogenic and teratogenic in rodents in extremely small amounts; however, the quantities ingested by humans are far lower than the lowest amounts that have been shown to cause cancer and reproductive damage in rodents (Ames, 1990a).

One reason why herbs may have a reputation for lack of toxicity may be that the concentrations of pharmacologic compounds in herbs are frequently very low, that is, very little of the active ingredient in an herbal preparation is actually delivered; all toxic effects are dose related. Regardless, drug receptors in an animal's body cannot distinguish whether a molecule comes from a chemical laboratory or from the plant kingdom. The toxic potential of an herbal remedy does not depend on its origin; rather, it is related to the pharmacologic characteristics and dose levels of its active ingredients.

MODERN HERBALISM—A NEW AND INVENTIVE FRONTIER

Current usage of botanicals is quite different from historical usage. Historically, even if they were unable to assist in the resolution of a disease process, herbal medicines may have served to make the patient feel cared for, and perhaps even helped to relieve some symptoms. However, when compared with modern usage, herbs were historically used in lesser amounts, for specific disease indications (as opposed to the modern practice of using herbs prophylactically, in an effort to prevent health problems), in crude form (as opposed to concentrated extracts), and by themselves, that is, not in association with other medications, such as pharmaceuticals, thereby obviating concerns about herb–drug interactions (Huxtable, 1999).

Although modern herbalism in the treatment of patients with disease conditions or symptoms may differ from historical usage, it also differs from conventional pharmacotherapy in its prescription. Whereas conventional medications are given primarily to treat disease, herbal medications may be offered for many more indications, including the treatment of healthy individuals. Herbal prescriptions may be offered for maintenance, well-being, or health, and may be prescribed to support, enhance, or stimulate various body processes (although the precise nature of such herbal activity is undefined but generally assumed to be good). Prescribing substances to improve health, rather than to treat disease, allows for an entirely different medical paradigm—one that is largely free of the constraints of evidence and objectivity.

Indeed, the English language appears to have been stretched to its ingenious limits in the attempt to ascribe health benefits to herbal products. The creative linguistics used to promote herbal medications appears to be designed solely for marketing the products—often ignoring truth in the process. For example, it cannot be said that the herb Echinacea, commonly used to treat or prevent the human cold, has ever been shown to be effective; indeed, there is good evidence that it is ineffective (Bent, 2004). However, it may be claimed that Echinacea has natural antibiotic actions and is considered an excellent herb for infections of all kinds. Ginseng—a genus with many different species—has long been promoted as an energy booster, for example, yet the military, in studies of possible energy enhancements for troops, has found it worthless (Lieberman, 2001). As such, the veracity of modern herbal marketers who may ignore such real data and continue to make prescriptions under false pretenses must be questioned. Furthermore, it is curious that even though herbal medications may be promoted as "natural," in fact, advocating the concept of regular ingestion of substances to promote health in individuals in whom no disease is apparent could be construed as anything but natural.

However, in addition to such philosophical differences and linguistic legerdemain, herbal prescribing diverges from modern pharmacotherapy primarily in three important areas:

1. **Use of whole plants.** Herbalists may use unpurified plant extracts that contain several different constituents, as opposed to purified agents that contain measured quantities of active ingredients. The rationale for such prescription asserts that the use of the whole plant allows the plant to work synergistically, that is, the effect of the whole herb is greater than the summed effects of its components. Modern herbalists may also claim that toxicity is reduced when whole herbs are used instead of isolated active ingredients ("buffering"). Although they may acknowledge that two samples of a particular herbal drug may contain constituent compounds in different proportions, in general, modern herbal practitioners claim that this does not cause clinical problems, although there is essentially no evidence by which such claims can be evaluated. Although some experimental evidence suggests synergy and buffering in certain whole plant preparations (Williamson, 2001), how far this can be generalized to all herbal products is not known.
2. **Herb combinations.** In some cases, several different herbs with similar proposed effects are used together simultaneously. Practitioners who engage in such practice may say that the principles of synergy and buffering apply to combinations of plants, claiming that combining herbs improves efficacy, provides multiple mechanisms of action, and reduces adverse effects (Table 9-1) (Vickers, 1999). This contrasts with conventional medical practice, whereby the use of multiple agents with the same effects or mechanisms of action is generally avoided, at least to the extent possible, so as to reduce the possibility of adverse effects.

TABLE 9-1

Example of an Herbal Prescription for Osteoarthritis

Herb	Function
Turmeric *(Curcuma longa)*	For anti-inflammatory activity and to improve circulation at affected joints
Devil's claw *(Harpagophytum procumbens)*	For anti-inflammatory activity and general well-being
Ginseng (*Panax* spp)	For weakness and exhaustion
White willow *(Salix alba)*	For anti-inflammatory activity
Licorice *(Glycyrrhiza glabra)*	For anti-inflammatory activity and to improve palatability and absorption of herbal medicine
Oats *(Avena sativa)*	To aid sleep and for general well-being

3. **Diagnosis.** Herbal practitioners may use different diagnostic principles that diverge from conventional practice. Thus, they may make diagnoses or prescribe treatments on the basis of vague rationales for which they have no proof. For example, when treating a patient with arthritis, a modern herbalist might observe under functioning of a patient's systems of elimination and may decide that the arthritis results from an accumulation of metabolic waste products. A diuretic, choleretic, or laxative combination of herbs might then be prescribed alongside herbs with anti-inflammatory properties. Herbal products might also be prescribed to support various body systems, even though the term "support" is vague and ill defined. No evidence may be available to suggest that such systems are in need of support or that the prescribed plant has the desired function.

SCIENCE AND HERBAL MEDICINES

At this point in time, it can be said that herbal medications are the treatment of choice in the treatment of no conditions in animals or humans. Nonetheless, with the promise, real or imagined, of such products, it behooves practitioners of scientific medicine to look for scientific data in support of the therapies that they provide to their patients.

In other countries, herbal and botanical products constitute an important market. For example, Germany has a long tradition in the use of herbal preparations marketed as drugs. In the United States and the United Kingdom, herbal medicinal products are marketed as "food supplements" or "botanical medicines." Traditional healers in the Third World commonly employ herbs (Bodeker, 1996). However, modern herbalists appear to have ceded to the pharmaceutical industry the use of most obvious pharmacologically active herbs (such as belladonna, ergot, and colchicum), possibly because plants with significant bioactivity have a narrow therapeutic window and misuse can be deadly (Eisenberg, 2000). The plant preparations that are in common use generally have neither the therapeutic potency nor the toxicity profile of botanicals such as foxglove.

Mechanisms of Action

Both raw plant materials and botanical extracts may contain intricate mixtures of organic chemicals, which may include fatty acids, sterols, flavonoids, alkaloids, glycosides, tannins, saponins, and terpenes (Rotblatt, 2002). In laboratory settings, certain plant extracts have demonstrated a variety of pharmacologic activities, including anti-inflammatory, vasodilatory, antimicrobial, anticonvulsant, sedative, and antipyretic effects. This should not be particularly surprising. Many plants contain pharmacologically active ingredients.

However, although they may be "natural," the pharmacologic compounds that occur in plants are not necessarily benign. Rather, they are apparently produced as a defense mechanism for the plants in which they are found. For example, one important subset of "natural" chemicals includes plant toxins that appear to protect plants against fungi, insects, and animal predators. Thousands of such compounds are known, and individual species may contain a few dozen toxins, including numerous carcinogens and mutagens (Ames, 1990b). So, for example, kava kava, for which there is evidence of usefulness in the treatment of humans with anxiety, depression, and insomnia (Pittler, 2002), may also be hepatotoxic (Centers for Disease Control and Prevention, 2003). As the toxicity of a particular compound is certainly dose dependent, so is pharmacologic activity, and, accordingly, so is the medical clinical relevance of such activity. Still, because of the obvious fact that some herbal and botanical remedies *do* contain pharmacologically active ingredients, and because not all drugs have been discovered, the development of drugs from plants continues, and many drug companies engage in large-scale pharmacologic screening of herbs.

On the other hand, some products do not contain *any* useful substances. It has been asserted that the more expensive the plant material, the more likely it is to be inferior (Tyler, 1994). Studies have shown that many ginseng products contain no active ingredients (Cui, 1994; Liberti, 1978). Herbs such as burdock root, "cleavers" (derived from a climbing plant that is common in England), oregano, and dandelion have no currently known therapeutic value (Natural Medicines Comprehensive Database, 2004), although all of these are ingredients in an over-the-counter herbal "anti-itch" preparation sold to horse owners. For such products, given that they work as advertised, either the mechanism of action is unknown or the product has a significant treatment effect on the owner of the animal.

Lack of Quality Control

Botanical agents intended for preventive or therapeutic use are not regulated as drugs under federal laws in the

United States. Instead, these products are marketed for humans as "foods" or "dietary supplements," but without specific health claims. Because they are not regulated as drugs, no legal standards exist for the processing, harvesting, or packaging of botanicals. Labels of herbal remedies generally do not list information about adverse effects, dangers, and contraindications, nor do they discuss dosages. In many cases, contents and potency are not accurately disclosed on the label. The lack of regulations regarding good manufacturing practices for these products and the lack of requirements for disclosure of all ingredients make it virtually impossible for the practitioner to know what an animal is actually receiving when it has been given a botanical remedy.

Because of the complexity of the mix of chemicals in plants, it can be difficult to determine which, if any, herbal product or component thereof has any biological activity. Reliable and reproducible assessments of activity are made even more difficult by the fact that processing of herbal products through techniques such as heating or boiling may alter the pharmacologic activity of their components. In addition, many environmental factors, such as soil type, altitude at which the plant is grown, seasonal variations in temperature, humidity, day length, rainfall, shade, dew, and frost, may affect the levels of components in any given lot of plant materials. Finally, other factors, such as insects, infections, planting density, plant species, and plant genetic factors, have important roles in the variability of herbal products (Wijesekera, 1991).

A basic problem associated with all clinical research in herbal medicines is the question of whether different products, extracts, or even lots of the same extract are comparable and equivalent [See Chapter 7 for a more detailed discussion]. Quality assurance is necessary to ensure that a particular herbal product has the expected effect; it is also an important determinant of product safety. For example, echinacea products may contain other plant extracts, may use different plant species *(Echinacea purpurea, E. pallida,* or *E. angustifolia)* or different parts (herb, root, both), or may have been produced in very different ways (i.e., hydrophilic or lipophilic extraction). In addition, the concentration of active ingredients can vary dramatically, depending on where the plants were grown or when they were harvested (Mrlianova, 2002). For example, glycyrrhizic acid, one of the primary pharmacologic agents in licorice root, occurs naturally in concentrations that range on average from 2% to 7%, with some rare plants having concentrations as high as 27%. Glycyrrhizic acid can be toxic; in addition, differing concentrations of the active ingredient make accurate dosing impossible, even though the glycyrrhizic acid may be removed, as in deglycyrrhizinated (DGL) licorice.

Even if the practitioner can obtain accurate information and determine the proper dosage and route of administration of an herbal or botanical product, another obstacle to its responsible administration remains. Very few herbal medicines have both the scientific name of the herb and an expiration date marked on the bottle. Several herbs may share common names, only one or two of which may be medicinal. For example, the name *snakeroot* can be applied to at least six very different plants. Also, ginseng is available in quite a few subspecies that have somewhat different properties and vary widely in cost. Wild ginseng has been shown to have immunomodulating effects that are absent in the cultured root (Mizuno, 1994). If only the common name is used, a less effective or even completely nonmedicinal herb may be substituted for the medicinal one.

Even a claim of "standardization" does not mean that the preparation is accurately labeled, nor does it indicate less variability in concentration of constituents of the herb (Gilroy, 2003). One common method of standardization involved blending several batches of the same herb that contained different amounts of the desired marker. Although this may produce a standardized single component, the effect on other, nonstandardized components is unclear. Some herbal manufacturers have tried to address the problem by adding purified active ingredients to batches of herbs (e.g., adding hyperforin to a batch of Saint John's Wort). This may give a batch a standardized content of active ingredients, but the original "balance" that some herbalists assert is necessary may be lacking (Bent, 2004). Thus, extrapolation of the results of any one study to any particular product may not be possible.

It is disturbing but true that cases of outright fraud in the herbal industry have been reported. For example, in 2003, the Australian regulatory body suspended the product license of Pan Pharmaceuticals, which produced 70% of the country's nutraceuticals and herbs and had a substantial overseas market (Pan Pharmaceuticals, 2004). At the same time, investigation proceeded into alleged fixing of safety data. In the United Kingdom, the British General Medical Council (GMC) determined that a company that produced evening primrose oil was guilty of falsifying clinical trials and offering inducements to researchers (Dyer, 2003). Perhaps worse was the fact that the products that contained the oil were found to be useless (Takwale, 2003).

Product Adulteration

Herbal products may be contaminated, adulterated, or misidentified. This appears to be a particular problem in herbal preparations from Asian sources (But, 1994; Chan, 1993; Lau, 2000); in 1998, the California Department of Health reported that 32% of Asian patent medicines sold in that state contained undeclared pharmaceuticals or heavy metals (Ko, 1998). Aplastic anemia has been reported with the use of an herbal medication adulterated with phenylbutazone (Nelson, 1995), and acute interstitial nephritis has occurred with another herbal preparation that was adulterated with meclofenamic acid (Abt, 1995). Cases of severe and even fatal poisoning have occurred after the use of medication with herbs containing aconitine, podophyllin, heavy metals, and anticholinergic substances (Chan, 1993; Chan, 1995; Chan, 1996; But, 1994). One survey of Chinese herbal medications found that on average, 23.7% of these were adulterated with everything from numerous nonsteroidal anti-inflammatory drugs to caffeine. More than half of the adulterated products contained two or more adulterants (Huang, 1997). Similarly, PC-SPES was a patented herbal preparation designed for the treatment of men with prostate problems; positive reports appeared even in major medical journals. However, chemical analysis of the product revealed the presence of diethylstilbestrol, indomethacin, warfarin, or a combination of these drugs (Sovak, 2002), and it was subsequently removed from the marketplace; lawyers for the victims claim that hundreds of people were harmed, and that some even died (Gillis, 2004). In perhaps the most notorious instance of adverse effects of herbal substitution in human medicine, rapidly progressive interstitial renal fibrosis and urothelial carcinoma have been reported in women taking Chinese formulas containing *Aristolochia* for weight reduction (Vanherweghem, 1998). Because of such problems, calls for tighter regulation of botanical products have been made with increasing regularity (Marcus, 2002).

SAFETY

Historical Aspects

The history of herbal medicine in general suggests a lack of efficacy. However, the long history of the use of herbal products should not be taken as an indication that such medications have been safe. It is probably reasonable, as a rule, to assume that an herb that enjoyed wide use for a considerable period is not *acutely* toxic *when used in the traditional manner*. The manner of preparation is important; traditional preparation of the raw tubers of the Oriental *Aconitum* species made the herb minimally poisonous, but modern manufacturing processes generated a hazardous product (Hikino, 1977); perhaps failure to adhere to traditional methods of preparation and usage caused the problems that resulted from use of *ma huang* (ephedra). In general, the effect that modern processing has on traditional remedies is largely unknown.

That said, assumptions about the lack of acute toxicity beg larger questions of chronic toxicities. Indeed, such products as comfrey, which is hepatotoxic and carcinogenic (Huxtable, 1986; Ridker, 1985), and tobacco were widely used for hundreds of years; tobacco was even endorsed by the medical profession. Concerns about long-term adverse effects may have been irrelevant in light of the short life spans of previous cultures—they are certainly not irrelevant today. However, even if concerns about chronic toxicities had been noted, they would likely not have resulted in limited use of botanical medicines because no real alternatives were available.

Direct Health Risks

Potent bioactive substances may exist in plants, and they have caused harm. Thus, for example, the US Food and Drug Association (FDA) attempted to ban the sale of dietary supplements containing ephedra; by January of 2003, kava extracts had been banned in the European Union and Canada and were subject to cautions and advisories ordered by the FDA as a result of 11 cases of hepatic failure that led to liver transplants, four of which resulted in death (Clouatre, 2004) [see Chapters 12 and the kava monograph in Chapter 24 for a more detailed discussion of this event]. Epidemiologic studies from various parts of the world show that certain "natural" chemicals in food may be carcinogenic risks to humans. Chewing of betel nuts with tobacco has been correlated with oral cancer (International Agency, 1988; Hirono, 1987). The phorbol esters present in Euphorbiaceae, some of which are used as folk remedies or herb teas, are potent mitogens and are thought to be a cause of nasopharyngeal cancer in China and esophageal cancer in Curacao (Hirayama, 1981; Hecker, 1981) and have been shown to cause signs of general poisoning in lactating goats and their milk-fed kids (Nawito, 1998). Pyrrolizidine toxins are mutagens that are found in comfrey tea, various herbal medicines, and some foods; they are hepatocarcinogens in rats and may cause liver cirrhosis and other diseases in humans. Allergic reactions, toxic reactions, possible mutagenic effects, adverse effects related to an herb's desired pharmacologic actions, and drug interactions have been reported with various herbal preparations (Bateman, 1998; Ernst, 1998b). However, the true extent of the direct risks posed by various herbal products is essentially unknown because currently no mandatory reporting mechanism for adverse reactions related to botanical products is in place. In addition, if the situation in veterinary medicine is analogous to that in human medicine, clients may not report to their veterinarians the use of herbal remedies or adverse reactions; this leads to an underreporting of important data.

Legal Obstacles and the Limitations of Experience

In the United States, the main barrier to ensuring safe and effective dietary supplements is the federal law that regulates these products. Unlike the laws governing prescription and over-the-counter drugs, which must be proved safe and effective before they are marketed, the Dietary Supplement Health and Education Act (DSHEA), passed in 1994, allows supplements to be marketed without any safety testing or proof of effectiveness (US FDA Web site, 2004b). This law does not require manufacturers to tell the FDA when their products are linked to serious injuries or death; it instead relies on a voluntary system that likely has resulted in significant underreporting of information on harmful reactions to herbal product supplements. Furthermore, the FDA can ban a supplement only if it can show that it poses "a significant or unreasonable risk of illness or injury."

Although many herbs have been used for thousands of years and folk healers and traditional herbalists have accumulated quite a bit of empiric information, these facts may lead to a false sense of security about herbal products. In fact, such information is not much help to practitioners in detecting effects that occur years after an herb is used (such as cancer) or in only a small percentage of individuals. Experience may be useful to clinicians in identifying obvious and predictable acute toxicities; however, it is a much less reliable tool for helping them detect reactions that are inconspicuous, rare, develop gradually, or have a prolonged latency period.

The risk that infrequently occurring adverse reactions to herbal remedies will remain unnoticed is illustrated by the statistical "rule of three." This rule dictates that the number of patients treated must be three times as high as the frequency of an adverse reaction if there is to be a 95% chance that the reaction will actually occur in the studied population. Thus, if an adverse reaction occurs 1 in 1000 times, the healer would have to treat at least 3000 patients to be 95% sure that he or she will see *one* reaction. However, the healer may need to see more than one reaction before a mental connection with the remedy is made. To have a 95% chance of seeing a reaction three times, the healer would have to treat 6500 patients with the same remedy, or approximately one patient a day for almost 25 years (DeSmet, 1993).

Reactions and Interactions

Although most herbal medicines are generally considered safe, herbal medicine probably presents a greater risk of adverse effects and interactions than is associated with any other "alternative" therapy. Allergic reactions, toxic reactions, adverse effects related to an herb's desired pharmacologic actions, and possible mutagenic effects have been identified (Ernst, 1998b). Reported adverse effects include germander with acute hepatitis, ephedra with fatal cardiovascular events, and comfrey with veno-occlusive disease (Essler, 2000).

Reports show that severe adverse effects and relevant interactions with other drugs can occur with herbal preparations. For example, hypericum (Saint John's Wort) extracts can decrease the concentration of a variety of other drugs through enzyme induction (Ernst, 1999). Other interactions include papaya extract with warfarin and evening primrose oil with epileptogenic drugs (increased likelihood of seizures). However, an interaction between two compounds is not always as expected. One would expect that the combination of ginkgo biloba and a thiazide diuretic would cause a hypotensive crisis. However, an elderly human patient taking this combination was found to have elevated blood pressure, which returned to normal when both agents were stopped (Shaw, 1997). Herbal remedies have also been shown in some instances to reduce the effectiveness of concurrently administered conventional medications. For example, co-administration of phenytoin with an Ayurvedic syrup called "Shankhapushpi" was reported to result in reduced concentrations of phenytoin and loss of seizure control (Dandekar, 1992). Several reviews summarizing adverse effects and interactions have been published (DeSmet, 1995; Miller, 1998; Fugh-Berman, 2000; Ernst, 2000a; Ernst, 2000b).

In veterinary medicine, the fact that some herbs have active pharmacologic ingredients has been a problem for unsuspecting animal owners and handlers. Numerous reports have described positive drug tests resulting from the administration of commercially available herbal products to animals. For example,

- Spinach octacosanol tablets were shown to be contaminated with phenylpropanolamine after a horse that was racing at Santa Anita racetrack in Los Angeles tested positive for phenylpropanolamine.
- Numerous trainers in the United States have been penalized for positive tests for caffeine after they had administered to their horses various herbal products containing guarana. (Guarana, made from the crushed seed of a climbing shrub native to Brazil and Uruguay, is used in the preparation of a hot beverage in those countries.) Some of these products are labeled "No added caffeine," although guarana is the obvious source of caffeine.
- Some ginseng-containing herbal products are known to contain sufficient caffeine to produce a positive test.
- Various herbal products contain alkaloids derived from ephedra. Some of these, such as "Herbal Ecstasy," also contain caffeine. Horse racing officials have received laboratory reports indicating positive tests for substances such as ephedrine, phenylpropanolamine, pseudoephedrine, norpseudoephedrine, and caffeine (Sams, 1998).
- Cases of melaleuca oil ("tea tree oil") toxicosis have been reported by veterinarians to the National Animal Poison Control Center when the oil was applied to the skin of dogs and cats (Villar, 1994). Indeed, essential oils of a number of plants can be problematic for both dogs and cats (Means, 2002).
- Accidental ingestion of a supplement containing guarana and *ma huang* led to a potentially lethal condition that required prompt detoxification and supportive treatment in 47 dogs (Ooms, 2001).
- Depression, epistaxis, lethargy, and diarrhea have been reported in cats that ingested chamomile (Means, 2002).
- Dogs dosed with 1.25 mL of garlic extract per kilogram of body weight developed oxidative injury to erythrocytes, including Heinz bodies and eccentrocytes (Lee, 2000).

The public and governmental agencies appear to be taking note of problems regarding the safety of herbal medications. In May of 2004, *Consumer Reports* magazine released its list of 12 supplements to avoid, which included 10 herbal products. These products—aristolochia, comfrey, chaparral, germander, kava, bitter orange, lobelia, pennyroyal oil, skullcap, and yohimbe—are listed as "definitely hazardous, very likely hazardous, and likely hazardous" (Dangerous Supplements, 2004). In 2001, the FDA and Congress were given recommendations from a committee asked to outline a science-based process for assessing supplement ingredients (Dietary Supplements, 2004). This report, issued by the Institute of Medicine and the National Research Council of the National Academies, suggested that federal laws should be modified to require supplement makers and distributors to inform the FDA of serious adverse health reactions associated with various supplements. The committee also recommended that before it is marketed, manufacturers and distributors of a particular product should be required to provide the FDA with both favorable and unfavorable information about that product's safety. In South Africa, in 2004, the government proposed a change to the Medicines Control Act that would mean that all complementary medicines, including self-treatments, nutritional supplements, vitamins, herbal supplements, energy drinks, homeopathic remedies, aromatherapy oils, and flower remedies, would have to undergo strict trials, like those already required for pharmaceuticals (Peters, 2004).

Indirect Risks

Even in the absence of direct adverse effects caused by herbal preparations, indirect risks result from their use when an unproven herbal remedy delays or replaces an effective form of conventional treatment. This may happen when the provider of therapy is overly optimistic about his or her abilities, or when a true believer puts too much faith in the healing powers of nature. An example of indirect health risk in animals is that which results when any number of natural remedies, in lieu of conventional antiparasitic agents, are advocated for the prevention and treatment of animals with internal or external parasites (e.g., garlic). Unfortunately, no herbal or botanical remedy has been shown to be effective in the control of internal or external parasites. Of course, harm does not always mean harm to animals. Botanical remedies may be harmful to a client if they necessitate additional expenditures for interventions of unknown benefit (Eisenberg, 1997).

Clinical Evidence

The quality of medical evidence that supports the practice of herbal medicine is highly variable, and critical examination of such evidence is almost completely lacking in literature provided by proponents of such approaches. Although numerous studies have investigated a variety of plant products or derivatives, much available information comes from in vitro studies on effects that may or may not have clinical relevance. Additional information provided in support of herbal therapies is generally heavily weighted toward books (in many cases, books by various authors on the subject of "alternative" medicine, both human and veterinary) and conference proceedings, uncontrolled case studies, or bench studies. Sorely lacking are high-quality, controlled clinical investigations, either human or animal. However, the general trend that is apparent in veterinary herbal medicine appears to be that if any, possibly beneficial, result of a selected intervention has appeared in *some* source, it provides sufficient grounds for the intervention to be considered "promising" enough to be tried in clinical cases.

In human and veterinary medicine, only relatively few of the medicinal plants that may be employed in herbal therapies have been tested in controlled trials. No matter how promising the laboratory experiments or anecdotal experiences, such results often fail to stand up to rigorous clinical investigation. Examples of these failures are numerous. For example mistletoe extract, which was reputed to have anticancer properties and has shown some interesting properties in in vitro research, did not affect disease-free survival or the quality of life in human patients with cancer of the head and neck (Steuer-Vogt, 2001). Similarly, evening primrose oil, which has been used for the treatment of humans with eczema and related skin conditions, failed to show a clinical effect in a well-designed study of 140 patients with eczema who took a high dose of gamma-linolenic acid (GLA) or placebo for 12 weeks (Takwale, 2003).

A number of systematic reviews on herbal medicines are available. In most cases, reviewers of herbal medicines have considered the available evidence as promising but only very rarely as convincing and sufficient to provide a firm basis for clinical decisions. Of the ten most commonly used herbs in the United States, a 2004 systematic review concluded that only four are *likely* to be effective, and that evidence by which the efficacy of approximately 20,000 other available herbal products can be evaluated is limited (Bent, 2004).

Reviewers have criticized the methodologic quality of documented primary studies (Linde, 2001). Trials using firm endpoints are very rarely available, and periods of observation are usually short. Nor is the clinical relevance of the observed effects always clear. Reviews most often show that the reported effects of herbal products are rather limited, need further confirmation by well-designed trials, or both. Data that directly compare herbal remedies with well-established pharmaceutical products are often not available or do not provide much useful information, for example, data may be derived from studies that failed to include a placebo group (Temple, 2000). In light of these considerations, there is little reason for practitioners to encourage use of an "alternative" herbal remedy if a safe and effective pharmaceutical already exists.

Herbal medicinal products are not, in general, subject to patent protection. Thus, drug companies may not be motivated to invest in trials of crude plant preparations, even though drug companies routinely engage in large-scale pharmacologic screening of herbs. Instead, many existing herbal medicine manufacturers are comparatively small companies. Perhaps this may help explain why the quality of many herbal medicine trials is low. Still, such an explanation is unconvincing, given estimates that expenditures by consumers on "alternative" remedies equal or exceed those for regulated pharmaceuticals (Richardson, 2001). It is also reasonable to consider that negative trials, which could threaten the company's survival, might not be published; indeed, the failure to report "negative" trials and the biased presentation of results by investigators and sponsors are problems that beset all medicine that aspires to be evidence based (Julian, 2003).

VETERINARY HERBAL AND BOTANICAL MEDICINE

The caveats and concerns regarding human applications of herbal and botanical veterinary medicines would be expected to be identical to those related to human medicine (Means, 2002). However, applying the findings of individual trials in human medicine to animal patient care may be problematic. With few exceptions, controlled studies on the clinical effects of herbal or botanical preparations in veterinary medicine appear to be essentially nonexistent. [See Chapter 24, Materia medica, for a review of studies and trials supporting the use of various herbs]. Doses are generally proportionate to those used in human herbal medicine; however, it should be kept in mind that experience with pharmaceuticals has shown that extrapolating dosage or toxicity data from one species to another can be dangerous. Because of their inherent toxicity, some herbal remedies should not be used under any circumstances. Others, such as tea tree oil, although it is safe at some dilutions, can cause significant adverse effects (Villar, 1994). In addition, because some herbal remedies contain multiple biologically active constituents, interaction with conventional drugs is also a concern (Poppenga, 2002).

ETHICAL CONCERNS

Although the body of scientific literature on herbs is growing, studies undertaken to determine whether particular compounds are teratogenic or carcinogenic are exceedingly rare. It is virtually impossible to find research that compares different quantities of a particular herb to find the optimum treatment dose. Very few herbs have been tested to determine the plasma peaks or the half-lives of their active ingredients. Studies or reports on the interactions of herbs with drugs, foods, or other herbs in animals are virtually unknown. Thus, the veterinary practitioner who intends to use herbal remedies is in the position of looking at the herb's primary mechanism of action, making assumptions about product content, extrapolating the dosage, then using his or her general pharmacology knowledge to try to spot potentially hazardous interactions while hoping for the best. The layperson who is trying to self-treat is left completely in the dark. This approach is likely to be troubling to science-minded veterinarians, as it essentially converts the clinical interaction from one whereby the animal may be prescribed treatment based on results gained from controlled testing on a number of patients, with documented results, to a series of uncontrolled experiments with an *n* of 1, with the subjects in the experiment often being attracted by false and/or unproven claims. Clinical veterinary medicine should be more than an exercise in trial and error performed on a case-by-case basis. Animal patients deserve much better, and clients deserve to be informed.

RECOMMENDATIONS FOR THE USE OF BOTANICAL REMEDIES

Consumers of veterinary herbal medicine must be alerted to the fact that herbal remedies are held to a standard that is lower than that applied to standard medicines. It is not acceptable to use products for which documentation of safety and efficacy is inadequate without the informed consent of a client. Certainly, botanical products that are known to have lethal or damaging adverse effects, either acutely or over an extended period, should be avoided. No matter what the inclination of a client or veterinarian, appropriate care must be given. Prescribing an unproven or disproven herbal therapy in cases where an acceptable and effective treatment already exists, or when the patient is at risk for greater suffering if the unproven treatment fails, would be unethical, in spite of the beliefs of the individual practitioner (Rollin, 1995). For example, even if an individual herbalist might assert that antibiotics are "unnatural" or "overprescribed," in the case of an animal that is sick with a bacterial infection, prescription of an unproven botanical remedy in lieu of antibiotics might cause harm and almost certainly will fall short of commonly accepted standards of care. Similarly, if animals are in pain, prescribing a plant product instead of an effective pain-relieving drug results in the risk that the animal may experience further suffering, which is morally reprehensible and represents a substandard method of care. Similarly, prescribing an herbal "tonic" to promote "wellness" is simply false advertising when evidence for such an effect (or even a definition of "wellness") is lacking. Although the well-being of an animal must be kept at the forefront of any consideration of therapy, even if a therapy is harmless, if it is not needed and a client must pay for it, there is no ethical basis for its prescription.

Currently, in the United States, botanical remedies are not required to meet any labeling standards [See Chapter 8 on Regulation for further information about labeling and production standards]. Clearly, this should be changed. Plant sources should be identified by their scientific names, rather than their common names, so that substitution with cheaper, ineffective, or possibly toxic ingredients can be avoided. Known active ingredients in a botanical remedy should be quantitatively and qualitatively identified on the label, and amounts of pharmacologically active substances should be sufficient for the product to perform as expected. Even the research priorities of the US National Center for Complementary and Alternative Medicine have placed an increased emphasis on studies of the mechanisms of action of botanical products (Centers for Research on Complementary and Alternative Medicine, 2004). Only those expectations that can be supported by science should be permitted on labels.

CONCLUSION

Herbal medicine exists, and may arguably deserve to exist, in the same way that other forms of "alternative" medicine do; that is, there appears to be some consumer demand for and satisfaction with it; therefore, the veterinary community might be well served, at least from a financial standpoint, to try to respond to that demand. Almost certainly, trying to eliminate modalities that are not supported by science would be quite incomprehensible to members of the public, politicians, regulators, or even veterinarians who have little grasp of the scientific issues and the complexities of patient/healer interactions. It might be possible to find some way of guarding the public from dangerous extremes, and of keeping medicine securely grounded in science, while still accommodating some more pragmatic considerations, but this delicate balance has so far not been achieved.

The needs of human beings for various therapies, or at least the demands that modern man has placed on "healers," are much more complex than modern scientific medicine may generally consider them to be. Apparently successful treatment for some of the less life- and limb-threatening conditions with which veterinarians are presented can likely be provided through any flavor of medical attention, regardless of rationality or intrinsic efficacy. It is the ongoing attention to the animal and the animal owner that counts. Consumers—and to some extent, professionals—have shown that they will exert their right to choose such attentions, regardless of anything that science, ethics, and rational considerations might say. Moreover, if veterinarians are unable to cure animals with vague illnesses of complex origin, or with vague complaints that have no obvious physiologic cause, the market is likely to be ready for those who can espouse novel, unsupported, or speculative theories and treatments that might "help."

The rise of herbal medicine and other alternative medical approaches should provide the animal and human medical community with occasion to reflect. The popularity of such remedies is clearly *not* based on constraints imposed by science and evidence, nor, in some cases, even by truth. The increase in use of botanical preparations would appear to indicate that members of the public—and all too frequently, veterinarians—fail to truly understand biomedical science and, as a result, fear and distrust what they do not understand. Such people are likely to eagerly embrace an alternative, particularly if that alternative is couched in vague, soothing, and evocative terminology. Indeed, if veterinary clients perceive scientific veterinary care as expensive, inconvenient, uncaring, dangerous, or ineffective, they may be very anxious to find an alternative (Eisenberg, 1997). However, enhancing such perceptions through false claims—even to the point of creating fear about modern scientific medicine and mistrust of those who practice it—is unethical, wrong, and ultimately, harmful to the veterinary profession.

The current practice of herbal medicine simply does not fit into scientific boundaries. At least in the United States, no generally objective standards have been devised for its use, no quality control has been put in place over its manufacture, and no follow-up has been provided after its distribution [See Chapter 8, Regulation and Quality Control, for more information]. Veterinary herbalists rely on the legislatively granted stamp of "professionalism" to protect their status, asserting that their unique knowledge of animal anatomy and physiology makes them the most ideally suited group to provide herbal medications to animals. However, as these herbalists endorse unscientific practices that may be equally well applied by nonveterinary professionals (some of whom are even trained by veterinarians), the concept of professionalism becomes diminished. Without standards of science and evidence, no distinction can be easily made between good medicine and quackery. As a result, the public is currently being victimized by unfounded, exaggerated, and false claims, glitzy advertising, and anecdotal and nontestable testimonials (some of which are currently being made by healthcare professionals themselves).

It may be argued that all of veterinary medicine is not science based, so to use such a stringent standard to evaluate a nonconforming therapy such as herbal and botanical medicine is inconsistent. This line of reasoning is the logical fallacy *tu quoque*. Such an argument tries to make the case that not following scientific standards is acceptable for herbal and botanical medicine because it is not uniformly the case in veterinary medicine. However, "two wrongs don't make a right," and, even if veterinary medicine were to be completely hypocritical in advocating and ignoring scientific standards for evaluation, this does not mean that such advocacy is not sound. Even if all of veterinary medicine were not science based, this would not justify the integration of herbal or other unconventional modalities with a similar dearth of supporting scientific evidence in mainstream medical practice. *Some* objective standard is necessary by which the profession can be evaluated and regulated, and science lays legitimate claim to being the *best* standard. Regardless, at least in human medicine, an assertion that medicine is not science based is not accurate (Imrie, 2000). Ultimately, the veterinary professional should insist that all therapies must be judged according to a consistent set of rules.

Clients come to veterinarians with any number of ideas and frames of mind, some of which may be quite different from those of the attending veterinarian. However, rather than attempting to pander to every frame of mind, veterinarians have the ability—indeed, the obligation—to explain and offer scientifically supported medicine to clients. There is no reason why this cannot be done in a manner that does not conflict with clients' beliefs. On the other hand, simply offering—even advertising—unsupported medical approaches is an affront to clients, patients, and veterinarians who may choose to eschew herbalism and other alternative approaches on reasonable grounds. Ultimately, such pandering cheapens the practice of veterinary medicine.

Veterinary medicine must strive to determine the best paths that can be used in the prevention and cure of animal diseases. Failing that, it must attempt to relieve an animal's suffering. Although the particular method used to achieve such goals is not important, this does not mean that the door is open to every conceivable approach. Veterinarians are obliged to not only "do no harm," but also to do some good (and to demonstrate that they *are*, in fact, doing good). Veterinarians must regulate themselves, so as to avoid external regulation by people with lesser expertise, as well as to protect the profession from an influx of untrained, albeit well-intentioned, laypeople. This goal can probably best be achieved through reliance on scientific methods designed to facilitate the search for empiric proof.

The late Varro E. Tyler, PhD, former dean of Purdue University School of Pharmacy and a leading authority on pharmacognosy, observed that more misinformation about the safety and efficacy of herbs is reaching the public currently than at any previous time, including the turn-of-the-20th-century heyday of patent medicines. In

1993, Dr. Tyler warned that consumers are "less likely to receive value for money spent in the field of herbal medicine than in almost any other" (Tyler, 1993). Such an admonition still rings true. In cases where treatment is not needed, veterinarians have an obligation to say so, and for real medical conditions associated with real pathology for which safe and effective pharmaceutical products are available, treatment with botanical preparations rarely makes sense.

References

Abt A, Oh J, Huntington R, et al. Chinese herbal medicine induced acute renal failure. Arch Intern Med 1995;155: 211–212.

Ackernecht EH. The American Medical Association and the cultivation of the cinchona tree in the United States. JAMA 1943;123:375.

Akerele O. Nature's medicinal bounty: don't throw it away. World Health Forum 1993;14:390–395.

Ames B, Profet M, Gold L. Nature's chemicals and synthetic chemicals: comparative toxicology. Proc Natl Acad Sci 1990a; 87:7782–7786.

Ames B, Profet M, Gold LS. Dietary pesticides (99.99% all natural). Proc Natl Acad Sci 1990b;87:7777–7781.

Angell M, Kassirer JP. Alternative medicine—the risks of untested and unregulated remedies. N Engl J Med 1998;339:839–841.

Balint GA. Artemisinin and its derivatives: an important new class of antimalarial agents. Pharmacol Ther 2001;90:261–265.

Bateman J, Chapman R, Simpson D. Possible toxicity of herbal remedies. Scott Med J 1998;43:7–15.

Bent S, Ko R. Commonly used herbal medicines in the United States: a review. Am J Med 2004;116:478–485.

Blanton WP. *Medicine in Virginia in the Seventeenth Century*. Richmond, Va: William Byrd Press; 1930.

Bodeker GC. Editorial. J Altern Complement Med 1996;3: 323–326.

But PP. Herbal poisoning caused by adulterants or erroneous substitutes. J Trop Med Hyg 1994;97:371–374.

Cairns J. In: Fortner JG, Rhoads JE, eds. *Accomplishments in Cancer Research in the United States*. Philadelphia, Pa: JB Lippincott; 1986:86.

Caldwell JC. Good health for many: the ESCAP region, 1950–2000. Asia-Pacific Population Journal 1999;14:21–38.

Centers for Disease Control and Prevention. Hepatic toxicity possibly associated with kava-containing products—United States, Germany, and Switzerland, 1999–2002. JAMA 2003;289: 36–37.

Centers for Research on Complementary and Alternative Medicine Program Fiscal Year 2004 Research Priorities. National Center for Complementary and Alternative Medicine. Available at: http://nccam.nih.gov/research/priorities/index.htm Accessed August 2, 2004.

Chan TY. Anticholinergic poisoning due to Chinese herbal medicines. Vet Hum Toxicol 1995;37:156–157.

Chan TY, Chan JC, Tomlinson B, et al. Chinese herbal medicines revisited: a Hong Kong perspective. Lancet 1993;342:1532–1534.

Chan TY, Critchley JA. Usage and adverse effects of Chinese herbal medicines. Hum Exp Toxicol 1996;15:5–12.

Chang H, But P. *Pharmacolocy and Applications of Chinese Materia Medica*, vol 1 and 2. Singapore: World Scientific; 1987.

Clouatre DL. Kava kava: examining new reports of toxicity. Toxicol Lett 2004;150:85–96.

Cui J, Garle M, Eneroth P, et al. What do commercial ginseng preparations contain? Lancet 1994;344:134.

Dandekar UP, Chandra R, Dalvi S, et al. Analysis of a clinically important interaction between phenytoin and Shankhapushpi, an Ayurvedic preparation. J Ethnopharmacol 1992;35: 285–288.

Dangerous supplements: still at large. *Consumer Reports*, 2004. Available at: http://www.consumerreports.org/main/content/display_report.jsp?FOLDER%3C%3Efolder_id=419337&bmUID=1091468673222. Accessed August 2, 2004.

DeSmet P. An introduction to herbal pharmacoepidemiology. J Ethnopharmacol 1993;38:197–208.

DeSmet P. Health risks of herbal remedies. Drug Safety 1995; 13:8193.

Dietary supplements. Available at: http://www.nap.edu/html/dietary_supplements/NI000760.pdf. Accessed August 2, 2004.

Duran-Reynals ML. *The Fever-Bark Tree*. Garden City, NY: Doubleday; 1946.

Dyer O. GMC reprimands doctor for research fraud. BMJ 2003; 326:730.

Eisenberg D. Advising patients who seek alternative medical therapies. Ann Intern Med 1997;127:61–69.

Eisenberg D, Kaptchuk T. The herbal history of digitalis: lessons for alternative medicine (response). JAMA 2000;283:884.

Ernst E. Patients' perception of complementary therapies. Forsch Komplementarmed 1995a;2:326–329.

Ernst E. Complementary medicine: common misconceptions. J R Soc Med 1995b;88:244–247.

Ernst E, DeSmet P, Shaw D, et al. Traditional remedies and the "test of time." Eur J Clin Pharmacol 1998a;54:99–100.

Ernst E. Harmless herbs? A review of the recent literature. Am J Med 1998b;104:170–178.

Ernst E. Second thoughts about safety of St John's wort. Lancet 1999;354:2014–2015.

Ernst E. Possible interactions between synthetic and herbal medicinal products. Part 1: A systematic review of the indirect evidence. Perfusion 2000a;13:415.

Ernst E. Possible interactions between synthetic and herbal medicinal products. Part 2: A systematic review of the direct evidence. Perfusion 2000b;13:60–70.

Essler D. Cancer and herbs. N Engl J Med 2000;342:1742–1743.

Fugh-Berman A. Herb-drug interactions. Lancet 2000;355: 134–138.

Gillis J. Herbal remedies turn deadly for patients. *Washington Post*, September 5, 2004. Available at: http://www.washingtonpost.com/ac2/wp-dyn/A62671-2004Sep4?language=printer. Accessed September 30, 2004.

Gilroy CM, Steiner JF, Byers T, et al. Echinacea and truth in labeling. Arch Intern Med 2003;163:699–704.

Haas KB. Animal therapy over the ages: 4. Early botanical medicine. Veterinary Heritage 2000;23:6–8.

Haller JS Jr. *Kindly Medicine*. Kent, Ohio: Kent State University Press; 1997.

Hecker E. Cocarcinogenesis and tumor promoters of the diterpene ester type as possible carcinogenic risk factors. J Cancer Res Clin Oncol 1981;99:103–124.

Hikino N, Yamada C, Nakamura K, et al. Change of alkaloid composition and acute toxicity of *Aconitum* roots during processing. Yakugaku Zasshi 1977;97:359–366.

Hirayama T, Ito Y. A new view of the etiology of nasopharyngeal carcinoma. Prev Med 1981;10:614–622.

Hirono I, ed. *Naturally Occurring Carcinogens of Plant Origin: Toxicology, Pathology and Biochemistry, Bioactive Molecules*, vol 2. Tokyo/Amsterdam: Kodansha/Elsevier Science BV; 1987.

Hiscox GD, Sloane TO, Eisensen HE, eds. *Fortunes in Formulas for Home, Farm and Workshop*. New York, NY: Books, Inc; 1957.

Huang W, Wen K, Hsiao M. Adulteration by synthetic therapeutic substances of traditional Chinese medicines in Taiwan. J Clin Pharmacol 1997;37:344–350.

Huxtable R. A brief history of pharmacology, therapeutics and scientific thought. Proc West Pharmacol Soc 1999;42:181–223.

Huxtable R. Safety of botanicals: historical perspective. Proc West Pharmacol Soc 1998;41:1–10.

Huxtable RJ, Luthy J, Zweifel U. Toxicity of comfrey-pepsin preparations. N Engl J Med 1986;315:1095.

Imrie R, Ramey D. The evidence for evidence based medicine. Comp Ther Med 2000;8:123–126.

International Agency for Research on Cancer. *IARC Monographs on the Evaluation of Carcinogenic Risks to Humans. Overall Evaluations of Carcinogenicity: An Updating of IARC Monographs*, vol 1-44, suppl 7. Lyon, France: IARC; 1988.

Itoh S, Marutani K, Nishijima T, et al. Liver injuries induced by herbal medicine, Syo-saiko-to (ziao-chai-hu-tang). Dig Dis Sci 1995;40:1845–1848.

Julian DG. What is right and what is wrong about evidence-based medicine? J Cardiovasc Electrophysiol 2003;14(9 suppl):S2–S5.

Kleiner SM. The true nature of herbs. Phys Sports Med 1995; 23:13–14.

Ko RJ. Adulterants in Asian patent medicines. N Engl J Med 1998;339:847.

Lau KK, Lai CK, Chan AW. Phenytoin poisoning after using Chinese proprietary medicines. Hum Exp Toxicol 2000;19: 385–386.

Lee K, Yamato O, Tajima M, et al. Hematologic changes associated with the appearance of eccentrocytes after intragastric administration of garlic extract to dogs. Am J Vet Res 2000; 61:1446–1450.

Liberti LE, Der Marderosian A. Evaluation of commercial ginseng products. J Pharm Sci 1978;67:1487–1489.

Lieberman HR. The effects of ginseng, ephedrine, and caffeine on cognitive performance, mood and energy. Nutr Rev 2001; 59:91–102.

Lilienfeld A. The evolution of the clinical trial. Bull Hist Med 1982;56:1–18.

Linde K, ter Riet G, Hondras M, et al. Systematic reviews of complementary therapies—an annotated bibliography. Part 2: Herbal medicine. BMC Complement Altern Med 2001;1:5.

Marcus DM, Grollman AP. Botanical medicines—the need for new regulations. N Engl J Med 2002;347:2073–2076.

Means C. Selected herbal hazards. Vet Clin North Am Small Anim Pract 2002;32:367–382.

Merillat LA, Campbell DM. *Veterinary Military History of the United States*. Kansas City, Mo: Haver-Glover Laboratories; 1935.

Miller LG: Herbal medicine. Selected clinical considerations focusing on known or potential drug-herb interactions Arch Intern Med 1998;158:2200–2211.

Mizuno M, Yamada J, Terai H, et al. Differences in immunomodulating effects between wild and cultured *Panax* ginseng. Biochem Biophys Res Commun 1994;200:1672–1678.

Mrlianova M, Tekelova D, Felklova M, et al. The influence of the harvest cut height on the quality of the herbal drugs *Melissae folium* and *Melissae herba*. Planta Med 2002;68: 178–180.

Natural Medicines Comprehensive Database. Available at: http://www.naturaldatabase.com. Accessed October 1, 2004.

Nawito M, Ahmed Y, Zayed S, et al. Dietary cancer risk from conditional cancerogens in produce of livestock fed on species of spurge (Euphorbiaceae). II. Pathophysiological investigations in lactating goats fed on the skin irritant herb *Euphorbia peplus* and in their milk-raised kids. J Cancer Res Clin Oncol 1998;124:179–185.

Nelson L, Shih R, Hoffman R. Aplastic anemia induced by an adulterated herbal medication. J Toxicol Clin Toxicol 1995;33: 467–470.

Ooms TG, Khan SA, Means C. Suspected caffeine and ephedrine toxicosis resulting from ingestion of an herbal supplement containing guarana and ma huang in dogs: 47 cases (1997–1999). J Am Vet Med Assoc 2001;218:225–229.

Osol A, Farrar GE, eds. *The Dispensatory of the United States of America*. 25th ed. Philadelphia, Pa: JB Lippincott; 1955: 444–460.

Pan Pharmaceuticals Limited, Australian Government. Regulatory action and product recall information. Available at: http://www.tga.health.gov.au/recalls/pan.htm. Accessed August 2, 2004.

Peters M. Sickening blow for alternative medicines. *Sunday Independent Online*, South Africa, September 26, 2004. Available at: http://iol.co.za/index.php. Accessed September 27, 2004.

Pittler MH, Ernst E. Kava extract for treating anxiety. Cochrane Database Syst Rev 2002;2:CD003383.

Poppenga R. Herbal medicine: potential for intoxication and interactions with conventional drugs. Clin Tech Small Anim Pract 2002;17:6–18.

Ramey D, Buell P. Equine medicine in sixth century China: *Qiminyaoshu*. In: Rossdale P, Green R, eds. *Guardians of the Horse II*. Suffolk, UK: Romney Publications; 2001:154–161.

Richardson MA. Biopharmacologic and herbal therapies for cancer: research update from NCCAM. J Nutr 2001:131(11 suppl):3037S–3040S.

Ridker PM, Ohkuma S, McDermott WV, et al. Hepatic venocclusive disease associated with the consumption of pyrrolizidine-containing dietary supplements. Gastroenterology 1985;88: 1050–1054.

Rollin B. An ethicist's commentary of the case of a veterinarian utilizing homeopathic therapy. Can Vet J 1995;36:268–269.

Rotblatt M, Ziment I. *Evidence-Based Herbal Medicine*. Philadelphia, Pa: Hanley and Belfus; 2002:388.

Sams R, Professor, Analytical Toxicology Department, College of Veterinary Medicine, The Ohio State University, personal communication, 1998.

Shaw D, Leon C, Kolev S, et al. Traditional remedies and food supplements. A 5-year toxicological study (1991–1995). Drug Safety 1997;17:342–356.

Sovak M, Seligson AL, Konas M, et al. Herbal composition PC-SPES for management of prostate cancer: identification of active principles. J Natl Cancer Inst 2002;94:1275–1281.

Steuer-Vogt MK, Bonkowsky V, Ambrosch P, et al. The effect of an adjuvant mistletoe treatment programme in resected head and neck cancer patients: a randomised controlled clinical trial. Eur J Cancer 2001;37:23–31.

Takwale A, Tan E, Agarwal S, et al. Efficacy and tolerability of borage oil in adults and children with atopic eczema: randomised, double blind, placebo controlled, parallel group trial. BMJ 2003;327:1385–1388.

Temple R, Ellenberg SS. Placebo-controlled trials and active-control trials in the evaluation of new treatments. Part 1: Ethical and scientific issues. Ann Intern Med 2000;133: 455–463.

Tyler V. *The Honest Herbal*. New York, NY: Pharmaceutical Products Press; 1993:7.

Tyler V. *Herbs of Choice: The Therapeutic Use of Phytomedicinals*. New York, NY: Pharmaceutical Products Press; 1994:5.

Unschuld P. *Medicine in China: A History of Pharmaceutics*. Berkeley, Calif: University of California Press; 1986.

Unschuld P. *Chinese Medicine*. Brookline, Mass: Paradigm Publications; 1988:69–81.

US FDA Web site. Available at: http://www.fda.gov/oc/initiatives/ephedra/february2004/. Accessed August 1, 2004a.

US FDA Web site. Available at: http://vm.cfsan.fda.gov/~dms/dietsupp.html. Accessed August 2, 2004b.

Vanherweghem LJ. Misuse of herbal remedies: the case of an outbreak of terminal renal failure in Belgium (Chinese herbs nephropathy). J Altern Complement Med 1998;4:9–13.

Vickers A, Zollman CE. ABCs of complementary medicine: herbal medicine. BMJ 1999;319:1050–1053.

Villar D, Knight MJ, Hanen SR, et al. Toxicity of melaleuca oil and related essential oils applied topically on dogs and cats. Vet Hum Toxicol 1994;36:139–142.

Vogel VJ. *American Indian Medicine.* Norman, Okla: University of Oklahoma Press; 1970.

Wijesekera ROB, ed. *The Medicinal Plant Industry.* Boca Raton, Fla: CRC Press; 1991.

Williamson EM. Synergy and other interactions in phytomedicines. Phytomedicine 2001;8:401–409.

Wynn SG, Marsden S. *Manual of Natural Veterinary Medicine.* St. Louis, Mo: Mosby, Inc.; 2003.

PART III

The Plants

Medical Botany

Robyn Klein

CHAPTER

WHAT IS MEDICAL BOTANY?

Medical botany is an expert field of study once consigned to the past and now summoned to serve the herbal renaissance. In the early 1900s, this discipline was known as pharmaceutical botany, with books such as *Textbook of Pharmaceutical Botany,* written by Heber W. Youngken and published from 1914 to 1938. These texts focused primarily on the botanical aspects of medicinal plants rather than their bioactivity. Alternately, pharmacognocists published textbooks throughout the 19th century on the chemistry and bioactivity of medicinal plants. The most well known is *Trease and Evans Pharmacognosy,* now in its 15th edition.

Today, medical botany is often simplified to the study of *materia medica,* natural substances that possess medicinal properties, as reflected in the newly revised edition of *Medical Botany* by Lewis and Elvin-Lewis (2003). This medically erudite treatment concentrates on the systems of the body and the herbs that affect these systems. Owing to a reliance on both conventional medicine and reductionistic ethnobotanical and natural products research, misinterpretations are common. Worse, a peculiar blindness to traditional medicine is sorely evident.

Medical botany is treated according to the eye of the beholder, and this chapter is no exception. From this author's view, medical botany is, first and foremost, a subset of biology called plant biology, or botany. Specialists within plant biology include plant scientists, taxonomists, systematicists, and botanists. The study of plants involves the evolution and taxonomic ordering of plants such as the vascular divisions of pteridophyte, gymnosperm, and angiosperm species, and the use of a plant key or flora to identify plants. This latter skill requires knowledge of plant anatomy and morphology (form and structure). Plant biology additionally covers the physiology, pathology, and metabolism of plants, encompassing photosynthesis, reproduction, growth, development, defense, nutrition, population, and the ecology of plants. One classic text on botany is *Biology of Plants* (2003) by Peter H. Raven.

The study of plant constituents is not well covered in plant biology. Students must therefore turn to chemistry and biochemistry texts. Plant metabolism investigates how plant compounds are synthesized and the role these compounds play in the plant itself. A beginning understanding of plant metabolism and biosynthesis is covered in *Biochemistry & Molecular Biology of Plants* (2000) by Buchanan, Gruissem, and Jones. A more thorough approach is found in *Medicinal Natural Products* (2002) by Paul M. Dewick.

Medical botany requires the study of medicine, including mammalian physiology, biochemistry, pathology, and pharmacy. Medical botany can be considered a subset of botany with a primary focus on the bioactivity of plants in humans and animals. A medical botanist would be familiar with not only a vast materia medica (the tools) of herbal medicine and medical science (conventional and traditional), but also of plant biology.

Several problems plague the study of medical botany. As mentioned, modern medical botany texts tend to be written within the scope of conventional science, ignoring the traditional herbal medicine paradigm. Medicinal plant research applied to medical botany is also couched within conventional scientific methods. This poses a dilemma because the therapeutic application of plant products greatly affects their efficacy and safety. Thus, it is important to appreciate that the history of using plants for medicine originates in the realm of indigenous wisdom or traditional medicine. According to the World Health Organization (2000), traditional medicine

> ". . . is the sum total of the knowledge, skills, and practices based on the theories, beliefs, and experiences indigenous to different cultures, whether explicable or not, used in the maintenance of health, as well as in the prevention, diagnosis, improvement, or treatment of physical and mental illnesses. The terms complementary/alternative/nonconventional medicine are used interchangeably with traditional medicine in some countries."

These two models of knowledge—traditional (indigenous) wisdom and conventional science—often do not

TABLE 10-1

Examples of Conventional Drugs Derived From Plants

Drug	Activity	Plant Source
Digoxin	Cardiovascular	*Digitalis purpurea* L., Scrophulariaceae
Reserpine	Cardiovascular	*Rauvolfia verticiliata* (Loureiro) Baillon, Apocynaceae
Scutellarin	Cardiovascular	*Scutellaria baicalensis* Georgi, Lamiaceae
Synephrine	Cardiovascular	*Citrus aurantium* L., Rutaceae
Camptothecine	Anticancer	*Camptotheca acuminata* Decne, Nyssaceae
Taxol	Anticancer	*Taxus chienensis* (Pilg.) Rehder, Taxaceae
Vinblastine	Anticancer	*Catharanthus roseus* (L.) G. Don, Apocynaceae
Huperzine A	Nervous system	*Huperzia serrata* (Thunb.) Rothm., Lycopodiaceae
Levodopa	Nervous system	*Mucuna cochinensis* (Lour.) A. Chev., Fabaceae
Scopolamine	Nervous system	*Scopolia japonica* Maxim., Solanaceae
Codeine	Respiratory system	*Papaver somniferum* L., Papaveraceae
Allicin	Antimicrobial	*Allium sativum* L., Liliaceae
Berberine	Antimicrobial	*Berberis julianae* C.K. Schneid., Berberidaceae
Silymarin	Digestive system	*Silybum marianum* (L.) Gaertn., Asteraceae
Arteannuin	Parasiticide	*Artemisia annua* L., Asteraceae

agree. Conventional medicine, considered "evidence based," uses concentrated chemicals with the therapeutic strategy of suppressing symptoms by inhibiting enzymes involved in normal metabolic and pathologic processes. However, the therapeutic strategy of traditional herbal medicine is to strengthen and resolve the underlying causes of pathology through gentle modulation of normal and pathologic processes. Additionally, traditional herbal products embrace complex forms of whole plant products, sometimes concentrated, but not to the degree found in conventional pharmacology (Table 10-1).

Although the practices of traditional medicine vary by culture, several ubiquitous themes are present. One ubiquitous theme is a belief in the wisdom of the body, *the vital force,* which some consider an untestable philosophy akin to string theory in physics. Nonetheless, *vital force* is somewhat synonymous to the traditional paradigms, *prana* in India, and *qi* in China. Additionally, traditional medicine focuses on the unique constitution and physiology of the patient, whereas the focus of conventional medicine is on pathology and treatment protocol. Energetics of the patient, pathology, and the herbs themselves are also important components common to models of traditional medicine.

As an example, the use of *Ephedra sinensis* in traditional Chinese medicine is very different from the reductionistic use of the alkaloid, ephedrine, by companies marketing it in weight loss products. The tool is *not* the same as the model. Herbal medicine is a model of healing that is regulated separately from the production and sale of herbal products (the tools). In the United States, healing modalities are regulated by each state through a medical board of practitioners. Herbal products are regulated by the federal government (US Food and Drug Administration and Federal Trade Commission) as dietary supplements under the Dietary Supplement and Health Education Act (DSHEA), passed by Congress in 1994. Botanical supplements are a new category that is currently under review.

To appropriately apply knowledge gained through the discipline of medical botany, the therapeutic model must be clearly delineated. A common mistake of new herbal medicine practitioners is to confuse the model with the tool. A conventional practitioner is not practicing traditional herbal medicine if he or she is using the herb product as a drug to inhibit an enzyme. *How* a tool is used affects the therapeutic outcome. Thus, the study of medical botany must reflect the model of medicine and must strive to keep such distinctions obvious. Most medical botany texts today are biased toward the conventional scientific model, which is a late player in the renaissance of herbal products. Traditional models are at the core of herbal products, and, if marginalized, the efficacy and safety of these products can drastically change. Although it may be appropriate to apply an herbal product through the use of conventional pharmacology, can it be said that herbal medicine is being practiced?

An additional problem plaguing medical botany is the preferential attention to animals and lack of interest in plants. This apparent blind spot in our society is believed to be due to the human visual process and to a zoocentric attitude among our educators. *Plant blindness* has been defined as

> "the inability to see or notice the plants in one's own environment—leading to (a) the inability to recognize the importance of plants in the biosphere, and in human affairs; (b) the inability to appreciate the aesthetic and unique biological features of the life forms belonging to the Plant Kingdom; and (c) the misguided, anthropocentric ranking of plants as inferior to animals, leading to the erroneous conclusion that they are unworthy of human consideration" (Wandersee & Schussler, 1998).

Veterinarians are in a unique position to observe fascinating similarities among three major groups of organisms if they add medical botany to their expertise. Herbal medicine requires an understanding of both traditional therapeutic models and the botany and chemistry of medicinal plants—the tools employed by these models. Medical botany encompasses this latter study, although it must compete with many other disciplines important to herbal medicine practitioners. Medical botany is deeply woven throughout ethnobotany, economic botany, entomology (study of insects), plant pathology, horticulture, microbiology, mycology (fungi), molecular cell biology, and toxicology. Most practitioners can barely keep up with their own specialty! Therefore, this chapter attempts to provide a basic overview for the veterinary herbalist, while revealing the extraordinary depth of plants and explaining their role in the health of all living creatures on our planet.

TAXONOMY

Plants are multicelled organisms placed in the Eukaryote domain, which includes Protista, Fungi, and Animalia. Plants are first divided into nonvascular and vascular groups. Nonvascular plants fall into two major categories: green algae, including diatoms and slime molds; and bryophytes, including liverworts, hornworts, and mosses. These are nonvascular because they lack xylem and phloem—water- and food-conducting tissues present in vascular plants. Vascular plants are divided into pteridophytes (horsetails and club mosses), gymnosperms (pines, junipers, *Ephedra*), and angiosperms (monocots and dicots). Most medicinal plants are found among the 250,000 angiosperm species, supporting the theory that plants have been developing more complex chemistry, along with their more intricate morphology (Gottlieb, 2002).

Taxonomy is a branch of biology that is concerned with naming and classifying forms of life. Plants are organized into groups such as classes, orders, families, and genera according to evolutionary ancestry. Nomenclature, or the naming of plant species, is set by the International Code of Botanical Nomenclature (ICBN). These naming "rules," which are updated periodically and published by the International Botanical Congress, are the result of agreement between taxonomists based on research and cannot be forced upon any botanist, or herbalist, for that matter. In fact, it may take decades for these changes to become accepted.

Taxonomy allows authorities to group plants according to any rule they choose. Thus, many classifications have been suggested for flowering plants. Taxonomists, systematicists, and botanists write floras based on the interpretation of their favored taxonomic authority. This is why no one can say for sure just how many plant families exist. Some authorities maintain that there are 350 plant families; others (fondly referred to as "splitters") have divided plant genera into 520 families (Cullen, 1997). The important thing for herbalists to remember is that they must not mix up authorities. One should stick to one authority, usually the author of the flora (list of plants) of your region.

Division Spermatophyta (plants with seeds)
  Class Angiospermae (angiosperms)
    Subclass Dicotyledoneae (dicots)
      Order Papaverales
        Family Papaveraceae (poppy)
          Genus *Papaver*
            Species *somniferum* (opium poppy)

Figure 10-1 System of taxonomic nomenclature.

The International Code of Botanical Nomenclature has set some basic rules. A plant name (or binomial) has two parts: a genus that is grouped into a family and a species that is grouped under that genus. For example, peppermint *(Mentha piperita)*, spearmint *(M. spicata)*, and field mint *(M. arvensis)* are grouped under the genus *Mentha*. Genera (plural) are placed in families, which are placed in orders, which are placed in subclasses, classes, and, finally, a division. This system gives a specific plant species the same Latin name for use all over the world. New name changes turn old names into synonyms. Latin names are always italicized as indicated. Figure 10-1 gives an example of the nomenclature scheme.

Each Latin bionomial is followed by a shortened acronym for the author who named that particular species. For example, *Cannabis sativa* L. was first named by Linnaeus. When a species name is changed, the original author is placed in parentheses, with the new author following, such as *Cimicifuga racemosa* (L.) Nutt. This is black cohosh, a species formerly named *Actaea racemosa* L. Recently, *Cimicifuga racemosa* (L.) Nutt. was returned to the genus *Actaea* L. (Compton, 1998)! It will take decades for this new name to become accepted in the literature. Herbalists may want to use this new name but many botanists will continue to employ *Cimicifuga*. It does not matter which name is used, as long as we all understand which plant species is being referred to. History suggests that herbalists have to be bilingual. Black cohosh can be found in old Eclectic texts as *Macrotys*. Burdock *(Arctium lappa)* was once named *Lappa major*, and *Echinacea* was once *Brauneria*.

The use of Latin names becomes even more important for Chinese herbs that can be referred to either in pinyin, Mandarin, Korean, or Japanese. Pharmaceutical names of plants and their medicinal parts must also be mastered, such as *Taraxaci folium* (dandelion leaf), *Salicis cortex* (willow bark), or *Valeriana radix* (valerian root). In short, herbalists must be proficient in the many ways of naming medicinal plants. From these examples, it is easy to see why common names are moot and even dangerous to rely on.

Many changes have recently been made to the names of plants because it was discovered that some plants are not related after all. This is because plants were originally classified by morphology. We now know that many plants with similar anatomic structure are actually not closely related. Similar-looking species sometimes achieve their design through convergent, or parallel, evolution. For example, both seals and penguins possess flippers. However, seals are mammals and penguins are birds. Both organisms developed flippers through independent means, not through common ancestral traits. Chloroplast and mitochondrial DNA provide stronger evidence than physical alikeness, which can be more subjective. Thus, many plant species have been moved to other families, causing some confusion and frustration among botanists and herbalists alike.

For example, most plant species once belonging to the Scrophulariaceae (figwort family) have now been moved to other families. New DNA evidence has revealed mistakes assumed by similar morphology. For instance, *Pedicularis* (lousewort) and *Euphrasia* (eyebright) are now placed in the Orobanchaceae, along with other parasitic genera such as *Orobanche* (broomrape). Similarly, *Veronica, Gratiola, Digitalis, Bacopa,* and *Chelone* have been moved to the Plantaginaceae (plantain family). Science, similar to nature, is in constant flux. Herbalists should understand that these changes are the result of important new discoveries, not an attempt to make botany more complicated.

Along with changes to the names of plant species and replacement into new families, the Latin names of some plant families have been changed. The most common family changes are as follows (new then old): pea family (Fabaceae/Leguminosae), parsley family (Apiaceae/Umbelliferae), grass family (Poaceae/Graminae), mustard family (Brassicaceae/Cruciferae), mint family (Lamiaceae/Labiatae), and aster family (Asteraceae/Compositae).

It should be no surprise that plant species with similar medicinal properties are found in the same or closely related families. Plant species in the rose family (Rosaceae) commonly possess an astringent property caused by tannins and flavonoids common to this family. Glucosinolates are common in the mustard family (Brassicaceae). Species in the mint family (Lamiaceae) are often antimicrobial owing to essential oils and tannins. The nightshade family (Solanaceae) contains tropane alkaloids in many of its species, such as belladonna *(Atropa belladonna),* black henbane *(Hyoscyamus niger),* jimsonweed *(Datura stramonium),* nightshade *(Solanum dulcamara),* and mandrake *(Mandragora officinarum).*

PLANT IDENTIFICATION

The identification of plant material is crucial to the safety and efficacy of an herbal product. In the present manufacturing arena, plant material is often identified microscopically (cell level) but also chemically through expensive techniques such as chromatography. Adulteration, contamination, and misidentification have plagued the medicinal plant industry in the past, but such events are rarer as quality and safety procedures are put into place.

Raw plant material arrives from growers and wildcrafters in many forms: fresh, uncut, cut, sifted, and powdered. If herbal practitioners do not make their own herbal products, they must trust manufacturers to correctly identify the plant material and process and preserve the material into a product that is consistent and effective. The skills of plant identification are valuable, yet not required of herb practitioners. However, whether the practitioner is collecting the plant or relying on a harvester, the responsibility of correct identification lies with the practitioner. Thus, plant identification skills are particularly necessary.

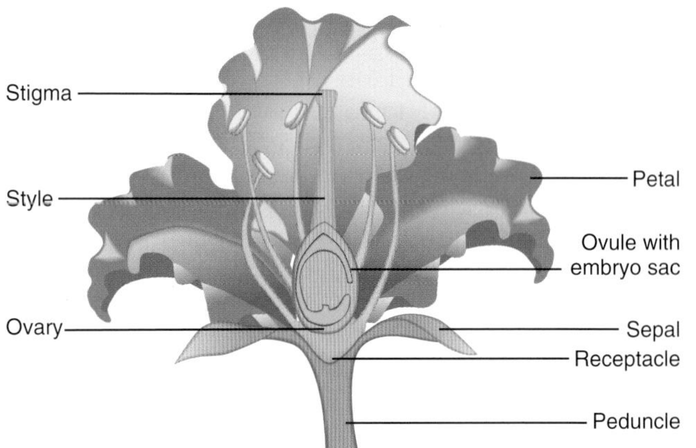

Figure 10-2 Parts of a flower.

Wild plants are identified with a plant key or flora for the local area in which the plant is found, although floras are not available for all states. Some floras, such as *Manual of Vascular Plants,* by Gleason, or *Vascular Plants of the Pacific Northwest,* by Hitchcock and Cronquist, encompass many states. Floras give lengthy, erudite descriptions of plant species employing scholarly terminology. To identify the flora or plant key for a particular country or state, one should make inquiries to a university herbarium or native plant society in the community. An illustrated glossary is essential, such as *Plant Identification Terminology,* by Harris and Harris. A plant cannot be keyed out unless it is in the flowering stage because most floras are based on the parts of a flower (Figure 10-2). The main parts of a flower consist of (from outside to inside) sepals, petals, stamens, and pistil. Floral diagrams (Figure 10-3) are commonly used to show the morphology and number of flower parts.

The diagram in Figure 10-3 illustrates a flower with three sepals in the outer whorl, three petals in the next inner whorl, six stamens (with paired anthers), and a three-parted pistil. This particular diagram thus shows a monocot species, possessing flower parts in 3's and 6's.

Floral formulas are commonly used. However, one must first become familiar with the meaning of the symbols in the formula. The four floral series—calyx, corolla, androecium, and gynoecium (see Glossary on p. 156)—are represented as follows:

K = calyx
C = corolla
A = androecium
G = gynoecium

As an example, the floral formula, K5 Cz 1+(2) + 2 A 9 + 1 $\underline{G}$ 1, denotes the following:

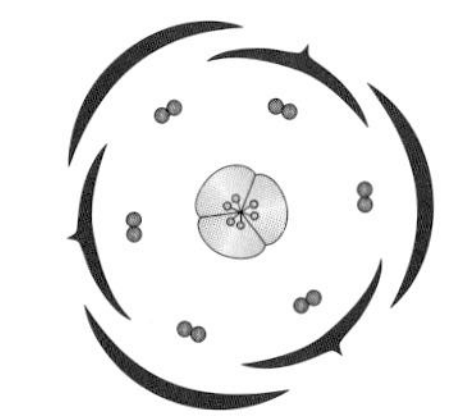

Figure 10-3 A floral diagram.

- Calyx of 5 separate sepals
- Corolla zygomorphic of 5 petals, 2 joined together, 2 free and forming a pair, and a fifth that is different
- Androecium of 10 stamens, 9 joined by their filaments, the 10th free; and
- Gynoecium unicarpellate, the ovary superior

For each floral formula, one must be familiar with the meaning of the terms used or consult a glossary. Practice is required to become proficient.

Flowers are arranged into inflorescences such as cymes, spikes, racemes, umbels, and heads. Every part of a plant can be described, including leaves, which comprise unique shapes, margins, tips, and bases. Plant identification involves the description of dozens, if not hundreds, of terms; thus, this section can go no farther. Suffice to say that keying plants is a skill gained from practice and patience, but it is very rewarding, once mastered.

PLANT ANATOMY

In a basic biology class, one learns that animal and plant cells share a common basic structure (Figure 10-4). All cells are bounded by a plasma membrane with cytoplasm inside, along with membrane-bound organelles such as a nucleus, mitochondria, peroxisomes, ribosomes, endoplasmic reticulum, and golgi complex. These organelles perform many of the same functions, whether in animal or plant cells. For example, the principal function of mitochondria is to generate energy in the form of adenine triphosphate (ATP). The main differences, seen in Box 10-1, are that animal cells contain lysosomes, centrioles, and sometimes flagella (organelles that provide locomotion for the cell, such as in sperm cells). Plant cells, on the other hand, are unique in that they possess a cell wall, plastids, a vacuole, and plasmodesmata.

The cell wall is the most distinctive feature of plant cells that is absent in animal cells. Cell walls are rich in cellulose, pectin, hemicelluloses, glycoproteins, and lignin, a structural compound that gives plants strength and rigidity (not to be confused with lignan, a bioactive compound found in many medicinal herbs). The cell wall is external to the plasma membrane of the cell. Thus, it is a layer that is not found in animal cells.

Plastids are the next most distinctive feature of plant cells. Plastids reproduce by fission and are semiautonomous. Three types of plastids are found in plant cells: chloroplasts, responsible for photosynthesis and production of many secondary compounds; chromoplasts, responsible for pigment coloration of plant tissues; and amyloplasts (leucoplasts), responsible for the formation of starch grains in storage tissues such as roots. These plastids can morph into each other, depending on environmental and developmental conditions. Think of the green coloration on the tops of carrots when they are exposed to sunlight in the garden. Chloroplasts are able to synthesize some amino acids, as well as some fatty acids. We will see later that chloroplasts also produce monoterpenes, diterpenes, carotenes, phytol, and ubiquinone.

BOX 10-1

The Major Differences Between Animal and Plant Cells

ANIMAL CELLS	PLANT CELLS
Lysosomes	Cell wall
Centrioles	Plastids
Flagella	Vacuole and tonoplast
	Plasmodesmata

Vacuoles are found only in plant cells. They are surrounded by a single membrane (the tonoplast) and can take up much of the cell volume. They are filled with cell sap (mostly water) and store hydrophilic compounds such as anthocyanins, alkaloids, nonprotein amino acids, saponins, glycosides, flavonoids, tannins, cyanogens, amines, glucosinolates, and some primary compounds.

Just as in animals, plant cells have a plasma membrane that regulates the exchange of substances within the cell and also controls the passage of materials into and out of the cell. Chemical homeostasis is just as important in a plant cell as in an animal cell. However, it must be remembered that the major difference is the cell wall. Therefore, passage of materials through the cell wall requires different strategies than those used in animal cells.

Plant cells are connected together by the plasmodesmata, which provide a cytoplasmic pathway for transport between cells of substances such as viruses, RNA, and transcription factors. The plasmodesmata are similar to the gap junctions of animal cells in that they allow movement of constituents from one cell to the next.

Signal transduction and secondary messaging also occur in plant cells. External and internal stimuli activate receptor proteins and provide signals that trigger complex signal transduction processes. Many plant signaling pathways are very similar to those found in animals. GTPases, phospholipids, calcium signaling networks, and protein kinases are important components of plant signaling processes that are also found in animal systems. Despite the major differences between plant and animal cells, the laws of energy and the processes of glycolysis and the citric acid cycle are similar in plants. Although plants can

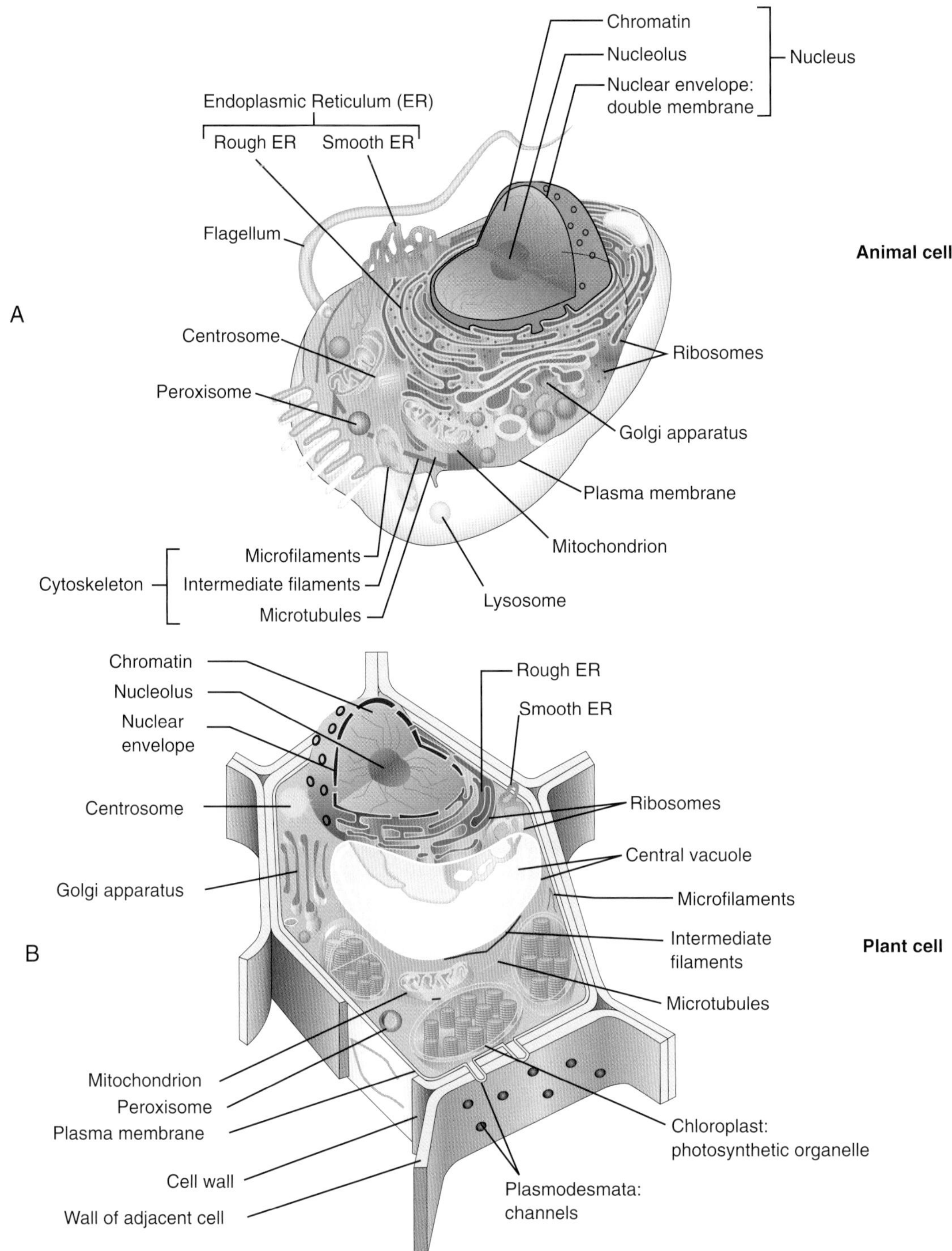

Figure 10-4 The major similarities and differences between animal **(A)** and plant **(B)** cells.

synthesize unique substances, plants contain many of the same enzymes that are found in animals. This is one reason why plants can be used to produce vaccines and human proteins such as antibodies.

The vascular system of plants is made up of the xylem and the phloem. Water traverses upward in the plant through the xylem. Food manufactured in the photosynthetic parts of the plant is transported through the phloem and is stored as starch, whereas animals store food as glycogen and fat.

Similar to animals, plants synthesize hormones that have roles in growth and development, as well as in defense and immunity. Plant scientists do not know as much about plant hormones as medical scientists know about human hormones. This is unfortunately due to both emphasis in the science and funding. It is interesting to note that some plants manufacture hormones that are also found in animals, such as serotonin, melatonin, and acetylcholine. The section on similarities in communication, defense, and detoxification elaborates on this subject.

Medicinal plant products originate from various parts of a plant. Knowing where the medicinal compounds are stored in a plant and how plant material should be handled, so as to preserve those compounds, is of great value to an herbalist. Bioactive compounds are not found uniformly through a plant but may exist only in the roots or may be highest in the flower. In some cases, a different part of the plant becomes an important source of bioactive compounds, such as in the leaf of *Echinacea purpurea,* instead of the root. Bioactive constituents often vary with specific parts of a plant. For example, the hypocotyle is the bioactive part of maca *(Lepidium meyenii),* the inflorescence is the part most valued for *Arnica,* and the leaf is most highly prized for green tea *(Camellia sinensis).*

Some plant compounds do not become active until they are broken down by enzymes stored in a different area within the plant. Some defense compounds are safely stored next to a vesicle that contains the enzymes needed to transmute them to the defense form. Crushing these tissues, whether by an herbivore or by collection, drying, or processing procedures, often combines the necessary ingredients. In garlic, allinase combined with alliin forms allicin, a potent antimicrobial. Young leaves of *Catharanthus roseus* (Madagascar periwinkle) accumulate glucoalkaloid strictosidine in the vacuole. Surrounding this vacuole are high levels of an enzyme that, when mixed with strictosidine, turns into a strong, protective antimicrobial compound (Verpoorte, 1998).

Plants commonly store volatile oils in glandular hairs on the surfaces of leaves and flowers. Powdering leaves may cause bioactive volatiles to escape, thus reducing the potency of the plant material. Therefore, storing dried leaves in as large a form as possible and not powdering until the last possible moment may be the best strategy for assuring potency. Understanding where plant compounds are stored also suggests which plant parts and what time of the year is best to collect plants.

Plant compounds are made in specific parts of the cell and are transported and stored in specific areas of the plant cell based on their polarity (Figures 10-5 and 10-6; Box 10-2). The choice of where these compounds are stored depends greatly on the hydrophobicity and hydrophilicity of the compound. For example, hydrophilic compounds such as flavonoids and tannins tend to be stored in the vacuoles, laticifers, and apoplasts of plant tissues. Lipophilic compounds such as terpenes, waxes, and anthraquinones tend to be stored in resin ducts, oil cells, and trichomes (Figure 10-6). It may be surprising to the reader that plant scientists understand little of how plant compounds are transported to storage compartments such as trichomes, far from their source of manufacture. In fact, scientists only recently discovered what triggers flowering! Plant chemistry and natural product research trudges rather slowly behind human and mammalian biochemistry and physiology.

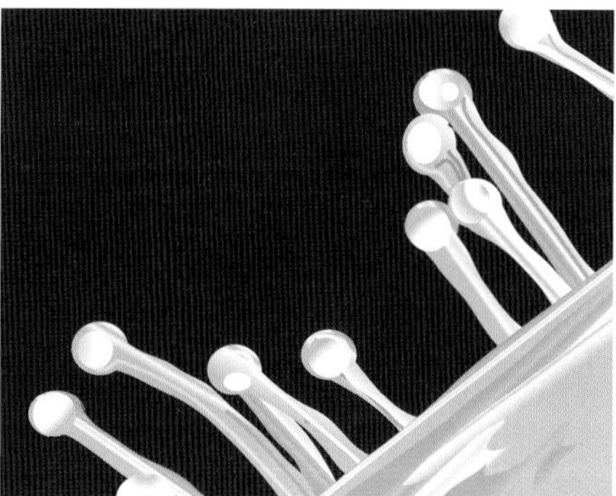

Figure 10-5 Trichomes on the surfaces of leaves store lipophilic compounds such as volatile oils.

BOX 10-2

Hydrophilic and Hydrophobic Plant Compounds and Their Storage Compartments

HYDROPHILIC COMPOUNDS

Vacuole
- Alkaloids, nonprotein amino acids, saponins, terpenoids
- Glycosides, flavonoids, tannins, anthocyanins, glucosinolates, cyanogens, amines

Lacticifer
- Nonprotein amino acids, alkaloids, cyanogens, cardiac glycosides

Apoplast
- Tannins

HYDROPHOBIC COMPOUNDS

Cuticle
- Waxes, lipophilic flavonoids

Trichomes
- Monoterpenes, sesquiterpenes

Resin Ducts
- Terpenes (C10, C15, C20, C30), Lipophilic flavonoids

Lacticifers
- Polyterpenes, diterpenes (phorbol esters), quinones, lipophilic flavonoids

Oil Cells
- Anthraquinones, terpenoids

Plastid Membranes
- Ubiquinones, tetraterpenes

PHOTOSYNTHESIS

Photosynthesis uses energy from the sun to produce building blocks for the synthesis of primary and secondary compounds. The photosynthetic process involves two phases: the light reaction phase, which produces oxygen, ATP, and nicotine adenine dinucleotide phosphate (NADPH); and the carbon-linked reactions (also

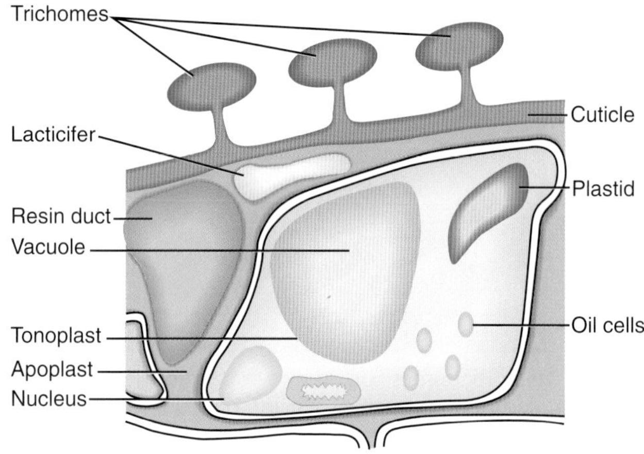

Figure 10-6 Plant compartments used for storage of various compounds.

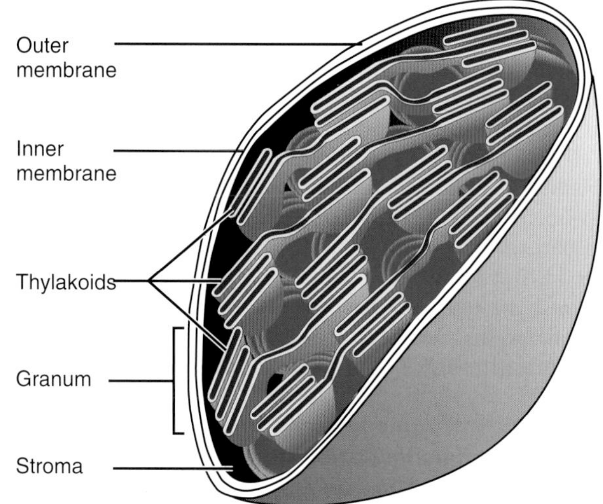

Figure 10-8 Thylakoids stacked into grana in the chloroplast.

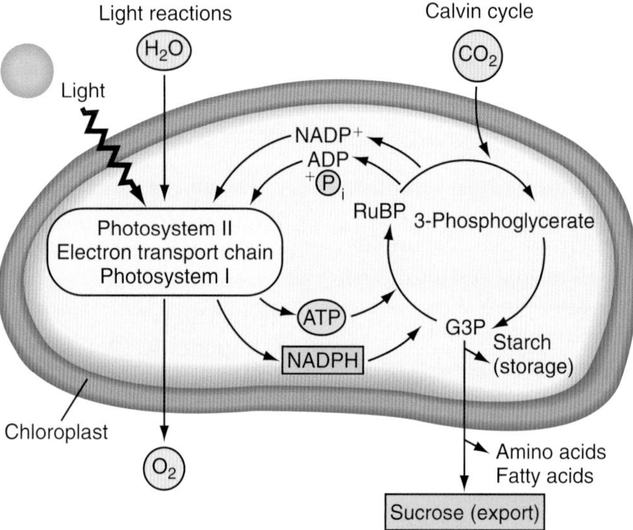

Figure 10-7 The two processes of photosynthesis: light reactions and the Calvin Cycle.

called the Calvin cycle), which reduce carbon dioxide to carbohydrate (Figure 10-7). These two phases occur in different regions of the chloroplast.

The energy compounds, ATP and NADPH, along with carbon, in the form of sugars, are the building blocks for medicinal compounds. Animals and humans cannot make most of these bioactive compounds, which number now in the tens of thousands (Wink, 1999). Plants are also an important dietary source of carbohydrates (e.g., potatoes, rice, wheat, cassava), fiber, and micronutrients, such as carotenoids, biotin, folate, lipoic acid, trace minerals, and vitamins. Deficiencies in these micronutrients have been shown to damage DNA through the same mechanism used by radiation. Degenerative diseases, such as heart disease, cancer, and cognitive dysfunction, have been linked to diets low in fruits and vegetables. All life is intricately tied to both plant macronutrients and micronutrients, and therefore, to photosynthesis.

Chloroplasts are unique to the Plant Kingdom. Similar to mitochondria, chloroplasts are hypothesized to have originated from a single-cell photosynthetic symbiont from the prokaryote domain (i.e., Bacteria and Archaea). Chloroplasts and mitochondria each possess their own genetic and protein synthesis machinery (Buchanan, 2000), that is, both plastids and mitochondria contain DNA that encodes various genes for proteins needed for functioning of those organelles, as well as for synthesis of some secondary compounds. Chloroplasts produce both primary and secondary compounds, such as monoterpenes, diterpenes, tetraterpenes (carotenoids), ubiquinone, and phytol. The chloroplast is surrounded by an outer and an inner membrane. Within the chloroplast are a series of tissues called thylakoids, which are stacked into grana (Figure 10-8).

The light reaction phase of photosynthesis occurs in the thylakoid double membrane, in which electron carrier complexes and proteins are embedded (Figure 10-9). These complexes, which are embedded in the plasma membrane of the thylakoids, contain chlorophylls and carotenoid pigments. Chlorophylls are carriers of electron transport and are made up of two parts—a porphyrin ring and a phytol tail (Figure 10-10). Porphyrin molecules are found elsewhere in the animal kingdom. In animals, heme is bound to proteins, forming hemoglobin, the part of red blood cells that reversibly binds oxygen. Several steps in the synthesis of chlorophyll and heme are shared. The main differences are that the heme in hemoglobin contains an iron molecule in the center, but magnesium is in the center of chlorophyll and a hydrocarbon chain is attached.

Phytol is a terpenoid compound that is made in the chloroplast. It provides the hydrocarbon chain "tail" of the chlorophyll molecule. Carotenoids are tetraterpenes made only in chloroplasts and closely related to monoterpenes, which are commonly found in essential oils. These carotenoids protect the chloroplast membrane proteins from oxidation damage during photosynthesis.

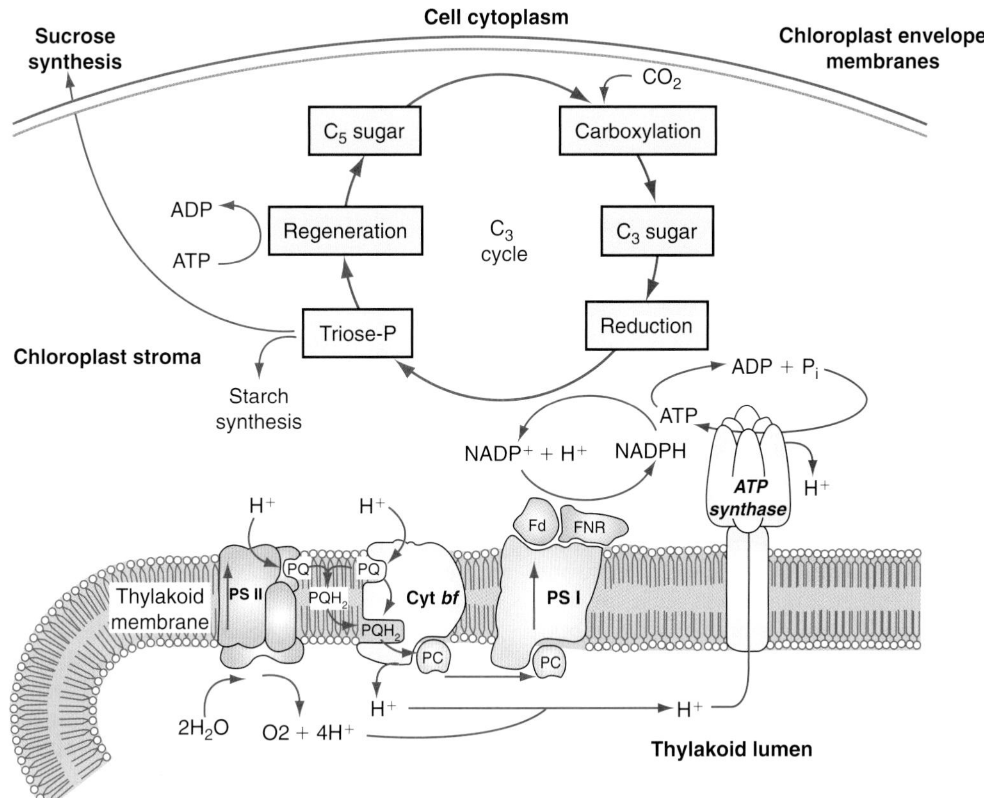

Figure 10-9 Photosynthetic complexes embedded in the thylakoid membrane.

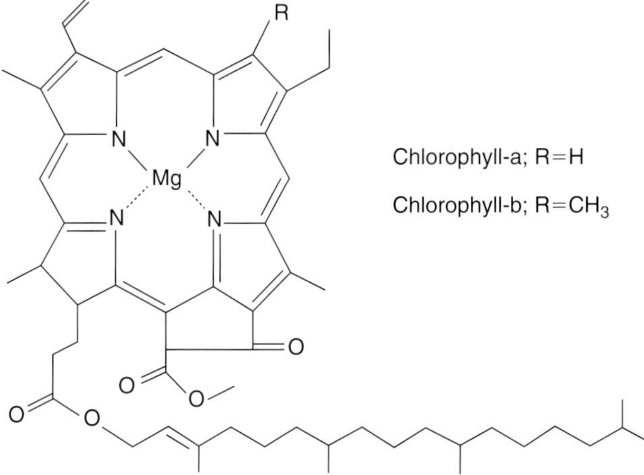

Figure 10-10 Chlorophyll a and b.

There are two kinds of chlorophyll—chlorophyll a and chlorophyll b. The difference is a hydrogen group or a methyl group that is attached to the corner of the porphyrin ring. The chlorophylls are found in two of the proteins—photosystem II and photosystem I (named backward because of their order of discovery, but placed in appropriate order of photosynthetic process).

Chlorophyll is green because it absorbs the red and blue regions of the light spectrum and reflects the green regions. Chlorophyll channels photons of light, turning these into chemical energy through photosynthesis. Chlorophyll transforms carbon dioxide and water into carbohydrates, oxygen, and the energy compound, NADPH, which drives biochemical reactions in the plant, represented here by the photosynthetic reaction:

$$CO_2 + H_2O \rightarrow (CH_2O) + O_2$$

When chlorophyll absorbs light energy, an electron is excited from a lower energy state to a higher energy state. This makes the electron more easily transferred or handed on to the next molecule in the process of electron transfer. In the end, the electron is transferred to carbon dioxide in the Calvin cycle, the second phase of photosynthesis. These complexes and proteins transfer electrons from sunlight through a chain of events that results in the production of energy compounds used in the second half of the photosynthetic process, the Calvin cycle.

The Calvin cycle converts carbon dioxide (CO_2) into carbohydrates (sugars), using an important protein called Rubisco (ribulose-1,5-biphosphate carboxylase/oxygenase). Rubisco is probably the most abundant soluble protein in the world and is a major source of nitrogen, which is recycled by perennial plants that lose their leaves at the end of the growing season. This recycling results in colorful fall leaves, denoting the carotenes that remain after the chlorophyll is broken down and the nitrogen is exported from the leaves to storage tissues in growing organs, seeds, and underground parts (Matile, 2000).

The important products of the two phases of photosynthesis are the energy compounds that fuel biosynthetic processes and the sugars that provide carbon units for the synthesis of primary and secondary compounds.

PRODUCTION OF PRIMARY AND SECONDARY COMPOUNDS

Plant compounds (metabolites) have been traditionally divided into two main types: primary and secondary. Sunlight, water, nitrogen, phosphate, and sulfur are used to make primary compounds such as carbohydrates, lipids, amino acids, and proteins. Primary compounds provide the building blocks for secondary compounds, such as flavonoids, terpenes, alkaloids, and anthraquinones.

Initially, secondary plant compounds were believed to be waste products of metabolism. Dogma then suggested that primary compounds performed metabolic roles essential to growth and development, and secondary plant compounds were responsible for plant defense and communication with other organisms, such as that involved in attracting pollinators. Today, the roles of both categories are blurred because it has been discovered that some primary compounds are involved in plant defense and some secondary compounds have roles in growth and development.

Some primary compounds have an important role in defense. Pathogenesis-related (PR) proteins elicit the biosynthesis of degrading enzymes, which then attack the exterior structures of fungal pathogens (Huang, 2001). Stimulation of these proteins produces short-term systemic resistance to many pathogens. Other proteins in the cell walls of plants defend the plant by inhibiting pathogen-produced enzymes themselves (Albersheim, 1971). Plants can sometimes perceive the presence of a fungal pathogen by sensing wax on the surfaces of leaves or by sensing glucans (sugars) in the cell walls of fungi; this sets off an alarm, thereby upregulating defense systems.

Sitosterol, campesterol, and stigmasterol are the most common sterols found in plants. These primary compounds provide structural components of plant cell and organelle membranes, regulating the fluidity and permeability of these membranes. They also act as hormonal growth regulators in plants and are involved in membrane-associated processes, such as vesicle trafficking and signaling, as well as regulation of transcription and translation, cellular differentiation, and cell proliferation (Piironen, 2000).

Phytosterols have bioactive properties in mammals and humans. They are particularly well known for (1) inhibiting both absorption of cholesterol and lowering of serum cholesterol through preferential uptake in the gut for plant sterols versus cholesterol, and (2) promoting the elimination of cholesterol. Beta sitosterol has been found to have anticancer, antiulcer, antidiabetic, anti-inflammatory, antipyretic (Gupta,1980; Bouic, 2002), and antivenom properties (Mors, 2000). It has been suggested that beta-sitosterol can enhance secretion of interleukin (IL)-2 and gamma-interferon, helping to promote natural killer cells and prime TH1 helper cells to steer the focus away from TH2 helper cells (Bouic, 2001). It has been suggested that in low doses, phytosterols may be involved in regulation of gene expression (Orzechowski, 2002). The lipophilicity of phytosterols allows them to easily diffuse through lipid membranes. It is possible that these compounds can prime the tissues, increasing sensitivity to other mediators and cofactors. Phytosterols are likely synergistic with secondary compounds. The sedative activity of *Perilla frutescens* is suggested to be caused by a combined effect of secondary and primary compounds (perillaldehyde and stigmasterol).

Other primary plant compounds are bioactive in mammals and humans. Omega-3 fatty acids are anti-inflammatory, and chlorophyll is suspected to be antioxidant (Ma, 1999). It is more surprising that phytol metabolites (the hydrocarbon tail of chlorophyll) have been shown to bind to the retinoic X receptor (RXR) and can pair with a host of other receptors, many of which are lipid sensors (Barsony, 2002). Thus, it can no longer be said that the only bioactive substances in plants are secondary compounds.

Secondary compounds can assist the growth and development of the plant by providing signals to attract pollinators and seed dispersers; communicating with symbiotic microorganisms; and protecting the plant against ultraviolet (UV) light and other stressors in the environment (Wink, 1999). It is estimated that more than 100,000 secondary plant compounds are at work in nature (Verpoorte, 1998). This should not be surprising, considering that plants have to negotiate survival in a world with 30 million species of insects and 1.5 million species of fungi, many of which attack and consume plants. Plants have also had eons of time to adapt to specific environmental conditions in response to temperature and soil nutrients.

Plant compounds are synthesized in both the cytosol and the chloroplast. In some cases, DNA from both the nucleus and the chloroplast is needed to form a product. Once made, metabolites are transported to storage areas throughout the plant. Most plant secondary compounds are derived from four main pathways: the acetate, shikimate, mevalonate, and deoxyxylulose phosphate pathways. Alkaloids are derived from amino acids in many different pathways.

SIMILARITIES IN CHEMICAL COMMUNICATIONS, DEFENSE, AND DETOXIFICATION

The search for nutrients, the need to detoxify and eliminate waste products, and need for protection against enemies are just a few of the challenges that all organisms face. Most organisms have done so using similar themes, evidenced by comparisons of gene sequences from organisms of all kingdoms. Elements for transcriptional activation of genes can be seen in organisms that evolved 2 billion years ago. Genetic ancestry strongly suggests that higher organisms borrowed survival and metabolic strategies from lower organisms (Baker, 1998). Homology, or similarity in characteristics resulting from a shared ancestry, is particularly relevant to the effects of phytochemicals on mammals and humans. Many plant compounds that are used by the plant for communication, defense, and detoxification are able to mimic mammalian hormones and neurotransmitters. The process by which chemicals selected for one function are subsequently employed by chance in an extension of that initial function is called exaptation (Stoka, 1999). Table 10-2 lists some examples of similar strategies and active chemicals between plants and mammalian organisms.

One theme among organisms is to use the same compound for multiple purposes. One role for a compound may have been extended to multiple roles because of the extraordinary energy costs involved in producing metabolic chemical signals and receptor proteins, as well as the biosynthetic enzymes needed to produce them. Costly compounds would not likely survive evolution (Wink, 1999). Thrifty strategies, such as using the same compound for many purposes, are more advantageous. The plant hormone, ethylene, is responsible for triggering the ripening of fruit (primary role); it also causes the formation of special root cells to allow growth in submerged environments (primary role), stem elongation (primary role), and resistance to fungal pathogens (secondary role) (Buchanan, 2000). Salicylic acid is involved in the generation of heat in flowers to release insect attractant compounds (primary role) and in disease resistance (secondary role) (Buchanan, 2000).

TABLE 10-2

Examples of Exaptation Between Plant, Microorganism, and Mammalian Systems, by Which Chemicals Selected for One Function Are Subsequently Employed by Chance in an Extension of That Initial Function

Lower Organisms (Bacteria, Fungi, Insects, Plants)	Higher Organisms (Mammals, Humans)
Synergy of defense chemicals against pathogens and herbivores (Zhou, 2005)	Synergy of phytochemicals in cancer prevention (Liu, 2004); in *Staphylococcus aureus* infection (Stermitz, 2000)
Flavonoids have hydroxyl group positions on molecular structures (Havsteen, 2002)	Estrogen has similar hydroxyl group positions on molecular structures (Havsteen, 2002)
Plant dihydroflavonol 4-reductase, which synthesizes some flavonoids, shares a common ancestor with . . .	. . . human 3 beta-hydroxysteroid dehydrogenase, an enzyme that converts pregnenolone to progesterone (Baker, 1998)
NodG, a bacterial gene product stimulated by nodulating flavonoid signals (Baker, 1998) . . .	. . . is homologous to human enzymes, mammalian 11β- and 17β-hydroxysteroid dehydrogenase and 15-hydroxy-prostaglandin dehydrogenase (Baker, 1992)
Isoflavonoid compounds act as signaling messengers in nodulation process with soil bacteria (Fox, 2004)	Isoflavonoids bind to estrogen receptors ERα and ERβ (Setchell, 1999); stimulate transcriptional activity of both ERα and ERβ (Dornstauder, 2001); induce changes in signaling pathways of transforming growth factor in cancer cells (Kim, 1998)
Flavonoid compounds prevent the nodulation process in nearby competing plants; insecticides inhibit nodulation (Fox, 2004)	Tamoxifen inhibits binding of estrogen to receptors; endocrine-disrupting chemicals affect estrogen system (Welshons, 2003)
Plant 5α-reductase metabolizes plant steroid hormones (Rosati, 2003)	Human 5α-reductase converts testosterone into 5α-dihydrotestosterone; 5α-reductase can metabolize brassinosteroids, a plant hormone (Baker, 1998)
Some isoflavones preferentially inhibit the enzyme, 3-βHSD II (Ohno, 2002)	3-βHSD II involved in synthesis of glucocorticoids (cortisol) and other steroid hormones such as progestin, mineralocorticoids, androgens, estrogens, and neurosteroids in the brain (Ohno, 2002)
Endophytic fungi (e.g., powdery mildew) become pathogenic under conditions of plant senescence	*Candida* yeast become pathogenic in states of immune deficiency
Carotenes protect against infection and UV exposure and repair DNA damage; involved in immunocompetence (Van Der Veen, 2005)	Dietary carotenes protect against free radicals and influence immunity
Oxidation of compounds (free radicals) used as defense by releasing nitric oxide to inhibit or kill pathogens and herbivores (Zhao, 2005)	Macrophages release nitric oxide to produce free radicals to stop invasion of pathogens (Zhou, 2005)
Plant defense systems sense glucans in the cell walls of pathogenic bacteria and fungi (Zhao, 2005)	Glucans in medicinal fungi trigger mammalian immune response (Stamets, 2002)
Phytoecdysteroids are synthesized by plants for defense against insects (Lafont, 2003)	Phytoecdysteroids stimulate the synthesis of proteins in animals and humans (Lafont, 2003)

Extra physiologic functions of chemicals may have developed from an evolutionary opportunism that originated as chemicals providing signals for food and danger to hormones and neurotransmitters in higher animals (Stoka, 1999). The ancient function of carotenoids in bacteria originally evolved as a mechanical function to protect cell membranes and the outer shells and eggs of mollusks and crustaceans. Carotenes became capable of transferring energy and protecting proteins involved in photosynthesis. Carotenes are now known to have crucial roles in color vision and coloration in animals (e.g., masking, attracting, warning); they act as hormones that regulate epidermal growth and defend against cancer (Vershinin, 1999). Anthocyanins also cause coloration in flower petals, attracting pollinators. Some of the enzymes responsible for producing anthocyanins share a common ancestor with mammalian enzymes that convert pregnenolone to progesterone (Baker, 1998). This suggests that compounds that bind to plant enzymes may be able to bind to mammalian enzymes, thereby affecting steroid hormones in mammals.

Communication

Insects are compelled to have a relationship with plants because they themselves cannot synthesize hormones without a dietary sterol precursor (Lafont, 2000). Plants provide insects with pollen, wax, and pheromone substances. Many insects require plants for feeding, mating, and reproducing. Some volatile plant compounds induce the release of pheromones in certain insects and often synergize or enhance insect responses to sex pheromones (Harrewijn, 2001).

Microbes have also devised beneficial associations with plants throughout millennia, having followed plants out of the oceans and onto land. Fungi and bacteria live on the surfaces of plant leaves and roots, as well as inside these tissues. These endophytes are mostly mutualistic, although some, such as powdery mildew (fungi), can become pathogenic once the leaf senesces at the end of the season. Similarly, *Candida* yeast endogenous to healthy human tissues can become pathogenic in states of immune weakness.

Plant compounds are believed to provide communication in endophytic relationships. For example, plant flavonoids act as signaling molecules in the formation of root nodules for nitrogen fixation. Plants entice soil bacteria to trade nitrogen for plant sugars by first releasing chemicals from their roots: flavones, isoflavonoids, flavanones, betaines, and chalcones. These chemicals turn on gene expression in bacteria—binding to receptors and signaling a genetic chain reaction—sending an invitation to bacteria to come live in nodules on the plant roots. Plants also use flavonoids to prevent the nodulation process in nearby competing plants. It is notable that endocrine-disrupting insecticides can also inhibit nodulation (Fox, 2004).

This ancient relationship between plants and bacteria is mirrored in the bioactivity of flavonoids on mammalian systems. Isoflavonoids can bind to estrogen receptors ER-α and ER-β; stimulate transcriptional activity of both ER-α and ER-β (Dornstauder, 2001); and induce changes in the signaling pathways of transforming growth factor in cancer cells (Kim, 1998). It is notable that flavonoids and estrogen have similar hydroxyl group positions on their molecular structures (Havsteen, 2002).

Not only can plant compounds mimic mammalian receptor ligands, but bacterial and plant enzymes have similar characteristics to mammalian enzymes. This is due to homology or shared genetic ancestry. NodG, a bacterial gene product stimulated by nodulating flavonoid signals in plants, is homologous to the human enzymes, mammalian 11β- and 17β-hydroxysteroid dehydrogenase (regulate androgen and estrogen action) and 15-hydroxyprostaglandin dehydrogenase (inactivates prostaglandin E2) (Baker, 1998). These enzymes regulate intercellular signals. Conversely, plant 5α-reductase can metabolize animal steroids, and human 5α-reductase can metabolize brassinosteroid, a plant hormone (Baker, 1998). Some isoflavones can also inhibit the enzyme, 3-beta-hydroxysteroid dehydrogenase (3-βHSD), which is responsible for synthesizing cortisol and other steroid hormones (Ohno, 2002).

Defense

Similarity between plants and mammals is also evident in strategies of defense. Plants are masters at employing a host of strategies—attracting enemies of insects; deterring, stimulating, and inhibiting feeding; disrupting major metabolic pathways; and retarding, accelerating, and interfering in growth and development. Many pathogens and herbivores have learned to rapidly outmaneuver plant defenses. Plants have countered by manufacturing tens of thousands of protective chemicals.

Oxidation can be used as a defense by the release of nitric oxide and free radicals to inhibit or kill pathogens and herbivores. This is complementary to the release of nitric oxide by macrophages, which inhibits invasion of pathogens (Zhou, 2005). Alternately, plants must defend themselves against free radical reactive oxygen species that are constantly generated during daily metabolism and by environmental factors such as ultraviolet sunlight, soil toxins, and damage from pathogenic microorganisms. Plants quench these oxidants with flavonoids and carotenes. Plants are thrifty, and rarely do the compounds that are so expensive to produce have only one purpose. Flavonoids and carotenes also perform other functions, including coloration of flowers and fruits, antifungal defense, and insect feeding attractant roles.

Flavonoids and carotenes are an important dietary source of antioxidants for mammals. Antioxidants are used to quench free radicals, which are produced by oxidation and detoxification processes. Yet, recent research suggests that flavonoids cannot possibly quench free radicals because they are present in such low levels in the circulation. Instead, flavonoids are more likely to influence gene expression and interact with signaling cascades within the cell (Williams, 2004). This theory is more analogous to the signaling roles of flavonoids in plant–rhizobia communication.

Figure 10-11 Substances made by animals and humans compared with plant compounds that mediate stress.

Precursor	Plant	Mammalian
isoprene unit	triterpenes, phytosterols, phytoecdysteroids	cortisol
tyrosine	flavonoids and lignans	adrenaline
fatty acids	oxylipins	cytokines

Many chemicals that were originally employed for defense seem to have become bioregulators in higher organisms. Some evidence for this can be found in the vertebrate-type steroid hormones present in insects and the fact that mammalian sterols and steroidal hormones can inhibit the growth of both microbes and parasites. This phenomenon is particularly applicable for herbal medicine in the use of phytoecdysteroids found in dietary supplements. Phytoecdysteroids are synthesized by plants for defense against phytophagous (plant-eating) insects. These compounds are exact replicas of ecdysteroids, hormones that are used by the arthropod (insect) and crustacean (crab/lobster) families in the molting process known as ecdysis. Insects not yet adapted to this defense lose weight, fail to molt, and die (Lafont, 2003). Curiously, phytoecdysteroids have been shown to stimulate the synthesis of proteins in animals and humans and to have adaptogenic, antimutagenic, hypocholesterolemic, immunostimulating, nutritive, and tonic properties (Kholodova, 2001; Lafont, 2003). *Rhaponticum carthamoides* (syn. *Leuzea carthamoides)* and *Serratula coronata* are both cultivated as sources of these compounds for the manufacture of dietary supplements. Hundreds of products containing ecdysone are marketed to weight lifters and sports enthusiasts as pseudosteroidal muscle enhancers (Lafont, 2003). The parallel activity between plant defense and remedy suggests that higher organisms adapted ancient ligands and enzymes for their needs.

Stress is a daily challenge for every organism. Plants use a mechanism for resisting stress called systematic acquired resistance (SAR), which uses salicylic acid as a defense against infection by pathogens. Salicylic acid is the most universally used natural product. A synthetic version, acetylsalicylic acid (aspirin), inhibits the production of prostaglandins. Prostaglandins are hormone-like chemicals that stimulate target cells, such as those involved in inflammation, vasoconstriction, and platelet aggregation, into action. Again, a similar hormonal action has been noted between plant defense and mammalian hormone communication.

Hormones and neurotransmitters (e.g., cortisol, adrenaline) are used by mammals to mediate extreme stress. The adaptogens, *Eleutherococcus senticosis* and *Rhodiola rosea,* have been shown to increase resistance to stress in both animals and humans. It is the triterpenes, flavonoids, and oxylipins that are believed to be the active compounds in adaptogens (Panossian, 2003). Some of these chemical compounds are synthesized in similar mammalian biosynthetic pathways with the use of the same precursors as those associated with plant biosynthesis (Figure 10-11). Adaptogens are believed to alleviate stress diseases by mimicking hormones and neurotransmitters involved in the response to stress (Panossian, 2003; Klein, 2004). Plant triterpenes and mammalian steroid hormones are made in the same biosynthetic pathway. Plant flavonoids and adrenaline are made with the same starting compound, tyrosine. Plant oxylipins and cytokines such as leukotrienes are made in the acetate pathway. Researchers who study adaptogens suggest that the mechanism of action of these plant compounds is a mimicking of the hormones and neurotransmitters that have gone awry during dysregulation of the stress resistance process (Panossian, 2003; Klein, 2004).

The defense strategy of raising the defenses by sensing glucans in the cell walls of pathogenic bacteria or fungi (Zhou, 2005) is also mirrored in mammals and humans. Certain types of glucans found in medicinal fungi are shown to trigger mammalian immune responses (Stamets, 2002).

Nitrogen is easily available to legumes to synthesize nitrogen-containing defense compounds because they are able to fix nitrogen. Thus alkaloids, non-protein amino acids, cyanogens, protease inhibitors, and lectins are common in the pea family. These compounds defend the plant against insects and animals via neurosignaling disruption and thus many plant alkaloids are agonists or antagonists of neurotransmitters and neuroreceptors, such as caffeine and atropine (Wink, 2003). Most hallucinogenic plants contain alkaloids that tend to be derivatives of the aromatic amino acids—tryptophan, phenylalanine, and tyrosine—and precursors of some brain hormones (Figure 10-12).

The amino acid, tyrosine, is the precursor not only for the neurotransmitters, dopamine, norepinephrine, and epinephrine, but also for the alkaloids, mescaline in *Lophophora williamsii* (peyote), and myristicin from *Myristica fragrans* (nutmeg) (Table 10-3). Mescaline and myristicin both enhance norepinephrine neurotransmission.

Tryptamines are made from the amino acid, tryptophan, and are synthesized by both plants and mammals (Figure 10-13). The amino acid, tryptophan, is the precursor not only for serotonin and melatonin, but also for the alkaloids, ergotamine in ergot fungus *(Claviceps purpurea),* 5-methoxy-N,N-dimethyltryptamine (DMT) in *Virola theiodora* (epená snuff), psilocybin in psilocybe mushrooms *(Psilocybe* spp*),* bufotenine in Bufo toad, and D-lysergic acid (LSD) in morning glory *(Convolvulus tricolor).* Psilocybin and DMT enhance serotonin.

The Fly Agaric mushroom, *Amanita muscaria* var. *muscaria,* contains ibotenic acid, which binds to glutamic

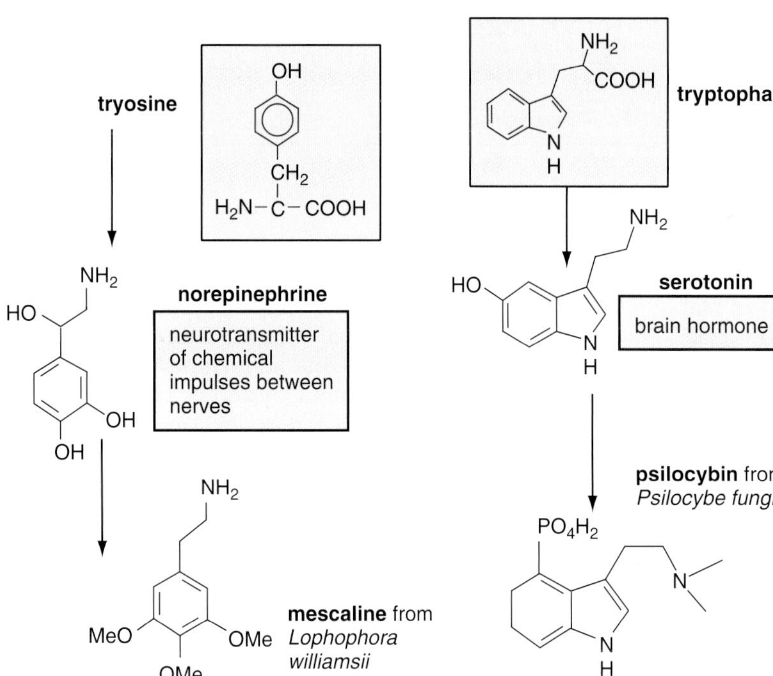

Figure 10-12 Plant hallucinogens often have chemical structure similar to that of brain hormones.

TABLE 10-3

Precursors of Plant Hallucinogenic Compounds and Mammalian Hormones and Neurotransmitters

Precursor	Plant Hallucinogenic Compound	Hormone/Neurotransmitter
Tryptophan	Ergotamine *(Claviceps purpurea)*	Serotonin
	DMT *(Virola theiodora)*	Melatonin
	Psilocybin (*Psilocybe* spp)	
	Bufotenine (*Bufo alvaris*, toad)	
	LSD *(Convolvulus tricolor)*	
Tyrosine	Mescaline *(Lophophora williamsii)*	Dopamine
	Myristicin *(Myristica fragrans)*	Norepinephrine
		Epinephrine
Glutamine	Ibotenic acid *(Amanita muscaria* var. *muscaria)*	Gamma-aminobutyric acid
Acetyl-CoA	Tropane alkaloids	Acetylcholine
Fatty acids	THC (cannabinoid, terpeneophenolic)	Anandamide

acid sites and inhibits gamma-aminobutyric acid (GABA), a neurotransmitter found in inhibitory pathways. This inhibition affects the concentrations of other neurotransmitters, such as norepinephrine, serotonin, and dopamine, in the same manner as LSD (Hobbs, 1995). The tropane alkaloids in *Datura* and other genera in the Solanaceae inhibit acetylcholine by binding to the nicotinic and muscarinic receptors (Schmeller, 1995).

Both the endogenous hormone, anandamide, and the cannabinoids in *Cannabis sativa* bind to opioid receptors in the brain. Anandamide, from *ananda* (Sanskrit for "bliss"), is a messenger molecule in the brain that participates in regulating pain, anxiety, hunger, and vomiting. Eating fatty foods increases production of anandamide and probably contributes to the feeling of satiety and somnolence associated with such a meal. Anandamide has been found in small amounts in chocolate and cocoa powder. N-acylethanolamines in cocoa block the breakdown of anandamide. Part of the pleasure of chocolate may come from anandamide and the anandamide-preserving N-acylethanolamines. Delta-9-tetrahydrocannabinol (THC), the cannabinoid in *Cannabis sativa,* binds to the same receptors in neurons as anandamide. Cannabinoids from *Cannabis sativa* have been shown to decrease serotonin; reduce corticotropin releasing hormone (CRH); cause short-term memory loss (similar

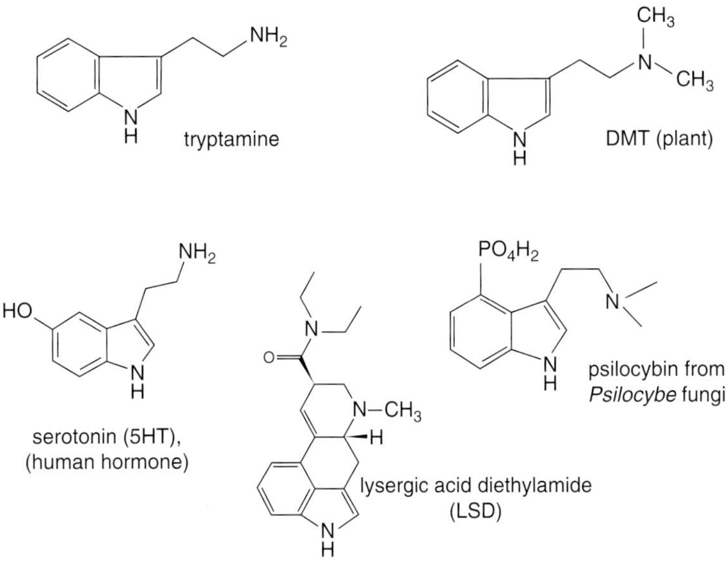

Figure 10-13 Tryptamines are synthesized by both plants and mammals.

to anandamine); and alter gonadal hormones (e.g., decrease sperm count, reduce size of testes, increase breast growth).

Some secondary compounds are elicited or induced only after infection with microorganisms or attack by herbivores. Biosynthesis of primary and secondary compounds may often be the result of the plant's responding to infection by a fungus or attack by a pathogen or herbivore. It is suspected that in many cases, one compound is not enough to cause a bioactive response against pathogens, that is, it has been shown that synergy between several or many compounds has an additive and successful effect.

Many of the same chemicals made by mammals and humans are also found in plants (see Table 10-2 and Table 10-3). Many plant metabolites, especially alkaloids, are poisonous or toxic to mammals and humans. Some perennial ryegrass and tall fescue produce an alkaloid called peramine, which deters the Argentine stem weevil. It is not known whether the fungal symbiont of the grasses is making the compound, or whether the compound requires the synergy of the fungus and the grass host together. Nonetheless, many other grasses cause diseases in livestock, such as fescue toxicosis and ryegrass staggers. These plants are defending themselves from ruminant herbivory. The compounds that cause toxicity are often ergot alkaloids, produced by fungi in the family Clavicipitaceae (Bacon, 1996). Just as ergot has been used for migraine headaches, other fungi can be the sources of important medicinal compounds.

Detoxification

The laws of nature have shown us that all organisms can adapt to toxins in their environment. Mammals render toxic compounds inactive through the Phase I, II, and III detoxification processes (oxidation, reduction, and hydrolysis; conjugation with endogenous compounds; and pumping out of cell via a cell pump protein). Plants may have taught these strategies to mammals, for they employ the same techniques.

Just as pathogens and cancer cells have developed resistance to antibiotics and chemotherapy, weedy plants have become resistant to herbicides through the very same detoxification processes. The P450 monooxygenases of Phase I are ancient enzymes found in all living organisms. Some herbicide-resistant weeds simply increase their production of glutathione and use conjugation to detoxify herbicides and toxic metals in soils. Multidrug pump inhibiting (MDR) systems of Phase III pump herbicides out of the plant cell.

Spraying glyphosate (Roundup®) has led to stimulation of a fungal disease in plants called *Fusarium* head blight. According to Heap (2002), more than 155 angiosperms have become resistant to various herbicides. This occurs primarily because of natural selection. All plants within a population are not the same. Some have unique abilities, such as outwitting an herbicide. Once the susceptible weeds die, the resistant ones can grow. The weed itself doesn't change—the population of the weed changes.

Many communication, defense, and detoxification strategies of higher organisms employ protective substances that had a primitive role in early evolution. Peptides, sterols, and steroids were once sources of nutrition and now act as growth factors in higher organisms. Foods, such as lipids, originally provided a metabolic role for lower organisms but act in higher organisms as regulatory messengers. The detoxifying substance, glutathione (GSH), is a feeding response activator in *Hydra littoralis,* a very ancient multicellular organism (Stoka, 1999). The origin and homology of both enzymes (proteins that catalyze metabolism of substances) and receptors suggest a close association between plants and animals. Table 10-4 illustrates metabolic substances utilized by both plants and humans. Plants really are our green relatives!

TABLE 10-4

Substances Synthesized by Both Plants and Humans

Substance	Role in Plants	Role in Humans
Heat-shock proteins	Stress resistance	Stress resistance
Lipoic acid	Redox signaling	Redox signaling
Glutathione	Detoxification	Detoxification
Antioxidants	Antioxidant	Antioxidant
Free radicals	Defense	Defense
CYP 450 monooxygenases	Detoxification, defense	Detoxification
Nitric oxide	Defense; signal hormone	Defense; neuronal; relaxes blood vessels
Melatonin	Precursor defense	Pineal gland hormone
GABA	Precursor defense	Neurotransmitter
Acetylcholine	Tropane alkaloid	Parasympathetic hormone
Serotonin	Precursor defense	Hormone
Phosphoenolpyruvate carboxykinase	CO_2 fixation enzyme	Tumor-suppressing gene

Medicinal Fungi

Fungi are not plants. They have been recently classified as relatives of animals (Raven, 2003). Similar to plants and animals, fungi are eukaryotic organisms. They have cell walls as plants do, but they contain chitin (similar to insects) instead of cellulose. Similar to animals, fungi are heterotrophs (i.e., they eat other organisms and their by-products). However, instead of ingesting and then digesting as animals do, fungi digest their food first and then absorb it. Instead of storing energy as starch as plants do, fungi store energy as glycogen, similar to animals. Fungi also produce a type of sterol called ergosterol, whereas animals produce cholesterol and plants produce phytosterols. Fungi do not contain chloroplasts as plants do and therefore cannot photosynthesize.

Fungi are everywhere—floating in the air; on hair, feathers, bones, horn, dung, and leaf litter; and in the digestive tracts of humans, animals, insects, fish, and other organisms. They can even be found digesting other fungi. Similar to bacteria, fungi existed long before the development of Angiosperms. Their relationship with plants dates back to 395 million years ago. Some of these relationships are parasitic or pathogenic, but many are mutualistic. Endomycorrhizae and ectomycorrhizae are fungi that grow on or inside plant roots that trade phosphates from the soil for carbohydrates made from photosynthesis by the plant. Mutualisms with fungi provide other clever survival strategies for plants. Fungi have been shown to protect plants. The fungus *Curvularia* spp provides thermal protection on extremely hot soils in Yellowstone National Park for hot springs panicgrass, *Dichanthelium lanuginosum* (Elliott) Gould (Redman, 2002).

Fungi are an important source of pharmacologic products such as penicillin from *Penicillium chrysogenum* Thom., cyclosporin A (an immune-suppressant drug) from *Beauveria nivea* (Rostrup) Arx, and lovastatin from *Aspergillus terreus* Thom. *Claviceps purpurea,* a smut fungus, attacks grasses and produces ergotamine that has been synthesized into a drug for migraines. Chemicals produced by fungi can be harmful to animals and humans. Ergotamine is hallucinogenic and can cause abortion. *Aspergillus flavus* produces aflatoxins that are carcinogenic. House moulds cause sick building syndrome. Despite their amazing bioactivity, research on fungal chemicals is in its infancy. Only 1% of the 1.5 million fungal species thought to exist have been screened for secondary compounds (Nisbet, 1991).

BOX 10-3

Examples of Fungi Commonly Used in Herbal Medicine Materia Medica

Phylum Ascomycota (yeasts, saprobes, cup fungi)
- *Cordyceps sinensis* (caterpillar fungus)

Phylum Basidiomycota (cap fungi and gilled mushrooms)
- *Inonotus obliquus* (chaga)
- *Auricularia auricular* (wood ear)
- *Ganoderma applanatum* (artist's conk)
- *Ganoderma lucidum* (reishi)
- *Grifola frondosa* (maitake)
- *Trametes versicolor* (turkey tails)
- *Lentinula edodes* (shiitake)
- *Flammulina velutipes* (enokitake)
- *Schizophyllum commune* (split gill)

The materia medica of most models of traditional medicine includes fungi. Many cap fungi, such as shiitake *(Lentinula edodes),* maitake *(Grifola frondosa),* and reishi *(Ganoderma lucidum)* (Basidiomycetes), are used for their antitumor and cancer preventative properties (Box 10-3). A more obscure fungus is one that is involved in the formation of a substance with centuries of use in Russia and India for stress, called Mumie or Shilajit (Schepetkin, 2003). This extraordinary black substance is thought to be produced from an association with a plant, a fungus, and lichen (lichens are symbiotic fungal/algal organisms).

Fungi that grow between and inside plant cells are called endophytes. Along with bacteria, fungal endophytes entertain many symbiotic, mutualistic, and pathogenic relationships with plants. The bioactive potential of endophytes is ignored by most herbalists and natural product chemists. Yet, endophytes often stimulate plants to synthesize chemical compounds for defense or growth. In fact, symbiotic fungi have traded genes responsible for the manufacture of chemicals with plants. The anticancer compound, taxol, is a diterpene compound made by the North American yew, *Taxus brevifolia,* and separately, by the fungus found living in its needles, *Taxomyces andreana* (Stierle, 1993).

It is likely that the chemicals produced by medicinal plants may be dependent on their symbiotic relationships with fungi or bacteria. Cultivating some medicinal plants may depend on such relationships. The annual angiosperm, eyebright *(Euphrasia* spp, L.*)*, is partially parasitic on grasses. Although *Euphrasia* is a weedy species, the herb market must rely on sources from the wild because eyebright's life cycle involves a mycorrhizal fungus that is attached to a host grass that has not been duplicated in cultivation. Further, medicinal chemicals in *Euphrasia* may possibly originate from the grass host or from the fungus itself.

An understanding of the life cycle of fungi may directly impact the efficacy of herbal products. Dong chong xia cao, *Cordyceps sinensis* (Berk.) Saccardo Clavicipitaceae, is used in Chinese medicine to increase stamina and treat patients with impotence. *Cordyceps* is in the same family as ergot, which attacks and parasitizes grain crops. In this case, *Cordyceps* attacks the larvae of *Hepialus americanus* or *Holotrichia koraiensis* (Hepialidae). The stalked fruiting bodies of the fungi attached to the larva represent the traditional form of dong chong xia cao. Today, *Cordyceps sinensis* is often mass produced on grain, not on a larval host. Insect larva contains ecdysteroid compounds that have many pharmacologic activities. Whether ecdysteroids are a part of the bioactivity of *Cordyceps* products is not known. Nor is it known whether *Cordyceps* grown on grain contains ecdysteroids, or whether the fungi itself produce ecdysteroids. In any case, the larvae may be crucial to the bioactivity of the *Cordyceps* fungus.

Fungi should be a concern to all health practitioners because they can cause deadly infections and autoimmune diseases. A course in medical mycology is not the same as one in medicinal mushrooms. The former is a subfield of microbiology that investigates infections caused by pathogenic fungi. Mycology is a vast science that encompasses the biology of fungi and studies how they relate to our lives and to the lives of plants. Many facts from the study of fungi can be very useful to practicing herbalists and medical botanists alike.

FUTURE TRENDS

Functional Medicine

A watershed change in medicine is brewing. The healthcare system is not invested in keeping people healthy. It is a system that is starting to be seen as expensive both in economic terms and in human terms. Natural products and molecular biology research are bound to find each other because both are discovering the importance of diet, vitamins, and micronutrients to the most serious and common degenerative diseases of our time (Ames, 2001; Fenech, 2002). Science is now discovering the immense potential for modulating function with the use of substances found in nature. We are, after all, organisms that rely on nature.

Functional medicine includes thoughts, attitudes, beliefs, function, environment, psychosocial events, and spiritual experiences. It assesses function with the use of many techniques but asks questions about how the person got sick and how function can be influenced. Functional medicine improves function so as to restore the ability of the body to maintain homeostasis and increase resistance to stress. This new model uses functional agents to promote the proper function of organs and systems. The disciplines of metabolomics, pharmacogenomics, and nutrigenomics are being applied to medicinal plant compounds in an effort to discover how they might affect gene expression, and thus treatment of patients with disease (Wang, 2005). The idea is to make pharmaceutical drugs that fit the individual's own genetic makeup and that take into account the individual's response to environment, diet, age, lifestyle, and state of health. These factors can influence a patient's response to medicines and may be involved in the occurrence of adverse effects. It is now believed that exposure to low levels of various agents, whether harmful or beneficial, can alter gene expression.

Taking the individual into account, rather than treating all via a general protocol, is a common theme in traditional medicine. Herb remedies are often formulated according to the individual, not the pathology. However, one big difference is that the goal of conventional pharmacists is to produce more powerful drugs that target the problem while causing fewer adverse effects and less damage to healthy cells. These drugs are based on the proteins, enzymes, and RNA associated with genes and diseases. It is interesting to see the parallels in traditional medicine. Perhaps one day, the two will learn to understand one another.

Many in the field are predicting that our healthcare system will move away from treating disease to promoting healthy function (Gazell, 2004; Hyman, 2004; Go, 2004). Veterinary herbalists may benefit from an awareness of these coming changes.

SUMMARY

Medical botany is the sum of many other disciplines, including not just botany, but also evolution and ecology, traditional medicine (ethnobotany), and plant chemistry (pharmacognosy). The biosynthesis and chemistry of the primary and secondary plant compounds intersect the study of medical botany, as well as ethnobotany, history of medicine, complementary and alternative medicine, traditional herbal medicine, toxicology, and natural products research. Each one of these sciences and human endeavors can add to our understanding of how plants can remedy our health conditions.

The cellular biosynthetic processes, the relationship of genera to families, and the evolutionary ancestry of plant species all give us clues to potential bioactive compounds found in plants. What do the adaptogen species *Withania somnifera* (ashwagandha) in the Solanaceae family have to do with *Eleutherococcus senticosis* (Siberian ginseng) in the Araliaceae family? Can we find more adaptogenic species by looking at the related species of these plants?

As plant scientists investigate important problems such as pathogenic organisms in crops, they are finding that other organisms in the ecosystem are intricately involved. These organisms are often forgotten, yet they are crucially and intricately woven into the lives of plants. These include the millions of bacteria, fungi, nematodes, insects, and many other microorganisms found in the soil, in the air, and living within and on the surfaces of plants. Plants are definitely not alone! Consider the rhizosphere. The world in which the roots of plants survive can tell us much about their medicinal properties for our uses. There is also the phyllosphere, the world of the leaf surface, with its myriads of not only symbiotic organisms such as fungi, bacteria, and insects, but also trichomes, stomates, and glandular hairs. Certainly, this begs the question, "Just how similar are plants to animals and humans?"

How plants interact in their environment with other organisms can give herbalists added information by which to improve their practicum skills. How do plants detoxify toxic metals? Why are plants not susceptible to cancer? How do plants build resistance to viruses? What are the roles of plant hormones? How are secondary compounds transported from their biosynthetic origin to a storage compartment?

An appreciation of the biological sciences suggests that medical botany is more than simply a study of the tools of herbal medicine. The biological connections between plant chemicals and other living organisms are likely to give us clues about the use of herbal products. How plant chemicals affect various living organisms can help clinical herbalists to understand the mechanisms of action of medicinal plants and perhaps to discover other efficacious remedies. Studying only the human health sciences cannot afford this interconnected view, which medical botany can supply.

Can plants teach us how to heal if we investigate how they themselves use these compounds for their own health? As a plant scientist and an herbalist, I believe so. Medical botany is much more than simply stating which plant is good for what illness or condition.

The complexity of mammalian metabolism is just beginning to be recognized. Matching this complexity with herbal products that contain dozens to hundreds of chemical compounds is just beginning to happen. These advances are in stark contrast to the high cost and serious potential adverse effects of single chemicals.

Glossary

Androecium (an-'drE-shE-um, an-'drE-sE-um)
The aggregate of stamens in the flower of a seed plant.

Calyx
The outer whorl of a flower that consists of sepals, usually green in color.

Corolla
A part of a flower that consists of the separate or fused petals and constitutes the inner whorl of the perianth.

Endophytes
Fungi and bacteria that live on and inside plant tissues in mostly mutualistic relationships.

Enzymes
Proteins in biosynthetic processes that catalyze the formation of a product.

Eukaryote
Multicelled (except for protists, which are single-celled) organisms that contain a membrane-enclosed nucleus and membrane-enclosed organelles, such as mitochondria. Some protists and plants additionally contain chloroplast organelles.

Gynoecium (ji-'nE-shE-um, gI-nE-sE-um)
The aggregate of carpels or pistils within a flower.

Homology
Similarity in characteristics resulting from a shared ancestry.

Hypocotyl ('hI-pu-"kä-tul)
The part of the axis of a plant embryo or seedling below the cotyledon.

Metabolomics
The science that attempts to understand the physiologic status of an organism in light of its full biochemical physiologic potential.

Morphology
The study of form and its development.

Nutrigenomics
The science that relates how the molecular and metabolite inputs (some from food and herbs) influence and control gene expression.

Pharmacogenomics
The study of how an individual's genetic inheritance affects the body's response to drugs.

Prokaryote
Single-celled organisms that do not have a membrane-enclosed nucleus or membrane-enclosed organelles; found only in the domains Bacteria and Archaea.

References

Albersheim P, Anderson AJ. Proteins from plant cell walls inhibit polygalacturonases secreted by plant pathogens. Proc Nat Acad Sci 1971;68:1815–1819.

Ames BN. DNA damage from micronutrient deficiencies is likely to be a major cause of cancer. Review. Mutation Res 2001;475:7–20.

Anonymous. *WHO Traditional Medicine Strategy, 2002–2005.* Geneva, Switzerland: World Health Organization; 2002.

Bacon CW, Hill NS. Symptomless grass endophytes: products of coevolutionary symbioses and their role in the ecological adaptations of grasses. In: Redlin SC, Carris LM, eds. *Endophytic Fungi in Grasses and Woody Plants: Systematics, Ecology, and Evolution.* St. Paul, Minn: APS Press: The American Phytopathological Society; 1996.

Baker ME. Evolution of regulation of steroid-mediated intercellular communications in vertebrates: insights from flavonoids, signals that mediate plant-rhizobia symbiosis. Mol Cell Endocrinol 1992;175:1–4.

Baker ME. Flavonoids as hormones. A perspective from an analysis of molecular fossils. Adv Exp Med Biol 1998;439:249–276.

Barsony J, Prufer K. Vitamin D receptor and retinoid x receptor interactions in motion. Vitam Horm 2002;65:345–376.

Bouic PJD. The role of phytosterols and phytosterolins in immune modulation: a review of the past 10 years. Curr Opin Clin Nutri 2001;4:471–475.

Bouic PJD. Sterols and sterolins: new drugs for the immune system? Drug Discov Today 2002;7:775–778.

Buchanan BB, Gruissem W, Jones RL, eds. *Biochemistry and Molecular Biology of Plants.* Rockville, Md: American Society of Plant Physiologists; 2000.

Compton JA, Culham A, Jury SL. Reclassification of *Actaea* to include *Cimicifuga* and *Souliea* (Ranunculaceae): phylogeny inferred from nrDNA and cpDNA TRNL-F sequence variation. Taxonomy 1998;47:593–634.

Cullen J. *The Identification of Flowering Plant Families.* 4th ed. Cambridge, UK: Cambridge University Press; 1997.

Dewick PM. *Medicinal Natural Products: A Biosynthetic Approach.* New York, NY: Wiley; 2002.

Dornstauder E, Jisa E, Unterrieder I, et al. Estrogenic activity of two standardized red clover extracts (Menoflavon) intended for large scale use in hormone replacement therapy. J Ster Biochem Mol Biol 2001;78:67–75.

Fenech M. Micronutrients and genomic stability: a new paradigm for recommended dietary allowances (RDAs). Food Chem Toxicol 2002;40:1113–1117.

Fox JE. Chemical communication threatened by endocrine-disrupting chemicals. Environ Health Persp 2004;112:648–653.

Gazell KA. Functional medicine pioneer. Altern Ther Health Med 2004;10.

General Guidelines for Methodologies on Research and Evaluation of Traditional Medicine. Geneva, Switzerland: World Health Organization; 2000.

Go VLW, Wong DA, Wang Y, et al. Diet and cancer prevention: evidence-based medicine to genomic medicine. J Nutr 2004; 134:3513S–3516S.

Gottlieb OR, Borin MR, de Brito NRS. Integration of ethnobotany and phytochemistry: dream or reality? Phytochemistry 2002; 60:145–152.

Gupta, MB, Nath R, Srivastava N. Anti-inflammatory and antipyretic activities of beta-sitosterol. Planta Med 1980;39: 157–163.

Harrewijn P, van Oosten AM, Piron PGM. *Natural Terpenoids as Messengers.* The Netherlands: Kluwer Academic Publishers; 2001.

Havsteen BH. The biochemistry and medical significance of the flavonoids. Pharmacol Therapeut 2002;96:67–202.

Heap IM. International survey of herbicide resistant weeds, 2002. Available at: www.weedscience.com. Accessed February 15, 2002.

Hobbs C. *Medicinal Mushrooms: An Exploration of Tradition, Healing, & Culture.* Santa Cruz, CA: Botanica Press; 1995.

Huang JS. Pathogenesis-related proteins and disease resistance. In: *Biochemistry and Physiology of Plant-Microbe Interactions.* Boston, MA: Kluwer Academic Publishers; 2001.

Hyman M. Paradigm shift: the end of 'normal science' in medicine. Altern Ther Health Med 2004;10:10–15, 90–94.

Institute for Science in Society, 1995. Available at: http://www.i-sis.org.uk/

Kholodova YD. Phytoecdysteroids: biological effects, application in agriculture and complementary medicine. Ukr Biokhim Z 2001;73:21–29.

Kim H, Peterson TG, Barnes S. Mechanisms of action of the soy isoflavone genistein: emerging role for its effects via transforming growth factor beta signaling pathways. Am J Clin Nutr 1998;68:1418S–1425S.

Klein R. Phylogenetic and phytochemical characteristics of plant species with adaptogenic properties. Professional paper submitted in partial fulfillment of the requirements for the degree of Masters of Science in Plant Sciences and Plant Pathology. Bozeman, MT: Montana State University; 2004.

Lafont R. The endocrinology of invertebrates. Ecotoxicology 2000;9:41–57.

Lafont R, Dinan L. Practical uses for ecdysteroids in mammals including humans: an update. J Insect Sci 2003;3:7.

Lewis WH, Elvin-Lewis MPF. *Medical Botany: Plants Affecting Human Health.* 2nd ed. New York, NY: John Wiley & Sons; 2003.

Liu RH. Potential synergy of phytochemicals in cancer prevention: mechanism of action. J Nutr 2004;134:3479S–3485S.

Ma L, Dolphin D. The metabolites of dietary chlorophylls. Phytochemistry 1999;50:195–202.

Matile P. Biochemistry of Indian summer: physiology of autumnal leaf coloration. Exp Gerontol 2000;35:145–158.

Mors WB, do Nascimento MC, Pereira BMR, Pereira NA. Plant natural products active against snake bite—the molecular approach. Phytochemistry 2000;55:627–642.

Nisbet LJ, Fox FM. The importance of microbial biodiversity to biotechnology. In: Hawksworth DL, ed. *The Biodiversity of Microorganisms and Invertebrates: Its Role in Sustainable Agriculture.* Wallingford, Oxon, UK: CAB International; 1991.

Ohno S, Shinoda S, Toyoshima S, et al. Effects of flavonoid phytochemicals on cortisol production and on activities of steroidogenic enzymes in human adrenocortical H295R cells. J Steroid Biochem 2002;80:355–363.

Orzechowski A, Ostaszewski P, Jank M, Berwid SJ. Bioactive substances of plant origin in food—impact on genomics. Reprod Nutr Dev 2002;42:461–477.

Panossian AG. Adaptogens: a historical overview and perspective. Nat Pharm 2003;7:1, 19–20.

Piironen V, Linday G, Miettinen, TA, et al. Plant sterols: biosynthesis, biological function and their importance to human nutrition. J Sci Food Agr 2000;80:939–966.

Raven PH, Evert RF, Eichhorn SE. *Biology of Plants.* New York, NY: W.H. Freeman and Company/Worth Publishers; 2003.

Redman RS, Sheehan KB, Stout RG, Rodriguez RJ, Henson JM. Thermotolerance generated by plant/fungal symbiosis. Science 2002;298:1581.

Rosati F, Danza G, Guarna A, et al. New evidence of similarity between human and plant steroid metabolism: 5α-reductase activity in *Solanum malacoxylon.* Endocrinology 2003;144: 220–229.

Schepetkin IA, Khlebnikov AI, Ah SY, et al. Characterization and biological activities of humic substances from mumie. J Agric Food Chem 2003;51:5245–5254.

Schmeller T, Sporer F, Sauerwein M, et al. Binding of tropane alkaloids to nicotinic and muscarinic acetylcholine receptors. Pharmazie 1995;50:493–495.

Setchell KD, Cassidy A. Dietary isoflavones: biological effects and relevance to human health. J Nutr 1999;129:758S–767S.

Stamets P. *MycoMedicinals: An Informational Treatise on Mushrooms*. Olympia, Wash: MycoMedia, LLC; 2002.

Stermitz FR, Lorenz P, Tawara JN, Zenewicz LA, Lewis K. Synergy in a medicinal plant: antimicrobial action of berberine potentiated by 5′-methoxyhydnocarpin, a multidrug pump inhibitor. Proc Nat Acad Sci 2000;97:1433–1437.

Stierle A, Strobel G, Stierle D. Taxol and taxane production by *Taxomyces andreanae* an endophytic fungus of Pacific yew. Science 1993;260:214–216.

Stoka AM. Phylogeny and evolution of chemical communication: an endocrine approach. J Mol Endocrinol 1999;22:207–225.

Van der Veen IT. Costly carotenoids: a trade-off between predation and infection risk? J Evolution Biol 2005;18:992–999.

Verpoorte R. Exploration of nature's chemodiversity: the role of secondary metabolites as leads in drug development. Drug Discov Today 1998;3:232–238.

Vershinin A. Biological functions of carotenoids—diversity and evolution. BioFactors 1999;10:99–104.

Wandersee JH, Schussler EE. A model of plant blindness. Poster and paper presented at: 3rd Annual Associates Meeting of the 15th Laboratory, Louisiana State University; April 13, 1998; Baton Rouge, La.

Wang Y, Tang H, Nicholson JK, Hylands PJ, Sampson J, Holmes E. A metabonomic strategy for the detection of the metabolic effects of chamomile *(Matricaria recutita* L.*)* ingestion. J Agric Food Chem 2005;53:191–196.

Welshons WV, Thayer KA, Judy BM, Taylor JA, Curran EM, vom Saal FS. Large effects from small exposures. I. Mechanisms for endocrine disrupting chemicals with estrogenic activity. Environ Health Perspect 2003;10:54–94.

Williams RJ, Spencer JPE, Rice-Evans C. Flavonoids: antioxidants or signaling molecules? Free Rad Biol Med 2004;36:838–849.

Wink M, ed. *Biochemistry of Plant Secondary Metabolism. Annual Plant Reviews,* vol 2. Boca Raton, Fla: Sheffield Academic Press/CRC Press; 1999.

Wink M. Evolution of secondary metabolites from an ecological and molecular phylogenetic perspective. Phytochemistry 2003;64:3–19.

Zhou J, Davis LC, Verpoorte R. Elicitor signal transduction leading to production of plant secondary metabolites. Biotechnol Adv 2005;23:283–333.

Plant Chemistry in Veterinary Medicine: Medicinal Constituents and Their Mechanisms of Action

CHAPTER

Eric Yarnell

Botanical medicines owe their activity to their multitude of constituents. These constituents are generally broken up into the categories of primary and secondary, that is, those essential for life and those with nonessential functions, respectively. This chapter reviews the major categories of plant compounds and their mechanisms of action, when they are known. Notes about potential differences in the effects of various plant constituents on different animals are stated, to the extent that they are known.

Primary constituents include carbohydrates, amino acids and proteins, and lipids. These compounds are already well known to veterinarians and other practitioners because knowledge of these compounds is fundamental to an understanding of the biochemistry, metabolism, and nutrition of animals. However, some primary constituents have therapeutic relevance that is not usually touched on in medical programs. These are discussed in more depth here.

Secondary metabolites are those that are not necessary for day-to-day function in plant cells but that provide other important benefits to plants and fungi. They are known to act as antioxidants to protect against the free radicals generated during photosynthesis (carotenoids, flavonoids), to attract pollinators or seed dispersers (terpenoids), to ward off herbivores or insect pests (alkaloids), to inhibit competing plants (terpenoids), and to function as cellular signaling molecules, among other functions. The old view that these compounds are useless junk is now uniformly known to be false because all plants use energy to make all categories of secondary metabolites, and it simply does not make evolutionary sense for organisms to develop elaborate and ultimately highly wasteful metabolic processes.

Secondary metabolites can be categorized in many ways, none of which is completely satisfactory. For chemists and pharmacognocists, it is generally most useful to categorize them by their biosynthetic pathways and structure. This is only minimally helpful to the clinician and certainly to the student. A functional perspective is much more useful. This chapter uses a fundamentally biosynthetic classification but highlights the clinical relevance of these groupings.

Secondary metabolites clearly provide most of the therapeutic activity of medicinal plants and fungi (Yarnell, 2003). Concurrent evolution of animals, plants, and fungi helps explain why this is so. Animals that are able to make use of plant secondary metabolites would be better suited to survive and spread the genes that allow for the benefits gained. This can be viewed as creating a genetic arms race in which plants and fungi evolve secondary metabolites to interfere with animal predators that are successfully exploiting plant compounds. It can also be viewed cooperatively, for animals can be hijacked by plants or fungi in the process, as occurs when animals become seed or pollen dispersers. Regardless, knowledge of secondary metabolites is critical to an understanding and the effective application of modern herbal medicines.

POLYSACCHARIDES

Complex carbohydrates occur in all plants and fungi and account for important therapeutic properties in many of them. This discussion focuses on polysaccharides other than starch that do not serve as glucose sources for nonruminants. The role of polysaccharides in the ruminant digestive tract is different and it is sufficiently discussed in standard texts, so it is not reviewed here.

Polysaccharides are high-molecular-weight chains composed of monosaccharide units attached from the hemiacetal hydroxyl group on the first carbon of one and any other hydroxyl group on the next. Polysaccharides do not crystallize and are tasteless or mildly sweet at best. They are generally brown or white in color. Polyuronides are polysaccharides that also contain some uronic acid units. They have essentially the same properties as polysaccharides.

Although most complex carbohydrates are technically water insoluble, they do form gels to varying degrees when mixed with water. Basically, water adsorbs into the hydrophilic pockets within and among the polysaccharide chains, leading to partial weak association of chains

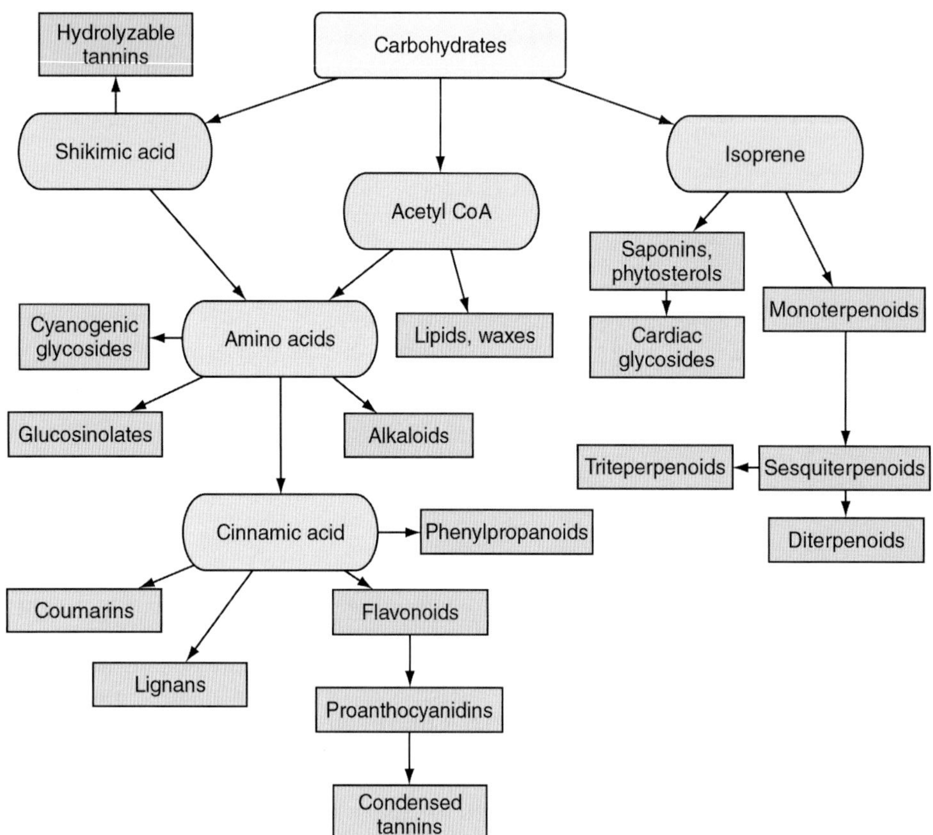

Figure 11-1 All pathways begin with carbohydrate formation via photosynthesis. Rounded rectangles represent key intermediate compounds. Rectangles represent major secondary metabolites. Arrows represent multiple metabolic steps.

Figure 11-2 Glucose. The primary structure of polysaccharides includes D-galacto-D-mannan, which is composed of beta-D-mannose units, with one alpha-D-galactose sidechain for every four mannose units.

Figure 11-3 Glucuronic acid.

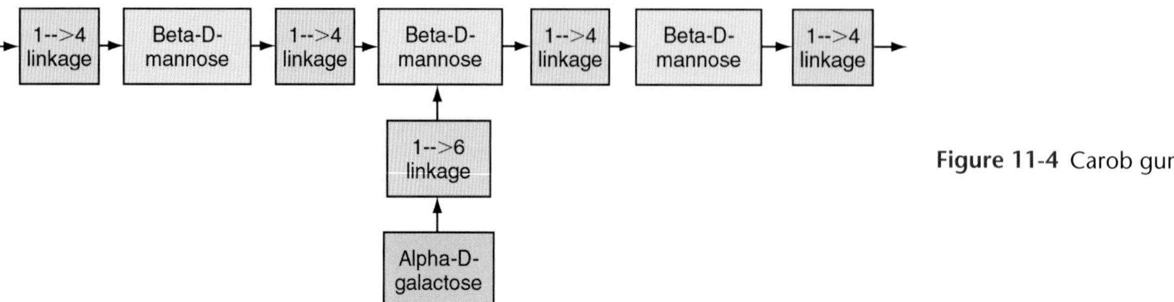

Figure 11-4 Carob gum structure.

via hydrogen bonding or coordination. These gels are generally reversible with addition of heat, although warm water is most effective in the creation of most gels. Some gel formation involves the formation of full covalent bonds and may be irreversible. These gels ultimately end up as insoluble precipitates.

The terms *mucilage* and *gum* are often used to describe the hydrocolloid gel that results when polysaccharides are mixed with water. The technically correct use of these terms is intermittent at best, although it is fortunate that this does not significantly affect therapeutic use. A mucilage is technically a heterogeneous branched polysaccharide (i.e., one made up of multiple different monosaccharide monomers) that is normally found in plant cells associated with special canals or cells; it is particularly common in external seed coats. A gum is a heterogeneous polyuronide that is usually formed in response to trauma.

Polysaccharides make up the main portion of dietary fiber, although these highly complex molecular mixtures also often contain lignins and other noncarbohydrate. Thus, dietary fiber and polysaccharides are not completely synonymous but are closely related. So-called soluble dietary fiber contains a higher percentage of gel-forming polysaccharides compared with insoluble dietary fiber.

The molecular mechanisms of action of polysaccharides and polyuronides have been most extensively studied as the dietary fiber portion of foods. Dietary fiber, likely through short-chain fatty acid breakdown products produced by gut microbes, decreases hepatic synthesis of fatty acids and thus reduces triglyceridemia (Delzenne, 1998). Fiber also increases bile acid turnover and modifies its synthesis, thus lowering systemic cholesterolemia (Levrat, 1994). Only soluble fibers have these effects consistently (Kay, 1980). Hypolipidemic effects generally require several weeks of treatment, as gene expression, microbial flora alterations, and other changes take time to occur after exposure to high-fiber diets (Delzenne, 1999).

Dietary fiber induces satiety and slow gastric emptying, apparently according to the viscosity of the material. In a normal nonruminant gut, fiber tends to reduce transit time, with variable strength depending on the type of fiber involved. When diarrhea is present, however, dietary fiber actually binds the stool and increases transit time. Fiber has also been shown in many studies to decrease formation of colon cancer in animals exposed to carcinogens, although much work remains to be done to elucidate the degree to which this effect is clinically relevant (Alabaster, 1993). The anticarcinogenic effects and many other properties of fiber may in part relate to its multifactorial effects on the gut flora, although at present, the exact effects of various types and amounts of fiber to be used for different durations of time have not been completely clarified (Woods, 1993). Fiber also reduces paracellular gut permeability in rodents (Mariadason, 1999).

Fiber in the gut delays absorption of glucose, which, in turn, reduces insulin responses (Kritchevsky, 1988). High-fiber diets have been extensively studied for their antidiabetic properties.

Gel-forming complex carbohydrates also act as demulcents or emollients. A demulcent is hydrating to the skin and moderately anti-inflammatory; it protects the gastric and esophageal epithelium from acid or other erosive materials. No research is available on the exact mechanisms involved in demulcent effects, other than the obvious mechanical barrier functions that they perform on tissue surfaces. The demulcent property is exploited clinically primarily to treat inflammatory conditions of the skin and digestive system. The immediate soothing effect of application of infusions of demulcent herbs has been demonstrated in clinical trials on humans with pharyngitis (Brinckmann, 2003).

Demulcents are believed to stimulate mucus production in the respiratory and urinary tracts via nerve reflexes, although this hypothesis has not been systematically assessed. One study of *Althaea officinalis* (marshmallow) root extract and polysaccharide isolate in cats showed that, at 100 and 50 mg/kg body weight doses, respectively, they acted as significantly more potent antitussives than the drug prenoxdiazine (Nosal'ova, 1992). Because complex polysaccharides are very unlikely to circulate in any quantity, it is difficult to imagine how they could act as antitussives, unless this occurs through some indirect mechanism.

Complex polysaccharides administered orally have repeatedly been shown to have immunostimulating effects. For example, polysaccharides from the root of *Rehmannia glutinosa,* an Asian medicinal herb, have been shown to inhibit complement (Tomoda, 1994). The polysaccharides of the root of *Glycyrrhiza uralensis* (gan cao), a close relative of licorice, and of the seed of *Plantago asiatica* (Asian plantain) have been shown to stimulate phagocytosis (Tomoda, 1990; Tomoda, 1991). Sulfated galactans from thallus of *Chondrus ocellatus,* a Chinese seaweed related to *Chondrus crispus* (Irish "moss," also actually a seaweed), have shown multiple complex effects on various components of the immune system (Zhou, 2004). Detailed molecular mechanisms for the immune effects of polysaccharides are largely unknown, although in the case of *Echinacea purpurea* leaf and flower polysaccharides, evidence suggests that its immune-stimulating effects are due to changes in levels of various interleukins (Parnham, 1999). Evidence for the proposed immunomodulating effects of polysaccharides, that is, their ability to both stimulate and suppress various immune cells depending on the milieu, was not located (Box 11-1).

Polysaccharides are extremely safe. They have no known toxic effects. Occasionally, some dietary fibers can cause loose stools in nonruminants. Highly gel-forming gums and mucilages can swell sufficiently to cause mechanical obstruction of the esophagus or small intestines, although this is very rare at usual levels of intake.

Polysaccharides can delay absorption of some drugs, such as digoxin, which is enterohepatically resorbed (Brown, 1978). Monitoring the blood levels of drugs in animals fed large amounts of polysaccharides may be necessary to ensure therapeutic effects in some cases (Box 11-2).

BOX 11-1

Actions of Gel-Forming Polysaccharides

- Decrease hepatic fatty acid synthesis
- Increase bile acid turnover
- Modify bile acid synthesis
- Reduce hyperlipidemia
- Slow gastric emptying
- Increase satiety
- Reduce transit time
- Bind diarrhea
- Have anticarcinogenic effects in the colon
- Modulate gut flora
- Reduce gut permeability
- Delay glucose absorption
- Provide demulcent/emollient effects—hydrate skin, act as anti-inflammatory topically, protect from stomach acid
- Antitussive
- Promote production of mucus in the respiratory and urinary tracts
- Act as immunostimulator

BOX 11-2

Select Polysaccharide-Rich Herbs

Angiosperms

- *Alcea rosea* (hollyhock)
- *Aloe vera* (aloe vera) gel
- *Althaea officinalis* (marshmallow)
- *Astragalus membranaceus* (astragalus)
- *Coix lachryma jobi* (Job's tears, yi yi ren)
- *Elymus repens* (couch grass)
- *Fucus vesiculosus* (bladderwrack)
- *Glycyrrhiza glabra* (licorice)
- *Glycyrrhiza uralensis* (gan cao)
- *Opuntia* spp (prickly pear)
- *Sphaeralcea parvifolia*
- *Symphytum officinale* (comfrey)
- *Ulmus rubra* (slippery elm)*
- *Zea mays* (corn, maize)

Fungi

- *Ganoderma lucidum* (shiitake)
- *Lentinula edodes* (reishi)
- *Trametes versicolor* (yunzhi, cloud mushroom)

Lichen

- *Cetraria islandica* (Icelandic "moss")

Red Algae

- *Chondrus crispus* (Irish "moss")

*Threatened in the wild. Use only cultivated sources.

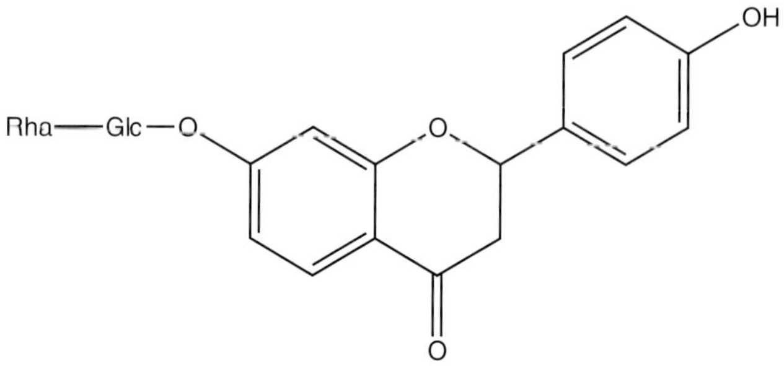

Rha—Glc—O (structure)

Figure 11-5 Naringin (or naringinoside), a flavonoid glycoside, illustrates the three major components of all glycosides. The glycone is composed of two sugars (Rha = rhamnose, Glc = glucose). The aglycone is the rest of the molecule. The glycosidic link extends between the glycone and the aglycone.

GLYCOSIDES

Glycosides consist of any of the many other categories of secondary metabolites discussed here that are bound to a monosaccharide or an oligosaccharide, or to uronic acid. The saccharide or uronic acid portion is referred to as the glycone, and whatever other molecule the glycone is attached to is referred to as the aglycone. For example, flavonoids frequently occur as glycosides, in which case, the flavonoid is the aglycone and whatever saccharide it is attached to is the glycone. The glycone and aglycone are attached via a glycosidic linkage. Although this usually involves a covalent bond to oxygen, it can also involve carbon, nitrogen, or sulfur, depending on the aglycone.

Because of the diversity of aglycones and glycosides, these compounds do not share a common biosynthetic pathway. The process of forming the glycosidic linkage is known as glycosylation and is accomplished via specialized enzymes that use a uridine diphosphosugar as the glycone source. The addition of the glycone usually renders the total glycoside more polar and thus more water soluble than the isolated aglycone. In most instances, it is believed that glycosides are formed to enhance ease of movement and storage of nonpolar or weakly polar aglycones within the plant.

The glycosidic linkage is relatively fragile. Several enzymes exist that can break the link, including beta-glucosidase and beta-galactosidase. It is unclear whether these enzymes exist in the gastrointestinal lumen of most animals but they almost always occur in their livers. Gut flora also typically possess these enzymes. Heat can break the bonds. According to one study of glycoside breakdown in leaves of *Senna alexandrina* (senna), 30° C (86° F) and 60% relative humidity and 40° C (104° F) and 75% relative humidity were sufficient to cause significant glycoside loss compared with 25° C (77° F) and 60% relative humidity (Goppel, 2004). A methanol extract of senna showed much less breakdown except at even higher temperatures. Ultraviolet light and extremes of pH can also break some of these bonds. Because of the changes in pharmacokinetics and possibly pharmacodynamics of herbs with intact glycosides versus free aglycones, many botanical practitioners believe that it is important for herbs containing glycosides to undergo minimal processing.

The pharmacokinetics of glycosides are complex but central to an understanding of their importance. A simple model is that of a built-in delayed release system, in which the hydrophilic glycoside delivers a hydrophobic aglycone to the large intestines. Most intact glycosides generally pass through the stomach and small intestines unchanged. However, some glycosides are absorbed, apparently by the intestinal epithelial intestinal Na+/glucose monosaccharide cotransporter, SGLT-1 (Wagner, 2003).

Once in the colon, the glycosidic bond is hydrolyzed by enzymes possessed by the gut flora. Some aglycones released by this process may also undergo enzymatic modification by gut bacteria. Aglycones are then absorbed via the large intestine, undergo first-pass metabolism in the liver, and circulate to varying degrees within the body. This process has been extensively studied, for example, with the glycosides in *Panax ginseng* (Asian ginseng) roots, known as ginsenosides (Hasegawa, 2000). Ginsenoside aglycones released by the action of gut flora have been shown to be more potent antineoplastic compounds compared with intravenously injected intact ginsenosides in mice (Wakabayashi, 1997). Some ginsenosides are esterified to fatty acids in the liver and may have prolonged half-lives as a result (Hasegawa, 2004).

Other properties of glycosides are highly dependent on the specific aglycone present. Some important types of glycosides are discussed in the following section to give the reader a sense of the wide range of therapeutic applications they can have.

Cardiac Glycosides

The aglycones in cardiac glycosides fall into one of two categories, both derived from a steroidal base. They can be the more common cardenolides, with a five-member ring attached to the steroidal base, or the much less common bufadienolides, with a six-member ring attached.

Regardless of their structure, all cardiac glycosides inhibit Na^+/K^+-ATPase pumps throughout the body. Because these pumps are most concentrated and critical in cardiac myocytes, they have their greatest effect on this tissue. When an action potential passes through a cardiac myocyte, the cardiac glycoside limits sodium outflow and potassium inflow from the cell. The linked Na^+/Ca^{2+} pump thus does not have sufficient sodium available to move calcium out of the cell. The higher than normal intracellular calcium concentration means that during the next action, potential contractility is increased. This is described as a positive inotropic action. Another consequence of this activity is a reduction in heart rate, described as negative chronotropic action. The glycosides also limit conduction velocity in the atrioventricular node, an action described as negative dromotropic.

All of these effects, combined with a mild tendency to reduce tubular resorption of sodium in the kidneys and a moderate vasoconstrictive effect, make cardiac glycosides

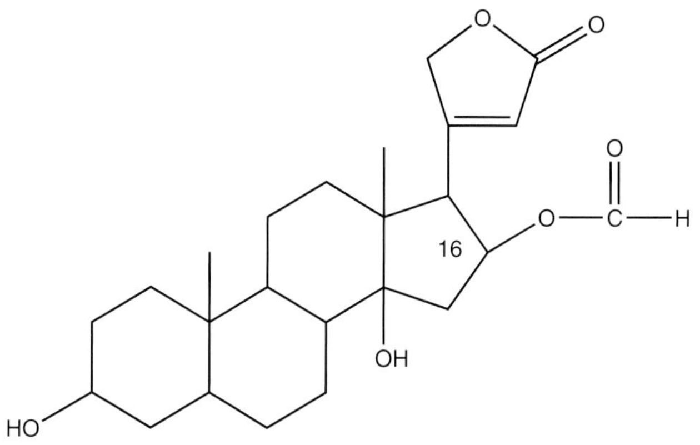

Figure 11-6 Digitoxigenin, a cardenolide aglycone.

best suited for relieving symptoms due to congestive heart failure (CHF). They can also reduce some atrial arrhythmias. However, these agents do not address the cause of CHF and do not appear to reduce CHF-induced mortality; they do, however, reduce the need for hospitalization, at least in humans (Hood, 2004).

The number of sugars or uronic acids attached to the aglycone affects the water solubility of the overall glycoside and can alter its bioavailability. A lesser degree of hydroxylation correlates with rapid oral absorption and rapid renal excretion; greater hydroxylation slows oral absorption and is associated with biliary excretion, significant enterohepatic recirculation, and long half-lives.

Cardiac glycosides with long half-lives (4 to 6 days in the case of digitoxin) accumulate in the body. This greatly increases the danger of toxicity. Those glycosides that are rapidly cleared, such as those found in *Convallaria majalis* (lily of the valley), do not accumulate and are of mild potency. Those that accumulate, such as those found in *Digitalis purpurea* (foxglove), are of strong potency and must be used cautiously. Major common adverse effects caused by overdose include anorexia, nausea, vomiting, arrhythmia, confusion, headache, depression, green or yellow tinting of the vision, blurred vision, and worsening CHF. The toxic and therapeutic doses of *Digitalis* and potent, isolated cardiac glycosides can be very close, and sometimes toxicity is noted before therapeutic benefit. These problems are rarely noted with milder herbs (Box 11-3). Because even mild potassium depletion can greatly increase the toxicity of all cardiac glycosides, it is critical for the practitioner to avoid combining these agents or herbs that contain them with potassium-depleting medications (Chung, 1969). Of particular concern are non–potassium-sparing diuretics, corticosteroids, and *Glycyrrhiza glabra* (licorice). Antibiotics may also unpredictably alter the effects of cardiac glycosides by changing the gut flora, thus altering enterohepatic recirculation. Any change in metabolism, such as fever, kidney failure, or intervening hyperthyroidism, can also dramatically alter the pharmacokinetics and thus the pharmacodynamics of these compounds.

BOX 11-3

Major Cardiac Glycoside–Containing Herbs*

- *Digitalis purpurea* (foxglove), *D. lanata* (woolly foxglove)
- *Strophanthus kombe* (stropanthus)
- *Adonis vernalis* (pheasant's eye)
- *Nerium oleander* (oleander)
- *Apocynum* spp (dogbane, Indian hemp)
- *Asclepias asperula* (inmortal)
- *Asclepias tuberosa* (pleurisy root)
- *Urginea maritima* (squill)
- *Convallaria majalis* (lily of the valley)

*Note: Arranged approximately from most toxic to least.

BOX 11-4

Major Anthraquinone Glycoside–Containing Herbs

- *Aloe vera* (aloe) latex
- *Frangula purshiana* (cascara sagrada)
- *Juglans cinerea* (butternut)*
- *Rhamnus frangula* (alder buckthorn)
- *Rheum palmatum* (Chinese rhubarb)
- *Rumex crispus* (yellow dock)*
- *Senna alexandrina* (senna)

*Mild effect.

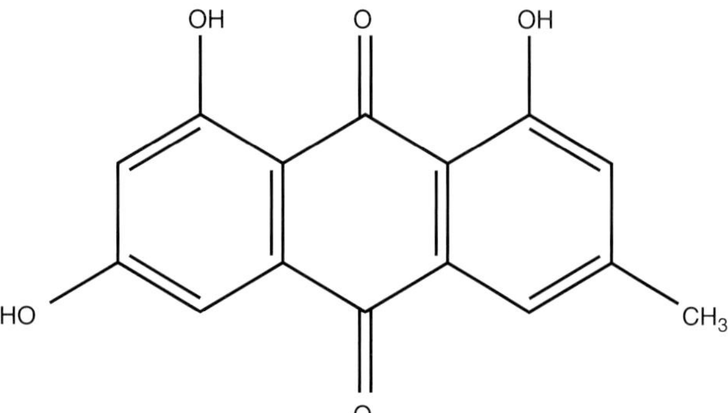

Figure 11-7 Emodin, an anthraquinone.

Anthraquinone Glycosides

Anthraquinone glycosides are generally orange, red, or brown-red compounds found in fairly limited distribution within the plant kingdom. Their solubility is similar to that of other glycosides with hydrophobic aglycones. Although some aglycones are absorbed within the small intestines, many of the intact glycosides make it to the colon before being hydrolyzed. In traditional Chinese medicine, this fact was exploited, although the rationale was explained differently. Herbs containing anthraquinone glycosides, particularly *Rheum palmatum* (rhubarb), were administered boiled if noncathartic properties were preferred because this would hydrolyze many of the anthraquinone glycosides. According to one review, boiling reduces the cathartic effects of rhubarb root 50% (Natori, 1981). Nonboiled forms of the herb were administered when catharsis was the desired outcome.

Anthraquinone glycosides can take 6 to 12 hours or longer to reach the colon, depending on gut motility and transit time of the patient. Once hydrolyzed in the colon, anthraquinones induce water and electrolyte secretion, as well as peristalsis, including catharsis. The contractions caused can be fairly strong and even painful (known as *griping*); thus, carminatives or antispasmodics are frequently administered simultaneously with anthraquinone glycosides. Use of anthraquinone glycosides for longer than 10 days consecutively can readily lead to induction of atonic constipation as the colon adapts to the cathartic impulses. Persistent use or abuse can also lead to diarrhea with fluid and electrolyte loss and, ultimately, rhabdomyolysis, renal failure, and other severe outcomes.

Some percentage of the anthraquinones are deposited in the colon wall, leaving dark brown or black patches referred to as *pseudomelanosis coli*. Most clinical research in humans confirms that this does not promote colorectal cancer (Yarnell, 2000). It is interesting to note that much research in fact shows that anthraquinones are antineoplastic. Emodin, found in rhubarb, is an apoptosis inducer (Lee, 2001).

Anthraquinones have other interesting properties. They are antifungal, inhibit excessive renal tubular cell proliferation, delay deterioration of patients in renal failure, modulate inflammation by partially inhibiting cyclooxygenase, and so forth (Agarwal, 2000; Guo, 1989; Sanada, 1996; Zheng, 1993). As far as is known, subcathartic doses or doses of noncathartic forms of herbs containing anthraquinone glycosides do not cause any serious adverse effects and will not cause pseudomelanosis coli. The aglycones can discolor the urine and feces red, brown, or black as they are excreted (Box 11-4).

Cyanogenic Glycosides

Cyanogenic glycosides have amino acid–derived aglycones that are mostly a safety concern in medicinal plants. The concerns about cyanogenic glycosides are twofold. First, these compounds interfere with iodine organification and thus can cause or promote goiter and hypothyroidism. However, this problem has been clearly documented to occur only in the setting of iodine deficiency or with massive overconsumption. Second, cyanogenic glycosides do spontaneously degrade to release potentially lethal hydrogen cyanide once the glycosidic linkage is hydrolyzed. However, unless massive and rapid intake of cyanogenic glycosides occurs, the cyanide is quickly and safely detoxified by hepatic thiosulfate sulfurtransferase. Smaller animals, juveniles, and herbivores that eat large amounts of *Prunus* spp leaves or white clover are potentially more susceptible. Other symptoms of acute cyanide exposure include headache, bronchial constriction, and weakness (Magnuson, 1997). Toxic effects, if any, of chronic, low-level exposure are unknown.

Evidence suggests that cyanogenic glycosides may have beneficial effects in animals that consume them. The most controversial evidence involves the cyanogenic glycosides from *Prunus* spp (cherry), particularly amygdalin (sold under the trade name Laetrile) and prunasin. These compounds do have anticarcinogenic activity in vitro according to recent research (Fukuda, 2003). Previous animal and human studies have, however, failed to show convincing clinical effectiveness of isolated injections of amygdalin (Hill, 1976; Moertel, 1982). Prunasin has also been shown to inhibit DNA polymerase in vitro (Mizushina, 1999).

GLUCOSINOLATES

Glucosinolates yield pungent, sulfur-containing, amino acid–derived aglycones, such as glucobrassicins, thiocyanates, and isothiocyanates, that give Brassicaceae, Capparidaceae, Resedaceae, and other families of plants their unique flavors. Similar to other glycosides, glucosinolates are water soluble, but their aglycones are hydrophobic. These aglycones have an oily consistency and are often known as mustard oils. Despite their strong odor and oily nature, these compounds are chemically very different from volatile oils and should not be confused with them. The sulfur-containing cysteine sulfoxides that give *Allium sativum* (garlic) and related plants their pungency and much of their activity are closely related to glucosinolate aglycones. Cysteine sulfoxides do not occur as glycosides.

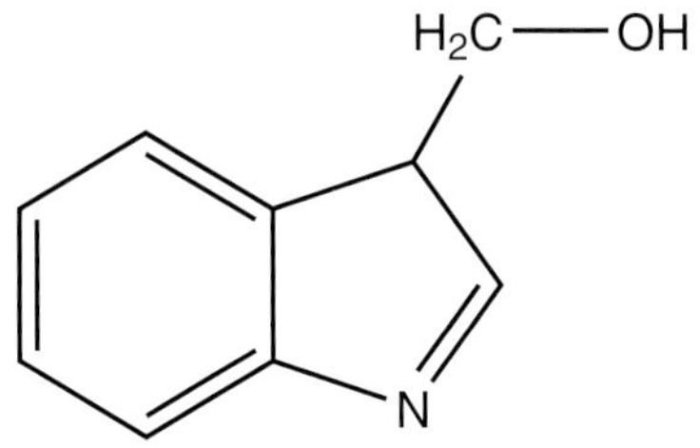

H_2C—OH

N

Figure 11-8 Indole-3-carbinol, a glucobrassicin-type glucosinolate.

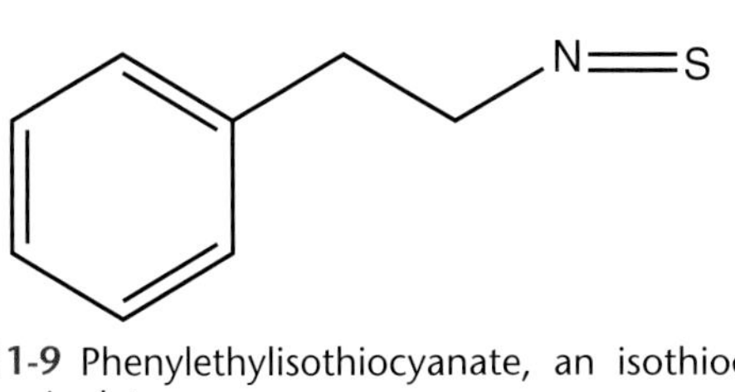

N═S

Figure 11-9 Phenylethylisothiocyanate, an isothiocyanate-type glucosinolate.

Isothiocyanate aglycones such as phenethyl isothiocyanate (PEITC) and sulforaphane and glucobrassicins indole-3-carbinol (I3C) and diindolylmethane (DIM) have been widely studied because of their presence in broccoli and other commonly consumed Brassicaceae vegetables. These compounds have complex effects on cytochrome P450 (CYP) isoforms 1A1, 1A2, and 2B1 in various parts of the body, but ultimately, they tend to decrease hepatic formation of carcinogenic metabolites from a wide variety of environmental chemicals (Smith, 2000; Shertzer, 2000). One of the best studied properties of I3C in particular is its ability to induce the 2-hydroxylation catabolic pathway for estradiol, which deprives the 16-alpha and 4-hydroxylation pathways of substrate and appears to greatly reduce the negative effects of estradiol (Bradlow, 1995). This is because 2-hydroxylation metabolites are vastly weaker estrogens than 16-alpha- or 4-hydroxylation metabolites (Bradlow, 1995).

Glucosinolate aglycones are traditionally used topically as rubefacients. They cause a warming sensation and reddening related to dilation of dermal capillaries. This is traditionally associated with relief from inflammation or pain in deeper or adjacent tissues, possibly caused by gating mechanisms in the spinal cord, although this has not been investigated. Empirically, they also provoke coughing when placed on the chest. If left in place too long, these compounds can cause minor or serious burns.

Glucosinolate aglycones are excreted by the kidneys after conjugation to glutathione by the action of glutathione-*S*-transferase (GST) or after conjugation to N-acetylcysteine. It has been shown that humans who have the GSTM-1 and GSTT-1 null genotypes do not excrete glucosinolate aglycones efficiently; thus, these stay in their bodies longer after ingestion. This correlates strongly with the anticancer effects of these compounds and helps explain why some people derive protection from cancer by eating Brassicaceae vegetables, while others do not (Lin, 1998; Spitz, 2000).

Glucosinolates can cause nausea and, in overdose, vomiting. This property is sometimes used in emergencies when no access to medical care is available, to induce vomiting through administration of large quantities of mustard powder. Other adverse effects resulting from internal use have not been documented. Because of their complex effects on CYP enzymes, their use with prescription drugs may cause relevant interactions. For example, it has been shown that reasonable doses of garlic reduce serum levels of protease inhibitors in healthy volunteers, consistent with CYP3A4 induction (Piscatelli, 2002).

FLAVONOIDS AND PROANTHOCYANIDINS

Flavonoids share a central three-ring structural motif and are all synthesized from cinnamic acid. Numerous subcategories of flavonoids exist, depending on the various functional groups present (Box 11-5). Note that the term *bioflavonoid* is redundant and thus should not be used. Proanthocyanidins are oligomers of flavonoids. Condensed tannins are large polymers of flavonoids. Thus,

BOX 11-5

Select Flavonoid-Rich Herbs

General Flavonoids
- *Calendula officinalis* (calendula)
- *Citrus paradisi* (grapefruit)
- *Fagopyrum esculentum* (buckwheat)
- *Ginkgo biloba* (ginkgo)
- *Glycyrrhiza glabra* (licorice)
- *Glycyrrhiza uralensis* (gan cao)
- *Hypericum perforatum* (Saint John's Wort)
- *Lespedeza capitata* (round-head lespedeza)
- *Matricaria recutita* (chamomile)
- *Nepeta cataria* (catnip)
- *Opuntia* spp (prickly pear) flowers
- *Orthosiphon stamineus* (Java tea)
- *Passiflora incarnata* (passionflower)
- *Rosmarinus officinalis* (rosemary)
- *Scutellaria baicalensis* (Baikal skullcap)
- *Scutellaria lateriflora* (skullcap)
- *Solidago canadensis* (goldenrod)

Isoflavones and Coumestans*
- *Psoralea carylifolia* (scurfy pea)
- *Pueraria montana* (kudzu)
- *Glycine max* (soy)
- *Iris germanica* (orris)
- *Medicago sativa* (alfalfa)
- *Trifolium repens* (red clover), *T. subterraneum* (subterranean clover)

Flavonolignans
- *Silybum marianum* (milk thistle)

*Coumestans are structually similar to isoflavones and also act as phytoestrogens.

Select Proanthocyanidin-Rich Herbs

- *Crataegus laevigata* (hawthorn), *C. monogyna* (hawthorn)
- *Croton lechleri* (dragon's blood)
- *Pinus sylvestris* (Scots pine)
- *Vaccinium corymbosum* (highbush blueberry)
- *Vaccinium macrocarpon* (cranberry)
- *Vaccinium myrtillus* (bilberry)
- *Vaccinium ovatum* (evergreen huckleberry)
- *Vitis vinifera* (grape)

these three categories of constituents are closely related biosynthetically, and, at least in the case of flavonoids and proanthocyanidins, chemically (Table 11-1). Condensed tannins develop very distinct properties from these other two types of molecules and thus are discussed in a separate section.

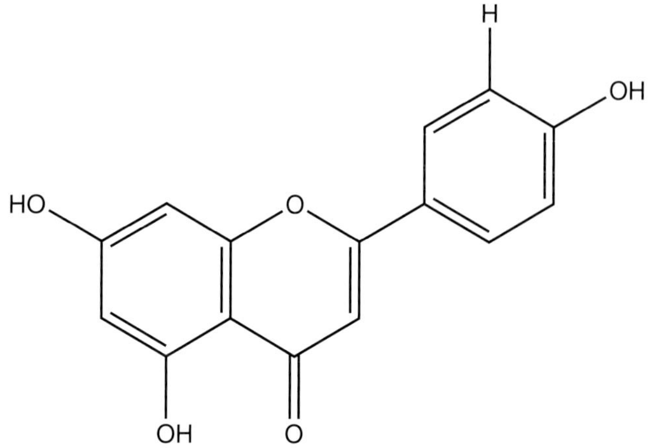

H
OH
HO
O
OH
O

Figure 11-10 Apigenin, a flavonoid.

Flavonoids and proanthocyanidins are almost universally antioxidant. They are believed to have this function in the plants or fungi in which they are found; thus, it is not surprising that they would do the same for anyone who consumes them. Many flavonoids and proanthocyanidins also generally tend to decrease capillary permeability and fragility, although at least one line of evidence suggests that the flavan-3-ol subgroup of flavonoids are the only ones that have this action, sometimes referred to as the "vitamin P [permeability]" effect (Roger, 1988). Lesions caused in blood vessels by vitamin C and flavonoid deficiencies in rodents are distinctive on a microscopic level (Casley-Smith, 1975).

Flavonoids, proanthocyanidins, and vitamin C have a complex and unclear relationship. Careful in vitro examination found that only dihydroquercetin, out of many flavonoids tested, could reduce oxidized vitamin C, contrary to the general belief that all flavonoids can do this (Bors, 1995). Another research group found that vitamins C and E were not synergistic antioxidants with various flavonoids in liposomes, but that their effects were merely additive (Vasiljeva, 2000). One in vitro study showed that some flavonoids, such as fisetin and quercetin, inhibited squamous cell carcinoma cells from growing only in the presence of ascorbic acid (Kandaswami, 1993). Much more research is clearly needed, but the strong link between flavonoids, proanthocyanidins, and vitamin C in the public mind is not solidly supported in the existing literature.

Other molecular actions of flavonoids and proanthocyanidins are extremely diverse, depending on the compound in question. For example, many flavonoids and proanthocyanidins are anti-inflammatory and antineoplastic. Numerous recent studies suggest that this is so because, at least in part, of the ability of these compounds to inhibit the NF-kappa-B signaling pathway that triggers inflammatory cascades (Moreira, 2004); they also inhibit mitogen-associated protein kinase (MAPK) and induce apoptosis, possibly through activation of c-Jun NH(2)-terminal kinase (JNK)–mediated caspase (Vayalil, 2004; Hou, 2004). Many flavonoids are also antiallergic. The aglycone of herperidin, hesperidin, released by action of

TABLE 11-1

Comparison of Flavonoids, Proanthocyanidins, and Condensed Tannins

Compound	Color	Flavor	Structure
Flavonoids	Yellow, orange	Nondistinctive	Tricyclic (see diagram)
Proanthocyanidins	Blue, red, purple	Slightly astringent	Flavonoid oligomers
Condensed tannins	Brown, black	Highly astringent	Flavonoid polymers

the gut flora, inhibited immunoglobulin E (IgE)-induced histamine release as effectively as the drug azelastine in vitro (Lee, 2004).

Isoflavones, which are structurally closely related to flavonoids, also occur as glycosides. Although these compounds have multiple activities, much research has focused on their function as phytoestrogens. Note that other constituents, notably some lignans, can also be phytoestrogenic. This means that they act as weak estrogen receptor (ER)-β agonists (Morito, 2001). Most phytoestrogens also bind and agonize ER-α, but much more weakly than ER-β; however, exceptions do exist (Kuiper, 1998). Because phytoestrogens are 100 to 100,000 times weaker agonists than estradiol, they are functional estrogen antagonists when ingested by animals with normal levels of estradiol (Bickhoff, 1962; Shutt, 1972). This interaction is particularly important to consider because many in vitro studies report that phytoestrogens stimulate ER-positive breast cancer cells, unless estradiol is added to the system, in which case, inhibition of breast cancer cells has been noted (Schmitt, 2001). The clinical effects of phytoestrogens thus depend on endogenous estrogen status; they can be conceptualized as balancing estrogen levels.

Sufficiently high levels of phytoestrogens can clearly induce reproductive changes in ruminants that are consistent with estrus (Nwannenna, 1995). A genistein dose of 0.7 mg daily in mice has shown osteoprotective effects, and 5 mg daily was sufficient to cause uterine hypertrophy, clearly indicating that levels of exposure within the system can cause very different effects (Ishimi, 2000). Contrary to the level of information available, the isoflavones genistein and daidzein are present at much higher levels in *Pueraria montana* (kudzu) root and several beans other than *Glycine max* (soy) fruit (Kaufman, 1997).

One of the great advantages of flavonoids and proanthocyanidins is that they are essentially nontoxic. Their widespread presence in foods means that most animals are exposed to gram quantities of total flavonoids and proanthocyanidins on a daily basis with no obvious signs of problems. The concern about carcinogenicity of some flavonoids, particularly quercetin, have not played out in animal studies unless absurdly high doses are used and do not fit with human epidemiologic data suggesting that diets rich in flavonoid- and proanthocyanidin-containing foods are protective against cancer (Hertog, 1996; Hertog, 1994). Part of the safety lies in the relatively short half-lives of most compounds, which, for example,

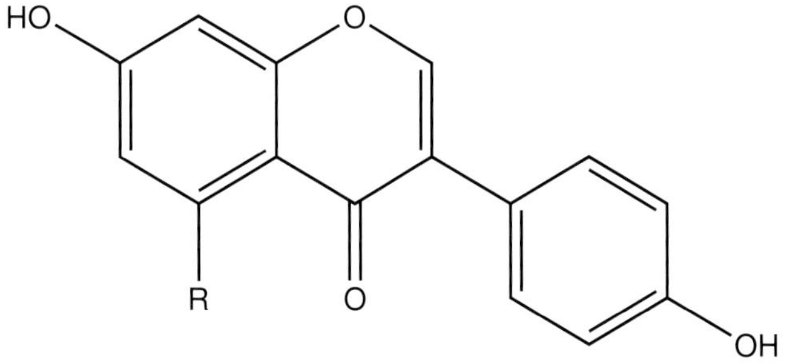

HO O R O OH

Daidzein, R = H
Genistein, R = OH

Figure 11-11 The isoflavones daidzein and genistein.

were found to be 2 to 3 hours in one human study of the anthocyanidin glycosides from *Hibiscus sabdariffa* (roselle) (Frank, 2005).

The pharmacokinetics of flavonoids and proanthocyanidins is similar to that of glycosides, as has been discussed. The flavonoids genistein and apigenin have been shown to undergo enterohepatic recycling, which actually appears to partially account for their relatively low systemic bioavailability (Chen, 2003). As has been mentioned in the discussion of actions of flavonoids, the action of the gut flora on flavonoid glycosides may be imperative for their activity. Some flavonoid aglycones are water soluble, depending on the degree of hydroxylation. The presence of five or more hydroxyl groups correlates with water solubility. One very preliminary clinical trial found that vitamin C was better absorbed from a citrus extract than was isolated vitamin C in humans, although this did not prove to be a clinically relevant outcome (Vinson, 1988).

TANNINS

Two distinct types of tannins have been identified on the basis of structure. Condensed tannins are composed of many flavonoids or proanthocyanidins joined together. However, the properties of condensed tannins are distinct from their building blocks. Hydrolyzable tannins are composed of a glucose (or rarely, other monosaccharide or polyol) core with several catechin derivatives attached. These medium to large polymers are very widely distributed in the plant and fungus kingdoms. Condensed and larger hydrolyzable tannins have most properties in common, although hydrolyzable tannins are less stable (being susceptible to hydrolysis) and have greater potential to cause toxicity.

Smaller tannins are hot water soluble, but as the molecules get larger, they become less and less soluble in any solvent. Tannins are generally much less soluble in cold water. Thus, relatively tannin-free extracts can usually be made through cold infusion of crude herbs.

Tannins generally possess an astringent flavor and activity, which relates to their ability to indiscriminately bind proteins. Only triester and larger hydrolyzable tannins are astringent. Tannins draw tissues together as proteins congeal, causing a peculiar puckering sensation in the mouth. This also tends to inactivate bound proteins. Tannin-rich herbs are frequently used to slow proteinaceous discharges of all types, most notably, transudates such as those associated with atopic dermatitis skin lesions, diarrhea, and hemorrhages from the skin or in the gastrointestinal tract.

In vitro, condensed tannins inhibit a wide variety of enzymes, in keeping with their ability to bind and inactivate proteins. For example, various tannins have been shown to partially inhibit angiotensin-converting enzyme and aldose reductase, as well as human immunodeficiency virus (HIV) integrase, protease, and reverse transcriptase (Liu, 2003; Suryanarayana, 2004; Notka, 2004). However, their bioavailability is extremely low, so it is unknown to what extent they have relevant activity systemically, as opposed to on the skin or in the gastrointestinal tract. Nevertheless, tannin-rich herbs are commonly used in traditional herbalism to quell internal bleeding and for a variety of actions, such as modulation of systemic inflammation, that suggest that they are circulating and active.

Tannins tend to bind or chelate many other types of molecules besides proteins, most notably, divalent cations and alkaloids. This can render the bound agents inactive and insoluble. Thus, tannins generally should not be administered simultaneously with any medication or nutrient because of the potential for reduced absorption and activity. Tannin-rich herbs do not tend to mix well with other herbs in formulas, although sometimes, this may reduce the potential toxicity of some herbs.

Tannins can cause nausea fairly readily, perhaps as a result of protein binding within the stomach and duodenum (Box 11-6). Consumption of tannins with food reduces this problem. For herbs that contain tannins and other beneficial constituents, but with which the tannins are causing nausea or otherwise are interfering, cold infusions are recommended to produce low-tannin extracts. Tannins also tend to be mildly constipating. High levels of tannins absorbed into the bloodstream can cause serious constipation and hepatotoxicity, as well as damage to other organs. Ruminants are particularly susceptible to these effects.

BOX 11-6

Major Tannin-Rich Herbs

- *Agrimonia eupatoria* (agrimony)
- *Arctostaphylos uva-ursi* (uva-ursi)
- *Arctostaphylos pungens* (manzanita)
- *Camellia sinensis* (green tea)
- *Ceanothus greggii* (red root)
- *Cinnamomum zeylanicum* (cinnamon), *C. cassia* (cassia)
- *Cola nitida* (cola)
- *Croton lechleri* (dragon's blood)
- *Ephedra sinica* (ma huang)
- *Ephedra nevadensis* (Mormon tea)
- *Filipendula ulmaria* (meadowsweet)
- *Geranium maculatum* (cranesbill)
- *Hamamelis virginiana* (witch hazel)
- *Jatropha cineria* (sangre de drago)
- *Krameria* spp (rhatany)
- *Morella cerifera* (bayberry)
- *Paullinia cupana* (guaraná)
- *Polygonum bistorta* (bistort)
- *Potentilla* spp (tormentil, cinquefoil)
- *Punica granatum* (pomegranate)
- *Quercus* spp (oak)
- *Rheum palmatum* (Chinese rhubarb)
- *Rosa* spp (rose)
- *Rubus* spp (raspberry, blackberry)
- *Theobroma cacao* (cocoa, chocolate)
- *Trillium ovatum* (bethroot)
- *Vaccinium* spp (bilberry, cranberry, blueberry)

Families Associated With Presence of Tannins

- Ericaceae
- Fagaceae
- Polygonaceae
- Rosaceae

LOW-MOLECULAR-WEIGHT TERPENOIDS, PHENYLPROPANOIDS, AND VOLATILE OILS

Terpenoids are synthesized via the mevalonate and deoxyxylulose pathways with the use of a five-carbon building block known as isoprene. This family of constituents has many different members, each with five more carbons than the last as another isoprene is added (Table 11-2).

Monoterpenoids, made up of two isoprene units, are the smallest and simplest type of terpenoids (Box 11-7). They are of sufficiently low molecular weight that they tend to volatilize readily. Their close cousins are the sesquiterpenoids, with three isoprene units. They are also of sufficiently light molecular weight as to be volatile. Monoterpenoids and sesquiterpenoids are referred to as low-molecular-weight terpenoids (LMWT). LMWT are generally found only in vascular plants, although occasionally, they may occur in simpler organisms and in some insects.

Although they are synthetically and structurally distinct, phenylpropanoids have most of the same properties as LMWT. Phenylpropanoids are synthesized via the shikimic acid pathway by way of cinnamic acid. This category of constituents, based on a nine-carbon skeleton, is not as diverse as LMWT. All statements that follow here

TABLE 11-2

Types of Terpenoids

Terpenoid Class	Basic Structure	Number of Isoprene Units	Miscellaneous Notes
Monoterpenoid	$C_{10}H_{16}$	2	Usually volatile
Iridoid	$C_{10}H_{16}$ (bicyclic)	2	Subclass of monoterpenoids
Sesquiterpenoid	$C_{15}H_{24}$	3	Usually volatile
Sesquiterpene lactone	$C_{15}H_{24}$ (cyclic ketone)	3	Subclass of sesquiterpenoids
Diterpenoid	$C_{20}H_{32}$	4	Not usually volatile. Often in resins
Triterpenoid	$C_{30}H_{48}$	6	Nonvolatile
Tetraterpenoid (carotenoid)	$C_{40}H_{64}$	8	Nonvolatile
Polyterpenoids	$>C_{40}$	10+	Nonvolatile

Modified with permission from Yarnell E. *Phytochemistry and Pharmacy for Practitioners of Botanical Medicine.* Wenatchee, Wash: Healing Mountain Publishing; 2004.

BOX 11-7

Select Low-Molecular-Weight Terpenoid-Rich Herbs

Monoterpenoids and Sesquiterpenoids

- *Hyssopus vulgaris* (hyssop)
- *Juniperus communis* (juniper)
- *Lavandula officinalis* (lavender)
- *Melissa officinalis* (lemon balm)
- *Mentha x piperita* (peppermint)
- *Mentha crispa* (curly mint)
- *Mentha pulegium* (pennyroyal)
- *Mentha spicata* (spearmint)
- *Origanum* spp (marjoram, basil)
- *Orthosiphon stamineus* (Java tea)
- *Pinus* spp (pine)
- *Piper nigrum* (black pepper)
- *Rosmarinus officinalis* (rosemary)
- *Salvia apiana* (white sage)
- *Salvia officinalis* (sage)
- *Santalum albium* (sandalwood)*
- *Stachys betonica* (betony)
- *Thymus serpyllum* (wild thyme)
- *Thymus vulgaris* (thyme)
- *Zingiber officinale* (ginger)

Sesquiterpene Lactones

- *Achillea millefolium* (yarrow)
- *Arnica* spp (arnica)
- *Artemisia annua* (sweet Annie)
- *Artemisia absinthium* (wormwood)
- *Cichorium intybus* (chicory)
- *Ginkgo biloba* (ginkgo)
- *Inula helenium* (elecampane)
- *Lactuca serriola* (wild lettuce)
- *Marrubium vulgare* (horehound)
- *Tanacetum parthenium* (feverfew)

Iridoid Glycosides

- *Erythraea centaurium* (common centaury)
- *Gentiana lutea* (yellow gentian)
- *Harpagophytum procumbens* (devil's claw)
- *Menyanthes trifoliata* (bogbean)
- *Morinda citrifolia* (noni)
- *Picrorhiza kurroa* (picrorhiza)
- *Plantago lanceolata* (English plantain)
- *Swertia chirayita* (chiretta)
- *Verbena* spp (vervain)

*Threatened in the wild. Use only ethically cultivated sources.

about LMWT terpenoids apply equally to phenylpropanoids. However, phenylpropanoids are much less common than LMWT (Box 11-8).

LMWT represent the most diverse category of plant constituents, with more than 25,000 individual compounds identified so far. This structural diversity gives rise to chemical and therapeutic variety. Generalizations about their actions are not as useful as with some other categories of constituents.

The vast majority of LMWT and phenylpropanoids share many chemical properties. They are lipophilic with marginal water solubility. They generally have strong odors and flavors and, in fact, form the basis of the flavor and perfume industries. The family best known for its LMWT is the Lamiaceae or mints, with its strong aromas and tastes. LMWT are flammable. Many are optically active, and different isomers can have completely different properties. They are almost always colorless.

BOX 11-8

Select Phenylpropanoid-Rich Herbs

- *Acorus calamus* (sweet flag)
- *Alpinia galanga* (galangal)
- *Cinnamomum* spp (cinnamon, cassia)
- *Eleutherococcus senticosis* (eleuthero)
- *Foeniculum vulgare* (fennel)
- *Melissa officinalis* (lemon balm)
- *Nigella sativa* (black seed)
- *Ocimum basilicum* (basil)
- *Pimpinella anisum* (anise)
- *Rhodiola rosea* (rhodiola)
- *Sassafras albidum* (sassafras)
- *Syzygium aromaticum* (clove)

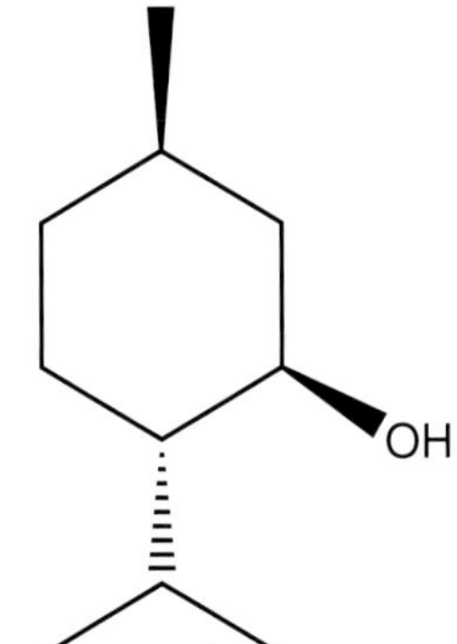

Figure 11-12 (–)-Menthol, a monoterpenoid.

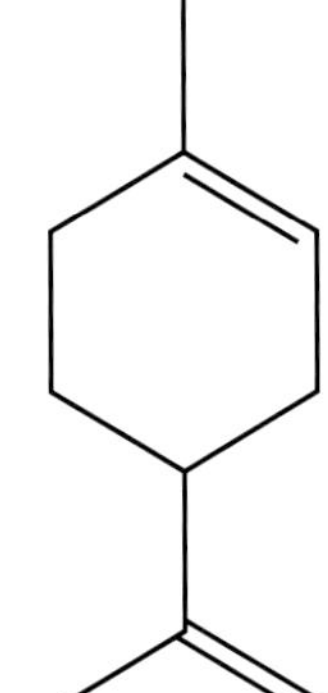

Figure 11-13 Limonene, a monoterpenoid.

The medicinal properties of LMWT are nearly as diverse as the molecules themselves. A small sampling will suffice to highlight this variability. D-Limonene solubilizes cholesterol from bile stones (Igimi, 1976) and has recently gained great acclaim as an antineoplastic and apoptosis stimulator, which it accomplishes through mechanisms that are not yet fully understood (Lu, 2004). Menthol is a calcium channel–blocking smooth muscle relaxant (Hawthorn, 1988). Linalool, cineole, geraniol,

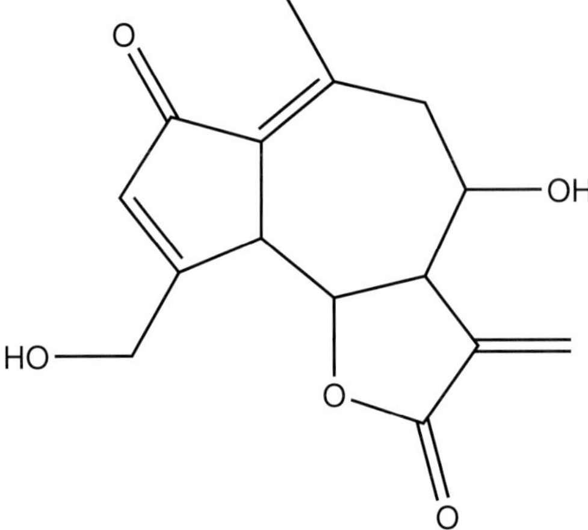

Figure 11-14 Lactucin, a sesquiterpene lactone.

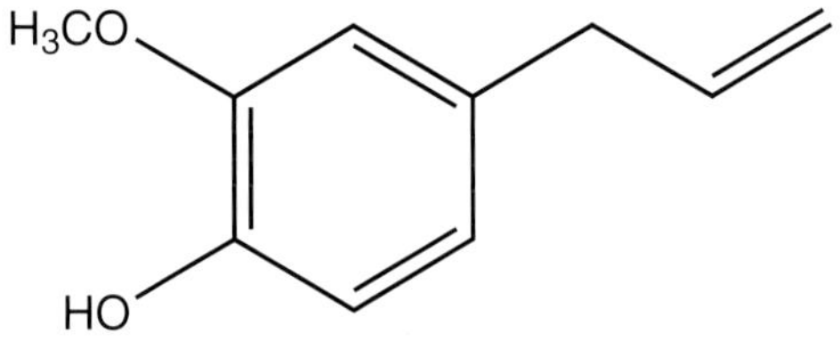

Figure 11-15 Eugenol, a phenylpropanoid.

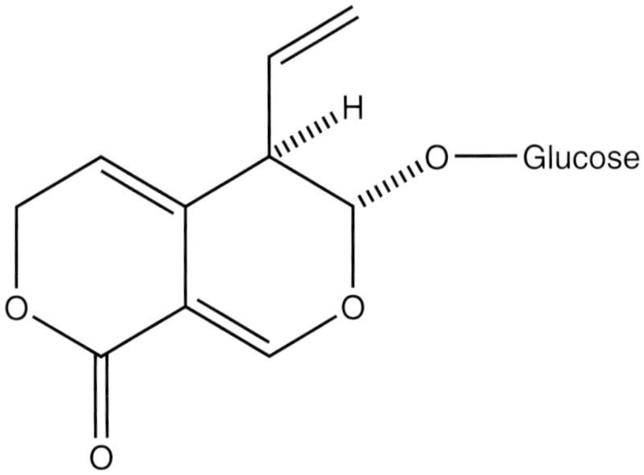

Figure 11-16 Gentiopicroside, an iridoid glycoside.

menthol, and citral were found to be antibacterial and antifungal to varying degrees (Pattnaik, 1997).

Iridoids are cyclic monoterpenoids that are almost uniformally bitter in taste. They often occur as glycosides. Their bitter flavor makes them general gastrointestinal stimulants. A quintessential example of a bitter iridoid glycoside–containing plant is *Gentiana lutea* (gentian) root. This can help remedy any number of conditions related to gastrointestinal atony, such as gastric ulcer, dyspepsia, and hypochlorhydria, but it may exacerbate conditions associated with gastrointestinal hyperactivity, such as duodenal ulcer, gastroesophageal reflux, and hyperchlorhydria. Iridoids can have other properties besides bitterness.

Sesquiterpene lactones are cyclic sesquiterpenoids that have a bitter flavor and activity, as iridoids do. A quin-

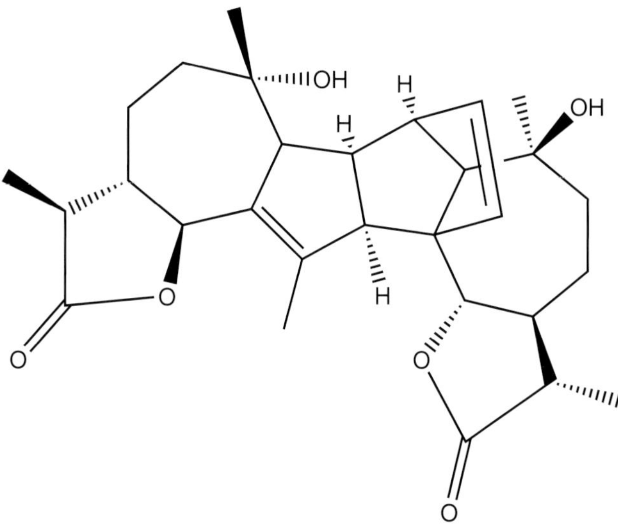

Figure 11-17 Absinthin, a sesquiterpene lactone.

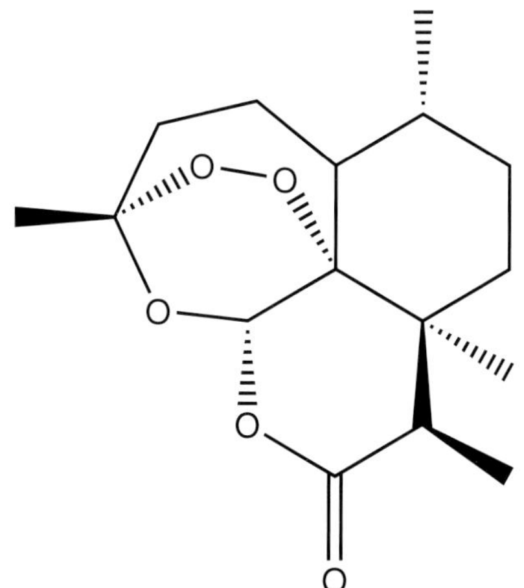

Figure 11-18 Artemisinin, a sesquiterpene lactone.

tessential example here is the compound absinthin found in *Artemisia absinthium* (wormwood). Sesquiterpene lactones can also have many other properties, and these have been widely investigated. Most important among these is the antineoplastic and antimalarial activity of artemisinin from *Artemisia annua* (sweet Annie) leaf (Beekman, 1998; Krungkrai, 1987). Sesquiterpene lactones in general can act as haptens and are responsible for the phenomenon in some animals of cross-sensitivity within the Apiaceae or Asteraceae family, as opposed to true allergies to multiple plants within these families.

The phenylpropanoids are as diverse in their effects as are LMWT. Eugenol has recently been shown to be a potent inhibitor of metastasis of melanoma cells and to strongly induce apoptosis in them, apparently through inhibition of a transcription factor dubbed E2F1 (Ghosh, 2005). It also inhibits adenosine triphosphate (ATP) production and may alter membrane permeability in many different pathogenic microbes, which helps to explain the antimicrobial activity of eugenol-rich herbs (Gill, 2004). Vanillin is a singlet oxygen-quenching antioxidant (Kamat, 2000).

LMWT and phenylpropanoids are well absorbed orally and transdermally. Evidence also suggests that they are absorbed via the olfactory nerve and transit directly to the brain after inhalation. After oral administration, the half-lives of those LMWT that have been studied, such as menthol, can be as long as 14 hours (Kaffenberger, 1990). This is not surprising, given their lipophilicity. LMWT and phenylpropanoids are excreted by the kidneys, as well as the lungs, making them particularly useful for conditions that affect those organs.

LMWT and phenylpropanoids occur in very small quantities in herbs (often <1%) and are not usually associated with any toxicity. The only problem with their use occurs when they are concentrated as volatile oils.

Volatile or essential oils are traditionally prepared from herbs by steam distillation or, in the case of *Citrus* spp (e.g., orange), by direct expression. Steam distillation was first developed by the Arabs approximately 1000 years ago; thus, volatile oils have been known for only that long. These oils are extremely concentrated mixtures of multiple LMWT and phenylpropanoids (depending on the herb in question). In the case of steam-distilled volatile oils, compounds are often chemically different from those found in the crude herb because of their exposure to heat. A classic example is the formation of chamazulene, a light blue sesquiterpenoid lactone not present in the crude herb, from matricin during steam distillation of *Matricaria recutita* (chamomile) flowers.

A newer type of volatile oil has also become available over the past few years; it is extracted with the use of supercritical carbon dioxide. Because no heat is needed in this process, the volatile oils produced are not the same as steam-distilled volatile oils, although they are the same as those oils obtained by expression. These extracts are certainly safer and superior to various volatile oils and related products (e.g., resinoids, concretes, absolutes) obtained by means of a variety of toxic organic solvents. Their relative activity compared with steam-distilled volatile oils is largely unknown because of a lack of comparative research and a very short clinical track record.

Volatile oils have the same properties as LMWT and phenylpropanoids because they are composed entirely of them. However, the concentration of these compounds is increased hundreds or thousands of times, greatly amplifying their potency and toxic potential compared to the crude plant material. All volatile oils must be treated as potentially lethal and administered only in low doses. They are readily absorbed through the skin and after ingestion. Depending on the individual and the concentration applied, they can cause cutaneous inflammation and sensitization. Partially for this reason and because of expense, volatile oils are almost always diluted at least 50% with fixed oils (fatty acids) before application.

DITERPENOIDS

Diterpenoids are 20 carbon terpenoids composed of 4 isoprene units. Although they are widely distributed and

BOX 11-9

Select Diterpenoid-Rich Herbs

- *Coffea arabica* (coffee)
- *Montanoa tomentosa* (zoapatle)
- *Plectranthus barbatus* (forskohlii, coleus)
- *Taxus brevifolia* (Pacific yew)
- *Teucrium chamaedrys* (germander)*
- *Vitex agnus castus* (chaste tree)

*Contains potentially hepatotoxic neoclerodane diterpenoids.

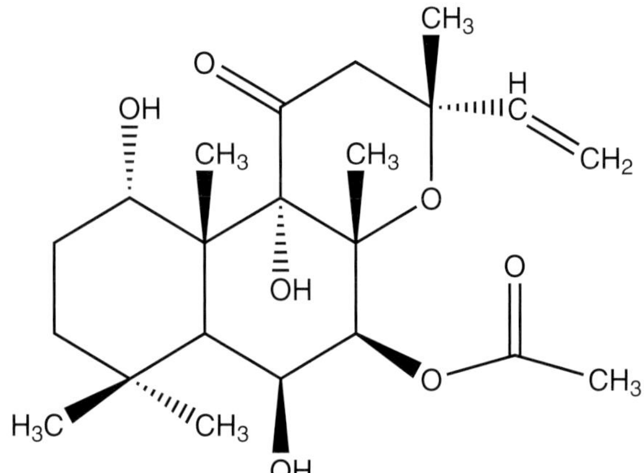

Figure 11-19 Forskolin, a diterpenoid.

clearly biologically active, much less is known about diterpenoids as a class. The discovery of paclitaxel, a taxane diterpenoid from *Taxus brevifolia* (Pacific yew), has sparked renewed interest in this family of compounds.

Diterpenoids are of sufficiently high molecular weight compared with LMWT that they are not volatile; thus, they are odorless. They are very lipophilic and tend to have strong flavors. They are typically found in resins in plants, as is discussed later. They do not tend to occur as glycosides. Little is known of their pharmacokinetics, although presumably, they are well absorbed orally, given their lipophilicity.

Diterpenoids show a wide range of activity, as do LMWT. (Box 11-9) Paclitaxel promotes tubulin assembly into stable microtubules, which tends to cause death in cancer cells (Schiff, 1979). Many other diterpenoids have been shown to have antineoplastic activity, and a few isolated examples, like iridoids or sesquiterpene lactones, have bitter properties (Sticher, 1977). Too little is known of the pharmacokinetics and toxicology of these compounds for general statements to be made about them.

RESINS

Resins are complex, lipid-soluble mixtures of various compounds. Usually, a resin is made up of a diterpenoid- and triterpenoid-containing nonvolatile fraction, as well as a volatile fraction. In the more common terpenoid resins, monoterpenoids and sesquiterpenoids predominate in the volatile fraction. Oleoresins are resins that contain a particularly high terpenoid volatile fraction, making them particularly fluid. In the less common phenolic resins, hydrophobic flavonoids and phenylpropanoids predominate. Resins are usually secreted by specialized structures in woody angiosperms. All resins are sticky and harden when exposed to the air. They produce fragrant smoke when burned and thus are commonly used as incense (frankincense and myrrh are resins used for this purpose). Amber is fossilized resin. Balsams are highly fragrant resins that tend to stay relatively soft at room temperature.

Gums and mucilages are not resins but instead are thick, sticky mixtures of polysaccharides. Sometimes, gums and resins intermix to form gum resins, but these are formed separately and are chemically distinct. Latex is also not a resin but is instead an even more complex chemical mixture produced by distinct secretory tissues within the plant that are separate from resins.

It is not surprising that given their diverse chemical makeup, the medicinal actions of resins vary enormously. Generally speaking, most resins are antimicrobial and wound healing in animals and in the plants that secrete them. This has been shown, for example, with balsam of Peru, the resin of *Myroxylon balsamum* var. *perierae* (Carson, 2003; Ondrovcik, 1995). Balsam of Peru also speeds healing of radiation burns when applied topically (Nikulin, 1980). Topical application of pine resin to wounds and burns has been shown to stimulate local immune function, normalize wound hemodynamics, and stimulate squamous epithelialization (Khmel'nitskii, 2002). Beyond this, resins from different plants can have a wide array of effects. For example, frankincense, the gum resin of *Boswellia serrata,* is well documented as an inflammation modulator that is helpful in asthma and ulcerative colitis; this is attributed at least in part to its inhibition of 5-lipoxygenase (Gupta, 1997; Gupta, 1998). The gum resin of *Commiphora molmol* (myrrh) is antiparasitic, analgesic, and antineoplastic (Massoud, 2001; Dolara, 1996; Qureshi, 1993). Resins also find widespread use outside of medicine as varnishes, lacquers, waterproofing agents, adhesives, and precursor materials for industrial chemical production.

Resins are generally safe (Box 11-10). Contact allergy to balsams is relatively common. In one series, roughly 1 in 100 human patients patch-tested positive to tincture of benzoin, with 1 in 400 having an intense reaction (Scardamaglia, 2003). More problematic are the resins of the Anarcardiaceae family, such as the all-too-familiar *Toxicodendron radicans* (poison ivy), which can cause severe type 4 hypersensitivity reactions in susceptible animals.

TRITERPENOID AND STEROIDAL SAPONINS

Triterpenoids or triterpenoid saponins are pentacyclic molecules that are ultimately synthesized from isoprene. Steroidal saponins are tetracyclic molecules that are ultimately synthesized from acetyl coenzyme A (CoA).

BOX 11-10

Select Resin-Rich Herbs

- *Abies* spp (fir)
- *Boswellia serrata* (frankincense)
- *Bursera microphylla* (elephant tree)
- *Cannabis sativa* (marijuana)
- *Commiphora molmol* (myrrh)
- *Commiphora mukul* (guggul)
- *Dryopteris fillix-mas* (male fern)
- *Grindelia* spp (gumweed)
- *Larrea tridentata* (chaparral)
- *Pinus* spp (pine)
- *Pistachia lentiscus* (mastic)
- *Zingiber officinale* (ginger)

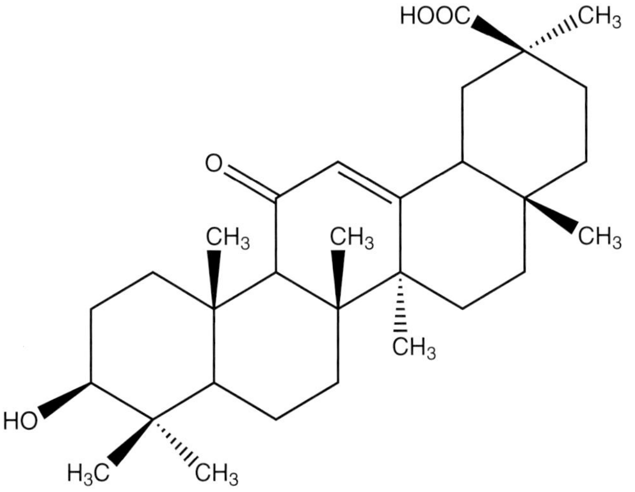

Figure 11-20 Glycyrrhetinic acid, a triterpenoid.

Although they are structurally distinct, molecules of both types have most properties in common. The only other major differences between these two groups of constituents is that triterpenoids tend to be acidic in pH and occur more commonly in dicots than in monocots, and steroidal saponins tend to be neutral in pH and occur more commonly in monocots than in dicots.

Triterpenoids and steroidal saponins are inherently lipophilic. However, these molecules tend to occur as glycosides. Because of the large size of the saponin molecules, what results is that one end of the molecule (where the glycone is attached) is hydrophilic and the other end (the head of the aglycone) is hydrophobic. As a result of this, saponins act as emulsifying agents and detergents. When placed in water and shaken, they form foamy colloids and allow lipophilic and hydrophilic molecules to mix. Saponins can act as mild soaps by removing dirt particles, which gives them a soapy or acrid flavor. This property also seems to improve the absorption of certain botanical constituents (including other saponins) from

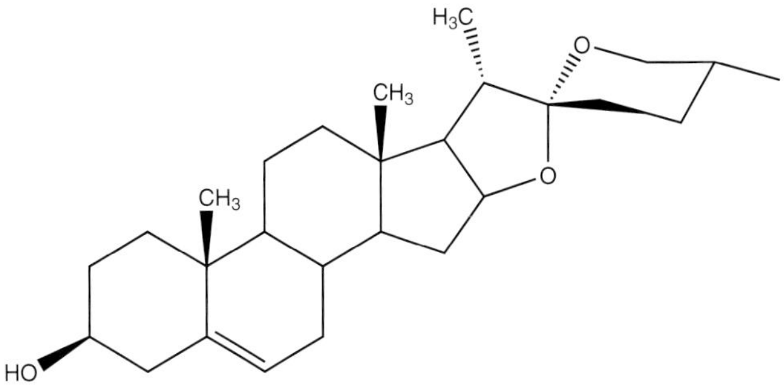

Figure 11-21 Diosgenin, a saponin.

the gut, when they are ingested simultaneously with saponins. The best published research on this effect confirms the traditional Chinese medical approach of frequently including saponin-rich plants in formulations, such as *Panax ginseng* (Asian ginseng) root (Watanabe, 1988; Yata, 1988).

Saponins can cause gastrointestinal distress through an unknown mechanism. Taking them with food tends to eliminate the problem. This same effect is theorized to be responsible for the reflex expectorant effect of saponins. When saponin-rich herbs, such as *Hedera helix* (ivy), are consumed orally, they tend to cause an increase in the production of mucus in the lungs, as well as coughing (Shin, 2002). This effect can be helpful for patients with coughs of all sorts, but particularly for those with dry cough. The reflex effect is believed to be neurologically mediated, but this has not been rigorously proved, and it is possible that saponins act directly within the lungs to provoke this effect.

Saponins, particularly those steroidal saponin-like molecules referred to as phytosterols, decrease cholesterol absorption from the gut, increase cholesterol excretion, and inhibit hepatic synthesis of cholesterol (de Jong, 2003). All saponins tend to be immune modulating and have consistently shown antineoplastic effects (Singh, 1984; Bouic, 1999; Awad, 2000). A wide range of other effects beyond these general properties of the group have been demonstrated with various specific saponins. A small sampling of this diversity can be seen with the saponins of *Glycyrrhiza* spp (licorice) root, particularly glycyrrhizin and its aglycone glycyrrhetinic acid. These molecules are anti-inflammatory and antiviral, inhibit cortisol catabolism, and have many other effects (Davis, 1991).

Saponin glycosides can cause hemolysis of red blood cells (Box 11-11). This primarily occurs when most saponins are injected intravenously or when they are hyperabsorbed from an abnormal gut. Some saponins have been successfully injected. Normally, saponins are not well absorbed orally, and the slow rate at which they are absorbed is more than sufficient to allow the body to adapt to them. This hemolytic effect does not appear to be related to the detergent properties of saponins but instead seems to be due to increasing cell membrane permeability. Overall, oral saponins appear to be extremely safe.

BOX 11-11

Select Triterpenoid and Saponin-Rich Herbs

Triterpenoid Glycosides
- *Actaea racemosa* (black cohosh)
- *Azadirachta indica* (neem)
- *Centella asiatica* (gotu kola)
- *Ganoderma lucidum* (reishi)
- *Glycyrrhiza glabra* (licorice)
- *Glycyrrhiza uralensis* (gan cao)
- *Panax ginseng* (Asian ginseng)
- *Panax quinquefolium* (American ginseng)
- *Zizyphus jujuba* (jujube)

Saponin Glycosides/Phytosterols
- *Aesculus hippocastanum* (horse chestnut)
- *Asparagus racemosa* (shatavari)
- *Commiphora mukul* (guggul)
- *Dioscorea villosa* (wild yam)
- *Hedera helix* (ivy)
- *Ononis spinosa* (spiny restharrow)
- *Ruscus aculeatus* (butcher's broom)
- *Smilax officinalis* (sarsparilla)
- *Withania somniferum* (ashwagandha)
- *Yucca* spp (yucca)

ALKALOIDS

These compounds are heterocyclic, contain nitrogen, generally have potent activity, and are of limited distribution in nature. Pseudoalkaloids are terpenoids that contain nitrogen or are derived from acetate, such as coniine. Protoalkaloids contain an amine structure but not within a heterocyclic ring, such as ephedrine. The chemical and biological properties of pseudoalkaloids and protoalkaloids are sufficiently similar to those of heterocyclic alkaloid that they are included in this category.

Alkaloids are synthesized from amino acids (Box 11-12). This is the basis of the biosynthetic and structural groupings of alkaloids commonly referred to in the literature. Certain alkaloid groups tend to be confined to certain plant families. Therapeutic differences may be extensive within a class of alkaloids, so these categories do not necessarily provide a good clinical basis for an understanding of these molecules.

Precursors	Alkaloids Included
Ornithine, putrescine, proline	Pyrrole, pyrrolizidine, tropane
Lysine	Pyridine, norlupinane
Tyrosine, phenylalanine	Protoalkaloids, isoquinoline
Tryptophan, tryptamine	Quinoline, indole
Histidine, threonine	Imidazole
Adenine, purine, xanthine, hypoxanthine	Purine
Acetate or mevalonic acid	Steroidal and terpenoid pseudoalkaloids

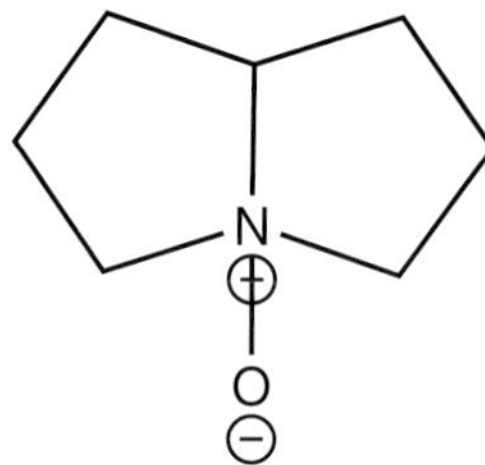

Figure 11-22 Pyrrolizidine skeleton N-oxide.

The nitrogen in alkaloids generally acts as a weak base, although this varies according to other functional groups and the exact configuration of the alkaloids. Primary, secondary, and tertiary amines (the nitrogen connected to one, two, or three carbons, respectively), as well as saturated, heterocyclic amines, are the most basic alkaloids. Aromatic and aniline heterocyclic amines are slightly basic. Amides and quaternary amines are neutral, and phenolics are actually acidic.

Alkaloids, particularly amines and other basic alkaloids, are usually found as salts in plants. They remain in salt form when placed in an acidic solution, and any free alkaloid generally becomes salt. This is critical because the salt forms are water soluble and the free alkaloids generally are not. For example, free quinine is 0.1% water soluble, and quinine hydrochloride is 99% water soluble. Acidic and neutral free alkaloids, such as caffeine, tend to be hydrophilic and may not form salts.

Alkaloids are variably bioavailable. They tend to be oxidized by the cytochrome P450 system to form *N*-oxide compounds, which are water soluble and nontoxic (Bickel, 1969; Mattocks, 1971). The *N*-oxides can be reduced in the body to their parent alkaloids and may cause problems or bring benefits (Mattocks, 1972). Alkaloids are irreversibly bound and are precipitated by tannins, making them almost totally unabsorbable. The two should generally be kept separate to avoid this interaction, although tannins can also serve as a useful immediate treatment for acute alkaloid overdose.

Alkaloids generally have a strong bitter taste. They tend to act as digestive stimulants, as was previously discussed with sesquiterpene lactones and iridoid glycosides. Otherwise, they have extremely diverse clinical properties. Several examples are given here to illustrate this diversity. The only rule that is generally true and inherent to the definition of these compounds is that they tend to be potent, meaning that small doses are all that are necessary to produce significant effects.

Atropine [a racemic mixture of (–)- and (+)-hyoscyamine] and scopolamine are tropane alkaloids found in *Atropa belladonna* (belladonna), *Datura* spp (thornapple), and *Hyoscyamus niger* (henbane). These alkaloids are muscarinic receptor antagonists that give these herbs strong anticholinergic activity. They are used to treat smooth muscle spasm, hypersecretion, and pain.

Pyrrolizidine alkaloids (PA) have no clear therapeutic benefit (although at least one, indicine *N*-oxide, is being studied as an anticancer agent [Powis, 1979]) but are important for their potential toxicity. Actually, only unsa-

BOX 11-12

Select Alkaloid-Rich Plants

Aporphine Alkaloids
- *Peumus boldus* (boldo)

Indole Alkaloids
- *Banisteriopsis* spp (ayahuasca)
- *Catharanthus roseus* (Madagascar periwinkle)
- *Claviceps purpurea* (rye ergot)
- *Gelsemium sempervirens* (gelsemium)
- *Pausinystalia yohimbe* (yohimbe)
- *Physostigma venenosum* (ordeal bean)
- *Psilocybe* spp
- *Rauvolfia serpentina* (Indian snakeroot)
- *Strychnos nux vomica* (nux vomica)
- *Tabernanthe iboga* (iboga)

Isoquinoline Alkaloids
- *Berberis* spp (barberry)
- *Cephaelis ipecacuanha* (ipecac)
- *Chelidonium majus* (greater celandine)
- *Coptis* spp (goldthread)
- *Corydalis yanhusuo* (yan hu suo)
- *Eschscholzia californica* (California poppy)
- *Fumaria officinalis* (fumitory)
- *Hydrastis canadensis* (goldenseal)
- *Jateorhiza palmata* (calumba)
- *Mahonia aquifolium* (Oregon grape)
- *Papaver somniferum* (opium)
- *Sanguinaria canadensis* (bloodroot)
- *Xanthorrhiza simplicissima* (yellow root)
- *Zanthoxylum clava-herculis* (prickly ash)

Norlupinane Alkaloids
- Sarothamnus scoparius (Scotch broom)

Protoalkaloids
- *Colchicum autumnale* (autumn crocus)
- *Catha edulis* (khat)
- *Ephedra sinica* (ma huang)
- *Lophophora williamsii* (peyote)

Purine Alkaloids (methylxanthines)
- *Camellia sinensis* (tea) folia
- *Coffea arabica* (coffee) semen
- *Cola nitida* (kola) semen
- *Paullinia cupana* (guaraná) semen
- *Ilex paraguayensis* (maté) folia
- *Theobroma cacao* (chocolate) semen

Pseudoalkaloids
- *Cicuta virosa* (water hemlock)
- *Conium maculatum* (hemlock)

Pyridine Alkaloids
- *Lobelia inflata* (lobelia)
- *Nicotiana tabacum* (tobacco)
- *Piper longum* (long pepper)
- *Piper nigrum* (black pepper)
- *Trigonella foenum-graecum* (fenugreek)

Quinoline Alkaloids
- *Cinchona* spp (Peruvian bark)
- *Galipea officinalis* (Angostura)

Tropane Alkaloids
- *Atropa belladonna* (deadly nightshade)
- *Datura stramonium* (Jimson weed, thornapple)
- *Erythroxylum coca* (Bolivian coca)
- *Hyoscyamus niger* (henbane)
- *Mandragora officinarum* (mandrake)

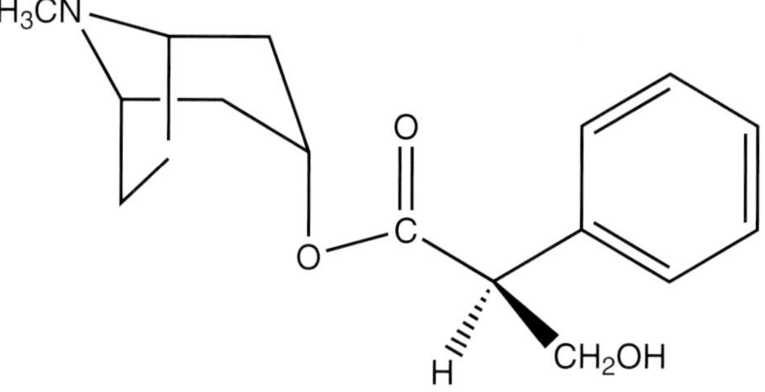

Figure 11-23 (–)-Hyoscyamine, a tropane alkaloid.

tured PA are toxic, and only those structures that are converted, in this case, to more toxic *N*-oxide forms by hepatic cytochrome P450 enzymes (Röder, 1995). Thus, although most members of the Asteraceae and Boraginaceae families (and a few other scattered members of various other families) contain PA, only a small number definitely contain the unsaturated type that may cause concern (Smith, 1981). Because these alkaloids do not cause widespread hepatic necrosis (except when extraordinary doses are ingested), monitoring of serum liver enzymes is not an effective screening test (Allen, 1979). It should also be noted that because unsaturated PA readily induce fibrosis, the damage that they cause is cumulative.

Different animal species show wide variation in susceptibility to induction of cirrhosis, hepatic veno-occlusive disease, and cancer because of unsaturated PA ingestion (Box 11-13) (Cheeke, 1998). Even though horses and cows are said to be highly susceptible, *Symphytum officinale* (comfrey) leaf has been safely and effectively used as fodder for these animals in large quantities, possibly because of low unsaturated PA levels in the feed (Hills, 1976). Differences in susceptibility may result from differences in gut flora, differences in hepatic conversion, differences in hepatic glutathione production, and differences in doses ingested (Huan, 1998). If unsaturated PA-containing herbs are to be used medicinally or as food, it is recommended that alkaline aqueous, glycerin, or dilute ethanol (<30%) extracts be prepared from aerial

BOX 11-13

Unsaturated Pyrrolizidine Alkaloid–Containing Medicinal Herbs

Asteraceae
- *Eupatorium perfoliatum* (boneset), *E. purpureum* (Joe Pye weed)
- *Petasites frigidus* (butterbur)
- *Psacalium decompositum* (matarique)
- *Senecio* spp (ragworts)
- *Tussilago farfara* (coltsfoot)

Boraginaceae
- *Borago officinalis* (borage)
- *Cynoglossum officinale* (hound's tongue)
- *Lithospermum ruderale* (gromwell)
- *Symphytum officinale* (comfrey)

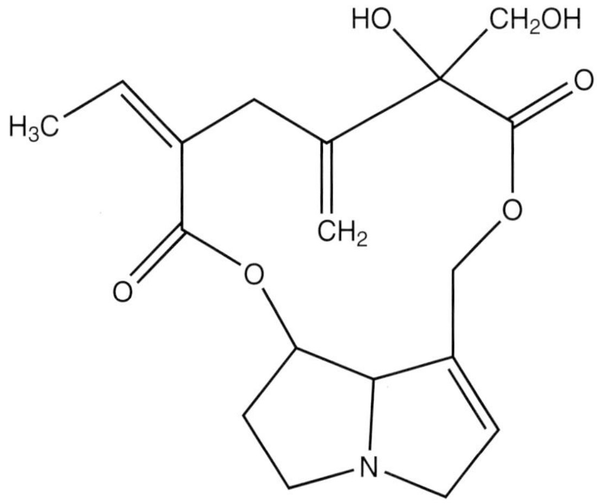

HO CH₂OH O H₃C O CH₂ O O N

Figure 11-24 Riddelliine, an unsaturated pyrrolizidine alkaloid.

OH O O N OH

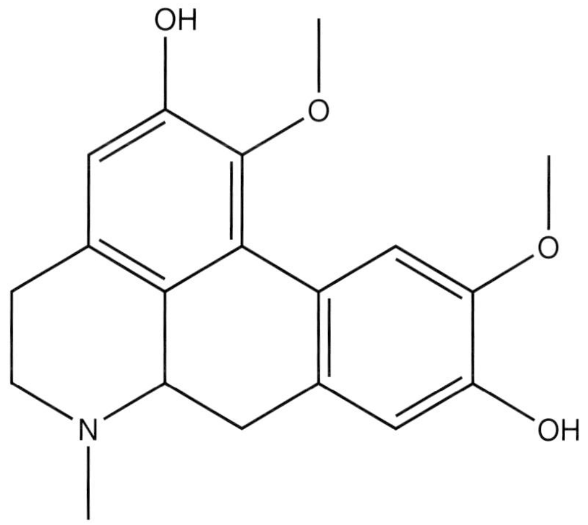

Figure 11-25 Boldine, an aporphine alkaloid.

parts. This method generally reduces the amount of PA extracted. Also, many supplement companies now provide extracts that are made from strains bred to contain low PA levels, or that have documented low PA levels caused by extraction methods.

Berberine, berbamine, hydrastine, and sanguinarine are isoquinoline alkaloids found in various combinations in several species, including but not limited to *Mahonia aquifolium* (Oregon grape), *Berberis vulgaris* (barberry), *Hydrastis canadensis* (goldenseal), *Coptis* spp (goldthread), *Xanthorrhiza simplicissimia* (yellow root), and *Sanguinaria canadensis* (bloodroot). These alkaloids have been shown in various study systems and clinical trials to have actions including inhibiting oxidation, indirect inhibition of phospholipase A2, killing bacteria and inhibiting their adhesion to cell surfaces, stimulation of bone marrow leukocyte production inhibition of arrhythmias, strengthening of myocardial contractility, inhibition of blood vessel formation by cancer cells, and apoptosis induction in cancer cells (Akiba, 1995; Cernakova, 2002; Eun, 2004; Ju, 1990; Kuo, 1995; Li, 1994; Sun, 1988; Zeng, 2003). It is important to note that complex, crude extracts of plants containing these alkaloids frequently show activity that is as good as or better than that seen in the alkaloids in isolation (Mahady, 2003).

Alkaloids and herbs that contain significant amounts of them should generally be treated as potentially toxic. This is not always the case, but many alkaloids are extremely potent and overdose is a possibility. No generic reaction to alkaloid overdose can be anticipated—the exact effects depend entirely on the properties of the specific alkaloid in the body.

LIGNANS AND LIGNINS

Lignans are composed of two phenylpropanoid units joined together to form an 18-carbon skeleton. Many other functional groups can then be added by the plant to modify this base structure. Generally, these molecules are lipophilic and function within plant cell membranes to provide rigidity, strength, and water impermeability. Most lignans are relatively safe. Few generalizations can be made about this class of compounds beyond these statements, in part because of the lack of research. As interest in lignans grows, more information will surely become available.

Several lignans have demonstrated intriguing and important clinical activity. Podophyllotoxin from *Podophyllum peltatum* (mayapple) acts as a cathartic laxative that is distinct from the anthraquinone glycosides; it inhibits human papillomavirus (HPV) and is antineoplastic (Kelly, 1954). The semisynthetic chemotherapy drugs teniposide and etoposide are derived directly from this molecule.

The lignans in *Linum usitatissimum* (flax), such as secoisolariciresinol, are transformed by the gut flora to enterodiol and enterolactone, known phytoestrogenic constituents that clearly are active in vivo (Haggans, 1999). Flax seeds have definite anticancer effects, as has been documented in the results of clinical trials (Thompson, 2000). Flaxseed oil (which is low in lignans) has not shown these same benefits as consistently; this supports

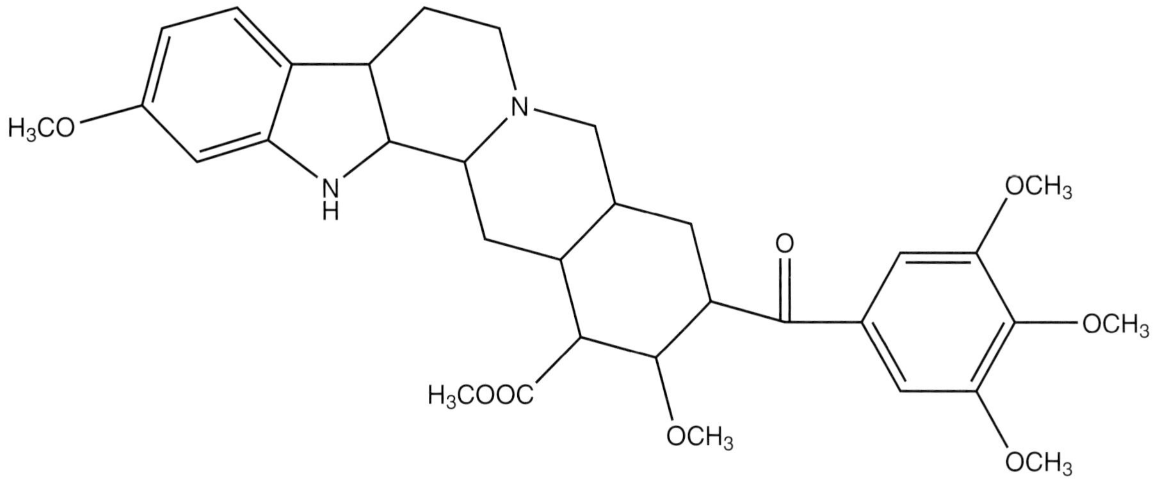

Figure 11-26 Reserpine, an indole alkaloid.

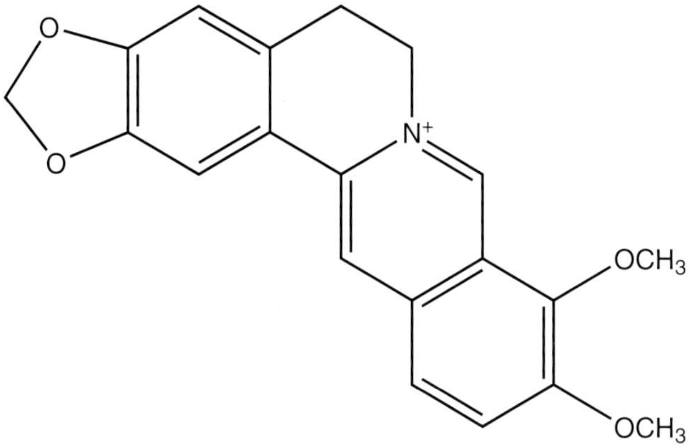

Figure 11-27 Berberine, an isoquinoline alkaloid.

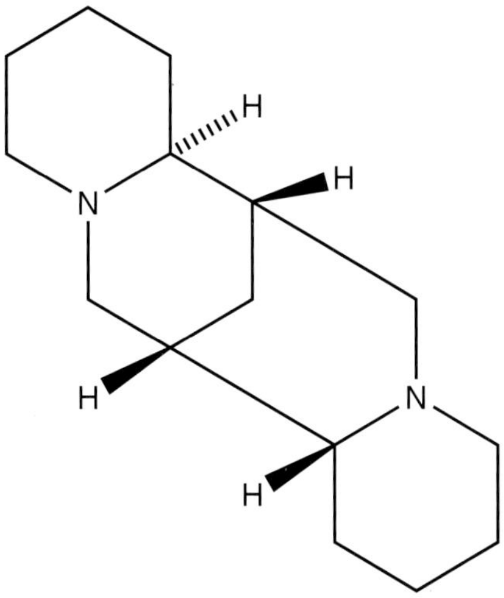

Figure 11-28 Sparteine, a norlupinane alkaloid.

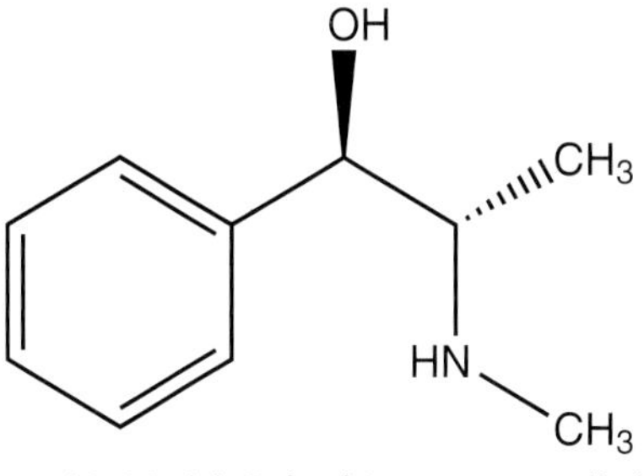

Figure 11-29 (–)-Ephedrine, a protoalkaloid.

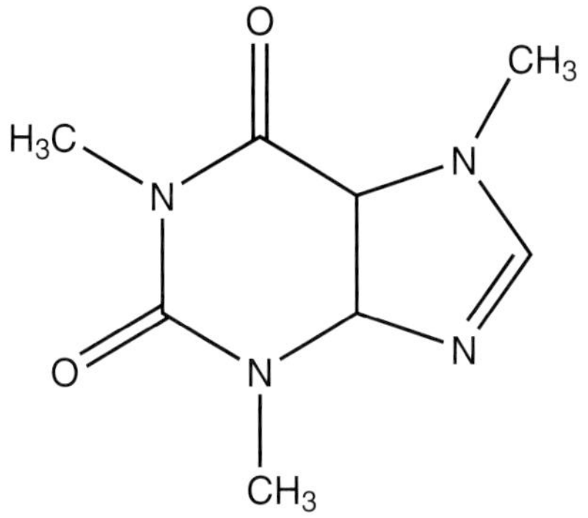

Figure 11-30 Caffeine, a purine alkaloid.

the contention that the lignans are critical to these effects when flax seeds are consumed.

Lignins are larger phenylpropanoid polymers that are a component of dietary fiber and thus may provide some benefits in this form, as was discussed earlier under polysaccharides. Otherwise, they are considered relatively unimportant as botanical constituents (Box 11-14).

LIPIDS AND WAXES

This category is touched on only partially here because lipids are primary constituents that are most often discussed in terms of their nutritional effects. Fatty acids, contained in fixed oils, are important therapeutic elements in many plants, particularly in their seeds. Omega-3 and -6 essential fatty acids from numerous species, including flax and *Oenothera biennis* (evening primrose), have been repeatedly shown to be inflammation- and

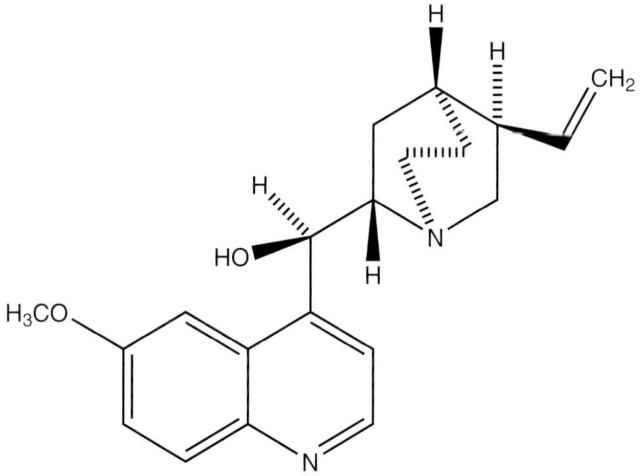

Figure 11-31 Quinine, a quinoline alkaloid.

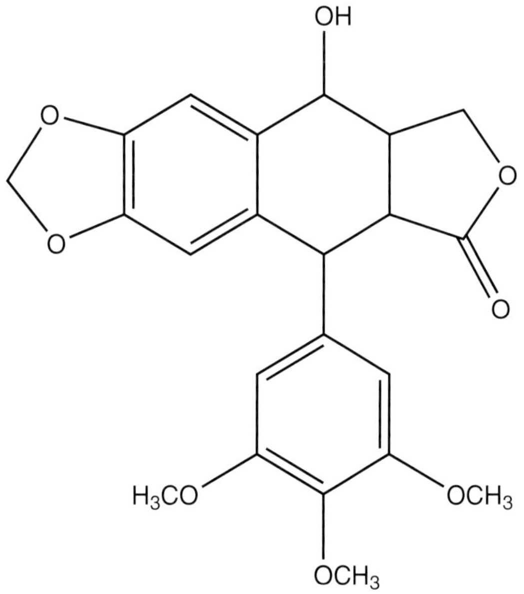

Figure 11-32 Podophyllotoxin, a lignan.

BOX 11-14

Select Lignan-Rich Herbs

- *Linum usitatissimum* (flax)
- *Podophyllum peltatum* (mayapple)
- *Schisandra chinensis* (schisandra, wu wei zi)

TABLE 11-3

Summary of Solubility

Constituent Class	General Solubility
Polysaccharides	Water*
Glycosides	Water (most aglycones are lipophilic)
Flavonoids	Variable
Proanthocyanidins	Water
Tannins	Water (especially hot)
Low-Molecular-Weight Terpenoids	Lipid†
Phenylpropanoids	Lipid
Volatile Oils	Lipid
Diterpenoids	Lipid
Resins	Lipid
Triterpenoids and Steroidal Saponins	Water and lipid (detergent)
Alkaloids	Lipid‡
Alkaloid Salts	Water
Lignans	Lipid
Lipids and Waxes	Lipid

*Water-soluble constituents will generally extract into water, glycerin, and <30% ethanol.
†Lipid-soluble constituents will generally extract into nonglycerin organic solvents, lipids, and 60% to 90% ethanol.
‡Extract in acidic solvent, typically with addition of a weak acid such as vinegar, converts alkaloids to their salt form or keeps them in that form.

immune-modulating agents (Horrobin, 1990; Kelley, 1992). The fatty acids from *Ricinus communis* (castor) seeds act as cathartic laxatives when taken internally but have intriguing inflammation- and immune-modulating properties and act to stimulate labor when applied topically to the skin or cervical os, respectively (Grady, 1997; Davis, 1984). Such effects generally require higher doses of the oil and thus are of little relevance in many crude plant extracts (particularly aqueous ones) that are used predominantly in modern botanical medicine.

Waxes are similar to fatty acids but have longer backbones than glycerin; in addition, the esterified hydrocarbon chains are generally much longer. These are mostly solid at room temperature, although a few, such as wax from *Simmondsia chinensis* (jojoba) seeds—a misnomer because it is native to the southwestern United States and northern Mexico—are liquid. These highly lipophilic compounds prevent water loss from leaf and other plant tissues. Although they generally have no known therapeutic effects, they do serve an important role in the manufacture of ointments for topical delivery of other lipophilic plant constituents, as well as for other commercial and industrial purposes (Table 11-3).

Useful Internet Resources

Lisa Ganora's Herbalchem
http://www.herbalchem.net
Dr. James Duke's Phytochemical and Ethnobotanical Databases
http://www.ars-grin.gov/duke/
American Society of Pharmacognosy Links
http://www.phcog.org/links.html
Ethnomedicinals.com Pharmacognosy Links
http://ethnomedicinals.com/pharmacognosy.htm

References

Agarwal SK, Singh SS, Verma S, Kumar S. Antifungal activity of anthraquinone derivatives from *Rheum emodi*. J Ethnopharmacol 2000;72:43-46.

Akiba S, Nagatomo R, Ishimoto T, Sato T. Effect of berbamine on cytosolic phospholipase A2 activation in rabbit platelets. Eur J Pharmacol 1995;291:343-350.

Alabaster O, Tang ZC, Frost A, Shivapurkar N. Potential synergism between wheat bran and psyllium: enhanced inhibition of colon cancer. Cancer Lett 1993;75:53-58.

Allen JR, Robertson KA, Johnson WD, Carstens LA. Toxicological effects of monocrotaline and its metabolites. In: Cheeke PR, ed. *Symposium on Pyrrolizidine (Senecio) Alkaloids: Toxicity, Metabolism, and Poisonous Plant Control Measures*. Proceedings of a Symposium Held at Oregon State University, February 23-24, 1979:37-42.

Awad AB, Fink CS. Phytosterols as anticancer dietary components: evidence and mechanism of action. J Nutr 2000;130:2127-2130.

Beekman AC, Wierenga PK, Woerdenbag HJ, et al. Artemisinin-derived sesquiterpene lactones as potential antitumour compounds: cytotoxic action against bone marrow and tumour cells. Planta Med 1998;64:615-619.

Bickel MH. The pharmacology and biochemistry of N-oxides. Pharmacol Rev 1969;21:325-355.

Bickhoff EM, Livingston AL, Hendrickson AP, Booth AN. Relative potencies of several estrogen-like compounds found in forages. J Agric Food Chem 1962;10:410-412.

Bors W, Michel C, Schikora S. Interaction of flavonoids with ascorbate and determination of their univalent redox potentials: a pulse radiolysis study. Free Radic Biol Med 1995;19:45-52.

Bouic PJD, Clark A, Lamprecht J, et al. The effects of β-sitosterol (BSS) and β-sitosterol glucoside (BSSG) mixture on selected immune parameters of marathon runners: inhibition of post marathon immune suppression and inflammation. Int J Sports Med 1999;20:258-262.

Bradlow HL, Sepkovic DW, Telang NT, Osborne MP. Indole-3-carbinol: a novel approach to breast cancer prevention. Ann NY Acad Sci 1995;768:180-200.

Brinckmann J, Sigwart H, van Houten Taylor L. Safety and efficacy of a traditional herbal medicine (Throat Coat) in symptomatic temporary relief of pain in patients with acute pharyngitis: a multicenter, prospective, randomized, double-blinded, placebo-controlled study. J Altern Complement Med 2003;9:285-298.

Brown DD, Juhl RP, Warner SL. Decreased bioavailability of digoxin due to hypocholesterolemic interventions. Circulation 1978;58:164-172.

Carson SN, Wiggins C, Overall K, Herbert J. Using a castor oil-balsam of Peru-trypsin ointment to assist in healing skin graft donor sites. Ostomy Wound Manage 2003;49:60-64.

Casley-Smith JR, Foldi-Borcsok E, Foldi M. A fine structural demonstration that some benzopyrones act as vitamin P in the rat. Am J Clin Nutr 1975;28:1242-1254.

Cernakova M, Kostalova D. Antimicrobial activity of berberine—a constituent of *Mahonia aquifolium*. Folia Microbiol 2002;47:375-378.

Cheeke PR. *Natural Toxicants in Feeds, Forage, and Poisonous Plants*. Danville, Ill: Interstate; 1998.

Chen J, Lin H, Hu M. Metabolism of flavonoids via enteric recycling: role of intestinal disposition. J Pharmacol Exp Ther 2003;304:1228-1235.

Chung EK. *Digitalis Intoxication*. Baltimore: Williams & Wilkins Co; 1969.

Davis EA, Morris DJ. Medicinal uses of licorice through the millennia: the good and plenty of it. Molec Cell Endocrinol 1991;78:1-6.

Davis L. The use of castor oil to stimulate labor in patients with premature rupture of the membranes. J Nurse Midwifery 1984;9:366-370.

de Jong A, Plat J, Mensink RP. Metabolic effects of plant sterols and stanols (Review). J Nutr Biochem 2003;14(7):362-369.

Delzenne N. The hypolipidaemic effect of insulin: when animal studies help to approach the human problem. Br J Nutr 1999;82:3-4.

Delzenne N, Kok N. Effect of non-digestible fermentable carbohydrates on hepatic fatty acid metabolism. Biochem Soc Trans 1998;26:1997-1999.

Dolara P, Luceri C, Ghelardini C, et al. Analgesic effects of myrrh. Nature 1996;379:29.

Eun JP, Koh GY. Suppression of angiogenesis by the plant alkaloid, sanguinarine. Biochem Biophys Res Commun 2004;317:618-624.

Frank T, Janssen M, Netzel M, et al. Pharmacokinetics of anthocyanidin-3-glycosides following consumption of *Hibiscus sabdariffa* L. extract. J Clin Pharmacol 2005;45:203-210.

Fukuda T, Ito H, Mukainaka T, et al. Anti-tumor promoting effect of glycosides from *Prunus persica* seeds. Biol Pharm Bull 2003;26:271-273.

Ghosh R, Nadiminty N, Fitzpatrick JE, et al. Eugenol causes melanoma growth suppression through inhibition of E2F1 transcriptional activity. J Biol Chem, January 18, 2005. [Epub ahead of print]

Gill AO, Holley RA. Mechanisms of bactericidal action of cinnamaldehyde against *Listeria monocytogenes* and of eugenol against *L. monocytogenes* and *Lactobacillus sakei*. Appl Environ Microbiol 2004;70:5750-5755.

Goppel M, Franz G. Stability control of senna leaves and senna extracts. Planta Med 2004;70:432-436.

Grady H. Immunomodulation through castor oil packs. J Nat Med 1997;7:84-89.

Guo CY, Zhao SY, Lin CR. [Effects of rhubarb on arachidonic acid metabolism of the renal medulla in the rabbit.] Zhong Xi Yi Jie He Za Zhi 1989;9:161-163, 134. [Chinese]

Gupta I, Gupta V, Parihar A, et al. Effects of *Boswellia serrata* gum resin in patients with bronchial asthma: results of a double-blind, placebo-controlled, 6-week clinical study. Eur J Med Res 1998;3:511-514.

Gupta I, Parihar A, Malhotra P, et al. Effects of *Boswellia serrata* gum resin in patients with ulcerative colitis. Eur J Med Res 1997;2:37-43.

Haggans CJ, Hutchins AM, Olson BA, et al. Effect of flaxseed consumption on urinary estrogen metabolites in postmenopausal women. Nutr Cancer 1999;33:188-195.

Hasegawa H. Proof of the mysterious efficacy of ginseng: basic and clinical trials: metabolic activation of ginsenoside: deglycosylation by intestinal bacteria and esterification with fatty acid. J Pharmacol Sci 2004;95:153-157.

Hasegawa H, Lee KS, Nagaoka T, et al. Pharmacokinetics of ginsenoside deglycosylated by intestinal bacteria and its transformation to biologically active fatty acid esters. Biol Pharm Bull 2000;23:298-304.

Hawthorn M, Ferrante M, Luchowski E, et al. The actions of peppermint oil and menthol on calcium channel-dependent processes in intestinal, neuronal and cardiac preparations. J Aliment Pharmacol Ther 1988;2:101-108.

Hertog MGL, Feskens EJM, Hollman PCH, et al. Dietary flavonoids and cancer risk in the Zutphen elderly study. Nutr Cancer 1994;22:176-184.

Hertog MGL, Hollman PCH. Potential health effects of the dietary flavonol quercetin [review]. Eur J Clin Nutr 1996;50:63-71.

Hill GJ 2nd, Shine TE, Hill HZ, et al. Failure of amygdalin to arrest B16 melanoma and BW5147 leukemia. Cancer Res 1976;36: 2102-2107.

Hills LD. *Comfrey: Fodder, Food and Remedy.* New York: Universe Books; 1976.

Hood WB Jr, Dans AL, Guyatt GH, Jaeschke R, McMurray JJ. Digitalis for treatment of congestive heart failure in patients in sinus rhythm: a systematic review and meta-analysis. J Card Fail 2004;10:155-164.

Horrobin DF. Gamma linolenic acid. Rev Contemp Pharmacother 1990;1:1-45.

Hou DX, Fujii M, Terahara N, Yoshimoto M. Molecular mechanisms behind the chemopreventive effects of anthocyanidins. J Biomed Biotechnol 2004:321-325.

Huan JY, Miranda CL, Buhler DR, Cheeke PR. Species differences in the hepatic microsomal enzyme metabolism of the pyrrolizidine alkaloids. Toxicol Lett 1998;99:127-137.

Igimi H, Hisatsuga T, Nishimura M. The use of d-limonene as a dissolving agent in gallstones. *Dig Dis* 1976;21:926-939.

Ishimi Y, Arai N, Wang X, et al. Difference in effective dosage of genistein on bone and uterus in ovariectomized mice. Biochem Biophys Res Commun 2000;274:697-701.

Ju HS, Li XJ, Zhao BL, et al. Scavenging effect of berbamine on active oxygen radicals in phorbol ester-stimulated human polymorphonuclear leukocytes. Biochem Pharmacol 1990;39: 1673-1678.

Kaffenberger RM, Doyle MJ. Determination of menthol and menthol glucuronide in human urine by gas chromatography using an enzyme-sensitive internal standard and flame ionization detection. J Chromatogr 1990;527:59-66.

Kamat JP, Ghosh A, Devasagayam TP. Vanillin as an antioxidant in rat liver mitochondria: inhibition of protein oxidation and lipid peroxidation induced by photosensitization. Mol Cell Biochem 2000;209:47-53.

Kandaswami C, Perkins E, Soloniuk DS, et al. Ascorbic acid-enhanced antiproliferative effect of flavonoids on squamous cell carcinoma in vitro. Anticancer Drugs 1993;4:91-96.

Kaufman PB, Duke JA, Brielmann H, Boik J, Hoyt JE. A comparative survey of leguminous plants as sources of the isoflavones genistein and daidzein: implications for human nutrition and health. J Altern Compl Med 1997;3:7-12.

Kay RM, Truswell AS. Dietary fiber: effects on plasma and biliary lipids in man. In: Spiller GA, Kay RM, eds. *Medical Aspects of Dietary Fiber.* New York: Plenum; 1980:153-173.

Kelley DS. Alpha-linolenic acid and immune response. Nutrition 1992;8:215-217.

Kelly MG, Hartwell JL. The biological effects and the chemical composition of podophyllin: a review. J Natl Cancer Inst 1954; 14:967-1010.

Khmel'nitskii OK, Simbirtsev AS, Konusova VG, et al. Pine resin and Biopin ointment: effects on cell composition and histochemical changes in wounds. Bull Exp Biol Med 2002;133:583-585.

Kritchevsky D. Dietary fiber. Annu Rev Nutr 1988;8:301-328.

Krungkrai SR, Yuthavong Y. The antimalarial action on *Plasmodium falciparum* of qinghaosu and artesunate in combination with agents which modulate oxidant stress. Trans R Soc Trop Med Hyg 1987;81:710-714.

Kuiper GGJM, Lemmen JG, Carlsson B, et al. Interaction of estrogenic chemicals and phytoestrogens with estrogen receptor beta. Endocrinology 1998;139:4252-4263.

Kuo CL, Chou CC, Yung BY. Berberine complexes with DNA in the berberine-induced apoptosis in human leukemic HL-60 cells. Cancer Lett 1995;93:193-200.

Lee HZ. Effects and mechanisms of emodin on cell death in human lung squamous cell carcinoma. Br J Pharmacol 2001;134:11-20.

Lee NK, Choi SH, Park SH, Park EK, Kim DH. Antiallergic activity of hesperidin is activated by intestinal microflora. Pharmacology 2004;71:174-180.

Levrat MA, Favier ML, Moundras C, et al. Role of dietary propionic acid and bile acid excretion in the hypocholesterolemic effects of oligosaccharides in rats. J Nutr 1994;124: 531-538.

Li SY, Jei W, Seow WK, Thong YH. Effect of berbamine on blood and bonemarrow stem cells of cyclophosphamidetreated mice. Int J Immunopharmacol 1994;16:245-249.

Lin HJ, Probst-Hensch NM, Louie AD, et al. Glutathione transferase null genotype, broccoli, and lower prevalence of colorectal adenomas. Cancer Epidemiol Biomark Prev 1998;7:647-652.

Liu JC, Hsu FL, Tsai JC, et al. Antihypertensive effects of tannins isolated from traditional Chinese herbs as non-specific inhibitors of angiontensin converting enzyme. Life Sci 2003;73:1543-1555.

Lu XG, Zhan LB, Feng BA, et al. Inhibition of growth and metastasis of human gastric cancer implanted in nude mice by d-limonene. World J Gastroenterol 2004;10:2140-2144.

Magnuson B. Cyanogenic glycosides. University of Idaho Department of Food Science and Toxicology, ExtoxNet FAQ, 1997. Available at: www.ace/orst/edu/info/extoxnet/faqs/natural/cya.htm. Accessed March 5, 2005.

Mahady GB, Pendland SL, Stoia A, Chadwick LR. In vitro susceptibility of *Helicobacter pylori* to isoquinoline alkaloids from *Sanguinaria canadensis* and *Hydrastis canadensis*. Phytother Res 2003;17:217-221.

Mariadason JM, Kilias D, Catto-Smith A, Gibson PR. Effect of butyrate on paracellular permeability in rat distal colonic mucosa ex vivo. *J Gastroenterol Hepatol* 1999;14(9):873-879.

Massoud A, El Sisi S, Salama O, Massoud A. Preliminary study of therapeutic efficacy of a new fasciolicidal drug derived from *Commiphora molmol* (myrrh). Am J Trop Med Hyg 2001;65:96-99.

Mattocks AR. Hepatotoxic effects due to pyrrolizidine alkaloid N-oxides. Xenobiotica 1971;1:563-565.

Mattocks AR. Acute hepatotoxicity and pyrrolic metabolites in rats dosed with pyrrolizidine alkaloids. Chem Biol Interact 1972;5:227-242.

Mizushina Y, Takahashi N, Ogawa A, et al. The cyanogenic glucoside, prunasin (D-mandelonitrile-beta-D-glucoside), is a novel inhibitor of DNA polymerase beta. J Biochem (Tokyo) 1999;126:430-436.

Moertel CG, Fleming TR, Rubin J, et al. A clinical trial of amygdalin (Laetrile) in the treatment of human cancer. New Engl J Med 1982;306:201-206.

Moreira AJ, Fraga C, Alonso M, et al. Quercetin prevents oxidative stress and NF-kappaB activation in gastric mucosa of portal hypertensive rats. Biochem Pharmacol 2004;68:1939-1946.

Morito K, Hirose T, Kinjo J, et al. Interaction of phytoestrogens with estrogen receptors alpha and beta. Biol Pharm Bull 2001;24:351-356.

Natori S, Ikekawa N, Suzuki M, eds. *Advances in Natural Products Chemistry: Extraction and Isolation of Active Compounds.* New York: John Wiley & Sons; 1981.

Nikulin AA, Krylova EA. [Comparative evaluation of the treatment of radiation skin injuries with oxycort ointment and Peruvian balsam.] Farmakol Toksikol 1980;43:97-100. [Russian]

Nosal'ova G, Strapkova A, Kardosova A, et al. [Antitussive action of extracts and polysaccharides of marsh mallow *(Althea officinalis* L, var robusta*).*] Pharmazie 1992;47:224-226. [German]

Notka F, Meier G, Wagner R. Concerted inhibitory activities of *Phyllanthus amarus* on HIV replication in vitro and ex vivo. Antiviral Res 2004;64:93-102.

Nwannenna AI, Lundh TJ, Madej A, Fredriksson G, Bjornhag G. Clinical changes in ovariectomized ewes exposed to phytoestrogens and 17beta-estradiol implants. Proc Soc Exp Biol Med 1995;208:92-97.

Ondrovcik P, Bravo C, Votava M. [Antibacterial effects of antiseptics in vitro and in an experiment in vivo.] Epidemiol Mikrobiol Imunol 1995;44:78-80. [Czech]

Parnham MJ. Benefit and risks of the squeezed sap of the purple coneflower *(Echinacea purpurea)* for long-term oral immunostimulant therapy. In: Wagner H, ed. *Immunomodulatory Agents from Plants*. Basel: Birkhäuser Verlag; 1999:119-135.

Pattnaik S, Subramanyam VR, Bapaji M, Kole CR. Antibacterial and antifungal activity of aromatic constituents of essential oils. Microbios 1997;89:39-46.

Piscatelli SC, Burstein AH, Welden N, et al. The effect of garlic supplements on the pharmacokinetics of saquinavir. Clin Infect Dis 2002;34:234-238.

Powis G, Ames MM, Kovach JS. Metabolic conversion of indicine *N*-oxide to indicine in rabbits and humans. Cancer Res 1979;39:3564-3570.

Qureshi S, al-Harbi MM, Ahmed MM, et al. Evaluation of the genotoxic, cytotoxic, and antitumor properties of *Commiphora molmol* using normal and *Ehrlich ascites* carcinoma cell-bearing Swiss albino mice. Cancer Chemother Pharmacol 1993;33:130-138.

Röder E. Medicinal plants in Europe containing pyrrolizidine alkaloids. Pharmazie 1995;50:83-98.

Roger CR. The nutritional incidence of flavonoids: some physiological and metabolic considerations. Experientia 1988;44:725-733.

Sanada H. [Study on the clinical effect of rhubarb on nitrogenmetabolism abnormality due to chronic renal failure and its mechanism.] Nippon Jinzo Gakkai Shi (Jpn J Nephrol) 1996;38:379-387. [Japanese]

Scardamaglia L, Nixon R, Fewings J. Compound tincture of benzoin: a common contact allergen? Australas J Dermatol 2003;44:180-184.

Schiff PB, Fant J, Horwitz SB. Promotion of microtubule assembly in vitro by taxol. Nature 1979;277:665-667.

Schmitt E, Dekant W, Stopper H. Assaying the estrogenicity of phytoestrogens in cells of different estrogen sensitive tissues. Toxicol In Vitro 2001;15:433-439.

Shertzer HG, Senft AP. The micronutrient indole-3-carbinol: implications for disease and chemoprevention. Drug Metab Drug Interact 2000;17:159-188.

Shin CY, Lee WJ, Lee EB, et al. Platycodin D and D3 increase airway mucin release in vivo and in vitro in rats and hamsters. Planta Med 2002;68:221-225.

Shutt DA, Cox RI. Steroid and phytoestrogen binding to sheep uterine receptors in vitro. Endocrinology 1972;52:299-310.

Singh V, Agarwal SS, Gupta BM. Immunomodulatory activity of *Panax ginseng* extract. Planta Med 1984;50:462-465.

Smith LW, Culvenor CCJ. Plant sources of hepatotoxic pyrrolizidine alkaloids. J Nat Prod 1981;44:129-152.

Smith TJ, Yang CS. Effect of organosulfur compounds from garlic and cruciferous vegetables on drug metabolism enzymes. Drug Metab Drug Interact 2000;17:23-49.

Spitz MR, Duphorne CM, Detry MA, et al. Dietary intake of isothiocyanates: evidence of a joint effect with glutathione S-transferase polymorphisms in lung cancer risk. Cancer Epidemiol Biomark Prev 2000;9:1017-1020.

Sticher O. Plant mono-, di- and sesquiterpenoids with pharmacological and therapeutical activity. In: Wagner H, Wolff P, eds. *New Natural Products and Plant Drugs with Pharmacological, Biological or Therapeutical Activity.* Proceedings of the First International Congress of Medicinal Plant Research, Section A; University of Munich, Germany; September 6-10, 1976. Berlin: Springer-Verlag; 1977:137-176.

Sun D, Courtney HS, Beachey EH. Berberine sulfate blocks adherence of *Streptococcus pyogenes* to epithelial cells, fibronectin, and hexadecane. Antimicrob Agents Chemother 1988;32:1370-1374.

Suryanarayana P, Kumar PA, Saraswat M, et al. Inhibition of aldose reductase by tannoid principles of *Emblica officinalis:* implications for the prevention of sugar cataract. Mol Vis 2004;10:148-154.

Thompson LU, Li T, Chen J, Goss PE. Biological effects of dietary flaxseed in patients with breast cancer. [Abstract #157.] Breast Cancer Res Treat 2000;64:50.

Tomoda M, Miyamoto H, Shimizu N. Structural features and anti-complementary activity of rehmannan SA, a polysaccharide from the root of *Rehmannia glutinosa.* Chem Pharm Bull (Tokyo) 1994;42:1666-1668.

Tomoda M, Shimizu N, Kanari M, Gonda R, Arai S, Okuda Y. Characterization of two polysaccharides having activity on the reticuloendothelial system from the root of *Glycyrrhiza uralensis.* Chem Pharm Bull (Tokyo) 1990;38:1667-1671.

Tomoda M, Takada K, Shimizu N, Gonda R, Ohara N. Reticuloendothelial system-potentiating and alkaline phosphatase-inducing activities of *Plantago*-mucilage A, the main mucilage from the seed of *Plantago asiatica,* and its five modification products. Chem Pharm Bull (Tokyo) 1991;39: 2068-2071.

Vasiljeva OV, Lyubitsky OB, Klebanov GI, Vladimirov YA. Effect of the combined action of flavonoids, ascorbate and alpha-tocopherol on peroxidation of phospholipid liposomes induced by Fe2+ ions. Membr Cell Biol 2000;14:47-56.

Vayalil PK, Mittal A, Katiyar SK. Proanthocyanidins from grape seeds inhibit expression of matrix metalloproteinases in human prostate carcinoma cells, which is associated with the inhibition of activation of MAPK and NF kappa B. Carcinogenesis 2004;25:987-995.

Vinson JA, Bose P. Comparative bioavailability to humans of ascorbic acid alone or in a citrus extract. Am J Clin Nutr 1988;48:6014.

Wagner B, Galey WR. Kinetic analysis of hexose transport to determine the mechanism of amygdalin and prunasin absorption in the intestine. J Appl Toxicol 2003;23:371-375.

Wakabayashi C, Hasegawa H, Murata J, Saiki I. In vivo antimetastatic action of ginseng protopanaxadiol saponins is based on their intestinal bacterial metabolites after oral administration. Oncol Res 1997;9:411-417.

Watanabe K, Fujino H, Morita T, et al. Solubilization of saponins of bupleuri radix with ginseng saponins: cooperative effect of dammarane saponins. Planta Med 1988;405-408.

Woods MN, Gorbach SL. Influences of fiber on the ecology of the intestinal flora. In: Spiller GA, ed. *CRC Handbook of Dietary Fiber in Human Nutrition.* 2nd ed. Boca Raton, Fla: CRC Press; 1993:361-370.

Yarnell E. Do anthraquinone glycoside laxatives increase the risk of colorectal cancer? HealthNotes Rev Compl Integr Med 2000;7:209-210.

Yarnell E. *Phytochemistry and Pharmacy for Practitioners of Botanical Medicine.* Wenatchee, Wash: Healing Mountain Publishing; 2003.

Yata N, Tanaka O. The effects of saponins in promoting the solubility and absorption of drugs. Oriental Healing Arts Intern Bull 1988;13:13-22.

Zeng XH, Zeng XJ, Li YY. Efficacy and safety of berberine for congestive heart failure secondary to ischemic or idiopathic dilated cardiomyopathy. Am J Cardiol 2003;92:173-176.

Zheng F. [Effect of *Rheum officinalis* on the proliferation of renal tubular cells in vitro.] Chung Hua I Hsueh Tsa Chih (Chinese Med J) 1993;73:3435, 3801. [Chinese]

Zhou G, Sun Y, Xin H, Zhang Y, Li Z, Xu Z. In vivo antitumor and immunomodulation activities of different molecular weight lambda-carrageenans from *Chondrus ocellatus*. Pharmacol Res 2004;50:47-53.

Herbal Medicine: Potential for Intoxication and Interactions With Conventional Drugs

12

CHAPTER

Robert H. Poppenga

The use of herbal remedies for the prevention and treatment of a variety of illnesses in small animals has increased tremendously in recent years. Although most herbal remedies, when used as directed and under the supervision of knowledgeable individuals, are safe, the potential for adverse effects or intoxications certainly exists. Because of inherent toxicity, some herbal remedies should not be used under any circumstance. Also, because nearly all herbal remedies contain multiple biologically active constituents, interaction with conventional drugs is a matter of concern. It is incumbent upon clinicians to be aware of those herbs that can cause intoxication and to be cognizant of potential herb–drug interactions. A number of evidence-based resources are available to assist clinicians in the safe use of herbal remedies.

Broadly defined, herbs are plants that are used for medicinal purposes or for their olfactory or flavoring properties. Herbs, along with vitamins, minerals, and amino acids, are also defined as dietary supplements by the Dietary Supplement Health and Education Act (DSHEA) of 1994.

Both veterinarians and animal owners are expressing an increased interest in learning about and using herbs and other "natural" products to treat medical problems (herbal medicine). The reasons underlying this increased use of herbal and other "alternative" medical modalities in human health have been investigated extensively and are multifactorial (Astin, 1998; Blais, 1997; Elder, 1997). Social, economic and philosophical reasons often underlie the decision by an individual to turn to alternative modalities such as herbal medicine. Unfortunately, similar investigations into the motivation of pet owners to employ such modalities for the treatment of their pets have not been conducted. However, it is likely that the same motivations apply.

Plants have been used by people for medicinal purposes since the beginning of recorded history and undoubtedly well before. In the West, many modern medicines, developed in the form of a "parent" compound or a synthetic derivative, originated from plants. Examples of "parent" compounds include salicylates (from *Salix* spp or willow bark), digitoxin and digoxin (from *Digitalis* spp or foxglove), quinine (from *Cinchona* spp or cinchona bark), and morphine (*Papaver* spp or opium poppy). The pharmaceutical industry continues to search for new and effective plant-derived compounds. Herbs are important components of traditional Chinese medicine, Ayurvedic medicine, and the medical practices of many indigenous cultures. Herbs were important components of both human and veterinary medicine in Europe and North America before the advent of purified natural and synthetic drugs.

Herbal medicine and conventional pharmacology differ in three fundamental ways (Vickers, 1999). First, herbalists use unpurified plant extracts that contain several different constituents in the belief that the various constituents work in coordination, additively, or synergistically (the effect of the whole herb is greater than the summed effects of its individual components). In addition, herbalists believe that toxicity is reduced when the whole herb is used instead of its purified active constituents; this is called "buffering." Secondly, several herbs are often used together. The theories of additivity, synergism, and buffering are believed to be applicable when herb combinations are employed as well. In conventional medicine, polypharmacy is generally not considered to be desirable because of increased risks of adverse drug reactions or interactions. Finally, herbalists, as well as many other alternative medical practitioners, approach patients in a more "holistic" way than do many conventional medical practitioners, who tend to focus more narrowly on the disease and exclude consideration of other conditions and propensities of the patient.

ACTIVE HERBAL CONSTITUENTS

The following broad classes of active chemical constituents are found in plants: volatile oils, resins, alkaloids, polysaccharides, phenols, glycosides, and fixed oils (Hung, 1998). Volatile oils are odorous plant ingredients. Examples of plants that contain volatile oils include catnip, garlic, and citrus. Ingestion or dermal exposure to volatile oils can result in intoxication. Resins are complex chemical mixtures that can be strong gastrointestinal irritants. Alkaloids are a heterogeneous group of alkaline, organic, and nitrogenous compounds. Often, these compounds are the most pharmacologically active plant constituents. Glycosides are sugar esters that contain a sugar (glycol) and a nonsugar (aglycone). In some cases, the glycosides are not toxic. However, hydrolysis of the glycosides after ingestion can release toxic aglycones. Fixed oils are esters of long-chain fatty acids and alcohols. Herbs that contain fixed oils are often used as emollients, demulcents, and bases for other agents, and, in general, these are the least toxic of the plant constituents.

Many of these plant-derived chemicals are biologically active and, if exposure is of sufficient magnitude, potentially toxic. Numerous case reports in the medical literature document serious and potentially life-threatening adverse effects following human and animal exposure to herbal preparations. It is worth noting that in several instances the incidence of animal intoxication from an herb, herbal preparation, or dietary supplement seems to parallel its popularity (Ooms, 2001; Gwaltney-Brant, 2000). However, it must be noted that, considered as a group, herbal products do not appear to be associated with a higher incidence of serious adverse effects than is associated with ingestion of conventional prescription or over-the-counter (OTC) pharmaceuticals. Serious adverse drug reactions (ADRs) to conventional pharmaceuticals in hospitalized people have been estimated at 6.7% (Lazarou, 1998). An approximately equal incidence of hospital admissions due to ADRs has been reported (Pirmohamed, 2004). A recent study estimated that approximately 25% of all herbal remedy and dietary supplement calls to a regional human poison control center could be classified as ADRs (Yang, 2003). The most common ADRs were associated with zinc (38.2%), echinacea (7.7%), chromium picolinate (6.4%), and witch hazel (6.0%). Only 3 of 233 ADRs were considered to be serious enough to warrant hospitalization. It is likely that ADRs are underreported for both conventional drugs and herbal remedies. Unfortunately, almost no information is available regarding the overall incidence of ADRs with conventional drugs or herbal remedies in veterinary medicine.

Poisoning of an animal might occur in various ways. Use of a remedy that contains a known toxin is one possibility. For example, long-term use of an herbal remedy that contains hepatotoxic pyrrolizidine alkaloids (PAs) may result in liver failure. Pennyroyal oil containing the putative hepatotoxin, pulegone, was responsible for the death of a dog after it was applied dermally to control fleas (Sudekum, 1992). Alternatively, administration of a misidentified plant may result in poisoning. Contamination of commercially prepared herbal remedies with toxic plants has been documented in the medical literature (DeSmet, 1991; Vanherweghem, 1998). Seeds of poison hemlock *(Conium maculatum)* have been found in anise seed. Recently, plantain sold as a dietary supplement was found to contain cardiac glycosides from *Digitalis* spp. Just as with traditional prescription medications, pet intoxication following accidental ingestion of an improperly stored remedy may occur. This is particularly true with dogs because of their indiscriminant eating habits. The author was involved in a case in which a miniature poodle ingested several tablets of its owner's medication containing rauwolfia alkaloids and developed clinical signs within 2 hours of ingestion. Reserpine was detected in the medication and the urine of the dog.

Some herbal remedies, particularly Chinese patent medicines, may contain inorganic contaminants such as arsenic, lead, or mercury or intentionally added pharmaceuticals such as nonsteroidal anti-inflammatories, corticosteroids, caffeine, or sedatives (Ko, 1998). Commonly found natural toxins in Chinese patent medicines include borneol, aconite, toad secretions *(Bufo* spp, Ch'an Su*)*, mylabris, scorpion, borax, acorus, and strychnine *(Strychnos nux-vomica)* (Ko, 1998).

Because herbal preparations contain numerous biologically active compounds, the potential exists for diverse drug interactions when they are used in conjunction with conventional pharmaceuticals. In addition, many naturally occurring chemicals found in herbal remedies cause induction of one or more liver P-450 metabolizing enzymes (see Table 12-5). For example, eucalyptus oil induces liver enzyme activity (Blumenthal, 1998a). This can cause altered metabolism of other drugs or chemicals, resulting in enhanced or diminished drug efficacy or toxicity. Coexisting liver or renal disease can alter the metabolism and elimination of herbal constituents, thus predisposing to adverse reactions. Apparent idiosyncratic reactions with herbal remedies have been documented in people. Such reactions might be due to individual differences in drug-metabolizing capacity (Stedman, 2002; Zhou, 2004).

Of particular concern to veterinarians is the possibility of species differences in susceptibility to the toxic effects of herbal constituents. For example, cat hemoglobin is quite susceptible to oxidative damage. The volatile oil in garlic contains oxidants such as allicin. Thus, one can hypothesize that oxidant-induced Heinz body anemia would be more likely to occur in cats given garlic than in other species. However, no information substantiates or refutes such a hypothesis. Unfortunately, little evidence-based information exists on which informed judgments about potential hazards of specific herbs to different species can be based.

According to annual surveys of herbs sold in the United States, the most commonly used herbs include coneflower *(Echinacea* spp*)*, garlic *(Allium sativa)*, ginseng *(Panax* spp*)*, gingko *(Ginkgo biloba)*, Saint John's Wort *(Hypericum perforatum)*, saw palmetto *(Serenoa repens)*, goldenseal *(Hydrastis canadensis)*, aloe *(Aloe* spp*)*, astragalus *(Astragalus* spp*)*, cayenne *(Capsicum* spp*)*, bilberry *(Vaccinium myrtillus)*, and cat's claw *(Uncaria tomentosa)*. Presumably, these herbs are those to which pets are most likely to be exposed. According to the recently published *Botanical Safety Handbook*, coneflower, saw palmetto, aloe (gel used internally), astragalus, and cayenne (used internally) should be considered safe when used appropriately. Garlic, ginseng, gingko, Saint John's Wort, goldenseal, aloe (gel used externally, dried juice used externally), and cayenne (used externally) have some restrictions regarding their use (McGuffin, 1997). For example, in humans, garlic should not be used by nursing mothers, and cayenne should not be applied to injured skin or near the eyes. Both gingko and Saint John's Wort are contraindicated in individuals taking monamine oxidase inhibitors because of the potential for herb–drug interactions. Only insufficient data are available on which clinicians can base a determination regarding the safety of bilberry and cat's claw, although bilberry is safe enough that it is also used as a food. Of interest is a recent study that listed the most common herb-related calls to a regional human poison control center (Haller, 2002). The most frequent calls, in descending order of frequency, involved Saint John's Wort, ma huang, echinacea, guarana, ginkgo, ginseng, valerian, tea tree oil, goldenseal, arnica, yohimbe, and kava kava. Not all of the calls could be categorized as ADRs.

SUMMARIES OF THE SAFETY OF COMMON HERBS

Not all of the following herbs, essential oils, and dietary supplements are used in herbal medicine because of well-recognized risks of intoxication. However, they are included in the following discussion precisely because of their inherent toxicity. Unless otherwise specified, the following information is taken from three primary sources: *The Botanical Safety Handbook, The Complete German Commission E Monographs: Therapeutic Guide to Herbal Medicines,* and *The Review of Natural Products* (McGuffin, 1997; Blumenthal, 1998b; DerMarderosian, 2001a).

Absinthe (Wormwood)

The name *wormwood* is derived from the ancient use of the plant *(Artemisia absinthium)* and its extracts as an intestinal anthelmintic. Wormwood was the main ingredient in absinthe, a largely banned, toxic liqueur whose chronic consumption was associated with absinthism. Absinthism was characterized by mental enfeeblement, hallucinations, psychosis, delirium, vertigo, trembling of the limbs, digestive disorders, thirst, paralysis, and death. α- and β-Thujone are the toxins found in wormwood. In rats, intravenous injection of thujone at 40 mg/kg and 120 mg/kg induces convulsions and death, respectively. According to the German Commission E, indications for the use of wormwood include loss of appetite, dyspepsia, and biliary dyskinesia. Thujone-free plant extract is used as a flavoring agent in alcoholic beverages such as vermouth. The US Food and Drug Administration (FDA) classifies the plant as an unsafe herb. The American Herbal Products Association indicates that the herb should not be used during pregnancy or lactation or on a long-term basis.

Aconite

Traditionally, aconite *(Aconitum* spp*)* root was used for topical analgesia, neuralgia, asthma, and heart disease. It contains several cardioactive alkaloids, including aconitine, aconine, picraconitine, and napelline. These act on the heart by increasing sodium flux through sodium channels. Acute toxicosis can be induced following the ingestion of 5 mL of aconite tincture, 2 mg of pure aconitine, or ~1 g of the plant. Clinical signs include burning sensation of the lips, tongue, and throat and gastrointestinal upset characterized by salivation, nausea, and emesis. Cardiac arrhythmias with unusual electrical characteristics have been observed following intoxication. Death can occur from minutes to days following ingestion. Although little used in the United States, aconite root continues to be used in traditional medicine in Asia and Europe. The most common herb-related adverse reaction in China involves aconite root (Ko, 1998). The American Herbal Products Association (AHPA) suggests that the herb should be taken only under the advice of an expert qualified in its appropriate use.

Aloe

Mucilaginous leaf gel (aloe gel) from parenchymatous leaf cells of *Aloe* spp is used as an emollient and for wound healing. Dried juice or latex (aloe resin) from cells below the leaf skin has been used as a laxative. The gel is the product most frequently used by the cosmetic and health food industries. Although commonly used internally, the gel is not approved by the FDA for internal use. External use of the gel on intact skin is generally considered safe and not associated with adverse reactions. The latex contains a number of chemicals of which the anthraquinone, barbaloin (a glucoside of aloe-emodin), is the most abundant. Aloe-emodin and other anthraquinones are gastrointestinal irritants that exert a strong purgative effect and cause severe cramping.

Aristolochia

Traditionally, the plant *(Aristolochia* spp*)* has been used as an anti-inflammatory agent and for the treatment of snakebites. Recently, it was found to be a contaminant of a weight loss preparation (Vanherweghem, 1998). The active ingredient in aristolochia is aristolochic acid, which is carcinogenic, mutagenic, and nephrotoxic. The rodent intravenous dose that kills 50% of the population (LD_{50}) is 38 to 203 mg/kg. In rats, doses as low as 5 mg/kg for 3 weeks have been associated with various neoplasias. This herb is not recommended for use.

Blue-Green Algae

Blue-green (BG) algae are single-celled organisms that have been promoted for their nutritional properties. Several BG algal species produce potent toxins. *Microcystis aeruginosa* produces the hepatotoxic microcystins. *Anabaena flos-aquae* produce the neurotoxins anatoxin-a and antoxin a_s. *Aphanizomenon flos-aquae* produce the neurotoxins saxitoxin and neosaxitoxin. Efforts are under way to better define the risks associated with ingestion of potentially toxigenic BG algae and to establish safe concentrations of total microcystins in marketed products. *Spirulina* has also been promoted as a nutritional supplement and is not considered a toxigenic BG algae genus. However, some products have been found to be contaminated with mercury, and microbial contamination could possibly be a concern if harvested algae grow in water contaminated with human or animal wastes.

Chapparal

Traditionally, a tea made from this plant *(Larrea tridentate)* has been used to treat acne, abdominal cramps, bronchitis, common colds, chicken pox, and snakebites. Additionally, the plant was believed to have analgesic, anticarcinogenic, and antiaging properties. Currently, this plant is not recommended for use because of its hepatotoxic properties, carcinogenicity, and ability to cause contact dermatitis; it was removed from the "generally recognized as safe" category by the FDA in 1970. Despite this regulatory action, it is sold for human and veterinary use. Nor-dihydroguaiaretic acid (NDGA) is believed to be responsible for most of the biological activity of the plant. Several human case reports associated the ingestion of chapparal tablets or capsules for 6 to 12 weeks with reversible hepatotoxicity.

Comfrey

Long-term consumption of *Symphytum* spp has been associated with hepatotoxicity because of the presence of PAs in the plant. PA metabolites form adducts with proteins DNA and RNA in hepatocytes, resulting in cell damage and death. In addition, several PAs in comfrey are carcinogenic to rats. Traditionally, the plant has been used externally to promote wound healing and treat hemorrhoids, and internally to treat gastric ulcers and as a blood purifier. Even when applied externally to rat skin, PAs have been detected in urine. Comfrey may be unsafe for use in any form.

Digitalis

Digitalis spp contain several cardiac glycosides, including digitoxin, gitoxin, and lanatosides, that inhibit sodium-potassium adenosine triphosphatase (ATPase). All parts of the plant are toxic. Toxic doses of fresh leaves are reported to be ~6 to 7 oz for a cow, ~4 to 5 oz for a horse and <1 oz for a pig. Children have been intoxicated by sucking on the flowers or ingesting seeds and leaves of the plant. Ornamental varieties of digitalis contain significantly lower concentrations of glycosides. Clinical signs of intoxication include gastrointestinal upset, dizziness, weakness, muscle tremors, miosis, and potentially fatal cardiac arrhythmias. Digitalis glycosides have a relatively long half-life and may accumulate, leading to intoxication. Poisoning by digitalis is one of the few plant intoxications for which a specific antidote is available. Digoxin-specific Fab antibodies are effective in treating patients with acute intoxication (Roberts, 2001). A number of other plants contain cardiac glycosides, including *Nerium oleander, Thevetia peruviana, Convallaria majalis, Taxus brevifolia, Strophanthus* spp, *Acokanthera* spp, and *Urginea maritima.*

Ephedra or Ma Huang

The dried young branches of ephedra *(Ephedra* spp*)* have been used for their stimulating and vasoactive effects. In addition, ephedra has been employed in several products promoted for weight loss. The plant constituents responsible for biological activity include the alkaloids, ephedrine, and pseudoephedrine. In commercial use, dried ephedra should contain no less than 1.25% ephedrine. Ephedrine and pseudoephedrine are sympathomimetics, and acute intoxication is associated with insomnia, restlessness, tachycardia, and cardiac arrhythmias. Nausea and emesis are also reported to occur. A case series involving intoxication of dogs following ingestion of a weight loss product containing guarana (caffeine) and ma huang (ephedrine) was recently reported (Ooms, 2001). Estimated doses of the respective plants associated with adverse effects were 4.4 to 296.2 mg/kg and 1.3 to 88.9 mg/kg. Symptomatology included hyperactivity, tremors, seizures, behavioral changes, emesis, tachycardia, and hyperthermia. Ingestion was associated with mortality in 17% of cases. North American species of ephedra (also called Mormon tea) have not been shown to contain any pharmacologically active alkaloids.

The use of ephedra in humans has been associated with a greatly increased risk for adverse effects compared with other commonly used herbs. One study reported that products containing ephedra accounted for 64% of all reported adverse effects from herbs, although they accounted for only 1% of herbal product sales (Bent, 2003). The actual frequency of adverse effects in patients using ephedra could not be determined because the study was based on calls received by human poison control centers. However, on the basis of such studies, the FDA initiated a ban on ephedra-containing products in April of 2004. This marked the first time that the FDA banned the sale of a dietary supplement since the passage of the DSHEA Act in 1994.The ban was later overturned by the federal courts because the FDA did not adequately demonstrate that low doses of ephedra posed a significant or unreasonable risk.

Garlic

Allium sativum is a member of the onion family. The plant contains 0.1% to 0.3% of a strong-smelling volatile oil containing allyl disulfides such as allicin. Extracts from garlic are reported to have a number of biocidal activities, to decrease lipid and cholesterol levels, to prolong clotting times, to inhibit platelet aggregation, and to increase fibrinolytic activity (Siegers, 1991; DerMarderosian, 2001a). Acute toxicity of allicin for dogs and cats is unknown; its LD_{50} for mice following subcutaneous or intravenous administration is 120 mg/kg and 60 mg/kg, respectively. Oral LD_{50}s for garlic extracts, given by various routes to rats and mice, range from 0.5 mL/kg to 30 mL/kg. In chronic toxicity studies with garlic oil or garlic extracts, anemia has been observed in dogs. A single 25-mL dose of fresh garlic extract has caused burning of the mouth, esophagus and stomach, nausea, sweating, and light-headedness (DerMarderosian, 2001b). Topical application of garlic oil causes local irritation, which can be severe. The sensitivity of cat hemoglobin to oxidative damage may make cats more sensitive to adverse effects.

Germander

Germander *(Teucrium chamaedrys)* contains polyphenol derivatives, diterpenes, flavonoids, and tannins. Plant constituents are hepatotoxic; perhaps requiring metabolism to toxic metabolites. The toxicity of germander is not well defined. It is categorized as a class 3 herb by the AHPA, which indicates that it should not be administered except under the advice of an individual qualified in its appropriate use.

Guarana

Guarana is the dried paste made from the crushed seeds of *Paullinia cupana* or *P. sorbilis,* a fast-growing shrub native to South America. Currently, the most common forms of guarana include syrups, extracts, and distillates used as flavoring agents and as a source of caffeine for the soft drink industry. Recently, it has been added to weight loss formulations in combination with ephedra. Caffeine concentrations in the plant range from 3% to 5%, which compares with 1% to 2% for coffee beans. Oral lethal doses of caffeine in dogs and cats range from 110 to 200 mg/kg body weight and 80 to 150 mg/kg body weight, respectively (Carson, 2001). See Ephedra for a discussion of a case series involving dogs that ingested a product containing guarana and ephedra (Ooms, 2001).

Kava Kava

The root and rhizome of *Piper methysticum* was recommended for the treatment of nervous anxiety, stress, and restlessness by the German Commission E; it is recognized as an effective anxiolytic in a Cochrane collaboration review. The plant contains at least 18 kava pyrones that are possible dopaminergic receptor antagonists.

The toxicity of kava kava is not well defined, although long-term use in humans is associated with dry, flaking, discolored skin and reddened eyes (kawaism). Recently, kava kava has undergone increased scrutiny because of its potential hepatotoxicity, and kava extracts have, in fact, been banned by Canada and some countries in Europe (Clouatre, 2004). A total of 78 cases of possible hepatotoxicity following use of the herb are available from a variety of databases. Relatively few of these cases can be reliably linked to kava kava use, and hepatotoxicity appears to be idiosyncratic. Postulated mechanisms of hepatotoxicity include inhibition of P-450 enzymes, reduced liver glutathione concentrations, and inhibition of cyclooxygenase enzyme activity (Clouatre, 2004; Anke, 2004). Overall, the safety of extracts of kava kava is good and compares favorably with the safety of conventional anxiolytics (Clouatre, 2004). Kava kava has the potential to interact with a number of other drugs and exacerbate the toxicity of other hepatotoxic agents. When kava kava extracts are still available, they should not be used during pregnancy, lactation, or clinical depression. In humans, the duration of use should be limited to 3 months to avoid habituation.

Khat

In humans, severe adverse effects such as migraine, cerebral hemorrhage, myocardial infarction, and pulmonary edema have been associated with khat *(Catha edulis)* use. Khat contains tannins that are potentially hepatotoxic. The active constituents in khat include cathine and cathinone; both have stimulant properties with potency of stimulation between those of caffeine and amphetamine. Animal studies indicate that cathinone can depress testosterone levels, cause testicular tissue degeneration, and decrease sperm numbers and motility. Khat use by pregnant humans has been associated with significantly lower birth rates. It may also be teratogenic and mutagenic.

Lobelia

Traditionally, *Lobelia inflata* has been used as an antispasmodic, respiratory stimulant, relaxant, emetic, and euphoriant. The plant contains pyridine alkaloids such as lobeline, lobelanine, and lobelanidine. Lobeline has nicotinic agonist properties (~5% to 20% the potency of nicotine). Toxicity has been associated with ingestion of 50 mg of dried herb, 1 mL of a tincture, and 8 mg of pure lobeline. Clinical signs of intoxication include hypothermia, hypertension, respiratory depression, paralysis, seizures, euphoria, nausea, emesis, abdominal pain, salivation, tachycardia, and coma. It is not recommended for use by the German Commission E, but the AHPA suggests that no evidence of severe symptoms or death following use of the plant has been substantiated. The AHPA suggests that the plant not be used during pregnancy or taken in large doses.

Mistletoe

Mistletoes are grouped into two broad categories: the European mistletoe *(Viscum album)* and the American mistletoe *(Phoradendron serotinum).* The European mistletoe is suggested for use in degenerative joint disease and as a palliative for malignant tumors. Plant constituents include β-phenylethylamine, tyramine, and structurally related compounds. In addition, European and American mistletoes contain proteins called viscotoxins and phoratoxins, respectively, with similar toxicity to abrin and ricin (found in *Abrus precatorius* and *Ricinus communis,* respectively). These compounds produce dose-dependent hypertension or hypotension, bradycardia, and increased uterine and gastrointestinal motility. All parts of the plant are considered toxic, and prompt gastrointestinal decontamination and symptomatic and supportive care should be instituted following ingestion. However, a review of the human toxicity of mistletoe indicated that most patients who ingested the plant remained asymptomatic, and no deaths were reported (Hall, 1986). Ingestion of up to three berries or two leaves is unlikely to produce serious human toxicity.

Nutmeg and Mace

Nutmeg is derived from the seed of *Myristica fragrans;* the spice, mace, is derived from the seed coat. Current uses of the plant include the treatment of gastrointestinal disturbances such as cramps, flatulence, and diarrhea. It has been investigated as an antidiarrheal medication in calves (Stamford, 1980). It has potential anticancer and biocidal activities. The toxicity of nutmeg is uncertain, although case reports suggest that if ingested doses are sufficient, acute toxicity can occur. Two tablespoons of ground nutmeg, one to three whole nutmegs, or 5 g of powdered nutmeg may cause clinical signs of hallucinations, nausea, and severe emesis. The German Commission E lists the plant as an unapproved herb, and the AHPA suggests that it be used at medicinal doses only under the supervision of an individual who is knowledgeable about its potential effects.

Oleander

Despite its toxicity, oleander *(Nerium oleander)* has been used for its medicinal properties for centuries. The plant contains a number of cardiac glycosides with activities similar to those of digitalis. In birds, ingestion of as little as 0.12 to 0.7 g of the plant can be fatal. Ingestion of as little as 0.005% of an animal's body weight in dry oleander leaves can be fatal (~10 to 20 leaves for an adult horse) (Kingsbury, 1964). Ingestion of oleander should be considered serious, and prompt medical attention should be sought. Digoxin-specific Fab fragments are antidotal. The extreme toxicity of the plant precludes its use in any form.

Pleurisy Root

Asclepias tuberosa root traditionally has been used to ease the pain and facilitate breathing in patients with pleurisy. The toxicity of the plant is not well defined; cardiac glycosides and neurotoxic resinoids are found in many *Asclepias* spp. The glycosides inhibit sodium-potassium ATPase. Clinical signs of intoxication include fatigue, anorexia, emesis, cardiac arrhythmias, bradycardia, and hypokalemia. This plant is best avoided by those not trained in its use.

Pokeweed

Phytolacca spp are ubiquitous in the United States and have a long history of use in folk remedies for rheumatism and arthritis and as an emetic and a purgative. Active plant constituents include triterpene saponins, a tannin, a resin, and a protein called *pokeweed mitogen.* All parts of the plant are toxic, except the above-ground leaves that grow in the early spring, which can be eaten after proper preparation. Toxic components are highest in the rootstock, less in the mature leaves and stems, and least in the fruit. Ingestion of poisonous plant parts causes severe stomach cramping, nausea, emesis, persistent diarrhea, dyspnea, weakness, spasms, hypotension, seizures, and death. Severe poisonings have been reported in adult humans who ingested mature pokeweed leaves and as little as 1 cup of tea brewed with ½ tsp of powdered pokeroot.

Saint John's Wort

A number of chemical constituents have been isolated from Saint John's Wort *(Hypericum perforatum),* including anthraquinone derivatives (hypericin and pseudohypericin), the phoroglucinols hyperforin and adhyperforin, flavonoids, phenols, tannins, and a volatile oil. External indications for use include acute injuries or contusions, myalgia, and first-degree burns. Taken internally, it is used to treat depression, anxiety, or nervous unrest. Assessment of possible antiviral properties is ongoing. Hyperforin is the most neuroactive component of the plant and is believed to be responsible for its central nervous system (CNS) effects. It modulates neuronal ionic conductances and inhibits serotonin reuptake. Hypericin is a photodynamic agent and, when ingested, it can induce photosensitization. Most reports of photosensitization in humans are associated with excessive intake of the plant. Other adverse effects are usually mild. As an aside, considerable variations in active constituent concentrations have been documented in different brands of Saint John's Wort.

Senna

Species of *Cassia* have been used for their laxative effects because anthraquinone glycosides (sennosides) are present in the plant. These compounds increase gastrointestinal motility, induce fluid movement in the lumen, and have direct irritant effects. Catharsis can result from ingestion of teas that contain 1 to 2 tsp of dried senna leaves. Long-term use of laxatives, including senna, can cause a laxative dependency syndrome, which is characterized by poor gastrointestinal motility in the absence of their use. Appropriate use of senna may be associated with mild abdominal cramping. More prolonged use can cause electrolyte disturbances, especially hypokalemia.

White Willow

Active constituents in willow *(Salix* spp*)* include salicylates (primarily in the form of glycosides salicortin and salicin) and tannins. Current indications for plant use include fever, rheumatism, and conditions that benefit from an anti-inflammatory agent. Therapeutic as well as adverse effects occur through inhibition of prostaglandin synthesis. In addition, salicylates inhibit oxidative phosphorylation and Krebs cycle enzymes. In cats, acetylsalicylic (AS) acid is toxic at 80 to 120 mg/kg given orally for 10 to 12 days. In dogs, AS administered at 50 mg/kg given orally twice a day is associated with emesis; higher doses can cause depression and metabolic acidosis. A dose of 100 to 300 mg/kg orally once daily for 1 to 4 weeks is associated with gastric ulceration; more prolonged dosing is potentially fatal (Osweiler, 1996). Cats are particularly vulnerable to overdose because of an inability to rapidly metabolize salicylates. (See Salicylates and Cats, p. 190.) Presumably, salicylates in willow have approximately equivalent toxicity. Most standards for medicinal willow bark require that salicylates be present at >1% dry weight, although this is difficult to achieve with many source species. A number of other plants contain salicylates, including *Betula* spp (birch), *Filipendula ulmaria* (meadowsweet), and *Populus* spp. (See "Oil of Wintergreen" later.)

Yohimbe

Pausinystalia yohimbe bark contains the alkaloid, yohimbine, at ~6%. Yohimbine is an α_2-adrenergic receptor blocker that has purported aphrodisiac and hallucinogenic properties. Yohimbine causes peripheral vasodilatation and CNS stimulation. In intoxication, yohimbine causes severe hypotension, abdominal distress, and weakness. CNS stimulation and paralysis have been reported. An acutely toxic dose for dogs is 0.55 mg/kg given intravenously. The drug or crude product should never be given without adequate medical supervision. Human formulations have been combined with other purported sexual stimulants such as strychnine, thyroid, and methyltestosterone.

Other herbs of toxicologic concern are listed in Table 12-1.

TABLE 12-1

Additional Herbs of Toxicologic Concern

Scientific Name	Common Names	Active Constituents	Target Organs
Acorus calamus	Acorus, calamus, sweet flag, sweet root, sweet cane, sweet cinnamon	β-Asarone (procarcinogen)	Liver—potent hepatocarcinogen
Aesculus hippocasteranum	Horse chestnut, buckeye	Esculin, nicotine, quercetin, rutin, saponins, shikimic acid	Gastrointestinal Nervous
Arnica montana, A. latifolia	Arnica, wolf's bane, leopard's bane	Sesquiterpene lactones	Skin—dermatitis
Atropa belladonna	Belladonna, deadly nightshade	Atropine	Nervous—anticholinergic syndrome
Conium maculatum	Poison hemlock	Coniine, other similar alkaloids	Nervous—nicotine-like toxicosis
Convallaria majalis	Lily of the valley, mayflower, conval lily	Cardiac glycosides	Cardiovascular
Cytisus scoparius	Scotch broom, broom, broom tops	l-sparteine	Nervous—nicotinic-like toxicosis
Datura stramonium	Jimsonweed, thornapple	Atropine, scopolamine, hyoscyamine	Nervous—anticholinergic syndrome
Dipteryx odorata	Tonka, tonka bean	Coumarin	Hematologic—anticoagulant
Euonymus europaeus, E. atropurpureus	European spindle tree; wahoo, eastern burning bush	Cardiac glycosides	Cardiovascular
Eupatorium perfoliatum, E. purpureum	Boneset, thoroughwort; joe pye weed, gravel root, queen of the meadow	Pyrrolizidine alkaloids	Liver
Heliotropium europaeum	Heliotrope	Pyrrolizidine alkaloids	Liver
Hyoscyamus niger	Henbane, fetid nightshade, poison tobacco, insane root, stinky nightshade	Hyoscyamine, yoscine	Nervous—anticholinergic syndrome
Ipomoea purga	Jalap	Convolvulin	Gastrointestinal
Mandragora officinarum	Mandrake	Scopolamine, hyoscyamine	Nervous—anticholinergic syndrome
Podophyllum peltatum	Mayapple, mandrake	Podophyllin	Gastrointestinal—gastroenteritis
Sanguinaria canadensis	Bloodroot, red puccoon, red root	Sanguinarine	Gastrointestinal
Solanum dulcamara, other *Solanum* spp	Woody, bittersweet, or climbing nightshade	Numerous glycoalkaloids, including solanine and chaconine	Gastrointestinal, nervous, cardiovascular
Tussilago farfara	Coltsfoot	Pyrrolizidine alkaloids, senkirkine	Liver
Vinca major, V. minor	Common periwinkle, periwinkle	Vincamine	Immune system

Salicylates and Cats

One of the most common cautions in small animal practice is the use of salicylate and salicin–containing herbs in cats due to their sensitivity to a salicylate derivative, acetylsalicylic acid (aspirin). This sensitivity to aspirin extends to phenolic compounds in general. Aspirin dose rates in cats for various conditions range from 10 mg/kg to 40 mg/kg body weight. Qualitative metabolism in cats is similar to that in other species involving hydrolysis of the parent compound in plasma, liver, and some other organs to salicylic acid, followed by formation of salicyluric acid, salicyluric glucuronide, salicyl ester glucuronide, salicyl phenol glucuronide, gentisic acid, and gentisuric acid. One of the reasons for the dosage interval (every 2 to 3 days) is the delayed metabolism of aspirin, which is due to decreased uridine diphosphate (UDP) glucuronyl transferase activity in the cat liver. How do we compare the risk of using herbs that contain unacetylated salicylate and salicins? If we consider that the dose of aspirin for a cat starts at 10 mg/kg, then a 5-kg cat would require 50 mg of acetylsalicylate acid. If we treat a cat with 1 mL of a 1:2 meadowsweet extract (containing one of the highest concentrations of salicins), the cat receives 0.388 mg of salicylate in a dose of 1 mL. This is 0.00776 times the dose of aspirin. Or, another way of expressing this is that the cat would need to receive 128.9 mL of the extract to receive a similar dose of 50 mg. Another example is willow bark *(Salix alba)* that contains 1% salicins. A 1:2 extract contains 500 mg of willow in 1 mL; 1% is 5000 micrograms or 5 milligrams. A 1-mL dose would provide 5 mg of salicins or 10% of the normal dose of aspirin. So, the risk of reaching toxic levels in normal doses in cats is very low. We know that cats detoxify drugs that contain salicylate much more slowly than do humans and dogs. However, perhaps with the exception of *Salix* species, most herbs have relatively low concentrations of salicylate acid when compared with aspirin, and accumulation, even on a daily dosing basis, is unlikely (Fougere, 2003).

ESSENTIAL OILS

Essential oils are the volatile, organic constituents of fragrant plant matter that contribute to plant fragrance and taste. They are extracted from plant material by distillation or cold pressing. A number of essential oils are not recommended for use because of their toxicity or potential for toxicity (Tisserand, 1999). These are listed in Table 12-2. These oils have unknown or oral LD_{50} values in animals of 1 g/kg or less. Most toxicity information has been derived with the use of laboratory rodents or mice; such data should be used only as a rough guide because they cannot always be extrapolated to other species. These oils are best avoided for aromatherapy or for dermal or oral use. Essential oils that are more difficult to assess for safety but that are best avoided are listed in Table 12-3, along with their oral LD_{50} values (between 1 and 2 g/kg). *Essential Oil Safety: A Guide for Health Care Professionals* is an excellent reference for in-depth discussions of general and specific essential oil toxicity. The following essential oils are of particular concern.

Camphor

Camphor is an aromatic, volatile, terpene ketone derived from the wood of *Cinnamomum camphora* or synthesized from turpentine. Camphor oil is separated into four distinct fractions: white, brown, yellow, and blue camphor (Tisserand, 1999). White camphor is the form used in aromatherapy and in over-the-counter (OTC) products (brown and yellow fractions contain the carcinogen, safrole, and are not usually available). OTC products vary in form and camphor content; external products contain 10% to 20% semisolid forms or 1% to 10% in camphor spirits. Camphor is used as a topical rubefacient and antipuritic agent. Camphor is rapidly absorbed from the skin and gastrointestinal tract, and toxic effects can occur within minutes of exposure. In humans, signs of intoxication include emesis, abdominal distress, excitement, tremors, and seizures, followed by CNS depression characterized by apnea and coma. Fatalities have occurred in humans who ingested 1 to 2 g of camphor-containing products, although the adult human lethal dose has been reported to be 5 to 20 g (Tisserand, 1999; Emery, 1999). One teaspoon of camphorated oil (~1 mL of camphor) was lethal to 16-month-old and 19-month-old children. Long-term ingestion in children can result in hepatotoxicity and neurotoxicity.

Citrus Oil

Citrus oil and citrus oil constituents such as D-limonene and linalool have been shown to have insecticidal activity. Although D-limonene has been used safely as an insecticide on dogs and cats, some citrus oil formulations or use of pure citrus oil may pose a poisoning hazard (Powers, 1988). Fatal adverse reactions have been reported in cats following the use of an "organic" citrus oil dip (Hooser, 1986). Hypersalivation, muscle tremors, ataxia, lateral recumbency, coma, and death were noted experimentally in three cats following use of the dip according to label directions.

Melaleuca Oil

Derived from the leaves of the Australia tea tree *(Melaleuca alternifolia)*, melaleuca oil is often referred to as tea tree oil. This oil contains terpenes, sesquiterpenes, and hydrocarbons. A variety of commercially available products contain the oil and shampoos, and the pure oil has been sold for use on dogs, cats, ferrets, and horses. Tea tree oil toxicosis has been reported in dogs and cats (Villar, 1994; Bischoff, 1998). A recent case report describes the illness

TABLE 12-2

Potentially Toxic Essential Oils

Oil	Genus/Species	Oral LD_{50} (g/kg)	Toxic Component
Wintergreen	*Gaultheria procumbens*	1.20	Methyl salicylate 98%
Cornmint	*Mentha arvensis* var. *piperascens*	1.25	*l*-menthol 35%–50% Menthone 15%–30% Pulegone 0.2%–5%
Savory (summer)	*Satureia hortensis; S. montana*	1.37	Carvacol 3%–67% Thymol 1%–49% *Para*-cymene 7%–26%
Clove leaf	*Syzygium aromaticum*	1.37	Eugenol 70%–95% *Iso*eugenol 0.14%–0.23%
Basil	*Ocimum basilicum*	1.40	Estragole 40%–87% Methyleugenol 0.3%–4.2% Linalool 0.5%–6.3%
Hyssop	*Hyssopus officinalis*	1.40	Pinocamphone 40% *Iso*-pinocamphone 30%
Sassafras (Brazilian)	*Ocotea pretiosa*	1.58	Safrole 85%–90%
Myrrh		1.65	Unknown
Birch (sweet)	*Betula lenta*	1.70	Methyl salicylate 98%
Bay leaf (W. Indian)	*Pimenta racemosa*	1.80	Eugenol 38%–75%
Oregano	*Origanum vulgare;* *Coridothymus capitatus,* others	1.85	Thymol—varies Carvacrol—varies
Sassafras	*Sassafras albidum*	1.90	Safrole 85%–90%
Tarragon	*Artemesia dracunculus*	1.90	Estragole 70%–87% Methyleugenol 0.1%–1.5%
Tea tree	*Melaleuca alternifolia*	1.90	Terpenes 50%–60% Cineole 6%–8%
Savin	*Juniperus sabina*	?	Sabinyl acetate 20%–53% Sabinene 20%–42%

From Tisserand, 1999.

TABLE 12-3

Most Toxic Essential Oils

Oil	Genus/Species	Oral LD_{50} (g/kg)	Toxic Component
Boldo leaf	*Peumus boldus*	0.13	Ascaridole 16%
Wormseed	*Chenopodium ambrosioides*	0.25	Ascaridole 60%–80%
Mustard	*Brassica nigra*	0.34	Allyl isothiocyanate 99%
Armoise	*Artemisia herba-alba*	0.37	Thujone 35%
Pennyroyal (Eur.)	*Mentha pulegium*	0.40	Pulegone 55%–95%
Tansy	*Tanacetum vulgare*	0.73	Thujone 66%–81%
Thuja	*Thuja occidentalis*	0.83	Thujone 30%–80%
Calamus	*Acorus calamus* var. *angustatus*	0.84	Asarone 45%–80%
Wormwood	*Artemisia absinthium*	0.96	Thujone 34%–71%
Bitter almond	*Prunus amygdalus* var. *amara*	0.96	Prussic acid 3%
Tree wormwood, Large wormwood	*Artemesia arborescens*	?	Iso-thujone 30%–45%
Buchu	*Barosma betulina; B. crenulata*	?	Pulegone 50%
Horseradish	*Cochlearia Armoracia*	?	Allyl isocyanate 50%
Lanyana	*Artemisia afra*	?	Thujone 4%–66%
Pennyroyal (N. Am.)	*Hedeoma pulegoides*	?	Pulegone 60%–80%
Southernwood	*Artemisia abrotanum*	?	Thujone
Western red cedar	*Thuja plicata*	?	Thujone 85%

From Tisserand, 1999.

of three cats exposed dermally to pure melaleuca oil for flea control (Bischoff, 1998). Clinical signs in one or more of the cats included hypothermia, ataxia, dehydration, nervousness, trembling, and coma. Moderate increases in serum alanine aminotransferase (ALT) and aspartate aminotransferase (AST) concentrations were noted. Two cats recovered within 48 hours following decontamination and supportive care. However, one cat died approximately 3 days after exposure. The primary constituent of the oil, terpinen-4-ol, was detected in the urine of the cats. Another case involved the dermal application of 7 to 8 drops of oil along the backs of two dogs as a flea repellent (Kaluzienski, 2000). Within approximately 12 hours, one dog developed partial paralysis of the hind limbs, ataxia, and depression. The other dog displayed only depression. Decontamination (bathing) and symptomatic and supportive care resulted in rapid recovery within 24 hours.

Pennyroyal Oil

A volatile oil derived from *Mentha pulegium* and *Hedeoma pulegiodes,* pennyroyal oil has a long history of use as a flea repellent and has been used to induce menstruation and abortion in humans. In one case report of pennyroyal oil toxicosis in the veterinary literature, a dog was dermally exposed to pennyroyal oil at approximately 2 g/kg (Sudekum, 1992). Within 1 hour of application, the dog became listless and within 2 hours began vomiting. At 30 hours after exposure, the dog exhibited diarrhea, hemoptysis, and epistaxis. Soon thereafter, the dog developed seizures and died. Histopathologic examination of liver tissue showed massive hepatocellular necrosis. The toxin in pennyroyal oil is thought to be pulegone, which is bioactivated to a hepatotoxic metabolite called menthofuran.

Oil of Wintergreen

Derived from *Gaultheria procumbens,* this oil contains a glycoside that, when hydrolyzed, releases methyl salicylate. The oil is readily absorbed through the skin and is used to treat muscle aches and pains. Salicylates are toxic to dogs and cats. Because cats metabolize salicylates much more slowly compared with other species, they are more likely to be overdosed. Intoxicated cats may present with depression, anorexia, emesis, gastric hemorrhage, toxic hepatitis, anemia, bone marrow hypoplasia, hyperpnea, and hyperpyrexia (see "Willow" earlier).

Sassafras Oil

Sassafras is the name applied to two trees native to eastern Asia and one native to eastern North America *(Sassafras albidum).* All parts of the tree are aromatic, and the oil is obtained from the peeled root. The main constituent of the oil is safrole (up to 80%). Sassafras has been used as a sudorific and flavoring agent and for the treatment of eye inflammation. The oil has been used externally for relief of insect bites and stings and for removing lice. Because safrole is carcinogenic, the FDA has banned the use of the oil as a food additive. Long-term administration of safrole at 0.66 mg/kg is considered hazardous for humans (Segelman, 1976). Tea samples, prepared as recommended in commonly used herbal medicine information sources or on product labels, contained between 0.09 mg and 4.66 mg per cup (Carlson, 1997). One product that contained 2.5 g of sassafras bark per tea bag was estimated to provide up to a 200-mg dose of safrole (Segelman, 1976). The actual amount of safrole ingested is dependent on the safrole content, the duration of the infusion, and the amount of tea consumed. Oil of sassafras is toxic to adult humans in doses as small as 5 mL (Grande, 1987). Because of toxicity, carcinogenicity, and lack of therapeutic benefit, the use of this plant cannot be recommended under any circumstances.

PRODUCT ADULTERATION

Chinese patent medicines, especially those originating from Hong Kong, have had a long history of being adulterated with metals and conventional pharmaceuticals or containing natural toxins (Ko, 1998; Au, 2000; Ernst, 2002; Dolan, 2003). Sedatives, stimulants, and nonsteroidal anti-inflammatory drugs (NSAIDs) are common conventional pharmaceuticals that are added to patent medicines without labels to indicate their presence. Commonly found natural toxins in Chinese patent medicines include borneol, aconite, toad secretions (*Bufo* spp, Ch'an Su), mylabris, scorpion, borax, acorus, and strychnine *(Strychnos nux-vomica)* (Ko, 1998).

The motivation for adulterating patent medicines is unclear. Perhaps it is believed that conventional pharmaceuticals are necessary to provide immediate relief to the patient while he or she is waiting for the herbs, with a slower onset of action, to have their desired effect, or that the combination provides a synergistic effect. It is also possible that without the addition of potent conventional drugs, the herbal preparations would not be efficacious.

Chinese patent medicines often contain cinnabar (mercuric sulfide), realgar (arsenic sulfide), or litharge (lead oxide) as part of the traditional formula. Recently, dietary supplements, purchased largely from retail stores, were tested for arsenic, cadmium, lead, and mercury (Dolan, 2003). Eighty-four of the 95 products tested contained botanicals as a major component of the formulation. Eleven of the 95 products contained lead at concentrations that would have caused lead intake to exceed recommended maximum levels in children and pregnant women, had the products been used according to label directions.

Serious adverse health effects have been documented in humans who used adulterated Chinese herbal medicines (Ernst, 2002). No cases have been published in the veterinary literature, although the author is aware of one case in which a small dog ingested a number of herbal tea "balls," which were prescribed to its owner for arthritis. The dog presented to a veterinary clinic in acute renal failure several days after the ingestion. Analysis of the formulation revealed low-level heavy metal contamination (mercury and lead) and rather large concentrations of caffeine and the NSAID, indomethacin. The acute renal failure was most likely due to NSAID-induced renal damage.

DRUG–HERB INTERACTIONS

Drug–herb interactions refer to the possibility that an herbal constituent may alter the pharmacologic effects of a conventional drug given concurrently, or vice versa. The result may be either enhanced or diminished drug or herb effects, or the appearance of a new effect that is not anticipated from use of the drug or herb alone. Although several ways of categorizing drug–herb interactions have been proposed, the most logical would seem to characterize interactions from either a pharmacokinetic or a pharmacodynamic perspective (Blumenthal, 2000). Possible pharmacokinetic interactions include those that alter the absorption, metabolism, distribution, or elimination of a drug or herbal constituent, resulting in an increase or decrease in the concentration of active agent at the site of action. For example, herbs that contain dietary fiber, mucilages, or tannins might alter the absorption of another drug or herbal constituent. Herbs containing constituents that induce liver enzymes might be expected to affect drug metabolism or elimination. Induction of liver-metabolizing enzymes can increase the toxicity of drugs and other chemicals via increased production of reactive metabolites. The production of more toxic reactive metabolites is called *bioactivation* (Zhou, 2004). Alternatively, enhanced detoxification of drugs and other chemicals can decrease their toxicity. Long-term use of herbs and other dietary supplements can induce enzymes associated with procarcinogen activation, thus increasing the risk of some cancers (Ryu, 2003; Zhou, 2004). The displacement of one drug from protein-binding sites by another agent increases the concentration of unbound drug available to target tissues. Pharmacodynamic interactions or interactions at receptor sites can occur; these can be agonistic or antagonistic.

The quality of evidence documenting various herb–drug interactions varies. Some interactions are documented in clinical trials, some are inferred from in vitro experiments, and others are suspected only on theoretical grounds. In one study that evaluated the reliability of published reports of drug–herb interactions, only 13% of reports were considered to be well documented, and 68% could not be evaluated because of poor or incomplete information (Fugh-Berman, 2001).

Table 12-4 lists potential drug–herb interactions based on conventional drug therapeutic class. Obviously, some therapeutic classes of drug are not used in veterinary medicine, such as antiparkinsonism drugs, but these are included in an effort to provide as complete an overview as possible. Table 12-5 lists specific drug–herb interactions. The information in Table 12-5 does not indicate whether an interaction is more or less likely to result in an adverse effect. If an interaction is listed, the reader should consult more detailed sources of information to determine its clinical relevance. It is important to point out that information regarding drug–herb interactions is expanding rapidly.

Several references can be consulted for in-depth information about specific drug–herb interactions (McGuffin, 1997; Blumenthal, 1998a and b; American Botanical

Text continued on p. 205

TABLE 12-4

Potential Drug–Herb Interactions Based on Drug Therapeutic Class

Therapeutic Class	Potential Herb Interactions	Possible Adverse Effects
Analgesics	Herbs with diuretic activity (e.g., corn silk, dandelion, juniper, uva ursi)	Increased risk of toxicity with anti-inflammatory analgesics
	Herbs with corticosteroid activity (e.g., licorice, bayberry)	May induce reduction of plasma salicylate concentration
	Herbs with sedative effects (e.g., calamus, nettle, ground ivy, sage, borage)	Possible enhancement of sedative effects
Anticonvulsants	Herbs with sedative effects (e.g., calamus, nettle, ground ivy, sage, borage)	Possible increase in sedative adverse effects; increase risk of seizure
	Herbs containing salicylates (e.g., poplar, willow)	Potentiation of phenytoin action
	Ayurvedic Shankapuspi	Decrease phenytoin half life
Antidepressants	Herbs with sympathomimetic amines (e.g., agnus castus, calamus, cola, broom, licorice)	Increase risk of hypertension with MAOIs; may potentiate sedative adverse effects
	Gingko biloba	Use with tricyclic antidepressants or other medications that ↓ seizure threshold not advised
Antiemetic and antivertigo drugs	Herbs with sedative effects (e.g., calamus, nettle, ground ivy, sage, borage)	May increase sedative effect
	Herbs with anticholinergic effect	Antagonism

Continued

TABLE 12-4

Potential Drug–Herb Interactions Based on Drug Therapeutic Class—cont'd

Therapeutic Class	Potential Herb Interactions	Possible Adverse Effects
Antiparkinsonism drugs	Herbs with anticholinergic effect	Potentiation of effects
	Herbs with cholinergic effect	Antagonism
Antipsychotics	Herbs with diuretic activity (e.g., corn silk, dandelion, juniper, uva ursi)	Potentiation of lithium action; increased risk of intoxication
	Herbs with anticholinergic effect	Reduction of phenothiazine concentrations; increased risk of seizures
	Ginseng, yohimbine, and ephedra	Concomitant use with phenelzine and MAOIs may result in increased adverse effects
Anxiolytics/hypnotics	Herbs with sedative effects (e.g., calamus, nettle, ground ivy, sage, borage)	Potentiation
Phenobarbital	Thujone-containing herbs (e.g., wormwood, sage) or gamolenic acid–containing herbs (e.g., evening primrose oil, borage)	May lower seizure threshold
NSAIDs	Feverfew	Reduce effectiveness of feverfew
	Herbs with antiplatelet activity (e.g., gingko, biloba, ginger, ginseng, garlic)	May increase risk of bleeding due to gastric irritation by NSAIDs
Stimulants	Ginseng	Increased risk of adverse effects
Antiarrhythmics	Herbs with cardioactive effects	Antagonism
	Herbs with diuretic activity (e.g., corn silk, dandelion, juniper, uva ursi)	Antagonism if hypokalemia occurs
Anticoagulants	Herbs with coagulant or anticoagulant activity (e.g., alfalfa, red clover, chamomile, gingko)	Antagonism or potentiation
	Garlic	Decrease platelet activity
	Ginger	Inhibit thromboxane synthetase activity, thus increasing bleeding time
	Herbs containing salicylates (e.g., poplar, willow)	Potentiation
Antihyperlipidemic drugs	Herbs with hypolipidemic activity (e.g., black cohosh, fenugreek, garlic, plantain)	Additive effect
Antihypertensives	Herbs containing hypertensive (blue cohosh, cola, ginger) or mineralocorticoid (e.g., licorice, bayberry) action	Antagonism
	Herbs with hypotensive action (e.g., agrimony, celery, ginger, hawthorn)	Potentiation
	Herbs with high levels of amines or sympathomimetic action (e.g., agnus castus, black cohosh, cola, mate, Saint John's Wort)	Antagonism
	Herbs with diuretic activity (e.g., corn silk, dandelion, juniper, uva ursi)	Potentiation
β blockers	Herbs containing cardioactive constituents	Antagonism
	Herbs with high levels of amines or sympathomimetic action (e.g., agnus castus, black cohosh, cola, mate, Saint John's Wort)	Risk of severe hypertension
Cardiac glycosides	Herbs with cardioactive constituents (e.g., broom, squill, mistletoe, cola nut, figwort)	Antagonism or potentiation
	Hawthorn, Siberian ginseng, Kyushin, uzara root	Increased risk of bleeding
Diuretics	Herbs with diuretic activity (e.g., corn silk, dandelion, juniper, uva ursi)	Increased risk of hypokalemia
	Herbs with hypotensive action (e.g., agrimony, celery, ginger, hawthorn)	Difficulty controlling diuresis

TABLE 12-4

Potential Drug–Herb Interactions Based on Drug Therapeutic Class—cont'd

Therapeutic Class	Potential Herb Interactions	Possible Adverse Effects
Nitrates and calcium channel blockers	Herbs with cardioactive constituents (e.g., broom, squill)	Antagonism
	Herbs with hypertensive action (e.g., bayberry, broom, blue cohosh, licorice)	Antagonism
	Herbs with anticholinergic effects (e.g., corkwood tree)	Reduced buccal absorption of nitroglycerin
Sympathomimetics	Herbs containing sympathomimetic amines (e.g., aniseed, capsicum, parsley, vervain)	Increased risk of hypertension
	Herbs with hypertensive action (e.g., bayberry, broom, blue cohosh, licorice)	Increased risk of hypertension
	Herbs with hypotensive action (e.g., agrimony, celery, ginger, hawthorn)	Antagonism
Antifungals (ketoconazole)	Herbs with anticholinergic effects (e.g., corkwood tree)	Decreased absorption of ketoconazole
Antidiabetic agents	Herbs with hypoglycemic or hyperglycemic principles (e.g., alfalfa, fenugreek, ginseng)	Antagonism or potentiation
	Herbs with diuretic activity (e.g., corn silk, dandelion, juniper, uva ursi)	Antagonism
	Chromium, karela	Effect on blood glucose levels, altering drug requirements
Corticosteroids	Herbs with diuretic activity (e.g., corn silk, dandelion, juniper, uva ursi)	Risk of increased potassium loss
	Herbs with corticosteroid activity (e.g., licorice, bayberry)	Increased risk of adverse effects such as sodium retention
	Herbs with immunostimulant effects	Antagonize immunosuppressive effect
Sex hormones	Herbs with hormonal activity (e.g., alfalfa, bayberry, black cohosh, licorice)	Potential antagonism or potentiation
Estrogens	Herbs containing phytoestrogens (e.g., dong quai, red clover, alfalfa, licorice, black cohosh, soybeans)	Hyperestrogenism
Drugs for hyperthyroidism or hypothyroidism	Herbs with high concentrations of iodine	Interferes with therapy
	Horseradish and kelp	Interferes with therapy
Oral contraceptives	Herbs with hormonal activity (e.g., black cohosh, licorice)	May reduce oral contraceptive effectiveness
Methotrexate	Herbs with salicylates (e.g., meadowsweet, poplar, willow)	Potential for toxicity
Drugs with immunostimulant or immunosuppressive action	Herbs with immunostimulant effects (e.g., boneset, echinacea, mistletoe)	Antagonism or potentiation
Probenecid	Herbs with salicylates (e.g., meadowsweet, poplar, willow)	Inhibition of uricosuric effect of probenecid
Acetazolamide	Herbs with salicylates (e.g., meadowsweet, poplar, willow)	Potential for toxicity
General anesthetics	Herbs with hypotensive constituents (e.g., black cohosh, goldenseal, hawthorn)	Potentiation of hypotension
Muscle relaxants	Herbs with diuretic action (e.g., broom, buchu, corn silk)	Possible potentiation if hypokalemia
Depolarizing muscle relaxants	Herbs with cardioactive constituents (e.g., cola, figwort, hawthorn)	Risk of arrhythmias

From Review of Natural Products, 2000a and b.
MAOI, monoamine oxidase inhibitor; NSAID, nonsteroidal anti-inflammatory drug.

TABLE 12-5

Potential Drug–Herb Interactions

Herb/Supplement	Common Name	Potential Drug Interactions
Acacia	*Acacia senegal*	↓ intestinal absorption of drugs
Aceitilla	*Bidens pilosa*	Insulin and oral hypoglycemic agents
Ackee apple seed	*Blighia sapida*	Insulin and oral hypoglycemic agents
Agar	*Gelidium and Gracilaria* spp	↓ intestinal absorption of drugs
Agrimony	*Agrimonia* spp	Alkaloidal drugs, anticoagulants, insulin, and oral hypoglycemic agents
Alfalfa	*Medicago sativa*	Potential photosensitizing drugs, insulin and oral hypoglycemic agents, lipid-lowering drugs, oral contraceptives/estrogen replacement therapy, vitamin K antagonists
Aloe gel	*Aloe* spp	Corticosteroids
Aloe (dried juice or leaf)	*Aloe* spp	↓ intestinal absorption of drugs, antiarrhythmics, corticosteroids, digoxin, diuretics, insulin, and oral hypoglycemic drugs
Andrographis	*Andrographis paniculata*	APAP, anticoagulants, antihypertensives, immunosuppressants, insulin, and oral hypoglycemic drugs
Angelica	*Angelica* spp	Anticoagulants, potential photosensitizing drugs
Anise	*Pimpinella anisum*	Anticoagulants, anticonvulsants, oral contraceptives/ estrogen replacement therapy, iron, MAOIs
Annatto	*Bixa orellana*	Insulin and oral hypoglycemics
Arnica	*Arnica montana*	Anticoagulants
Ashwagandha	*Withania somnifera*	Azathioprine, barbiturates, benzodiazepines, CNS depressants, cyclophosphamide, immunosuppressants, insulin and oral hypoglycemic agents, paclitaxel, prednisolone, thyroid replacement therapy
Astragalus	*Astragalus membranaceus*	Acyclovir, anticoagulants, cyclophosphamide, immunosuppressants, interferon α_1, interleukin-2
Autumn crocus	*Colchicum autumnale*	Fluoxetine, MAOIs
Bai zhi	*Angelica dahurica*	Drugs metabolized by CYP2C, CYP3A, and CYP2D1 P-450 enzymes
Bai zhu	*Atractylodes* spp	Insulin and oral hypoglycemic agents
Baikal skullcap	*Scutellaria baicalensis*	Drugs metabolized by CYP1A1/2 P-450 enzyme, 5-fluorouracil, anticoagulants, benzodiazepines, CNS depressants, cyclophosphamide, insulin, and oral hypoglycemic agents
Balloon cotton	*Asclepias fruticosa*	Digoxin or other cardiac glycosides
Balloon flower	*Platycodon grandiflorum*	APAP, CNS depressants
Banana	*Musa sapientum*	Aspirin, NSAIDs, insulin and oral hypoglycemics, prednisolone, cysteamine, enteral nutrition, insulin, and oral hypoglycemic agents
Banyan stem	*Ficus bengalensis*	Insulin and oral hypoglycemic agents
Barberry	*Berberis vulgaris*	Drugs metabolized by P-450 enzymes, APAP, α-adrenergic agents, antiarrhythmics, antibiotics, antihypertensives, CNS depressants, cyclophosphamide, cardiac glycosides, general anesthetics, MAOIs, potential photosensitizers, pyrimethamine, and tetracyclines
Barleria plant	*Hygrophilia auriculata*	APAP, thioacetamine
Bay leaf	*Laurus nobilis*	Drubs metabolized by CYP2B P-450 enzyme
Bayberry	*Myrica cerifera*	Corticosteroids
Belladonna	*Atropa belladonna*	Anticholinergic drugs

TABLE 12-5

Potential Drug–Herb Interactions—cont'd

Herb/Supplement	Common Name	Potential Drug Interactions
Betel nut	*Areca catechu*	Alkaloidal drugs, anticholinergic drugs, cholinergic drugs, procyclidine, and thyroid medications
Bilberry	*Vaccinium myrtillus*	Alkaloidal drugs, anticoagulants, insulin, and oral hypoglycemic agents
Bishop's weed	*Ammi visnaga*	Drugs metabolized by P-450 enzymes, antihypertensives, calcium channel blockers, cardiac glycosides, and drugs with potential hepatotoxic and photosensitizing effects
Bitter melon	*Momordica charantia*	Insulin and oral hypoglycemics
Bitter orange	*Citrus aurantium*	Ephedrine, drugs metabolized by CYP3A4 P-450 enzyme, MAOIs, and potential photosensitizers
Black currant	*Ribes nigrum*	Anticoagulants, diuretics
Black hellebore	*Helleborus niger*	Cardiac glycosides, quinidine, quinine
Black pepper	*Piper nigrum*	Drugs metabolized by P-450 enzymes, coenzyme Q10, barbiturates, NSAIDs, phenytoin, propranolol, methylxanthines, and zoxazolamine
Black seed	*Nigella sativa*	Anticoagulants, antihypertensives, cisplatin, and doxorubicin
Black walnut	*Juglans nigra*	Alkaloidal drugs
Blackberry	*Rubus fruticosus*	Insulin and oral hypoglycemics
Blazing star	*Aletris farinosa*	Oxytocin
Blessed thistle	*Cnicus benedictus*	Alkaloidal drugs
Blue cohosh	*Caulophyllum thalictroides*	Nicotine
Bogbean	*Menyanthes trifoliata*	Anticoagulants
Boldo leaf	*Peumus boldus*	Drugs metabolized by CYP1A and CYP3A P-450 enzymes, anticoagulants
Borage	*Borago officinalis*	Anticoagulants, drugs with hepatotoxic potential, and tamoxifen
Brahmi	*Bacopa monniera*	Barbiturates, phenothiazines
Bromelain	*Ananas comosus*	Antibiotics, anticoagulants, chemotherapeutic drugs, and cyclosporine
Buckthorn	*Rhamnus frangula*	↓ intestinal absorption of other drugs, corticosteroids, cardiac glycosides, and diuretics
Bugleweed	*Lycopus virginicus*	Thyroid drugs
Burdock	*Arctium* spp	APAP, insulin, and oral hypoglycemics
Butcher's broom	*Ruscus aculeatus*	α-adrenergic agonists
Calendula	*Calendula officinalis*	Acyclovir, CNS depressants
California poppy	*Eschscholzia californica*	Analgesics, barbiturates, benzodiazepines, CNS depressants, and MAOIs
Carrageenan gum	*Gigartina mamillosa*	↓ intestinal absorption of other drugs
Cascara sagrada	*Rhamnus purshiana*	↓ intestinal absorption of other drugs
Castor oil	*Ricinus communis*	Cardioactive glycosides
Castor-aralia tree	*Kalopanax pictus*	Insulin and oral hypoglycemic agents
Catnip leaf	*Nepeta cataria*	CNS depressants, barbiturates
Cat's claw	*Uncaria tomentosa*	Drug metabolized by CYP3A4 P-450 enzyme, antihypertensives, chemotherapeutic drugs, immunosuppressive drugs, and NSAIDs
Cayenne	*Capsicum* spp	Drugs metabolized by P-450 enzymes, ACE inhibitors, antihypertensives, anticoagulants, aspirin, barbiturates, CNS depressants, ethylmorphine, insulin and oral hypoglycemic agents, MAOIs, NSAIDs, and methylxanthines
Celery	*Apium graveolens*	APAP, anticoagulants, drugs with photosensitizing potential, thioacetamine, thyroxine

Continued

TABLE 12-5

Potential Drug–Herb Interactions—cont'd

Herb/Supplement	Common Name	Potential Drug Interactions
Cereus	*Selenicereus grandiflorus*	Cardiac drugs, cardioactive glycosides, and MAOIs
Chamomile	*Matricaria recutita, Chamomilla recutita*	Drugs metabolized by CYP1A2 and CYP3A4 P-450 enzymes, anticoagulants, aspirin, benzodiazepines, CNS depressants, iron, and chemotherapeutic agents
Chan su		Cardiac glycosides
Chaparral	*Larrea tridentate*	Potentially hepatoxic drugs, MAOIs
Chard	*Beta vulgaris*	Insulin and oral hypoglycemic agents
Chaste tree	*Vitex agnus castus*	Bromocriptine, dopamine agonists, oral contraceptives, and estrogen replacement therapy
Chicory	*Chichorium intybus*	Insulin and oral hypoglycemic agents
Chinese cinnamon	*Cinnamomum aromaticum, C. cassia*	Drugs metabolized by P-450 enzymes, metacycline, and tetracycline
Cinchona bark	*Cinchona* spp	Anticoagulants, digoxin, mefloquine, and neuromuscular blocking agents
Cloves	*Syzgium aromaticum*	Anticoagulants
Cocoa	*Theobroma cacao*	APAP, anticoagulants, aspirin, benzodiazepines, cimetidine, clozapine, disulfiram, ephedrine, ergotamine, fluvoxamine, furafylline, grapefruit juice, ibuprofen, idrocilamide, insulin and oral hypoglycemic agents, iron, lithium, MAOIs, methotrexate, methoxsalen, mexiletine, oral contraceptives, phenylpropanolamine, quinolone antibiotics, terbinafine, theophylline, and verapamil
Cola	*Cola nitida*	Benzodiazepines, β-adrenergic agonists, methylxanthines, cimetidine, clozapine, disulfiram, ephedrine, furafylline, grapefruit juice, NSAIDs, idrocilamide, insulin and oral hypoglycemic agents, lithium, MAOIs, methotrexate, methoxsalen, mexiletine, oral contraceptives, phenylpropanolamine, propranolol, pseudoephedrine, quinolone antibiotics, terbinafine, theophylline, and verapamil
Coltsfoot	*Tussilago farfara*	Alkaloidal drugs, antihypertensives, cardiovascular drugs, and drugs with hepatotoxic potential
Coriander	*Coriandrum sativum*	Insulin and oral hypoglycemic agents
Cranberry	*Vaccinium* spp	Omeprazole
Crucifer	*Brassica* spp	Anticoagulants, drugs metabolized by CYP1A2 P-450
Cumin	*Cuminum cyminum*	Anticoagulants, insulin and oral hypoglycemic agents
Damiana	*Turnera diffusa*	Insulin and oral hypoglycemic agents
Dan shen	*Salvia miltiorrhiza*	Anticoagulants, cardiac glycosides
Dandelion	*Taraxacum officinale*	Drugs metabolized by CYP1A2 and CYP2E P-450 enzymes, anticoagulants, quinolone antibiotics, diuretics, insulin and oral hypoglycemic agents, and lithium
Devil's claw	*Harpagophytum procumbens*	Antiarrhythmics, anticoagulants, antihypertensives, cardiac drugs, and antihypertensives
Dogbane	*Apocynum cannabinum*	Cardiac glycosides
Dong quai	*Angelica sinensis*	APAP, anticoagulants, oral contraceptives, and estrogen replacement therapy
Echinacea	*Echinacea* spp	Drugs metabolized by CYP3A4 P-450 enzymes, chemotherapeutic agents, econazole, and immunosuppressants

TABLE 12-5

Potential Drug–Herb Interactions—cont'd

Herb/Supplement	Common Name	Potential Drug Interactions
Elder	*Sambucus nigra*	Insulin and oral hypoglycemic agents
Elder, American	*Sambucus Canadensis*	Drugs metabolized by CYP3A4 P-450 enzymes
Ephedra	*Ephedra sinica*	Anticonvulsants, antihypertensives, antacids, β blockers, bromocriptine, bupropion, methylxanthines, corticosteroids, cardiac glycosides, diuretics, urine-alkalizing drugs, entacapone, epinephrine, ergotamine, general anesthetics, guanethidine, insulin and oral hypoglycemic agents, linezolid, MAOIs, methyldopa, methylphenidate, methylxanthines, morphine, oxytocin, pseudoephedrine, reserpine, sibutramine, sympathomimetics, stimulants, thyroid replacement therapy, and tricyclic antidepressants
Eucalyptus	*Eucalyptus globules*	Drugs metabolized by P-450 enzymes, insulin, and oral hypoglycemic agents
Evening primrose oil	*Oenothera biennis*	Anticoagulants, general anesthetics, phenothiazines, and tamoxifen
Fennel	*Foeniculum vulgare*	ACE inhibitors, antihypertensives, ciprofloxacin, and diuretics
Fenugreek	*Trigonella foenum-graecum*	May alter drug absorption; anticoagulants, insulin, and oral hypoglycemic agents
Feverfew	*Tanacetum parthenium*	Anticoagulants, paclitaxel
Figwort	*Scrophularia nodosa*	Cardiac glycosides
Flaxseed	*Linum usitatissimum*	Alter drug absorption; anticoagulants, insulin and oral hypoglycemic agents, and hormone replacement therapy
Foxglove	*Digitalis* spp	Albuterol, amiodarone, aminoglycosides, amphotericin B, antacids, anticoagulants, antiarrhythmics, bleomycin, calcium channel blockers, carmustine, cholestyramine, colestipol, cyclosporine, cytarabine, cardiac glycosides, diuretics, doxorubicin, erythromycin, flecainide, hydroxychloroquine, NSAIDs, itraconazole, macrolide antibiotics, tetracycline, nefazodone, penicillamine, phenytoin, procarbazine, propafenone, quinidine, sulphasalazine, stimulant laxatives, trozodone, verapamil, and vincristine
Frangipani	*Plumeria rubra*	Cardiac glycosides
Fucus	*Fucus* spp	Altered drug absorption; anticoagulants, diuretics, hyperthyroid medications, iodine-containing drugs, lithium, and thyroid replacement therapy
γ-Linolenic acid	NA	Anticoagulants, paclitaxel, and tamoxifen
Garlic	*Allium sativum*	Drugs metabolized by CYP3A, CYP2B1, CYP2C, CYP2D, and CYP2E1 P-450 enzymes; APAP, antacids, anticoagulants, antihypertensives, doxorubicin, insulin and oral hypoglycemic agents, isoprenaline, and saquinavir
Genipap	*Genipa americana*	Drugs metabolized by P-450 enzymes
Ginger	*Zingiber officinale*	Anticoagulants, aspirin, chemotherapeutic agents, barbiturates, NSAIDs, insulin and oral hypoglycemic agents, and SSRIs

Continued

TABLE 12-5

Potential Drug–Herb Interactions—cont'd

Herb/Supplement	Common Name	Potential Drug Interactions
Gingko	*Gingko biloba*	5-FU, drugs metabolized by CYP3A4 and CYP2D6 P-450 enzymes, anticoagulants, anticonvulsants, cyclosporine, doxorubicin, fluoxetine, general anesthetics, gentamicin, haloperidol, insulin and oral hypoglycemic agents, MAOIs, meclofenoxate, SSRIs, thiazide diuretics, trazodone, and trimipramine
Ginseng, American	*Panax quinquefolius*	Cyclophosphamide, doxorubicin, insulin and oral hypoglycemic agents, methotrexate, morphine, oral contraceptives and hormone replacement therapy, paclitaxel, and tamoxifen
Ginseng, Asian	*P. ginseng*	Drugs metabolized by CYP2D6 P-450 enzymes, anticoagulants, antihypertensives, anxiolytics, methylxanthines, cardiac glycosides, immunosuppressants, insulin and oral hypoglycemic agents, kanamycin, MAOIs, monomycin, morphine, stimulants, and zidovudine
Globularia	*Globularia alypum*	Insulin and oral hypoglycemic agents
Goat's rue	*Galega officinalis*	Anticoagulants and insulin and oral hypoglycemic agents
Goldenrod	*Solidago virguarea*	Diuretics and lithium
Goldenseal	*Hydrastis canadensis*	Drugs metabolized by CYP3A4 P-450 enzymes, APAP, α-adrenergic agonists, anticoagulants, antiarrhythmics, antihypertensives, CNS depressants, cyclophosphamide, cardiac glycosides, general anesthetics, NSAIDs and other highly protein-bound drugs, isoprenaline, MAOIs, paclitaxel, barbiturates, potential photosensitizers, pyrimethamine, and tetracycline
Goldthread, coptis	*Coptis* spp	Chemotherapeutic agents, MAOIs
Gossypol	*Gossypium* spp	Drugs metabolized by P-450 enzymes, alkylating agents, cardiac glycosides, diuretics, isoproterenol, barbiturates, stimulant laxatives, and thyroid replacement therapy
Gotu kola	*Centella asiatica*	Aspirin, CNS depressants, insulin, and oral hypoglycemic agents
Grape	*Vitis vinifera*	Drugs metabolized by P-450 enzymes, APAP, anticoagulants, idarubicin, and cyclophosphamide
Gravel root	*Eupatorium purpureum*	Drugs with hepatotoxic potential
Guar gum	*Cyamopsis tetragonolobus*	Alter drug absorption, provide enteral nutritional support
Guarana	*Paullinia cupana*	APAP, alkaloidal drugs, anticoagulants, aspirin, benzodiazepines, β-adrenergic agonists, cimetidine, clozapine, disulfiram, ephedrine, ergotamine, fluvoxamine, furafylline, NSAIDs, idrocilamide, insulin and oral hypoglycemic agents, lithium, MAOIs, methotrexate, methoxsalen, mexiletine, oral contraceptives, phenylpropanolamine, propranolol, quinolones, terbinafine, methylxanthines, and verapamil
Guava	*Psidium* spp	Alkaloidal drugs, insulin, and oral hypoglycemic agents
Guggul	*Commiphora mukul*	Diltiazem, propranolol, and thyroid replacement therapy

TABLE 12-5

Potential Drug–Herb Interactions—cont'd

Herb/Supplement	Common Name	Potential Drug Interactions
Hawthorn	*Crataegus oxyacantha*	Anticoagulants, antihypertensives, cardiac drugs, CNS depressants, and vasodilators
Hellebore, American	*Veratrum verde*	Antihypertensives
Henbane	*Atropa belladonna*	Anticholinergic agents
Hops	*Humulus lupulus*	Drugs metabolized by CYP2B and CYP1A P-450 enzymes, CNS depressants, oral contraceptives, and hormone replacement therapy
Horehound	*Marrubium vulgare*	Antihypertensives, insulin, and oral hypoglycemic agents
Horse chestnut	*Aesculus hippocastanum*	Anticoagulants, diuretics, insulin, and oral hypoglycemic agents
Horseradish	*Armoracia rusticana*	Thyroid replacement therapy
Horsetail	*Equisetum arvense*	Cardiac glycosides, diuretics, and lithium
Iboga	*Tabernanthe iboga*	Drugs altering serotonin concentrations in CNS, morphine
Iceland moss	*Cetraria islandica*	Alter drug absorption
Indian snakeroot	*Rauvolfia serpentina*	Drugs that are substrates of PGP, anticoagulants, antihypertensives, barbiturates, benzodiazepines, CNS depressants, cardiac glycosides, diuretics, general anesthetics, MAOIs, neuroleptics, quinidine, sympathomimetics, and tricyclic antidepressants
Ivy	*Hedera helix*	Anticoagulants
Java tea	*Orthosiphon* spp	Diuretics
Jimsonweed	*Datura stramonium*	Anticholinergic drugs
Juniper	*Juniperus* spp	Anticoagulants, insulin, and oral hypoglycemic agents
Kava	*Piper methysticum*	Alprazolam, antipsychotics, barbiturates, benzodiazepines, CNS depressants, estrogens, and drugs with hepatotoxic potential
Kelp	Various species	Anticoagulants, iodine-containing drugs, lithium, and thyroid replacement therapy
Khat	*Catha edulis*	Amoxicillin, amphetamines, ampicillin, guanethidine, indoramin, MAOIs, sympathomimetics, and thyroid replacement therapy
Kudzu	*Pueraria lobata*	Drugs metabolized by P-450 enzymes
Lagerstroemia	*Lagerstroemia speciosa*	Insulin and oral hypoglycemic agents
Lavender	*Lavandula* spp	Alkaloidal drugs, barbiturates, and CNS depressants
Lemon balm	*Melissa officinalis*	Barbiturates, CNS depressants, and thyroid replacement therapy
Lemongrass	*Cymbopogon citratus*	Drugs metabolized by CYP2B P-450 enzymes
Licorice	*Glycyrrhiza glabra*	Drugs metabolized by CYP1A2, CYP2B, and CYP3A4 P-450 enzymes; APAP, amiloride, amphotericin B, anticoagulants, antihypertensives, aspirin, cimetidine, corticosteroids, cyclophosphamide, cardiac glycosides, diuretics, oral contraceptives and estrogen replacement therapy, NSAIDs, insulin and oral hypoglycemic agents, MAOIs, spironolactone, stimulant laxatives, and sympathomimetics
Lily of the valley	*Convallaria majalis*	Calcium, corticosteroids, cardiac glycosides, quinidine, saluretics, and stimulant laxatives
LIV 100	Ayurvedic formulation	Isoniazid, pyrazinamide, and rifampicin
Long pepper	*Piper longum*	Drugs metabolized by P-450 enzymes, aspirin, coenzyme Q10, barbiturates, NSAIDs, phenytoin, propranolol, methylxanthines, and zoxazolamine

Continued

TABLE 12-5

Potential Drug–Herb Interactions—cont'd

Herb/Supplement	Common Name	Potential Drug Interactions
Lovage	*Levisticum officinale*	Anticoagulants
Lycium	*Lycium barbarum*	Anticoagulants
Madagascar periwinkle	*Catharanthus roseus*	Insulin and oral hypoglycemic agents, cardiac glycosides, vincristine, and vinblastine
Maté	*Ilex paraguariensis*	Drugs metabolized by CYP1A2 P-450 enzymes, alkaloidal drugs, APAP, aspirin, benzodiazepines, β-adrenergic agonists, cimetidine, clozapine, disulfiram, ephedrine, ergotamine, fluvoxamine, furafylline, NSAIDs, idrocilamide, insulin and oral hypoglycemic agents, lithium, MAOIs, methotrexate, methoxsalen, mexiletine, oral contraceptives, phenylpropanolamine, quinolones, terbinafine, methylxanthines, and verapamil
Milk thistle	*Silybum marianum*	Drugs metabolized by CYP3A4 and CYP2C9 P-450 enzymes, drugs transported by PGP, APAP, aspirin, butyrophenones, cisplatin, cyclosporine, doxorubicin, general anesthetics, insulin and oral hypoglycemic agents, oral contraceptives, phenothiazines, tacrine, and vincristine
Mistletoe	*Viscum album*	Chemotherapeutic agents, MAOIs, and radiotherapy
Motherwort	*Leonurus cardiaca*	Alkaloidal drugs, anticoagulants, CNS depressants, and cardiac glycosides
Myrrh	*Commiphora molmol*	Cyclophosphamide, NSAIDs
Neem	*Azadirachta indica*	Insulin and oral hypoglycemic agents, glyburide/glibenclamide, and thyroid replacement therapy
Nettle, stinging	*Urtica dioica folia*	Antihypertensives, anticoagulants, CNS depressants, diuretics, insulin, and oral hypoglycemic agents
Noni	*Morinda* spp	Oral hypoglycemic agents
Nutmeg	*Myristica fragrans*	Drugs metabolized by CYP1A1, CYP1A2, and CYP2E1 P-450 enzymes, flunitrazepam, and MAOIs
Oats	*Avena sativa*	Alter drug absorption; morphine and protease inhibitors
Olive	*Olea europaea*	Antihypertensives, insulin, and oral hypoglycemic agents
Onion	*Allium cepa*	Drugs metabolized by CYP1A, CYP2B, and CYP2E1 P-450 enzymes; anticoagulants, insulin, and oral hypoglycemic agents
Opium poppy	*Papaver somniferum*	CNS depressants
Oregon grape	*Berberis aquifolium*	Drugs metabolized by P-450 enzymes; APAP, α-adrenergic agonists, antiarrhythmics, anticoagulants, antihypertensives, cyclophosphamide, cardiac glycosides, general anesthetics, MAOIs, potential photosensitizing drugs, pyrimethamine, and tetracycline
Papaya extract/papain	*Carica papaya*	Anticoagulants, cyclophosphamide, and diuretics
Passion flower	*Passiflora incarnate*	Anticoagulants, anxiolytics, CNS depressants, and barbiturates
Pau d'Arco	*Tabebuia* spp	Anticoagulants
Pennyroyal oil	*Mentha pulegium*	Drugs with hepatotoxic potential, iron
Peppermint	*Mentha piperita*	Drugs metabolized by CYP1A2 and CYP2E P-450 enzymes, drugs ↓ gastric acid secretion, and iron
Periwinkle	*Vinca minor*	Cardiac glycosides, vincristine, and vinblastine

TABLE 12-5

Potential Drug–Herb Interactions—cont'd

Herb/Supplement	Common Name	Potential Drug Interactions
Pheasant's eye	*Adonis vernalis*	Albuterol, amiodarone, aminoglycosides, amphotericin B, antacids, antiarrhythmics, bleomycin, calcium, calcium channel blockers, carmustine, cholestyramine, colestipol, cyclophosphamide, cyclosporine, cytarabine, cardiac glycosides, diuretics, doxorubicin, erythromycin, flecainide, glucocorticosteroids, hydroxychloroquine, NSAIDs, itraconazole, laxatives, macrolide antibiotics, tetracycline, nefazodone, penicillamine, phenytoin, procarbazine, propafenone, quinidine, quinine, saluretics, trazodone, verapamil, and vincristine
Phyllanthus	*Phyllanthus* spp	Cyclosporine
Plantain	*Plantago* spp	Alter drug absorption
Pleurisy root	*Asclepias tuberose*	Cardiac glycosides
Prickly pear	*Opuntia* spp	Insulin and oral hypoglycemic agents
Psyllium	*Plantago* spp	Alter drug absorption; calcium, carbamazepine, cholestyramine, colestid, cardiac glycosides, estrogen, insulin and oral hypoglycemic agents, lithium, and protease inhibitors
Quercetin	Found in many herbs	Drugs metabolized by CYP1A2 P-450 enzymes, cisplatin, and tamoxifen
Raspberry	*Rubus idaeus*	Alkaloidal drugs
Red clover	*Trifolium pretense*	Drugs metabolized by CYP3A4 P-450 enzymes, estrogen, and oral contraceptives
Red sandalwood	*Pterocarpus santalinus*	Insulin and oral hypoglycemic agents
Reishi	*Ganoderma lucidum*	Acyclovir, anticoagulants, antihypertensives, antibiotics, cefazolin, immunosuppressants, insulin and oral hypoglycemic agents, and interferon
Rhubarb	*Rheum officinale*	Alter drug absorption; antiarrhythmics, cisplatin, corticosteroids, cardiac glycosides, diuretics, laxatives, and quinidine
Roman chamomile	*Chamaemelum nobile*	Drugs metabolized by P-450 enzymes; CNS depressants, insulin, and oral hypoglycemic agents
Rosemary	*Rosmarinus officinalis*	Drugs metabolized by CYP1A, CYP2E, and CYP3A P-450 enzymes, PGP substrates, cyclophosphamide, diuretics, insulin and oral hypoglycemic agents, and iron
Rue	*Ruta graveolens*	Anticoagulants
Sacred basil	*Ocimum sanctum*	Anticoagulants, barbiturates, bromocriptine, doxorubicin, insulin and oral hypoglycemic agents, isoproterenol, and thyroid medications
Safflower	*Carthamus tintorius*	Anticoagulants
Sage	*Salvia officinalis*	Alkaloidal drugs
Saiboku-to	Herb mixture	Benzodiazepines, prednisolone
Sairei-To TJ-114	Contains glycyrrhizin	Gentamicin
Sarsaparilla	*Smilax* spp	Bismuth, cardiac glycosides, and hypnotics
Sassafras	*Sassafras albidum*	Drugs metabolized by P-450 enzymes
Saw palmetto	*Serenoa repens, Sabal serrulata*	Drugs metabolized by CYP3A4 P-450 enzymes; alkaloidal drugs, anticoagulants, doxazosin, estrogens, finasteride, immunomodulatory drugs, oral contraceptives, and terazosin

Continued

TABLE 12-5

Potential Drug–Herb Interactions—cont'd

Herb/Supplement	Common Name	Potential Drug Interactions
Scopolia	*Scopolia carniolica*	Amantadine, quinidine, and tricyclic antidepressants
Scotch broom	*Cytisus scoparius*	Drugs metabolized by CYP2D6 P-450 enzymes, MAOIs, and sympathomimetics
Skullcap	*Scutellaria lateriflora*	CNS depressants
Senega snakeroot	*Polygala senega*	Insulin and oral hypoglycemic agents
Senna	*Cassia* and *Senna* spp	Alter intestinal absorption of drugs; antiarrhythmics, corticosteroids, cardiac glycosides, and diuretics
Shankhapushpi	Herb mixture	Phenytoin
Shiitake mushrooms	*Lentinula edodes*	Anticoagulants, chemotherapeutic agents, and didanosine
Sho-saiko-To TJ-9	Herb mixture containing glycyrrhizin	Drugs metabolized by CYP3A4 and CYP1A2 P-450 enzymes, insulin and oral hypoglycemic agents, lamivudine, interferon-α, prednisolone, and tolbutamide
Siberian ginseng	*Eleutherococcus senticosis*	Drugs metabolized by CYP3A4 P-450 enzymes, barbiturates, CNS depressants, cytarabine, cardiac glycosides, insulin and oral hypoglycemic agents, kanamycin, and monomycin
Slippery elm	*Ulmus* spp	Alter drug absorption
Soybeans	*Glycine max*	Cisplatin, estrogen, oral hypoglycemic agents, MAOIs, tamoxifen, and thyroid replacement therapy
Squill	*Urginea maritima*	Cardiac glycosides, laxatives, quinidine, and saluretics
Saint John's Wort	*Hypericum perforatum*	Anticoagulants, drugs metabolized by CYP3A4 P-450 enzymes, drugs transported by PGP, alprazolam, amsacrine, amitriptyline, amphetamines, methylxanthines, carbamazepine, cyclosporine, dextromethorphan, cardiac glycosides, etoposide, fexofenadine, general anesthetics, L-tryptophan, lithium, MAOIs, mianserin, midazolam, moclobemide, morphine, nevirapine, nifedipine, NNRTIs, nortriptyline, offenfluramine, oral contraceptives, phenprocoumon, potential photosensitizing drugs, protease inhibitors, reserpine, drugs that alter serotonin concentrations, sildenafil, simvastatin, tramadol, SSRIs, tolbutamide, trazodone, tricyclic antidepressants, and venlafaxine
Stephania	*Stephania tetrandra*	Anticoagulants, calcium channel blockers
Strophanthus	*Strophanthus* spp	Anticoagulants, cardiac glycosides
Sweet basil	*Ocimum basilicum*	Drugs metabolized by P-450 enzymes
Sweet clover	*Melilotus officinalis*	Anticoagulants
Tarragon	*Artemisia dracunculus*	Benzodiazepines
Tea	*Camellia sinensis*	Alter drug absorption, drugs metabolized by CYP1A1, CYP1A2, and CYP2B1 P-450 enzymes; anticoagulants, APAP, aspirin, drugs used for atopic dermatitis, benzodiazepines, β-adrenergic agonists, cimetidine, cisplatin, clozapine, disulfiram, doxorubicin, ephedrine, ergotamine, estrogen, fluvoxamine, furafylline, NSAIDs, idrocilamide, insulin and oral hypoglycemic agents, iron, lithium, MAOIs, methotrexate, methoxsalen, metoprolol,

TABLE 12-5

Potential Drug–Herb Interactions—cont'd

Herb/Supplement	Common Name	Potential Drug Interactions
		mexiletine, oral contraceptives, phenylpropanolamine, propranolol, quinolones, terbinafine, methylxanthines, and verapamil
Thorny burnet	*Sarcopoterium spinosum*	Insulin and oral hypoglycemic agents
Tonka	*Dipteryx* spp	Anticoagulants
Trikatu	Herb mixture	Drugs metabolized by P-450 enzymes; aspirin, coenzyme Q10, barbiturates, NSAIDs, isoniazid, phenytoin, propranolol, rifampicin, methylxanthines, and zoxazolamine
Tumeric	*Curcuma longa*	Drugs metabolized by CYPA1, CYP1a2, and CYP2B1 P-450 enzymes; anticoagulants, cyclosporine, NSAIDs, and reserpine
Uva ursi	*Arctostaphylos uva ursi*	β-Lactam antibiotics, alkaloidal drugs, corticosteroids, and NSAIDs
Valerian root	*Valeriana officinalis*	Drugs metabolized by CYP3A4 P-450 enzymes; barbiturates, benzodiazepines, and CNS depressants
Vervain	*Verbena officinalis*	Anticoagulants, iron
Watercress	*Nasturtium officinale*	Anticoagulants, drugs metabolized by CYP1A1/2 and CYP2E1, APAP, and chlorzoxazone
Wild carrot	*Daucus carota*	Antihypertensives
Willow	*Salix* spp	Alter drug absorption; salicylates
Wintergreen	*Gaultheria procumbens*	Anticoagulants, salicylates
Witch hazel	*Hamamelis virginiana*	Alter drug absorption
Wormwood	*Artemisia absinthium*	APAP, alkaloidal drugs, and barbiturates
Yellow oleander	*Thevetia peruviana*	Cardiac glycosides
Yi mu cao	*Herba leonuri*	Drugs metabolized by CYP3A4 P-450 enzymes
Yin yang huo	*Herba eppimedii*	Drugs metabolized by CYP3A4 P-450 enzymes
Yohimbe	*Pausinystalia yohimbe*	α-Adrenergic antagonists, antihypertensives, β blockers, benzodiazepines, clonidine, CNS stimulants, insulin and oral hypoglycemic agents, levodopa, MAOIs, morphine, phenothiazines, reserpine, SSRIs, sympathomimetics, tricyclic antidepressants, venlafaxine, and xylazine
Yoko	*Paullinia yoko*	Drugs metabolized by CYP1A2 P-450 enzymes

From Review of Natural Products, 2000a and b; Herr, 2002.

NA, not applicable; APAP, acetaminophen; MAOI, monoamine oxidase inhibitor; CNS, central nervous system; ACE, angiotensin-converting enzyme; SSRI, selective serotonin reuptake inhibitor; 5-FU, 5-fluorouracil; PGP, p-glycoprotein; NNRTI, nonnucleoside reverse transcriptase inhibitors.

Council, 1998; Brinker, 1998; Blumenthal, 2000; Review of Natural Products, 2000a and b; Herr, 2002).

DIAGNOSIS OF INTOXICATION

Without a history of exposure to an herbal remedy, the diagnosis of intoxication is difficult. Clinical signs are often nonspecific, and the animal may have concurrent signs caused by an underlying disease condition. Vomitus or gastric lavage material should be examined for the presence of plants or other possible herbal formulations. Essential oil exposure might be suspected on the basis of odor of stomach contents or skin. In some instances, a constituent of an herbal remedy may be detected in a biological specimen. For example, pulegone was found in liver tissue from a dog intoxicated by pennyroyal oil (Sudekum, 1992). Some laboratories have the capability to detect potential patent medicine adulterants. However, many veterinary diagnostic laboratories do not have such broad capabilities to detect natural products, and laboratory confirmation of exposure or intoxication is often impossible. In suspected herbal poisonings, a veterinary toxicologist should be consulted about available laboratory procedures and appropriate tissue samples for submission.

TREATMENT OF INTOXICATION

Treatment is directed toward undertaking appropriate decontamination procedures such as inducing emesis and administering activated charcoal with or without a cathartic (Poppenga, 2004). Indications and contraindications for decontamination procedures should be followed. In general, other treatment is symptomatic and supportive. In rare cases, an antidote might be available (e.g., digoxin Fab fragments for cardiac glycosides). The adage "treat the symptoms and not the patient" is appropriate in most suspected poisonings due to herbal preparations.

SOURCES OF INFORMATION

Because of the increased interest in natural products, there has been an explosion of information regarding their use and potential hazards of use. It is important for individuals to have access to objective, science-based information so they can make rational decisions regarding the safety and efficacy of plant-derived chemicals. Three excellent resources are *The Botanical Safety Handbook,* prepared for the Standards Committee of the American Herbal Products Association (AHPA); the German Commission E monographs, which have recently become available in English; and, more recently, *The Review of Natural Products* (McGuffin, 1997; Blumenthal, 1998; DerMarderosian, 2001a). An excellent lay-oriented reference is entitled *The Honest Herbal: A Sensible Guide to the Use of Herbs and Related Remedies* (Tyler, 1993). In addition, excellent chapters regarding risks associated with the use of natural products can be found in several human-oriented toxicology textbooks (Hung, 1998; Ko, 1998; Palmer, 2001). Essential oil toxicology is extensively covered in a text by Tisserand and Balacs and a chapter by Vassallo (Tisserand, 1999; Vassallo, 2001).

A relatively recent study suggested that six commonly used herbal references contained insufficient information for the assessment and management of suspected ADRs of herbal remedies (Haller, 2002). The Natural Medicines Comprehensive Database (www.naturaldatabase.com) was considered by the authors to be the most complete and useful reference source.

Finally, several other internet Web sites provide herb-related information and links to other herb information resources. These include the American Botanical Council (www.herbalgram.org), the Herb Research Foundation (www.herbs.org), and the American Society of Pharmacognosy (www.phcog.org) Web sites. Unfortunately, membership or a subscription is required for individuals to fully access information on these sites. The FDA (www.fda.gov) and the National Institute of Health's National Center for Complementary and Alternative Medicine (NCCAM) (nccam.nih.gov) are two government-sponsored sites that provide free information. The FDA site provides consumer alerts and advisories about herbs/dietary supplements and mechanism for reporting possible adverse effects related to herb/dietary supplement use. The NCCAM site, in addition to providing alerts and advisories, provides suggestions for evaluating medical resources on the Web for objectivity and accuracy. HerbMed® (www.herbmed.org) is an interactive, electronic herbal database sponsored by the Alternative Medicine Foundation that provides hyperlinked access to evidence-based data on the use of herbs for health. A subscription is required if one is to obtain all of the information provided on the site. For access to the scientific literature, PubMed (www.pubmed.org), sponsored by the National Library of Medicine, contains more than 14 million citations from the biomedical literature dating back to the 1950s.

References

American Botanical Council. Herb Reference Guide (pamphlet). Austin, Tex: American Botanical Council; 1998.

Anke J, Ramzan I. Kava hepatotoxicity: are we any closer to the truth? Planta Med 2004;70:193–196.

Astin JA. Why patients use alternative medicine: results of a national study. JAMA 1998;279:1548–1553.

Au AM, Ko R, Boo FO, et al. Screening methods for drugs and heavy metals in Chinese patent medicines. Bull Environ Contam Toxicol 2000;65:112–119.

Bent S, Tiedt TN, Odden MC, Shlipak MG. The relative safety of ephedra compared to other herbal products. Ann Intern Med 2003;138:468–471.

Bischoff K, Guale F. Australian tea tree *(Melaleuca alternifolia)* oil poisoning in three purebred cats. J Vet Diagn Invest 1998;10:208–210.

Blais R, Maïga A, Aboubacar A. How different are users and non-users of alternative medicine? Can J Public Health 1997; 88:159–162.

Blumenthal M. Perspectives on the safety of herbal medicines. in Leikin JB, Paloucek FP, eds. *Poisoning and Toxicology Compendium.* Cleveland, Ohio: Lexi-Comp, Inc.; 1998a: 845–851.

Blumenthal M. Interactions between herbs and conventional drugs: introductory considerations. HerbalGram 2000;49: 52–63.

Blumenthal M, Busse WR, Goldberg A, et al, eds. *The Complete German Commission E Monographs.* Boston, Mass: Integrative Medicine Communications; 1998b.

Brinker FJ. *Herb Contraindications and Drug Interactions.* 2nd ed. Sandy, Ore: Eclectic Medical Publications; 1998.

Carlson M, Thomspon RD. Liquid chromatographic determination of safrole in sassafras-derived herbal products. JAOAC 1997;80:1023–1028.

Carson TL. Methylxanthines. In: Peterson ME, Talcott PA, eds. *Small Animal Toxicology.* Philadelphia, Pa: WB Saunders; 2001:563–570.

Clouatre DL. Kava kava: examining new reports of toxicity. Toxicol Lett 2004;150:85–96.

DerMarderosian A, ed. *Review of Natural Products.* St. Louis, Mo: Facts and Comparisons; 2001a.

DerMarderosian A, ed. *Garlic, Review of Natural Products.* St. Louis, Mo: Facts and Comparisons; 2001b:237–239.

DeSmet PAGM. Toxicological outlook on the quality assurance of herbal remedies. In De Smet PAGM, Keller K, Hansel R, Chandler RF, eds. *Adverse Effects of Herbal Drugs.* Berlin: Springer-Verlag; 1991:1–50.

Dolan SP, Nortrup DA, Bolger M, Capar SG. Analysis of dietary supplements for arsenic, cadmium, mercury, and lead using inductively coupled plasma mass spectrometry. J Agr Food Chem 2003;51:1307–1312.

Elder NC, Gillcrist A, Minz R. Use of alternative health care by family practice patients. Arch Fam Med 1997;6:181–184.

Emery DP, Corban JG. Camphor toxicity. J Paediatr Child Health 1999;35:105–106.

Ernst E. Adulteration of Chinese herbal medicines with synthetic drugs: a systematic review. J Intern Med 2002;252:107–113.

Fougere B. Cats and Salicylates: Using Suspect Herbs Safely, Veterinary Botanical Medicine Association Symposium 2003 Proceedings, Durham, NC.

Fugh-Berman A, Ernst E. Herb-drug interactions: a review and assessment of report reliability. J Clin Pharmacol 2001;52: 587–595.

Grande GA, Dannewitz SR. Symptomatic sassafras oil ingestion. Vet Human Toxicol 1987;29:447.

Gwaltney-Brant SM, Albretsen JC, Khan SA. 5-Hydroxytryptophan toxicosis in dogs: 21 cases (1989–1999). J Am Vet Med Assoc 2000;216:1937–1940.

Hall AH, Spoerke DG, Rumack BH. Assessing mistletoe toxicity. Ann Emerg Med 1986;15:1320–1323.

Haller CA, Anderson IB, Kim SY, Blanc PD. An evaluation of selected herbal reference texts and comparison to published reports of adverse herbal events. Adverse Drug React Toxicol Rev 2002;21:143–150.

Herr, SH: *Herb-Drug Interaction Handbook* (2nd ed.), Nassau, NY: Church Street Books, 2002.

Hooser SB, Beasley VR, Everitt JI. Effects of an insecticidal dip containing D-limonene in the cat. J Am Vet Med Assoc 1986;189:905–908.

Hung OL, Lewin, NA, Howland, MA. Herbal preparations. In: Goldfrank LR, Flomenbaum NE, Lewin NA, et al, eds. *Goldfrank's Toxicologic Emergencies.* 6th ed. Stamford, Conn: Appleton and Lange; 1998:1221–1241.

Kaluzienski M. Partial paralysis and altered behavior in dogs treated with melaleuca oil. J Toxicol Clin Toxicol 2000;38:518.

Kingsbury JM. *Poisonous Plants of the United States and Canada.* Englewood Cliffs, NJ: Prentice-Hall; 1964:264–267.

Ko RJ. Herbal products information. In: *Poisoning and Toxicology Compendium.* Cleveland, Ohio: Lexi-Comp, Inc.; 1998: 834–844.

Lazarou J, Pomeranz BH, Corey PN. Incidence of adverse drug reactions in hospitalized patients. A meta-analysis of prospective studies. JAMA 1998;279:1200–1205.

McGuffin M, Hobbs C, Upton R, et al, eds. *Botanical Safety Handbook.* Boca Raton, Fla: CRC Press; 1997.

Ooms TG, Khan SA, Means C. Suspected caffeine and ephedrine toxicosis resulting from ingestion of an herbal supplement containing quarana and ma huang in dogs: 47 cases (1997–1999). J Am Vet Med Assoc 2001;218:225–229.

Osweiler GD. Over-the-counter drugs and illicit drugs of abuse. In: *The National Veterinary Medical Series: Toxicology.* Philadelphia, Pa: Williams and Wilkins; 1996:303–313.

Palmer ME, Howland MA. Herbals and other dietary supplements. In: Ford MD, Delaney KA, Ling LJ, et al, eds. *Clinical Toxicology.* Philadelphia, Pa: WB Saunders; 2001:315–331.

Pirmohamed M, James S, Meakin S, et al. Adverse drug reactions as a cause of admission to hospital: prospective analysis of 18,820 patients. BMJ 2004;329:15–19.

Poppenga R. Treatment. In: Plumlee KH, ed. *Clinical Veterinary Toxicology.* St. Louis, Mo: Mosby; 2004:13–21.

Powers KA, Hooser SB, Sundberg JP, Beasley VR. An evaluation of the acute toxicity of an insecticidal spray containing linalool, d-limonene, and piperonyl butoxide applied topically to domestic cats. Vet Human Toxicol 1988;30:206–210.

Review of Natural Products. Potential Herb-Drug Interactions. St. Louis, Mo: Facts and Comparisons; 2000:653–657.

Review of Natural Products: Specific Herb-Drug Interactions. St. Louis, Mo: Facts and Comparisons; 2000:658–665.

Roberts DJ. Plants: cardiovascular toxicity. In: Ford MD, Delaney KA, Ling LJ, et al, eds. *Clinical Toxicology.* Philadelphia, Pa: WB Saunders; 2001:922–928.

Ryu S, Chung W. Induction of the procarcinogen-activating CYP1A2 by an herbal dietary supplement in rats and humans. Food Cosmet Toxicol 2003;41:861–866.

Segelman AB, Segelman FP, Karliner J, Sofia RD. Sassafras and herb tea. Potential health hazards. JAMA 1976;236:477.

Siegers CP. *Allium sativum.* In: DeSmet PAGM, Keller K, Hänsel R, Chandler RF, eds. *Adverse Effects of Herbal Drugs.* Berlin: Springer-Verlag; 1991:73–75.

Stamford IF, Bennett A. Treatment of diarrhea in calves with nutmeg. Vet Rec 1980;106:389.

Stedman C. Herbal hepatotoxicity. Semin Liver Dis 2002;22: 195–206.

Sudekum M, Poppenga RH, Raju N, et al. Pennyroyal oil toxicosis in a dog. J Am Vet Med Assoc 1992;200:817–818.

Tisserand R, Balacs T. *Essential Oil Safety: A Guide for Health Care Professionals.* Edinburgh, UK: Churchill Livingstone; 1999.

Tyler VE. *The Honest Herbal: A Sensible Guide to the Use of Herbs and Related Remedies.* 3rd ed. New York: Pharmaceutical Products Press; 1993.

Vanherweghem LJ. Misuse of herbal remedies: the case of an outbreak of terminal renal failure in Belgium (Chinese herbs nephropathy). J Altern Complement Med 1998;4:9–13.

Vassallo S. Essential oils. In: Ford MD, Delaney KA, Ling LJ, et al, eds. *Clinical Toxicology.* Philadephia, Pa: WB Saunders; 2001: 343–351.

Vickers A, Zollman C. ABC of complementary medicine: herbal medicine. BMJ 1999;319:1050–1053.

Villar D, Knight MJ, Hansen SR, Buck WB. Toxicity of melaleuca oil and related essential oils applied topically on dogs and cats. Vet Hum Toxicol 1994;36:139–142.

Yang S, Dennehy CE, Tsourournis C. Characterizing adverse events reported to the California poison control system on herbal remedies and dietary supplements: a pilot study. J Herb Pharmacother 2003;2:1–11.

Zhou S, Koh H, Gao Y, Gong Z, Lee EJD. Herbal bioactivation: the good, the bad and the ugly. Life Sci 2004;74:935–968.

Herbal Energetics: A Key to Efficacy in Herbal Medicine

CHAPTER

Steven Paul Marsden

EXPLORING HERBAL MEDICINE

Benjamin Franklin defined insanity as "doing the same thing over and over and expecting different results." The desire of veterinarians to explore herbal medicine is therefore quite cogent, since it varies inversely with their tolerance for continuing disappointments in conventional treatment of chronic disease.

Despite the allure of possibly improved therapeutic outcomes, veterinarians are still aware that conventional medicine is the acknowledged standard of practice for their profession. The ample body of research into its methods offers some certainty about the anticipated therapeutic outcome, however unsatisfactory it may be. In no way, however, are these outcomes sufficient to justify a self-righteous stance that herbal medicine should not be pursued until conventional medicine validates it.

Individuals interested in herbal medicine may hesitate to explore it because its efficacy has not been demonstrated. There is no lack of anecdotal reports of success, but what is needed to sway the profession as a whole is unbiased clinical evidence. The dearth of clinical trials in herbal medicine is a product of the phase of development that veterinary herbal medicine is currently in. It is only from the field research that is currently ongoing in examination rooms around the world that testable hypotheses regarding herbal medicine will be developed. In the meantime, evidence of efficacy must be sought personally, the same way the field observations are being recorded, on an individual case-by-case basis.

Albert Einstein stated, "We can't solve problems by using the same kind of thinking we used when we created them." Pathophysiology and pharmacology thus seem an inadequate basis for prescribing herbal formulas, in that a complete pathophysiologic understanding of most chronic diseases still eludes us, leading to the current frustration with conventional medical efforts. Other methods of prescribing must be explored for maximum efficacy with the use of herbal medicine.

METAPHORIC MEDICINE

This is not the first time that humans have faced the prospect of treating serious diseases in the absence of definitive knowledge about them. The near-universal cultural taboos against human dissection resulted in a lack of definitive knowledge of the human body, forcing most societies to develop instead a schematic understanding of internal physiology and anatomy.

In their attempt to frame models of anatomy and physiology in more familiar terms, Chinese medicine practitioners chose to equate the internal environment of the human body with the external one. The choice seemed logical, in that humans resonate so much with their environment that it seems to invade and dominate them. Patients could "catch a cold," or echo the same heat and desiccation of any desert that surrounded them. The internal landscape seemed subject to the same laws and phenomena of the external landscape.

The resultant climatic model seemed accurate enough to be validated almost daily by human experience, leaping over the wide gaps in medical knowledge. These same models are being explored today when, once again, we lack definitive knowledge of chronic disease, such that the best efforts of modern medicine are palliative at best.

It is surprising to note that other cultures took a similar approach to grappling with the mysteries of inner space. The close agreement among these medical systems is stunning and supports the validity of the metaphoric approach, however abstract it may be. Despite the fact that there is no evidence of significant cultural exchange between the citizens of ancient Greece and their contemporaries in China, congruencies between the two medical systems run the gamut from diagnosis to treatment. The importance of "phlegm" and its elaboration in the digestive tract as a major cause of disease; the existence of four obvious phases of life and the "climatic influences" that tend to dominate them; the use of pulse and tongue diagnosis in patient evaluation; the crucial importance of diet in preventing disorders; and even the medical application of specific herbs—all were salient features of both bodies of work. Even between ancient China and 19th century America, the indications of any globally distributed plant species were synonymous long before cultural exchange occurred.

Eventual information exchange served only to deepen the accord between traditions. When knowledge was shared freely between India and China, and between China and Japan, agreement about use of a multitude of plants and formulas became nearly universal. The translation, preservation, and assimilation of ancient Greek texts by Muslim nations during Europe's Dark Ages likewise ensured the propagation and survival of some of mankind's most important empirical advances, including the specific medicinal use of hundreds of herbs.

Each of these medical systems is thus a candidate for the veterinarian who is contemplating a different approach to prescribing herbs. Chinese medicine is, however, favored by many veterinary herbalists because resources available for study and reference are abundant, detailed, and sophisticated enough to warrant a place on a health professional's bookshelf. Many of the most important of these references were originally published 2 millennia ago, but since the Chinese language has barely changed during that period, herbalists can read verbatim the notes of a physician such as Sun Si Miao of the 6th century and, through his characteristically detailed description of symptoms, determine exactly what condition was being treated. Recipes, indications, and dosing instructions were precise, allowing us to re-create and study in the 21st century the efficacy of these ancient approaches to disease.

Before an herbal therapy could be prescribed in Chinese medicine, it had to be understood in the same climatic frame of reference as the patient. This broad understanding of a plant's climatic effect, together with knowledge of the region of the body where this effect is exerted, constitutes what many modern authors refer to as the "energetic" of an herb.

As a simple example, then, a therapy that is capable of relieving the superficial aches and chills associated with "catching a cold" had to be able to "expel cold pathogens invading the neck and back." The diagnosis of the patient implies a general blueprint for an effective treatment. Of all potentially antimicrobial, immune-stimulating, or antiviral herbs, the only ones that would suffice in this instance are those that could be understood to be warming and to provide some sort of outward push to a pathogen that invades the periphery of the body. Perspiration following ingestion of a plant was considered tangible evidence of its outward push. Herbs most appropriate for our patient would thus include the spicy pungent diaphoretics, such as garlic. Although diaphoresis does not itself resolve a cold, it is an associated effect of plants with abundant volatile oil content, which, in turn, are often strongly antimicrobial.

Modern practitioners have the benefit of knowing both the pharmacologic makeup of herbs and their energetic. It is important, however, to consider the pharmacologic appropriateness of an herb as the last step. First, the practitioner must "suspend their disbelief" of metaphoric medical models and use them to rapidly remove from consideration a host of therapies, then home in quickly on just a few highly and generally appropriate candidates. Rather than being a fumbling process of guesswork (trial and error), metaphoric schemata allow the prescription of herbal medicines by even a novice herbalist to be specific, rapid, and incisive.

THE BEDROCK OF DISEASE

The process of prescribing Chinese herbs accurately begins with understanding the patient in metaphoric terms. Very frequently, the same general diagnosis would be rendered for most of the different diseases a patient might suffer over time. Like the land they live upon, humans and animals seem to be subject to the same repetitive sequence of climatic patterns.

The bedrock of a mountain provides a good metaphor by which an understanding of this consistent recurrent predisposition in a patient can be facilitated. Mountains often have a completely different appearance when viewed from neighboring valleys, yet the same bedrock creates both topographies. Likewise, a consistent general metaphoric predisposition in a patient can give rise to two seemingly unrelated illnesses. The idea of an enduring weakness that could "outcrop" any time if not mitigated is similar to the notion of constitutional predisposition embraced by homeopaths. It also corresponds roughly to genetic predisposition. Herbal therapies cannot, of course, change genetic makeup but can certainly play a role in deciding whether and to what extent genes are expressed, allowing outcroppings of the patient's own particular bedrock to retreat to the interior.

Despite the resources expended in the development and mastery of tools of disease intervention such as acupuncture, herbal medicine, surgery, or gene therapy, the tie that binds most of the world's medical systems together is the belief that nothing is more important than an ideal diet, exercise, adequate rest, and a healthy lifestyle in the treatment and prevention of disease. If these factors are not addressed, responses to treatment are often incomplete or are followed by another problem that materializes in the near future. Only preventive lifestyle measures are considered powerful enough in the long term to keep the bedrock of disease concealed.

The importance of prevention in furthering therapeutic outcomes makes Chinese medicine an extremely powerful tool; such measures are never ignored or eclipsed by the intricacies involved in diagnosing and treating a condition. Sooner or later, the Chinese medical clinician turns his or her attention to determining which specific lifestyle factors might have precipitated the illness; in some cases, the diagnosis itself hinges upon an identification of these factors. For example, if a patient experienced problems following overwork or overexercise, Kidney Qi deficiency would be far more likely to function as an underlying cause of illness than, say, a "pathologic excess" such as Damp Heat.

Lifestyle factors facilitate not only diagnosis but treatment; indeed, Chinese herbal medicine was originally itself a form of dietary therapy, with a few herbs added to enhance the therapeutic effectiveness of certain dishes. This practice is still common in China to this day with, for example, medicinal herbs such as Dang Gui root and White Peony root served routinely as tea or added to dishes served in restaurants.

Sometimes, no obvious lifestyle factors are suggested as the cause of an illness during questioning of the patient. Even then, however, Chinese medicine has a unique advantage over conventional medicine in that it is able to postulate and institute preventive diets long before conventional medicine eventually identifies and verifies them as effective.

This ability comes from a metaphoric approach to medicine, and it is one of the many reasons why Chinese medicine was not abandoned, even as definitive knowledge of the body was later acquired.

In general, once a metaphoric diagnosis has been validated by a response to an appropriate treatment, other modalities with the same effect are immediately suggested as suitable preventive measures. Thus, when a patient responds to anti-inflammatory drugs in conventional medicine, no particular preventive strategy is implicated. When, on the other hand, a patient with inflammation responds to a strategy that "drains damp and clears heat" (regardless whether a drug, herb, or surgery was the treatment), a "dampening and heating" diet, or one that is too calorically dense, is immediately suggested as a likely contributing cause.

Although these conclusions were drawn centuries ago by Chinese medical practitioners, it is only in the 20th century that, for example, overnutrition was identified by conventional medicine as a contributing factor to arthritis and pancreatitis. Such is the power of a metaphoric approach to medicine.

A corollary of the precept that one underlying predisposition governs all manifestations of illness in a patient is that every episode of illness and every clinical finding in each of those episodes is reflective of that one core disorder. Diagnosis is thus a process of triangulation, where all salient features of the history and all readily apparent physical features are analyzed until one common denominator is found—the one and only problem, or bedrock, that might underlie them all.

Technically, finding the common denominator behind as many clinical findings as possible is also the ideal of conventional medical diagnosis. For example, if a patient has polyuria, polydipsia, weight loss, hyperglycemia, and glycosuria, the best treatment is not a separate therapy for each of these findings, but rather, one that addresses the common denominator of diabetes mellitus at its core. To this extent, then, both conventional and Chinese medicines are equally "holistic"; they both attempt to understand and treat the whole patient. The main difference between them is the extent to which they can identify relationships between diverse symptoms and signs. The inability of conventional medical analysis to explain relationships between concomitant findings becomes a very important indicator to the practitioner that another system of medicine, one that can weave all salient features of a case into a single assessment, may be better suited to treating a given patient.

An interesting implication arises from the idea that a diagnosis involves finding the common denominator of divergent findings. In general, and in direct contrast to conventional medicine, the implication is that the more complicated a patient's case is, the easier it is to diagnose. Conversely, when symptoms and signs are vague, general, and nondescript, any number of core disorders may conceivably have given rise to them. Diagnosis becomes much the same as a verdict in a courtroom—the fewer the witnesses and the more absent the physical evidence, the more it is possible that anybody could have committed the crime. In circumstances in which symptoms are vague or nondescript, meticulous attention to the physical nuances of the patient—pulse, complexion, even the timber of the voice—becomes all important in exposing the bedrock of disease at the patient's core. Chinese medicine refers to this cataloging of the physical data of a patient as The Four Examinations.

THE FOUR EXAMINATIONS

Questioning

It has been said that a good history in conventional medicine will give the clinician the diagnosis of a patient 75% of the time. The same is also true of Chinese medicine, where Questioning—the first of the Four Examinations—will suggest a likely Chinese medical diagnosis if it is thorough enough. A thorough history in Chinese medicine includes approximately the same information as a complete history in conventional medicine. General areas of inquiry include the following:

- History of present illness
- Review of complaints in other systems
- Past medical history
- Prior treatments and response
- Diet and lifestyle
- Family history
- Appetite, thirst, and temperature preferences
- Sleep patterns

It is especially important during questioning that the practitioner should not settle for an interpretation offered by the client or the patient, but instead should seek out raw data and draw his or her own conclusions. For example, during an inquiry about complaints in other organ systems, the subject of behavior comes up. In response to the question, "How would you describe your dog's personality?" An owner might reply, "He's very dominant—very protective of me." This is an interpretation and is not suitable in itself for interpretation from a Chinese medical perspective. An appropriate follow-up question would therefore be, "What is it about your dog's behavior that makes you think he is dominant or protective?" If the owner replies that the dog tries to intimidate other strange dogs, or barks furiously when people come to the door, only to slink away if they enter, the dog is likely more fearful than protective.

Historical data can be interpreted according to a number of perspectives. One of the simplest and most useful methods used by the author is to decide whether the information gathered is most reflective of a Hot, Cold,

BOX 13-1

Common Signs of Heat

- Yellow tongue coat or discharges
- Redness of skin, eyes, or tongue
- Heat radiation
- Sweating
- Aggravated and unsettled at night
- Thirst
- Excitability
- Agitation, restlessness
- Aggression
- Heat intolerance
- Dryness
- Hunger

BOX 13-2

Common Signs of Cold

- Cold intolerance
- Profuse, clear water discharges (includes urine)
- White mucoid discharges
- Cold to touch
- Seeking of heat
- Lethargy
- Pain aggravated by exposure to cold damp weather
- Cold tongue
- Stiffness and immobility
- Low thirst

BOX 13-3

Common Signs of Stasis

- Generally better from movement
- Mental agitation manifesting as pacing
- Pain in general indicates stasis; permanent loci of pain are more severe forms of stasis than temporary fleeting pains
- Deficient stasis—pain relieved by pressure and massage
- Often induced by overexertion or trauma
- Increased muscle tone and spasm
- Resonant cough
- May be hot, cold, excessive, or deficient
- Pain causing restlessness and pacing
- Excess stasis—intolerant of touch in painful area
- Even if the patient is excessively warm, pain from stasis is often relieved by the application of warmth
- Obstructions to circulation may be autogenous, arising from accumulation of pathologic excesses (Dampness, Phlegm)
- Bloat
- Persistent lesions, such as tumors or perianal fistulae

Excess, Deficient, or Stasis syndrome, or some combination of these. Boxes 13-1 through 13-5 list typical historical and physical findings for each category, although a patient may have traits of more than one.

Listening

Listening is another of the Four Examinations. Listening refers here not to taking a history, but rather, to taking note of sounds from patients' bodies. Do they have borborygmi? Are their voices weak or loud? When they cough, does it sound moist, weak, or resonant? Rales would be a sign of Excess, Phlegm in particular. Resonant coughs are a sign of circulatory stasis; a weak voice or cough is indicative of Deficiency. Other notes made from listening to the patient are similarly interpreted to define the patient's bedrock of disease.

BOX 13-4

Common Signs of Deficiency

- Weight loss
- Fatigue in the morning
- Faint voice
- Small bowel diarrhea
- Mild intensity of symptoms
- Timidity
- Territorial; avaricious
- May be hot or cold
- Weakness; flaccidity
- Loss of appetite
- Feeble cough
- Muscle wasting and loss of tone
- Mild mannered
- Fear
- Fine, powdery dander
- Hair thinning

Looking

The Looking method of the Four Examinations is employed during the Questioning phase. As the clinician is recording the history, the patient's posture, body composition, movements, and complexion are all being studied for further clues as to whether they can best be described as Hot, Cold, Excess, Deficient, Stagnant, or some combination of these. For example, a very overweight animal is far more likely to suffer from an Excess syndrome, at least in part. An animal that is restless and therefore relieved by pacing and moving may best be classified as having a Stasis syndrome. Animals with injected mucous membranes are much more likely to be Hot than Cold.

Included in the Looking phase is tongue diagnosis. Use of the tongue as a general barometer of what is happen-

BOX 13-5

Common Symptoms and Signs of Excess

- Weight gain
- Foul odor (halitosis, flatus, skin, ears)
- Confidence
- Lichenification
- Abundant exudation
- Large areas of alopecia
- Extreme symptoms and presentations
- Greasy skin and ears
- Tumors, nodules
- Edema
- May be hot or cold
- Rounded belly

BOX 13-6

Interpretation of Tongue Color

COLOR	INTERPRETATION
Pale	Deficient, Cold
Red	Hot
Lavender	Impaired circulation
Purple	Severe circulation impairment

BOX 13-7

Interpretation of Tongue Features

TRAIT	INTERPRETATION
Moisture	Body moisture content
Size	Tendency to tissue abundance or engorgement
Location	Location of disorder

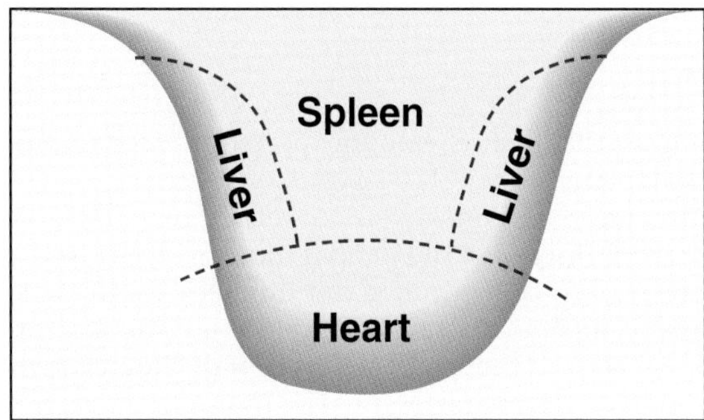

Figure 13-1 Representative areas of major organs in Chinese tongue diagnosis.

ing in other tissues that are concealed from view was rather ingenious. The tongue was easily accessed and had a transparent coating, lending it to easy inspection and interpretation of its degree of perfusion. Although it is easily observed, the tongue was protected from the elements, allowing moisture to build up on the tongue if there was a surfeit in the body. It was also freely movable yet loosely contained, allowing increases in size to occur, yet its condition was betrayed by the indentations of teeth along its edges. Many medical systems stumbled upon the technique of tongue diagnosis and made the same logical assumptions about the body as a whole on the basis of its appearance. Some key interpretations are recorded in Boxes 13-6 and 13-7.

Use of the location of a lesion on a tongue to identify where a lesion might be located in the body (Figure 13-1) bears special mention because the logic may not be immediately obvious. Chinese medicine practitioners believed, for example, that redness on the tip of the tongue was reflective of heat disorders in the organs of the upper body such as the brain, heart, and lungs; a lavender color in the center indicated that stasis was affecting the digestive organs (the spleen). The edges of the tongue were associated with liver, which in Chinese medicine is the organ that facilitates smooth laminar flow of circulation to the periphery of the body.

Such assignments of these functions to specific regions of the tongue make sense once they are contemplated from a hemodynamic perspective. For example, the head may be considered an extremity as far as hemodynamics is concerned, similar to an arm or a leg. The more a patient tends to be hot, the stronger is the peripheral blood flow to the head, limbs, and even tongue, reflecting itself in a flushed complexion, an easily located radial pulse, and full perfusion of the tip of the tongue. Likewise, the more extensively peripheral circulation is inhibited, the greater is the quantity of blood that is shunted to the splanchnic vasculature. Peripheral circulation to the tongue edges is also inhibited, with a gathering of blood at the point of vasoconstriction, which is in the body of the tongue. A correlation can be made between poor peripheral circulation and a pale tongue edge; and between congestion in the digestive organs and a purple tongue center.

Touch

Touch is the final of the Four Examinations. It refers in part to palpation of painful, swollen, or warm acupuncture points, which can generally be counted upon to be the most effective ones for inclusion in a prescription. In addition, both acupuncturists and herbalists use touch to interpret the pulse of the patient.

Chinese medical practitioners are famous for the mysterious art of pulse diagnosis, but pulse diagnosis has been employed by most medical traditions worldwide throughout human history. Although skeptics may be quick to dismiss it as a dubious practice, agreement on the interpretation of the pulse has been considerable among medical traditions, suggesting that the practice is underpinned by an empiric logic. As with tongue

BOX 13-8

Interpretation of Pulse Parameters

TRAIT	INTERPRETATION
Depth	Heat, Stasis
Force	Vitality
Rate	Heat or Cold
Width	Deficiency
Tone	Stasis
Rhythm	Stasis
Amplitude	Stasis

diagnosis, that logic is, not unexpectedly, based on simple hemodynamics.

Any pulse is considered to reflect on the internal bedrock of disease of the patient, but smaller vessels that can be broken down into seven different parameters are generally superior. Listed in Box 13-8 are the interpretations for each of these parameters or traits, some of which are immediately self-evident. For example, most practitioners would evaluate cardiac function in an animal with an irregular rhythm, with a view to ruling out heart disease, or circulatory stasis. They would also expect a hot patient who is running a high fever to have a rapid pulse and a hypothermic hypothyroid, and therefore, a cold dog would be expected to have a slow pulse. Association of the force of the pulse with the overall vigor or vitality of the patient also seems intuitive.

Basic hemodynamics are used to explain remaining pulse correlations. For example, an animal with a slightly reduced (or deficient) circulating blood volume would be expected to have a thinner pulse. It would also be expected that a response to prolonged reduction in blood volume would be peripheral vasoconstriction, resulting in an increase in vessel wall tone with resultant impairment of blood flow (stasis). Failure of the blood column to move forward results in increased back pressure, causing the vessel wall to push more forcibly outward with each heartbeat, thereby establishing the correlation between stasis and pulse amplitude.

Pulse depth is the relative depth to which the finger must be pushed into the skin for the maximum beat intensity of the pulse to be felt. The lighter the digital pressure that needs to be exerted, the more superficial the pulse and the stronger the peripheral circulation. Increased blood flow to the periphery is often reflective of an attempt by the body at thermoregulation through the dissipation of heat. Conversely, the deeper the pulse, the greater the degree of Stasis, or lack of circulation to the periphery, that is suggested.

The 28 different pulses described by Chinese medicine are not inconsistent with this method of pulse diagnosis but are merely labels applied to different collections of individual traits. For example, a wiry pulse has increased tone and often increased amplitude. A sinking pulse is one that has increased vessel wall tone but is also very deep. The classical interpretation of a wiry or a sinking pulse is in complete accordance with the logical interpretation of each of the individual traits; a wiry pulse is associated with Qi stagnation (stasis), and a sinking pulse is associated with stagnation of Qi deep in the interior of the body (stasis). Only memorization of the implications of each basic pulse parameter is required for a patient's condition to be accurately diagnosed through their pulse.

ASSESSING THE ENERGETIC OF AN HERB

The metaphoric diagnostic methods of traditional medical systems require that patients and treatments be classified in broad strokes, according to the same frame of reference. We have discussed how patients are analyzed and classified by means of the Four Examinations.

Understanding how herbs are classified requires a brief exploration of how the medicinal effects of herbs were determined in the first place.

Doctrine of Signatures

A popular but usually uninformed opinion is that herbal actions have been determined through a deadly process of trial and error. A random approach to investigation is much more in keeping, however, with the mindset of a modern researcher who is more interested in probabilities and statistics than with the mindset of an early clinician who believed divergent phenomena are linked on a metaphoric level. Early herbal practitioners believed in patterns, not randomness, and can be trusted to have tried to induce the general action of a plant in the same way that they diagnosed a patient's condition—by trying somehow to interpret the subject's physical traits to gain an overall sense of the metaphoric dynamic that infuses it.

One of the most popular theories of how the actions of plants were discovered through inductive reasoning is the Doctrine of Signatures. The gist of the theory is that the physical appearance of the plant gives strong clues about its medicinal effect. Yellow coloration, particularly inside the roots and bark, suggested the plant "cleared heat" or treated fevers; a notable example is Peruvian Bark, from which quinine would later be extracted and isolated. Plants with vivid red components were considered to help with circulation or stasis; an obvious example is *Carthamus tinctoria* or Carthamus (*Hong Hua*, literally, "Red Flower"), which has been employed as a blood mover in Chinese medicine. Plant shape was also believed to provide clues to a plant's effects. For example, spicy Capsicum was commonly used in the West to promote circulation; internally, it is chambered, similar to the heart.

The problem with the Doctrine of Signatures is that the physical traits of plants do not have predictive value in revealing the effects of plants and are only evident in hindsight. Bell peppers are also chambered, but they do not have any obvious ability to improve circulation. Tulips are often red or yellow but are not used medicinally to clear heat or move blood.

One forward-looking correlation that is surprisingly reliable is the association between the part of a plant that is used and its medicinal effect. Flowers and the outer bark of plants typically act to "disperse" pathogens from the outer layers of the body that are most prone to external invasion. Thus, the bark of Chinese wolfberry *(Lycium chinense)* is indicated to treat hemoptysis associated with tuberculosis, and dandelion flowers are used to treat bacterial infection of the mammary glands and skin. Roots, on the other hand, in keeping with their location, are often used to provide fundamental support in deficient patients. *Panax ginseng* root, as a Heart Qi tonic, is a potent adaptogen that helps to strengthen patients by fostering optimal adrenal function. The immune polysaccharides of Astragalus *(Astragalus membranaceus)* root, another Qi tonic, enhance immune function and resistance to infection.

At least some of the explanation of the correlation between plant part and medicinal effect has to do with the importance of each respective part to the plant itself. Flowers and bark are exposed to invading pathogens just as the skin and lungs are in people and would thus be expected to contain a relatively high concentration of antimicrobial compounds. Roots, on the other hand, provide sustenance to perennials, allowing the aerial parts to die off but be replaced the following spring. They would thus be expected to have a high concentration of polysaccharides and other nutritive compounds.

The Importance of Taste

The only rule of thumb in inducing a plant's effects that would have been reliable enough to have been discovered through experience by every herbal culture is one with a chemical basis. Although chemical differences most likely account for the predictable effects of different plant parts, by far the most obvious and accessible plant trait with a chemical basis is its taste. If the physiologic effect of a particular taste was rapid enough, resultant symptoms would have been rapidly interpreted and the general effect of the plant quickly induced.

An obvious example is Juniper berries, known by modern herbalists to increase renal filtration by causing glomerular hyperemia. Lesser known, however, is the use of Juniper berries in earlier traditions for the treatment of stasis conditions such as arthritis. This benefit is immediately suggested, however, as soon as a Juniper berry is sampled. At the same time that the strong pungency of the berry is released into the mouth and nasal passages, a wave of "lubricating warmth" associated with increased peripheral blood flow is felt to diffuse through the body all the way out into the arms and legs. Both chronic inflammation and stasis conditions are benefited by improved circulation. If a person who sampled the berry centuries or even millennia ago happened to have an arthritic or stasis condition, for at least a brief time some relief would have been experienced, building an immediate association between Juniper berries and the treatment of musculoskeletal pain.

Even more important, however, would have been the suggestion of an association of a warm pungent taste with an ability to relieve pain. Corroboration of this relationship would have been found when other plants such as Aconite root, Corydalis root, Boswellia resin, and Prickly Ash bark were tasted. There is no lack of herbs with an obvious taste that can be linked to a rapid, strong chemical effect. The diaphoresis following a heavy dose of hot pungent garlic and the catharsis following a large dose of bitter Cascara sagrada bark are matters of common knowledge even in conventional medicine; an immediate link between those tastes and those actions would undoubtedly have been noted in the minds of traditional herbalists.

Once taste became associated with action, early herbalists also had their first means of quality control. The use of taste as a crude method for testing the strength and likely efficacy of a preparation of, for example, Echinacea, persists today; this method can even be used to help identify the ideal times for harvesting medicinal plants. Taste was heavily relied upon by the Eclectic herbalists of 19th century America who, although they were pioneers involved in chemically isolating, characterizing, and standardizing the active ingredients, still relied heavily on taste as a field method of confirming the identity and chemical content of plants before the harvest.

The flurry of inductive reasoning sparked in the traditional herbalist's mind by the association of a physiologic effect with a particular taste would have had one more logical extension—the development of a model of physiology, or how the body works in health, and how a breakdown in that physiology leads to the development of certain diseases. Naysayers attempt to diminish herbal medicine by claiming that the application of herbs in Chinese medicine is a recent phenomenon with no long track record of safety and efficacy. In reality, however, early experimentation with herbs appears to have helped give rise to Chinese medicine in its earliest stages.

Herbal medicine inspired the earliest understanding of how the body works because it is an empiric and experiential pursuit. Imagine once again an individual with intestinal cramping who then samples one of the many spices commonly used in food preparation even to this day. Many of these culinary herbs, including fennel and ginger, have antispasmodic effects on the intestinal tract, and commonly have a pungent and warm taste. As cramps were eased, an association would have been made between proper digestion and warming, pungent herbs. This relationship could later have been canonized in the medical literature as a dependence of the spleen (digestion) on adequate Yang energy (warmth).

The importance of taste as both the main source of information on an herb's effects and the inspiration for all of Chinese medicine comes from Shen Nong, the Divine Farmer of ancient China (circa 3494 BC). Shen Nong appears to have been a tribal leader and is credited with fueling the development of China's earliest agricultural methods. He is also believed to have spawned the development of herbal medicine, and he explored the actions of plants on the body by tasting them. The first forays into an empiric exploration of the physiologic effects of plants must certainly have been risky, with Shen

Nong reputedly "tasting a hundred herbs in a day and meeting seventy toxins." He apparently survived the experience, however, and a summary of observations credited to him were eventually recorded in the *Shen Nong Ben Cao Jing* (Shen Nong Herbal Medicine Classic) about 500 AD.

The seminal text in Chinese medicine is the *Huang Di Nei Jing (Yellow Emperor's Inner Classic)* first written in 200 BC and based on conversations purported to have occurred between the Yellow Emperor and his physician. Similar to Shen Nong, the Yellow Emperor appears to have been a tribal leader and warrior, most likely of the Hong Shan culture in Northern China. He is believed to have conquered and united several clans to become a de facto emperor. He is also credited with several advances in Chinese culture, including construction of its first boats and vehicles (carts) and the development of history's first medical model, which is recorded in the *Huang Di Nei Jing*. Although the text discusses the treatment of a few specific diseases with the use of plants, it poetically summarizes in several locations the major impact of each of the five herb tastes on the body, proving that an exhaustive knowledge of herbal medicine had already been acquired, most likely from Shen Nong, but long before the *Ben Cao Jing* was ever written down.

A few centuries after the *Nei Jing* was written, in approximately 200 AD, the detailed knowledge of herbal medicine that existed at the time finally materialized in the *Shang Han Lun (Treatise on Cold Febrile Disease)*, a discussion of how to use more than 100 different formulas to treat various types of "pathogen invasion." The symptomatic indications for these formulas are abundantly detailed and the recipes precise. Most of the formulas are still in common use today for their original indications, underscoring their safety and effectiveness, the incredible length of time that current Chinese medical practices have been used, and the likelihood that herbal medicine was practiced in a sophisticated form well before 200 AD. Given its complexity, it is highly unlikely that herbal medicine as a discipline suddenly materialized at the time of writing of the *Shang Han Lun*. Scholars instead believe that medical lore was simply transmitted orally for centuries until writing systems were finally developed. Even today, memorization and recitation of poems on Chinese medicine is a primary method used by clinicians to recall Chinese medical precepts. The body of knowledge memorized and recalled in this rote fashion is known as the "heart transmission of medicine."

The Five Tastes and the Four Natures

Shen Nong's classic describes four temperatures or natures of herbs (hot, warm, cool, cold), whose clinical indications are patently obvious—warm or hot herbs for cold patients, and cool or cold herbs for hot patients. The nature of a plant as warming or cooling was determined not only by the sensation created by physical contact with the plant, but also by the nature of the symptoms relieved. If a bitter plant was observed to reduce the perspiration and rapid heart rate associated with high fever in a hot patient, its nature was obviously cooling.

BOX 13-9

The Five Flavors and Their Actions

TASTE	FUNCTION
Sour	Contains and moistens
Bitter	Cools, dries, moves, descends
Pungent	Moves, expands, dries
Salt	Moistens and descends
Sweet	Relaxes, nourishes, supports, leeches

In addition to the Four Natures, both the *Huang Di Nei Jing* and the *Shen Nong Ben Cao Jing* focus on Five Tastes and their medicinal effects. These flavors—Sour, Bitter, Salty, Pungent, and Sweet—are the reason why metaphoric systems of medicine work. Although they determine the overall appropriateness of a plant to the metaphoric assessment of a patient, allowing a short list of herbal treatment candidates to be compiled, they also are indicative of the chemicals within a plant and its physiologic effects. Taste then is what closes the gap between Eastern and Western medicine.

Box 13-9 lists the Five Flavors and their general effects on the body—the tendency of chemicals with these distinct tastes to always produce one of the listed effects is remarkably consistent. Following is a more detailed discussion of the effects of the five tastes, along with some familiar chemical examples.

The sour taste

Most sour-tasting compounds are organic acids. In a nutshell, they have the effect of "marshalling fluids," that is, of gathering and astringing fluids into one location. The natural facial reaction after sucking on a lemon epitomizes this effect. The entire countenance is drawn together even as the mouth fills with saliva in response. A gathering effect can be very helpful when healthful fluids are being lost or excessively secreted, such as in hemorrhage or chronic diarrhea. Glycopyrrolate, through its reduction in gastric acid secretion, is an excellent example of the astringing effects of organic acids.

In the metaphoric view of Chinese medicine, the gathering of blood together in one place facilitates more powerful and steady flow, serving to enhance circulation. Ginkgo leaf is a sour herb that is believed to have the effect of enhancing cerebral blood flow. Sour-tasting ascorbic acid gathers blood and prevents hemorrhage by facilitating collagen cross-linkages. Citric acid is likewise recognized as a hemostatic.

In addition, sour herbs can promote the release of digestive juices, such as saliva in the mouth and gastric acid in the stomach, and can increase smooth muscle tone, resulting in sour foods such as lemon acquiring a reputation as digestive aids.

The bitter taste

The bitter taste is described as "draining fire," such as occurs with the high fever, perspiration, and inflammation associated with acute infection in Excess patients. Many anti-inflammatory and antimicrobial compounds thus have an intense bitter taste. Bitter compounds were also considered to be strongly drying as a consequence of their draining effect, resulting in, for example, the elimination of exudation.

A rapid heart rate is also a symptom of severe heat. Bitter-tasting plant compounds that slow heart rate and are therefore cooling include cardiac glycosides such as digitalis. Bitter-tasting substances were considered to drain other things besides fire, including stool. Aloe-emodin is an example of a bitter plant chemical with a very strong cathartic effect. Bitter descending herbs also are known for their strong calming effects. Chemical examples of strong plant-derived sedatives include the isoquinolone opiates.

The pungent taste

Most pungent plant compounds contain aromatic rings, and anybody who has eaten a little too much Cayenne pepper or horseradish is familiar with their invigorating effects. The pungent taste behaves like a strong dry wind blowing through the body, moving everything in its path and invigorating circulation. Aromatic or pungent plant compounds with an obvious effect of promoting circulation include the anticoagulant coumarins of the Clover family. Camphor, a pungent bark extract, was once popular as a highly potent stimulant for use in shock. It is used today topically as a decongestant to mobilize respiratory secretions.

A relatively new discovery about aromatic compounds is their strong antimicrobial effect. Their efficacy as antimicrobial agents is enhanced by the fact that they can easily cross most cell membranes to whatever place an infection may be located. Antimicrobial pungent herbs were used to induce diaphoresis in patients with acute cold and flu. Perspiration induced by the use of pungent herbs such as garlic is not in itself helpful in eliminating a cold but is caused by the same compounds that kill microbes, allowing diaphoresis from ingestion of an herb to be an indicator of its anti-infective properties.

The salty taste

Chinese medicine described the taste of bones, shells, and high–mineral content plants as salty. The *Nei Jing* provides the first recorded association between salt consumption and increased blood volume. It was believed that many other minerals could also attract water, resulting in their addition to formulas to emolliate nodules. More than likely, some of these masses were goiters that were responsive to iodine contained in shells of marine origin. Other minerals are used for an emolliating effect in conventional medicine as well, including magnesium sulfate to soften stool masses, sodium iodide for lumpy jaw in cattle, and potassium iodide as a topical application for fibrocystic breast disease.

The other major indication of the salty taste was the facilitation of descent of Yang energy in the body. Yang energy is considered to be hot and powerful with a tendency to move upward and outward. In the body, ascendant Yang manifests clinically as hypertension, seizures, tremors, and even psychosis. In conventional medicine, there is no lack of minerals that can be used to address these conditions, with lithium remaining the treatment of choice for patients with bipolar disorder, potassium bromide being prescribed to manage idiopathic epilepsy in dogs, and calcium carbonate being used in humans to counter hypertension, relieve anxiety, and help promote sleep.

The sweet taste

Sweet describes both overtly sweet herbs and those with a more neutral or bland taste. Vitamins, lipids, and polysaccharides are usually responsible for the sweet taste, which is not surprising in that it is reflective of an ability to strengthen and nourish the body. Sweet herbs are thus strongly indicated in deficient patients.

Sweet and neutral-tasting constituents not only can be metabolized as fuel sources but have physiologic effects that can be broadly described as strengthening. Polysaccharides, for example, are responsible for the immune-stimulating effects of Reishi and Maitake mushrooms. Vitamins important for normal cell division, maturation, and development commonly have a neutral taste; these include folic acid and retinoic acid. Beta sitosterol has a multitude of effects in the body, including an adrenal-sparing effect, making it of interest in the treatment of Addison's disease.

In addition to its nutritive value, the sweet taste was regarded as able to promote softening and relaxation of tissues. From a conventional medical viewpoint, it has a smooth muscle–dilating effect. An example is saw palmetto, noted by naturalists on the southeast coast of the United States to have androgenic effects in animals, but used medicinally in humans for the management of benign prostatic hypertrophy (BPH). Some of the relief provided to patients with BPH is due not to inhibition of the effects of testosterone on prostate growth, but rather to a spasmolytic effect on the urethra conferred by beta sitosterol-d-glucoside. Saw palmetto is used by some veterinary herbalists as a rapid and effective means of promoting urethral dilation in cats prone to obstruction.

Combining tastes

Research into botanical medicine has resulted in significant progress in identification of the active ingredients associated with certain clinical effects. It has only barely begun, however, to explore the daunting question of how these active ingredients interact with each other.

The few studies that have been done are commonly able to demonstrate a synergistic interaction between plant constituents, such that the physiologic effect of the whole plant is measurably stronger than a much larger quantity of its active ingredient. This potential for synergy exists not only between compounds in the same plant, but also between compounds of different plants combined in the same formula.

Synergy between plant ingredients has exciting implications; it increases not only efficacy but also safety. Because a lower quantity of an active ingredient is required to create a clinical effect, the chances of toxicity from that ingredient are also lowered. The risk of adverse effects is lowered further if the adverse effects of some compounds in plant mixture are antidoted by the effects of others. At the same time, the use of compounds in different plants can provide a broader range of clinical effect compared with the use of one plant alone.

An everyday example for most veterinarians of the very real benefits of synergy is the use of multiple drugs to induce general anesthesia. Drugs are chosen carefully, such that the adverse effects of one drug are compensated for by the effects of another. In addition, each drug contributes something different to the goals of inducing unconsciousness and analgesia. The result is a surgical plane of anesthesia with minimal risk. The same synergy that can be easily established between synthetic drugs can also be achieved among naturally occurring plant compounds.

The miracle of synergy in herbal medicine is not that it exists, but rather how often traditional cultures were able to attain it, given the astronomically high number of possible plant combinations. Once again, though, instead of just proceeding randomly, early herbalists developed a very empiric and logical approach that continues to be used to this day. They made the assumption, borne out in practice, that the effects of an herbal combination would once again be dictated by taste. If, for example, sweet herbs added fluids to the body and sour herbs gathered what was already present, sweet and sour might be especially hydrating and strongly indicated in deficient patients. It merely remained then to see which of the possible sweet and sour combinations actually had that effect in patients, and which did not.

Certain taste combinations were common within plants and were especially popular as goals for the combining of herbs. Their effects are also logically derived from the effects of individual tastes:

Sweet and Pungent

- Nourishing and invigorating; potently tonifying
- In addition, the sweet taste is moistening and the pungent taste moving, allowing the combination of sweet and pungent to soften and break apart masses and accumulations

Bitter and Pungent

- The most common form of herbal synergy
- Both bitter and pungent tastes can precipitate movement. With the bitter taste, this movement is usually in a downward (draining) direction
- When the two are combined, the descending action of bitter harnesses the expanding power of pungent to create a dilating or opening effect that is important in inducing bronchodilation and regulating peristalsis. In addition, this opening effect seemed to affect blood vessels, resulting in improved circulation and relief of chronic inflammation. If the pungent herb was also hot, analgesia would be accentuated

Pungent, Warm, and Mildly Sweet to Neutral

- The pungent warm or hot herb was essentially considered to embody Yang, or power, and could be used to boost the power of milder herbs. When combined with the mildly sweet plants that facilitated urination, the effect seemed to be a more powerful form of diuresis

Detractors of herbal medicine claim that long-standing use of herbs does not at all ensure their safety, speculating that early herbalists had no systematic method of recording adverse effects and were thus blissfully unaware of them. The *Nei Jing*, written in 200 BC, disproves this notion, because it poetically summarizes experiences to date not only as the effects of the Five Tastes, but also with a view toward how they could be used to antidote each other. Sour herbs were used to contain the otherwise explosive and scattering power of pungent herbs. Sweet herbs were used to avoid excessive draining and weakening of the patient with the use of bitter herbs. Warm pungent herbs were used to counteract the vigorous cooling effects of bitter herbs.

HOW TO PRACTICE HERBAL MEDICINE

Modern botanical medical prescribing tends to revolve around treating patients with disease as defined in textbooks. Plants are chosen from among a myriad of possibilities that have similar pharmacologic effects, although it is generally unknown whether any synergistic reactions can be expected. Nuisance adverse effects are likewise somewhat unpredictable.

Although taste determines action, specific actions are not necessarily the exclusive domain of a particular taste. Compounds that relieve musculoskeletal pain may be sour, pungent, or bitter, but a patient who experiences pain relief from a sour herb is generally much more deficient than a patient who benefits from a strongly bitter or pungent herb. Indeed, if a patient is deficient, the forceful draining and moving properties of a bitter pungent herb are probably contraindicated and likely to cause adverse effects. Prescription that is based on symptomatic, pharmacologic, and physiologic principles alone may thus end up providing an herb that is inappropriate from an overall metaphoric, or "energetic," perspective.

In contrast to the modern biomedical approach, the traditional approach is to work at a general level first, before worrying about specific symptomatic and pharmacologic effects. The steps involved are as follows:

- Diagnose the patient's condition in metaphoric terms starting by characterizing the patient as either "Hot", "Cold", "Excess", or "Deficient"
- Determine general desired plant actions on the basis of the metaphoric diagnosis of the patient
- Determine general plant tastes that fulfill this requirement
- From within this group, choose a subset that have the desired symptomatic effects

In modern prescribing, a final step is added—the selection of herbs that have desired specific physiologic and pharmacologic effects, when known. It should be noted, though, that choosing plants according to taste already ensures that the chemical content is broadly appropriate. Thus, if specific chemical requirements for the treatment of a disease are unknown, the traditional prescriber can still proceed with confidence, whereas the modern botanical prescriber cannot.

To illustrate the process, consider a patient with constipation. If diagnosed as hot and excessive, strongly bitter herbs are called for. Sweet oily emollients would play only a minor role in the formula because the intense physical presentation of the patient would require that the dominant plants in the formula must be cathartic. The pharmacologic goal of therapy would be to vigorously stimulate peristalsis.

Now, consider a constipated patient who is cold and deficient. Bitter herbs would be contraindicated, except when used in very small amounts. The reason is that peristaltic contractions are present, but they are simply too weak to expel stool. Sweet emollient formulas and herbs that have a lubricating action and generally strengthen peristaltic contractions are now more appropriate.

If cathartics were used in a cold deficient constipated patient, the patient might certainly respond but may be more likely to manifest adverse effects such as vomiting and dehydration. In addition, the draining effects of cathartics might weaken the patient further, resulting in a perpetuation of the problem as an apparent laxative addiction. Dependence on laxatives would be resolved only after moistening and strengthening herbs are introduced. Ironically, Chinese medicine would be much more likely than conventional medicine to view laxative dependency as an adverse effect of inappropriate treatment, reminding us again just how aware traditional herbal prescribers really were of the potential for adverse effects of their treatments.

In summary, the prescription of herbs first according to their energetics ensures overall appropriateness and minimizes adverse effects. Ratios of herbs in a formula can even be adjusted to create the ideal overall taste that exactly matches the metaphoric presentation of the patient. Because taste is determined by chemical content, intensity of taste correlates with the pharmacologic activity of the formula. More severe or acute disease calls for stronger tasting formulas and herbs with a higher amount of the active ingredient. Strong tastes are used more sparingly or are diluted out with the inclusion of other herbs in formulas for chronically ill and deficient patients.

A good general strategy is to select herbs that enhance each other's actions and reduce each other's adverse effects. Focusing on taste helps one to identify herbs that are likely to interact synergistically. Emphasis on taste allows adverse effects to be specifically anticipated and prepared for. For example, if a strong bitter herb were necessary for use in a cold deficient patient, symptoms consistent with further weakening would be anticipated, unless the formula was modified with the inclusion of a sweet, warm, pungent herb.

Possibly because of this emphasis on taste as a guide to avoiding adverse effects, adverse reactions and drug–herb interactions are rarely reported and often merely speculative. Despite this, veterinarians should not become complacent and instead should place a priority on using a centralized adverse event reporting system. Until that time, however, the matching of patients and herbs first on a metaphoric level, and only then on a conventional medical level prevails as the best defense against unwanted adverse effects.

As veterinarians begin to identify consistently effective therapies for typical small animal disorders, it behooves them as a profession to explore the implications of these treatments from a pharmacologic perspective. When the pathophysiology of the condition that is being treated is not known, the pharmacology of the herbs should be characterized, and the means by which they could resolve the problem hypothesized. Hypotheses could then be tested and, when they are not disproved, used to drive the development of new conventional medical stratagems.

For example, the routine success, in my practice, of high doses of saw palmetto berry in aborting urethral obstruction in cats, even when urine pH is 6.0 or less and crystalluria is not observed, strongly suggests that saw palmetto is behaving as a spasmolytic. Within the saw palmetto berry, beta sitosterol-6-glucoside (BSS6G) may to be the main spasmolytic.

The next step would be to test the hypothesis that BSS6G has a spasmolytic effect on the urethra; a negative finding would not disprove the hypothesis but would require that a potential synergistic reaction between BSS6G and some other component of saw palmetto must be identified. If BSS6G was recognized as a urethral spasmolytic effective in cats with urethral obstruction, the way would be paved for a pharmaceutical company to attempt to enhance its effectiveness and produce a new drug for the condition. Ironically, small animal veterinarians with no interest in or even patience for herbal medicine would then directly benefit from the work of veterinary herbalists.

It may be that the effects of saw palmetto cannot be improved upon. In this instance, the benefits of BSS6G in urethral obstruction would be accessed only through administration of the herb, highlighting a curious irony. Herbs may well contain the most powerful drugs in the world but may be forever doomed to suffer the disdain of herbal medicine critics, because their chemical constituents cannot be improved upon sufficiently to warrant the expense of clinical trials and patents.

Veterinary herbal medicine has arrived at an important data-gathering stage. Observations are now being made in the field of veterinary herbal medicine that will very likely be published in the near future, barring editorial bias. These case series will then serve as fodder for studies undertaken to confirm a treatment's effectiveness and its pharmacologic basis. Without the reporting of these field observations, such advancement might never occur, underscoring the need for tolerance of the work and traditions of veterinary herbalists by members of the conventional medical community.

Herb Manufacture, Pharmacy, and Dosing

CHAPTER

Barbara J. Fougère and Susan G. Wynn

A plethora of products is available on the market. Why wouldn't we simply recommend that our clients go and buy one off the shelf for their animal? Quite apart from the standard practice of prescribing according to individual needs, one of our main concerns is whether the practitioner can be confident of product quality. Is it safe? Will it be effective? Quality control is covered in Chapter 8, and integral to this is the matter of how herbs are manufactured. This chapter looks at how herbs are made into various useful forms and how they can be dispensed and dosed appropriately.

HERB VARIABILITY

It is well established that the same species of herb can vary widely depending on cultivation practices. Differences in water availability, fertilizer type, temperatures, and other factors can make for more or less concentrated herbs. The sophisticated quality control procedures that are needed to monitor these variations are not available to veterinarians but may be used by some companies. The best advice for minimizing the effect of this variability on patients is to find a reputable herbal pharmacy or supplier and to use herbal products consistently.

GOOD MANUFACTURING PRACTICE

To know which herbs a patient is receiving, practitioners must make their own or purchase good-quality herbal medicines and formulate from these. Manufacture of herbal medicinal products should be undertaken according to Good Manufacturing Practice (GMP), with the goal of providing quality assurance and safety in all manufactured products. It is important to know that the chosen manufacturer complies with these standards, which ensure that the right species is being used, that it is being produced and stored properly, and that it is not contaminated or adulterated.

Compared with well-defined synthetic drugs, herbal medicines exhibit some marked differences, namely,

- They are defined biologically rather than chemically
- The active principles are frequently unknown
- Standardization, stability, and quality control are feasible but problematic
- The availability and quality of raw materials are frequently problematic

It is no surprise that manufacture of herbal products under GMP is more complex than that of conventional drugs. However, GMP is not applied to growing, harvesting, drying, or sifting of herbs, nor is it related to preliminary processing of herbal oils. So, the sources of raw material and the good practices of manufacturing processes are certainly essential steps in the quality control of herbal medicines. One critical issue for safety and efficacy is identification of the right plant species. Substitution of one herbal raw material for another can be a serious problem when it is a subspecies, the wrong species (e.g., Aristolochia for Stephania causing renal failure), or a less active plant part, or when an herb is contaminated by another species (e.g., digitalis in comfrey).

Therefore, it is important that material specifications for crude herbs should include information on source, part used, description, and identification, as well as reports on contamination with pesticides, microbes, mould, pests, or foreign matter and on purity or potency. Herbs have been contaminated with heavy metals (e.g., cadmium and arsenic) and have been adulterated with drugs (e.g., nonsteroidal anti-inflammatory drugs). Any contamination could compromise the safety and efficacy of an herbal preparation, even when the practitioner decides to make his or her own herbs in practice; a specification form should be requested when bulk purchases are made.

In the first instance then, the source and quality of raw materials play a pivotal role in the quality and stability of herbal preparations. Other factors such as use of fresh or dried plants, season, light exposure, water availability, nutrients, period and time of collection, storage and transportation of raw material, age and part of the plant collected, and methods of collecting, drying, and packing can greatly affect the quality and consequently the therapeutic value of herbal medicines. These factors also account for variability of individual constituents or markers in herbal preparations. This variability is not a feature of conventional drug manufacture.

STANDARDIZATION

The American Herbal Products Association (AHPA) defines standardization very broadly as "the complete body of information and controls that serves to optimize the batch-to-batch consistency of a botanical product. Standardization is achieved by reducing the inherent variation of natural product composition through quality assurance practices applied to agricultural and manufacturing processes."

Standardized extracts are common in trade and are prepared by maceration, percolation, or distillation (volatile oils). Ethanol, water, or mixtures of ethanol and water are used for the production of fluid extracts. Solid or powdered extracts are prepared by evaporation of solvents used in the process of extraction of the raw material.

Advances in the processes of purification, isolation, and measuring of certain phytochemicals have made possible the establishment of appropriate strategies for the analysis of quality and the process of standardization of herbs toward maintaining as much as possible the homogeneity of the plant extract. Among others, gas chromatography, high-performance liquid chromatography, thin-layer chromatography, mass spectrometry, infrared spectrometry, and ultraviolet/visible spectrometry, used alone or in combination, can be successfully used for standardization and to control the quality of the raw material and the finished herbal products.

However, plants contain several hundred constituents, and some of them are present at very low concentrations; despite these technologically advanced chemical analytical procedures, rarely do phytochemical investigations succeed in isolating and characterizing all secondary metabolites present within a plant extract. Also, marker substances used in standardization and quality control tests may not really account for the therapeutic action reported for an herbal product.

As well, marker compounds may exhibit wide variation, for example, *Echinacea purpurea* products in Australian products have demonstrated wide variation in such markers as alkylamides and caffeoyl phenols. Thus, standardization and quality control of raw material and herbal preparations are challenging compared with these processes in standard drug manufacturing, and their relevance to therapeutic value may be questionable. Standardization can enhance only the reproducibility of a preparation—not its quality.

The AHPA white paper on standardization notes that the concept of standardization has been misunderstood to describe the "control or isolation of particular constituents. On the contrary, standardization is a complex, multifaceted process that relies primarily on appropriate controls of raw materials and the manufacturing process. Quantitative testing such as bioassays or measurement of specific constituents may be used in addition to, but never in place of, these other measures, because analytical measurements by themselves can only confirm, not control, "batch-to-batch consistency."

SOURCES OF HERBS

Commercial herbal preparations draw plant material from two main sources: wildcrafting and cultivation. Wildcrafting involves the harvesting of plants from the wild by trained collectors; these herbs are preferred by many herbalists. Cultivated plants are specifically grown for the trade and are the best sources of endangered or threatened herbs. Herbalists and especially herb pharmacies have voiced concern that plants in cultivation are not of the same quality as wildcrafted herbs. Herb pharmacies are investigating this issue in partnership with academic centers; no clear answers have been revealed as yet.

Wildcrafting has led to the endangerment of a number of herbs, including goldenseal and ginseng. There is concern about others—even wild echinacea in the United States and thyme in Europe. Some herbs have very limited habitats, and although they are not now endangered, they are subject to trends and shifts in popularity. When herbs are bought from a supplier who wildcrafts, the purchaser should make sure that the label says "ethically wildcrafted." This means that the wildcrafter protects the herbs by harvesting only a small percentage. It is MUCH better for practitioners to find an organic cultivated source for these herbs.

A third source of herbs may be your own garden. Home production of locally endangered plants lightens the strain of commerce in that plant and provides the herbalist with an opportunity to better study his or her medicine from germination to patient administration. Even if regulatory pressures discourage veterinarians from assuming liability for their home-prepared herbal medicines, the use of home-grown plants in their own personal family pharmacy supports the learning process and is highly recommended for recreation and exercise. An excellent reference for home medicine-makers is Cech (2000).

BOX 14-1

Types of Herbal Preparations

- Water extractions
  - Infusions
  - Decoctions
- Oil extractions
- Tinctures
  - Alcohol
  - Glycerin
  - Vinegar
- Fresh or dried herb for direct feeding
- Succi (fresh pressed juice)
- Herbal syrups and honey
- Special preparations (Pao Zhi)

FORMS OF HERBAL MEDICINES

Veterinarians are usually too busy to make their own herbal medicines, but it is important that they know how the herbs are prepared. Herbal products begin as fresh or dried plant, or as plant extracts (Box 14-1). These preparations form the basis for capsules, tablets, pills, salves, oils, liniments, juices, and tinctures.

Which form is commercially available or preferred depends upon whether the main constituents of an herb are lipid or water soluble, as well as on their palatability and level of patient acceptance. Whole fresh or dried plant is obviously the form that keeps all constituents intact, but it is the form that requires greater volume and may result in poor taste and potentially poor bioavailability; however, for ruminants and horses, this form may be the most acceptable.

Dried Forms

Dried herbs

Dried bulk herb has been harvested, dried, and sometimes powdered. Dried powdered herb may be supplied as a dried bulk herb, as loose powder, or in capsules. Gardeners may dry herbs from their own plots with basic knowledge of the plant part used and the correct harvest time. Aerial parts may be cut and bundled together to be hung on a rafter in a dry spot or on drying screens until dehydrated. A gentle air current can speed drying time, which cuts down on microbial contamination. The herb must be protected against excessive heat and light and not left exposed for long after it is dried. Once the herb is completely dried, it can be stripped from the stalks and stored in jars with lids, or in tins. This form can be used for teas or decoctions, or can be fed directly mixed in the animal's food, which is probably ideal. Dried herbs are best stored under cold conditions (less than 11° C) to limit the hatching of insect eggs, which inevitably infest organic herbs.

US Pharmacopoeia (USP) Definitions

Fluid extract: Alcoholic or hydroalcoholic preparation providing a dry herb : liquid strength ratio of 1 : 1. These very concentrated extracts require vacuum equipment.

Fresh plant fluid extract: Alcoholic or hydroalcoholic tincture prepared using 1 part fresh herb by weight for 1 part liquid by volume. This weight : volume relationship takes into account the water content in fresh plants. (The AHPA adds that fluid extracts are also sometimes 1 : 2 biomass : solvent, and that traditionally dried herb is used.)

Soft extract: An extract that has the consistency of a thin to thick liquid or paste.

Solid extract: A USP fluid extract that has been evaporated or vacuum extracted to 4 parts herb for every 1 part extract.

Powdered extract: A powdered version of a USP solid extract or fluid extract, prepared by evaporation to remove liquid. The concentration can range from 1 : 1 to 10 : 1, or greater.

Standardized extract: A powdered extract prepared by any of the previous methods, with certain constituents (either a particularly active ingredient or a marker compound) standardized to a specific preset level in every batch of extract. These extracts may or may not change the ratio of constituent ingredients within the plant to each other, depending on which compound is chosen and how the plant is standardized.

Galenical extract: A pharmacopoeial extract prepared according to guidelines from various pharmacopoeias, such as the British Pharmaceutical Codex, that dictate the method of preparation, the solvent used (usually alcohol and water), and the ratio of herb material to final extract. In modern times, this extract is often formed into a tablet or capsule.

Dried extracts

The herb has been concentrated by simmering in water (see Infusions and Decoctions, later) removing the residue, and spraying the concentrated "tea" in a vacuum chamber, resulting in powder or granules of remaining concentrated herbal constituents. One caution in the use of this form of herb is that because the solvent used is water, the extract may miss active constituents that are only alcohol soluble. A commonly provided form is a 4 : 1 or 5 : 1 extract, which allows veterinarians to recommend fewer capsules than if powdered herb is used. Dried extracts may also be available as loose powders or granules, encapsulated powders or granules, or pressed tablets.

Tinctures and Liquid/Fluid Extracts

These are the most commonly dispensed liquid forms of herbs; combining liquids makes formulation and prescribing easy. The advantages of tinctures include the following:

- Alcohol based (good solvent and preservative at 25%–100%)
- Concentrated
- Good shelf-life
- Convenient

Alcohol is a useful solvent and forms tinctures with nearly unlimited shelf-life, unless precipitation occurs over time. For extraction of water and lipid-soluble herb components, alcohol and water proportions may range from 20 : 80 to 40 : 60 (vodka is conveniently made this way) up to 100% alcohol. The percentage of alcohol needed varies according to the constituents to be dissolved, and good manufacturers vary the alcohol:water ratio to reflect the ideal extract for each individual herb (Table 14-1). For instance, mucilage does not dissolve well in ethanol, so a low alcohol percentage is best at 15% to 25%, and resinous herbs dissolve only in high-alcohol menstruum (90%+). Many herbs extract well in plain 80 proof (40% alcohol) vodka. Tinctures must contain at least 24% to 26% pure alcohol to be well preserved. Some manufacturers decoct herbs that are traditionally used this way (concentrated through multiple boiling water extractions), then preserve with alcohol.

One interesting variation on this theme is to extract some of the herb in 100% alcohol and decoct the other

TABLE 14-1

Solubility of Herb Components

Component	Example Plants	Solubility
Alkaloids	Goldenseal, lobelia, bloodroot, corydalis	High solubility in alcohol, low water solubility. Vinegar may enhance extraction
Essential oils	Peppermint, lavender, thyme, tea tree	High solubility in alcohol, low water and glycerin solubility. Extract well into fixed oils
Glycosides	Hawthorn, licorice, milk thistle, gentian	Soluble in water and alcohol
Mucilage	Slippery elm, marshmallow, purslane	Water soluble only and best extracted in cold water; will precipitate if alcohol is added. Usually used fresh or simply dried
Polysaccharides	Astragalus, mushrooms, boneset, echinacea	Water soluble only, will precipitate if alcohol is added
Resins	Kava, rosemary, grindelia, propolis, sweetgum	Soluble in alcohol and hot oil; not soluble in water. To make an ointment, use tincture in 95%—100% alcohol; add oil, then gently heat to evaporate the alcohol
Saponins	Ginseng, wild yam, yucca	Water soluble
Tannins	Witch hazel, blackberry leaf, self heals	Water and glycerin soluble

portion of herb, then add the two together at an optimal proportion; presumably, this allows maximal extraction of both water- and alcohol-soluble ingredients. It is wise to know what the concoction smells and tastes like when it is first made, so that one can check for spoilage later.

Alcohol extracts are concentrated and are believed by herbalists to have the most rapid gastrointestinal absorption rate and bioavailability of active components. It is likely that alcohol acts to keep these active components in solution after ingestion, thus facilitating their absorption into circulation. Alcohol extracts taste terrible to most dogs and cats, but the small amount required, in addition to the ease with which they can be combined by the herbalist, makes liquid extracts popular.

Strength of tinctures and fluid extracts

The concentration of a tincture (TR) or a fluid extract (FE) is expressed as a weight : volume ratio (w : v), that is, the weight of dried herb used to the volume of menstruum (or solvent) added.

Technically,

- FEs are concentrated 1 : 1 or 1 : 2 w/v
- TRs are concentrated 1 : 3 or weaker (e.g., 1 : 4, 1 : 5, 1 : 10)

In practice though, herbalists tend to refer to their alcohol-based extracts as tinctures, no matter the strength.

Making tinctures and fluid extracts

The folk method of preparing tinctures is simply to loosely pack a jar with fresh or dried cut herb, then to pour solvent over it to cover completely. To make a more standardized extract, the weight : volume method is used to describe the concentration of a tincture. The herb is weighed and the volume of the solvent is added in some proportion to the weight (grams of herb to milliliters of solvent, for instance), and typical proportions are 1 : 2 for fresh herb and 1 : 5 for dried herb. For example, 2 ounces by weight of an herb may be placed in a small jar, then covered with 4 oz of vodka, to produce a 40% alcohol 1 : 2 tincture. Strong herbs, such as lobelia and pokeweed, are often tinctured at lower concentrations (1 : 10) to guard against overdoses.

Tinctures are prepared with use of the herb (the "marc") and a solvent (the "menstruum"). The herb is prepared before it is tinctured. Fresh herb should be minced finely to destroy as many cell walls as possible. Because fresh herbs contain variable amounts of water, they should be tinctured in the higher percentages of alcohol. Fresh roots should be sliced thinly or chopped finely. Some are very tough and require pruning shears for cutting (use of a meat cleaver is effective, but root pieces fly all over the place). Roots are best used fresh in the home pharmacy because when dried, they become too hard to be chopped without commercial equipment. Dried herb aerial parts are simply crushed, ground in a food mill or coffee grinder, or pressed through a screen before tincturing. Dried herbs swell with water when the menstruum is added, so room must be left in the macerating jar to account for this. The herb is usually "moistened" overnight before the menstruum is poured, to minimize any change in volume. If seeds are used, they should be dried for a few hours and separated from any chaff, then ground or bruised before tincturing.

The blender method is very effective—put menstruum and chopped herb into a blender, and begin blending. Keep adding pieces of herb until the blender can take no more. This method produces a stronger tincture, but it is more difficult to squeeze the menstruum from at completion of the tincturing process.

In the industry, two main methods are used to make TRs and FEs: percolation and maceration.

Maceration: Dried herb is soaked (macerated) in the desired menstruum at room temperature for a time. To prepare an herbal tincture, one should loosely fill a wide-mouthed glass bottle or jar with herbal parts. Plastic may be acceptable but could adsorb certain plant components, and metal should be avoided. If fresh herbs are used, they should be cut into manageable pieces. If dried herbs are used, they should be crumbled into the container. Pure spirits, such as vodka or a calculated ethanol:water combination, should be added to cover the herbs. The container should be sealed and the tincture allowed to stand in a warm place for 2 weeks. During the time that the tincture is maturing, the container should be shaken daily. After 2 weeks, the herbs (marc) should be strained out (in an herb press or a fine sieve, or wrapped in muslin by hand) and the residue squeezed out so that as much liquid as possible is retrieved. The final menstruum is allowed to settle, decanted and filtered through cheesecloth, a coffee filter, or laboratory filter paper. Dark glass bottles should be sealed well and stored out of direct sunlight. This process is suitable for small-scale production of tinctures and can easily be done in the practice. Fluid extracts can also be made by means of multiple maceration, a process that involves a series of macerations by which constituents are concentrated. For the home pharmacy, wine bottles are convenient for storage.

Percolation: Ground dried herb is soaked in the menstruum (solvent) for several hours. The swollen plant material is then packed into a percolator, which is a tall metal or glass cylinder. More menstruum is added to cover the plant material, and this is left to macerate for 24 to 48 hours, and sometimes for weeks, depending on the herb. A tap at the bottom of the percolator is then opened to allow a slow drip, and the percolate is collected in a closed container. This process of simple percolation is suitable for the preparation of home tinctures. A number of complicated processes are used commercially to make more concentrated extracts.

Dilution: Some manufacturers make very concentrated extracts by reducing the volume of liquid under partial vacuum, then diluting in another liquid. This usually involves heat; therefore, extracts made in this way are generally considered to be of inferior quality because of the potential for heat damage to some of the constituents. TRs and FEs made by diluting these concentrated extracts are therefore of poorer quality than those made by maceration or percolation.

Glycerin Extracts, Glycerites, and Glycetracts

Glycetracts use glycerin and water as solvents. They were traditionally made with mucilaginous herbs like marshmallow *(Althea officinalis)* and licorice *(Glycyrrhiza glabra)*, but now many herbs are available in this form. The following is true of glycetracts:

- They are sweet tasting
- More palatable than alcohol extracts
- Sweet taste of glycerin may hide the taste of the herbs, but some herbs may taste bad enough that animals do not accept glycerin extracts readily
- Are dispensed in the same way as FEs and TEs
- Can be mixed with alcohol-based extracts

Fresh plant extracts are best used with glycerin because it is better at preserving fresh plant juice as opposed to extracting components from the plant cells. Glycerin extracts tannins well and may help protect them from precipitation in mixed alcohol tinctures. One limitation to using glycerin tinctures is the potential for microbial contamination, especially from fresh plant starting material. Glycetracts can be made through maceration or percolation, as described; however, glycerin is not as good a solvent as water or alcohol. This problem is overcome by the making of modern glycetracts by replacement.

Replacement

Replacement involves gentle heating of a fluid extract to evaporate off the alcohol (and sometimes water). When the desired volume is reached, glycerin is added to return the extract to its original volume.

Glycerites ideally should be kept capped and refrigerated because they can mould. Glycerin tinctures must consist of more than 55% pure glycerin if they are to have preservative capacity (vegetable glycerin contains 5% water, which must be factored into the calculation).

For herbs that are best extracted in glycerin (including mucilaginous herbs like marshmallow), generally 4 parts glycerin and 1 part water are used to extract the herbs. Glycerin can also be mixed with a small amount of alcohol for broader extraction and better preservation.

Vinegar Extracts

Vinegar may be added to alcohol, water, or glycerin tinctures to increase the extraction of certain constituents, especially alkaloids. Aceta are pure vinegar tinctures, and these are not as strong as alcohol tinctures.

Supercritical CO_2 Extracts

A newer type of concentrated herb extract is the *supercritical carbon dioxide (CO_2) extract.* CO_2 is generally recognized by the US Food and Drug Administration (FDA) as a safe solvent (GRAS). In this process, pressurized CO_2 gas is pumped into a chamber filled with plant matter. Pressurized CO_2 is very dense; it functions as a liquid and extracts lipophilic components from the herb. Reported advantages of supercritical CO_2 extracts include the following:

- They leave no chemical residue of their own in the extract
- No high temperatures are used, which means that plant constituents have not been heat stressed (extraction temperature is 95° F–100° F, as opposed to 140° F–212° F)
- They are environmentally safe, leaving no harmful residues that need disposal
- They are highly concentrated and require no preservation because water, proteins, and sugar required to support microbial growth are absent

The end result is a broad spectrum of lipophilic constituents in the herb, which also means that this is not the appropriate technology for all herbs.

Fresh Plant Extracts

Fresh plant tinctures (FPTs) are made from fresh rather than dried plants. Some herbalists prefer this because of the "vitality" aspect retained in the plant; in some cases, drying changes the chemistry of the herb, making it less useful. However, fresh plants are bulkier and contain more moisture; this means that more menstruum is needed to cover the material. Also, the water that is an innate part of the plant will add to the volume of the menstruum; therefore, it is difficult to make a concentrated extract of FPT.

By convention, the strength of FPT is based on the equivalent dried weight of the plant used, and the FPT product may state its dried weight equivalent (e.g., a 1 : 10 FPT is far less concentrated than a 1 : 10 liquid extract from dried herb). FDA regulations do not require that a dry equivalent must be stated on the label, however, which is sensible because no equivalent dried product may be available (e.g., in those cases where fresh plant extracts are more effective than dried plant extracts).

DISPENSING TINCTURES AND FLUID EXTRACTS

The beauty of stocking and dispensing TRs and FEs is that each is made from one species of medicinal plant and can be combined in limitless permutations, allowing for individualization of medicine according to patient needs.

In general, TRs and FEs can be mixed together with no problem. Some attention should be given to the relative alcohol percentages because these can affect the solubility of certain constituents. For example, mixing a mucilaginous extract with a high-alcohol extract causes the mucilage to precipitate out of solution and form a lump in the bottom of the bottle. Tannins and alkaloid extracts can also cause precipitation.

To remove some of the alcohol from a tincture, a suitable number of drops or volume of tincture must be added to 1 tablespoon of very hot water. Most of the alcohol evaporates away in about 5 minutes. This must be cooled and added to moist food.

Various flavoring agents can be used to improve palatability.

TANNIN/ALKALOID COMBINATIONS TO AVOID

Plants high in tannins and those high in alkaloids should not be mixed together. Tannins generally bind with alkaloids to form insoluble compounds (Boxes 14-2 and 14-3).

Specific classes of herb constituents frequently have similar biochemical characteristics that guide herb pharmacists in deciding on appropriate extraction techniques. It must be noted that exceptions to the guidelines that follow are frequent (see Table 14-1).

OTHER HERBAL EXTRACTS

Tinctures and fluid extracts are probably the most commonly dispensed liquid herbal medicines, but there are others.

BOX 14-2

Plants High in Tannins

- Agrimony
- Uva ursi
- Birch
- Cinnamon
- Geranium (Cranesbill)
- Guaiacum
- Witch hazel
- *Juglans* spp (walnut, butternut)
- Bayberry
- Potentilla
- Oak
- *Rubus* spp (blackberry, raspberry)
- *Vaccinium* spp (blueberry/bilberry)

BOX 14-3

Plants High in Alkaloids

- *Berberis* spp (barberry)
- *Coptis* spp (goldthread)
- *Corydalis* spp
- Gelsemium
- Goldenseal
- Lobelia
- Oregon grape
- Passionflower
- Bloodroot
- Tribulus
- *Vinca major* (periwinkle)

Infusions and Decoctions

These are water-based extracts that are sometimes called *herbal teas*. Some herbs are best extracted with cold water; these include mucilage-containing herbs or those with delicate volatile oils. Infusions and decoctions are recommended for administering diaphoretic herbs (because hot tea encourages sweating) and herbs used for increasing urine volume when urinary tract conditions are treated. They are also a good alternative when alcohol is contraindicated.

Infusions are made from delicate plant parts like leaves and flowers. It should be noted that to use plants by infusion or decoction usually requires a much higher dose by volume than is needed with the dried herb from which it is made; this is often a consideration when one is treating animals and children. The traditional dose is 10 g (1–2 tsp) of dried herb added to 1 cup (180–200 mL) water three times daily for people (animal doses may be scaled up or down from this starting point—see dosing guidelines below). Teas may be added to broths and foods and can be used as the basis for herbal washes and compresses.

TABLE 14-2

Common Herbs That Can Be Infused and Decocted

Herb	Process	Uses
Ginger	Infusion	Motion sickness, nausea
Chamomile	Infusion	Topically and orally for mild diarrhea
Slippery elm	Cold water infusion	Poultice, and orally for gastrointestinal disease
Peppermint	Infusion	Orally, for flatulence, bloating, colic, ulcerative colitis
Green tea	Infusion	Topically, cancer protective mix with food
Cinnamon	Decoction	Warming, flatulence, bloating, colic, diarrhea
Fennel	Infusion	Carminative, anorexia, pharyngitis
Fenugreek	Infusion/ decoction	Diabetes, anorexia, gastritis, convalescence
Linseed	Mix with warm water	To aid removal of foreign bodies, mucilage, constipation

Decoctions are made from tougher plant parts, such as roots, stems, bark, and sometimes leaves, by placing the plant material in cold water and bringing it to a boil, then simmering for 20 minutes or so. The combination is allowed to cook until it is reduced in volume, then the filtered liquid is added to more herb material and water, and the entire combination is cooked to concentration again. The continued simmering and boiling cycle releases volatile components like essential oils but has the advantage of concentrating some of the more stable constituents like minerals and alkaloids.

Infusions and decoctions can be preserved for 2 to 3 days by refrigeration or by freezing (Table 14-2). Freezing the liquid in ice cube trays aids dosing, and these blocks can be readily added to dog and cat food.

Succi

Succi are herb juices that can be made only from fresh plant material and from a limited range of plants with high water content, like cleavers *(Gallium aparine)*, chickweed *(Stellaria media)*, nettles *(Urtica dioica)*, gotu kola *(Centella asiatica)*, plantain *(Plantago major)*, calendula *(Calendula officinalis)*, and fumitory *(Fumaria officinalis)*. They are ground or mashed, and the juice is pressed by hand or under an herb press. Alternatively, they may be juiced in a blender. They should be used within 24 hours unless preserved with alcohol (25%–33%).

Syrups

Syrups can disguise bad-tasting herbs and allow for greater contact with oral mucosa because of their viscosity. They are made by concentrating sugar in aqueous herb extract, or by making a sugar solution and adding herbal extract to make the syrup. To make an herbal syrup, one must combine 1 part water-extracted herb (decoction or infusion) with 2 parts sugar over a gentle heat. The sugar acts as a preservative and improves the palatability of the herb. Another alternative is to use honey instead of sugar, and a liquid extract (water or alcohol). The alcohol may be reduced with heating.

Herb Pills, Capsules, and Troches

Dried herbs can be powdered and mixed with water and honey and some forms of mucilage or paste to make a consistency that can be rolled into pills, then dried. Herb pills may be useful because powdered herbs reduce palatability when added to an animal's food, or when pilling is an easy option for clients.

Capsules can be made by packing dried herb into capsule shells. When small doses are used, it is sometimes easier to add honey and flour than to fill capsules. It may be difficult to get a significant amount of dried herb into a capsule, although it will suit small to medium-sized dogs and cats. Some manufacturers overcome this problem by freeze-drying a concentrated liquid extract, then compressing the solid material into a tablet or granules.

Troches (similar to a lozenge) can be made by mixing dried herbs or concentrated granules with moist pet food or mince with a little bran to bind them, then forming balls and refrigerating them. This makes them easy to handle and administer. Some animals readily accept these as snacks, making dosing easy.

Infused Oils

Infused oils are made by macerating (meaning 'soak and separate') plant material in oil (e.g., olive, almond, or grapeseed) for 1 to 2 weeks. The dried herb is first ground (a coffee grinder is very useful), then placed in a container; oil is added to cover the dried material and to prevent mould formation. The mix is placed in sunlight and rotated daily to expose the plant to the oil. "Digesting" is macerating combined with gentle heat (around 40° C). The container is placed in a low-temperature oven, a low-temperature water bath, or a sand bath placed on a heated element. The idea is to provide gentle heat for 6 to 10 hours, which speeds the process of infusion. Oils are selective in that they will dissolve only oil-soluble constituents like essential oils and resins. When ready, the oil is filtered—often several times—to remove fine plant material. Infused oils can be used topically but, more commonly, they form the basis of ointments, lotions, creams, and salves. Essential oils that evaporate when heat is applied can be brought back later by adding a couple of drops to the oil infusion.

Lotions and Creams

Herbal lotions and creams are useful in the treatment of acute and chronic focal skin conditions and as a first aid measure. They are prepared by emulsifying an aqueous phase with an oily phase. The aqueous phase can be any of the liquid herb extracts (infusions, decoctions, or tinctures), and the oily phase can be an infused oil, so that both phases are medicated, which makes a stronger preparation. Emulsifying wax is probably the most effective and available emulsifier.

An alternative method is to use add herbal tinctures to a sorbolene or vitamin E cream base. This is quick and convenient; it means that one container can be made for a particular patient on the spot that addresses individual requirements.

Herbs commonly used include comfrey *(Symphytum officinale)*, marigold *(Calendula officinalis)*, lavender *(Lavendula* spp*)*, chickweed *(Stellaria media)*, gotu kola *(Centella asiatica)*, and Saint John's Wort *(Hypericum perforatum)*.

Ointments and Balms

Herbal ointments are similar to creams but contain no water. They are made by melting beeswax or other more solid oils or butters with an infused herbal oil. They seem to encourage licking but may be more useful in large animals, particularly in the form of liniments and chest rubs.

Ointments and balms are made by creating an oil infusion, then adding beeswax:

- Make oil infusion as described earlier
- Add beeswax—the amount depends on intended use
- Pour into tins or jars, cool with lid on loosely, tighten lid, then store in a dark place
- Shelf-life is short—probably 2 to 3 months, longer with refrigeration

Balms contain relatively more wax compared with ointments. Balms are meant to provide a barrier on the skin and are thicker. Ointments are lighter and contain more oil, so they can be absorbed through the skin.

To find the right consistency, one should start by using a final concentration of 10% beeswax for an ointment and 25% for a balm. A small amount of the infused oil should be used for the test run; then, the product should be refrigerated and the consistency checked in a minute or two. If needed, more infused oil or more beeswax is added, depending on the desired result. Infused oils can be augmented with glycerin tinctures, alcohol tinctures, and infusions. The more aqueous the mixture, the more like a light cream or lotion the end result will be. If a mistake is made, the ointment mixture may be reheated so that the hardness can be adjusted with more infused oil or more wax. The final ointment is then tested and poured into jars.

Liniments

Liniments are easy to make in an oil or spirit base. They are most often liquid based but may be semisolid, as in a liniment ointment. A variety of herbal extracts may be suitable, for example, cinnamon, clove, ginger, pepper, rosemary, and peppermint as oils or extracts.

Herbal Baths

An herbal bath can be very useful for pruritus. An herbal bath can be prepared in several ways.

- If a soluble ingredient, such as aloe vera gel, is used, one should simply dissolve it in hot water, then add to lukewarm bath water
- If oatmeal is used, it should be bagged. Oatmeal seems soft, but it does not release active constituents unless it has first been very finely milled. Instant oatmeal works well
- If fresh herbs are used, they should be bagged in a square of cheesecloth, a knee-high stocking, or a thin sock. A loose weave permits maximum release of the herbal essence, yet keeps the parts from floating free in the bath water. Approximately 6 or more ounces of dried or fresh herbs should be used. To fill the tub, one should place the bagged herbs under a forceful stream of hot water. The herbs should then be allowed to sit in a small volume of hot water (infuse); lukewarm water should be added, so that the end result is water at body temperature
- If a pruritic skin condition is treated, the bag should be gently rubbed across the affected areas, or liquid should be squeezed from the bag onto the skin

A pre-prepared herbal infusion can be made by soaking 6 tablespoons of dried or fresh herbs overnight in 3 cups of water. One should start with very hot water and allow it to cool naturally. The following morning, the residue should be strained out. No bag is needed; the strained infusion can be poured directly onto the patient or into bath water.

Pessaries and Suppositories

Commercial herbal pessaries and suppositories are not readily available. They have many potential uses in veterinary medicine, including administration of herbs when vomiting prevents oral administration, when rectal or anal conditions are treated, and when analgesic herbs are administered.

A traditional method of making herbal suppositories was to stiffen an infused oil with beeswax. They are not difficult to make. The two most commonly used bases include:

- Cocoa butter as a fatty base—this is useful for carrying fat-soluble herbal extracts. This base has an emollient action on the tissue with which it is in contact
- Glycerin and gelatin—this is an aqueous base, so it can be used to carry water-soluble herbal extracts. The glycerin is slightly drying to tissues

Herbs commonly used include marigold *(Calendula officinalis)*, slippery elm powder *(Ulmus fulva)*, and witch hazel *(Hamamelis virginiana)*.

Enema

Herbal extracts may be given in diluted form as a tea or extract (with alcohol evaporated away) via enema, particularly in large animals and animals that cannot take medication orally. This is particularly useful when the patient is dehydrated and is vomiting, for example, in acute pancreatitis or renal failure. The starting dose for a high enema is 5 mL/lb of body weight.

Poultices and Compresses

These are applied to the skin and can be used to treat the skin or deeper tissues. They are generally very effective and simple to make. Poultices are made by crushing fresh or dried plant material and adding small amounts of water to create a thick paste before applying to the affected area.

Compresses are made by soaking a soft cloth in an herbal extract and applying the moist cloth to the area. Both poultices and compresses can be used hot or cold for a number of conditions. For example,

- A comfrey poultice is vulnerary on ulcerated tissue
- A chamomile eye compress is soothing for conjunctivitis
- Grated potatoes can be used for minor burns
- Slippery elm or linseed can be used as a drawing agent
- Oatmeal poultice can be applied for pododermatitis

Herbal Vapor

An herbal inhalation treatment is very helpful for respiratory and sinus conditions. It opens up congested sinuses and lung passages, helping the patient to discharge mucus, breathe more easily, and heal faster. A bucket or sink should be filled with very hot water and 2 to 5 drops of essential oil added. The patient should be enclosed in a small space (stable or bathroom, or a covered cage or crate) and should inhale the steam for at least 5 minutes.

Choosing the Best Preparation

Some herbs lose potency when they are dried, and they should be used fresh—usually, as a tincture, unless fresh material is available to the practitioner. Others, such as *Astragalus*, must be decocted before they are preserved with alcohol because straight tincturing of the dried root seems to result in a very weak medicine. Ginger is used both fresh and dried, and each preparation has distinct medicinal characteristics. Although the information needed to make the best preparation is available in old dispensatories, personal experience is important as well. A good herb pharmacy usually knows the best way to prepare each individual herb.

*Herbs better used fresh or tinctured fresh**

- Skullcap
- Cleavers
- Corn silk
- Cactus
- Eyebright
- Stillingia
- Collinsonia

*From Winston, 2003.

*Herbs better used in dried form**

- Blue cohosh
- Buckthorn bark
- Ganoderma
- Culvers root
- Codonopsis

*From Winston, 2003.

PAO ZHI

Pao zhi refers to traditional Chinese techniques for processing and preparing medicinal herbs. These methods may range from simple washing, chopping, and drying to fermentation to stir frying with other foods or herbs. In the Chinese energetic system, this processing changes the properties of the herbs significantly. One example described by Philippe Sionneau involves the formula *Bu Zhong Yi Qi Tang* (Sionneau, 1995). If the ingredients in this combination were used in unprepared form, the final actions of the formula would be to secure the exterior, disinhibit urination and stool, clear heat and resolve toxin, and dry dampness. However, we use *Bu Zhong Yi Qi Tang* to supplement the center and to boost and upbear *Qi*. This activity occurs only when prepared herbs are used. *Pao Zhi* confers a number of changes to the herbs processed, including the following:

- Lessens toxicity, moderates drastic actions, or diminishes adverse effects
- Modifies energetic properties
- Reinforces therapeutic effects
- Modifies tropism
- Reduces disagreeable odors or flavors
- Facilitates storage, production, and assimilation
- Eliminates foreign substances

Methods of preparation are as follows:

- Washing and rinsing
- Pulverizing
- Cutting
- Defatting—used most often to extract oils from seeds and grains, usually to lessen toxicity such as that found in croton seed oil
- Moistening and soaking—removes debris (such as seed coats), facilitates cutting, and may lessen toxicity
- Aqueous trituration (usually used for hard, insoluble minerals so that a fine powder is obtained)
- Stir frying without additions
- Stir frying until yellow—reinforces actions of some herbs, lessens toxicity, and moderates actions of others
- Stir frying until scorched—primarily to lessen toxicity but may also strengthen some actions
- Stir frying until carbonized—reinforces hemostatic activity, based on an old saying that "when blood sees black, bleeding is stopped"
- Stir frying with additions—each addition confers its own properties to the combination to change the nature of the original herb. Liquids or solids may be fried together with the herb.

  - Wheat bran—sweet, bland, and neutral; lessens drastic actions, protects stomach, and supplements spleen; harmonizes middle burner and deodorizes
  - Rice—sweet and neutral, eliminates dampness, reinforces antidiarrheal herbs, supplements spleen and *Qi*, harmonizes stomach, eliminates vexation, stops sweating, and lessens toxicity
  - Terra flava usta (medicinal earth)—acrid and warm—harmonizes and warms the middle burner, stops diarrhea
  - Powdered conch—salty and cold, eliminates dampness and oily substances, clears heat, transforms phlegm, softens hard masses
  - Powdered alum—sour and cold, lessens toxicity, eliminates phlegm, expels parasites, dries dampness, reinforces astringent herbs
  - Honey—sweet and cool but warm if cooked; calms spasms, stops pain, moistens dryness, stops cough, supplements the middle burner, lessens toxicity, and harmonizes medicinal herbs
  - Rice vinegar—bitter, sour, and warm; directs therapeutic effects to the liver, rectifies the *Qi*, quickens the blood and stops pain, lessens toxicity, reinforces astringent herbs, deodorizes
  - Rice wine—sweet, acrid, very hot; frees the flow of channels and quickens network vessels; moderates cold, directs therapeutic effects to the upper body, and deodorizes
  - Salt water—salty and cold, directs therapeutic effects to kidneys, softens hard masses, clears heat and cools blood, supplements Yin, and drains empty fire
  - Ginger juice—acrid and warm; stops vomiting, expels phlegm, warms middle burner, resolves exterior, lessens toxicity, controls cold
  - Animal fat—promotes penetration of bones, supplements spleen and kidneys
  - Licorice solution—sweet and neutral; harmonizes the center, calms spasms, moistens lungs, supplements spleen, lessens toxicity, harmonizes other herbs
  - Black soybean juice—sweet and neutral; quickens blood, disinhibits urination, supplements liver and kidneys, nourishes blood, dispels wind, lessens toxicity
  - Bile—clears liver heat, brightens eyes, rectifies the gallbladder, frees stool, resolves toxins, disperses swelling, moistens dryness
  - Sand—reduces toxicity of some herbs, facilitates pulverization, eliminates disagreeable tastes and odors
  - Conch—reduces risk of total carbonization, draws out fat from some remedies, lessens disagreeable odors and tastes, reinforces heat clearing action and transformation of phlegm
  - Talc—reduces toxicity, reduces risk of carbonization, lessens disagreeable tastes and odors, facilitates pulverization
- Calcination—cooking in an open or sealed pot
- Roasting—reduces fat, lessens adverse effects, reinforces astringent effects
- Blast frying—herbs are fried and continuously stirred until they are burnt but not completely carbonized; this lessens toxicity and modifies an herb's nature
- Baking, stone-baking—used primarily to slowly dehydrate herbs to facilitate storage
- Steaming—modifies herb actions, lessens adverse effects, facilitates cutting and storage
- Boiling—reinforces herb actions, reduces toxicity; may be boiled with other substances such as vinegar and licorice
- Scalding—blanching eliminates non-medicinal parts (such as seed coats) and facilitates drying and storage
- Dip calcining—mineral-type remedies such as shells and scales are heated until red hot, then dipped into water or vinegar; this process is repeated until the material is friable enough to be pulverized
- Distilling—used to obtain essential oils from aromatic plants
- Fermentation—plants are humidified until they ferment. This confers new actions on the herbs
- Germination—grains and seeds are watered or humidified and kept at a kindly temperature until they germinate; this transforms the remedy to have new actions

All of the above information comes from the excellent book, *An Introduction to the Use of Processed Chinese Medicinals*, by Philippe Sionneau (Sionneau, 1995).

STABILITY

Dried herbs are fairly delicate and should be stored away from heat and light to preserve their potency. Spent dried herbs lack the strong aroma and color of newly dried herbs, and because of oxidative processes may not be as potent. Visual and olfactory assessment is a good way to assess their therapeutic potential. Capsules protect dried herbs somewhat, but should still be used in less than 1 year. Dried extracts have a longer shelf-life, the expiration date of which should be provided by manufacturers. Water extracts have a shelf-life of only about 24 hours but can be frozen. Aceta (pure vinegar extracts) may last about 6 months. Glycerin tinctures are more prone to bacterial/fungal contamination (which can be minimized by storage in sterilized glass containers and kept in refrigeration), and these tinctures can last for 1 to 2 years. Alcohol tinctures last for 2 years or longer (many herbalists claim that 10 years is a reasonable shelf-life as long as precipitation has not occurred). Alcohol-preserved succi may last up to 2 years.

Stability is also important in herbal manufacturing from preparation of raw materials to creation of the end product. Some plant constituents are heat labile, and the plants that contain them need to be dried at low temperatures. Also, other active principles are destroyed by enzymatic processes that continue for long periods after plant collection has been completed. The final product can be tested for stability with the use of analytic markers, as well. For some active ingredients, however, it would be impossible to test for all phytochemicals in the product; these could degrade at different rates. These are important considerations because these factors can also account for differences in the therapeutic value of an herbal medicine.

PHARMACY

Starting and maintaining an herbal dispensary in the practice can be relatively straightforward and can range from a few bottles of herbal tinctures and tablets to full dispensaries with equipment and the facility to custom-blend formulas for patients. The herbal dispensary is not that different from a veterinary pharmacy. Similar principles apply.

Quality control is needed for both storage of herbs (shelf-life, expiry dates, stock rotation, storage conditions, appropriate containers) and processing of formulas (accurate weighing and measuring, sterile containers, lids, droppers).

Stock control is essential to avoid over ordering and stock wastage, as well as the inconvenience of under ordering. Ideally, one should choose suppliers with short delivery times. Stock should be checked each quarter for expiry and glycetracts monitored for contamination. One should develop a relationship with a local herbalist to obtain less frequently used herbs in small quantities.

Dispensed items require clear and precise labels and instructions that include patient identification and dosing. Good record keeping is essential; as with drugs, herb dosage, contraindications, and adverse events must be understood and managed appropriately.

The dispensing area and pharmacy should be maintained at a level of cleanliness that is suitable for the dispensing of medicines. All equipment and surfaces with which the herbs will come into contact should be appropriately cleaned after use. Staff should be trained in stock control and ordering procedures so that it should be possible to trace a particular batch of herbs if needed. Stock rotation and management of expiry dates is also important. An appreciation of storage conditions is essential.

Herbs should be organized alphabetically by common name or Latin (botanical) name, or, if one is using Chinese herbs, by Pin Yin or Latin (botanical) name.

DISPENSING PROCEDURES

Staff should be fully trained in the procedures of dispensing for each of the available forms of herbal medicines, whether tinctures, fluid extracts, dried herbs, powders, pills and capsules, or external preparations. A procedure for following a formula through dispensing should be employed to ensure that no duplications or omissions occur. The formula should be recorded in the patient notes and on the prescription label, along with dosage.

Each formula should be labeled and dated and should include the name of the patient, along with dosage and preparation instructions. In the case of multiple packets of dried herbs, each packet should be individually dated for identification and the whole prescription put in a packet with patient and instruction details. Other additions to the label, such as hospital contact information, should be included, in keeping with state or federal law.

Accurate weighing and measuring apparatus should be used. A scale that measures in grams is essential for formulating Chinese formulas. Accurate measuring is defined as having the ability to measure consistently within 1 g for crude herbs, and to within 0.1 g for concentrated powders. Measuring flasks, graduated in milliliters, are needed for dispensing liquid herbs. Staff should be able to fill capsules and should have knowledge of the production of external preparations, if such products are available from the dispensary, so that all products are consistently produced.

Scheduled herbs, if used, should be recorded in a drug ledger that is put aside for this purpose.

If any herb is out of stock, staff must inform the prescribing practitioner, who will advise accordingly. Also, if staff are at all concerned about any aspect of the prescription or the method of dispensing herbs, they should not issue the formula until the prescribing practitioner has cleared it.

Dispensing staff should sign each finished formula, either on the label or on the accompanying instructions, for quality control tracking and to signify that it is completed and ready for collection.

Dispensary Requirements

A small dispensary needs a number of basic supplies. Most herbal manufacturers and wholesalers have these items available, as do most kitchen suppliers:

- Reference books
- Paper towels
- Measuring cylinders (25 mL, 50 mL, 100 mL, 250 mL)
- Bottles (25 mL, 50 mL, 100 mL, 200 mL [in the United States, 2 oz, 4 oz, 8 oz])
- Containers with lids for dried herbs to hold 50 g and 100 g, or 2-oz or 4-oz jars
- Lids and droppers
- Medicine measures (30 mL plastic) and syringes for clients to use in measuring doses
- Labels
- Funnels for pouring herbs into bottles
- Bottle brushes for cleaning
- Jars (50 g amber) for creams
- Container in which to mix creams
- Tongue depressors with which to mix creams
- Weighing scales for powdered and dried herbs and for measuring creams
- Shelving for storage

The size and design of the dispensary are critical because they affect workflow, manufacturing, and communications.

Optional supplies include the following:

- Spatulas
- Mortar and pestle
- Spritzer bottles
- Heating tray and pans with which to make ointments
- Beeswax
- Jars (200 mL–500 mL) for use in making oil infusions

The practitioner should visit a number of herbal pharmacies before investing to set one up, to see the available options and decide what will work best in his or her practice.

DOSING

Posology (Greek *posos* meaning "how much" + *logos* meaning "science") in modern veterinary botanical medicine is in its infancy. Factors that influence dosage include route, frequency, degree of absorption, age and condition of patient, unique physiologic characteristics of various domestic species, and tolerance and idiosyncrasy of individuals. Fortunately, many proprietary brands of herbal formulas for veterinary use have instructions for usage; however, even these doses have not been proved optimal. Veterinary herbalists who make their own prescriptions are faced with the challenges of determining the appropriate dose for an individual patient. This can be a challenge because of the scarcity of scientific data and recorded traditional data on animals.

Liquid extracts are widely used, especially for the ease of preparation of formulations for the individual patient. As well, if properly prepared, extracts involve minimal processing and reflect the chemical characteristics of the herb in a compact, convenient form. They also confer considerable dosing flexibility, which is especially relevant for small animals.

Comparing Doses

The dried herb equivalent of a given amount of extract or product can be calculated. For example, a dried herb equivalent of 1 g might be

- 5 mL of a 1 : 5 liquid extract
- 2 mL of a 1 : 2 liquid extract
- 1 mL of a 1 : 1 liquid extract
- 200 mg of a 5 : 1 spray dried powder

Some General Considerations

The rule adhered to by most herbalists is as follows: When not sure, begin with the smallest dose first and work upward if needed. An understanding of the energetics of each formula or herb, along with its pharmacology, uses, contraindications, potential toxicity, drug–herb interactions, and speed of action, assists the practitioner in determining dose. Generally speaking, herbs are remarkably safe and user friendly. However, some are strong and may cause adverse effects if dosed inappropriately, or for certain individuals. Therefore, the patient's vitality, disease condition, concurrent medications, and age and maturity, as well as the condition of the organs in metabolizing, using, and eliminating herbs, are important considerations. It also must be acknowledged that herbs work on physical, energetic, subtle, and gross levels; this may be why herbs have traditionally been used in many different ways and yet have still proved to be effective.

Historical Veterinary Doses

Veterinary pharmacology books published from 1860 to 1950 are the best sources of information about herb dosing. Notes from these books and from veterinary school lectures suggest this dosing scheme:

The dose for a horse consists of

- Fluid extract: 1 dram (3.7 ml; can be rounded up to 4 ml)
- Powder: ½–1½ dram
- Tincture: 1 oz
- Injection: about ½ the amount given by mouth
- Enema: about twice as much as that given by mouth

Using the horse as a standard, other animals receive the following:

- Cattle: 1½ times that dose
- Sheep and goats: ⅕
- Pigs: ⅛
- Dogs: 1/16 (about the same as a human for medium to large dogs)
- Cats: 1/32

With human doses used as the standard, proportionate doses according to veterinary lectures from the 1920s were as follows:

- Dogs: equal to humans but proportionate to their size
- Pigs: 2×
- Sheep and goats: 3×
- Horses: 16× (*Note:* Modern herbalists consider this a very high dose; these levels are not presently used in equine practice)

Guidelines

- Acute conditions: Stronger herbs can be used; simples (single herbs) are often effective. Larger doses should be used every 2 to 4 hours until symptoms subside. If improvement does not occur quickly, the formula or herb selection should be reevaluated. A tonic formula given afterward for a short period time might be indicated
- Chronic conditions: Formulas are usually given for extended periods (weeks to months) because most chronic conditions develop over long periods of time. As the condition changes, formulas might change too. Slower-acting herbs and more gentle herbs may be used. Herbal treatment should be combined with the holistic approach to diet, environment, exercise, and so forth
- Adverse events: Some animals may have idiosyncratic reactions to some herbs. When this occurs, the herb should be discontinued and recommenced, perhaps at a lower dose, when the symptoms have subsided. If these symptoms stop suddenly, one should consider changing the formula. Also, the practitioner should document the reaction and report it to the manufacturer and to the Veterinary Botanical Medicine Association (VBMA) at www.vbma.org
- Rest periods: For long-term use of herbal formulas, rest periods are traditionally recommended. A schedule of 5 days on, 2 days off or 3 weeks on, 1 week off provides an opportunity for the body to return to an unassisted state. It also provides rest periods for the owner and the animal

DOSE RECOMMENDATIONS

A number of veterinary dosing recommendations have been published. They vary considerably. The main ones are outlined as follows:

Drop Dosing

Drop dosages are preferred by some herbalists, irrespective of the size of the animal. Drop doses of 1 : 5 tinctures or even more dilute tinctures are suggested, along with (usually) the use of one plant at a time. For example, 2 to 3 drops of a tincture may be given for animals of any size. The difficulty with this system is that it probably does not provide a pharmacologically active "dose"; however, it may work on a more subtle level. The other issue is that the drop is an inherently imprecise measure of volume. The number of drops to be given per milliliter varies with dropper bore size, viscosity of liquid, and alcohol strength.

The following recommendation, which is based on the size of an animal, is suggested by Dr. Ihor Basko:

1–2 drops* per 2 lb, or 1 kg (Schoen, 1998)

A common way of dispensing drop doses is through the use of a 25-mL or 1-oz dropper bottle.

This approach does not take into account differences in potency of extracts. For example, a 1 : 5 extract contains 0.2 g in 1 mL, and a 1 : 2 extract contains 0.5 g in 1 mL. However, it does take into account strength and safety because more toxic herbs are usually provided in less concentrated forms than 1 : 1, 1 : 2, or 1 : 5 tinctures (1 : 10 is common). More toxic herbs are dosed at the lower end of the scale. A formula that consists of more than one herb is presumably dosed at the same rate, meaning that each herb is diluted. Dropper sizes vary and the amount delivered by a dropper varies when dispensed by the client (up to 50% variation with between 20 and 30 drops per milliliter). However, this is a very easy and convenient method by which the practitioner can work out dosage for an individual animal.

One recommendation provided by Drs. Susan Wynn and Steve Marsden that takes into account size of the patient and different strengths and potential toxicity of individual herbs is the following:

0.25–5 drops per 1 lb or 0.5 kg (Wynn, 2003)

When more than one herb is included in a formula, the easiest way to dose is to combine the herbs in the same ratio as occurs with individual doses of the herbs. For example, an herb at 1 drop per pound plus another at 2 drops per pound, and another at 3 drops, will be combined in a ratio of 1 : 2 : 3. The dose is the sum of these ratios and 6 drops per pound; the volume to be made up is a multiple of 6. This is a relatively easy system to use.

Wynn and Marsden additionally present herb doses that are derived from a proportional dosing system as well (see Proportionate Dose, later).

*1 mL is equated with approximately 20 to 30 drops.

Standard Dose

A common prescription recommended by Dr. Steve Marsden (Wynn, 2003) is 0.2 mL per 5 lb body weight for a simple or for a formula.

0.2 mL is equal to approximately 4 to 6 drops per 5 lb, or is very close to 1 drop per pound. This guideline means that if five herbs are used in a formula, the dose is the same as if one herb is used. The individual contribution and phytotherapeutic effect of each herb contained within a formula are potentially diluted. Provided the energetics of the formula is in concordance with that of the patient, this may, however, be appropriate. This recommendation provides a volume measurement that is more accurate than drop dosing.

Square Root Formula

Another recommended system is outlined by Dr. Are Thoresen as follows:

2 drops per lb (1 per kg) per herb divided by the square root of the number of herbs used (Thoresen, 2003)

For example, a four-herb combination would contain equal parts. The dose would be

$$\frac{2\,(\text{drops per pound}) \times 4}{\sqrt{4}} = 4 \text{ drops per pound}$$

This is another low-dose strategy that takes into account the possible synergies in a formula.

Clarke's Rule

This is a standard approach to dosing children that may be applicable to animals. It determines the fraction of an adult human dose.

To determine dosage, one must divide the weight of the child (animal) by 150 pounds (or 70 kg), which is the weight of an average adult; this value will equal the fraction of the adult dosage (Martindale, 1941).

$$\frac{\text{Weight of child}}{150\,(\text{adult weight})} = \text{Fraction of adult dosage}$$

For example, assuming that the adult human dose is 30 mL per week of a single and that a dog weighs 50 lb, the dose is $^{50}/_{150}$, or $^{1}/_{3}$ of the adult dose, which is equivalent to 10 mL per week.

Meeh's Formula*

The rate of catabolism of an animal is not proportionate to size or weight but is approximately proportionate to body surface. Surfaces of their solids of the same shape

*From Martindale's The Extra Pharmacopeia.

are proportionate to the two-thirds power of their volumes (i.e., the cube root of the square of the volumes). Because the specific gravity of animals varies only slightly, their body surface is a function of the two-thirds power of their weight. This relationship is expressed in Meeh's formula:

$$S = k(W)^{2/3}$$

where S is the surface in square centimeters, W is the weight in grams, and k is a factor that is nearly constant for all animals of the same shape.

Values for k:

- Human 12.3
- Dog 10.1–11.2
- Rabbit 12.0–12.9
- Cat 10.4
- Guinea pig 10.5

If the doses for human and animals should be proportionate to their rates of catabolism (i.e., to their body surface), then

$$\frac{DH}{DA} = \frac{SH}{SA} = \frac{k(WH)^{2/3}}{k(WA)^{2/3}}$$

DH = Human dose in grams or milliliters.
DA = Animal dose in grams or milliliters.
SH = Body surface of human.
SA = Body surface of animal.
WH = Weight of human in grams.
WA = Weight of animal in grams.

Thus,

$$DA = \frac{(WA)^{2/3}}{(WH)^{2/3}} \times DH = (WH)^{2/3}$$

Thus, if the dose for a 70-kg human is 3 mL of a 1 : 2 tincture per day, then for a 10-kg dog, the dose is as follows:

$$\text{Dose for dog} = \frac{k\,10000^{2/3}}{k\,70000^{2/3}} \times 3$$

$$\text{Dose for dog is } \frac{10.1 \times 10000^{2/3}}{12.3 \times 70000^{2/3}} \times 3$$

Dosing equivalents based on this formula follow.

Cat kg/Human Dose Equivalent	1 g	3 mL/d	20 mL/wk
1	60 mg	0.18 mL	1.20
2	100 mg	0.29 mL	1.91
3	130 mg	0.38 mL	2.51
4	150 mg	0.46 mL	3.04
5	180 mg	0.53 mL	3.53
6	200 mg	0.6 mL	3.99

Dog kg/Human Dose Equivalent	1 g	3 mL/d	20 mL/wk
1	0.06 mg	0.18 mL	1.17
5	0.17 mg	0.51 mL	3.43
10	0.27 mg	0.82 mL	5.46
15	0.36 mg	1.07 mL	7.17
20	0.43 mg	1.3 mL	8.69
30	0.57 mg	1.71 mL	11.4
40	0.69 mg	2.07 mL	13.83
50	0.8 mg	2.41 mL	16.06

Proportionate Dose

On the basis of efficacy, potential toxicity, and clinical trials, the doses of many Western herbs have been determined for human use (Mills, 2000). One approach involves the use of 20 mL per herbal extract per week, on the assumption that this is a pharmacologic dose of a nontoxic herb (this dose will vary from herb to herb). It is commonly prescribed as 1 to 3 mL given once to three times daily. A dose of 3 mL of a single herb per day is equivalent to 21 mL per week. Herbs used in higher volumes might be used at high doses for short periods, for example, *Echinacea purpurea* might be used at 3 mL three times daily or more. More toxic herbs are used in the 5- to 10-mL range per week according to a formula. Also, herbs like gentian are used in much smaller quantities because the effect of the taste (bitters) is enough to stimulate change, and a dose per se may not be required. So, when combined in a typical formula of five to seven herbs (to make 100 mL), the dose is 7.5 mL twice daily or 5 mL three times per day (or 105 mL per week). This is convenient for adult humans.

Extrapolating a similar system for cats and dogs, the daily dose per kilogram can be calculated for an individual herb on the basis of a given human dose per week.

	Proportionate Dose Per Day for Small Animals (kg)							
Human Dose mL/wk	Dose/Kg	5 kg	7.5 kg	10 kg	15 kg	20 kg	30 kg	40 kg
5.0	0.05	0.05	0.1	0.1	0.15	0.2	0.3	0.4
10.0	0.1	0.1	0.2	0.2	0.3	0.4	0.6	0.8
20.0	0.3	0.2	0.3	0.4	0.6	0.8	1.2	1.6
30.0	0.4	0.3	0.5	0.6	0.9	1.2	1.8	2.4
40.0	0.6	0.4	0.6	0.8	1.2	1.6	2.4	3.3
50.0	0.7	0.5	0.8	1.0	1.5	2.0	3.1	4.1

Human Dose mL/wk	Proportionate Dose Per Day for Small Animals (lbs)							
	Dose/lb	10 lb	15 lb	20 lb	30 lb	40 lb	60 lb	80 lb
5.0	0.05	0.05	0.1	0.1	0.15	0.2	0.3	0.4
10.0	0.1	0.1	0.2	0.2	0.3	0.4	0.6	0.8
20.0	0.1	0.2	0.3	0.4	0.6	0.8	1.1	1.5
30.0	0.2	0.3	0.4	0.6	0.9	1.1	1.7	2.3
40.0	0.3	0.4	0.6	0.8	1.1	1.5	2.3	3.0
50.0	0.3	0.5	0.7	1.0	1.4	1.9	2.9	3.8

This approach can be extrapolated to take into account the various sizes of veterinary patients on the basis of therapeutic doses established in human patients, assuming that the dose rate would be similar in humans and in animals. This could well be a spurious assumption; however, in the authors' experience, this system works well.

For example, a cat of 5 kg/10 lb is given a formula that contains five herbs—all nontoxic:

Assume equal proportions of herbs 1 : 1 : 1 : 1 : 1 : 1; dosing per herb on the basis of a human dose of 20 mL per week would require 0.2 mL of each herb per day (a total of 1 mL of the formula per day or 7 mL per week). A 25-mL bottle containing equal proportions would supply a cat for 3 to 4 weeks.

Mother Tinctures–Potentized Herbs

Homeopathic preparation of herbs offers another dosing choice. This may be an appropriate method for animals that are in a weakened state for which more potent herbs may be excessive for the vitality of the patient. The dilutions used in homeopathic medicine may also provide a safer dose of very strong herbs, such as Nux vomica *(Strychnos nux-vomica)* or Gelsemium *(Gelsemium sempervirens)*. For some animals, dosing may be difficult because of the palatability of the herbs or formula. Herbs can be diluted in water for application. They might also be homeopathically prepared so that the putative benefits of a homeopathic preparation, as along with a diluted phytopharmacologic action, can be attained.

The process of homeopathic herbal preparation is based on the concept of potentization or potentiation. Mother tincture (also referred to as "Ø") refers to a crude homeopathic compound that is usually 1 part herbal extract to 9 parts alcohol, distilled water, or lactose as the dilution matrix (this is a 1× potency). The use of this dilution process to prepare a homeopathic herbal preparation is controversial. It is thought that the "molecular impressions" that remain in the dilution, often referred to as energy or power, are sufficient for the treatment of ailments with a minimal adverse event potential. The animal may be dosed in a drop form, with the assumption that it is the "vital energy" of the herb, rather than the phytochemical action, that is important.

COMPARISON OF DIFFERENT DOSING GUIDELINES

A simple exercise can demonstrate the different dosing strategies outlined earlier. Assume that a 20-lb dog will receive the following formula:

1 part dandelion root (1 : 2), 1 part milk thistle (1 : 2), 1 part licorice (1 : 2), 1 part fennel (1 : 2), and 1 part Globe artichoke (1 : 2)

Comparisons of Dosing Strategies

Dose Strategy	Assume	Per Herb	Total Dose	mL Equivalent 20 drops/mL	Dried Herb Equivalent of Dandelion 1 : 2 extract (500 mg in 1 mL dandelion)
1–2 drops* per 2 lb	1 drop	10 drops	50 drops (2.5 mL)	0.5	250 mg
0.25–5 drops per 1 lb	1 drop	20 drops	100 drops (5 mL)	1.0	500 mg
0.2 mL per 5 lb	Formula	0.16 mL	0.8 mL	0.2	100 mg
2 dr/lb/sq root 5	40 drops each × 5/2.2	18 drops	90 drops (4.5 mL)	0.9	450 mg
Wt/150 × adult dose	15 mL/day formula	0.4 mL	2.0 mL	0.4	200 mg
Meeh's formula	Human dose 3 mL each herb per day	0.82 mL	4.1 mL	0.82	410 mg
Proportionate dose		0.4 mL	2.0 mL	0.4	200 mg
Mother tincture	10 mL in 90 mL, 1-mL dose	0.02 mL	1 mL	0.02	10 mg

From this exercise (excluding a potentized homeopathic formula), it can be seen that a fivefold difference may occur in the total herb provided in a given formula. This will vary, depending on what assumptions are made. It is important for the practitioner to realize that this can have a considerable impact on the potential toxicity and efficacy of a given herb. What seems to be observed in veterinary herbal medicine is a variety of strategies that are used consistently and that provide consistent results—consistent enough for them to be published or taught. Flexibility and variability might make it difficult for a new herbalist; however, subscribing to published human dose rates that are based on clinical trial work would seem to provide a dose at the *lower* end of the scale across all strategies and therefore would be expected to be a safe and efficacious practice.

For weights and measures conversions, please refer to Appendix A.

DOSING TIPS

Animals vary in their reactions to treatment: Some individuals are more intolerant of herbs than others. It may be a palatability issue or the act of dosing. It is useful to start with a smaller dose and see what the effect is going to be. One can then increase slowly, remaining on each level for 2 to 3 days, to observe for unusual reactions.

For other dose formats (e.g., tablets, capsules) one should divide the pet's weight by 150 (the assumed average adult weight in pounds). Example: A dog weighs 50 pounds. This is $\frac{1}{3}$ the weight of the adult (of 150 pounds). Therefore, this dog should be given $\frac{1}{3}$–$\frac{1}{2}$ of the recommended dose.

Most herbs have not been studied in pregnant animals. If the practitioner determines that they are safe for use, smaller doses are given and the response observed. Mild and nutritive herbs are best. Many herbs (including diuretics, purgatives, and emmenagogues, all of which are active in the pelvic area) should not be given during pregnancy.

Caution is required in older animals or those that might have hypertension. The practitioner should avoid herbs that stimulate the heart or constrict the blood capillaries and arteries (e.g., licorice root, ephedra, lily of the valley). However, prickly ash, cayenne, and garlic can be used in normal amounts.

One must be aware of herb combinations and drug–herb interactions. Some herbs may overpower or neutralize the effects of others.

The formula can be diluted with water or stock or added to food. Many formulas are bitter, but the bitter property and taste provide a therapeutic benefit, particularly in gastrointestinal conditions. Flavoring agents such as meat flavors, sweet honey, licorice, fennel, sarsaparilla, and aniseed might be tolerated well in some animals. For hints on administering herbs to animals see Appendix E.

References

Cech R. Making Plant Medicine. Williams, Ore: Horizon Herbs LLC; 2000.

Marsden S. In: Wynn S, Marsden S, eds. *Manual of Natural Veterinary Medicine*. Sydney, Australia: Mosby; 2003.

Martindale's The Extra Pharmacopeia, vol 1. 22nd ed. London, United Kingdom: The Pharmaceutical Press; 1941.

Mills S, Bone K. *Principles & Practice of Phytotherapy in Modern Herbal Medicine*. Sydney, Australia: Churchill Livingstone; 2000.

Schoen A, Wynn S, eds. Ihor Basko's protocols. In: *Western Herbal Medicine Clinical Applications, Complementary and Alternative Medicine Principles and Practice*. Sydney, Australia: Mosby; 1998.

Sionneau P. An Introduction to the Use of Processed Chinese Medicinals. Boulder, Colo: Blue Poppy Press; 1995.

Thoresen AS. Proceedings of the Annual Conference of the Australian Veterinary Acupuncture and Holistic Medicine Association; September 2003; Durham, North Carolina.

Winston D, Washington, NJ. Communication to Herbalhall listserv, 2003.

Wynn S, Marsden S. *Manual of Natural Veterinary Medicine*. Sydney, Australia: Mosby; 2003.

Designing the Medicinal Herb Garden

Ellen Zimmermann

CHAPTER

A GARDENER'S PERSONAL ACCOUNT

St. Fiacre—patron saint of gardeners—was a 6th century monk whose gardens grew as his herbal/medical practice for the poor grew. Many of us find our gardens growing as our knowledge and love of herbal medicine deepen, and this nourishes our appreciation for our environment and our relationship to it. Herbal medicine presumes that our cells have a natural relationship with plant chemicals. However, as our medicinal herbs are endangered by their growing popularity, our relationship with the environment becomes much more global, and we are invited—no, required—to learn about and become active in conservation movements—Which brings us back to our gardens.

Many nights in early spring, I awaken at 3 or 4 AM *and cannot wait to get outside and begin working in the garden. I am infected with spring fever. In Texas, where I live, I am also afflicted with fall fever, as that is our best gardening season. I love to garden. I love being outside with the plants, listening to the birds, smelling sweet, fresh air, and communing with the quiet, the stillness, and the activities of nature. Working the soil and feeling how it has changed and improved since last season feels like a blessing. Planning new garden beds, planting seeds and small transplants and even weeding the garden is work that gives me such pleasure and serenity; I want to share some of that with you.*

I am in the garden every day, even on the days I do not touch the soil, I walk through the garden checking plants, perhaps watering a bit and maybe stooping down to pick off some yellowed leaves. Gardening is a practice of mindfulness. If you listen with your heart, the plants communicate their needs. You instinctively know whom to water, whom to transplant, whom to prune, and when to just walk by, heart full of joy, and smile. Gardening is learning and practicing nurturance. I am a mother of two grown children and have realized I am a woman who is meant to nurture and care for others. Those others are not only people, but also dogs, cats, fish, chickens, and all of my dear, green friends. I have a 4000 square foot garden and care for it myself. My sweet husband helps at times when the occasional hard, manual labor is needed to build and maintain a garden space.

Gardening employs many health benefits for both the gardener and the recipients of the harvest. The health benefits derived from planting an herb garden include physical, nutritional, and medicinal benefits. The therapeutic benefits include the feeling of thankfulness and appreciation for the sheer beauty of the plants, the excitement felt as a new seedling emerges to be part of creation, continuous new beginnings, and feeling a sense of community and connectedness to Nature.

Throughout this chapter, you will learn about garden design, conditions of the environment that need consideration, and how to maintain your garden by employing organic gardening techniques. You will also discover how to research and acquire appropriate herbs from your local environment, and how to harvest and store herbs. My thoughts regarding the deeper and intrinsic nature of the plants and their relationship to us are included as well.

While reading this chapter, you will follow the life cycle of one very popular herb, Echinacea purpurea, *and will enjoy learning when and how to seed and maintain this important herb, and when and how to tincture it.*

Welcome to my world of gardening! My hopes are that by the end of this chapter, you will be eager to go outside, get your hands in the soil, and begin a garden of your own.

GARDEN DESIGN

Looking out at a blank canvas of land and planning your herb garden can be a challenging and sometimes overwhelming task for many beginning gardeners. "Start small" is the best advice I can give to the eager, enthusiastic herb grower. When designing your garden space, it is best, I believe, to incorporate what naturally preexists. You will need a sunny spot to grow most herbs, although some will grow in shade, which will be discussed later. It may be necessary to remove trees or large branches to get the sun you need. Save the removed trees for building fences, gates, benches, and other creative homemade carpentry projects.

When assessing your garden site, you will need to consider the following:

- The topography of the land—Does the land slope? Is it flat? Are you on a hillside?
- Exposure—Most gardens do best when they have exposure to the sun for most of the day. Morning sun is the most advantageous for plants; however, some afternoon shade is a welcome relief for many herbs, especially in the warmer climates. Remember, when planning your garden site, to consider the difference in summer and winter sun exposure.
- Soil quality—Assess what you have, take notice of what presently grows there. Adding appropriate amendments will be discussed in detail later.
- Drainage—Check your garden site after a rainstorm, and see how well the rainwater drains. Are there areas where the water pools? Most herbs require good drainage and do not like to have their feet wet. An exception to this would be Horsetail *(Equisetum arvense)*, which likes to grow in a pond or bog.

Gardens have been evolving for centuries. Examples include formal knot gardens, sprawling rose gardens, classical circular herb gardens, practical garden plots, and natural, personal herb gardens. Determining what type of garden you would like is one of your first decisions. The veterinary herbalist who chooses to grow medicinal herbs might wish to forego a formal design and plan a garden with consideration of the following organizational plans.

Which Herbs Would You Like to Grow?

Choose herbs that you use for yourself and your family, so you can have fresh herbs to harvest for your personal health and nutritional needs. Also, choose the herbs that you most often recommend for the animals you treat. Knowing what plants you want to use and grow will help you determine your garden design more efficiently.

Design by Plant Uses

Many herbalists plan their gardens by grouping plants by their uses and functions. This design has been referred to as a Pharmacy Garden or a Physic Garden. If you are in Europe, you will often notice a Physic Garden in the back of the local pharmacy or herb shop. One design possibility would be to group together digestive herbs, respiratory herbs, and so forth. This design, however, does not take into account the specific needs of the plants. If you are planning to create a teaching or research garden, grouping herbs by their function may work well for you (Table 15-1).

TABLE 15-1

Design by Body Systems

System	Herbs
Digestive system	Fennel, Dill, Anise, Gentian Root, Senna, Peppermint, Ginger, Cascara Sagrada
Immune system	Echinacea, Garlic, Chaparral, Burdock Root, Golden Seal, Ashwagandha, Ho Shou Wu
Nervous system	Chamomile, Saint John's Wort, Passionflower, Valerian, Skullcap, Lemon Balm, Oatstraw
Reproductive system	Nettles, Red Clover, Red Raspberry, Vitex, Motherwort, Black Cohosh, Blue Cohosh
Respiratory system	Comfrey, Horehound, Mullein, Pleurisy Root, Sage, Licorice Root, Slippery Elm, Elecampane
Urinary system	Uva Ursi, Cleavers, Chickweed, Cornsilk, Dandelion Leaf, Juniper Berries, Goldenrod

Design for Beauty

Aesthetically minded gardeners may wish to design a garden by considering the colors of the flowers, the texture and shape of the foliage, and the types of plants (i.e., shrubs, perennials, and annuals). For example, a white garden uses very light green-leafed plants such as the Artemesias, Mullein, and some Sages. Some gardeners like to group their color patterns. Other gardeners like to design while thinking ahead of what is blooming in the spring and summer and what will bloom in fall. It is wonderful to have colorful blossoms painting your garden for as much of the year as possible. Some of your herbs may be deciduous, loosing their leaves in the winter; some will die back to the ground, ready to bloom again in spring; and some herbs may be evergreen. So when thinking of the beauty of your garden, remember to consider these previous concepts. Tables 15-2 and 15-3 suggest a few herbs for seasonal bloom and identify flower colors.

TABLE 15-2

Herbs in Bloom

Spring Blooming Herbs	Summer Blooming Herbs	Fall Blooming Herbs
Borage	Saint John's Wort	Betony
Calendula	Echinacea	Roses
Crocus	Vitex	Goldenrod
Dandelion	Salvias	Angelica
Elder	Chamomile	Chicory
Motherwort	Asclepias	Burdock
Nasturtium	Passiflora	Gentian
Poppies	Comfrey	Hops
Roses	Monardas	Lemon Balm

Specific Plant Needs Design

Conserving water is becoming more and more important in many parts of the world. A practical method of planning your garden design is to group your herbs according to their needs, particularly water and sun requirements. For example, many Mediterranean herbs, such as Rosemary, Thyme, and Sage require dry soil, so they are

TABLE 15-3

Flower Colors

Cool Colors Pink, Purple, Blue	Warm Colors Red, Orange, Yellow	White
Borage	Agrimony	Basil
Echinacea	Arnica	Black cohosh
Garden sage	Bee balm	Catnip
Germander	Calendula	Datura
Joe Pye Weed	California poppy	Elder
Lavender	Dill	English and French thyme
Motherwort	Fennel	Horehound
Passionflower	Goldenrod	Marjoram
Rosemary	Mullein	Mugwort
Scutellaria	Pleurisy root	Nettles
Vitex	Rue	Oregano
Wild bergamor	Saint John's Wort	Valerian

Conditions for Growing Echinacea

Echinacea purpurea likes to be in the sun and enjoys some water, particularly at the beginning of its growth cycle. Once the plant is established, reduce watering. Echinacea prefers a well-drained soil, as do most herbs, but it will grow well in most soils. You should place your plants 1 to 2 feet apart because they will likely grow to a height of 2 to 3 feet. Echinacea is a perennial herb that will return and multiply each year. It can also be planted in partial shade but will not flower as readily. If Echinacea is planted by seed, be sure to acquire fresh seeds, either commercially or from a friend. Scatter the seeds on the ground, lightly step on them, and water them in. At least three times each day, spray the planted area with a misting spray. The ground must be kept moist, so the seedlings will emerge. If you miss a misting, do not worry, especially if it is cloudy or cool outside. When the seedlings emerge, you can begin to limit your watering.

grouped together. Sun-loving plants, shade-loving varieties, and plants that require more frequent moisture are planted together. You will be surprised that this practical method is quite beautiful. Conserving our water sources is a great gift to the planet, the people, and future generations.

Cottage Garden Design

My favorite way of gardening is the English style of cottage gardening. Herbs and flowers are planted instinctively, with consideration of specific needs and uses, but the plant, or seeds, along with the voice of your heart, will tell you where to plant your herbs. The garden matures looking a bit wild and beautiful, and full of many colors, textures, and styles. The plants will naturally tell you if they're in the wrong spot, and every gardener knows that moving plants around is just part of your gardening day. I like this method best because it simulates Nature. Plants are often found together in Nature, grouped by their specific needs and also by their uses. For example, I often see Mullein *(Verbascum thapsus)* and Horehound *(Marrubium vulgare)* near one another in open fields. Both of these herbs are used for respiratory problems. Another example is Jewelweed *(Impatiens capensis)*, which is often found near poison ivy *(Toxicodendron radicans)* and is used as a remedy for that pesky plant.

A variety of considerations and thoughts are part of your garden design. It is most important that you go deep inside yourself and discover which design works for you. When I designed my garden, I just went out to the area close to the back of our house, walked around quietly, and began arranging white limestone rocks as borders for garden beds. I knew I wanted large paths in between the beds, and I incorporated many of the native trees and shrubs that were already in the garden space. I feel that it is wise and important to use native and local material that you already have either on your property or near your home. Using native and local material is cost effective, provides a continuum of design, and is consistent with the philosophy of "What we need is all around us." Patronizing local organic nurseries and community plant organizations is essential to consider and will be discussed in greater detail further in the chapter.

CONDITIONS TO CONSIDER

In addition to deciding how you want to design your garden, you must evaluate several important factors before you begin planting your herbs—the SAWS, that is, Soil, Air, Water, and Sun. Be familiar with your climate and which zone you live in. In the United States, we have a US Department of Agriculture (USDA) zone chart. The country is divided into zones, and plants are sold and labeled by the zone in which they grow best. Know the average temperature of your area, when you have your first and last freezes of the seasons, and how much average rainfall you receive. These factors will help you determine which plants you choose to grow.

Soil

It is vital to determine what type of soil you have in your garden space. If you are lucky, you will have soft, viable soil that drains well and is easy to dig in. The gardeners I know in Texas strive to amend their soil to the consistency of a devil's food cake (a very rich, dark chocolate cake). It is important to get your soil tested by a local agriculture extension office or a private company that provides soil testing. This inexpensive test will give you information regarding the ph level of your soil, which minerals are present, and what is lacking. Always inform the service of your objective in the garden—to plant herbs! If your soil is rocky, you might wish to build raised beds for planting. If your soil is hard packed clay, you may want to add sand. Whatever the consistency of your soil, you will want to add good-quality compost (either homemade or purchased locally) at least twice each year. Spring and fall are great times to add compost to your existing soil; over time, any garden soil can be amended until you have "chocolate cake."

Compost is not only beneficial to your plants and your garden soil, it also conserves waste and promotes recycling of organic matter. Every time you prepare a meal, keep your vegetable and fruit scraps, eggshells, coffee grounds, and other meatless products in a plastic container or compost bucket near your sink. I gather enough organic material to bring out to my compost pile or to feed my chickens almost daily. A compost pile is composed of fallen leaves and grass clippings, organic scraps from your kitchen and garden, and some type of manure. I have used horse manure, cow manure, chicken manure, and llama manure. Just about any herbivorous animal manure will do.

It's fun to layer leaves, manure, and organic scraps in your compost pile. It is good practice to turn the pile every 2 weeks and keep it moist. I have used blood meal to get the compost cooking (heating occurs during the bacterial degradation process). After a few months, you will be delighted with rich organic matter called "compost" that you will need to strain and use generously in your garden. Composting feels good. You recycle your waste, help keep our Mother Earth's cycle continuing, and create rich, healthy plant material that is useful for food and medicine. The Cycle of Life continues.

Where and When to Plant Echinacea?

A friend has given you some viable *Echinacea purpurea* seeds for your garden. *Echinacea* is a wildflower, grows naturally in North America, and can be grown easily in many parts of the world. Plant your seeds by just scattering them in the fall or very early spring. With natural rainfall and perhaps some weeding around the seedlings, your Purple Coneflower (one of *Echinacea's* common names), will emerge in the spring, grow strong and sturdy, and flower beautifully for you in the summer. *Echinacea* does like full sun the best but will tolerate some shade; it just won't bloom as much. *Echinacea* is a perennial herb and will return and multiply every year. *Echinacea* provides a great lesson for the herbalist, and that is the lesson of patience. You need to wait 3 years before harvesting your *Echinacea* root for medicine. Harvesting will be discussed later in the chapter.

Air

Herbs and most other plants need good air circulation around them if they are going to thrive. Many new gardeners make the mistake of planting their new transplants too close together. We want to fill in the space because that is quite appealing, but it is important to give your herbs space in which to grow. Again, it is the ultimate lesson of patience. If plants are overcrowded, they will not grow to their full potential and they may become more prone to disease. Remember to do your research and know the potential size of your plant, and give it the proper space.

Water

All plants need water to grow. It is important to discover the watering requirements for your individual herbs and then plan accordingly. Most herbs, however, after they are established, require less water than other types of garden plants. Many people use overhead sprinkler systems for their gardens. This is really not the best method of watering your garden. I feel strongly that using a drip irrigation system or soaker hoses is a more efficient, economical, and practical way of irrigating. The water that evaporates into the air from a sprinkler is a waste of water resources. With a drip irrigation system, you can place an emitter (the device from which the water flows) at the base of each plant. You can use emitters of different sizes, depending on the needs of the plants. For example, in my garden, I place a 2-gallon emitter (that means the plant will receive 2 gallons of water each hour) on my large rose bushes, but the Rosemary plant gets only a ½-gallon emitter because it requires much less moisture. Of course, if you live in an area where you get abundant rainfall, you might not need a watering system at all. Most likely, you will need to supplement by watering by hand periodically. It is remarkably therapeutic to go out into the garden in the morning or evening, turn on the hose, and walk around the garden spraying liquid nourishment on your plants. It is mindful, relaxing, and calming to the soul. You also get the opportunity to check out each plant and evaluate its immediate needs.

Sun

The last condition in SAWS is the sun. Most herbs require at least 6 to 8 hours of sunshine per day, so you will need to accommodate them. Some herbs, however, prefer shade, or at least partial shade. Some of those include Comfrey, Self-Heal, Gotu kola, Ginger, Hoja Santa, some Monardas and various Mints. Shade-loving plants can also be planted in clay pots on a patio or porch or can be used as a hanging basket. Herb gardens planted in a variety of artistic clay pots are beautiful and lush, and can be delightfully attractive as well as useful (Table 15-4).

PLANTING AND MAINTAINING YOUR HERB GARDEN

Your garden beds are designed and you've worked your soil sufficiently enough to begin planting. Perhaps you are incorporating your herbs into an existing garden bed.

TABLE 15-4

Shade Plants versus Sun-Loving Plants

Shade Plants	Sun-Loving Plants
Ashwagandha	Asclepias
Black Cohosh	Basil
Bloodroot	Calendula
Blue Cohosh	Catnip
Chelidonium	Chamomile
Comfrey	Comfrey
Geranium	Costmary
Ginger	Dandelion
Ginseng	Datura
Goldenseal	Echinacea
Gotu Kola	Elecampane
Hoja Santa	Geranium
Ho Shou Wu	Honeysuckle
Lily of the Valley	Hops
Mayapple	Joe Pye weed
Mitchella	Lavender
Monarda	Lemon Balm
Pipsissewa	Ma Huang
Self-Heal	Meadowsweet
Smilax spp	Mints
Solomon's Seal	Monarda
Trillium	Motherwort
Usnea	Mullein
Valerian	Nettles
	Parsley
	Passiflora
	Plantain
	Pokeweed
	Elder
	Poppies
	Prunella
	Rose
	Rosemary
	Saint John's Wort
	Salvias
	Scutellaria
	Sheep Sorrel
	Thyme
	Vitex
	Yerba Mansa
	Yucca

I feel it is best to take your transplant to the spot where you think you would like it to grow. Leave the herb there for a while, and soon you will discover whether this is the right spot. Usually, it is. Your intuition guides you correctly. Dig a hole that is suitable for the plant. I like to add some starting amendments of bat guano and a local product that adds phosphate to the soil. I lovingly and carefully take the transplant out of its container and plant it. I add some compost around the plant and water it in with some liquid seaweed or root stimulator.

If you are planting seeds, you have two options. You can direct seed right into the garden soil, or you can start your seedlings in seed starting trays (I use recycled, black plastic plant trays from the nursery). If you are starting seeds in trays, first make or purchase a good seed-starting soil mixture. My inexpensive version of potting mix is recycled soil taken from various pots lying around, some compost, a small amount of vermiculite and perlite (for aeration), and perhaps some sand. I plant my seeds and mist with the hose at least three times a day. I am lucky enough to perform this very pleasurable task in a greenhouse. Determined seedling starters can do this indoors in a warm, well-lighted area.

If you are direct seeding, that's easier. Once the last danger of frost has passed (for most plantings), just determine where you want these plants, and use a garden fork to loosen the soil. Add your starting amendments, sprinkle out, or place your seeds to the correct depth and cover them with soil. I like to add some compost on top and water them in. It's essential to keep seeds watered several times a day in hot climates. Remember to ease up on the watering once the seedlings emerge.

I love planting seeds because it is wonderfully exciting to go out in the morning and discover that a tiny little green plant being has arisen from this soil, the water, and your love. Watching a seedling grow so quickly is fun, interesting, and remarkably rewarding. I also love purchasing unusual herbs, herbs for replacement in my garden, and native plants and flowers. My favorite way of acquiring new plants for my garden is getting "Pass-Along Plants" from my gardening friends. I have a few friends who willingly share plants and seeds from their gardens. I belong to the local Herb Society, where each month, people bring extra plants and seeds. Sometimes, plants just appear on my front porch, and that is the greatest gift of all. "Pass-Along Plants" grow and thrive the best in my garden. As I walk by these green friends, I am reminded of the special person who shared his or her plant with me. I feel warm, happy, and blessed.

One of the most unique and interesting parts of my garden, and the one that is recognized and commented upon by others, is my collection of garden art. Beginning gardeners especially notice my collection, which includes St. Francis, fairies, a dragon, a tiny chair or two, angels, Buddha, Quan Yin, birdhouses, chickens, and chimes. One of my favorite stone statues is St. Fiacre, the Patron Saint of Gardeners. Living near Mexico is a plus because I have conveniently acquired many colorful Mexican plaques, terra cotta clay pots, and a hand-painted fountain to adorn my garden. Adding meaningful garden art makes a garden uniquely yours. As you invite guests into your garden, it is such fun to point out and talk about the plants; viewing colorful, mystical, or playful garden art gives people many ideas with which they can begin creating their own special place. Many people use garden plaques with spiritual sayings, fun handmade objects of art, and the very popular flowers and bugs on tall wrought iron sticks, adding whimsical delight to an already beautiful, colorful, and inspiring garden.

Maintaining *Echinacea purpurea*

Once you have planted your Echinacea seeds and they have sprouted, water them occasionally depending on the amount of local rainfall. Echinacea does not need a lot of water once it is established and growing. You will notice it growing quite rapidly when the weather warms up. Soon you will have tall, elegant Purple Coneflower blooming gloriously everywhere you planted it. Echinacea does not seem to need much fertilizer; however, a little seaweed or fish emulsion once or twice a season is always a good idea. Also, some compost scratched in around the base of the plant helps it keep blooming all summer long. If you deadhead a spent flower, you might get another bloom in the same place. If you cut the stem farther down on the plant, this will most likely ensure another blossom before the end of the summer.

ORGANIC GARDENING TECHNIQUES

As an herbalist, gardener, and lover of the Planet Earth, I believe that there is only one way to garden, and that is organically or naturally. Gardening organically means that you plant and use methods to maintain your garden space that comprise only natural fertilizers, natural soil amendments, and organic insect control products. There is absolutely no use for chemical pesticides or chemical fertilizers. The use of chemicals can harm wildlife; nearby streams and other water sources, and even your own pets and children. There is some concern about pesticide residues being concentrated as various herbal extraction techniques are used. If you are growing herbs and possibly vegetables and fruits for your own consumption, be assured that you do not want to use anything but organic techniques. Organic gardening is smart, economical, and safe. It fits the lifestyle and practices of most herbalists, health practitioners, and garden lovers.

Two of my favorite organic fertilizers include liquid seaweed and fish emulsion. These products are easily available at quality nurseries and are best purchased by the gallon. You will use them frequently, and they maintain an excellent shelf-life. I use liquid seaweed when I transplant a container plant and as a foliar spray at least once a month. To foliar spray your garden, you need to get a hose-end sprayer, fill it with liquid seaweed, attach it to your hose, and spray all the foliage in your garden early in the morning. The seaweed enters the leaves through the stomata and nourishes the plant as the xylem and phloem of the plant carry the water and seaweed throughout the plant. I have noticed that regular foliar feeding helps to maintain a healthy, vibrant, green garden. I also like to use a liquid fish emulsion product, which is thick and heavy but also very nourishing for your plants. Other recommended products include soil activators, molasses, and the nitrogen-rich bat guano.

Above all, the best organic fertilizer is compost. You can purchase good-quality compost from a soil yard or garden center, or you can create and use your own compost. Just find a shady place; recycle all of your organic waste from your kitchen (including vegetable scraps, fruit peels, eggshells, and coffee grounds). I do not use any meat products or very large or hard items, such as avocado pits. I usually make compost lasagna, which includes layers of leaves, manure, kitchen and garden scraps, grass clippings, and so forth. It's good to add some blood meal to begin the heating process. It is also good to moisten your compost pile occasionally and turn it at least once or twice a month. After just a few months, you can strain it and use it in your garden. It is best to use composted manure and not fresh manure directly on your garden. Compost truly is your very best fertilizer and can be used on all of your plants; including herbs, trees, shrubs, flowers, and vegetables. See Table 15-5 for a list of some frequently used soil amendments, their nitrogen, phosphorous and potassium content, and suggested rates of application.

A universal problem shared by the gardeners of the world is the problem of insect control. How frustrating it is to get up early one morning, walk through your garden, and notice that the bugs have had a huge midnight snack of your tomatoes or passionflower vines, or the lovely

TABLE 15-5

Soil Amendments

Soil Additive	Nitrogen	Phosphorus	Potassium	Rate to Apply	Comments
Bat guano	11	4	1	1–2 tsp per plant	Use sparingly; good for herbs and vegetables
Compost	1	1	1	1 inch thick around entire garden	Apply Spring and Fall
Fish emulsion	5	2	2	2 T per gallon of water	Apply once a month or as needed
Liquid seaweed	1	0	1	1 oz per gallon of water	Apply to transplants and as needed
Blood meal	11	0	0	1 T per plant	High in nitrogen, good to promote flowering
Cow manure	2	1	1	Add to compost pile	When composted, apply as fertilizer
Poultry manure	5	3	3	Add to compost pile	When composted, apply as fertilizer, or let chickens roam the garden

zinnias you just planted. Yes, insects live in your garden. They will be there every day in differing numbers, and we need to learn to better tolerate their ever-lasting presence. There are, however, methods that you can employ that might deter their presence or keep them to a minimum.

A few years ago, we had a huge grasshopper infestation that was very damaging to my garden. The best natural solution for me was to build a chicken coop and let my hens free-range in the garden. Within 1 week, the chickens had the grasshopper problem under control and then began to provide me with fresh eggs every day and wonderful fertilizer for my plants. I now have eight chickens and they are a pleasure to observe and easy to care for, and they lay the best eggs you could ever want. They eat several different types of insects and scratch and soften the earth and fertilize as they go. What a fun organic method!

Attracting other types of birds to your garden is also important. Many birds eat insects and help minimize the ill effects of too many insects in your garden space. Setting up birdbaths and bird feeders and birdhouses around your garden will help attract your feathered friends. It is also a good idea to employ the beneficial insects, including ladybugs, green lacewings, and praying mantises. These insects will eat the nonbeneficial insects and will help keep your garden healthy. Many of the herbs that you plant in your garden such as Dill, Fennel, and Parsley act as host plants that will help keep your ladybug population in the garden.

Being a natural gardener might mean that you do not purchase any organic amendments or fertilizers but instead use the plants themselves to fertilize and nourish each other and to keep those bugs at bay. A friend of mine from India taught me to place yellowed and eaten leaves next to thriving plants. The yellowed leaves eventually break down and feed the plant, and additionally serve as food for the insects. If you use plants discarded after weeding, make sure they are free of viable seeds. If you are on a strict budget or would like to go the completely natural route, give this method a try. You will be surprised at the splendid results.

COMMUNITY RESOURCES

Now that you have adequately planned your garden space and are ready to plant herbs for your purposes, it is important that you research which herbs are most appropriate for your local area. Herbs that are native to your area, those that are naturalized, and those herbs that have needs for which your environment will provide are best suited for you to grow in your garden. For example, where I live the climate is hot and dry and the soils are mostly rocky. This area is similar to the climate and terrain in the Mediterranean area; hence, many of the herbs that are endemic to the Mediterranean do very well here.

There are many ways that you can begin researching which herbs are native and locally grown. One place to begin is your closest city, county, or state botanical garden. Most communities have a local botanical garden of some size. You can visit this garden, notice the plants growing there, and then research organizations or clubs that are affiliated with the botanical garden. Joining local gardening clubs provides you with a vast amount of information regarding growing and using your herbs. Native plant societies, master gardener programs, local herb societies, and organic gardening clubs have memberships available for enthusiastic gardeners.

In most US states, the Department of Agriculture has extension offices that maintain paid or volunteer staff who are available to answer gardening questions. They offer help with soil analysis, help with retaining rebates for xeriscape gardens (low water use), and are particularly useful to the beginning gardener. Taking time to use this resource can provide you with much horticultural information for your local area.

When I first became interested in gardening, I would drive to one of our local nurseries and just walk around taking notice of the plants I was attracted to and which plants were grown locally and discovering which soil amendments (i.e., organic and nonorganic) were available. I soon decided that the few organic nurseries and the ones that sold a large variety of native and locally grown plants would be the businesses I would frequent. I recommend finding those nurseries in your area. Many areas also have local farmer's markets, particularly on the weekends, where local growers sell fresh produce, herbs, and flowers, as well as potted plants and more. Getting to know local herb growers and local farmers is an excellent way to learn more about growing herbs. State and national herb grower's associations are available for membership. Every gardener and herbalist I know owns a large library of herb books, magazines, and seed and plant catalogues. Every bookstore has a section on gardening, and many carry a good selection of herb books. Also, local health food stores often have excellent herb books for sale. Many seed catalogues provide useful cultivation information as well.

My favorite and richest source of information is networking and socializing with other gardeners and herbalists. Sharing information, sharing plants and seeds, and "Sharing the wisdom of the plants" (EZ Herbs, this author's tagline) fills my heart and soul with incredible satisfaction and contentment. "Pass-Along Plants" are the plants that grow best in my garden, and they are the plants I talk about the most on my garden tours.

HARVESTING AND STORING HERBS

Growing medicinal plants is pleasurable and good for the soul, and having the herbs on hand to harvest when needed is an added bonus. My foremost belief is that you should harvest your herbs when you need them. For example, if I've cut myself working in the garden, I wouldn't wait to harvest some Yarrow *(Achillea millefolium)*, chew it a bit, and place it on my cut to arrest the bleeding and begin the healing process. However, it is best to harvest your herbs at around 10:00 AM, after the morning dew has evaporated and before the sun shines brightly. It is also best to harvest plants when they are in robust health and are looking very alive, vibrant, and full of energy. Many new gardeners are hesitant to cut their herbs, but herbs love to be pruned. They grow fuller and healthier when you harvest and use them.

For centuries, our gardening ancestors have given thanks to their plants at harvest time. I continue this tradition by offering thanks to the plant before gathering, while speaking aloud my intended purpose of the harvest. For example, if I am using the herb for medicinal purposes, or for educational reasons, I let the plant know my intention. Grateful gathering of herbs has been practiced by cultures across the globe since the beginning of time. Some traditions of indigenous peoples will be discussed later in this chapter.

Most of the herbs I harvest are the aerial parts of the plant. I do harvest some roots, which I will discuss later in the section on harvesting *Echinacea purpurea.* If I am harvesting tall stands of herbs, like Motherwort *(Leonurus cardiaca)* or long stalks of Rosemary *(Rosmarinus officinale)*, I simply tie the bundles together and hang them upside down in a dry room in the house. After a few days, depending on the humidity and time of year, I simply garble (run my fingers over the stems) and pull off the dried herb. If I am harvesting a small amount of herb, such as Lemon Balm *(Melissa officinalis),* I cut the leaves directly off the plant and place them on a drying rack, or even on a straw tray with a paper towel on it. This primitive method of drying actually works very nicely. I watch the herbs closely for several days, and when they are dry to the touch and crumble between my fingers, they are ready to be stored. Be careful not to dry your herbs too long, or handle them too much, as they may lose some potency.

You can also place your cut herbs on stacked drying racks in a room with a dehumidifier. Drawing moisture from the air will help your herbs dry more quickly, while maintaining their freshness and medicinal properties. I have witnessed great success with this method by herbalists who are drying large amounts of plant material for their herbal practice.

After your herbs have dried, storing them properly is of great significance. I recommend that you store all your dried herbs in air-tight, glass containers. Herbs must be completely dry, as any moisture still present may result in mould. If your dried herbs are kept in a dark closet or pantry, they will stay fresh for at least 1 year. Some herbs may last for up to 2 years. After that, I think it is best if they are discarded. Herbs should maintain their color, smell strongly, and work in the way they are intended. For instance, properly dried Peppermint leaves *(Mentha piperita)* maintain a dark green color and have a strong and fresh fragrance. Before purchasing dried herbs, rather than drying them yourself, ensure that they are still colorful and have the intense smell of freshly harvested and dried herbs.

Once you have a viable garden growing, you will want to occasionally harvest seeds to grow again, or to trade, or just to give to others as gifts. I frequently harvest favorite plant seeds to give away to fellow herbalists and gardeners. When the flowers on your plant are spent and the seeds have formed and dried, it is generally the right time to harvest. I simply stroll about the garden, gather seeds in my hand or in a small container, and package them in small manila envelopes. I have found handy envelopes (2 ¼″ × 3 ½″) at a local office supply store that work well and are very economical. You can seal these envelopes and label them with content, date of harvest, and your name. Most seeds stay viable for several years. Archeologists have been known to find seeds hundreds of years old that when planted, still grow—one of the miracles of the Green World!

Dried herbs or, even better, fresh herbs can be used to make your herbal preparations for personal use or that of your patients. A very brief introduction to making herbal teas is presented in Table 15-6.

Harvesting, Preparing, and Storing *Echinacea purpurea* Tincture

HARVESTING ECHINACEA	PREPARING ECHINACEA	STORING ECHINACEA TINCTURE
For a whole plant medicine: • In the summer, harvest robust Echinacea flowers, seed pods, and leaves (which are fresh-wilted/dried for several hours). • In the fall, harvest 3-year-old Echinacea roots.	• Place your flowers, seed heads, and leaves in a 50% alcohol solution (such as good-quality vodka). • In the fall, add freshly harvested roots that are cleaned and dried. • Add roots to Echinacea tincture solution. • Macerate (soak) the herbs in alcohol for 8 weeks. • Shake the jar every day.	• After 8 weeks, strain the herbs from the liquid. • Bottle in dark glass (amber or cobalt blue) tincture bottles or larger storage bottles such as wine bottles. • Keep in a dark closet or pantry. • Properly made tinctures will last up to 10 years.

TABLE 15-6

Preparing your Herbal Tea

An Herbal Infusion	An Herbal Decoction
Made with the soft, aerial parts of the plant:	Made from the hard parts of the plant:
Leaves, flowers, soft stems	Roots, berries, stems
Use 1 tsp dried herb per 8 oz water or	Use 2 tbsp dried herbs per quart of water
Use 2 tsp of fresh herb per 8 oz water	1. Measure your herb and water.
1. Measure your herb and water.	2. Place herb in water and bring to a boil.
2. Place herb in water and bring to a boil.	3. While covered, lower to simmer and gently boil the herbs for at least 20 minutes.
3. Remove from heat.	4. Strain the herbs, and serve your decoction.
4. Cover and infuse for at least 15 minutes.	
5. Strain herbs, and serve your infusion.	

Common Medicinal Plants Poisonous to Pets in Low Doses*

- Castor bean
- Many lilies
- Aconite
- Crocus
- Senna
- Comfrey
- Datura, Atropa
- Jessamine
- Privet
- Daphne
- Dumbcane
- Daylily
- Elder
- English ivy
- Bittersweet
- Flax
- Foxglove
- Horsechestnut
- Mayapple
- Milkvetch
- Mistletoe
- Morning glory
- Mustards
- Oaks
- Oleander
- Pokeweed
- Rhubarb

*There are many listings of "toxic plants" that include strong medicinal plants, and this is an incomplete list. These may include plants that the overwhelming majority of pets would never eat on their own (unless starved or deranged), and that are not readily available to the public to be administered by capsule. The list above includes those that are common garden and houseplants, those that animals may or may not eat, and those that have medicinal properties when used appropriately.

ANIMAL-FRIENDLY GARDENS*

Susan G. Wynn

Most veterinarians have pets, and pets may not always respect the priorities of the medicinal herb gardener. A number of main considerations are presented here for gardeners with pets (Butcher, 1994):

1. Select robust plants—delicate endangered species, succulent plants with easily ruptured stems, and annual plants of any sort are not likely to bounce back from animal damage as easily as perennials, shrubs, and so forth. Alternatively, fierce protection in the form of fences may need to be employed.
2. Exclude pets—either fence judiciously or distract pets. Sandpits and catnip may keep cats focused on a single area away from the garden. Chickens, other birds, and squirrels tend to graze on seeds (fallen naturally or those you planted) and young plants. It may be best to protect plants grown from seed until they are mature and ready for transplanting.
3. Consider becoming a beekeeper—bees increase yields of fruits and vegetables and are threatened by pesticides and parasites such as the Varroa mite (which is the reason organic honey is so hard to find). Find a beekeeper group in your area, and learn about keeping bees to make your garden healthier and improve the health of the bee population.

Dogs can be very destructive in a garden, yet we love to have their company while we enjoy the work of gardening. A few hints here may help preserve your relationship later. If you are placing a garden in a spot where the dog is accustomed to playing or sleeping, consider designing *around* the dog's favorite spots. If the dog has a usual path from the door to a favorite spot, respecting that path by using lawn or other types of walkways may help. Walkways should be comfortable on the dog's feet, or he may avoid them! Active dogs may need more play space than older or naturally mellow dogs. Cats really enjoy hanging around the garden, and if you want to make sure he or she doesn't wander, cat enclosures are ideal. These should be enclosed with chicken wire or wire mesh on all sides, including the roof. If roofing isn't possible, fences can be designed that cave inward at the top, preventing the cat from scaling the summit. An additional feature is a double-door safety entry, so that you can enter an enclosed entry cubicle before entering the enclosure—just in case the cat is faster than you!

Raised beds present a natural visual barrier that may discourage a dog from jumping into plant beds. A single plant with a reputation of repelling dogs and cats has become available; this is *Coleus canina,* or the Scaredy cat plant. You may wish to entice a dog away from plant beds with his own personal playground—a splash pool or digging pit might work for some. For cats, the catnip should be placed well away from spots you want left undisturbed. Finally, if your pets will hang out in the garden, be aware of poisons that may endanger their health—these include poisonous plants, as well as soil amendments, fertilizers, and pesticides (especially pest bait systems).

In barns where hanging baskets can be used decoratively, horsemen may consider growing certain medicinal herbs in the basket next to a horse's stall. Herbs to consider include red clover, dandelion, chamomile, chickweed, and meadowsweet (if the basket is large). Hang the basket where horses can occasionally nibble or nose plants that are mature enough to overhang the basket, so they can't eat everything in one go.

*From Smith, 2003; Butcher, 1994.

CONSCIOUS AND RESPECTFUL HERBALISM

I am not a professional gardener, or even a Master Gardener, nor have I had any formal training in gardening, other than taking several local classes. I belong to the local Herb Society and do most of my learning from friends and fellow gardeners. I began gardening when I was 5 years old by helping my father weed the tomato garden. I fell in love with feeling the dirt run through my fingers, and until this day, I maintain dirty fingernails. I do clean up well for special occasions!

I am an intuitive gardener, using my instincts and my heart while listening to the needs of the plants. I have developed a deep, true love of the Green World, and the plants in my garden know this. They respond to my nurturing and care by growing well, providing me with much abundance, and every day showing me their beauty in many different ways. Every day is new; every day is another surprise. Gardening has so many rewards and gifts that there are too many to mention. Ancient and indigenous people knew the gifts of the Earth better than we do today. Many indigenous people created elaborate ceremonies when harvesting their herbs. They always honor the Earth and its bounty, and express sincere gratitude for every harvest. To elaborate on the previously mentioned time-honored spiritual Gardening traditions, Native Americans ask permission of the plant when harvesting for food or medicine, and they give back to the Earth by making an offering of cornmeal or tobacco. This is a beautiful and easy practice to incorporate into your harvesting regime. My suggestion is to buy a lovely, small pouch for yourself and fill it with tobacco or cornmeal. Keep this pouch in your harvesting basket and each time you go into your garden to collect some leaves, flowers, or roots, you will have your offering with you. Simply ask the plant if it is agreeable to take some of its energy for whatever purpose you need it (e.g., medicine, food, teaching purposes). Offer a sprinkling of tobacco back to the Earth with gratitude and appreciation. I believe that plants are here to say yes to our requests and are most happy to oblige our harvesting and uses. It's that simple and that beautiful.

I am an avid supporter of plant conservation and living lightly on our land. Many herbs today are listed "At Risk" by a grassroots conservation group entitled "United Plant Savers." This organization began in the United States with several dedicated herbalists who worked diligently to educate the public regarding the effects of the devastation of valuable plants. Because herbalism has gained so much popularity over the past 15 years, some very useful herbs have become scarce in their natural environments. Some of these "At Risk" herbs include Ginseng, Echinacea, Golden Seal, and Slippery Elm. Some overzealous gatherers might have unethically overharvested some of these plants. Additionally, because of the vast amount of development that is taking place in this country, wild plants have lost much of their natural habitat. Whatever the reason, or combination of reasons, the United Plant Savers encourage their members and other plant lovers to be conscious of this unsettling occurrence. It is important to encourage people to grow their own herbs for medicine and conservation, and to purchase herbs that are cultivated, rather than wildcrafted. (Wildcrafting is the practice of harvesting herbs and plants from their natural habitat to be sold and used as medicine.) Wildcrafting can be performed ethically by always leaving an abundance of plant material after harvesting. This author feels that so much damage has already been done to our environment that the practice of wildcrafting should be greatly minimized, if practiced at all. Many organic farms specialize in growing medicinal herbs; plants are cultivated, cared for, harvested, dried, and sold in quantities suitable for use in making herbal medicines. I believe that our efforts now need to be placed toward supporting these growers or, better yet, growing our own medicines in our personal medicinal herb gardens.

The plants are our allies, friends, benefactors, and spiritual guides. Take time to grow your own herbs, flowers, trees, shrubs, vegetables, and fruits. Do it with joy, honor, and mindfulness. Helping to maintain the integrity of our planet is the responsibility of all of us. One way you can do this well is by having a garden of your own, maintaining it beautifully, and sharing with others the abundance it provides. I have no doubt that once you start your garden; you will become infatuated, fall in love, and begin a lifetime practice of gardening. I am grateful to be able to share some of my enthusiasm with others who are considering taking this "Green Path." I hope that this chapter may serve as the soul of this textbook.

I will see you in the garden.

References

Butcher D. *Pets in Your Garden.* Chatswood, NSW: Reed (part of William Heineman Australia); 1994.

Smith CS. *Dog Friendly Gardens, Garden Friendly Dogs.* Wenatchee, Wash: Dogwise Publishing; 2003.

Other Resources

Gardening Books

Cech R. *Growing At-Risk Medicinal Herbs: Cultivation, Conservation and Ecology.* Williams, Ore: Horizon Herbs; 2002.

De La Tour S, De La Tour R. *The Herbalist's Garden: A Guided Tour of 10 Exceptional Herb Gardens: The People Who Grow Them and the Plants That Inspire Them.* North Adams, Mass: Storey Books; 2001.

Fletcher K. *Themes for Herb Gardens.* Victoria, Australia: Viking Penguin Books Australia; 1996.

Gladstar R, Hirsch P. *Planting the Future: Saving our Medicinal Herbs.* Rochester, VT: Healing Arts Press; 2000.

Harrisson J, Shapiro HY. *Gardening for the Future of the Earth.* New York, NY: Bantam Publishers; 2000.

Hartung T. *Growing 101 Herbs That Heal: Gardening Techniques, Recipes and Remedies.* North Adams, Mass: Storey Books; 2000.

McDowell CF, Clark-McDowell T. *The Sanctuary Garden, Creating a Place of Refuge in Your Yard or Garden.* Simon & Schuster, New York, NY; 1998.

Streep P, Glover J. *Spiritual Gardening.* Alexandria, Va: Time-Life Books; 1999.

Sturdivant L, Blakley T. *The Bootstrap Guide to Medicinal Herbs in the Garden, Field and Marketplace.* Friday Harbor, Wash: San Juan Naturals; 1999.

Tenenbaum F, ed. *Taylor's Guide to Shade Gardening*. New York, NY: Houghton Mifflin Company; 1994.

Organizations

American Botanical Council: http://www.herbalgram.org/
Herb Society of America: http://www.herbsociety.org//library//links.htm
Internet Directory for Botany: http://public.srce.jr/botanic/cisb/Edo/flora/subject/botsoc.html
United Plant Savers: http://unitedplantsavers.org/
US Department of Agriculture Zone Map: http://www.usna.usda.gov/Hardzone/ushzmap.html

Plant and Seed Suppliers

Horizon Herbs
P.O. Box 69
Williams, OR 97544-0069
http://www.horizonherbs.com

Seeds of Change
P.O. Box 15700
Santa Fe, NM 87592-1500
1-888-762-7333
www.seedsofchange.com

Sandy Mush Nursery
316 Surrett Cove Rd
Liecester, NC 28748-5517
828-683-2014
Herb and other plants

Richters Herbs
Goodwood, Ontario
LOC 1AO
Canada
Phone: 1-905-640-6677
FAX: 1-905-640-6641
www.richters.com

16 CHAPTER

Commercial Production of Organic Herbs for Veterinary Medicine

Terrence S. Fox

The resurgent interest in herbal medicine in the Western world can be characterized as an herbal renaissance. Over the past 20 years, the increasing depth and breadth of rekindled interest in traditional herbal medicine has placed the market near full circle. Although practitioners are strongly dependent on pharmaceutical drugs, a move is taking place toward the herbal remedies that are derived from plants that grow in meadow, plain, field, lot, roadsides, and household backyards. These plants offer efficacy, minimal adverse effects, and wide availability, and their activities are increasingly understood with scientific investigation. Advocates believe that not only is botanical medicine an important part of the future of veterinary medicine, but it is fast becoming the "leading edge" of veterinary medicine.

Because of this growing interest and increasing demand, veterinarians must be aware of the sources of the medicines they use. A lot of the world's herbs are produced in developing countries, where labor is inexpensive and chemical usage is high. Prices paid to these growers are usually low, resulting in high volumes but low quality. Many imported herbs are fumigated and irradiated, which makes them not necessarily ideal raw ingredients for medicines.

Domestically, one of the concerns associated with increased demand for botanical medicines is that it will soon bring about the extinction of some species. A widely held belief among growers is that through cultivation of threatened plants, pressure from wildcrafting will be removed and all will be well. Some growers have entered the herb farming business, believing that herbal manufacturers would pay a premium because of this conservation-oriented business philosophy. However, most have discovered that it is difficult to cultivate and market herbs profitably. A number of reasons have been proposed for this situation.

First, a very small farm can at present produce adequate supply for the most popular herbs. Second, the market has historically been supplied by wildcrafters, who do not need to plow, plant, irrigate, harvest, clean, and ship product, much less suffer the expense of land, taxes, tractors, plowing, planting, and irrigating. Third, some herbal manufacturers publicly, and for political reasons, agree that wildcrafting is inherently unsustainable but continue to purchase from wildcrafters.

However, sustainability is a key issue, and with rapidly declining wild stocks, herb farming and domestic production constitute an increasingly necessary industry. The market demand for "clean" high-quality herbs has given farming of quality medicinal herbs a niche for commercial production.

WHAT IS A SUSTAINABLE HERB FARM?

Potential growers must carefully plan crops—not simply sell what already grows on their land. After assessing veterinary market needs, the grower should consider these questions:

1. Can I grow what is needed on my land? And will it flourish in my climate zone?
2. Can I compete with others in the market?
3. Is the demand high enough?
4. What quality standards can I maintain?
5. Can I sustain a profitable enterprise?

The market for botanicals for veterinary medicine is in its infancy. At this time (2006), a small market has been established, but new growers may be able to create a market for a particular product.

Following are some factors that growers should consider when they choose crops to grow:

A. Which conditions are presented to veterinarians most frequently?
B. What conditions are not satisfactorily treated with conventional therapies?
C. Does a potential botanical treatment exist?
D. Can the required plants be grown on the land that is available?

The decision-making process starts here. The considerations listed above are represented as circles in Figure 16-1. In the area where there exists a mutually inclusive

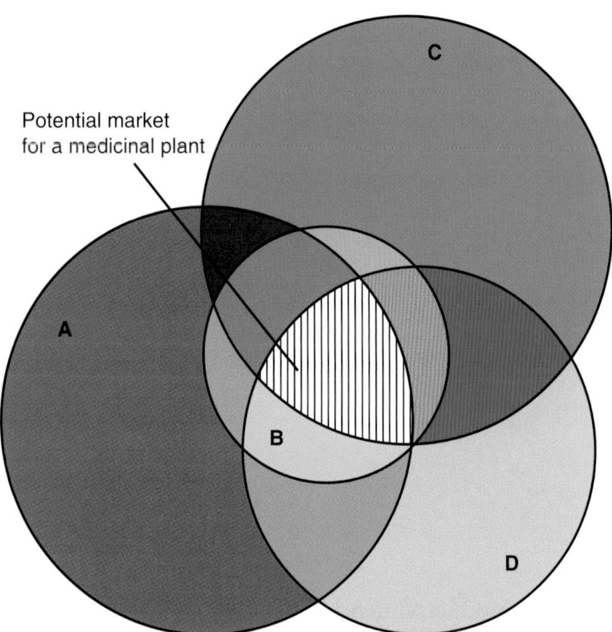

Figure 16-1 Market growing considerations.

overlap of all four circles, a potential market awaits exploration. The overlap area set of conditions is ideal: a potential herbal remedy exists for an important clinical condition, conventional treatment is not satisfactory or problematic, and the herb can be grown on the land that is available. When the market is still small, these conditions allow for its growth.

KEY ISSUES FOR HERB GROWERS

To grow any horticultural crop requires an understanding of timing, soil care, and water management. Several other factors affect the chemistry of a plant, including variability in plant genetics, growth rate, age at harvest, availability and chemistry of water and its unavoidable adulterants, use of fertilizers, and other additives. These principles apply to large growers as well as to backyard growers.

Growing for quality requires the following:

- Plants that are suitable for local growing conditions
- Knowledge of the requirements of individual herbs. For example, *Echinacea angustifolia* is best when grown slowly and while under stress for adequate water
- Care in ensuring the correct species and variety of plant. This should be obvious; however, incorrect plant material is selected by growers all too often
- Growing organically without the use of pesticides or herbicides
- Avoiding the use of animal manure. It cannot be confirmed that source animals are organic, or even if they are organic, that the food they consumed was organic and without adulterants that could find their way into the crop
- Use of manure or compost that is organic and contains no seed, if it is available
- Weed control, which allows the growth of healthy herbs and roots without competition for resources

> **Growing Opportunity**
>
> Of special clinical importance is the undisputed need to avoid overuse of antimicrobials because of the development of ever more resistant pathogens. The use of natural antiviral, antifungal, and antibacterial botanicals when they are effective is desirable. This argument alone provides reason for the grower to expect success in the commercial production of botanical antimicrobials.

When the grower maintains consistency in the factors that affect crop chemistry and the manufacturer does the same, then herbal quality and chemistry are more consistent. This is important from a clinical viewpoint. However, the variability in a botanical preparation from plant to plant, from region to region, and from year to year is probably no greater than the variability in response from patient to patient, and from condition to condition.

WHAT IS A HIGH-QUALITY HERB?

High-quality raw herbs have these distinguishable features:

- Grown by means of organic culture methods and certified as organic
- Present with good color and vibrance
- Display no discolored leaves or impurities
- Offer a clear, distinctive flavor
- Have been correctly harvested, cleaned, dried and processed

CROPPING MEDICINAL BOTANICALS

Reliance on a single crop increases vulnerability in the present veterinary botanical medicine market. Land that provides a variety of soil, shade, moisture, and drainage conditions is ideal for supporting more diverse plantings, and growers who add greenhouses increase their capacity to grow a diverse variety of herbs. It may take 5 years to produce the first crops of goldenseal, bloodroot, arnica, and echinacea, for example. To provide an annual harvest, along with cash flow, the herbal grower must plant an additional area each year and must harvest and plant on a rotation basis.

One quarter of an acre for each of these plant species is a reasonably sized plot for a single annual harvest. Two and one-half acres of hardwoods and the same in sun-drenched open field would provide for an annual harvest that is worth a respectable sum—approximately $250,000 at premium prices in 2006. However, for all of these plants, longer than 4 years is required from planting to harvest, so this income is delayed while the crops mature.

A small but growing portion of the market is organic. Organic certification provides some regulatory protection for the herb farmer against the wildcrafter.

Arnica

Arnica likes full sun and moist, well-drained soil. It tolerates a lot of clay but does not like sandy or gravelly soil. Seeds should be started in flats early in the spring and transplanted to rows. Plants should be spaced 8 to 12 inches apart in rows that are 18 to 24 inches apart. The plants, when established, will spread to form a continuous mat; further plantings can be done by separating the mat and transplanting to a newly prepared bed. Arnica needs regular water and when stressed, it does not bloom. It wilts and yellows easily but responds immediately to water. Arnica plantings grow slowly and yield repeated flowers for many years. These flowers are harvested and must be kept cool and promptly delivered to customers because they decompose easily and very quickly.

Bloodroot and Goldenseal

Bloodroot is more easily cultivated when it is planted from division rather than from seed. Bloodroot likes rich humus soil and shade. It should be well drained but should have continuous moisture. It can be planted in the spring or fall, but plants prosper more if planted in the fall. The plants produce a mat like arnica and can be propagated by division.

Goldenseal likes the same conditions of humus-enriched soil, shade, and moisture that bloodroot prefers. Goldenseal is best planted through division of mature plants in the fall.

Echinacea

Echinacea purpurea is easy to grow but is a poor second to *Echinacea angustifolia* medicinally. However, *E. angustifolia* is difficult to germinate. Seeds of *E. angustifolia* must be stratified, then planted very shallowly in flats under greenhouse conditions, to encourage germination. The flats must be deep—4 inches minimum—because the taproot will be otherwise constrained. Plants should be transplanted into deeply cultivated *weed-free* fields before the taproots are compromised and should be watered sparingly during the hot season. Growers who have fertilized and irrigated, then harvested after 3 years, have produced an extract that is green—not brown—and the market does not like it. Plants that are grown too quickly because of overwatering weigh 3 to 6 ounces each within 3 years. This is large for an *E. angustifolia* plant, but the quality and color of the end product suffer. Superior *E. angustifolia* root can be grown by watering very sparingly and waiting 6 to 10 years before harvest.

ORGANIC FARMING

Organic farming means different things to different people. To many, organic farming is simply the production of crops in accord with the rules of a certifying organization. To purists, organic farming is a way of life. It is the application of agricultural policies and procedures that complement and sustain the land. It is a method that is in tune with nature, a stewardship that enriches the land and ensures sustainability of the harvest.

Untouched by the hand of man, the entire world was once organic. Technology has provided herbicides, pesticides, and other synthetic aids, in addition to mechanized methods, that contribute to air, water, and soil pollution. If land has been isolated from nonorganic farming and is free of pollution (i.e., remotely located), then obtaining certification for organic farming will be relatively easy. If the land has been intensively farmed, is located along a busy highway in town, or is the site of a toxic spill, dump, or other pollution, attaining organic certification will be much more difficult.

The Importance of Organic Farming

Nature, through evolution, has created a marvelous ecologic system that is in biological balance. Agriculture is the alteration of natural biological activity to achieve specific production objectives. Alterations may introduce mineral elements and synthetic compounds that are designed to influence yield, control pests and weeds, and alter characteristics of a particular plant or animal crop. These alterations, if modest, may be designated organic, but if they involve drastic modifications such as the use of herbicides, pesticides, or chemical fertilizers, the activity is deemed nonorganic.

A flow of water, nutrients, and catalysts occurs between the soil, the plant or animal, and the atmosphere. Unnatural and potentially undesirable contaminants in this system may, and usually do, get carried over into the products processed from contaminated nonorganic produce.

It is the objective of the organic farmer to eliminate contamination of agricultural products by chemicals or mixtures of compounds that have been shown to be, or are potentially, detrimental to the health, well-being, and longevity of those who use or come into contact with these products. Organic farming does not guarantee freedom from unnatural toxic or potentially toxic exposure. It does, however, minimize the risks.

Organic Techniques

Weed control is best handled by disking the ground every month for at least a year before planting ensues. This activity kills the vast majority of existing cover and sets the stage for the most effective herbicides available today—the hoe and the human hand. It is vital for the caretaker to hoe and weed a crop before the undesirable plants make seed or send out root stalks. Without weed control, yields can be reduced by 50% to 80%. An experienced hoer can deweed 1 acre per day. Usually, hoeing twice a season is sufficient.

Conventional literature recommends that composting and soil enrichment through addition of composted materials should be accomplished; this practice is implemented widely. The technique is rooted in long-established agricultural practices that do not qualify as organic by modern standards. All biodegradable vegetation is suitable for composting, but contaminants must not be introduced.

It is very difficult for the farmer to obtain raw vegetation that is seed free and contaminant free. For instance, kitchen waste is generally considered to be proper compost material. If it is not of organic origin, however, it is disqualified. Manure is another common compost material that is also routinely added directly to the soil; however, it is impossible for the grower to ensure that it is free of residue and seeds.

Because of the serious practical difficulties involved in obtaining seed-free, contaminant-free composting materials, and the significant effort that is required to compost materials and then till these into the farm soil, this author does not compost unless organic compost materials can be obtained.

Cover crops are another frequently used technique for soil enrichment and nitrogen fixation. Obtaining unadulterated seed is a nearly insurmountable difficulty, and a cover crop takes the ground out of production unnecessarily for a year with only marginal improvement in fertility. Alternatively, the deliberate harvesting of certified organic materials such as grasses, leaves, forbs, twigs, and chipped wood for tilling directly into the soil each fall is the favored technique. For perennial garden plots (e.g., arnica, goldenseal, bloodroot), these materials make a great mulch and become tilled into the soil through routine cultivation.

Pests and disease are a fact of life. Most plants have developed efficient pest and disease resistance strategies. Fences work well to prevent grazing by rabbits, deer, and other large wildlife. When such techniques are not satisfactory, as in the case of insects, herb gardeners have used a variety of approaches to protect their gardens, including soap sprays, garlic sprays, dead bug sprays, and a host of other potentially contaminating materials. Insect traps and the introduction of predator insects have also been routinely used.

The problem with these so-called natural pesticides and control strategies is that not only do most not work well enough to be broadly effective or even practical, but many have adverse effects that belie the term *natural*. Following are some examples:

- Predatory or beneficial insects upset the balance of nature, and their adverse effects can be detrimental.
- Insect traps are not practical even on a small scale.
- Dead bug rinses introduce animal tissue and disease to herbs.
- Soap, garlic, and so forth, are contaminants and do not work well on a wide spectrum of insects; also, their application consumes a lot of the grower's time.

None of the above—insects (dead or alive), soaps, garlic rinses—are organic and contaminant free. Therefore, their use is not consistent with certified organic medicine purity. In spite of the fact that they have been routinely recommended and widely used, they do not qualify for use in production of certified organic medicine. Therefore, the recommended technique is to plant enough to accommodate losses due to pests and disease. Should this approach fail, some herbal remedies minimize contamination, which differentiates them from soaps and dead bug rinses.

Neem, yarrow, and fossil diatom—all in fine powder formulation—are very effective, in this author's experience, against almost all garden insects, including aphids, leaf hoppers, cabbage moths, potato beetles, ants, and so forth. Neem is nontoxic and nonmutagenic to mammals, fish, and birds. Yarrow is generally regarded as safe, and diatom powder is edible. The grower should keep in mind that all materials have an LD_{50} (dose that kills 50% of a sample population), so the use of even the most benign herbal remedy should be kept to a minimum. A little goes a very long way, and nontarget insects and spiders are also eliminated with the use of neem, yarrow, or diatom powder.

Certification of growers by an accredited organization is required by law in most countries. The laws vary from country to country, however, and organic farmers must review their own specific regulations.

Organic Certification in the United States

As of February 2004, the US Department of Agriculture (USDA) had accredited 54 domestic certifying agents and 36 foreign agents. Details of this information are readily available from local USDA field offices or local libraries, or on the Internet. The National Organic Standards (NOS) are recorded in the Federal Register 7 CFR Part 205; they are easy to find, read, and understand. References for many countries are available from USDA field offices and on the Internet.

After reading the NOS and obtaining a list of accredited certification agents, the grower should contact one or more of these agents at a state, regional, national, or international level. The greater the umbrella of the agent, the more bureaucratic inflexibility it seems to have. Therefore, growers may have an easier time working with one of the more local agencies, such as a state organization. Many agencies have local chapters that meet regularly; these meetings may be open for growers to attend. Most are focused on the development of national and international markets and on making sales contacts for their chapter members. They view growers as sources of new revenue for meeting chapter expenses and are likely to be very helpful by providing paperwork and guidance throughout the certification process.

Completion of certification documents requires effort and coordination with others. The grower is required to create a production plan that details the flow of production from seed or seedling source through delivery of finished product. Log books are required to allow the organic inspector to pick a product at any point in its growth or processing and trace it to the source of its planting, thereby determining from whence the seed or seedling may have come. After the application has been submitted, it is common for growers to receive requests for clarification and additional information.

Ultimately, an inspector contacts the grower to schedule an inspection of the farm and facility. The inspector reviews the production plan in detail and queries the grower on all aspects of farming and production processes. He or she then creates a report and files it with the agent. The agent reviews the report, and the grower is notified of his or her qualification to be certified organic. Noncompliance items may relate to the farm or may simply represent administrative vehicles that must be put in place so that compliance with standards can be facilitated.

WILDCRAFTING

Wildcrafting of medicinal plants should never be endorsed unless the wildcrafter has total control of the land on which the activity is focused. Sustainable harvesting is a matter of great concern that requires substantial knowledge and experience. Land that is open to multiple wildcrafters is certain to be plundered. Even responsible wildcrafters who take 20% of a stand can decimate it in two or three seasons if they are followed by just two equally conservative wildcrafters.

After four seasons, the once-plentiful stand is only 10% of what it had been. Any disease, drought, or infestation can eliminate the colony completely. This sad story occurs repeatedly; coupled with overgrazing and loss of habitat due to urban sprawl, wildcrafting is leading to a world in which cultivation offers the only sensible alternative.

On the other hand, a sustainable system consists of a wildcrafter who owns the land and harvests less than is produced by the natural reproduction rate. The harvest is limited to natural annual colony expansion through reproduction; thus, the colony is not decreased and may even increase. Under these circumstances, wildcrafting is not only reasonable but is a most pleasurable activity that puts the wildcrafter in tune with the natural environment.

HARVESTING FOR QUALITY

In commercial herbal enterprises, harvesting for quality involves the following:

- Harvesting only what can be handled with regard to drying space and time
- Harvesting at mid morning, when the dew is off the plants, to minimize mold and keep oil content optimal
- Being aware of possible contaminants such as weeds and insects
- Harvesting only fresh, vibrant-looking plant material
- Ensuring correct postharvesting management of plants

DRYING HERBS

Growers need a drying room that is designed to allow maximum ventilation, while at the same time protecting products from vermin to prevent soiling and contamination. Herbs may be hung to dry or may be placed on drying screens. Drying herbs should be kept out of direct sunlight because anecdotal information indicates that chemical degradation and loss of volatile oils occurs with direct heating (Figure 16-2).

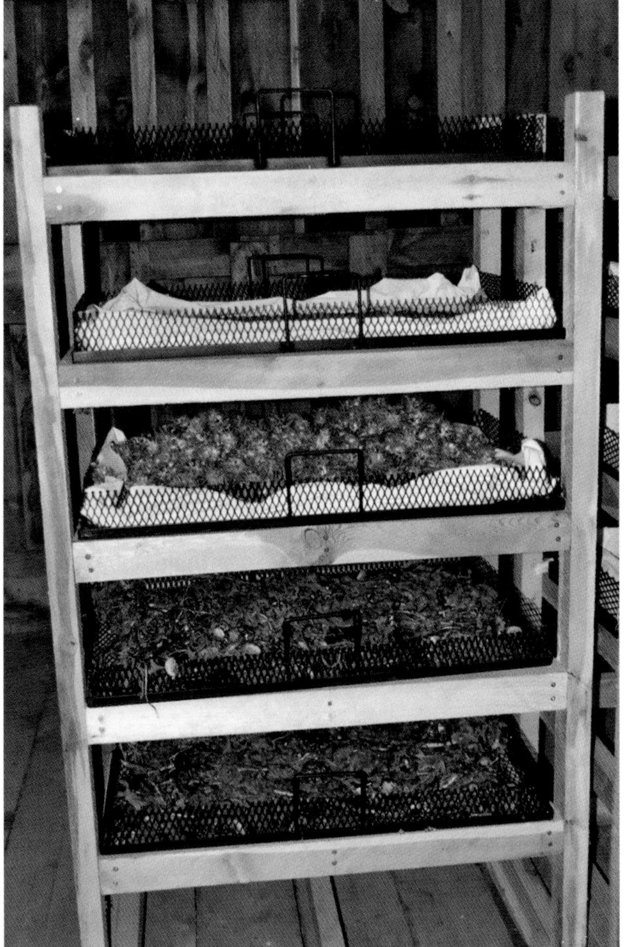

Figure 16-2 Drying herbs.

Processing of Dried Herbs

The dryness of the herb is important. If it is too wet, the herb will mildew. A total of 5% to 7% moisture is about correct and has been attained when the stem or root breaks clean upon being bent. If the herb is too dry, the stems may break into pieces that are too small to be easily removed from the batch, resulting in lower quality. The finished herb is placed into bags that are not airtight and are correctly labeled (e.g., species, date of harvest). Herb material should be placed in dry storage or frozen for 4 days so that insect eggs and larvae are destroyed. If frozen, the material should be redried to prevent mildew. Finally, the herbs should be stored in vermin-proof, waterproof containers, away from direct sunlight and temperature fluctuations.

HERBAL MEDICINE FOR THE VETERINARIAN

Dozens of growers now supply organic herbal products for animal use. In some countries, regulation of the growing and manufacturing of herbal products is sophisticated; in others, standards are still being developed. For meaningful standards to occur, the way in which herbal medicines work must be understood. It is not just a matter of controlling the concentration of more than one chemical constituent (called *standardization*). The whole plant is important. For the present, it is essential that herbal medicines be sourced from a grower and a manufacturer who begin with the proper species and document processing for quality control. To have confidence in herbal medicine, veterinarians must understand the production process from soil to pharmacy shelf.

Worldwide Organic Agriculture Resources

IFOAM—http://www.ifoam.org/
International Foundation for Organic Agriculture description and annotated links.

Soil Association—http://www.soilassociation.org/
Campaigning for organic food and farming and sustainable forestry. Site includes extensive document library that covers organic issues.

Organic Farming Research Foundation—http://www.ofrf.org/
To foster improvement in and widespread adoption of organic farming practices.

Organic Trade Association—http://www.ota.com/
The mission of the Organic Trade Association is to encourage global sustainability by promoting diverse organic trade.

Organic Crop Improvement Association (OCIA)—http://www.ocia.org/
Offers certification and accreditation for this type of farming. Includes a download of regulations, a newsletter, and a list of related links.

International Society of Organic Agriculture Research (ISOFAR)—http://www.isofar.org/
Gives the aims and a list with supporters and pictures from the foundation in June 2003.

United States

California Certified Organic Farmers (CCOF)—http://www.ccof.org/
Links, news, FAQs, and descriptions useful to organic buyers and growers.

The Organic Materials Review Institute—http://www.omri.org
List materials approved for organic use in the United States.

Northeast Organic Farming Association of New Jersey—http://www.nofanj.org/
Includes a calendar of events and information for consumers and growers.

Northeast Organic Farming Association of Vermont (NOFA VT)—http://www.nofavt.org/
The home page of the Northeast Organic Farming Association of Vermont. This is where you can find out all about the NOFA Vermont.

Hawaii Organic Farmers Association—http://www.hawaiiorganicfarmers.org/
Home page of HOFA, the premier organic certifier in Hawaii.

Northeast Organic Farming Association of New York, Inc—http://nofany.org
An organization of farmers, gardeners, and consumers who work to promote organic growing in the United States Northeast. Includes details of certification, links, and forums.

Northeast Organic Farming Association of Connecticut—http://www.ctnofa.org/
Includes a calendar of events, membership information, and a list of farms.

Oregon Biodynamics Group—http://oregonbd.org
A nonprofit group that promotes biodynamic farming and gardening.

Northeast Organic Farming Association of Rhode Island—http://www.nofari.org/
Includes a list of farms and a calendar of events.

OEFFA—Ohio Ecological Food & Farm Association—http://www.oeffa.org/
The Ohio Ecological Food & Farm Association is a grassroots coalition of food producers and consumers formed in 1979.

Worldwide Organic Agriculture Resources—cont'd

Florida Organic Growers—http://www.floridaplants.com/FOG/Default.htm
Directory and information.

Northeast Organic Farming Association of Massachusetts—http://www.nofamass.org/
Includes membership application, news, and food guide.

United Kingdom
Organic Farmers and Growers Ltd—http://www.organicfarmers.uk.com
Offers certification for UK growers.

Soil Association of Scotland—http://www.soilassociationscotland.org
Aims to lead and support the development of the organic food and farming sector in Scotland.

The Yorkshire Organic Centre—http://www.yorkshireorganiccentre.org
Aims to lead and support the development of the organic food and farming sector in the Yorkshire and Humber regions.

Canada
Alberta Organic Producers Association—http://www.albertaorganicproducers.org
AOPA membership details, including guidelines and requirements, fees, and rules.

Canadian Organic Growers—http://www.cog.ca/
A national information network for farmers, gardeners, and consumers. COG promotes organic foods through national publications and events, and through memberships in local chapters.

Southwest Saskatchewan OCIA Chapter #8—http://www.ocia8.sk.ca
The members of this organic growers organization have listed their contact information and the previous year's production.

Certified Organic Associations of British Columbia—http://www.certifiedorganic.bc.ca/
Umbrella group of local certified organic grower associations. Includes definition of organic farming, promotional resources, member associations, contact details, and certification information.

Ireland
Irish Organic Farmers & Growers Association—http://www.irishorganic.ie/
IOFGA aims to aid the production, marketing, and promotion of organic food in Ireland.

Australia
Canberra Organic Growers Society—http://www.netspeed.com.au/cogs/cogs.htm
Information about the society, including membership details, and photograph gallery. State location: Australian Capital Territory.

The Organic Herb Growers of Australia Inc—http://www.organicherbs.org/
Established in 1987 in Northern New South Wales, to promote the growing, processing, and marketing of herbs and herbal products.

Organic Farming/Product Certification with Biological Farmers of Australia—http://www.bfa.com.au/
Organic and biodynamic certification for all categories of organic and biodynamic farming and food production.

India
Indian Organic Certification of Agriculture—http://www.indocert.org
Certification authority, with details of standards, downloadable forms, and news.

Europe
ENOF—http://www.cid.csic.es/enof/index.html
European Network for Scientific Research Coordination in Organic Farming.

Research Institute of Organic Agriculture (FiBL)—http://www.fibl.ch/english/index.php
Swiss-based coordinating group of researchers for organic agriculture in Europe. Details of research, publications, services, and training.

New Zealand
Organic (Ltd)—http://organic.com.au
A nonprofit organization that promotes organic and sustainable agriculture in Australia and New Zealand.

Conserving Medicinal Plant Biodiversity

CHAPTER

James Martin Affolter and Andrew Pengelly

Current patterns of exploitation threaten the commercial future, as well as the biological survival, of many species of medicinal plants. This chapter discusses the global dimensions of this issue and the problems associated with biodiversity loss. Bringing wild-collected species into cultivation is one solution, but this approach has many limitations. Market forces, socioeconomic considerations, and ecologic factors suggest that most medicinal plants will continue to be wild-harvested. As the global market for herbal medicines increases, supply chains and production methods are in a state of flux. Medical practitioners, consumers, and vendors must be well informed so they can use their influence to steer the industry in a direction that promotes environmental stewardship, as well as improved product quality and availability.

GLOBAL DIMENSIONS AND CAUSES OF BIODIVERSITY LOSS

The work of cataloguing the world's flora is still far from complete. So far, scientists have named and described more than 250,000 species of "higher" plants—a group that includes flowering plants, conifers, ferns, and horsetails. Yet many species remain unknown to science, particularly those in the richly diverse tropical regions. We can only make an educated guess, but recent estimates of the number of flowering plant species that exist worldwide range from 270,000 to 422,000 (Bramwell, 2002; Govaerts, 2001).

Loss of medicinal plant biodiversity reflects the general decline in plant diversity that is occurring globally. The current rate of plant and animal extinction is estimated to be 100 to 1000 times greater than previous average levels (Tuxill, 1999). Many researchers of biodiversity agree that we are entering a phase of mass extinction that has been unprecedented since the meteorite that struck off the coast of the Yucatan ended the age of the dinosaurs 65 million years ago (Wilson, 2002). In North America, the Heritage Program considers approximately one third of the continent's flowering plant species to be at risk (Stein, 2000).

Human cultures in every region of the world have identified and used native species of plants for their medicinal value. The diversity of these regional pharmacopoeias is remarkable. Estimates for the number of species used medicinally worldwide include 35,000 to 70,000 (Farnsworth, 1991) and 53,000 (Schippmann, 2002). The great majority of medicinal plant species are used only in traditional or folk medicine. Schippmann and colleagues (2002) estimate that the total number of medicinal and aromatic plant species in international trade is about 2500. Only a fraction of these—probably no more than a few hundred—are in formal cultivation for commercial purposes.

No reliable estimate is available for the number of medicinal plants that are globally threatened, but the number has been variously calculated as 4160 or 10,000 (respectively, Schippmann, 2002, and Vorhies, 2000). Medicinal plants known to be globally extinct are very few (Hamilton, 2004).

The principal causes of the general decrease in plant diversity are well known. They include habitat destruction, competition from alien species, mortality from introduced diseases, pollution, and overexploitation. Natural populations of medicinal plants are subject to all of these pressures, but the fact that they are selectively targeted and collected poses special problems for those working to conserve them. For example, one strategy that is frequently included in species recovery plans for federally protected plants in the United States is the carrying out of "reintroductions." This involves propagating plants off-site, then planting them out to establish new populations of a species in areas of suitable habitat within its historical range. This approach can work well for little-known species that are not likely to attract much attention from the public. However, in cases of native medicinal species with commercial value (e.g., ginseng, goldenseal), the creation of artificial populations amounts to little more than stocking the shelves for future wild-harvesters.

An example of this dilemma was witnessed during a visit to Karoo National Botanical Garden in South Africa in 1996. The Karoo Garden is located 120 km from Cape Town near Worcester, at the foot of the Brandwacht Mountains. It concentrates on plants from the semidesert areas of South Africa, which are some of the most unusual succulent species in the world. Many of these species overcome dry conditions by storing water in their leaves and stems, or in underground roots and bulbs. Some species are quite large, such as the colorful tree aloes; others, such as tiny stone plants, are nearly indistinguishable from the gravelly soils in which they grow. In addition to horticultural collections, the garden includes a 144-hectare nature reserve. When one of the authors (JA) visited the Karoo Garden, a staff member pointed to a row of large, coarsely textured bulbs that were lying on the ground. These were the underground storage structures of the Candelabra Lily—*Brunsvigia josephinae* (Amaryllidaceae)—which is a striking plant with the biggest bulb (8-inch diameter) and the greatest inflorescence of any of the South African geophytes. These plants had been taken from poachers who were discovered in the nearby nature reserve. A total of 49 plants were recovered. The papery tunic of the bulbs is used medicinally as a dressing. Among some native South Africans, a young man's passage to manhood is marked by a circumcision ritual. (In his autobiography, Nelson Mandela [1994] gives an account of his rite of passage ceremony.) The traditional bandage that is applied following circumcision is the cottony tissue of the Candelabra Lily, so the plant has great ritual significance and value. Staff members at the Karoo Garden were hesitant to return the bulbs they had seized to their original location in the reserve because they would surely be stolen again. They were looking for a safer place within the garden boundaries to reestablish them. This dilemma is encountered whenever reintroduced species are valuable and easily recognizable.

Although many medicinal plant species are under stress, others have become more common and more widely distributed, thanks to human activities. Some medicinal species have ecologic traits that preadapt them for easy dispersal and survival in disturbed habitats. Many, such as dandelion *(Taraxacum officinale)*, various plantains *(Plantago* spp), Saint John's Wort *(Hypericum perforatum)*, and *Artemesia annua*—the source of the antimalarial drug artemesinin—have become cosmopolitan weeds. Recent analyses of herbal use in Mexico and North America indicate that plants with weedy traits are overrepresented in these traditional pharmacopoeias (Stepp, 2001). The distribution and abundance of medicinal plants reveal the same two trends that currently dominate the plant kingdom as a whole: (1) a mixing or homogenization of the global flora, as aggressive species become transported and established around the globe, and (2) a reduction in biodiversity and abundance of many species, as habitats are destroyed and exploitation pressures increase.

PROBLEMS ASSOCIATED WITH BIODIVERSITY LOSS AND OVEREXPLOITATION

From a commercial standpoint, the most obvious consequence of the disappearance of medicinal plant populations is a dwindling supply of wild-harvested plants, but this is only the tip of the iceberg. Unwise patterns of harvest and usage have led to numerous biological and environmental problems; have negatively affected product quality and availability; and have increased socioeconomic tensions within local communities that are involved in the collection and use of native species of medicinal plants.

The harvest pressure on wild populations of medicinal plants appears to be increasing (Hamilton, 2004; Sheldon, 1997), and many species have suffered reductions in the number and size of populations, as well as in overall geographic range. This trend has had serious biological and evolutionary consequences for individual species. In small populations, genetic factors such as changing demographic structure, inbreeding, genetic isolation, and genetic drift have led to smaller effective population sizes (Ellstrand, 1993), which, in turn, can increase the risks of local extirpation and extinction. Genetic diversity is often directly related to population size (Frankham, 2002), and reduced diversity can reduce individual fitness and decrease the likelihood of population persistence. Small populations tend to become increasingly unstable.

Threats to medicinal plant populations may affect ecologically related species. Removal of a plant species can affect the pollinators, herbivores, soil fauna, microorganisms, and other plants and animals that depend on that species and the physical environment it creates. Saw palmetto *(Serenoa repens)* is not a threatened species, but the manner in which it is used by wildlife illustrates the important role that a medicinal plant species can play within an ecosystem. Until recently, much of the scientific literature on saw palmetto focused on methods of eradicating the plant (Carrington, 2000). The fruits of this scrubby palm, which is native to the coastal plain of the southeastern United States, are valued in the treatment of benign prostatic hyperplasia. The plant grows densely in open fields and pine understories, and many landowners consider it a rangeland weed that transforms good pasture into an obstacle course for cattle. The fruits of saw palmetto have been likened in taste to "rotten cheese steeped in tobacco," but they were an important source of starch for the Seminole Indians, and they are consumed by many species of wildlife, including raccoons, foxes, gopher tortoises, whitetail deer, fish, and waterfowl. They are also a major food source for the state-threatened Florida black bear *(Ursus americanus* subsp *floridanus)*, and they provide cover for this species and for the endangered Florida panther (Bennett, 1998). Black bears often give birth under the cover provided by saw palmetto thickets. Although saw palmettos are common, the Florida black bear has experienced a significant population reduction. It prefers areas with dense understory vegetation, including pine flatwoods and other areas dominated by saw palmetto. Researchers in Florida are concerned that indiscriminate harvesting of saw palmetto fruits could adversely affect the black bear and other wildlife species, especially in low–fruit production years, when prices for saw palmetto berries may be high. Bears have reportedly shifted their ranges in search of fruits during the fall. Researchers plan to identify the extent of fruit harvesting in areas used by black bears to determine whether management practices should take the harvesting impact into account (University of Florida Web site: http://wfrec.ifas.ufl.edu/range/sawpalm/research.html).

Uncontrolled harvest of wild plants can also lead to erosion and other physical damage to the environment. This pattern was observed in an arid region of Argentina, where wild-harvest of medicinal plants is an important component of the local economy. Córdoba, a province in north central Argentina, is well known for its diversity of native herb species, many of which are collected from the wild for commercial use in herbal teas and medicines. In the mountainous western districts of the province, known as the Sierras de Córdoba, as many as 80% of families collect herbs as a primary source of income. Natural populations of many commercially harvested species in the region are declining in geographic distribution and abundance. This is a result of both indiscriminate collection and widespread habitat destruction. The arrival of railroads in the region during the 1930s resulted in large-scale deforestation. Mountain valleys that once possessed extensive hardwood forests now contain only small residual stands. Removal of the forest cover and burning of vegetation to control weeds and insects have hastened erosion of soils by wind and summer rains. Plant collectors in this region often harvest woody species by ripping up entire plants by the roots. Many species grow on the slopes of mountains and hillsides, and the erosional gullies that result are a frequent sight in such habitats (Lagrotteria, 1999).

Loss of medicinal plant species affects practitioners and consumers. Adulteration becomes more likely as wild-harvested plants become scarce. Substitution with different (and sometimes harmful) species may occur, but more often, less effective plant parts may be used (e.g., stems instead of leaves, leaves instead of roots). In addition, increasing scarcity makes desirable species less available, which drives prices up. Finally, as a species becomes rare, various chemotypes are lost, thus reducing the genetic variation and hence the potential range of phytochemicals that provide medicinal activity.

Loss of medicinal plant diversity has socioeconomic implications as well. Ethnobotanists have noted that as desired plant species disappear, local people have difficulty finding plants to satisfy their own health needs (Balick, 1996; Tuxill, 1999). The livelihoods of local wildcrafters may be threatened, and poaching and trespassing may increase (Hamilton, 2004). The negative impact of overcollection is often confined to the local level until such times as regional or global scarcity becomes critical. When the need to initiate horticultural production is finally recognized, tension may develop between local wildcrafters and "outsiders" who appear on the scene to encourage commercial production of plants.

WILD HARVEST VERSUS CULTIVATION OF MEDICINAL PLANTS

With relatively few species of medicinal plants in large-scale cultivation, it seems logical that horticultural production of additional species would relieve the pressure on wild populations and result in the availability of higher-quality products on the market. Although this is certainly a good strategy in some cases, the choice of which species to domesticate involves many variables, and the obstacles to profitable horticultural production can be formidable.

Which Types of Plants Are Most Vulnerable to Overharvest in the Wild?

Several factors determine the vulnerability of a plant species to overharvest in the wild. Plants with a wide geographic distribution and broad habitat tolerance are less vulnerable than are species with restricted ranges and highly specific habitat requirements. The frequency and intensity of harvest affect the resilience of natural populations. The life cycle of the plant and the part of the plant harvested are also of prime importance. Longer-lived species such as ginseng are far more vulnerable to destructive harvesting than are short-lived ones. Plants of slight stature such as partridge berry *(Mitchella repens)* may appear to be locally common; however, commercial harvest on any scale would severely deplete their populations.

Schippmann and associates (2002) summarized the relationship between a plant's life form and plant parts collected and its susceptibility to overcollection from the wild. Examples of highly susceptible species include annual plants whose seeds or fruits are collected and perennial species whose roots are harvested. Leaf, flower, or fruit collection from trees and shrubs is likely to be highly sustainable. Among the most at-risk species are those that are habitat specific, slow growing, and destructively harvested for their bark or roots, or for the whole plant.

Cunningham (2001) describes detailed field methods for assessing harvesting impact on a variety of wild-collected plants, including medicinal species. These techniques enable researchers to move beyond generalizations based on plant part harvested and life form, and to actually quantify the effects of defoliation, bark removal, and fruit collection on plant growth, reproduction, and survival. Accurate predictions require study on a species-by-species basis, or at least a detailed understanding of harvesting characteristics that can be acquired only through on-the-ground observations. For example, the physical accessibility of fruits and the timing of their release influence how destructively they are harvested. Tall plants that bear valuable but hard-to-reach fruits are often felled. On the other hand, if these same fruits fall to the ground at a stage of ripening at which they can be successfully collected, harvesting impact is likely to be low. Cunningham (2001) cites a survey by Phillips (1993) of more than 30 species of edible fruit–bearing trees in the Peruvian Amazon. When 10% or less of edible fruits fell onto the ground and fruit access height was between 8 and 23 meters, trees were felled. Examples of other factors that must be considered for an accurate estimation of harvesting impact include plant mating systems (Are flowers able to self-pollinate? Or, are male and female flowers on separate plants?), timing and frequency of defoliation, and patterns of bark removal (cutting of vertical strips and patches vs complete girdling). Cunningham provides numerous examples of field rating systems that can be used to measure harvest impact, but additional research is needed. For example, no rating scale is given for plant exudates (gums, resin, latex) other than for rubber tapping. Gums and resins constitute a major resource for medicinal products. For example, gum arabic trees *(Acacia senegal)* yield 250 g of gum per season, and one country alone (Sudan) exports more than 11,000 tons each year (Cunningham, 2001).

What Are the Comparative Benefits and Risks of Cultivation Versus Wild Harvest?

Although cultivation may appear to be the obvious solution for arresting the decline of wild populations, a range of factors must be considered, some of which favor retaining the status quo. Schippmann and colleagues (2002) have addressed this question by comparing the pros and cons from the viewpoints of (1) species and ecosystems, (2) market factors, and (3) the people who depend on the system to make their living (Table 17-1).

Schippmann discusses an example of genetic pollution that can occur through cultivation of species indigenous to the region. The ex situ gene pool is at risk for contamination because of cross-pollination by cultivated (cloned) stock. The concern is that offspring from such cross-fertilization can exemplify "hybrid vigor," with new dominant genes that mask inferior recessive genes weakening the overall gene pool over the longer term (Low, 2002). This risk can be minimized through the creation of small-scale, mixed-species plantations, or by the use of wind breaks and shelter breaks (McCarthy, 1998).

Under What Circumstances Is Cultivation a Realistic or Necessary Alternative?

1. Cultivated material must be able to compete economically with wild-harvested material. Wild-harvest requires little or no monetary investment. Domestication of a wild species requires time and capital (Schippmann, 2002). Commercial production involves risk, and producers require a measure of predictability in the market.
2. Obstacles to cultivation based on the biological or ecologic requirements of the species must be surmountable. Examples of potential obstacles include slow growth, unusual soil or nutrient requirements, susceptibility to pests or diseases, symbiotic relationships with other plants or fungi that are difficult to establish, absence of pollinators, and slow germination. Some of these can be overcome through research.

TABLE 17-1

Wild Harvesting Versus Cultivation of Medicinal and Aromatic Plants: A Summary of Advantages and Disadvantages From the Perspectives of Ecology, Market Demand, and People

Wild-Harvesting		Cultivation	
Advantages	Disadvantages	Advantages	Disadvantages
Ecologic			
Puts wild plant populations in the continuing interest of local people	Uncontrolled harvest may lead to the extinction of ecotypes and even species	Relieves harvesting pressure on very rare and slow-growing species, which are most susceptible to threat	Devalues wild plant resources and their habitats economically and reduces incentive to conserve ecosystems
Provides an incentive to protect and maintain wild populations, their habitats, and the genetic diversity of medicinal plant populations	Common access to the resource makes it difficult to adhere to quotas and the precautionary principle		Narrows genetic diversity (gene pool) of the resource because wild relatives of cultivated species become neglected
	In most cases, knowledge about the biology of the resource is poor and the annual sustained yields are unknown		May lead to conversion of habitat for cultivation
	In most cases, resource inventories and accompanying management plans do not exist		Cultivated species may become invasive and have a negative impact on ecosystems

TABLE 17-1

Wild Harvesting Versus Cultivation of Medicinal and Aromatic Plants: A Summary of Advantages and Disadvantages From the Perspectives of Ecology, Market Demand, and People—cont'd

Wild-Harvesting		**Cultivation**	
Advantages	Disadvantages	Advantages	Disadvantages
			Reintroducing plants can lead to genetic pollution of wild populations
Market demands			
Cheaper because it does not require infrastructure and investment	Greater risk of adulteration	Guarantees continuing supply of raw material	Successful cultivation techniques do not exist (e.g., for slow-growing, habitat-specific taxa)
Many species are required only in small quantities that do not make cultivation economically viable	Risk of contamination through nonhygienic harvest or poorly controlled postharvest conditions	Makes reliable botanical identification possible	More expensive than wild harvest
For some plant parts, extra large cultivation areas are required (e.g., *Arnica* production for flowers)		Genotypes may be standardized or improved	Needs substantial investment before and during production
No pesticides are used		Quality standards are easier to maintain, and better control over postharvest handling is possible	
Traditional beliefs hold that wild plants are more potent		Production volume and price can be agreed on for longer periods, and resource price is relatively stable over time	
		Certification as organic production is possible	
People			
Provides access to cash income without prior investment	Unclear land rights create ownership problems	Provides in-country value adding	Capital investment for small farmers is high
Provides herbal medicines for local healthcare needs	This income and healthcare resource is becoming scarce through overharvesting	Secures steady supply of herbal medicines (home gardens)	Competition from large-scale production puts pressure on small farmers and on wild-harvesters
Maintains the resources for rural populations on a long-term basis (if done sustainably)			Benefits are made elsewhere and traditional resource users have little or no benefit return (issues of intellectual and genetic property rights)

Modified from Schippmann U, Cunningham AB, Leaman DJ. *Impact of Cultivation and Gathering of Medicinal Plants on Biodiversity: Global Trends and Issues.* Rome, Italy: Inter-Department Working Group on Biology Diversity for Food and Agriculture, FAO; 2002.

3. Benefits to rural communities and livelihoods should outweigh the disruption brought about by implementation of new production and economic systems.
4. In some cases, cultivation may be essential from a conservation standpoint, even when it is not economically competitive. When plants become seriously threatened in the wild, subsidized intervention in the form of ex situ conservation (in botanical gardens or seed gene banks, or by government agencies or nonprofit groups) may be the only alternative to local extirpation or extinction (Hamilton, 2004; Sumner, 2000; Tuxill, 1999).

5. An "International Standard for Sustainable Wild Collection of Medicinal and Aromatic Plants" is being developed by the German Federal Agency for Nature Conservation, the World Conservation Union (IUCN), and the World Wildlife Fund (WWF)/Trade Records Analysis of Flora and Fauna in Commerce (TRAFFIC) (http://www.floraweb.de/proxy/floraweb/map-pro/). These standards are designed to bridge the gap between existing general guidelines and management plans tailored to specific projects.

REGULATING MEDICINAL PLANT HARVEST AND TRADE

Regulating the collection and commercial trade of wild-collected medicinal plants is a formidable task. Treaties, international guidelines, and local regulations have been developed for some species, but enforcement is difficult. Ultimately, local human populations must support conservation efforts if they are to be successful. Government agencies are simply understaffed, and the problem is too diffuse for tight control.

An important policy milestone for plant conservation occurred in 2002, when the Convention on Biological Diversity that emerged from the 1992 Rio Earth Summit adopted the Global Strategy for Plant Conservation (GSPC; Botanic Gardens Conservation International [BGCI] Web site: http://www.bgci.org.uk/conservation/strategy.html; Schippmann, 2002). This strategy addresses conservation and sustainable use goals for all plants and sets a series of general and specific targets for the year 2010. Examples of general goals include reversal of the decline in plant resources that support sustainable livelihoods, local food security, and health care; absence of species of wild flora that are subject to unsustainable exploitation because of international trade; and development of a widely accessible working list of known plant species as the first step toward a complete world flora. Some specific goals of the GSPC include making 90% of threatened plant species available in off-site collections and 20% included in recovery programs; having 70% of the genetic diversity of crops and other major socioeconomically valuable plant species conserved; and ensuring that 30% of plant-based products are derived from sources that are sustainably managed. Tremendous progress would be represented if these three goals could be achieved for wild-collected medicinal plants by the end of this decade.

The World Health Organization (WHO) has published a series of technical guidelines related to the quality assurance and control of herbal medicines. Its members acknowledge that adverse medicinal reactions to herbal medicines are often the result of poor-quality raw materials or unacceptable production practices. Guidelines on good agricultural and collection practices for medicinal plants (WHO, 2003) provide a summary of the techniques and measures required for appropriate collection and cultivation. Topics addressed include use of ecologically nondestructive collection systems (e.g., collecting strips of bark rather than completely girdling trees), training of field personnel, properly documenting the origin and identity of plant material, drying techniques, cleanliness standards for processing facilities, postharvest handling, packaging, and many more. However, the authors of these guidelines note that, even though progress has been made in developing standards, ". . . there is still considerable disparity between knowledge and implementation." Pharmaceutical companies are striving to meet higher standards of quality for herbal medicines; however, their products can be no better than the initial steps in the market chain that provides the raw materials; much training is therefore needed for harvesters and growers.

Only the European Union and a few countries such as China and Japan have developed regional and national guidelines for good agricultural practices for medicinal plants (WHO, 2003). China is a major global supplier of herbal medicines, but major concerns have been expressed about the quality, safety, and standardization of Chinese herbal exports. A new law passed in 2002 requires large producers in China to provide more information with each batch of herbal products, including botanical name, place of origin, time of harvest, and level of insect contamination. Material of cultivated origin requires information on the fertilizers and pesticides used, as well as on heavy metal content. Quotas have been established to prevent the overharvesting of wild species in certain areas (Hamilton, 2004).

The Convention on International Trade in Endangered Species (CITES) was established in 1973. More than 150 countries have signed the treaty, which seeks to control international traffic in threatened plants and animals. It prohibits trade of the most highly endangered species (listed in CITES Appendix I) and monitors vulnerable species (CITES Appendix II) by requiring permits for the export and import of these species among member countries. The only frequently traded medicinal plant species in Appendix I is *Saussurea lappa*, which is popular in Asia and the Middle East as an aphrodisiac and treatment for patients with skin disease. American ginseng *(Panax quinquefolius)* and goldenseal *(Hydrastis canadensis)* are among 15 Appendix II plant species that are listed specifically because of concerns about their trade as medicinals (Hamilton, 2004). Although CITES is generally recognized as a successful international agreement, Schippmann (2002) notes that it has a number of limitations as a conservation tool: Internal trade is not monitored; many plant products such as bark and extracts are difficult to identify by species, making it hard to track them; and many countries are reluctant to support the listing of species that bring needed international exchange.

Finding Information on the Conservation Status of Medicinal Plants

Where can you find information concerning the conservation status of a particular species? The nonprofit organization United Plant Savers has developed "At-Risk" and "To Watch" lists of medicinal plants native to North America (www.unitedplantsavers.org). Detailed information concerning the status of plants and animals native to North America (including distribution maps; state, national, and global ranks of conservation status; literature references; and management guidelines) can be accessed online at www.natureserve.org, a database maintained by the Natural Heritage Program. The most widely used system outside of North America for rating the conservation status of species has been developed by the Species Survival Commission of the IUCN. This group publishes red lists and red data books by country and region. The first worldwide red list for plants was published in 1998; the current list is available and searchable online at www.redlist.org.

CONCLUSION

Why is it worthwhile for a practitioner to develop an understanding of medicinal plant conservation issues and strategies? In the same way that users of herbal medicines must often employ a "buyer beware" approach when it comes to the quality and safety of individual herbal products, practitioners should not be too quick to accept the claims of suppliers that herbs have been sustainably produced or harvested and obtained from ethical sources. By developing a general understanding of strategies for conserving medicinal plants, the reader will be in a better position to evaluate claims regarding specific species and suppliers.

There may come a time when herbal markets and supply chains stabilize in such a way that practitioners and consumers can have greater confidence that the products they are using are sustainably harvested or produced, and that information concerning the conservation status of medicinal plants is more available and more reliable. In the meantime, practitioners should be aware of the species that are at greatest risk (see Chapter 18), so they can support efforts to protect the plants they use in their practice.

References

Balick M, Cox P. *Plants, People, and Culture: The Science of Ethnobotany*. New York, NY: Scientific American Library, HPHLP; 1996.

Bennett BC, Hicklin JR. Uses of saw palmetto *(Serenoa repens*, Arecaceae*)* in Florida. Economic Botany 1998;52:381–393.

Bramwell D. How many plant species are there? Plant Talk 2002;28:32–34.

Carrington ME, Mullahey JJ, Krewer G, Bowland B, Affolter J. Saw palmetto *(Serenoa repens):* an emerging forest resource in the southeastern United States. Southern Journal of Applied Forestry 2000;24:129–134.

Cunningham AB. *Applied Ethnobotany: People, Wild Plant Use, and Conservation*. London, United Kingdom: Earthscan; 2001.

Ellstrand CC, Elam DR. Population genetic consequences of small population size: implications for plant conservation. Annual Review of Ecology and Systematics 1993;24:217–242.

Farnsworth NR, Soejarto DD. Global importance of medicinal plants. In: Akerele O, Heywood V, Synge H, eds. *Conservation of Medicinal Plants*. Cambridge, United Kingdom: Cambridge University Press; 1991:25–51.

Frankham R, Ballou JD, Briscoe DA. *Introduction to Conservation Genetics*. Cambridge, United Kingdom: Cambridge University Press; 2002.

Govaerts R. How many species of seed plants are there? Taxonomy 2001;50:1085–1090.

Hamilton AC. Medicinal plants, conservation, and livelihoods. Biodiversity and Conservation 2004;13:1477–1517.

Lagrotteria M, Affolter J. Sustainable production and harvest of medicinal and aromatic herbs in the Sierras de Córdoba Region, Argentina. In: Nazarea VD, ed. *Ethnoecology: Situated Knowledge/Located Lives*. Tucson, Ariz: University of Arizona Press; 1999:175–189.

Low T. *The New Nature*. Melbourne, Australia: Viking; 2002.

Mandela N. *Long Walk to Freedom: The Autobiography of Nelson Mandela*. Boston, Mass: Little, Brown; 1994.

McCarthy J. Native foods and provenance. Presented at: Conference on Provenance; 1998; Greening Australia.

Phillips O. The potential for harvesting fruits in tropical rainforests: new data from the Peruvian Amazon. Biodiversity and Conservation 1993;2:18–38.

Schippmann U, Cunningham AB, Leaman DJ. *Impact of Cultivation and Gathering of Medicinal Plants on Biodiversity: Global Trends and Issues*. Rome, Italy: Inter-Department Working Group on Biology Diversity for Food and Agriculture FAO; 2002.

Sheldon JW, Balick MJ, Laird SA. *Medicinal Plants: Can Utilization and Conservation Coexist? Advances in Economic Botany*, vol 12. Bronx, NY: New York Botanical Garden; 1997.

Stein BA, Kutner LS, Adams JS. *Precious Heritage: The Status of Biodiversity in the United States*. Oxford: Oxford University Press; 2000.

Stepp JR, Moerman DE. The importance of weeds in ethnopharmacology. J Ethnopharmacol 2001;75:19–23.

Sumner J. *The Natural History of Medicinal Plants*. Portland, Ore: Timber Press; 2000.

Tuxill JT. Nature's cornucopia: our stake in plant diversity. Worldwatch Paper 148. Washington, DC: Worldwatch Institute; 1999.

Vorhies F. The global dimension of threatened medicinal plants from a conservation point of view. In: Honnef S, Melisch R, eds. *Medicinal Utilization of Wild Species: Challenge for Man and Nature in the New Millennium*. Hanover, Germany: WWF Germany/TRAFFIC Europe-Germany, EXPO 2000; 2000:26–29.

Wilson EO. Loss of biodiversity is a global crisis. In: Dudley W, ed. *Biodiversity: Current Controversies*. San Diego, Calif: Green Haven Press; 2002:24–28.

World Health Organization. *WHO Guidelines on Good Agricultural and Collection Practices (GACP) for Medicinal Plants*. Geneva, Switzerland: WHO; 2003.

Safe Substitutes for Endangered Herbs: Plant Conservation and Loss of Our Medicines

18

CHAPTER

Susan G. Wynn

THE PROBLEM—WHY YOU NEED TO CARE

The consumer-driven herbal products industry has reached $17 billion in international trade at the time of this writing. No reliable estimates are available for the number of endangered or threatened medicinal plants worldwide, but estimates range from 4160 to 10,000 species (Schippmann, 2002, Vorhies, 2000). Even when plants are not recognized by official conservation bodies as endangered, genetic erosion may be occurring because of diminished populations.

TRAFFIC (Trade Records Analysis of Flora and Fauna in Commerce) India, set up by the World Wildlife Fund (WWF) and the World Conservation Union (IUCN), monitors plant species endangerment and has set goals to correct the problem. TRAFFIC lists 33 plants from the Ayurveda/Tibetan/Unani/Siddha *Materia medica* as critically endangered and 17 as endangered. In Europe, TRAFFIC lists popular medicinal plants such as arnica, uva ursi, thyme, and licorice. *Panax quinquefolius* has been exported from the United States since the 1700s and has been regulated under the Convention on International Trade in Endangered Species (CITES) since 1975. Even so, the US Department of Agriculture (USDA) and the US Fish and Wildlife Service have reported a trend toward harvesting smaller and younger roots over the past 15 years.

Although no medicinal plants have become extinct in recent memory, it is believed that the first recorded species to succumb is silphion, a plant prized by Ancient Greeks and rendered extinct about 250 BC, probably because of overharvesting. The reasons for the increasing scarcity of once-common plants are many and include the following:

- The variety of commercially available herbs has diminished since herbs were dropped from official pharmacopoeias, and unpopular herbs are unprotected in the environment—some even depend on human cultivation.
- The United States has no strong traditional medicine culture and relies on scientific discovery, which is slow paced and has popularized very few herbs.
- Laypeople and less experienced herbalists do not know enough to differentiate among the properties listed for various herbs; for instance, they automatically use echinacea as an "immune stimulant" when medicinal mushrooms may be more appropriate in some cases.
- Deforestation and urbanization lead to loss of habitat.
- Unsustainable agricultural practices leave the land unsuitable for natural recolonization.
- Export and trade of some endangered plants have increased.
- Current monitoring and regulation of illegal trade are inadequate.
- Lack of information and scientific support leads to a lack of interest in conservation.

Another reason for concern is that increasingly scarce medicinal herbs have been found adulterated in international trade. Table 18-1 provides a list of these plants (Gladstar, 2000).

The effect of biodiversity loss on local populations may well be incalculable. Schubert (1999) describes a visit to an area of India where poor families could no longer afford a traditional tonic, *Withania,* for their families. The local wild populations of this plant had all been harvested and sold to the United States and Australia.

WORLDWIDE ENDANGERED MEDICINAL PLANTS: THE CITES INDEX

CITES is an international pact, with 145 member countries, that endeavors to prevent international trade of species threatened with extinction (Box 18-1).

Endangered Medicinal Plants of Australia

In Australia, CITES policies are recommended and implemented through the Wildlife Protection (Regulation of Exports and Imports) Act of 1982. The Australian Environment Protection and Biodiversity Conservation Act of 1999 lists endangered plants, including some common medicinal plants or those used in native medicine. *Pandanus spiralis* var. *flammeus* is used in Bush medicine as a

TABLE 18-1

Plant Products That Are Commonly Adulterated

Plant in Trade	Common Adulterant
Black cohosh	Baneberry *(Actaea* spp*)*
Black haw	Striped maple *(Acer pensylvanicum)*
Echinacea	Prairie dock *(Parthenium integrifolium)*
Goldenseal	Oregon grape root
Prickly ash	Bristly sarsaparilla *(Aralia spinosa)*
Sheep sorrel	Yellow dock leaf
Siberian ginseng	*Periploca* or *Acanthopanax* spp
Skullcap	Germander
Slippery elm	Rice flour

BOX 18-1

Medicinal Plants Listed by International Conservation Agencies

CITES Appendix I (These Are Critically Endangered)
Saussaurea costus

CITES Appendix II
Rauwolfia serpentina
Panax ginseng
Panax quinquefolius
Cistanche deserticola
Hydrastis canadensis
Picrorrhiza kurroa
Guaiacum spp

TRAFFIC European Species of Concern
Adonis spp
Arctostaphylos uva-ursi
Arnica montana
Cetraria spp
Drosera spp
Gentiana spp
Glycyrrhiza glabra
Gypsophila spp
Menyanthes spp
Orchids
Paeonia spp
Primula spp
Ruscus spp
Sideritus spp
Thymus spp

CITES, Convention on International Trade in Endangered Species; TRAFFIC, Trade Records Analysis of Flora and Fauna in Commerce.

poultice for joint or muscle pain, as a gargle for toothache and sore mouth, topically for scabies, skin sores, boils, and so forth, and as drops for eye disorders (Devanesen, 2000). *Amyema scandens* is listed as endangered; this is a species of mistletoe that may have been used for coughs and colds. A number of *Eucalyptus* species, used for coughs, colds, dysentery, and wounds, are also listed. Various *Melaleuca* species have been used topically and for colds, fever, and sinus problems. *M. biconvexa, M. deanei*, and *M. kunzeoides* are considered vulnerable species, and *M. sciotostyla* is endangered.

Historically, customs seizures in Australia have netted many endangered plant species from other countries, including ginseng, cactus, orchid, and cycad, as well as parts from endangered animals such as tigers, rhinos, bears, leopards, turtles, and cobras (Trimmer, 1999).

US Endangered Herbs: United Plant Savers (UPS) "At Risk"

- **American ginseng** *(Panax quinquefolius)*
- **Black cohosh** *(Actaea [Cimicifuga] racemosa)*
- **Bloodroot** *(Sanguinaria canadensis)*
- **Blue cohosh** *(Caulophyllum thalictroides)*
- **Echinacea** *(Echinacea* spp*)*
- **Eyebright** *(Euphrasia* spp*)*
- **Goldenseal** *(Hydrastis canadensis)*
- **Helonias root** *(Chamaelirium luteum)*
- **Kava kava** *(Piper methysticum)* (Hawaii only)
- **Lady's slipper** *(Cypripedium* spp*)*
- **Lomatium** *(Lomatium dissectum)*
- **Osha** *(Ligusticum porteri,* L. spp*)*
- **Peyote** *(Lophophora williamsii)*
- **Slippery elm** *(Ulmus rubra)*
- **Sundew** *(Drosera* spp*)*
- **Trillium, beth root** *(Trillium* spp*)*
- **True unicorn** *(Aletris farinosa)*
- **Venus fly trap** *(Dionaea muscipula)*
- **Virginia snakeroot** *(Aristolochia serpentaria)*
- **Wild yam** *(Dioscorea villosa, D.* spp*)*

Key Endangered Medicinal Herbs and Their Stand-ins

The information below is derived primarily from two sources. Chemical constituent data are derived from Dr. Duke's Phytochemical database (http://www.ars-grin.gov/duke/), and traditional indications are quoted directly from *King's American Dispensatory,* (Felter, 1898).

Eyebright (Euphrasia officinalis)

Cultivation: Difficult to grow; a saprophyte with sensitive environmental requirements. Certain other species of *Euphrasia* are equally threatened.

Traditional uses: "Acute catarrhal diseases of the eyes, nose, and ears; fluent coryza with copious discharge of watery mucus." "Secretion of acrid mucus from eyes and nose with heat and pain in frontal sinus" (Felter, 1898).

Unique or predominant chemical constituents: Tannins, gallotannin, aucubin (an iridoid glycoside that has antibacterial and anti-inflammatory properties), phenolic caffeic and ferulic acids (which have a wide variety of activities, including anti-inflammatory).

Veterinary indications: Conjunctivitis.

Suggested substitutes: Ragweed *(Ambrosia* spp*)*, purple loosestrife *(Lythrum salicaria* L.*)*, tea *(Camellia sinensis)*, chamomile *(Matricaria recutita),* galbanum *(Ferula galbaniflua),* calendula *(Calendula officinalis),* sage, Chinese coptis, yarrow.

Goldenseal (Hydrastis canadensis)

Cultivation: CITES Appendix II. Only 34% of marketed goldenseal was derived from cultivated sources in 1999.

Traditional uses: Bitter digestive stimulant, stomatitis, gastric ulcers/gastritis, sludging of bile with jaundice, chronic constipation, diarrhea, hemorrhoids and anal/rectal irritations, pharyngitis/tonsillitis, conjunctivitis, blepharitis, purulent otitis media, otitis externa, uterine diseases such as endometritis and abnormal hemorrhage, cystitis, topically for many cutaneous disorders, chronic fevers.

Unique or predominant chemical constituents: A variety of alkaloids, including berberine, berberastine, hydrastine, canadine, corypalmine, including some not reported in other plants (meconine, xanthopucine, hydrastidine).

Veterinary indications: Stomatitis, pharyngitis, conjunctivitis, otitis, gastritis, metritis, topically for skin inflammation.

Suggested substitutes: Using sustainably grown goldenseal only is preferred. One company in the forefront of this movement is Frontier Cooperative (Brainard, Nebraska), which switched from 100% wildcrafted goldenseal to 100% cultivated organic in just 3 years.

- *Stomatitis:* Barberry species (*Berberis vulgaris* and possibly other *Berberis* spp), *Mahonia aquifolium* (itself on the "to watch" list), *Coptis chinensis, Anemopsis californica* (yerba mansa), pokeweed, myrrh.
- *Cutaneous disorders (topically): Anemopsis californica* (yerba mansa), *Echinacea* spp, tea tree oil, basil *(Ocimum gratissimum).*
- *Cystitis:* Hydrangea, barberry species (*Berberis vulgaris* and possibly other *Berberis* spp), *Mahonia aquifolium* (itself on the "to watch" list), *Coptis chinensis, Eryngium yuccifolium* (rattlesnake master).
- *Ophthalmic disorders:* Eucalyptus tea, barberry *(Berberis vulgaris).*
- *Uterine disorders:* Partridgeberry *(Mitchella repens), Echinacea* spp, black haw *(Viburnum prunifolium),* barberry species (*Berberis vulgaris* and possibly other *Berberis* spp), *Mahonia aquifolium* (itself on the "to watch" list), *Coptis chinensis, Anemopsis californica* (yerba mansa).
- *Gastritis:* Bayberry *(Myrica cerifera),* cranesbill, barberry species (*Berberis vulgaris* and possibly other *Berberis* spp), *Mahonia aquifolium* (itself on the "to watch" list), *Coptis chinensis, Anemopsis californica* (yerba mansa).
- *Ear disorders:* Mullein *(Verbascum thapsus),* witch hazel, barberry species (*Berberis vulgaris* and possibly other *Berberis* spp), *Mahonia aquifolium* (itself on the "to watch" list), *Coptis chinensis, Anemopsis californica.*

Kava kava (Piper methysticum)

Culture: Lacks a complete sexual reproductive system, so kava is usually propagated by cutting or layering. Probably a cultigen of *Piper wichmannii,* developed over 2000 to 3000 years by man.

Traditional uses: Calms the mind, stimulates imagination, relieves muscle and joint pain, relaxes muscles, topically for treatment of skin problems, dental pain, dysuria.

Unique or predominant chemical constituents: Unique resinoids such as kawain, methysticin, and yangonin have anesthetic and antispasmodic activities.

Veterinary indications: Anxiety, pain, feline lower urinary tract disease, seizure disorders.

Suggested substitutes: The plant may contain some of the active constituents, so aerial parts may be tried.

- **Pain:** *Corydalis* spp, *Cannabis sativa,* California poppy *(Eschscholzia californica),* passionflower, lobelia, wood betony *(Pedicularis canadensis),* boneset in some cases, as well as some of the toxic herbs such as henbane, gelsemium, and bryonia.
- **Anxiety:** Valerian, skullcap, passionflower, wood betony *(Pedicularis canadensis)*
- **Dysuria, feline lower urinary tract disease:** Saw palmetto, rattlesnake master, couch grass *(Agropyron repens* or *Elymus repens)*

Slippery elm (Ulmus rubra)

Culture: This tree is fairly common in the United States; however, population growth has slowed while the trade in slippery elm bark has increased substantially over the past 10 years. Frontier Herbs (Norway, Iowa) alone sells 11,000 lb yearly. When the bark is harvested properly, the tree is unharmed, but there is suspicion among conservationists that this is not occurring, and the tree is not in cultivation at this time. The bark should be harvested in vertical strips, leaving the vital cambium to transport nutrients to the tree extremities.

Traditional uses: The Eclectics used slippery elm for inflammation of the lungs, bowels, stomach, bladder, or kidneys. As a tea, it is used for coughs, sore throat, diarrhea, and, to a lesser extent, cystitis. A Native American use of note was as a topical agent for inflammatory and traumatic skin conditions.

Unique or predominant chemical constituents: Sugars and mucilage; a complex soluble carbohydrate that decreases intestinal transit time; decreases absorption of drugs, sugar, and other digestible contents of the gastrointestinal tract; binds lipids; and benefits indigenous bacterial populations.

Veterinary indications: Chronic diarrhea, including inflammatory bowel disease and colitis; pharyngitis, tracheobronchitis.

Suggested substitutes: Other elm species, including *Ulmus pumila* (Siberian elm), have been used in a similar manner. Marshmallow *(Althaea officinalis),* psyllium *(Plantago ovata),* fenugreek *(Trigonella foenum-graecum),* and okra also contain mucilage.

American ginseng (Panax quinquefolius) Korean ginseng, red ginseng (Panax ginseng)

Culture: Cultivated American ginseng is grown in covered buildings in deforested areas such as Wisconsin. However, the cultivated variety requires herbicides due to mold problems and is only worth a small fraction of the wild variety (Appalachian Ginseng Foundation Web site [see Resources]). Raising wild ginseng demands hardwood forest canopy, something not present in the deforested

Orient, where a closely related and equally valuable variety *(Panax ginseng)* grows and has been prized for thousands of years for the number of its cures.

Traditional uses: Traditional Chinese use of these varieties is slightly different, *P. ginseng* being a Qi tonic and *P. quinquefolius* being a yin tonic. *P. ginseng* tonifies Lung and Spleen, and *P. quinquefolius* is said to tonify Lung, Stomach, Kidney, and Heart. *P. quinquefolius* was used by many Native American tribes for various purposes, including "female health," and as a mental health tonic and a physical and sports tonic. The Eclectics called *P. quinquefolius* a mild tonic and stimulant, indicated for "Nervous dyspepsia; mental and other forms of nervous exhaustion from overwork."

Unique or predominant chemical constituents: The two different species of plants both contain certain unique saponins known as *ginsenosides,* in addition to polysaccharides, polyacetylenic alcohols, and unique sesquiterpenes.

Veterinary indications: Specific indications as Qi or Yin tonic in veterinary traditional Chinese medicine patterns; as an adaptogenic tonic for chronically ill or debilitated animals; to improve glycemic control and lower blood glucose in those with diabetes mellitus.

Suggested substitutes:

- Adaptogenic function: *Eleutherococcus senticosis* (Siberian ginseng), *Smilax* spp (sarsaparilla), *Rhodiola rosea, Astragalus* spp.
- Diabetes mellitus: *Gymnema sylvestre, Momordica charantia* (bitter melon), *Trigonella foenum-graecum* (fenugreek).

Picrorrhiza (Picrorrhiza kurroa)

Culture: Used in both Ayurvedic and traditional Chinese medicine. Often sold with (and not differentiated from) *Neopicrorrhiza scrophulariifolia*; the IUCN estimates that up to 80% of internationally traded picrorrhiza is actually neopicrorrhiza. Recent work on this herb has concentrated on identifying the actual amount exported.

Traditional uses: Indigestion, bitter tonic, constipation, periodic fever, liver problems, upper respiratory tract disorders, diarrhea, scorpion sting, and snakebite.

Unique or predominant chemical constituents: Unique constituents of this plant include kutkoside, kutkin and picrorrhizin, and glycosidic picrosides, as well as cucurbitacin glycosides.

Veterinary indications: Asthma, rheumatoid arthritis, gastrointestinal tract problems, hepatoprotection, immune modulator, vitiligo.

Suggested substitutes:

- Gastrointestinal tract disorders: Gentian *(Gentiana lutea)*, quassia *(Picraena excelsa)*, barberry *(Berberis vulgaris)*, wormwood *(Artemisia* spp*)*.
- Asthma: Coleus *(Plectranthus barbatus)*, petasites *(Petasites formosanus)*, lobelia (itself on the UPS threatened list), English ivy, Ma huang *(Ephedra sinica)*, tylophora *(Tylophora indica, T. asthmatica)*, boswellia *(Boswellia serrata)*.
- Rheumatoid arthritis: Boswellia *(Boswellia serrata)*, devil's claw *(Harpagophytum procumbens)*, turmeric *(Curcuma longa)*, meadowsweet *(Filipendula ulmaria)*.
- Hepatoprotection: Milk thistle *(Silybum marianum)*, phyllanthus *(Phyllanthus niruri)*, turmeric *(Curcuma longa)*.

Mu xiang, Kuth, Costus (Saussurea lappa [Decne], Aucklandia lappa, Aplotaxis lappa [Decne], Saussurea costus)

Culture: Saussurea costus is the only common medicinal herb listed in Appendix I (critically endangered) of the CITES Index. *S. costus* and *S. lappa* are two species that are used interchangeably by herbalists as the medicinal mu xiang. Yun mu xiang is grown in China, and guang mu xiang is grown in India and Burma. Chuan Mu Xiang is actually the root of *Vladimiria souliei,* which is produced in China and Tibet. United Kingdom Customs Service reports that *S. costus* is the most frequently found plant in seizures of medicines.

Traditional uses: Traditionally used in India as an aphrodisiac, tonic, stimulant, and antiseptic. It is used in bronchitis, asthma, cough, cholera, and as a stimulant diuretic and a perfumery ingredient. In traditional Chinese medicine formulas as a *Qi* mover for gastrointestinal problems, it enters the Spleen, Stomach, Large Intestine, Gallbladder, and Triple Heater channels. This herb is included in the following common traditional Chinese medicine formulas: *Sha Xiang Liu Jun Zi, Shao Yao Tang, Shen Su Yin, Gui Pi Tang, Ju He Wan, Mu Xiang Bing Lang Wan, Shi Pi Yin, Shu Gan Wan,* and many patent formulas including Curing Pills. Acrid, sweet, and bitter; it is, in Western terms, carminative, emmenagogue, and antiseptic; used for swelling and fullness of stomach, irregular menses, pulmonary disorders, difficulty in swallowing, and wasting of muscle tissues. A modern study in humans shows that the herb reduces the frequency of angina.

Unique or predominant chemical constituents: This is a plant that is full of essential oils and inulin, which may be found in other plants, but it also has unique constituents that are not well investigated. Saussurine has antispasmodic activity. Some of the lactone fractions and delactonized oil exhibit hypotensive, antispasmodic, bronchodilating, and diuretic activities.

Veterinary indications: Gastroenteritis, gastrointestinal parasites, bronchitis, and asthma.

Suggested substitutes:

- GI upset, gastroenteritis: Elecampane *(Inula helenium)*, *Vladimiria souliei*, ginger, *Pogostemon patchouli*, boswellia, *Xiang Fu Zi (Cyperus rotundus)*
- Bronchitis/asthma: Elecampane, lobelia, boswellia.

Devil's claw (Harpagophytum procumbens)

Culture: Has been proposed for CITES Appendix II listing; although it has not yet made the list, it is believed to be threatened. African nations that produce the plant have resisted adding devil's claw to the CITES listing because it was believed that this would have a negative impact on local farmers of the product.

Traditional Uses: Southern Africans used this plant for digestive complaints and rheumatic pain. Studies show that it is anti-inflammatory, analgesic, and antioxidant, and that is effective in the treatment of patients with arthritis. It is used as a digestive bitter and has been shown to stimulate hepatic detoxification processes.

Unique chemical constituents: Iridoid glycosides, including harpagoside, procumbine, and harpagide, are anti-inflammatory and analgesic, and some have cardiovascular effects.

Veterinary indications: Arthritis, mild gastroenteritis (for short-term use), hepatic.

Suggested substitutes: Figwort *(Scrophularia nodosa),* meadowsweet *(Filipendula ulmaria),* willow *(Salix alba).*

See Table 18-2 for a list of other at-risk herbs and potential substitutes.

ZOOTHERAPY

The ethical considerations in zootherapy are twofold: One is whether we should endanger the survival of rare species by continuing to sacrifice them for our medicines when little proof of efficacy exists; the other is whether it is ethical to use sentient beings for the good of other sentient beings, whether as food, medicine, or clothing.

The Veterinary Botanical Medicine Association (VBMA) Working Group addressed the following concerns:

- What role should personal ethics (such as vegan lifestyle practices or cultural indoctrination into

TABLE 18-2

Other At-Risk Herbs and Potential Substitutes*

At-Risk Herbs	Substitutes
Arnica	Yerba del lobo *(Helenium hoopesii),* calendula, comfrey (musculoskeletal disorders), yarrow (bruising)
Black cohosh	Yucca (musculoskeletal problems), skullcap (headaches, mood swings, anxiety), pulsatilla, motherwort
Bloodroot	Celandine. For respiratory, dermatologic, and antibacterial uses, try rosemary
Blue cohosh	Motherwort
Calamus root	Centaury *(Centaurium* spp*),* wormwood, blue vervain. For carminative and antispasmodic effects, use dill and fennel
Cascara sagrada	Cultivated turkey rhubarb, buckthorn (and possibly other *Rhamnus* spp), possibly Japanese knotweed *(Polygonum cuspidatum)*
Echinacea	For antibacterial, antiviral, antifungal, and immune stimulating effects, spilanthes. Thyme and burdock also have some antibacterial effects
Goldthread	Barberry
Helonias, false unicorn *(Chamaelirium luteum)*	Motherwort
Lady's slipper	Valerian, cultivated California poppy, cultivated passionflower, lemon balm for antispasmodic and nervine properties; skullcap for antispasmodic, nervine, sedative, and anodyne actions
Lobelia	Thyme, hyssop
Lomatium	Cultivated echinacea, arborvitae *(Thuja occidentalis),* Saint John's Wort, lovage, angelica, and rosemary for respiratory problems and for antiseptic, diaphoretic, and antibacterial properties
Oregon grape	Dandelion, yellow dock, barberry
Osha	Thyme, elecampane, marshmallow, lovage, angelica, rosemary
Partridgeberry	Motherwort, catnip, raspberry, peppermint
Pipsissewa	Uva ursi, goldenrod, gravel root
Pleurisy root, asclepias	Elecampane
Slippery elm	Marshmallow, comfrey, mullein
Spikenard	Cultivated ginsengs, Siberian ginseng. For skin conditions, cleavers and chickweed
Stoneroot	European horse chestnut, red clover, sweet clover, garlic, parsley root
Sundew	Cultivated echinacea, mullein, elecampane. Spilanthes for respiratory conditions and for antimicrobial action. Sage for sore thoughts and antimicrobial activity. Thyme for antimicrobial and antifungal activities
Trillium	Raspberry leaf, motherwort, shepherd's purse
Venus fly trap	Echinacea, red clover
Virginia snakeroot	Blessed thistle, burdock. Yucca for joint problems. Dill, fennel, and ginger for digestive problems. Cultivated echinacea for snake/insect bites and poison ingestion
White sage	Garden sage *(Salvia officinalis),* sagebrush *(Artemisia tridentate),* mugwort *(Artemisia vulgaris)*
Wild indigo	Boneset, cultivated echinacea, spilanthes
Wild yam (American)	Chamomile, licorice, catnip, peppermint
Yerba mansa	Tormentil, self-heal
Yerba santa	Pine, elecampane, thyme, sage, grindelia

*From Gladstar, 2000.

widespread use of animals) play in the discussion of zootherapy?

- What methods do we use to determine which animals are sufficiently endangered to justify proscribing their use?
- What is the extent of tradition that makes "traditional use" an acceptable benchmark?
- How do we decide that a zootherapeutic product provides a unique pharmacologic effect as opposed to a nutritional effect that could be provided by other animal parts or herbs?
- In the presence of ethical or conservation concerns, what level of scientific evidence justifies use of an animal product in the natural product pharmacopoeia?

The VBMA white paper is available on the website (www.vbma.org). Initial conclusions may be read there. Endangered animal species and their products that should always be avoided include the following:

- Tiger
- Rhinoceros
- Pangolin
- Sea horse
- Chinese soft-shelled turtle
- Brown bear, Asiatic black bear

PROBLEMS TO SOLVE

We face multiple obstacles in establishing conservation programs for medicinal herbs. Herbalists, for instance, may be resistant to using cultivated crops because they are chemically different from wildcrafted plants. Wildcrafting (even "sustainable" wildcrafting) has historically been a job for some of the poorest local populations, and although some of these people depend on wildcrafting as a source of income, economic pressures have broken through attempts to preserve threatened plant populations. Educating local populations on the advantages of growing rather than wildcrafting herbs involves time and expense, but some cultural revival and charitable groups are working on sustainable community development initiatives (such as silviculture of crops) all over the world. Concerned herbalists have noted that clinical studies on herbs have driven the use of threatened herbs before conservationists could prepare for the increased trade. These authors have suggested that studies on threatened herbs should begin by investigating sustainable culture methods before focusing on clinical effects.

STRATEGIES FOR RESOLUTION

On a personal level, we can all be responsible consumers. It is good to know which plants are highly endangered and to be familiar with those that are threatened. Consumers and practitioners who purchase herbs should know the policies of their herb pharmacies well and should read labels on individual products purchased over the counter. Concerned herbalists may act globally by joining conservation or environmental groups, and locally by patronizing local growers and nurseries. When it is possible to grow threatened herbs locally, the herbalist may reduce his or her impact on the trade for that herb by using a different, less sensitive species or genus.

Although it is important to experiment with alternative medicinal plants when a threatened plant seems indicated, herbalists should know that popular substitutes are not chemically identical. Also, different species within a genus may have widely different properties, and we cannot expect to automatically find substitutes within a genus. Some herbalists are using different parts of a plant and are getting satisfactory results. For instance, the aerial parts of goldenseal contain more berberine than is found in the roots, and harvesting leaves does not kill the plant. Others are using echinacea seed and aerial parts as opposed to the root. Clinical experimentation must continue, so the best substitutes for disappearing medicinal plants can be discovered.

Groups such as Rural Action, Heifer International, the Appalachian Ginseng Foundation, and Slow Food International empower disenfranchised communities to grow their own crops and become good stewards of the land. Herbs may be grown in intensive monocultures, which decrease surrounding biodiversity and deplete the land, or growers may slowly wait for natural regeneration. Sustainable agriculture utilizes semi-intensive production, which involves multiple crops in a natural habitat. Indigenous people can make a living by selling herbs grown in a sustainable manner, so that their crops are assured for many years. They may then process those herbs for export with the use of cooperative structures. Co-ops may provide opportunities for research and education that benefit scientists and consumers worldwide. For example, the Appalachian Ginseng Foundation (AGF) has assisted its members in growing "virtually wild" ginseng, while saving the forest cover that is required to grow it. In addition, the AGF has developed ways to help market this ginseng to attain the best prices and to prevent illegal poaching of wild ginseng. The US Forestry Service has actually implanted microchips in ginseng plants to prevent poaching. Aveda, which is an Estee Lauder subsidiary, has hired Native American communities to plant new areas of sage and cedar for use in their products. At Rutgers University, one program has been developed to teach Madagascar farmers about overharvesting. In Pennsylvania, children in a Waldorf School are collaborating with Tis Mal Crow, a Native American herbalist, to plant and manage a 2-acre medicinal and aromatic garden.

According to Peter Purbrick of Mediherb (1999), Australian growers could potentially produce many threatened herbs, including butterfly weed, blue cohosh, black cohosh, wild yam, eyebright, goldenseal, uva ursi, arnica, helonias, cascara sagrada, trillium, aletris, baptisia, osha, lomatium, bloodroot, stillingia, and gentian. Growers already produce popular herbs that were formerly bought from their native countries, including echinacea, celandine, meadowsweet, passionflower, rue, valerian, and thyme. Consumers should be encouraged to purchase locally grown herbs for both economic and practical reasons—these herbs are likely to be fresher as well. Australian sourced plant extracts are also supported by the Australian Government Rural Industries Research and Development Corporation.

HOW TO FIND THE ENDANGERED PLANTS IN YOUR AREA

Local botanical gardens often emphasize local endangered species and are involved in efforts to conserve them. County extension offices, state departments of agriculture, and university horticulture departments may also be sources of information about endangered plants. Rosemary Gladstar's wonderful book, *Planting the Future: Saving Our Medicinal Herbs*, provides an extensive listing of botanical sanctuaries and seed and plant suppliers.

SUMMARY

It is good to remember that even if we find substitutes for these endangered plants, the indigenous populations that depend on them may not have the same resources. Although the richest countries in the world are responsible for the growth in herb trade, 70% to 80% of the world's population depends on plant medicine for its primary medical needs, and this need is driven largely by the poorest countries. We need to reevaluate our needs and our sources for their commitment to sustainable culture.

ACKNOWLEDGMENT

Special thanks to Andrew Pengelly for his assistance in preparing this manuscript.

References

Devanesen DAM. Traditional aboriginal medicine practice in the Northern Territory. Proceedings of the International Symposium on Traditional Medicine, World Health Organization; September 11–13, 2000; Awaji Island, Japan.

Felter HW, Lloyd JU. King's American Dispensatory, 1898. Available at http://www.henriettesherbal.com/eclectic/kings/index.html (Henriette Kress's Herbal Homepage), accessed January 30, 2006.

Gladstar R, Hirsch P, eds. *Planting the Future: Saving Our Medicinal Herbs*. Rochester, Vt: Healing Arts Press; 2000.

Ridgeway-Bissett C. Traditional medicine: environmental and resource management—an indigenous perspective. Medicinal Plants for the Future: Sustainability and Ethical Issues Conference (addressing perceived threats to the future supply of plant material for medicinal use); August 13–24, 1999; Byron Bay, NSW, Australia.

Schippmann, U.; Leaman, D.J. And Cunningham, A.B. Impact of Cultivation and Gathering of medicinal plants on Biodiversity: Global Trends and Issues. In: *Biodiversity and the Ecosystem Approach in Agriculture, Forestry and Fisheries*. FAO, 2002, 1-21.Available online at: http://www.fao.org/documents/show_cdr.asp?url_file=/DOCREP/005/AA010E/AA010E00.HTM

Schubert M. Stakeholders in the herbal renaissance in Australia. Medicinal Plants for the Future: Sustainability and Ethical Issues Conference (addressing perceived threats to the future supply of plant material for medicinal use); August 13–14, 1999; Byron Bay, NSW, Australia.

Trimmer M. The Wildlife Protection Act and medicinal plants. Medicinal Plants for the Future: Sustainability and Ethical Issues Conference (addressing perceived threats to the future supply of plant material for medicinal use); August 13–14, 1999; Byron Bay, NSW, Australia.

Vorhies F. The global dimension of threatened medicinal plants from a conservation point of view. In Medicinal utilization of wild species: challenge for man and nature in the new millennium. Honnef S, and Melisch R, Eds. Pp 26–29. WWF Germany/TRAFFIC Europe-Germany, EXPO 2000, Hannover, Germany.

Resources

Appalachian Ginseng Foundation: http://www.a-spi.org/AGF/

Australian Environment Protection and Biodiversity Conservation Act 1999: list of endangered species: http://www.deh.gov.au/cgi-bin/sprat/public/publicthreatenedlist.pl?wanted=flora

Australian Government Rural Industries Research and Development Corporation: http://www.rirdc.gov.au/programs/eop.html

Australian Network for Plant Conservation: http://www.anbg.gov.au/anpc/

Convention on International Trade of Endangered Species of Wild Fauna and Flora: http://www.cites.org

National Center for the Preservation of Medicinal Plants: http://home.frognet.net/~rural8/frames2.html

National Park Service Medicinal Plant Working Group: http://www.nps.gov/plants/medicinal/plants.htm

Rural Action: http://www.ruralaction.org

TRAFFIC: http://www.traffic.org

United Plant Savers: http://www.unitedplantsavers.org

PART IV

Veterinary Clinical Uses of Medicinal Plants

Approaches in Veterinary Herbal Medicine Prescribing

CHAPTER

Barbara J. Fougère

There is no one correct system of prescribing. Ten herbalists can prescribe different formulas and still achieve success in treating a patient. This chapter outlines the theories behind prescribing and introduces approaches to herbal prescribing that are useful in practice.

HERBAL PRESCRIBING DIFFERS FROM ORTHODOX MEDICINE

One of the key features of traditional systems of medicine that differentiates it from orthodox or conventional medicine is the method of matching a particular treatment to the constitution and auxiliary needs of the individual patient, rather than treating on the basis of a single diagnosis per se. This is particularly true for chronic or recurrent disease. Although conventional medicine plays a very important role in disease diagnosis and management and is well suited to acute conditions, the current limitations of modern medicine suggest that herbal medicine may have potential for more comprehensive treatment of patients with chronic disease.

Practitioners of conventional medicine are interested in the patient's diet, lifestyle, and potential contributing factors and attempt to address them; however, chronic disease remains a dilemma for most practitioners. Herbalists believe that part of this problem lies in the convention of prescribing identical treatments to individuals with the same diagnosis. Herbal medicine emphasizes accompanying conditions and predisposing or underlying causes of disease in every prescription. In general, more time is taken in understanding the individual patient and his or her lifestyle, diet, and seemingly unrelated signs. Although three patients may all have "osteoarthritis," for example, each may have a different set of signs. One patient may have severe pain on rising that improves with exercise (a cold lameness) but may also have chronic loose stools. Another may feel worse in humid weather, and yet another may feel worse after eating particular foods.

Herbalists are interested in the patient's unique signs as much as they are in the diagnosis. The unique features of an individual's condition give us clues as to predisposing factors and possibly related system dysfunction. This picture can provide clues about the vitality and constitution of the patient. What underlying factors can we reduce or remove to improve vitality and normal body functioning? The point of this comprehensive approach to patient signs is that it can direct us to the selection of herbs for an individualized formula to restore health. By its very nature, herbalism is vitalistic and holistic in its approach.

Another dilemma in orthodox medicine is the nature of the medicines used to treat patients with chronic disease. The conventional pharmacopoeia consists of a large number of drugs from a limited range of classes. Herbs, by contrast, can be targeted to supply vitamins and minerals that can enhance nutrition simultaneously, while pharmacologically active phytochemicals promote specific eliminative functions in the body, modulate multiple body systems and cellular functions, and enhance physiologic function when needed. The vast array of herbs and synergistic permutations of formulas offers much greater selection for the treatment of patients with chronic disease.

In using herbal medicine to treat those with chronic disease, herbalists assess the vital reserves of the patient. Many practitioners attempt to "detoxify" the body (i.e., enhance urinary, gastrointestinal, and skin elimination, along with liver detoxification activity). If the patient is extremely debilitated, a slower approach with the use of low doses, gentle herbs, and tonics may be necessary. Modern medicine does not usually modify treatment protocols on the basis of vitality, except by modifying dose rates, but the longer-term strategy of detoxification and physiologic support may provide better outcomes than are noted with the use of drugs alone. Herbal medicine practitioners may take into account less observable, but just as important, factors in the perpetuation of chronic disease.

When predisposing or perpetuating factors cannot be changed, herbal medicine may also be effective in the treatment of patients with chronic disease as an alternative or complementary medicine to long-term drug treatment. Herbs can be used when a conventional drug may be undesirable, to lower the dose of conventional drugs, or to reduce the adverse effects caused by conventional drugs.

TRADITIONAL APPROACHES TO PRESCRIBING

Traditional systems of herbal medicine consistently emphasize the importance of (1) maintenance of good health, (2) the nature of interrelationships between the individual and the environment, seasons, foods, and emotions, and (3) the healing process itself. Traditional Chinese medicine and Ayruvedic medicine both apply sophisticated approaches to medicine, and it is sometimes thought that Western herbal medicine lacks this philosophical sense of integration because it largely focuses on the *Materia medica* and on knowing which herbs work best for which condition. However, an underlying philosophy forms the basis of Western herbal medicine today. Western herbal medicine philosophy is derived from Greek humoral theory and the physiomedicalism of the Anglo-European–North American pioneers, and it continually incorporates pieces of other traditions as well as the evolving scientific literature. Although they are not always elucidated in the herbal literature, these influences are seen in most herbal prescriptions, which take into account the diagnosis, constitution, and energetics of patients while matching them to appropriate plant medicines.

Traditional Diagnosis

Elements of the human environment were seen as a reflection of the underlying belief that the microcosm mirrors the macrocosm—the interrelatedness of all things (Moore). For example, the impact of the "elements" on the patient was considered. In contemporary veterinary herbal medicine, it is no surprise that in summer, when the weather is hot and humid, dogs are prone to "hot spots," and in winter, dogs suffer more Bi syndrome, or an invasion of "cold" into their arthritic joints. Energetics diagnosis was both literal and metaphoric and was useful in prescribing. Heat experienced by the patient, or "hot" signs, would be balanced by "cooling" herbs. (See Chapter 13 on Chinese medicine for a more detailed explanation of the traditional Chinese approach to energetics of herbal medicine.

In the traditions of herbal medicine and in the absence of technology, use of the five senses—sight, sound, taste, feel, and listening—led to identification of patterns that formed the basis of treatment. Observation of symptoms and signs helped the practitioner to define the patient's constitution and his or her "vitality" or energy strength.

Diagnosis from a Western perspective is useful, but traditional physical diagnosis can also provide helpful information. For example, 10 dogs may have the Western diagnosis of inflammatory bowel disease, yet they may all be prescribed different herbal formulas. One patient may be chilly (seeks warm resting places, avoids drafty places, sleeps under the covers) and need warming herbs; another may be hot (rests on tile and near air vents, exhibits thirst), requiring cooling herbs. These herbs may demonstrate similar gastrointestinal actions of reducing gastrointestinal tract inflammation, although different mechanisms of action or different auxiliary effects may be at work. So although contemporary veterinary herbalists have the benefit of technology, a diagnosis, and even a scientific basis for the actions of herbs, the traditions remind us to use this information in the context of the much bigger picture of the individual patient. When the variables in the case are taken into account, rather than the similarities, the herbal formula can be tailored to meet individual needs.

In exploring this further, a review of traditional concepts helps to demonstrate why this has importance in prescribing today.

Traditional Concepts

Western herbal medicine today has evolved from the Chinese, Ayruvedic, Indian, and Greco-Roman cultures that developed with descriptions of similar systems for explaining human physiology. At the heart of them was and is an understanding of the Vital Force—the concordances of the elements and the interrelationships of all things.

The "Vital" Force

Vitalism has provided the foundation for medical thinking since the times of Hippocrates and Galen. The premise of Vitalism considers that living processes are animated by the Vital Force, which starts flowing at the moment of conception and ceases with death. This flow of vital energy in the body nourishes, heals, develops, and sustains the body. The flow of Vital Force is linked with the emotional experience of the being, wherein emotions have a direct effect on the body's physiologic function and thoughts affect emotion. Thus, Vitalism embraces the interrelationships of mental, emotional, and physical experience; and holistic thinking about the human (and animal) body has served as the basis for almost all traditional systems of medicine (Holmes 1997).

How is Vitalism relevant to modern-day prescribing? Whether or not the Vital Force exists from a scientific perspective, the relative "vitality" of the patient is important in prescribing. Extremely debilitated patients should be prescribed a different formula than would be given to a robust animal with strong vitality, even though they may have the same diagnosis. An example may be seen in the treatment of constipation in a debilitated 15-year-old dog that might be treated with a formula containing butternut, a gentle laxative, versus a 5-year-old robust dog that might be given cascara (a stronger laxative) in the formula instead.

"Thus, this view of the pathology of disease does not militate against our cardinal principle, 'that disease is an impairment of vitality'" (Scudder, 1874).

The Full Circle—Science and Tradition

Although science has become disconnected from Elemental theory, it is beginning to reexplore interrelationships through the science of ecology—the study of the relationships of living things to their environment and to other species. Ecology breathes new life into Elemental knowledge, but now, the Elements are called "ecological factors" and include light, heat, moisture, soil, and wind.

Guises of Vitalism and Elemental Knowledge still appear in Chinese, Indian (Ayurvedic), and Arabic traditional medicine today.

Traditional Chinese medicine

Traditional Chinese medicine (TCM) is based on the theories of Yin-Yang and the Five Elements, which have arisen from ancient Chinese observations of nature's cycles and changes (Figure 19-1). These theories held that wood, fire, earth, metal, and water are the basic substances constituting the material world. These five basic substances were considered an indispensable part of daily life. Each of these elements represents a category of related functions (concordances) and qualities pertaining to direction, season, climatic conditions, color, taste, smell, yin and yang organs, body opening, body tissue, emotion, and human sound.

Traditional Chinese Herbal Medicine Prescribing: In traditional Chinese medicine, the armamentarium against disease uses dietary therapy, exercise, meditation, massage, and acupuncture. Herbs are prescribed when dietary changes, meditation, and massage no longer address the disease condition. Herbs are combined into formulas to maximize additive and synergistic effects, and to minimize adverse effects.

Formulas are composed according to a traditional hierarchy. This arrangement is similar to the Chinese Imperial Court with a Principal (Emperor), Deputy, Envoy, and Assistants. Any herb can fill any of these roles. Which role is filled depends on which herbal formula includes the particular herb.

- The Chief or Emperor has the major therapeutic effect and is indispensable to the formula; it has the greatest effect on the primary pattern of the disease or syndrome.
- The Deputy or Minister is synergistic or additive to the chief herb and may have an effect on a coexisting condition, perhaps directed toward any secondary disease pattern. In modern scientific terms, this herb may also be directed toward the primary syndrome but with a different mechanism of action.
- Assistants help in making the formula more acceptable to the patient; they moderate the strength of the main herbs to guide the therapeutic outcome and can reinforce the main herb or treat a lesser symptom. They can also change the overall energy of the formula.
- Envoy Herbs or Guides make the formula easier to dispense or use; they usually focus the action of the formula and harmonize the actions of other ingredients. They can also direct the formula to particular organs or meridians. An example commonly used is licorice root.

The formula *Si Jun Zi Tang*, also called Four Gentlemen Tea, exemplifies these roles. It is prescribed for *Qi* deficiency. The Chief or Emperor is Ren Shen (ginseng), which tonifies source *Qi*, tonifies Lung and Spleen *Qi*, and generates fluids and slightly tonifies Heart *Qi*.

The Minister herb is bai zhu (white atractylodes). It tonifies Spleen *Qi* and resolves Damp. The assistant herb is fu ling (poria); it helps to drain Damp and tonify the

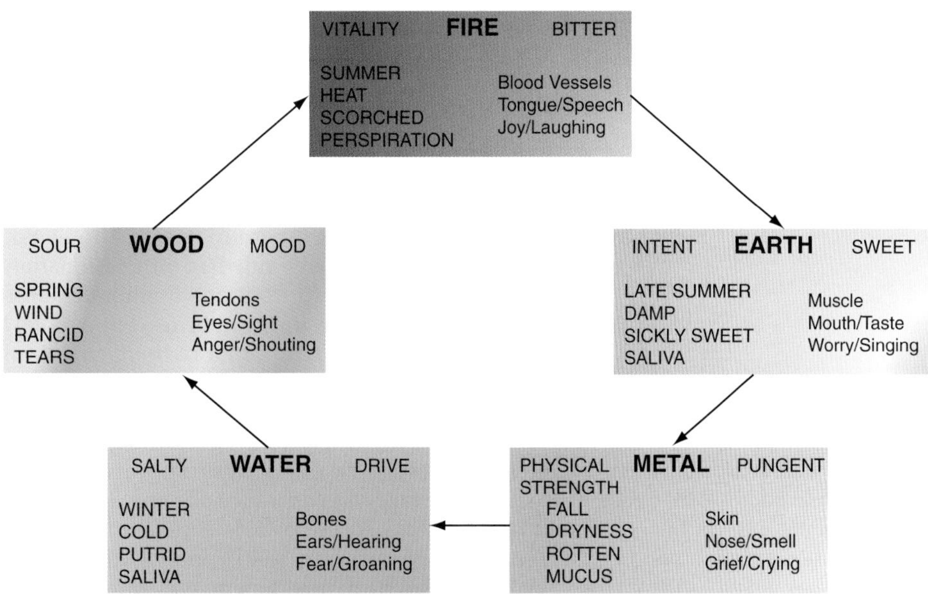

Figure 19-1 Five element concordances.

Spleen, helps resolve phlegm, and calms the Heart and the Shen. The Guide herb is Gan Cao (licorice), which harmonizes the herbal formula (reducing potential adverse effects) and guides the formula through all 12 main channels; it also tonifies the Spleen, Heart *Qi*, and Lung *Qi* and moderates the actions of the other herbs.

This basic TCM approach to herbal prescribing can be helpful to consider when one is formulating with Western herbs too. Most formulas contain four or more herbs. The reasons for this are that herbs can be used synergistically to strengthen the effects of the formula, as well as to deal with some of the secondary aspects of the patient. Herbs can also be added to balance the formula, thereby preventing adverse effects. The Emperor can be the main herb; for an animal that is debilitated and lethargic with inflammatory bowel disease, this herb might be *Withania somnifera*—an adaptogen, tonic, anti-inflammatory, and nervine sedative that assists with debility and convalescence. It is appropriate for chronic inflammatory disease associated with stress. The Minister might be a digestive strengthening herb such as *Chamomilla recutita* (chamomile), a carminative, anti-inflammatory, bitter tonic, spasmolytic, antiallergic, and cholagogue that is ideal for inflammation of the gastrointestinal tract and food intolerance. The Assistant might be Marshmallow *(Althaea officinalis)*, a demulcent and vulnery that is ideal for colitis. The harmonizing Guide might be licorice, which would improve the taste of the formula for the patient but would also provide some gastrointestinal anti-inflammatory effect. The formula might look like this:

Withania somnifera	40%
Chamomilla recutita	30%
Althaea officinalis	20%
Glycyrrhiza glabra	10%

Ayurveda: Ayurveda identifies three basic types of energy (called *doshas*) that are present in everybody and everything; these are *Vata*, *Pitta*, and *Kapha*. These *doshas* are in turn related to the elements of Air, Fire, Water, and Earth (*Vata*-Air, *Pitta*-Fire and Water, *Kapha*-Water and Earth). All people and animals have *Vata*, *Pitta*, and *Kapha*, but one is usually primary, one secondary, and the third least prominent. *Vata* is the energy of movement, *Pitta* the energy of digestion or metabolism, and *Kapha* the energy of lubrication and structure. The cause of disease in Ayurveda is viewed as the lack of proper cellular function because of an excess or deficiency of *Vata*, *Pitta*, or *Kapha*, or the presence of toxins. As with the humoral theory, balance and health are maintained through a variety of lifestyle, diet, and medicinal interventions. (See Chapter 6 for more information.)

Humoral theory

Humoral theory (originally developed by Hippocrates) describes the concept that a balance of qualities exists within a patient that include his or her fundamental nature, physical characteristics, behavior, and physiology.

The four humors are perceived within the blood through each of the four Elements in turn (Figure 19-2):

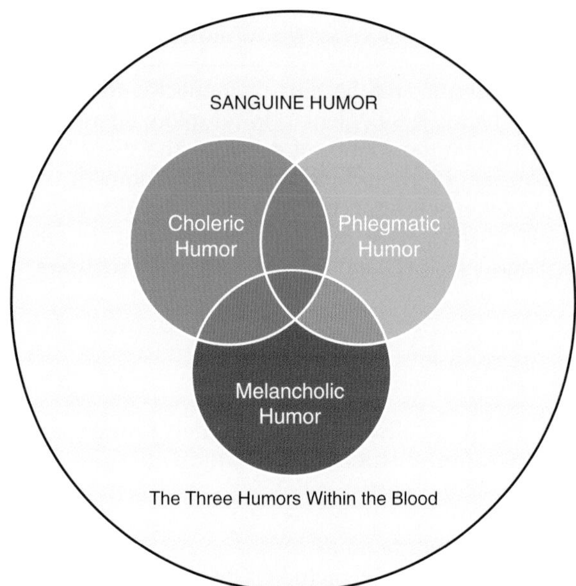

Figure 19-2 The sanguine humor (blood) containing the choleric, melancholic, and phlegmatic humors.

- Melancholic humor (Gk. *melanchole* = black bile) corresponds to Earth.
- Phlegmatic humor (Gk. *phlegma* = phlegm) corresponds to Water.
- Choleric humor (Gk. *chole* = bile) corresponds to Fire.
- Sanguine humor (L. *sanguineus* = bloody) corresponds to Air.

Samuel Thomson (1769–1843) developed a system of practice that recalled elements of this theory. He thought that all diseases are brought about by a decrease or change in vital fluids—the humors—"either by taking cold or the loss of animal warmth." He saw health as a balance within the body of four elements—earth, air, fire, and water. Accumulated wastes led to obstruction, lessening heat in the body and resulting in disease. With diffusion of heat throughout the body, the obstruction could be removed. Thomson saw fever and sweating as natural responses of the body designed to eliminate wastes via the skin. It was therefore logical to conclude that diaphoretics such as Capsicum would aid sweating during fever, thus assisting the innate healing power of the body (Griggs 1997).

Humor and Temperament: Each humor has its own temperament in terms of hot, cold, wet, and dry and is traditionally ruled by different planets. The humors can be explained from both symbolic and biochemical viewpoints, and they can be used to parallel biochemical medicine. The symbolism of the Elements also helps to reveal the nature of the humors (Table 19-1).

The particular humoral composition of a patient was called *temperament*, from the Latin *temperare*, meaning "to mingle or mix in due proportion." When the person was healthy, the balance or temper of the humors allowed the Vital Force to flow easily; this was accompanied by an inner clarity, peace, and harmony.

The temperament was often used as a starting point for evaluating health and disease and would serve as the

TABLE 19-1

Humoral Relationships

	Melancholy	Sanguine	Choleretic	Phlegmatic
Element	Earth	Air	Fire	Water
Temperature	Chilly, dry	Hot, moist	Hot, dry	Cold, moist
Coat	Rough, thin or alopecic	Smooth, soft	Rough, dry	Smooth, thin or alopecic
Build	Slender	Solid	Lean	Fat
Pulse	Slow	Full	Strong	Weak, low
Appetite	Good	Good, fast eater	Strong	Weak
Urine	Pale	Yellow	Yellow	Pale
Behavior	Fearful, timid	Hyperactive, sociable	Aggressive	Apathetic, anxious
Breed Example	Whippet	Border collie	Australian Cattle dog	Cavalier King Charles spaniel

basis of herbal prescribing. To determine temperament, herbalists would assess the color and shape of the body, as well as habits, personality, temperature, pulse, colors, odors, and consistency of excretions. For a representation of this in veterinary terms, see Table 19-1.

In disease, the harmonious temper is lost. When a particular humor dominates, this causes a characteristic "distemper." The humor was identified by the symptoms produced, whether they were hot or cold, dry or moist. The common cold is classically a phlegmatic condition—a cold and moist disease. The therapeutic objective was to counteract the predominating humor and restore temper. For example, a fever is a hot and dry condition. It can be visualized as a fire burning within the patient—pyrexia, coming from the Greek *pyr*, meaning "fire." The rise in body temperature and dehydration through perspiration illustrates its hot and dry nature. To counteract this fiery choleric condition, medicines of a cooling, moistening, and watery nature are needed—like willow (*Salix alba*).

In humoral terms, willow has an affinity with the cold, moist phlegmatic humor in the body. This is opposite to the hot and dry choleric humor, hence its particular reputation for treating fevers. It is interesting to note that willow is a source of salicylates that are used to treat fever—the fire of the fever is extinguished, restoring balance to the humors so that health returns.

The principles upon which humoral physiology are based are thus highly relevant to the perceptive skill of an herbalist. Even if the exact pathology is not known, we can use the energetic, elemental principles to guide us. If the patient is hot, one should use cooling herbs; if dry, moistening herbs should be used. There is no reason why humoral ideas cannot be juxtaposed alongside biochemical ideas. The potential benefit of using both is great.

Physiomedicalism

Physiomedicalism arose in the United States in the mid 19th century and became the primary basis for education of herbalists in England in the 20th century. The objective of physiomedicalism was to restore vitality and return the body's function to normal. Physiomedicalists delineated some fundamental therapeutic principles, including the promotion of elimination, the restoration of circulation, and the balance between the sympathetic and parasympathetic nervous system, as well as restoration of tissue function.

Physiomedical prescribing is directed toward resolving the underlying cause of a condition, thereby relieving symptoms without compromising the integrity of the Vital Force. The goals of treatment are to increase the vital capacity of the body, restore homeostasis, and eliminate obstructive conditions. These principles aid us in formulating and indicate the importance of including herbs that are specific to the actual condition, and that support weakened organ systems, ensure the proper function of eliminative organs, and support both the cardiovascular and nervous systems.

Modern physiomedical prescribing

Physiomedical concepts have evolved into a step-by-step process for developing a formula. This method has been described by Bone and allows the herbalist to set treatment goals, prescribe efficiently, and monitor the progress of patients (Mills 2000, Bone, 1994, 1996). It is especially useful in treating patients who present with a wide range of clinical signs and symptoms. The basic principle is to write balanced prescriptions by setting short-term and long-term goals that are appropriate for the individual patient.

The steps involved in physiomedical prescribing are described in the following sections.

Physiologic Enhancement: This step takes into account the constitutional state of the patient. The aim is to create a state of robust vitality, so the approach takes into consideration diet, exercise, and environment. Body chemistry can be optimized by improving nutrition and enhancing detoxification. This usually requires attention to the digestive system. Bitters, cholagogues, and hepatorestoratives for the liver, depuratives (alteratives), and sometimes laxatives are employed.

Body energy is also optimized, which can be accomplished through the use of tonics and adaptogens, which improve energy level and enhance the ability to cope with stress, thereby helping to conserve vitality. This may also require the enhancement of specific organs like the kidneys or adrenals.

Physiologic processes are enhanced through regulation or enhancement of digestive function, immunity, circulation, respiratory function, and function of the liver, kidneys, and so forth. Specific tissues are targeted, such as the exocrine pancreas, or functions may be enhanced, like bile secretion from the liver. Detoxification can be achieved both by stimulating detoxification processes with depuratives, and liver herbs and by facilitating elimination with diuretics, lymphatics, laxatives, and expectorants.

Physiologic Compensation: Sometimes an overstimulated function must be controlled directly, deficiencies must be compensated for, or the patient needs relief from symptoms. Depending on treatment goals, herbs are chosen for the patient on the basis of actions required. Herbs used in such cases have actions that begin with "anti-," including anti-inflammatory, antispasmodic, antiviral, and antiallergy.

Treat the Perceived Causes: What is the cause of disease in an individual patient? Physiologic enhancement or compensation should be directed at the perceived cause. Often, a chain of causal events occur. Factors involved in disease causation can be divided into predisposing, excitatory, and perpetuating.

- Predisposing causes include stress, poor vitality, inadequate diet, and inherited disorders, among others.
- Excitatory causes, such as infection or trauma, provoke the disease.
- Perpetuating causes or sustaining causes hinder resolution of the disease; an example is chronic inflammation.

Typically, predisposing causes can be treated through physiologic enhancement, and excitatory causes via compensatory mechanisms. Occasionally sustaining causes simply need physiologic compensation to break the cycle.

Treating the links in a causal chain involves the following steps (imagine a stray dog with parainfluenza virus who has been impounded for 2 weeks):

1. Stress
2. Lowered vitality
3. Weakened immunity
4. Viral infection
5. Catarrhal state of mucous membranes
6. Cough

Steps 1 through 3 are predisposing causes, 4 is the excitatory cause, 5 is the sustaining cause, and 6 is the symptomatic expression of disease. For steps 1 and 2, we would prescribe adaptogens (such as *Eleutherococcus senticosis*, which is adaptogenic and immunomodulatory). For step 3, immune modulators *(Eleutherococcus* and *Echinacea)* would be given; for 4, antiviral herbs *(Echinacea)*; for 5, anticatarrhal herbs *(Sambucus nigra)*; and for 6, antitussive herbs *(Glycyrrhiza glabra)* would be included. This approach can be taken in conventional medicine through the use of available drugs as well; however, such comprehensive disease management is not usually seen in conventional practice. An additional advantage of herbal medicine is that the herbalist can put all needed medications into a single combination formula by using herb tinctures.

A formula for this patient might be as follows:

Eleutherococcus senticosis	40%
Echinacea angustifolia	30%
Sambucus nigra	20%
Glycyrrhiza glabra	10%

Match the Treatment to the Patient: The herbal formula administered should be matched energetically and constitutionally to the patient (Table 19-2). "Warming" herbs are thought to aggravate "hot" patients, and "cooling" herbs may aggravate cold patients. Thus, if a cooling herb is indicated for a cold patient, warming herbs should be added to compensate for these potentially adverse energetic effects. This is one of the reasons why tonics (which are usually warming) theoretically should not be used in patients with acute infection.

In summary:

1. Use the case history and decide on treatment goals.
2. Link treatment goals to the choice of herbs through their actions.
3. Select herbs that demonstrate those actions (consider herbs with overlapping actions).
4. Combine the herbs in a formula with the use of appropriate doses.
5. Match the treatment and dosage energetically and constitutionally to the patient.

What Is the Herxheimer Reaction?

In traditional medicine there is a concept called aggravation that sometimes occurs when commencing treatment. Its important to explain this as a possible side effect. This phenomenon is recognized as the Jarisch-Herxheimer reaction (JHR), believed to be caused when injured or dead bacteria release endotoxins into blood and tissues at a faster rate than the body can handle them. This provokes a sudden, exaggerated inflammatory response and is associated with the systemic appearance of cytokines (Mangin, 2004). This means that symptoms may sometimes worsen temporarily after treatment has been initiated. If the reaction becomes difficult for the patient to tolerate, then the dose of herb should be reduced to half or even less, to allow the patient to gradually build up tolerance.

THE HOLISTIC VETERINARY FRAMEWORK

In Western herbal medicine, being able to effectively prescribe herbs to animals is a skill that lies somewhere between science and art. Much of veterinary herbal practice is empiric, adaptive, and experiential by nature. An herbalist must be able to interpret signs and diagnose conditions and must have strong knowledge of the *Materia medica*, including aspects of herbs that lie outside the scientific understanding of their constituents and their potential to alter pathophysiology. The energetics of plants, how they interact with other herbs, herb–drug

TABLE 19-2

Determining the Energetics of the Patient

Heat signs	*Cold signs*
Caused by dehydration, diet, extreme behaviors, hot weather, failure to eliminate toxins (constipation)	Result from lack of heat or vitality; exposure to cold weather, cold foods, some chronic illness
Red, sometimes dry, tongue	Pale tongue
Panting	Poor circulation
Red eyes	Diminished mental ability
Upper body affected (heat rises)	Catarrhal respiratory tract
Red, inflamed skin	Chills, shivering
Fever	White or clear discharge
Inflamed mucous membrane	Frequent urination
Dry cough	Large volumes of pale urine passed
Bleeding	Limbs often affected (colder parts of body)
Irritation	Slow, deep pulse
Dry eyes	Dislike of cold, tendency to seek heat
Pain	Aggravated by cold weather
Yellow discharge	Fatigue
Scant, dark urine; strong odor	Fixed pain, stiff joints
Thirst	Poor digestion, bloating
Worsening of symptoms in hot weather	Diminished appetite
Moist signs	*Dry signs*
(= Dampness of traditional Chinese medicine)	
Overeating, especially of certain types of food; humid weather, damp environment, sedentary lifestyle, emotional turmoil, inactivity, poor vitality	Windy weather, dry foods, lack of fluids, extreme emotions
Greasiness	Dry skin, cracked skin on nose
Ulcers, abscesses, blisters	Dry nails
Thick mucus	Dry and red eyes (heat)
Clear, white mucus (cold)	Inflamed, dry, itchy skin or mucous membranes (dry heat)
Offensive discharge (heat)	Wheezing, shortness of breath, dry cough
Moisture settling in lower part of body (cold)	Dry and red tongue (heat) or pale tongue (cold)
Cloudy urine, strong smell (heat)	Pulse rapid (heat), slow (cold), or indistinct
Slippery, rapid pulse (heat) or slow and deep pulse (cold)	Dislikes wind, worse in autumn
Wet tongue	Thirsty
Dislike of cold, wet places or weather	Muscle wasting and weakness
Sore joints, stiffness worse with rest, improvement with movement	Allergic conditions
Diminished appetite, poor digestion (especially fatty food) (heat)	Restlessness associated with heat
Copious diarrhea with mucus (cold) or with offensive odor (heat)	Dry stools
Poor resistance to infection	Poor resistance to infection of skin, mucous membranes, and respiratory tract
Constipated or with edema	Insatiable thirst; likes swimming, water
Diseases of liver, gallbladder often associated with moist hot disorders	
Phlegmatic individual (cold and moist) more dull	
Sanguine (hot and moist) less forceful	

Modified from Trickey R. The origins of disharmony. Modern Phytotherapist 1998;4:19–127.

interactions, and adverse effects are just as important as therapeutic potential and actions. Prescriptions should be formulated with aspects of the individual patient in mind. From a holistic perspective, the prescription is one part of the treatment; lifestyle, environmental factors, and diet should also be modified as necessary.

The Patient

Diagnosis is important but is not the only step that should precede prescribing. An understanding of the underlying pathophysiology of the condition is just as important as diagnosis in herbal prescribing. Such an

BOX 19-1

Signs of Health for Dogs*

Good Health Indicators

- Ability to exercise more than 30 minutes daily
- Abundant energy when exercising or playing
- Relaxed demeanor with other dogs, strangers, friends, and family
- Clean white teeth without yellow or brown staining or build-up of calculus
- Normal weight for breed
- No bad breath
- Shiny, full coat with minimal shedding, except at moult
- Itch-free and healthy skin; no odor, no spots, no lumps
- Firm, consistent bowel movements passed easily daily
- Clear urine, odor free; passed easily
- Free mobility with no stiffness or soreness
- Eyes that are bright and clear all the time
- Ears that are clean and odor free
- Good appetite and normal hunger
- Balanced desire for fluids; increases in hot weather and with exercise
- Sleep that is balanced with wakefulness
- Dreaming that does not disturb sleep
- Normal breathing; no abnormal sounds

*Fougère, 2003.

understanding helps the herbalist to identify the most useful herbs for treating patients with a particular condition. One of the easiest ways of prescribing is to treat according to herbal actions—for example, using anti-inflammatory herbs to relieve inflammation.

Sometimes, a conventional diagnosis is not forthcoming and pathophysiology is unclear. As veterinarians, we are not necessarily trained to treat "predisease" states, and we sometimes even wait to repeat a test to see whether we can now indeed diagnose the condition. However, nuances and subtleties can indicate an imbalance long before disease becomes apparent. Changes in stool quality and appetite, coat condition, behavior, drinking habits, cravings for particular foods, sneezing, flatulence, and altered sleep patterns may be relevant if day-to-day changes are ruled out and a trend is evident.

Herbal prescribing offers an advantage in that it can be used to treat a number of seemingly unrelated signs and problems, or a number of diagnoses within the same patient, without the problems associated with polypharmacy in conventional medicine. Combining herbs that deal with primary pathophysiologic features, as well as underlying causes, can be a safe and effective way to treat patients.

One way to detect early changes before diagnosis of disease is possible is to determine how far the patient deviates from robust vital health (Box 19-1). This means detecting and treating changes before they manifest as disease per se. This is one of the benefits of herbal medicine—that balance can be restored before problems become chronic and entrenched.

Formulating the Prescription

Diagnosis, history, and presenting signs and problems help the herbalist to make distinctions in determining a strategy for selecting herbs. A simple approach is to choose specific herbs that will target the condition, such as gymnema for diabetes, devil's claw for arthritis, or corydalis for smooth muscle pain. This requires familiarity with the *Materia medica*, which is the place to start when one is developing a formula. This is the way many herbalists begin. However, this simple approach to prescribing means essentially using the same formula or herbs for all "cases with the same diagnosis."

Another option is to formulate with the goal of meeting the needs of the individual patient. Herbs for a particular condition can still be incorporated, but now the aim of prescribing is not only to address the symptoms and signs, but at the same time, to strengthen the patient and support and tonify relevant tissues and organs. This approach is based on physiomedical prescribing and is considered holistic because it involves not simply treating the signs, but also restoring health and vitality through various agents, such as tonics, adaptogens, trophorestoratives, eliminatives, alteratives, and other categories of herbs that influence health on a much broader scale.

Decision Tree for Formulating a Prescription

One should first assess the patient. The diagnosis should be obtained, along with a problem list and an evaluation of patient vitality (general robustness). It should be determined whether the condition is an excess (generally warm to hot) or deficient one (generally cool or cold), and whether the signs reflect dryness or moisture, heat or cold, and so forth. This information guides the herbalist in deciding the nature of the formula, for example, whether it should be invigorating, sedating, tonifying, cleansing, warming, cooling, and so forth. It also allows the herbalist to select the best herb from a group with similar actions after he or she reviews the energetics of the herbs to be considered.

Treatment goals, both short-term and long-term (if necessary), must be clear. The aim of formulating the prescription is to select four or five herbs that will relieve the patient in the first instance, especially if the condition is acute. Many systems may be involved, and at first, the patient's condition may be overwhelming. What is the most important thing that can be done for the patient initially? Once this has been accomplished, the formula can be altered to help with less pressing issues.

- Does the patient have any gastrointestinal signs, or evidence of weak digestion? If yes, the gastrointestinal function should be treated first, so that any additional herbs given can be assimilated properly.
- Is the condition acute? This is one of the few times when herbal medicine is focused almost solely on the

BOX 19-2

Actions of Digestive Herbs

DIGESTIVE HERBS	EXAMPLES
Bitters improve digestion, assimilation, and elimination. One should select herbs that will also relieve other signs in the patient (assuming thorough knowledge of the *Materia Medica*). If uncertain, dandelion and chamomile are safe and effective in most cases.	Yarrow, horse chestnut, agrimony, andrographis, wormwood, oregon grape, barberry, bupleurum, corydalis, globe artichoke, gentian, devil's claw, goldenseal, chamomile, picrorrhiza, *Polygonum multiflorum*, baical skullcap, dandelion leaf, dandelion root, thyme
Carminatives assist in reducing bloating and flatulence and ease abdominal discomfort.	Yarrow, cinnamon quills, fennel, lavender, chamomile, lemon balm, peppermint, catmint, parsley, aniseed, rosemary, sage, goldenrod, thyme, valerian, chaste tree, prickly ash, ginger

disease, although it is still important to take into consideration the energetics of the patient. When a treatment regimen is adopted, it is usual to resolve an acute complaint before resolving a chronic one. Acute formulas are often given at high doses, repeated frequently, and given for short times. Constitutional formulas for chronic conditions are usually given at lower doses for extended periods, so they are not usually given at the same time. It is also important to note that many of the adaptogens used as tonics are contraindicated in acute complaints.

- Is the condition acute in a robust animal? If yes, then one should treat symptomatically using herbal actions that treat specific symptoms, such as anti-inflammatory, antitussive, and so forth.
- Is the condition acute, affecting a patient with less than good health? If yes, then one should treat the acute condition as described in the first bulleted entry above; then, the underlying constitution or chronic disease should be addressed.
- Is the condition chronic? If yes, then one should consider the need for tonics or eliminatives.
- Debilitated patients should be given tonics and should have their vitality (energy) restored before elimination regimens are considered.
- If the patient is not generally debilitated, eliminative herbs can be given at the same time as tonics.
- One should always formulate with the goal of avoiding potential adverse effects by using herbs that can offset any strong actions that might aggravate a patient.
- One should select herbs that achieve treatment goals and meet the needs of the patient. Herbs with overlapping clinical actions are ideal.

Strategies and Formulation

One can select from a number of categories of herbs when formulating. This becomes second nature when one is familiar with the *Materia medica,* and with experience, little time is required. Initially, however, the new herbalist should consider the need for the various categories of herbs and should decide on priorities according to patient presentation. These categories also offer strategies, and it is worthwhile for the practitioner to become familiar with these. Often, overlap between categories occurs, and herbs that serve a number of purposes for the individual patient become the core of a formula.

Digestives

If the patient is unable to absorb and assimilate herbs, or has a gastrointestinal tract condition that is the reason for presentation, this must be treated as a priority. Consideration is given to diet and to the method of administration of herbs (Box 19-2). If a patient is vomiting, enema administration of teas rather than tinctures should be considered, at least initially. Mixing herbs with food is the easiest way to treat dogs; however, cats may need to be administered a diluted tincture using a syringe. Palatability agents should be considered, if necessary, as should altering the form of the herb (i.e., powders, tablets, capsules). For information on treatment of patients with inflammatory bowel disease, colitis, or other diagnosed gastrointestinal tract disease, see the section on gastrointestinal disease in Chapter 20.

HERBAL ACTIONS

The simplest way to prescribe is to select herbs according to their actions, with the goal of addressing the pathophysiology that is evident in the patient (Table 19-3). This approach works well for the generally robust patient, but if the patient is debilitated and vitality is low, more specialized prescribing is required to restore vitality and the general health of the patient. Herbs discussed in the following sections are listed in no particular level of importance, but if one is looking for a particular action, these herbs are good places to start.

ADAPTOGENS AND TONIC HERBS

A recently proposed definition of plant adaptogens is as follows: "Smooth" pro-stressors that reduce the reactivity of host defense systems and decrease the damaging effects

TABLE 19-3

"Anti" Herbal Actions

Action	Herbs
Analgesic	Pulsatilla, corydalis, yellow jasmine, devil's claw, willow
Anodyne	Pulsatilla, corydalis, California poppy, hops, passionflower, kava, Jamaica dogwood, yellow jasmine, willow
Antacid	Meadowsweet
Anthelmintic	Garlic, wormwood, butternut, black walnut, thyme
Antiaging	He Shou Wu
Antiallergic	Albizia, dong quai, chamomile, peony, picrorrhiza, baical skullcap, feverfew, tylophora, butterbur
Antiarrhythmic	Dong quai, corydalis, hawthorn, devil's claw, Asian ginseng, dan shen, withania
Antiasthmatic	Adhatoda, ephedra, euphorbia, lobelia, tylophora
Anticancer	Garlic, green tea, greater celandine, turmeric, chaparral, baical skullcap, pau d'arco, thuja, red clover, violet leaves, withania
Anticatarrhal (lower respiratory tract)	Bryony, polygala, sage, mullein
Anticatarrhal (upper respiratory tract)	Garlic, eyebright, chamomile, elder flowers, goldenrod
Anticholesterolemic	Albizia, garlic, globe artichoke
Anticoagulant	Dan shen
Anticonvulsant	Peony, skullcap, ziziphus, bacopa, baical skullcap
Antidiarrheal	Cinnamon, Oregon grape root, chamomile, slippery elm
Antiemetic	Oregon grape root, fringe tree, cinnamon, peppermint, ginger, chamomile, meadowsweet
Antiepileptic	Bacopa, peony, kava, valerian
Antifibrinolytic	Garlic, gotu kola, dan shen
Antifibrotic	Gotu kola, dan shen
Antifungal (topical)	Pau d'arco, cat's claw, tea tree
Antigalactagogue	Sage, bilberry
Antiglaucoma	Forskohlii
Antihemorrhagic (systemic)	Yarrow, agrimony, ladies' mantle, shepherd's purse, codonopsis, horsetail, cranesbill, witch hazel, white dead nettle, rehmannia, beth root, yunnan pai yao
Antihemorrhagic (topical)/styptic	Yarrow, shepherd's purse, witch hazel, white dead nettle, nettle, yunnan pai yao
Antihemorrhagic (uterine)	Yarrow, ladies' mantle, horsetail, goldenseal, white dead nettle, beth root, nettle leaf
Antihyperprostatic	Epilobium, hydrangea, saw palmetto, nettle root
Anti-inflammatory	Andrographis, dong quai, Oregon grape, calendula, codonopsis, turmeric, wild yam, echinacea, ginkgo, meadowsweet, licorice, Saint John's Wort, chamomile, picrorrhiza, rehmannia, baical skullcap, sarsaparilla, feverfew, withania
Anti-inflammatory (circulation)	Ginkgo, butcher's broom
Anti-inflammatory (female reproductive system)	Dong quai, wild yam, peony
Anti-inflammatory (gastrointestinal)	Calendula, wild yam, meadowsweet, licorice, chamomile, chickweed
Anti-inflammatory (liver)	Bupleurum, picrorrhiza
Anti-inflammatory (musculoskeletal)	Celery seed, silver birch, gotu kola, black cohosh, turmeric, guaiacum, devil's claw, hemidesmus, rehmannia, willow, sarsaparilla, heartsease, ginger
Anti-inflammatory (respiratory tract)	Pleurisy root, goldenrod
Anti-inflammatory (topical)	Calendula, gotu kola, chamomile, chickweed, nettle, green tea
Anti-inflammatory (urinary)	Couch grass, marshmallow, silver birch, crataeva, licorice, ribwort, goldenrod, corn silk
Antilithic	Ladies' mantle, marshmallow, crataeva, horsetail, gravel root, hydrangea, tylophora, corn silk, uric acid–juniper, crataeva (calcium oxalate stones), vaccinium
Antimicrobial	Neem, Oregon grape, barberry, calendula, green tea, citrus seed extract, echinacea, fennel, goldenseal, elecampane, chamomile, lemon balm, olive leaves, propolis, dan shen, baical skullcap, pau d'arco, thyme
Antineoplastic	Mistletoe, violet leaves
Antiobesity	Forskohlii, myrrh, bladderwrack
Antiedematous	Horse chestnut, bilberry, sweet clover

TABLE 19-3

"Anti" Herbal Actions—cont'd

Action	Herbs
Antioxidant	Andrographis, green tea, hawthorn, turmeric, ginkgo, olive leaves, polygonum multiflorum, rosemary, baical skullcap, St. Mary's thistle, cat's claw, bilberry, grapeseed
Antiprotozoal	Chinese wormwood, propolis, barberry, goldenseal, euphorbia, pau d'arco, garlic, yucca, kava
Antiplatelet	Garlic, andrographis, dong quai, coleus, myrrh, turmeric, dan shen, ginger
Antipruritic	Neem, sarsaparilla, chickweed, chamomile
Antipruritic (topical)	Chickweed, green tea
Antipyretic	Ladies' mantle, andrographis, neem, wild indigo, rehmannia, willow, baical skullcap
Antirheumatic	Silver birch, blue cohosh, black cohosh, wild yam, gravelroot, meadowsweet, bladderwrack, guaiacum, poke root, poplar, willow, sarsaparilla, dandelion, heartsease, prickly ash, devils claw, ashwagandha
Antiseptic (gastrointestinal)	Yarrow, albizia, garlic, wormwood, wild indigo, calendula, cayenne, chili, citrus seed extract, myrrh, echinacea, juniper, peppermint, picrorrhiza, propolis, sage, baical skullcap, pau d'arco, thyme
Antiseptic (respiratory tract)	Pleurisy root, echinacea, elecampane, picrorrhiza, sage, goldenrod, thyme
Antiseptic (topical)	Calendula, echinacea, Saint John's Wort, propolis, pau d'arco
Antiseptic (urinary)	Couch grass, celery seed, uva ursi, buchu, crataeva, echinacea, meadowsweet, licorice, saw palmetto, goldenrod, thyme
Antispasmodic (muscle)	Forskohlii, wild yam, licorice, lavender, chamomile, lemon balm, peppermint, peony, kava, red clover, valerian, black haw, cramp bark
Antispasmodic (respiratory tract)	Adhatoda, pleurisy root, coleus, euphorbia, licorice, grindelia, elecampane, inula, lobelia, thyme
Antispasmodic (uterus)	Dong quai, blue cohosh, wild yam, licorice, inula, motherwort, peony
Antitumor	Green tea, cat's claw
Antitussive	Marshmallow, neem, bupleurum, black cohosh, wild yam, licorice, hops, elecampane, schisandra, thyme (on trachea)
Antiulcerogenic (gastrointestinal)	Meadowsweet, licorice, chamomile, propolis
Antiviral (systemic)	Garlic, neem, echinacea, Saint John's Wort, lemon balm, propolis, pau d'arco, thuja, cat's claw, andrographis
Antiviral (topical)	Calendula, licorice, hops, Saint John's Wort, lemon balm
Anxiolytic	Saint John's Wort, kava
Astringent	Yarrow, agrimony, ladies' mantle, uva ursi, calendula, green tea, myrrh, horsetail, eyebright, meadowsweet, cleavers, cranesbill, witch hazel, Saint John's Wort, black walnut, white dead nettle, peony, ribwort, oak, rosehips, raspberry, yellow dock, willow, sage, thuja, thyme, beth root, nettle, bilberry
Astringent, uterine	Calendula, shepherd's purse, cranesbill, goldenseal, nettle leaf

of various stressors by increasing the basal levels of mediators involved in the stress response (Panossian, 1999). Because of their effects on the body's ability to withstand stress, combined with their tonic activity, these herbs can be used for a wide range of conditions and for just about any form of chronic disease. They are especially valuable for patients for whom stress is a predisposing or perpetuating factor. Adaptogens are frequently tonics also; however, the primary purpose of adaptogens is to conserve adaptogenic activity; tonics essentially increase adaptation energy (Box 19-3).

Adaptogenic herbs can be used in the following situations: treatment for any chronic illness, convalescence, postsurgery care, relief of stress, boarding/kennel care, pound/rescue of animals, relief of travel stress, intensive training, chemotherapy and radiation therapy, reduction in debility, and enhancement of performance. The particular adaptogen selected for use in a formula varies according to the other actions attributed to the herb, as well as its energetics.

For patients with chronic conditions, one should establish which kinds of strengthening or tonifying herbs are appropriate. Tonic herbs are best employed when a patient shows evidence of deficiency in function and when energy is generally low. Restoring vital energy is important before increased function is encouraged through the use of eliminatives, because elimination is thought to require functioning tissues and organs. Thus, tonics improve function before activity is increased. Assessment of patient vitality helps the practitioner to determine which approach is best. If appropriate, adaptogens should be incorporated at the same time, or an adaptogen that serves both functions should be chosen. Table 19-4 can be used as a starting point for selection of appropriate herbs for each specific case.

ENHANCING ELIMINATION

Eliminatives are herbs that are used to facilitate or promote eliminative functions. These are usually prescribed as constitutional treatment rather than as acute treatment, and they are generally used when the patient is strong or robust and when "excess" signs are noted. These signs include excessive secretions, constipation, heat, pain, congestion, and irritability. When the patient is debilitated or vitality is low, but signs of excess are evident, eliminative herbs should be balanced with tonics.

Disease of the bladder and kidneys can be treated with diuretics, which encourage elimination of toxins and metabolites through the urine. Laxatives are employed for elimination of metabolites and toxins through the gastrointestinal tract. Expectorants are used to stimulate production of mucus and subsequent expectoration of phlegm. Choleretic herbs are used to promote elimination of bile (Box 19-4).

BOX 19-3

Adaptogenic Herbs

Herbs with well established adaptogenic activity include the following:

- *Panax ginseng*
- *Eleutherococcus senticosis*
- *Withania somnifera*
- *Astragalus membranaceus*

Others, with less well-established adaptogenic activity, include the following:

- *Schisandra chinensis*
- *Bupleurum falcatum*
- *Codonopsis pilosa*
- *Panax quinquefolius*
- *Glycyrrhiza glabra*
- *Cordyceps sinensis*

ALTERATIVES

The term *alterative* was common in veterinary texts until the mid 1900s. Alteratives are defined in Banham & Young's Veterinary Posology (1935) as drugs and other agents that "gradually change and correct the morbid condition of organs." Alterative treatments are often used in long-term, chronic conditions and are otherwise traditionally known as "blood cleansers," or depuratives. Alteratives are used to promote a gradual change in chronic disease states, especially skin, joint, and connective tissue disorders. These plants may work by improving the processes of detoxification and elimination, or by immune modulation. They act slowly, and progress is usually noted over months, rather than days or weeks. An alterative can also be an herb that is a rich source of nutrients (usually mineral) that assist the intermediate mechanisms of metabolism (Box 19-5).

NERVINES

Chronic stress, depression, and anxiety can delay healing and recovery (Cole-King, 2001). Sometimes, anxiety and depression can be attributed to chronic pain. In herbal

TABLE 19-4

Actions of Tonic Herbs

Tonic Target	Herbs
Qi tonic	Astragalus
Adaptogens	Asian ginseng, eleutherococcus, withania
Kidney/urogenital tonics	Rhemannia, damania, uva ursi, crataeva, astragalus, bupleurum, dan shen, schisandra, goldenrod
Heart	Hawthorn, astragalus, salvia miltiorrhiza, albizia, dong quai, coleus, motherwort, olive leaves, Asian ginseng
Liver	Milk thistle, bupleurum, dandelion, andrographis, Oregon grape, barberry, fringe tree, globe artichoke, Asian ginseng, picrorrhiza, dan shen, schisandra
Adrenal glands	Licorice (hypertensive), rehmannia (nonhypertensive)
Blood	Dong quai, codonopsis, polygonum, rehmannia, withania
Cognition	Bacopa, ginkgo, gotu kola, peony
Male reproduction	Asian ginseng, saw palmetto, sarsaparilla, damiana
Nervous system	Oat seed, bacopa, gotu kola, wild yam, Saint John's Wort, He Shou Wu, schisandra, baical skullcap, damiana, valerian
Postpartum	Partridge berry
Uterus	Ladies' mantle, dong quai, blue cohosh, false unicorn root, black cohosh, goldenseal, partridge berry, schisandra, beth root, chaste tree
Venotonic	Horse chestnut, lily of the valley, wild yam, ginkgo, witch hazel, grapeseed

BOX 19-4

Actions of Eliminative Herbs

Diuretics

- *Agropyron repens*
- *Althaea officinalis*
- *Apium graveolens*
- *Arctium lappa*
- *Astragalus membranaceus*
- *Atractylodes macrocephala*
- *Barosma betulina*
- *Centella asiatica*
- *Chelidonium majus*
- *Cynara scolymus*
- *Eupatorium purpureum*
- *Gallium aparine*
- *Hydrangea arborescens*
- *Iris versicolor*
- *Juniperus communis*
- *Mitchella repens*
- *Petroselinum crispum*
- *Plantago major*
- *Rosmarinus officinalis*
- *Ruta graveolens*
- *Scutellaria baicalensis*
- *Serenoa serrulata*
- *Taraxacum officinale folia and radix*
- *Tilia* spp
- *Urtica dioica folia*
- *Vitis vinifera*
- *Zea mays*

Laxatives

- *Aloe barbadensis*
- *Articum lappa*
- *Mahonia aquifolium*
- *Berberis vulgaris*
- *Cassia* spp
- *Chionanthus virginicus*
- *Fumaria officinalis*
- *Glycyrrhiza glabra*
- *Iris versicolor*
- *Juglans cinerea*
- *Taraxacum officinale radix*
- *Trigonella foenum-graecum*

Expectorants

- *Adhatoda vasica*
- *Angelica archangelica*
- *Asclepias tuberosa*
- *Glycyrrhiza glabra*
- *Grindelia camporum*
- *Hyssopus officinalis*
- *Inula helenium*
- *Lobelia inflate*
- *Petroselinum crispum*
- *Pimpinella anisum*
- *Plantago lanceolada*
- *Sanguinaria canadensis*
- *Stillingia sylvatica*
- *Thymus vulgaris*
- *Trigonella foenum-graecum*
- *Usnea barbata*
- *Verbascum thapsus*
- *Viola tricolor*

Cholagogues (Improve Bile Secretion)

- *Agrimonia Eupatorium*
- *Andrographis*
- *Artemisia vulgaris*
- *Berberis aquifolium*
- *Calendula officinalis*
- *Chelidonium majus*
- *Chamomilla recutita*
- *Chionanthus virginicus*
- *Curcuma longa*
- *Cynara scolymus*
- *Dioscorea villosa*
- *Gentiana lutea*
- *Iris versicolor*
- *Juglans cinerea*
- *Rumex crispus*
- *Taraxacum officinalis leaf and root*
- *Picrorrhiza kurroa*

Choleretics (Improve Bile Flow)

- *Andrographis paniculata*
- *Berberis vulgaris*
- *Calendula officinalis*
- *Chelidonium majus*
- *Curcuma longa*
- *Cynara scolymus*
- *Glycyrrhiza glabra*
- *Hydrastis canadensis*
- *Mentha piperita*
- *Picrorrhiza kurroa*
- *Silybum marianum*
- *Zingiber officinale*

medicine, nervines are important tools for addressing these influences. A nervine is a plant remedy that has a beneficial effect on the nervous system in some way (Box 19-6). Traditionally, they can be subdivided into three groups:

1. Nervine tonics (e.g., milky oats) strengthen and restore the nervous system.
2. Nervine relaxants (e.g., passionflower) ease anxiety and tension. These include hypnotics, strong antispasmodics, and anodynes (analgesics). These herbs act on visceral musculature, the central nervous system, and, indirectly, on skeletal muscle; they have relaxing or sedating effects. Nervine relaxant treatment is directed at reducing pain, tension, anxiety,

BOX 19-5

Alterative Herbs

- *Articum lappa*
- *Apium graveolens*
- *Trifolium pretense*
- *Taraxacum officinalis*
- *Gallium aparine*
- *Urtica urens*
- *Mahonia aquifolium*
- *Equisetum arvense*
- *Hydrastis canadensis*
- *Berberis vulgaris*
- *Aloe*
- *Cascara sagrada*
- *Centella asiatica*
- *Echinacea* spp
- *Iris versicolor*
- *Juglans cinerea*
- *Phytolacca decandra*
- *Rumex crispus*
- *Scrophularia nodosa*
- *Stillingia sylvatica*
- *Usnea barbata*

irritability, restlessness, and insomnia, all of which can be associated with physical signs such as shaking, spasms, cramps, and seizures.

3. Nervine stimulants (e.g., coffee and kola nut) directly stimulate nerve activity.

In cases of shock, stress, or nervous debility, nervine tonics strengthen and restore tissues directly. They can also contribute to the healing of damaged nerve tissue.

SPECIFIC SUPPORT FOR TISSUE AND ORGAN FUNCTION

Herbs may be targeted at a specific condition or toward other organs and tissues involved in the overall pathogenesis of a particular condition. The traditional understanding is that because of the integrated nature of the body, when one organ is not functioning efficiently, another organ has to compensate. Individual organ weaknesses, or weaker organs and tissues, may need to be supported with specific tissue tonics, in addition to treatment aimed at improving the overall constitution. *Trophorestorative* is a traditional term that refers to an herb that has a beneficial effect on the repair and biochemical functioning of a particular organ or tissue (Table 19-5). For more information, see "Adaptogens and Tonic Herbs," earlier.

TABLE 19-5

Herbs for Organ/Tissue Support

Organ/Tissue	Herbs
Cardioprotective	Andrographis, corydalis, hawthorn, Asian ginseng, dan shen
Circulatory stimulant	Dong quai, horseradish, oat seed, cayenne, chili, ginkgo, Asian ginseng, rosemary, prickly ash
Circulatory stimulant (cerebral blood flow)	Ginkgo, lesser periwinkle
Circulatory stimulant (systemic)	Horseradish, cayenne, chili, prickly ash, ginger
Connective tissue trophorestorative	Gotu kola, calendula
Mucous membrane trophorestorative	Eyebright, goldenseal, ribwort, goldenrod
Hepatoprotective	Andrographis, dong quai, bupleurum, turmeric, globe artichoke, Asian ginseng, picrorrhiza, dan shen, schisandra, milk thistle, sarsaparilla
Hypothalamic-pituitary-ovarian (HPO) regulator	False unicorn root, black cohosh, wild yam, licorice, peony, beth root, chaste tree
Immune stimulant	Andrographis, dong quai, astragalus, codonopsis, echinacea, Siberian ginseng, Szechuan lovage root, peony, Asian ginseng, poke root, picrorrhiza, propolis, pau d'arco, thuja, cat's claw
Lymphatic	Wild indigo, calendula, echinacea, cleavers, blue flag, poke root
Pancreatic trophorestorative	Oregon grape, gymnema
Renal protective	Astragalus, bupleurum, rehmannia
Thymoleptic	Asian ginseng
Thyroid stimulant	Forskohlii, bladderwrack, dan shen
Vasoprotective	Bilberry, blueberry
Vulnerary	Aloe, marshmallow, astragalus, calendula, gotu kola, myrrh, echinacea, horsetail, cranesbill, Saint John's Wort, white dead nettle, chamomile, partridge berry, ribwort, propolis, chickweed, cat's claw, mullein, many more (see section on topical herbs in Chapter 20)

BOX 19-6

Actions of Nervine Herbs

Nervine Sedatives/Relaxants
- *Matricaria recutita*
- *Lavandula officinalis*
- *Piper methysticum*
- *Passiflora incarnata*
- *Cimicifuga racemosa*
- *Valeriana officinalis*
- *Withania somnifera*

Nervine Stimulants
- *Camellia sinensis*
- *Rosmarinus officinalis*

Nervine Tonics
- *Avena sativa*
- *Bacopa monniera*
- *Centella asiatica*
- *Hypericum perforatum*
- *Schisandra chinensis*
- *Scutellaria baicalensis*
- *Scutellaria lateriflora*
- *Valeriana officinalis*
- *Dioscorea villosa*
- *Polygonum multiflorum*
- *Verbena officinalis*

Anxiolytics
- *Hypericum perforatum*
- *Piper methysticum*

Hypnotics
- *Passiflora incarnata*
- *Humulus lupulus*
- *Valeriana officinalis*
- *Ziziphus spinosa*
- *Piper methysticum*

Antispasmodics
- *Inula racemosa*
- *Leonurus cardiaca*
- *Lobelia inflata*
- *Melissa officinalis*
- *Mentha piperita*
- *Nepeta cataria*
- *Pimpinella anisum*
- *Rosmarinus officinalis*
- *Salvia officinalis*
- *Sanguinaria canadensis*
- *Stillingia sylvatica*
- *Valeriana* spp
- *Viburnum opulus*
- *Viscum album*
- *Paeonia lactiflora*
- *Chamomilla recutita*
- *Dioscorea villosa*
- *Piper methysticum*

Analgesics and Anodynes
- *Anemone pulsatilla*
- *Corydalis ambigua*
- *Gelsemium sempervirens*
- *Harpagophytum procumbens*
- *Ligusticum wallichii*
- *Salix alba*
- *Eschscholzia californica*
- *Passiflora incarnata*
- *Piscidia erythrina*

MINIMIZING ADVERSE EFFECTS

Adverse effects may occur because of incorrect combinations of herbs, use of herbs that are inappropriate for an individual patient, or, most commonly, administration of a formula that is dosed incorrectly. Methods for counteracting adverse effects are often built into the formula. Some examples include the following:

- Very bitter (and usually cooling) herbs are given with warming herbs, hot herbs with cooling herbs, drying herbs with moistening herbs, and so forth, to modify potential deleterious effects.
- Very hot herbs such as chili (rubefacient—increasing blood flow to the tissue) are given with gastrointestinal demulcents to prevent burning and gastrointestinal tract irritation.
- Toxic herbs are combined with certain specific herbs to offset the potential for poisoning and are given in smaller proportions in the formula. Gelsemium, for example, is extremely toxic and therefore makes up only 5% to 10% of any formula.
- Some bitter herbs are given with gastrointestinal spasmolytics or carminatives to prevent the tendency toward cramping.

By now, the themes involved in the herbal treatment of a patient should be apparent. Once four or five herbs have been selected, the formula is mixed and a dosing regimen decided.

CASE STUDY

Sarah is a 4-year-old, 10-kg (22-lb) cross-breed, owned for 2 months, but in a pound for 6 months, with a history of recurrent skin, tonsil, and bladder infections and one bout of contagious bronchitis. She has already had four courses of antibiotics—two of the courses for 6 weeks' duration. She is nonpruritic and currently free of cystitis and fleas, but debilitated; her tonsils are slightly inflamed, her coat condition is sparse and dry, and she is still underweight. She is thin and seeks warmth (cool and dry constitution). Her stools are inconsistent but have improved on a new diet. No other abnormalities have been detected. In this case, chronic stress and undernourishment have contributed to poor immunity. Emphasis is placed on improving immunity and reducing the effects of stress.

Patients with poor immunity or recurrent infection should receive treatment selected from the following priority groups:

- Immune-enhancing herbs, including *Echinacea, Astragalus, Picrorrhiza,* and *Andrographis. Astragalus* should not be prescribed during acute episodes; because *Picrorrhiza* and *Andrographis* are bitter, they should not be prescribed for a constitutionally cold animal.
- Tonic and adaptogenic herbs such as *Panax, Eleutherococcus,* and *Withania.*
- Digestive herbs, including bitters if the patient is undernourished or anemic; the cooling effect should be countered with warming herbs.

In this case, the following herbs were chosen:

- *Echinacea angustifolia* (warm, acrid, and sweet)—an immune stimulant, anti-inflammatory, antibacterial, and antiviral to provide nonspecific immune support.
- *Withania somnifera* (warm)—a tonic, adaptogen, and nervine (assuming this dog has been stressed physically and mentally) given to support convalescence, debility, and anemia.
- Burdock *(Arctium lappa)* (cold)—an alterative, nutritive herb that is mildly antiseptic for skin disease.
- *Crataeva nurvala* (cooling)—a bladder tonic.
- Licorice *(Glycyrrhiza glabra)* (neutral and moist)—an anti-inflammatory, adaptogen, and taste improver

The formula consisted of the following:

Echinacea	30 mL
Withania	40 mL
Burdock	15 mL
Varuna	15 mL
Licorice	10 mL
Total	110 mL

A full bottle contains 110 mL. The dose prescribed was 2 mL twice daily for 3 weeks. The formula overall was warming and slightly sweet. It was given twice over 6 weeks, and during that time, Sarah's coat condition and weight improved. She became more active, her stool quality improved, her tonsillitis resolved, and no infections have recurred at this point.

References

Banham GA, Young WJ, *Veterinary Posology*. Bailliere Tindall & Cox, London, 1935.

Bone K. A systematic approach to Western herbal therapeutics. Modern Phytotherapist 1996;2:10–17.

Bone K, Burgess N. Methodology for prescribing herbal medicines. Modern Phytotherapist 1994;1:12–13.

Cole-King A, Harding KG. Psychological factors and delayed healing in chronic wounds. Psychosom Med 2001;63:216–220.

Fougére B. Healthy Dogs: A Handbook of Natural Therapies 2003.

Griggs B. *New Green Pharmacy: The Story of Western Herbal Medicne*. New York, NY: Random House; 1997.

Holmes P. Vitalism in Western and Chinese medicine. Eur J Herb Med 1997;3:37–40.

Mangin M. Observations of Jarisch-Herxheimer Reaction in Sarcoidosis Patients. JOIMR 2004;2(1):1

Mills S, Bone K. *Principles and Practice of Phytotherapy: Modern Herbal Medicine*. Edinburgh: Churchill Livingstone; 2000.

Moore M. *Herbal Energetics in Clinical Practice* (self-published). Available online at: http://www.swsbm.com. Accessed July 2005.

Panossian A, Wikman G, Wagner H. Plant adaptogens. III. Earlier and more recent aspects and concepts on their mode of action. Phytomedicine 1999;6:287–300.

Scudder TM. *Specific Diagnosis*. Portland, Ore: Eclectic Medical Publications; 1994. [reprint of 1874 edition]

Trickey R. The origins of disharmony. Modern Phytotherapist 1998;4:19–127.

Veterinary Herbal Medicine: A Systems-Based Approach

CHAPTER

Susan G. Wynn and Barbara J. Fougère

This chapter reviews traditional and scientific approaches to the use of herbal medicine in treating an array of conditions by system. Clinically, it is common to find more than one system affected, so it is important to consider the whole patient and not just the diagnosis or system. In this section formulas are offered as starting points; however, it is intended that they should be modified to match the needs of the individual patient wherever possible (see Chapter 19).

Frequently treatment with orthodox medicine has already been implemented. In the authors' experience herbal medicines can frequently be used alongside the conventional approach but can also be used instead in many instances, particularly for complicated or chronic conditions. Care should always be taken to consider possible drug-herb interactions and herb-herb interactions, dosing, and the vitality of the patient. Inexperienced veterinary herbalists are advised to cross reference with the monographs and chapters pertaining to prescribing and pharmacology. In many cases below, studies are described that involve experimental animal models and herb extracts (as opposed to whole herbs). It is important to maintain proper perspective on if and how these studies relate to clinical patients, whether they are safe in the species of interest, and how dosing of an herb might differ from doses described in the studies.

HERBS FOR BLOOD AND IMMUNOLOGIC DISORDERS

Of all the systems discussed in this section, the immune system is at once the most difficult and the most self-evident to treat. Practitioners are frequently asked how to "stimulate the immune system," yet herbalists and scientists alike realize that the complexity of immune function makes this effort at least naïve and at best inadvisable. Immune function represents an ecologic balance within the body that is attained with contributions from endocrine and neurologic activities. It has even been recognized that the "invaders" fought by the immune system are not all bad—we may even need our viruses to help us fend off the development of tumors and our bacteria to maintain normal immune function.

So any attempt to modify immune function must take into account the relationship between the patient and all functions of the immune system, as well as the environment and its microbial influences that interface with the forward defenses of the immune system. In this sense, traditional concepts of clinical disease and empirically determined treatments may be even more useful than evidence-based guidance, simply because our knowledge of the complexities of immune function is so limited. We truly must treat an entire patient, instead of bone marrow and secondary immune organs.

Similarly, disorders of the blood are about more than just the bone marrow. For instance, hyperlipidemia in people is surely not just a problem with the blood—it is a lifestyle problem in many cases. Although this section is all about blood and immune disorders, every condition that is listed requires a global approach to treatment. Herbs inherently provide complex actions that address more than one deranged process in the body.

Mechanisms of Interest

Adaptogens

These plants have been noted both traditionally and in human clinical trials and animal studies to increase resistance to stress, which predisposes animals to disease, including infection. Adaptogens generally work by modulating the hypothalamic-pituitary-adrenal axis, but many have other effects as well, such as modulation of immune function.

ASIAN GINSENG *(PANAX GINSENG)*: Hundreds of scientific papers have established that *Panax ginseng* has numerous clinical effects. In laboratory animals, these include central nervous system (CNS) stimulation; protection against exogenous damage from radiation, toxins, and infection; protection from physical and psychological stress; and an influence on carbohydrate and lipid metabolism and immune stimulation. All of these may bear on an animal's response to stress. Recently, investigators have developed rat models of stress that have resulted in measurable physical and chemical changes. In these studies, pretreatment with ginseng attenuated the stress-induced rise in corticosterone, hyperglycemia, immune suppression, increased adrenal gland weight, gastric ulceration, and other signs of chronic stress (Rai, 2003b; Kim, 2003). The dose in rats used in one study was 100 mg/kg of ginseng root powder (Rai, 2003b). The saponin-rich fraction of ginseng also reduced the secretion of catecholamines from bovine adrenal medullary chromaffin cells (Tachikawa, 2004).

American ginseng *(Panax quinquefolius)*: This herb is biochemically similar to *Panax ginseng;* however, the plant has not been studied as extensively as *P. ginseng.*

Bacopa *(Bacopa monnieri)*: Rai and colleagues (2003a) showed that a dose of 40 mg/kg of a standardized extract reversed stress-induced ulcer development, and higher doses (80 mg/kg) additionally prevented increases in adrenal gland weight in rats.

Eleuthero *(Eleutherococcus senticosis)*: Water extracts high in isofraxidin and eleutherosides B and E (especially E) reduced corticosterone levels in stressed mice (Kimura, 2004). On the contrary, in human athletes, Eleuthero slightly worsened a hormonal indicator of stress after 6 weeks of training. The athletes were administered 8 mL daily of a 33% hydroethanolic extract (Gaffney, 2001).

Cordyceps *(Cordyceps sinensis)*: This herb is not a well known adaptogen; nonetheless, one laboratory animal study suggests that it may have antistress properties. A hot water extract was administered to stressed rats (150 mg/kg daily), and investigators found that stress-induced changes in adrenal and thyroid gland weights, as well as changes in cholesterol and alkaline phosphatase, were suppressed (Koh, 2003).

Ashwagandha *(Withania somnifera)*: A standardized extract given to rats at 25 mg/kg and 50 mg/kg suppressed stress-induced changes in blood glucose levels, glucose intolerance, corticosterone levels, gastric ulceration, immunosuppression, and mental depression (Bhattacharya, 2003). A single withanolide, as well as a withanolide-free fraction, has shown adaptogenic activity in stress models (Kaur, 2003; Singh, 2003a).

Rhodiola *(Rhodiola rosea)*: Russian studies have long suggested that the root of this plant has adaptogenic activity. Two double-blind, placebo-controlled human clinical trials used an extract of *Rhodiola* and found significant improvements in cognitive functions, fatigue, and "neuromotoric tests" (Spasov, 2000; Darbinyan, 2000).

Other herbs: Other adaptogens include *Andrographis paniculata,* gotu kola, *Codonopsis pilosa,* licorice, and *Schisandra.*

Anticoagulant Herbs

Anticoagulation is a less common therapeutic strategy in veterinary medicine than in human medicine. Herbs with anticoagulant activity may be considered for animals at risk for thrombosis, such as cats with cardiomyopathy or dogs undergoing heartworm treatment or possibly for animals that are immobilized for long periods.

Dan Shen *(Salvia miltiorrhiza)*: According to in vitro and animal studies, this herb may have multiple effects, including interference with extrinsic blood coagulation, antithrombin III-like activity, inhibition of platelet aggregation, and promotion of fibrinolytic activity.

Other herbs: Herbs with antiplatelet activity include garlic *(Allium sativum),* turmeric *(Curcuma longa),* ginger *(Zingiber officinale), Plectranthus forskholi,* and *Salvia miltiorrhiza.*

Anti-inflammatory Herbs

Herbs with anti-inflammatory properties probably work through a large variety of mechanisms. Some are recognized cyclooxygenase (COX)-2 inhibitors, and others are not as well defined. The mechanisms of inflammation are reviewed more completely in the section on musculoskeletal herbs. In autoimmune conditions, anti-inflammatory herbs should be directed toward the organ involved; this is explored further in relevant sections of this text.

Blood Tonics

These herbs are used both for frank anemia and for the traditional Chinese medicine signs of "Blood Deficiency," which include dry and itchy skin, dream-disturbed sleep, dry coat, and dry eyes.

Dang Gui, Dong Quai *(Angelica sinensis)*: This is a traditional Chinese herb that is used to tonify as well as "invigorate" the blood. A case report in a human kidney patient with anemia who was resistant to erythropoietin treatment indicated that treatment with this herb improved hematologic measures (Bradley, 1999). Wang (2001) found that dang gui improved measures of erythrocyte deformability and fragility.

Rehmannia *(Rehmannia glutinosa)*: In traditional Chinese medicine, this herb is used to "cool" the Blood and is an important herb in treating Yin deficiency, which is seen, for example, in patients with diabetes. However, one Chinese study suggested that in people with chronic aplastic anemia, Rehmannia root could improve symptoms and recovery (Yuan, 1998). In anemic mice, the root appeared to enhance replication of certain bone marrow progenitor cells (Yuan, 1992).

Rhodiola *(Rhodiola rosacea)*: This is a European and Asian plant that has been used traditionally to treat anemia. In vitro studies have suggested that it protects human erythrocytes from damage caused by glutathione depletion and hemolysis that occurs via oxidation (De Sanctis, 2004). An extract appeared to stimulate replication of mouse bone marrow cells in vitro as well (Udintsev, 1991).

Other herbs: Other herbs suggested by traditional herbalists include Codonopsis, Nettle, and Ashwagandha. Herbs especially used for iron deficiency anemia include yellow dock, nettle, and parsley.

Immune Modulators

A Medline search on "immune" and "herbal" would suggest that a legion of plants may stimulate some aspect of immune function. The problem here is that most studies have been conducted in vitro or at best in experimental animals and most of these plants have not been used traditionally for immune support. The herbs described below give researchers plenty to explore and are those that are deemed most useful by herbalists. Immune stimulant herbs have been implicated in reactivation or worsening of autoimmune disease, and they should be used with caution in these patients (Lee, 2004c).

Medicinal Fungi: These are very likely to work in similar ways. Individual fungi are listed here:

- Reishi *(Ganoderma lucidum)*
- Maitake *(Grifola frondosa)*
- Shitake *(Lentinula edodes)*
- Turkey tail *(Trametes versicolor)*
- Cordyceps *(Cordyceps sinensis)*
- Hime-matsutake *(Agaricus blazei)*
- Chaga *(Inonotus obliquus)*

All these fungi contain polysaccharide complexes and sterols that appear to enhance cell-mediated immune function and that may have antitumor activity as well (Ooi, 2000; Wasser, 1999; Zhu, 1998b). Still, structural differences have been noted in some of the primary constituents, and it is possible that their activities in vivo are somewhat different. As a rule, polysaccharide complexes such as those found in medicinal fungi are more likely to be completely extracted in aqueous or dried preparations than in alcohol extracts.

ECHINACEA *(ECHINACEA SPP)*: Extracts have been shown to increase phagocytic activity in human peripheral monocytic cells, to promote production of various cytokines, and to enhance natural killer cell function, all of which involve the innate immune system as opposed to specific, adaptive processes. Most clinical studies in humans have involved upper respiratory infection and, in fact, Echinacea may shorten the duration of the common cold (Percival, 2000), depending on the form administered. Echinacea is often recommended for chronic recurrent viral upper respiratory infection in cats, and some practitioners use Echinacea to treat patients with retroviral infection. Although some practitioners caution against the long-term use of Echinacea because toxicity or autoimmune conditions may result, this concern has not been well documented. However, immunostimulants are probably best used as pulsed treatments if they are administered on a long-term basis, because full response to treatment is probably reached in a few weeks and does not continue to increase. In a 4-day observational study conducted at the Ohio Eclectic College in 1935, students were administered Echinacea before meals and at bedtime. Leukocyte counts increased 24 to 48 hours after initiation of treatment. Short-term (2- to 4-week), on-off administration is most sensible. The Echinacea monograph (see Chapter 24) describes studies in swine and horses that suggest immune modulating effects in these species.

ASTRAGALUS *(ASTRAGALUS MEMBRANACEUS)*: This traditional Chinese herb has been shown to increase T cell–mediated immune function in vitro in mice, as well as in uncontrolled trials in humans (Zhao, 1990; Sun, 1983; Yoshida, 1997).

GINSENG POLYSACCHARIDES AND SAPONINS: These have shown immunostimulating capacity in vitro and in animal models (Kitts, 2000). In one study, rats with chronic *Pseudomonas aeruginosa* lung infection were administered extracts of *Panax ginseng;* the treated group exhibited higher bacterial clearance and lower serum immunoglobulin levels than did the untreated group, which suggests enhancement of cell-mediated immunity (Song, 1998).

THUNDER GOD VINE *(TRIPTERYGIUM WILFORDII)*: This herb appears to be a true immune suppressant. Extracts of this plant have been investigated in human clinical trials for the treatment of rheumatoid arthritis, myasthenia gravis, lupus erythematosus, graft rejection, asthma, and other immune-mediated problems, generally with positive results (Tao, 2000; Tao, 2002). Various trials have shown reductions in interleukin (IL)-6, IL-5, IL-2, NF-kappaB, and CD 4+ levels, caused by an extract or by single constituents such as triptolide. In one trial, it was effective for rheumatoid arthritis when applied topically (Cibere, 2003). The plant has some toxicity, most notably causing infertility in both males and females.

OTHER HERBS: Other herbs used traditionally as immune stimulants include Eleuthero *(Eleutherococcus senticosis),* Schisandra *(Schisandra chinensis),* Privet *(Ligustrum lucidum),* Usnea *(Usnea barbath),* Thuja *(Thuja occidentalis),* Lomatium *(Lomatium dissectum),* and Baptisia. However, many others, including *Andrographis paniculata, Codonopsis pilosa, Ligusticum wallichii, Paeonia lactiflora, Phytolacca decandra, Picrorrhiza kurroa, Poria cocos,* Propolis, and *Uncaria tomentosa,* are employed as immune enhancers. Other plants that have been used as immune stimulants tend to be high in vitamins such as vitamin C (rosehips) and flavonoids (beet root, black currant).

Hemidesmus indicus and *Tylophora indica* may also have immune suppressant activity. The effect of an ethanolic extract of each herb was studied on delayed-type hypersensitivity, humoral response to sheep red blood cells, skin allograft rejection, and phagocytic activity of the reticuloendothelial system in mice. *Tylophora indica* appeared to stimulate phagocytic function while inhibiting the humoral component of the immune system. *Hemidesmus indicus* suppressed both cell-mediated and humoral components of the immune system (Atal, 1986).

Antihyperlipidemics

GARLIC *(ALLIUM SATIVUM)*: This herb has shown modest efficacy in lowering cholesterol and triglyceride levels in laboratory animals and people (Ackermann, 2001). Garlic has the potential for causing Heinz body anemia in dogs and especially in cats. Many veterinarians, however, use garlic for their patients and monitor blood parameters.

RED YEAST RICE *(MONASCUS PURPUREUS)*: This is a natural statin that has been shown to reduce cholesterol and triacylglycerol concentrations in controlled trials in humans (Heber, 1999). Similar to other statins, it may cause rhabdomyolysis. This author (SW) has observed a case of rhabdomyolysis in a dog who was being treated with both red yeast rice and gemfibrozil.

GUGULIPID *(COMMIPHORA MUKUL)*: This herb contains resins that have been shown to have cholesterol- and triglyceride-lowering activity in humans (Singh, 1994) and laboratory animals. However, the overall effect is mild to moderate compared with cholesterol-lowering drugs used in people (Caron, 2001).

GLOBE ARTICHOKE *(CYNARA SCOLYMUS)*: This herb has been shown in human clinical trials to lower cholesterol and triglycerides, at doses ranging from 900 to 1920 mg per day. Globe artichoke leaf extract not only increases choleresis and, therefore, cholesterol elimination, but it also has been shown to inhibit cholesterol biosynthesis (Kraft, 1997b). It is suggested that a possible mechanism of action might be the indirect inhibition of hydroxymethylglutaryl–CoA reductase (HMG-CoA) (Gebhardt, 1998). In vitro studies have documented a concentration-dependent inhibition of de novo cholesterol biosynthesis in cultured rat and human hepatocytes for globe artichoke leaf extract given at 0.03 to 0.1 mg/mL (Petrowicz, 1997).

Hemostatics

Many hemostatics in Western herbal medicine are astringent and exert their effects through direct contact with skin or mucous membranes to stop bleeding via a styptic action. The concept is different in Chinese medicine, where bleeding may be due to Excess Heat in the blood (so it should be cooled) or Blood Stasis (which causes bleeding by allowing blood to back up and subsequently "overflow," or extravasate, around the area of stasis). A bruise is an example of Blood Stasis, and hematochezia and epistaxis are often due to Blood Heat.

YUNNAN PAI YAO *(WHITE MEDICINE FROM YUNNAN PROVINCE)*: This is the most popular Chinese herbal formula in veterinary medicine for the control of hemorrhage. The formula contains San qi *(Panax notoginseng)*, an herb that has a reputation for being able to stop bleeding anywhere in the body. Other herbs in the formula (according to the label on a box purchased in 2005) are *Ajuga patantha, Dioscorea opposita, Dioscorea nipponica, Erodium stephanianum, Alpinia officinarum,* and *Dryobalanops aromatica* (or *Blumea balsamifera*). The formula is often guarded, and labels don't always provide an ingredient list, but it always contains pseudoginseng (San Qi or Tienchi) *Panax pseudoginseng,* and variously Chinese yam *(Dioscorea opposita),* yam rhizome *(Dioscorea hypolglauca),* sweet geranium *(Erodium stephanianum)* and galangal rhizome *(Alpinia officinarum)* (Polesuk, 1973). Yunnan bai yao has been shown to decrease both clotting times and prothrombin times (Ogle, 1977) and to initiate platelet release (Chew, 1977).

OTHER HERBS: Other herbs used as hemostatics include Horsetail *(Equisetum arvense),* Witch hazel *(Hamamelis virginiana),* Oak bark *(Quercus robur),* Nettle leaf *(Urtica dioica),* Lesser periwinkle *(Vinca minor),* Grape *(Vitis vinifera),* Rehmannia, and Trillium. Astringent herbs include agrimony *(Agrimonia eupatoria),* cranesbill *(Geranium maculatum),* and yarrow *(Achillea millefolium).*

A Chinese herbal formula, Wen-She decoction (WSD), resolved acute upper digestive tract hemorrhage in an open sequential controlled trial. It was concluded that WSD was an excellent treatment for hemorrhage of the upper digestive tract. WSD consists of *Codonopsis pilosa, Atractylodes macrocephala, Poria cocos, Glycyrrhiza uralensis, Zingiber officinale, Os sepia, Halloysitum rubrum,* and *Astragalus membranaceus* (Gong, 1989).

REVIEW OF SPECIFIC HEMATOLOGIC AND IMMUNOLOGIC CONDITIONS

Anemia, General

Therapeutic rationale

Anemia must be addressed by determining the cause, such as immune-mediated destruction, blood loss, or bone marrow suppression. Blood tonics may offer temporary support while the cause is addressed, and may even stimulate hematopoiesis.

A formula to build on might consist of a combination of blood tonics (Rehmannia and Dang gui), adaptogens (such as Rhodiola or Ashwagandha), and herbs that address the conventional diagnosis as well. Red root *(Ceanothus americanus)* has an indication for use with an enlarged spleen, which may be seen in autoimmune hemolytic anemia.

A prescription for anemia might include the following:

Dang gui	33% (circulatory stimulant, anti-inflammatory, vasodilator, antiallergic, warming)
Rhodiola	33% (immune modulating, adaptogen)
System- or organ-specific herb	33% (such as an astringent for gastrointestinal tract bleeding)

Autoimmune Disorders, General

Therapeutic rationale

- Reduce inflammation and tissue destruction at target organs.
- Modulate the inappropriate immune response.

Aside from Thunder God Vine, which has significant toxicity and is not widely available, few herbs address autoimmune disorders as a general class of medicine. *Hemidesmus indicus, Tylophora indica,* and *Stephania tetrandra* are immune suppressants that must be used very carefully by experienced herbalists. Ideally, the prescription addresses the underlying or perpetuating factors that contribute to the pathophysiology. Autoimmune disease may be precipitated by viral infection, so antiviral herbs may need to be used. Prescriptions generally include anti-inflammatory herbs, as well as those that address specific organ involvement and "leaky gut" (see later section on dermatologic herbs for more information). Herbs that enhance elimination should also be included. Immune-modulating herbs described earlier as immune stimulant are not always inappropriate but should be chosen with special attention to all of their purported effects. Focusing on maintaining systemic health rather than on suppressing the immune system is a worthwhile strategy, and herbal medicine is particularly useful when combined with the conventional treatment of autoimmune disease.

A prescription for autoimmune disease support follows:

Rehmannia	40%
Bupleurum	20%
Milk thistle	20%
Bilberry	20%

Coagulopathy and Bleeding

Therapeutic rationale

- Identify specific clotting defect and treat accordingly.

When coagulation defects cause signs of bleeding, possibly the most important herb to choose is yunnan pai yao. Hemostatic and astringent herbs may also address bleeding from gastrointestinal tract mucous membranes; in traditional herbal medicine, they may have systemic effects. These include yarrow, agrimony, and shepherd's purse. Red root *(Ceanothus americanus)* is also astringent and is indicated when the spleen is enlarged, as is often seen in some immune-mediated coagulopathies. Cinnamon was valued by the Eclectics, primarily for postpartum hemorrhage, but also for hemoptysis and bleeding that occurs elsewhere.

Hyperlipidemia

Therapeutic rationale

- Identify predisposing factors such as endocrinologic disorders, liver disease, and pancreatitis.
- Reduce dietary fat.
- Clear excess serum lipids.

Formulas that contain garlic, globe artichoke, guggul, and red yeast rice may be effective but should be combined with herbs that address any predisposing cause. In addition, herbalists may prescribe aids to digestion and biliary function, such as globe artichoke, dandelion root, prickly ash *(Zanthoxylum americanum)*, and calamus *(Acorus calamus)*. Some medicinal fungi, including Reishi, have also been shown to have antihyperlipidemic properties.

A prescription for hyperlipidemia (1) follows:

Garlic	5%
Guggul	30%
Reishi	25%
Dandelion	15%
Calamus	15%
Prickly ash	10%

A prescription for hyperlipidemia (2) is presented here:

Globe artichoke	60%
Dandelion root	30%
Garlic	10%

Herbal Treatment of Bleeding

Nonspecific Sign	Herb
Bleeding gums	Bilberry, Witch hazel
Hematemesis	Cranesbill, Yunnan pai yao
Hematuria	Yunnan pai yao, Rehmannia, Trillium
Hemoptysis	Bugleweed, Yunnan pai yao, Cinnamon
Gastric hemorrhage	Yarrow, Atractylodes, Agrimony, Plantain, Shepherd's purse, Cranesbill

Immune Deficiency or Suppression

Therapeutic rationale

- Identify causative factors (e.g., retroviral or other chronic disorders).

Patients with poor immunity should be prescribed herbs from three main groups:

1. **Immune-enhancing herbs.** Selection can be based on traditional notions of organ or system affinity, or may be combined according to their other effects on the body. Herbs to consider include Echinacea *(Echinacea purpurea, E. angustifolia, E. pallida)*, Astragalus *(Astragalus membranaceus)*, *Ligusticum walchii*, Pau d'arco *(Tabebuia avellanedae)*, Usnea *(Usnea barbata)*, *Picrorhiza kurroa*, Ginseng (*Panax* spp), and medicinal fungi such as Reishi mushroom *(Ganoderma lucidum)*, Maitake mushroom *(Grifola frondosa)*, Shitake mushroom *(Lentinus edodes)*, Turkey tail *(Trametes versicolor)*, and Cordyceps *(Cordyceps sinensis)*.
2. **Tonic and adaptogenic herbs.** These include Panax, Eleutherococcus, and Ashwagandha. As a general guide, stimulating herbs should be avoided during the acute phase of an infection. This is perhaps derived from traditional Chinese medicine, wherein stimulating and tonic herbs are contraindicated in Deficient Yin patterns with Heat signs—typically, fever and inflammation or infection. One study on Eleutherococcus showed that administration before induced listeriosis infection in rabbits and mice increased resistance to infection. However, when administration occurred simultaneously with an induced infection, the severity of disease was exacerbated (Farnsworth, 1966). Despite this, Eleutherococcus is frequently found in low doses in formulations for acute infection such as cold and flu.
3. **Bitter herbs.** Gentiana or any of the bitters described under the gastrointestinal system should be considered; these are generally cooling herbs. If the patient is cool or cold, the cooling effect should be countered with warming herbs. One of the proposed theories for the benefit of bitters is the general improvement that occurs in digestive function, hence enhanced gut-associated lymphoid tissue function. Better immunity at the gut level (T helper 3 cell mediated) helps to moderate and regulate T helper 1 and T helper 2 cells, thereby improving immune balance systemically.

Echinacea and Astragalus are two of the most popular "immune" herbs in human herbal medicine. Echinacea improves phagocytosis and generally enhances immune surveillance. It must be used in high doses during acute infections, such as infected wounds or viral infections. In humans, doses of 20 to 30 mL per day can be taken; it takes about 3 days for phagocytic activity to peak. Many studies that detract from the benefits of Echinacea are flawed by incorrect dosing and improper extract type. Echinacea can be used for chronic bacterial and viral infections, postviral syndromes, acquired immunodeficiency syndrome resulting from feline leukemia virus (FAIDS), in the appropriate formulas, autoimmune disease and long-term allergies and intolerances. It can be used during chemotherapy or pneumonia, and for chronic purulent or pyodermic skin infection—at relatively high doses in all cases (in humans, 15 mL per day for serious chronic states of immune deficiency). Doses as high as 40 mL on the first day followed by 16 mL daily were used in one positive clinical trial (Goel, 2004). Astragalus, on the other hand, is more appropriately used as a preventive measure during disease outbreaks or for chronic immune incompetence and autoimmune disease (especially nephritis). The dose in humans is between 20 and 40 mL per week. High dosing in the case of Echinacea is an important consideration because it does influence efficacy.

A prescription for general immune support follows:

Echinacea	40%
Oregon grape root	20%
Astragalus	20%
Licorice	20%

Infection

Infections are addressed in this text within the sections on specific systems or organs in which they occur. Herbalists generally develop formulas that combine antimicrobial activity, organ support, and immune stimulation (where appropriate). For instance, a formula for pneumonia might include antimicrobials such as thyme and sage, immune support from Astragalus and Echinacea, and expectorants such as elecampane and horehound. It should be noted that some of these herbs have multiple indications that magnify their effects on the respiratory tract (Thyme is both antimicrobial and expectorant, Echinacea is an immune stimulant and an antimicrobial, and Astragalus is an immune stimulant that is specifically associated with the lung in traditional Chinese medicine).

Herbal management of infections should include the following:

- Immune-enhancing herbs, whether acute or chronic.
- Organ support herbs (Milk thistle for the liver, Saw palmetto for the prostate, etc.).
- Herbs that act against specific microbes (fungal, bacterial, protozoal), if known. The activity of most antiseptic herbs is mild and most effective for dermatologic (topically) or gastrointestinal tract infection. Hydrastis is particularly indicated for gastrointestinal tract infection.
- Viral infection can be treated with Saint John's Wort (for enveloped viruses such as herpes, hepatitis, poxvirus, paramyxovirus, retrovirus, coronavirus). Thuja may be helpful against a range of viruses such as papovaviridae, poxviridae, picornaviridae, and bunyaviridae viruses.

Thrombocytopenia

Therapeutic rationale

- Identify platelet pathology.
- Suppress immune-mediated damage, if autoimmune in origin.
- Give blood or platelet transfusions.
- Administer anabolics to enhance regeneration.

No herbs specifically address thrombocytopenia; however, anecdotally, yunnan pai yao is effective in controlling resultant hemorrhage. (See also the section on coagulation disorders, earlier.)

Sheng xue ling

One formula that may be useful in treating idiopathic thrombocytopenic purpura is Sheng xue ling (SXL). In an open study in China, 86 human cases of ITP were divided randomly into two groups. A total of 56 patients were treated with SXL, and 30 patients were administered prednisone, each for 3 months. In the SXL group, the "total effective rate" at 3 months was 85.71%, similar to prednisone (83.33%), but at 6 months, efficacy for SXL was greater (91.07%) than that of the prednisone group (53.33%), without adverse reactions. Bleeding was alleviated; blood platelet count was increased; platelet-associated immunoglobulin and IL-4 dropped; natural killer cell activity increased; and T lymphocyte subsets gradually returned to normal level. All differences described here were statistically significant. The mechanism by which the formula might work was not identified (Zhou 2005).

HERBS FOR CANCER

General Considerations

Cancer biology is yet to be fully understood. Cellular mutation may occur as a result of free radical damage (with activation of oncogenes or suppression of tumor suppressor genes) and genetic susceptibility and toxicity (e.g., hepatopathogenic toxins). In traditional herbal medicine, cancer is nearly always viewed as a sign of systemic toxicity. However, immune dysregulation has to be considered, and can occur with stress, toxin, heavy metal and pesticide exposure, dysbiosis, hormonal imbalance, nutrient imbalance, infection, inflammation, and radiation. Chemotherapy is also a major cause of immune dysregulation; for example, vincristine is weakly myelosuppressive, and cyclophosphamide and glucocorticoids are strongly myelopsuppressive.

Many chemotherapeutic drugs currently in use in medicine were first identified in plants, including taxol, vinblastine and vincristine, and etoposide and teniposide (Boik, 1996). Herbs offer a rational potential in the treatment of cancer in animals; however, it is important to note that herbs may be used for purposes other than direct antitumor activity. On the other hand, just about any selection of herbs prescribed to treat a patient will more than likely have some anticancer activity because of the presence of widely occurring anticancer constituents like flavonoids.

Although little research has been conducted in cats and dogs specifically, a plethora of research pertains to rats, mice, hamsters, and guinea pigs. At least pocket pets are amply catered to if they are diagnosed with cancer! Herbs can be used to help manage the effects of chemotherapy; to assist in recuperation after chemotherapy, radiation, or surgery; to complement conventional cancer treatment; to provide an alternative to conventional treatment in some cases; to assist in cancer prevention; and to support various systems that are affected by cancer. One of the approaches used by veterinary herbalists is to treat cancer as a chronic disease, with emphasis on improving the health of the whole body, regardless of the presence of cancer. Anecdotal evidence from veterinary herbalists indicates that herbs offer improved quality of life and may support remission in some cases.

The rational use of herbal medicine for the treatment of patients with cancer depends on a growing understanding of the biological mechanisms by which cancer cells proliferate, maintain life, and die. These include differentiation (the maturation process of cells), angiogenesis (the growth of new blood vessels into tumors), apoptosis (programmed cell death), invasion (the spread of the tumor mass into adjacent tissue), metastasis (the spread of tumor cells to distant locations), mitosis (the proliferation of cells), and evasion of the immune system. As these mechanisms have become elucidated, their weak points have been identified and have become the targets of research that is both conventional and complementary (Boik, 1996). The selection of several herbs that have different mechanisms of action provides a broad spectrum of anticancer activity. A holistic strategy that incorporates all elements discussed here is proposed under "Review of Strategies for Cancer Prescriptions" at the end of this section.

Targets Unique to Neoplastic Cells for Cancer Therapy

- Genetic instability
- Abnormal transcription factor activity
- Abnormal signal transduction
- Abnormal cell-to-cell communication
- Abnormal angiogenesis
- Invasion and metastasis
- Abnormal immune function

Mechanisms of Interest

Antineoplastic/cytotoxic actions

It is logical to select herbs is on the basis of cancer biology. An extremely comprehensive review of anticancer plants and natural compounds is provided in John Boik's book, *Natural Compounds in Cancer Therapy* (2001). This book explains in great detail the mechanisms of action of many plants and their constituents. It is important to note that most herbs have many actions, and this list is merely indicative of the wide range of such mechanisms that have been documented. (Search Medline for more information; use the herb name and cancer or activity as search terms.)

Boik highlights the importance of synergism as a strategy by which lower doses can be used without reduced efficacy; he also discusses the use of herbs with different antineoplastic mechanisms for targeting events that take place in the progression of cancer. Choosing compounds that have direct-acting, indirect-acting, and immune-stimulating activities is likely to inhibit procancer events. Constituents like flavonoids can target multiple aspects of tumor biology.

Adaptogens

This strategy recognizes that a patient can live with cancer as opposed to having to die of cancer. Many of our elderly animal patients, in particular, have never been in better health than when they are on herbal and nutritional treatment, even though they have cancer, because the prescriptions that they are given promote overall health. Herbs should be used to strengthen body resistance, and vitality is enhanced through the use of adaptogens. Most adaptogens also have anticancer activity.

ASTRAGALUS ***(ASTRAGALUS MEMBRANACEUS):*** Astragalus induces cell differentiation and cell death in vitro (Cheng, 2004) and exerts anticarcinogenic effects through activation of cytotoxic activity and the production of cytokines in mice (Kurashige, 1999).

ASHWAGANDHA ***(WITHANIA SOMNIFERA):*** The antitumor and radiosensitizing effects of *Withania* have been studied. Growth of carcinoma in mice was inhibited and survival increased with *Withania* treatment, especially when it was combined with radiation (Sharada, 1996). When given before irradiation, it synergistically increased survival, even in mice with advanced tumors (Devi, 1995). Complete regression of sarcoma in mice caused by *Withania* root extract was observed (Devi, 1992).

ELEUTHERO ***(ELEUTHEROCOCCUS SENTICOSIS):*** This herb was able to inhibit tumor growth and prolong survival time in tumor-bearing mice; these effects were significantly related to enhanced immune response (Xie, 1989). Siberian ginseng appeared to reduce the quantity of conventional antimetabolites that were needed to attain antiproliferative effects on tumor cells in vitro (Hacker, 1984).

ASIAN GINSENG ***(PANAX GINSENG):*** This herb induces cell differentiation, reduces the effects of chemical carcinogens, mitigates inflammatory carcinogenesis, induces apoptosis, inhibits proliferation, and has proved beneficial in the treatment of a number of cancers in humans (Helms, 2004).

Immune Modulators

Most conventional chemotherapeutic agents are immunosuppressant and cytotoxic in nature, and they exert a variety of adverse effects that are particularly evident in cancer chemotherapy. Botanically based immunomodulators and immune stimulators are employed as supportive or adjuvant therapy to overcome the adverse effects of these agents and to restore normal health. Many of these herbs also have anticancer activity.

Anticancer Mechanism of Selected Herbs and Constituents

Apoptosis Inducers
- Greater celandine *(Chelidonium majus)* (Note: This is a very strong herb that is usually administered topically.)
- Baical skullcap *(Scutellaria baicalensis)*
- Bupleurum *(Bupleurum falcatum)*
- Boswellia *(Boswellia serrata)*
- Turmeric *(Curcuma longa)*
- Saint John's Wort *(Hypericum perforatum)*
- Garlic *(Allium sativum)*
- Flavonoids (apigenin, luteolin, genistein, quercetin, reversatrol)

Differentiation Inducers
- Burdock *(Articum lappa)*
- Boswellia *(Boswellia serrata)*
- Berberine
- Flavonoids (reversatrol, apigenin, luteolin, genistein, quercetin)
- Emodin

Cytotoxic Agents
- Mistletoe *(Viscum album)*
- Limonene
- Emodium

Inhibitors of Angiogenesis
These include herbs and constituents that inhibit increased vascular permeability, or that beneficially affect prostanoid and leukotriene systhesis, or that inhibit mast cell degranulation.
- Butcher's broom *(Ruscus aculeatus)*
- Gotu kola *(Centella asiatica)*
- Horse chestnut *(Aesculus hippocastanum)*
- Garlic *(Allium sativum)*
- Turmeric *(Curcuma longa)*
- Siberian ginseng *(Eleutherococcus senticosis)*
- Ginkgo *(Ginkgo biloba)*
- Picrorrhiza *(Picrorrhiza kurroa)*
- Flavonoids (including proanthocyanidins, anthocyanidins, reversatrol, genistein, apigenin, luteolin, quercetin)
- Emodium

Inhibitors of Local Invasion
These are herbs or constituents that inhibit hyaluronidase and its assistant enzymes or elastase, or that affect collagen or cell migration.
- Gotu kola *(Centella asiatica)*
- Horse chestnut *(Aesculus hippocastanum)*
- Butcher's broom *(Ruscus aculeatus)*
- Turmeric *(Curcuma longa)*
- Panax *(Panax ginseng)*
- Hawthorn (*Crataegus* spp)
- Bilberry *(Vaccinium myrtillus)*
- Dong quai *(Angelica sinensis)*
- Flavonoids (proanthocyanidins, anthocyanidins, apigenin, reversatrol, genistein, luteolin, quercetin)
- Mushroom polysaccharides
- Emodin
- Boswellic acids

Inhibitors of Metastasis
These are herbs or constituents that have anticoagulant activity.
- Aloe succus *(Aloe vera)*
- Green tea *(Camellia sinensis)*
- Cordyceps *(Cordyceps sinensis)*
- Reishi mushrooms *(Ganoderma lucidum)*
- Garlic *(Allium sativum)*
- Panax *(Panax ginseng)*
- Astragalus *(Astragalus membranaceus)*
- Dong quai *(Angelica sinensis)*
- Feverfew *(Tanacetum parthenium)*
- Dan shen *(Salvia miltiorrhiza)*
- Turmeric *(Curcuma longa)*
- Flavonoids (including reversatrol, anthocyanidins, genistein, apigenin, luteolin, quercetin)
- Emodium

Immune-modulating herbs can also be employed when chemotherapy is not used. (See "Immune System Herbs" earlier in this chapter or refer to individual monographs in this book for additional details.)

CORDYCEPS *(CORDYCEPS SINENSIS):* Controlled, open-label clinical studies have found that Cordyceps appeared to restore immune cell function in patients with advanced cancer who were given conventional cancer therapies (Zhou, 1995; Zhu, 1998b). Of 59 patients with advanced lung cancer, 95% were able to complete chemotherapy and radiotherapy with the use of Cordyceps compared with 64% of controls. More than 85% of Cordyceps-treated patients showed more normal blood cell counts versus 59% of controls (Zhu, 1998b). A study in patients with various types of tumors found that a cultured mycelium extract of Cordyceps (6 g/d for over 2 months) improved subjective symptoms in most patients. White blood cell counts were maintained at $<3000/mm^3$, and tumor size was significantly reduced in approximately half of patients (Zhu, 1998b).

ECHINACEA *(ECHINACEA PURPUREA):* Mice who received dietary Echinacea daily throughout life, from youth until late middle age, demonstrated significant longevity/survival differences, as well as differences in various populations of immune/hematopoietic cells. Key immune cells, acting as the first line of defense against developing neoplasms and natural killer (NK) cells, were significantly elevated in absolute number in their bone marrow production site, as well as in the spleen. Cells of the myeloid/granulocyte lineages remained at control levels in the bone marrow and the spleen in Echinacea-consuming mice. Thus, it appears that regular intake of Echinacea may indeed be beneficial or prophylactic because it maintains elevated levels of NK cells, which are elements in immunosurveillance against spontaneously developing tumors (Brousseau, 2005).

ASTRAGALUS ***(ASTRAGALUS MEMBRANACEUS):*** The efficacy of this herb in enhancing quality of life and reducing the toxicity of chemotherapy in human patients with malignant tumors was investigated. Astragalus (by injection) supplemented by chemotherapy was noted to inhibit the development of tumors, decrease the toxic or adverse effects of chemotherapy, elevate immune function, and improve quality of life in treated patients (Duan, 2002).

ASHWAGANDHA ***(WITHANIA SOMNIFERA):*** This herb demonstrates antitumor properties in mice and protects against induced carcinogenic effects. It also reverses the adverse effects of a carcinogen (urethane) on total leukocyte count, lymphocyte count, body weight, and mortality (Singh, 1986). Significant increases in hemoglobin; red blood cell, white blood cell, and platelet count; and body weight were observed in cyclophosphamide-, azathioprine-, and prednisolone-treated mice that were given *Withania* versus controls (Ziauddin, 1996).

OTHER HERBS

- Siberian ginseng *(Eleutherococcus senticosis)*
- Cat's claw *(Uncaria tomentosa)*
- Pau d'arco *(Tabebuia avellanedae)*
- Shitake and Reishi mushrooms

Alteratives

In traditional herbal medicine, alteratives represent a key strategy for the treatment of cancer. Alteratives act through the lymphatic, blood, and eliminatory systems to facilitate and enhance the breakdown and removal of metabolic wastes. They are also used to improve the absorption and assimilation of nutrients. Alteratives are thus considered to be "blood purifiers" or "detoxifiers", believed to circulate and improve blood flow, while removing waste from blood and lymph. The function of these herbs is to optimize the body's eliminative functions performed via the liver, kidneys, lungs, and gastrointestinal system.

Ideally, these herbs are chosen according to their other actions and affinities for particular organs or systems, so as to maximize their benefit. For example, poke root and cleavers are specific for the lymphatic system. Many of these herbs contain alkaloids and flavonoids and have documented anticancer activity; many others have not been studied. Modifying prescriptions every 2 to 3 months reduces the risk of potential toxicity associated with some of these herbs.

Alteratives include the herbs listed here:

BURDOCK ***(ARTICUM LAPPA):*** Differentiation-inducing activities have been demonstrated against mouse myeloid leukemia cells. The most active derivative induced more than half of leukemia cells to become phagocytic cells (Umehara, 1996).

DANDELION ROOT ***(TARAXACUM OFFICINALE):*** In vitro antitumor activity has been documented for an aqueous extract of dandelion. The mechanism of action was thought to be similar to that of tumor polysaccharides such as lentinan (Baba, 1981).

SHEEP SORREL ***(RUMEX ACETOSELLA):*** One study found that *Rumex acetosella* polysaccharide displayed antitumor activity in mice that were implanted with sarcoma (180 solid tumors) (Ito, 1986).

OREGON GRAPE ***(MAHONIA AQUIFOLIUM):*** Berberine has anticancer activity and exhibits the ability to induce apoptosis in leukemia cells (Kuo, 1995; Yang, 1996). In addition, some protoberberines are highly effective as cytotoxic agents against several carcinoma lines; berberine consistently showed the highest cytotoxicity among the alkaloids tested (Cernakova, 2002).

OTHER HERBS

- Barberry *(Berberis vulgaris)*
- Echinacea *(Echinacea pupurea)*
- Stillingia *(Stillingia sylvatica)*
- Yellow dock *(Rumex crispus)*
- Poke root *(Phytolacca decandra)*
- Cleavers *(Gallium aparine)*
- Red clover *(Trifolium pratense)*

Antioxidants

Herbs with potent antioxidant activity generally have anticancer activity as well. Whether to use antioxidants concurrently with chemotherapy or radiotherapy has been questioned. Chemotherapy and radiotherapy cause DNA damage to both normal cells and cancer cells by causing free radical damage; one concern is that antioxidants will reduce the efficacy of treatment. On the other hand, antioxidants protect healthy tissue from damage, and after and between conventional treatment, antioxidants continue to offer benefit as anticancer agents themselves. Anecdotal evidence provided by veterinary herbalists indicates that herbal antioxidants can continue to be used alongside conventional treatment without adversely affecting the outcome.

GREEN TEA ***(CAMELLIA SINENSIS):*** Green tea polyphenols in mice increased antioxidant levels and glutathione peroxidase, catalase, and quinine reductase in skin, small bowel, liver, and lungs. These combined activities make green tea an effective chemopreventive agent against the initiation, promotion, and progression of multistage carcinogenesis (Katiyar, 1997). Human clinical trials suggest that the concentrated extract EGCG (epigallocatechin gallate), dosed at approximately 200 mg daily, is most efficient at improving blood antioxidant levels.

REDGRAPE ***(VITIS VINIFERA):*** Resveratrol, a phytoalexin found in red wine, inhibits the metabolic activation of carcinogens, has antioxidant and anti-inflammatory properties, decreases cell proliferation, and induces apoptosis (Bianchini, 2003; Granados-Soto, 2003). Oligomeric proanthocyanidins (OPCs) increased NK cell cytotoxicity, modulated levels of interleukins from immune compromised mice (including those infected with retrovirus) (Cheshier, 1996), and demonstrated antimutagenic activity in vitro (Seo, 2001).

HAWTHORN ***(CRATAEGUS SPP):*** Crataegus contains OPCs, and much of what is known about grape seed extract applies to Crataegus.

MILK THISTLE ***(SILYBUM MARIANUM):*** Silymarin and silibinin (silybin) are antioxidants that react with free radicals, transforming them into more stable, less reactive compounds (Morazzoni, 1995). The cancer chemoprevention and anticarcinogenic effects of silymarin have been shown to be caused by its major constituent, silibinin (Bhatia, 1999). Its antitumor effect occurs primarily at stage I tumor promotion; silymarin may act by inhibiting COX-2 and IL-1α (Zhao, 1999). Such effects may involve inhibition of promoter-induced edema, hyperplasia, the proliferation index, and the oxidant state (Lahiri-Chatterjee, 1999). Silibinin may also have anti-angiogenic effects (Yang, 2005; Singh, 2005).

TURMERIC ***(CURCUMA LONGA):*** The abilities of turmeric to scavenge radicals, reduce iron complex, and inhibit peroxidation may explain the possible mechanisms by which turmeric exhibits its beneficial effects in medicine (Tilak, 2004). The anticancer properties of curcumin have been demonstrated in cultured cells and animal studies. Curcumin inhibits lipoxygenase activity and is a specific inhibitor of COX-2 expression. It halts carcinogenesis by inhibiting cytochrome P450 enzyme activity and increasing levels of glutathione-S-transferase (Chauhan, 2002).

DAN SHEN ***(SALVIA MILTIORRHIZA):*** Dan shen is a potent antioxidant that demonstrates free radical scavenging activity (Xia, 2003). Recent studies showed that one of its tanshinone constituents possesses cytotoxic activity against many kinds of human carcinoma cell lines, induces differentiation and apoptosis, and inhibits invasion and metastasis of cancer cells. Its mechanisms are believed to be inhibition of DNA synthesis and proliferation of cancer cells; regulation of the expression of genes related to proliferation, differentiation, and apoptosis; inhibition of the telomerase activity of cancer cells; and change in the expression of cellular surface antigen (Yuan, 2003).

BILBERRY ***(VACCINIUM MYRTILLUS):*** The anthocyanosides in bilberry inhibit protein and lipid oxidation (Morazzoni, 1995). Components of bilberry have been reported to exhibit potential anticarcinogenic activity in vitro, as demonstrated by inhibition of the induction of ornithine decarboxylase (ODC) by the tumor promoter phorbol 12-myristate 13–acetate (TPA) (Bomser, 1996).

SCHISANDRA ***(SCHISANDRA CHINENSIS):*** Schisandra lignans act as free radical scavengers and inhibit iron-induced lipid peroxidation and superoxide anion production (Lu, 1992). Geranylgeranoic acid, a constituent of Schisandra, has been shown to induce apoptosis in a human hepatoma–derived cell line (Shidoji, 2004).

GINKGO ***(GINKGO BILOBA):*** This leaf extract has significant antioxidant activity because of its flavonoid and terpenoid components. Recent studies with various models show that the anticancer properties of Ginkgo are related to antioxidant, antiangiogenic, and gene-regulatory actions. Antiangiogenic activity may involve antioxidant activity and the ability to inhibit both inducible and endothelial forms of nitric oxide synthase. Exposure of human breast cancer cells to a Ginkgo extract altered expression of the genes involved in the regulation of cell proliferation, cell differentiation, or apoptosis. Exposure of human bladder cancer cells to a Ginkgo extract produces an adaptive transcriptional response that augments antioxidant status and inhibits DNA damage. Flavonoid and terpenoid constituents of Ginkgo extracts may act in a complementary manner to inhibit several carcinogenesis-related processes; therefore, the total extracts may be required for optimal effects (DeFeudis, 2003).

GINGER ***(ZINGIBER OFFICINALE):*** Some pungent constituents in ginger and other zingiberaceous plants such as gingerol have potent antioxidant and anti-inflammatory effects, and some of them exhibit antitumor promotional activity in experimental carcinogenesis (Surh, 1998). The chemopreventive effects are probably associated with antioxidative and anti-inflammatory activities (Surh, 1998).

ROSEMARY ***(ROSMARINUS OFFICINALIS):*** Several extracts and constituents of rosemary have exhibited antioxidant activity (ESCP, 1999). The volatile oil was reported to be toxic to leukemia cells (Ilarionova, 1992). Topical administration of a methanol extract 5 minutes before application of carcinogens to the dorsal surface of mice reduced the irritation and promotion of tumors. Application of rosemary extract before carcinogen application reduced the formation of metabolite–DNA adducts by 30% and 54%, respectively (Huang, 1994). In rats, dietary supplementation with 1% rosemary extract for 21 weeks reduced the development of induced mammary carcinoma in the treated group, compared with the control group (40% vs 75%, respectively) (Singletary, 1991).

Analgesics

Cancer patients suffering pain may be administered anti-inflammatory, antispasmodic, and analgesic herbs as necessary. A review of these herbs can be found in the section on neurology, pain, and behavior.

Platelet-Activating Factor Inhibitors

Platelet-activating factor (PAF) is an ether-linked phospholipid that has been postulated to be a stimulator of malignant tumor growth; it may be significant in the early stages of tumor development.

GINKGO ***(GINKGO BILOBA):*** Ginkgolides have been reported to competitively inhibit the binding of PAF to its membrane receptor (Braquet, 1987).

Anticachectic Activity

COPTIS ***(COPTIS CHINENSIS):*** This herb was investigated in mice bearing colon carcinoma cells that cause IL-6–related cachexia after cell injection. Coptis significantly attenuated weight loss in tumor-bearing mice compared with controls, without changing food intake or tumor growth. It was therefore shown to exert an anticachectic effect associated with tumor IL-6 production, and it was suggested that this effect might be due to berberine (Iizuka, 2002).

Anticancer Action by Organ/System

Following is a brief review of just some of the herbs that may be beneficial for the treatment of particular organ/system cancers. It is intended as a starting point rather than a comprehensive review. In vivo studies are discussed; herbs that are supported by in vitro studies are only listed.

Respiratory system: small cell lung carcinoma

CHASTE TREE ***(VITEX AGNUS-CASTUS):*** Metastasis (Ohyama, 2003).

GRAPE SEED ***(VITIS VINIFERA):*** Oral administration of grapeseed extract reduced the number of metastatic nodules induced in mice by 26.07% compared with a control group treated with ethanol (Martinez 2005).

GREEN TEA AND BLACK TEA ***(CAMELLIA SINENSIS):*** Consumption of tea (Camellia sinensis) has been suggested to prevent cancer, heart disease and other diseases. Animal studies have shown that tea and tea constituents inhibit carcinogenesis of the skin, lung, oral cavity, esophagus, stomach, liver, prostate and other organs (Lambert 2003). For example, mice were given decaffeinated green or decaffeinated black tea in their drinking water before, during, and after treatment with a carcinogen. Mice that received 0.63% or 1.25% green tea, or 1.25% black tea, exhibited a reduction in liver tumor numbers of 54%, 50%, and 63%, and a decrease in the mean number of lung tumors of 40%, 46%, and 34%, respectively, compared with controls (Cao 1996). In some experiments, reduction in tumor number and size has been observed in the tea-treated groups; in other experiments, decreased tumor incidence has also been observed (Yang 2005). Black tea preparations have been shown to reduce the incidence and number of spontaneously generated lung adenocarcinomas and rhabdomyosarcomas in mice; they also were noted to inhibit the progression of lung adenoma to adenocarcinoma. In many of these experiments, tea consumption resulted in reduced body fat and body weight; these factors may also contribute to the inhibition of tumorigenesis (Yang, 2005).

CRUCIFEROUS VEGETABLES: Feeding mice diets enriched in dried cruciferous vegetables (cabbage and collards) resulted in a significant decrease in the number of pulmonary metastases after the animals had been injected intravenously with mammary tumor cells. Cruciferous vegetables may be beneficial in cancer prevention (Scholar, 1989).

FLAXSEED ***(LINUM USITATISSIMUM):*** Mice were fed a basal diet, or the basal diet supplemented with 2.5%, 5%, or 10% flaxseed, for 2 weeks before and after an intravenous injection of 0.75×10^5 melanoma cells. The median number of tumors in mice fed the 2.5%, 5%, and 10% flaxseed-supplemented diets was 32%, 54%, and 63% lower, respectively, than that in controls. The addition of flaxseed to the diet also caused a dose-dependent decrease in tumor cross-sectional area and tumor volume. Flaxseed reduces metastasis and inhibits the growth of metastatic secondary tumors in animals (Yan, 1998).

Reproductive system: mammary carcinoma

CALENDULA ***(CALENDULA OFFICINALIS):*** In a study of mice fed for 3 weeks a diet containing a calendula extract (high in the carotenoid lutein), mammary tumor cells were infused into the mammary glands. Tumor latency increased and tumor growth was inhibited in a dose-dependent manner by dietary lutein. In addition, dietary lutein was reported to enhance lymphocyte proliferation (Chew, 1996).

CHASTE TREE ***(VITEX AGNUS-CASTUS):*** (Ohyama, 2003).

GARLIC ***(ALLIUM SATIVUM):*** Organosulphur compounds markedly inhibited growth of canine mammary cells in culture (Sundaram, 1993).

GRAPESEED: Procyanidins in grapeseed could be used as chemopreventive agents against breast cancer through suppression of in situ estrogen biosynthesis (Eng, 2003).

MILK THISTLE ***(SILYBUM MARIANUM):*** (Bhatia, 1999).

FLAXSEED ***(LINUM USITATISSIMUM):*** This herb is the richest source of lignans and α-linolenic acid; it was investigated regarding its effects on the growth and metastasis of established human breast cancer in a mice model. Compared with controls, those supplemented with 10% flaxseed showed a significant reduction in tumor growth rate and a 45% reduction in total incidence of metastasis. Lung metastasis incidence was 55.6% in the control group and 22.2% in the flaxseed group; the incidence of lymph node metastasis was 88.9% in controls and 33.3% in the flaxseed group. Metastatic lung tumor number was reduced by 82% in the flaxseed group. It was concluded that flaxseed inhibits human breast cancer growth and metastasis in a mouse model, and that this effect is due in part to the downregulation of insulin-like growth factor I and epidermal growth factor receptor expression (Chen, 2002).

Urogenital system

Kidney Cancer

BLACK CUMIN ***(NIGELLA SATIVA):*** This herb provides a chemopreventive effect against induced renal carcinogenesis. Treatment of rats orally with black cumin (50 and 100 mg/kg body weight) resulted in significant decreases in blood urea nitrogen and serum creatinine, as well as in the incidence of tumors (Khan, 2005).

MISTLETOE ***(VISCUM ALBUM):*** Extracts of mistletoe plant have been used for decades in cancer therapy for nonspecific stimulation of the immune system. Mistletoe lectin has been identified as the active principle with cytotoxic and immunomodulatory potencies. An aqueous mistletoe extract was investigated in renal cell carcinoma, colon carcinoma, and testicular carcinoma. After induction of these tumors, mice were treated with the extract at dose levels corresponding to 0, 0.3, 3, 30, or 300 ng mL/kg/d by the intraperitoneal or subcutaneous route for 4 consecutive weeks. Significant tumor growth inhibition was observed with these carcinomas at 30 and 300 ng mL/kg/d (Burger, 2001).

Astragalus (*Astragalus membranaceus*) and Cnidium (*Ligustrum lucidum*): Renal cell carcinomas were planted in mice. One group was treated intraperitoneally daily for 10 days with 100 microliters of phytochemicals that contained 500 micrograms each of *Astragalus membranaceus* and *Ligustrum lucidum;* the other group (controls) received saline. A "cure rate" of 57% was obtained with these phytochemicals, which may have exerted their antitumor effects via augmentation of phagocyte and lymphokine-activated killer (LAK) cell activities (Lau, 1994).

Bladder Cancer

Kava (*Piper methysticum*): Flavokawains identified in kava cause strong antiproliferative and apoptotic effects in human bladder cancer cells. The anticarcinogenic effects of flavokawain A were evident in the inhibitory growth (57% inhibition) of bladder tumor cells in a nude mouse model (Zi, 2005).

Garlic (*Allium sativum*): *Allium sativum* was investigated in induced transitional cell carcinoma in mice. Orally administered *Allium sativum* was tested at doses of 5 mg, 50 mg, and 500 mg per 100 mL of drinking water. Mice that received 50 mg/dl oral *Allium sativum* demonstrated significant reductions in tumor volume when compared with controls, and mice that received 500 mg/dl oral *Allium sativum* exhibited significant reductions in both tumor volume and mortality (Riggs, 1997).

Prostate Cancer

Saint John's Wort (*Hypericum perforatum*): The antiproliferative effects of serotonin reuptake inhibitors and serotonin antagonists have been demonstrated in prostate tumors. Because Saint John's Wort components act as serotonin reuptake inhibitors and exert cytotoxic effects on several human cancer cell lines, the effects of treatment with Saint John's Wort extract on the growth of human prostate cancer cells in vitro and in vivo were examined. This study highlighted a significant reduction in tumor growth and in the number of metastases, suggesting that Saint John's Wort may be useful in the treatment of patients with prostate cancer (Martarelli, 2004).

Milk Thistle (*Silybum marianum*): (Bhatia, 1999).

Red Clover (*Trifolium pratense*): (Jarred, 2002).

Neurologic system

Boswellia (*Boswellia serrata*): Two observational reports of patients undergoing treatment for brain tumor suggest that boswellia extract may assist in reducing cerebral edema (Streffer, 2001; Janssen, 2000). Experimental and in vitro studies showed that boswellia extract may slow growth and increase apoptosis of tumor cells implanted in the brains of experimental animals (Winking, 2000).

Cannabis (*Cannabis sativa*): Gliomas are brain tumors that are common in humans. Several studies have shown that cannabinoids—active components of the plant *Cannabis sativa* and their derivatives—slow the growth of different types of tumors, including gliomas, in laboratory animals. Cannabinoids induce apoptosis of glioma cells in culture and inhibit angiogenesis in vivo. It is remarkable that cannabinoids kill glioma cells selectively and can protect nontransformed glial cells from death (Velasco, 2004).

Aloe Vera and Melatonin: A clinical study evaluated whether the concomitant administration of aloe may enhance the therapeutic results of melatonin in patients with advanced solid tumor for whom no effective standard anticancer therapies are available. This study included 50 patients with lung cancer, gastrointestinal tract tumor, breast cancer, or brain glioblastoma, who were treated with melatonin alone (20 mg/d orally in the dark period) or melatonin plus *Aloe vera* tincture (1 mL twice/d). The percentage of nonprogressing patients was significantly higher in the group treated with melatonin plus aloe than in the melatonin group (14/24 vs 7/26). The 1-year survival percentage was significantly higher in patients treated with melatonin plus aloe (9/24 vs 4/26). Both treatments were well tolerated. The combination may produce some therapeutic benefits, at least in terms of stabilization of disease and survival, in patients with advanced solid tumor, for whom no other standard effective therapy is available (Lissoni, 1998).

Mistletoe (*Viscum album*): Patients with malignant glioma were prospectively enrolled in a clinical trial. The treatment group received a galactoside-specific lectin from mistletoe, called ML-1. Analyses of all patients revealed prolongation of relapse-free intervals/overall survival time for the treatment group as compared with the control group (Lenartz, 2000).

Musculoskeletal system

Osteosarcoma

Red Clover (*Trifolium pratense* L.): Extracts were tested for their ability to stimulate the activity and maturation of osteoblastic osteosarcoma cells. Alkaline phosphatase was chosen as a marker of osteoblasticity. In vitro data clearly suggest a role for red clover isoflavonoids (Chloroform extract) in the stimulation of osteoblastic cell activity and cell differentiation (Wende, 2004).

Diosgenin (Found in Trillium, Fenugreek, and Wild Yam): This phytochemical was investigated in vitro to determine its effects on proliferation rate, cell cycle distribution, and apoptosis in the human osteosarcoma cell line. Diosgenin treatment resulted in inhibition of cell growth, with a cycle arrest in G1 phase, apoptosis induction, and induced cyclooxygenase activity (Moalic, 2001).

Pokeweed (*Phytolacca americana*): The plant hemitoxin, pokeweed antiviral protein (PAP), was conjugated to pokeweed extract (TP-3) to produce an immunotoxin that was highly active against osteosarcoma. In vitro studies suggest that it may be useful in the treatment of patients with osteosarcoma and some soft tissue sarcomas (Anderson, 1995). In vivo, TP-3 elicits potent antitumor activity in a hamster cheek pouch model of human osteosarcoma. At nontoxic dose levels, it significantly delays the emergence and progression of leg tumors and markedly improves tumor-free survival in severe combined immunodeficient mice challenged with human osteosarcoma cells. Thus, it may be useful in the treatment of patients with osteosarcoma (Ek, 1998).

Fibrosarcoma

Wormwood *(Artemisia annua)*: This herb contains artemisinin, which has been shown to selectively kill cancer cells in vitro and retard the growth of implanted fibrosarcoma tumors in rats. In vitro, it rapidly induces apoptosis in cancer cells (Singh, 2004).

Aloe *(Aloe vera)*: Acemannan is the name given to the major carbohydrate fraction obtained from the gel of the *Aloe vera* leaf. Injection of acemannan has been shown to offer increased immune protection against implanted malignant tumor cells (Merriam, 1995). Acemannan in the presence of interferon-gamma (IFN-γ) induces apoptosis in cancer cells (Ramamoorthy, 1998). It is conditionally licensed by the US Department of Agriculture (USDA) for the treatment of dogs and cats with fibrosarcoma (King, 1995). A total of eight dogs and five cats with histopathologically confirmed fibrosarcoma were treated with acemannan in combination with surgery and radiation therapy. Following four to seven weekly treatments, tumor shrinkage occurred in 4 of 12 animals. Complete surgical excision was performed on all animals between 4 and 7 weeks after initiation of acemannan therapy. Radiation therapy was instituted immediately after surgery. Acemannan treatments were continued monthly for 1 year. In all, 7 of 13 animals were alive and tumor free (range, 440+ to 603+ days), with a median survival time of 372 days. Acemannan may be an effective adjunct to surgery and radiation therapy in the treatment of canine and feline fibrosarcomas (King, 1995). A total of 43 dogs and cats with spontaneous tumor were treated with acemannan by intraperitoneal and intralesional routes of administration. Tumors from 26 of these animals showed marked necrosis or lymphocytic infiltration. Moderate to marked tumor necrosis or liquefaction was noted in 13 animals. In all, 21 demonstrated lymphoid infiltration, and 7 demonstrated encapsulation. A total of 12 animals showed obvious clinical improvement, as assessed by tumor shrinkage, tumor necrosis, or prolonged survival; these included five of the seven animals with fibrosarcoma. It is believed that acemannan exerts its antitumor activity through macrophage activation and the release of tumor necrosis factor, IL-1, and interferon (Harris, 1991).

Rhabdomyosarcoma

Green Tea and Black Tea *(Camellia sinensis)*: Black tea preparations have been shown to reduce the incidence and number of spontaneously generated lung adenocarcinomas and rhabdomyosarcomas in mice (Yang, 2005).

Gastrointestinal tract

Asian Ginseng *(Panax ginseng)*: In case control studies, cancers of lip, oral cavity and pharynx, larynx, lung, esophagus, stomach, liver, pancreas, ovary, and colorectum were significantly reduced through Panax consumption. As to the type of ginseng, cancer was reduced in users of fresh ginseng extract, white ginseng extract, white ginseng powder, and red ginseng. *Panax ginseng* has non–organ specific cancer preventive effects against various cancers primarily because of its ginsenosides (Yun, 2003).

Oral Tumors

Black Tea *(Camellia sinensis)*: An open study in people with oral leukoplakia treated with black tea showed a treatment benefit. Several in vitro and animal studies have suggested the efficacy of tea in the chemoprevention of cancer (Halder, 2005).

Green Tea *(Camellia sinensis)*: In induced squamous cell carcinoma (SCC) in vivo in hamsters, 0.6% green tea powder as drinking fluid or 10 μmol curcumin or combination or nothing (control) was applied topically 3 times weekly for 18 weeks. The combination decreased the incidence, number, and size of SCC and precursor tumors. This activity may be related to suppression of cell proliferation, induction of apoptosis, and inhibition of angiogenesis (Li, 2002).

Turmeric *(Curcuma longa)*: This herb and its active principle, curcumin, have been extensively investigated for their antimutagenic and antioxidant effects in bacterial and animal systems. Turmeric or curcumin or a combination of the two was administered to hamsters in the diet or applied locally for 14 weeks, along with a carcinogen. Tumor number and tumor burden were significantly lower in the animals that received turmeric in the diet and had it applied locally. Histopathologic neoplastic grading was least in the animals fed or painted with curcumin. Turmeric or curcumin in the diet or applied as paint may have a chemopreventive effect on oral precancerous lesions (Krishnaswamy, 1998).

Black Raspberry *(Rubus occidentalis)*: Black raspberries were shown to inhibit oral cavity tumors in hamsters fed 5% and 10% lyophilized black raspberries (LBRs) in the diet for 2 weeks before treatment with a known carcinogen and for 10 weeks thereafter. A significant difference was observed in the number of tumors between the 5% LBR and control groups (27 tumors/14 animals and 48 tumors/15 animals, respectively); an intermediate number of tumors in the 10% berry-treated animals (39 tumors/15 animals) showed that dietary black raspberries inhibit tumor formation in the oral cavity (Casto, 2002).

Garlic *(Allium sativum)*: Administration of garlic (250 mg/kg orally, three times a week) effectively suppressed induced tongue carcinogenesis in rats, as revealed by the absence of carcinomas in the initiation phase and their reduced incidence in the postinitiation phase. Garlic may exert its chemopreventive effects by modulating lipid peroxidation and enhancing the levels of glutathione (GSH), GSH peroxidase, and GSH S-transferase (Balasenthil, 2001).

Ginkgo *(Ginkgo biloba)*: This extract induces apoptosis in oral cavity cancer cells (Kim, 2005).

Pokeweed *(Phytolacca americana)*: A pilot study of pokeweed mitogen immunotherapy in pets was conducted. One case reports 3-year remission and apparent cure of gum melanoma metastatic to regional and hilar lymph nodes and to the lungs in an aged dog following pokeweed mitogen therapy. A small total dose of

300 μg induced the remission. However, melanoma may be a uniquely responsive tumor (Wimer, 2000).

NEEM ***(AZADIRACHTA INDICA):*** This aqueous extract of neem leaf extract effectively suppressed induced oral carcinogenesis (squamous cell carcinomas in hamsters), as revealed by a reduced incidence of neoplasms. Neem may exert its chemopreventive effects in the oral mucosa through modulation of lipid peroxidation, antioxidants, and detoxification systems (Balasenthil, 1999).

TOMATO ***(LYCOPERSICON ESCULENTUM):*** Tomato paste containing lycopene at concentrations of 2.5, 5, or 10 mg/kg body weight was given to hamsters three times per week on days alternate to carcinogen application. Tomato paste containing 5 mg lycopene per kg of body weight exhibited chemopreventive effects that were caused by modulation of lipid peroxidation and enhancement of antioxidants in the target organ, as well as in the liver and erythrocytes (Bhuvaneswari, 2004a). Combined administration of tomato and garlic during induced SCC in hamsters significantly inhibited the development of carcinomas and induced apoptosis (Bhuvaneswari, 2004b).

Gastric Cancer

GINGER ***(ZINGIBER OFFICINALIS):*** This herb inhibits the growth of *Helicobacter pylori,* which is a causative agent associated with the development of gastric and colon cancers and may contribute chemopreventive effects (Mahady, 2003).

ASTRAGALUS ***(ASTRAGALUS MEMBRANACEUS):*** Root specifically inhibits gastric cancer cells growth in vitro and the mechanism is mainly cytostatic but not cytotoxic or inducing apoptosis (Lin 2003).

Colon Cancer

FENUGREEK ***(TRIGONELLA FOENUM-GRAECUM):*** These seeds in the diet inhibit colon carcinogenesis in rats by modulating the activities of β-glucuronidase and mucinase. Beneficial effects may be attributed to the presence of fiber, flavonoids, or saponins (Devasena, 2003).

GINSENG: The powder was investigated in an induced rat colon cancer model. Diets containing quercetin, curcumin, silymarin, ginseng, and rutin decreased the number of aberrant cells by 4-, 2-, 1.8-, 1.5-, and 1.2-fold, respectively, compared with controls. All herbal supplements, except silymarin, induced apoptosis, with quercetin being the most potent (3× increase compared with control). Furthermore, ginseng and curcumin were region specific in inducing apoptosis. Taken together, these results suggest that these herbs may exert beneficial effects on decreasing the number of precancerous lesions and inducing apoptosis in the large intestine (Volate, 2005).

Liver Cancer

WHITE PEONY ***(PAEONIA LACTIFLORA):*** This herb induced apoptosis in vitro in hepatoma cell lines (Lee, 2002).

CURCUMIN (EXTRACT OF ***CURCUMA LONGA***)***:*** Curcumin has been studied for its ability to suppress hepatic tumor growth and metastasis in laboratory animals. In a mouse model of hepatocellular carcinoma, daily oral curcumin administration (3000 mg/kg) significantly attenuated tumor capillary growth (Yoysungnoen, 2005). Rats bearing an ascites hepatoma were given curcumin (20 mcg/kg) and tumor growth appeared inhibited (Busquets, 2001). In animals implanted with hepatocellular carcinoma cells and administered curcumin, metastasis was suppressed dose dependently (Ohashi, 2003).

GREEN TEA AND BLACK TEA ***(CAMELLIA SINENSIS):*** (Yang, 2005).

PANAX ***(PANAX GINSENG):*** (Yun, 2003).

Haematopoietic system

Leukemia

ECHINACEA ***(ECHINACEA PURPUREA):*** Leukemia was induced in 4-week-old female mice predisposed to developing leukemia, and the animals were given powdered *Echinacea purpurea* leaves orally three times weekly for 8 weeks (7.5 mg/mouse/wk). Survival was significantly prolonged and enlargement of thymic lymphoma was significantly suppressed compared with controls. Proliferation of leukemia (MuLV) viruses in the thymus was markedly inhibited as compared with untreated controls after the first oral administration of the *E. purpurea* preparation. Endogenous IFN-γ was also effectively augmented with Echinacea; however, the production of other cytokines such as tumor necrosis factor (TNF)-α and IL-12 was minimal. Thus, suppressive effects on MuLV may depend on enhancement of nonspecific immune or cellular immune systems (or both) by Echinacea (Hayashi, 2001). Daily dietary administration of *E. purpurea* root extract to normal mice for as little as 1 week also resulted in significant elevations in NK cells (immune cells that are cytolytic to virus-containing cells and many tumor cells). Such boosting of this fundamental immune cell population suggests a prophylactic role for this herb in normal animals (Currier, 2001). *E. purpurea*–treated mice exhibited a 2.5-fold increase in the absolute numbers of NK cells in their spleens. By 3 months after leukemia induction, *E. purpurea*–treated mice still had 2 to 3 times the normal numbers of NK cells in their spleens compared with controls. No leukemic, untreated (control) mice remained alive at 3 months; however, at 3 months after tumor onset, all major hematopoietic and immune cell lineages in the bone marrow birth site were recorded at normal numbers in *E. purpurea*–consuming, leukemic mice. The survival advantage provided by administration of *E. purpurea* to these leukemic mice versus untreated mice was highly significant (Currier, 2001).

ACEMANNAN (EXTRACT OF ***ALOE VERA***)**:** Administration of acemannan for 6 weeks intraperitoneally to clinically symptomatic cats significantly improved both quality of life and survival rate. It was noted that 12 weeks after initiation of treatment, 71% of treated cats were alive and in good health (Sheets, 1991).

Myeloma

BAICAL SKULLCAP ***(SCUTELLARIA BAICALENSIS):*** (Ma 2005).

Lymphoma/Lymphosarcoma

MISTLETOE ***(VISCUM ALBUM):*** This extract given as subcutaneous applications (3 times per week for 14 consecutive days; 2, 20, 100, and 500 μg/injection per mouse) upregulated thymocyte and peripheral blood leukocyte counts in tumor-bearing mice. Tumor weight and tumor volume were reduced with doses greater than 20 μg. Injections protected against metastasis of introduced lymphosarcoma and sarcoma cells (Braun, 2002). In another study, non-Hodgkin's lymphoma was induced in mice. One group was fed mistletoe-containing diets (10 mg lectin daily); the other group, a control diet. Diet produced several identifiable changes in morphology and size of non-Hodgkin's lymphoma tumors. In 4 of 15 mice fed the mistletoe-containing diet for 11 days, no evidence of viable tumor was apparent. Results show that this lectin exerts powerful antitumor effects when provided by the oral route (Pryme, 2004).

CAT'S CLAW ***(UNCARIA TOMENTOSA):*** (Sheng 1998).

GOTU KOLA ***(CENTELLA ASIATICA, L.):*** Oral administration of crude extract retarded the development of solid and lymphoma ascites tumor and increased the life span of tumor-bearing mice (Babu, 1995).

CORDYCEPS ***(CORDYCEPS SINENSIS):*** This extract was given orally to mice implanted with lymphoma cells; it reduced tumor size and prolonged mouse survival time. Mice treated with cyclophosphamide (100 mg/kg) 3 and 5 days after tumor transplantation had their immune suppression restored through treatment (Yamaguchi, 1990).

TURKEY TAIL MUSHROOM ***(CORIOLUS VERSICOLOR):*** (Lau 2004).

BITTER MELON ***(MOMORDICA CHARANTIA):*** Studies have shown activity in various diseases, including numerous cancers (lymphoid leukemia, lymphoma, choriocarcinoma, melanoma, breast cancer, skin tumor, prostatic cancer, squamous carcinoma of tongue and larynx, human bladder carcinoma, and Hodgkin's disease). Few reports on clinical use in patients with cancer show promising results (Grover, 2004).

INDIAN LONG PEPPER ***(PIPER LONGUM):*** Alcoholic extract of *Piper longum* (10 mg/animal) inhibited solid tumor development in mice induced with lymphoma and increased the life span of mice bearing carcinoma to 37.3% and 58.8%, respectively (Sunila, 2004).

ASHWAGANDHA ***(WITHANIA SOMNIFERA):*** Ethanolic root extract provided a significant increase in life span and a decrease in cancer cell number and tumor weight in lymphoma tumor–induced mice. Hematologic parameters were also corrected by *Withania* in tumor-bearing mice (Christina, 2004). *Withania somnifera* possesses cell cycle disruption and anti-angiogenic activity, confirmed *in vitro* and *in vivo,* which may be a mediator for its anticancer action (Mathur 2006).

CURCUMIN ***(FROM CURCUMA LONGA):*** This herb inhibits cell proliferation and induces apoptosis in a dose-dependent manner in vitro in several primary effusion lymohoma cell lines (Uddin, 2005).

Popular "Anticancer" Herbal Remedies

Iscador, helixor, and eurixor *(Viscum album)*

The primary use of mistletoe is as a palliative cancer therapy. Iscador is a fermented aqueous extract of *Viscum album* that is marketed as IscadorM (from apple trees), IscadorP (from pine trees), IscadorQ (from oak trees), and IscadorU (from elm trees). Helixor is an unfermented aqueous extract of *V. album* L. that is standardized through its biological effects on human leukemia cells in vitro; it is marketed as HelixorA (from spruce trees), HelixorM (from apple trees), and HelixorP (from pine trees). Eurixor is an unfermented aqueous extract of *V. album* L. that is harvested from poplar trees *(V. album).* These extracts are administered parenterally and may cause inflammation at injection sites. The antineoplastic activity of *V. album,* Helixor, and Iscador is documented in vitro and in vivo, and mistletoe preparations have proved effective in fighting solid tumors in eight of ten animal studies (seven in mice, three in rats); in two studies, they significantly inhibited metastasis and reduced tumor volume. In two negative studies, ML did not inhibit chemically induced bladder cancer (Loeper, 1999).

Iscador is an injectable extract of mistletoe (SC 0.045 mg/kg equivalent to lectin concentration of 3.5 ng/kg) (Schramm, 2001). Although Iscador is regarded as a complementary cancer therapy, it is the most commonly used oncologic drug in Germany (Grossarth-Maticek, 2001). A prospective, nonrandomized and randomized, matched-pair study nested within a cohort study was conducted in Germany. A total of 10,226 human patients with cancer were involved in a prospective, long-term, epidemiologic cohort study that included 1668 patients treated with Iscador and 8475 who had taken neither Iscador nor any other mistletoe product (control patients). In the nonrandomized, matched-pair study, the survival times of patients treated with Iscador were longer for all types of cancer studied. In the pool of 396 matched pairs, mean survival times in the Iscador groups (4.23 years) were roughly 40% longer than in control groups. Iscador treatment can achieve a clinically relevant prolongation of survival time for patients with cancer and appears to stimulate self-regulation (Grossarth-Maticek, 2001).

Helixor has been in use since 1968. A number of components with different possible effects have been isolated, including lectins, viscotoxins, and alkaloids. Contraindications include pregnancy, hyperthyroidism, and intolerance. Depending on the type and stage of the tumor, treatment in humans is based on a specific schedule that can be lifelong. Local inflammatory reactions may occur. Fever is desirable (Kast, 1990).

A multicentric, randomized, open, prospective clinical trial was conducted in China. A total of 224 patients with breast, ovarian, and non–small cell lung cancer fulfilled the requirements for final analysis (n = 115 treated with Helixor A; n = 109 control group treated with Lentinan). All patients were provided with standard tumor destructive treatment schedules and were treated with standardized mistletoe extract or Lentinan during chemotherapy. The study showed that complementary treatment with Helixor can reduce the adverse effects of chemotherapy in patients with cancer, thereby improving quality of life (Piao, 2004).

An off-label veterinary protocol has been proposed by Dr. Chris Piper (New Zealand), who prefers to use HelixorP because it produces fever and local swelling at a level somewhere between the stronger HelixorM and the weaker HelixorA. Clinical effects include pyrexia, leukocytosis, and inhibition of tumor growth. It can be combined with chemotherapy with anecdotal evidence of enhanced well-being, reduced adverse effects of chemotherapy, and increased survival times (personal correspondence, 2005).

Hoxsey formula

The cancer treatment first popularized by Harry M. Hoxsey (1901-1974) is controversial, popular, and one of the longest-lived unconventional herbal therapies for cancer (Spain, 1988). Depending on the type and stage of cancer, and the individual patient's condition, Hoxsey would add to a basic solution of cascara *(Rhamnus purshiana)* and potassium iodide one or more of the following plant substances: poke root *(Phytolacca americana),* burdock root *(Arctium lappa),* barberry or berberis root *(Berberis vulgaris),* buckthorn bark *(Rhamnus frangula),* Stillingia root *(Stillingia sylvatica),* or prickly ash bark *(Zanthoxylum americanum)* (Spain, 1988).

Studies on individual herbs leave no doubt that Hoxsey's formula contains many plant constituents with potential therapeutic activity. Research has identified antitumor activity of one sort or another in all but three of Hoxsey's plants, and two of these three are purgatives; one of them *(Rhamnus purshiana)* contains the anthraquinone glycoside structure now recognized as predictive of antitumor properties (Kupchan, 1976). Whether Hoxsey's particular formula has therapeutic merit is still unsubstantiated by clinical data, despite provocative findings of antitumor properties in many of the individual herbs that he used. However, anecdotal evidence from veterinarians who have used various versions of the formula indicates that it improves quality of life and may inhibit growth of tumors in animals. It is difficult to evaluate the benefits of the traditional approach of detoxification through laxative effects, liver support, improved nutrition, and so forth, all of which may strengthen the immune system and favorably affect the cancer status of a human patient (Spain, 1988); Hoxsey proposed that this was how the formula worked.

A prospective study with no controls evaluated survival for 39 patients with a variety of histologically verified cancers treated at a Mexican clinic. Cancer types for six long-term survivors were lung, melanoma, recurrent bladder cancer and one labial vulva cancer. Twenty three patients were lost to follow-up, and 10 died after an average of 15.4 months. Six remained disease-free with an average follow-up of 48 months (Austin, 1994). A retrospective cohort study followed new cancer patients (n = 149) registered at the same clinic during the first quarter of 1992. At the end of 5 years, 17 (11.4%) were alive, 68 (45.6%) deceased and the status of 64 (43%) unknown. The large proportion lost to follow-up (45.6%) made comparison of the survival of this cohort to the survival of other cohorts of cancer patients reported in the literature impossible (Richardson, 2001).

Various versions of Hoxsey-like formulas are available commercially (Bergner, 1995). The original formula contained an herb identified as *Cascara amarga* (Honduran bark), which is apparently not available in commerce. Most companies substitute *Cascara sagrada* or another alterative in its place.

A Hoxsey-like formula for constitutional cleansing and cancer support is made up of the following (Bergner, 1995):

Licorice root *(Glycyrrhiza glabra)*	6 oz
Red clover *(Trifolium pratense)*	6 oz
Burdock root *(Arctium lappa)*	3 oz
Queen's root *(Stillingia sylvatica)*	2 oz
Oregon grape root *(Berberis aquifolium)*	3 oz
Poke root *(Phytolacca decandra)* (toxic)	2 oz
Cascara sagrada bark *(Rhamnus purshiana)*	2 oz
Buckthorn bark *(Rhamnus frangula)* (toxic)	2 oz
Prickly ash bark *(Zanthoxylum americanum)*	1 oz
Baptisia *(Baptisia tinctoria)*	2 oz
Potassium iodide	3/4 oz

Human dose: From 30 drops 2× per day to 1 tsp 3× per day

Caution on Phytolacca: This herb, used alone, can raise the white blood cell count, mimicking leukemia.

Another recipe (source unknown), per 5 mL:

Potassium iodide	150 mg
Licorice *(Glycyrrhiza glabra)*	20 mg
Red clover *(Trifolium pratense)*	20 mg
Burdock root *(Arctium lappa)*	10 mg
Stillingia root *(Stillingia sylvatica)*	10 mg
Barberry *(Berberis vulgaris)*	10 mg
Cascara *(Cascara sagrada)*	5 mg
Prickly ash bark *(Zanthoxylum americanum)*	5 mg
Buckthorn bark *(Rhamnus catharticus)*	20 mg
Pokeroot *(Phytolacca americana)*	10 mg

Author's note (BF): We do not include potassium iodide in our practice formula.

Essiac

Another controversial "unproven" herbal remedy is Essiac. Various formulas have been prepared on the basis of four herbs:

1. Burdock root *(Arctium lappa)*
2. Sheep sorrel *(Rumex acetosa)*
3. Turkey rhubarb *(Rheum palmatum)*
4. Slippery elm *(Ulmus fulva)*

Many commercial products consist of varying proportions of these herbs. The powdered formula is decocted over minutes to hours, depending on the supplier.

As with the Hoxsey formula, no controlled trials have substantiated the efficacy of Essiac; however, studies on the herb constituents support antineoplastic activity. In the early 1980s, the Canadian Bureau of Human Prescription Drugs conducted a retrospective review physician summaries about Caisse's patients. Eighty six patient histories were submitted. All had previously received conventional therapy. Of the 86 patients, 1 showed subjective improvement, 5 required fewer analgesics, and 3 remained stable (Office of Technology Assessment, 1990). In a survey of North American consumers of one brand of essiac, 50.6% of respondents reported improvement in their symptoms. 6.6 percent reported adverse events of nausea, vomiting and diarrhea, but 11.8% had exceeded the daily recommended dose (Richardson, 2000).

Antitumor activity has been demonstrated in vivo with burdock, with various fractions inhibiting induced sarcoma by as much as 61% in mice (Dombradi, 1966). Burdock seed contains a number of ligands, including arctigenin, which has been shown to induce differentiation in mouse myeloid leukemia cells. Arctigenin has also demonstrated potent cytoxic effects against a human leukemia cell line, while showing no toxicity toward normal lymphocytes (Hirano, 1994). Sheep sorrel contains emodin, which has antitumor activity; its polysaccharides have displayed antitumor activity in mice implanted with sarcoma (Ito, 1986). Some constituents of rhubarb (aloe, emodin, catechin, and rhein) have shown antitumor activity. Rhein has antitumor activity in vivo, increasing survival time in leukemia-bearing mice in one study, and inhibiting melanoma in mice by 76% in another (Konopa, 1957).

Other formulas

Other traditional cancer formulas include Scudder's alterative (equal parts of corydalis tubers *[Corydalis yanhusuo]*, black tag alder *[Alnus serrulata]*, figwort *[Scrophularia nodosa]*, and yellow dock *[Rumex crispus]*) and Compound Syrup of Scrophulara (figwort leaves and roots, Phytolacca root, *Rumex crispus* root, *Celastrus scandens* bark and root, *Corydalis formosa* root, Podophyllum root, juniper berries, prickly ash berries, and guaiacum wood). The recipes for these formulas are found in Eli Jones' classic, *Cancer: Its Causes, Symptoms and Treatment,* first published in 1911 and recently reprinted (Jones, 1911).

Review of Strategies for Cancer Prescriptions

One of the primary concerns of veterinarians is how to control cancer without weakening the host; herbal therapy offers a very practical and effective solution to this dilemma. In the authors' opinion, when conventional therapy offers a very good chance of curing or sending a cancer into remission, then conventional therapy is warranted, with herbal adjunctive therapy of paramount importance. However, when the outcomes are likely to be palliative, or when they are unknown, then herbal "chemotherapy" is a viable alternative to conventional chemotherapy after risks and benefits of treatment have been weighed. Even with grave prognoses, many cases have demonstrated that improvement in health and longevity is possible, despite the presence of cancer.

The known mechanisms of herbal actions can be integrated in a holistic approach to cancer care through a strategy that incorporates tradition and science. By using a variety of herbs with different anticancer activities, veterinarians are using, in effect, a form of "polyvalent herbal chemotherapy." At the same time, traditional herbal medicine treatment is aimed at treating the patient, rather than the disease. As has been discussed, the number of herbs that have demonstrated some form of anticancer activity is immense and may at first seem overwhelming, but this fact can be used to take advantage of both approaches.

The individual animal's diagnosis, stage of disease, history, presentation, vitality or debility, and system functioning will affect treatment strategy and herb selection. Traditional Chinese herbalists and Western herbalists have always used several herbs in combination and will change formulas over time as the needs of the patient change.

The author proposes that several herbs that treat the individual patient should be combined to obtain the following outcomes:

- Alleviation of signs and symptoms of the patient.
- Relief of possible pain, anemia, poor appetite, cachexia, depression, diarrhea, adverse effects of chemotherapy, bleeding, edema, leukopenia and so forth.
- Appropriate herbs that treat specific areas of the body should be selected, for example, renal herbs or liver herbs for renal or liver cancer.

Alteratives

Cancer is a very diverse disease that is considered by herbalists to be an expression of physiologic imbalance. Treatment seeks to improve physiologic functioning and waste removal through "detoxifying" with the use of gentle aperatives and laxatives, lymphatics, and "blood-cleansing" herbs (i.e., alteratives). Particular attention should be paid to herbs of the gastrointestinal system with concurrent actions, such as cholagogues, liver tonics, bitters, diuretics, and carminatives.

Immune support

Herbs that support the patient should be selected in the first instance, particularly if infection is present (previous high-dose prednisolone therapy is common with occult infections that have often been untreated). Antimicrobials and antiseptics should be considered, if necessary. Herbs that modify or stimulate immunity help the patient's own body to resist the effects of cancer.

Adaptogens

The practitioner seeks to reduce the physical effects of stress and assist "adaptive energy," particularly when the patient is debilitated, but also in an attempt to prevent debilitation. Most adaptogens have multiple actions, and selection must be made according to which is the best one for the patient. For example, a hyperactive young dog with lymphosarcoma would be better treated with *Withania* rather than *Panax;* however, an old, debilitated, sleepy dog might be better suited to *Panax*.

Tumor biology and tumor type

When possible, the practitioner should incorporate herbs that have known antineoplastic activity; often, these are the same herbs that fall into the other categories discussed earlier. When possible, and when the information is available, one should select herbs that have known activity against particular tumor types.

Antioxidants

Patients with cancer or that are on chemotherapy or radiation therapy will benefit from antioxidants. Reviews of the many in vitro, animal, and human studies have demonstrated the beneficial effects of antioxidants on oxidative damage reduction (Conklin, 2000; Labriola,

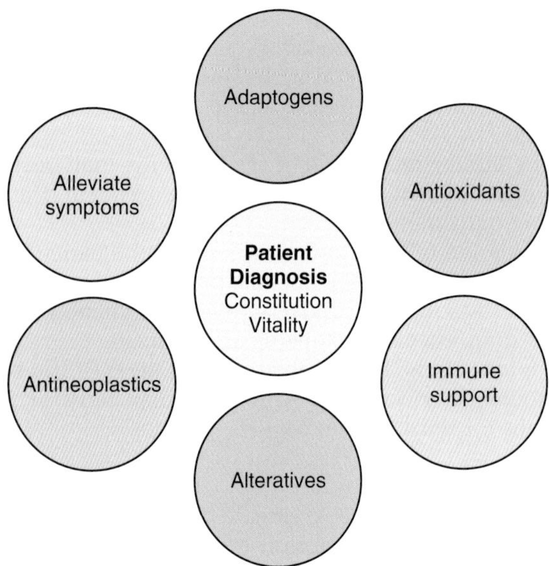

Figure 20-1 Schemata of herbal selection for cancer treatment. Choose herbs that cross provide more than one of these actions, tailored to the patient's needs.

1999; Lamson, 1999). Many herbs with antioxidant activities have antineoplastic activity, and similarly, many antineoplastic herbs have antioxidant activity. (See "Herbs and Chemotherapy" at the end of this section.)

In summary, a simple approach involves considering the effects or potential effects of the cancer on an individual patient with goals toward strengthening bodily resistance and overall health by improving immunity and physiology, alleviating symptoms, and using antioxidant and adaptogen herbs. If this is done, anticancer activity is usually inherent in the prescription. As well, specific herbs can be used for known activity against particular types of cancers. Many herbs exhibit overlapping actions that fulfill more than one action category (Figure 20-1).

Strategy for prescribing using key mechanisms of action focused on the patient

Example: An old dog with hepatic adenocarcinoma that is cold, arthritic, and overweight. Chemotherapy has been declined. (*Note:* This formula could be used concurrently with chemotherapy.)

- Burdock 25% (cold): Differentiation inducer, depurative (alterative), diuretic, mild laxative, mild antiseptic. Traditional use in arthritis, cancer.
- Turmeric 25% (warm): Inhibits metastasis, angiogenesis, local invasion. Is anti-inflammatory, antioxidant, antiplatelet, hepatoprotective, cholagogue. Traditional use in arthritis, cancer, and improved digestion and hepatic function.
- *Panax ginseng* 25% (neutral to warm, dry): Inhibits local invasion, adaptogenic, stimulant, tonic, hypoglycemic, immune stimulant, hepatoprotective, cardioprotective. Traditional use for cancer, chronic inflammation, improved resistance to infection, and minimization of adverse effects of chemotherapy.
- Astragalus 25% (sweet and slightly warm): Inhibits metastasis. An adaptogen, tonic, cardiotonic, immune enhancer, diuretic. Used for cancer, chronic debility, chronic hepatitis.

This formula provides antineoplastic activity; adaptogen, antioxidant, alterative, and immune-supporting herbs; and alleviates symptoms of chronic inflammation (arthritis). In addition, some hepatoprotective and tonic effects are given for this old dog. This formula could be altered with milk thistle, Schisandra, or Bupleurum over time. In addition, this diet should be supplemented with turmeric or green tea for further antioxidant and antineoplastic actions. Generally, the formula is also warming.

Herbs and Conventional Tumor Therapies: Many oncology drugs induce cellular toxicity and death through free radical generation; some concern exists that antioxidants may negate these cytotoxic properties. In a review of all English articles listed in Index Medicus between the years 1990 and 2000 that were related to antioxidants and interactions with anticancer drugs or radiation, the authors concluded, "There is a rational basis for the continued use of antioxidant agents as a therapeutic adjunct in cancer therapy, with such use also offering potential to abrogate the carcinogenic process and mutation-driven drug resistance, but convincing data and widespread acceptance of such a role [are] dependent on additional, appropriately relevant trials" (Block, 2001). Chemotherapeutic drugs that are best known for creating cellular damage by initiating free radical and reactive oxygen species (ROS) damage include the alkylating agents, such as cyclophosphamide, ifosfamide, and melphalan; the tumor antibiotics, such as doxorubicin, bleomycin, and epirubicin; and the platinum compounds, such as cisplatin (Conklin, 2000; Labriola, 1999; Lamson, 1999; Lamson, 2000). Radiation therapy uses ionizing radiation to produce cell kill through free radical generation (Lamson, 1999; Lamson, 2000). Unfortunately, a number of physiologic adverse effects of these therapies (e.g., doxorubicin-induced cardiotoxicity, cisplatin-induced nephrotoxity, bleomycin-induced pulmonary fibrosis) are related to oxidative damage (Conklin, 2000). Evidence is accumulating that antioxidants are helpful in attenuating these side effects (Ferreira, 2004), (Weijl, 2004). Careful selection of herbs that help reduce these adverse effects and protect these organs and systems (see relevant system herbs) can be used. Because antioxidant activity is inherent in many herbs, two options with chemotherapy and radiation therapy are available, if the theoretical concern exists. Herbal treatment should be stopped just before conventional treatment is begun (24-48 hours) and recommenced in approximately 5-7 days depending on the half life of the chemotherapeutic drug (or longer for radiation therapy); or herbal treatment should be continued concurrently. In the authors' experience, concurrent treatment helps to reduce the adverse effects of treatment and to maintain "wellness."

Much has been made in the medical literature of drug-herb interactions, and specifically the CYP450 hepatic microsomal system which is responsible for metabolizing many commonly prescribed drugs. While the list of *potential* interactions is very long, the evidence for real interference, by herbs, in the metabolism of most drugs is lacking. In many cases, medical experts warn that potentially useful herbs should not be administered on the basis of a single *in vitro* study of a single chemical contained within that plant. Food itself can alter the activities of CYP450 enzymes. Herbs taken orally must pass through the GI tract, be acted upon by digestive enzymes and gut bacteria, pass through portal circulation and get to the liver for whatever processes occur there.

As an example, isolated gingkolic acids from gingko and hyperforin from Saint John's Wort *inhibit* CYP2C19 activity in vitro (Zou, 2002). However, using more complete extracts of the herb of each in humans appears to *induce* CYP2C19 (Wang, 2004). To date, a small number of herbs have been examined in humans and animals for their influences on metabolism of a small number of drugs. Chapter 12 provides a listing of potential herb-drug interactions, and should be used by the practitioner as a starting point for an evidence-based approach to the subject.

HERBS FOR CARDIOVASCULAR DISEASE

General Considerations

Digoxin is the legacy of an herbal success story. Dr. William Withering was widely acclaimed for his discovery of foxglove for the treatment of patients with heart disease. However, Withering did not discover it at all, of course—he observed the treatment successes of a local "herb woman" (or witch, depending on the account one reads) who used foxglove in her formulas. Withering was able to divine which of her herbs was the most promising, and he commenced to chronicle *10 years* of his own experience of treating patients with this plant (published in 1785). This is the proper course of clinical herbal research—investigators should (1) note that a plant in long use may actually have clinical effects, (2) document these effects well, and (3) publish findings for others to put them to the test. Many of the plants discussed in this section have been used as traditional treatments for heart failure, and some have undergone scientific investigation. We know that some of these have interesting effects in vitro, yet they have not been tested clinically. It will be noted when no traditional database is available to guide practitioners in their prescription.

Congestive Heart Failure

Heart failure or congestive heart failure is a clinical syndrome—not a disease. It results from interaction among the heart and neuroendocrine and vascular systems. The heart may increasingly lose capacity to pump blood at a rate that can maintain tissue metabolism requirements, or it may do so at elevated filling pressures, resulting in impaired organ function. Therapy must address inciting causes (if known), improve myocardial function, reduce volume overload, or reduce pressure overload. Drug therapies for myocardial failure are "Band-Aid therapies" that palliate the effects of heart disease for a short duration but do little to address the primary disease process. Some goals of drug therapy are to reduce pulmonary venous pressure and augment systolic performance. In addition, therapy is increasingly targeting neurohormonal changes that hasten the progression of heart failure, including activation of the sympathetic nervous system and the renin-angiotensin system. It is worth noting that some herbs traditionally used for heart failure (such as hawthorn and linden) have mild anxiolytic activity, which may reduce sympathetic nervous system activity.

Mechanisms of Interest

Cardiotonic and cardioprotective herbs

Cardiotonic and cardioprotective herbs are generally rich in flavonoids, which may reduce oxidative stress and reduce capillary fragility. They may also exhibit vasorelaxant activity.

HAWTHORN ***(CRATAEGUS* SPP*):*** (Upton, 1999, Rigelsky, 2002). This herb may increase myocardial contractility and reduce peripheral vascular resistance. The mechanism is attributed to a slight inhibition of sodium/potassium adenosine triphosphatase (Na^+/K^+-ATPase), which might be responsible for the positive inotropic action. Evidence also reveals inhibition of angiotensin-converting enzymes (ACEs) and of interactions with the cyclic adenosine monophosphate (cAMP)-mediated β-adrenergic system, which may explain the vascular effects of the extract. Most trials indicate greatest effect after 6 to 8 weeks of use, and clinical trials in humans suggest that higher doses are more effective in severe cases. In patients with New York Heart Association (NYHA) Class II heart failure (see Table 20-1). 160 to 900 mg divided daily of a particular leaf and flower extract (WS 1442) was effective, but a dose of 1800 mg produced better results in people with Class III failure.

GINKGO ***(GINKGO BILOBA):*** Ginkgo appears to have vasodilatory effects on peripheral circulation and antioxidant capacity by virtue of the flavonoids it contains. Ginkgo extract and the terpenoid, bilobalide, have potent concentration-dependent vascular smooth muscle relaxant activity; other constituents of Ginkgo have variable effects on cardiomyocyte action potential duration, nitric oxide release in the endothelium and aorta, and Ca^{2+} channel flux (Satoh, 2004; Zhou, 2004a). Ginkgolides inhibit PAF; this may have additive effects for human

TABLE 20-1

New York Heart Association Functional Classification of Heart Failure for Humans

Class I	Heart disease without exercise intolerance or signs of heart failure
Class II	Signs of cardiac-related exercise intolerance exhibited.
Class III	Signs of heart failure during normal activity.
Class IV	Clinical signs at rest or with minimal activity.

TABLE 20-2

International Small Animal Cardiac Health Council Heart Disease Classification Scheme

Class I	Asymptomatic Ia: Signs of heart disease but no cardiomegaly Ib: Signs of heart disease and evidence of compensation (cardiomegaly)
Class II	Mild to moderate heart failure—clinical signs of heart failure are evident at rest or with mild exercise and adversely affect quality of life
Class III	Symptoms at rest—clinical signs of congestive heart failure are immediately obvious IIIa: Home care is possible IIIb: Hospitalization is recommended (cardiogenic shock, life-threatening edema, large pleural effusion, refractory ascites)

patients or cats taking anticoagulants to prevent thrombosis.

ASTRAGALUS *(ASTRAGALUS MEMBRANACEUS):* This Chinese herb is often used as a Qi tonic and has been studied for its therapeutic benefit in the treatment of patients with ischemic heart disease, myocardial infarction, and heart failure, and those who seek relief from anginal pain. Clinical studies have indicated that its in vitro antioxidant activity is the mechanism by which it affords cardioprotective benefit (Miller, 1998).

MOTHERWORT *(LEONURUS CARDIACA):* This herb is traditionally used for palpitations, arrhythmias, and the stress and anxiety that accompany those symptoms. One component, lavandulifolioside, causes significant negative chronotropism, prolongation of the P-Q and Q-T intervals and the QRS complex, and decreased blood pressure (Milkowska-Leyck, 2002). This herb has not been well investigated.

CACTUS *(SELENICEREUS GRANDIFLORUS):* Both the stem and flowers of this herb were very important as a heart remedy to the Eclectics, and yet it is almost never used by veterinary herbalists and has not been scientifically investigated. Ellingwood described the indications for it as "irregular pulse; feebleness of the heart's action; dyspnea; weight; oppression in the chest; violence of the heart's action depending upon atonicity or enervation." This plant has developed a reputation as a strong or toxic herb, but those who have used it most often and have written about it have declared it a safe tonic. A detailed monograph on this plant can be found at the Southwest School of Botanical Medicine Web site at: http://www.swsbm.com/ManualsOther/Selenicereus-Lloyd.PDF. The veterinary dose recommended by Milks (1949) is $^{1}/_{12}$ gr for a horse (0.005 g) and 1/60 gr for a dog (0.001 g), but he was clearly unconvinced of its efficacy at these doses. The previously mentioned monograph describes human doses as low as a fraction of a drop to 0.3 mL, and as high as 1.8 mL three times daily. It has commonly been combined with *Avena sativa* and should be used for several months before its effects are assessed.

COLLINSONIA *(COLLINSONIA CANADENSIS):* This herb has been recommended as a cardiac tonic that acts primarily to improve vascular tone.

OTHER HERBS: Other herbs include the following:

- Corydalis *(Corydalis ambigua)*
- *Panax ginseng*
- *Panax notoginseng*
- *Salvia miltiorrhiza*
- *Terminalia arjuna*

Cardioactive herbs

CACTUS *(SELENICEREUS GRANDIFLORUS):* As previously discussed, this herb is said to be a positive inotrope.

HAWTHORN *(CRATAEGUS OXYANCANTHA):* As was previously discussed, this is a positive inotrope.

LILY OF THE VALLEY *(CONVALLARIA MAJALIS):* Aerial parts contains 40 cardenolides (cardiac glycosides), which, like digoxin, inhibit N^+/K^+-ATPase pumps. King describes Convallaria thus: "Compared with digitalis, convallaria is generally as efficient, both as a heart tonic and as a diuretic, and in many cases, is said to act better. It is safer than digitalis, which may destroy life by paralyzing the heart—an effect never produced by convallaria. Moreover, it is freer from cumulative effects." The dose that kills 50% of a sample population (LD_{50}) in cats for a single constituent, convallatoxol, was 0.14 mg/kg given intraperitoneally. A human dose for this herb is 0.6 g of powdered herb or 5 to 10 drops of tincture, divided daily. A case report described a dog that had eaten lily of the valley in its fenced yard and died suddenly (Moxley, 1989).

BROOM *(CYTISUS SCOPARIUS OR SAROTHAMNUS SCOPARIUS):* This is a rarely used plant that is generally considered a poison and a noxious weed. Its traditional naturopathic uses are as a cardiac stimulant, peripheral vasoconstrictor, and diuretic. King claims that it is useful in "dropsy of the thorax" (pulmonary edema). Combining the herb with dandelion and juniper may reduce toxicity and lend synergistic effects. This author (SW) has no experience with the herb, but it is used by respected naturopaths and herbalists and appears to have potential as an acute or emergency medicine.

BUGLEWEED *(LYCOPUS EUROPAEUS):* This herb is usually recommended for people with thyrotoxic agitation and palpitations. It is considered a diuretic, a nervine, and a peripheral vasodilator. King's (Felter, 1898) describes the action of Lycopus on the heart thus: "Cardiac disease, both organic and functional, has been markedly impressed by lycopus. Administered to patients suffering from endocarditis and pericarditis, it quickly subdues the inflammation. It is a good remedy for cardiac palpitation . . . It is best adapted to those forms of heart disease characterized by irritability and irregularity, with dyspnea and precordial oppression. Lycopus powerfully increases the contraction of the unstriped muscular fibers, particularly those of the heart and arteries, hence its value in cardiac dilatation and hypertrophy, which have been known to undergo marked improvement under its administration. It quickly relieves the suffering and anxiety nearly always experienced in heart disease. It has favorably influenced exophthalmic goiter." Despite its previous popularity as a treatment for arrhythmia and cardiomyopathy, this herb has not been investigated in clinical trials.

TERMINALIA *(TERMINALIA ARJUNA):* This traditional Indian herb is used for heart problems. A double-blind crossover trial in people with NYHA Class IV congestive heart failure showed that people who received 500 mg three times daily of Terminalia had improved NYHA Class evaluation, end-systolic volume, left ventricular end-diastolic volume, left ventricular stroke volume index, and left ventricular ejection fractions, compared with those given placebo (Bharani, 1995).

FORSKOHLII *(PLECTRANTHUS BARBATUS):* Laboratory animal studies show that the forskolin extract increases myocardial contractile strength and peripheral vasodilation and may also reduce cardiac preload and afterload, possibly by activating adenylate cyclase (Baumann, 1990).

TRIBULUS *(TRIBULUS TERRESTRIS):* This Ayurvedic herb has many traditional uses, including its administration as a diuretic. In vitro studies on isolated heart muscle suggest that it has a positive inotropic effect (Seth, 1976).

BLOOD ROOT *(SANGUINARIA CANADENSIS):* This is considered a cardiotonic herb. In vitro studies confirm that sanguinarine, a benzophenanthridine alkaloid derived from blood root, produced a concentration-dependent positive inotropic effect and increased contractility (108%) that was comparable with the maximal inotropic effect of ouabain. Sanguinarine caused inhibition of Na^+/K^+-ATPase isolated from guinea pig myocardium (Seifen, 1979). Blood root is another strong herb that should be used carefully by trained herbalists.

Circulatory stimulants

CAYENNE *(CAPSICUM ANNUUM):* Capsaicin, a single extract of Capsicum, caused hypertension in dogs and cats when given intravenously. Peripheral vasoconstriction in anesthetized dogs (followed by hypotension) and isolated arterial strips appeared mediated through cholinergic mechanisms (Toda, 1972). The effect of oral ingestion of the whole herb in the treatment of cardiovascular disease is unknown.

PRICKLY ASH *(ZANTHOXYLUM AMERICANUM):* This herb has not been investigated, but the Eclectics valued its use for "sluggish circulation." King describes its effect as "Cardiac action is increased, the pulse becomes slightly accelerated, and the integumentary glands give out an abundant secretion."

GINKGO *(GINKGO BILOBA):* The effects of ginkgo leaf extract have been studied in normal rats and those with ischemic brain damage caused by middle cerebral artery occlusion. Oral administration of ginkgo extract at 100 mg/kg was reported to increase cerebral blood flow in normal rats, but the increase was less marked in rats with cerebral artery occlusion (Zhang, 2000).

OTHER HERBS: Other circulatory stimulants include the following:

- Dong quai *(Angelica sinensis)*
- Horseradish *(Armoracia rusticana)*
- Chuan xiong *(Ligusticum wallichii)*
- Bayberry *(Myrica cerifera)*

Agents that decrease peripheral resistance, hypotensives, and peripheral vasodilators

TERMINALIA: Laboratory animal studies suggest that it has antioxidant activity (Gupta 2001, Karthikeyan, 2003), reduces blood pressure, and demonstrates positive inotropic activity. An uncontrolled study in dogs suggests that it may also have β_2-adrenergic activity (Nammi, 2003).

HAWTHORN *(CRATAEGUS OXYACANTHA):* This herb may increase myocardial contractility and reduce peripheral vascular resistance. Most trials demonstrate greatest effect after 6 to 8 weeks of use. It may enhance the effects of cardiac glycosides (Jellin, 1999) and may have mild antihypertensive effects. In mildly hypertensive humans, 500 mg daily of hawthorn extract led to a reduction in diastolic blood pressure (Walker, 2002).

GARLIC *(ALLIUM SATIVUM):* This herb is popular in the management of human cardiovascular disease; evidence suggests that the primary focus of action involves modulating blood lipids and controlling atherosclerotic disease, although one study in dogs indicated the capacity to reduce diastolic blood pressure and heart rate (Martin, 1992; Nagourney, 1998). Multiple in vitro and ex vivo studies in rats suggest that garlic relaxes vascular smooth muscle through nitric oxide (NO)-mediated mechanisms (Kim-Park, 2000; Baluchnejadmojarad, 2003). Garlic has mild antihypertensive properties in humans, rats, and dogs (Wilburn, 2004; Sharifi, 2003a; Pantoja, 1991; Malik, 1981). Its mechanisms are unknown, but endothelium-derived relaxing and constricting factors, as well as prostaglandin-mediated and NO-mediated mechanisms, are suspected (Banerjee, 2002).

GINKGO *(GINKGO BILOBA):* In vitro studies show that ginkgo causes vasodilation in endothelium and aortic vascular muscles, possibly via Ca^{2+} influx through the Ca^{2+} channel and the activation of NO release (Satoh, 2004).

FORSKOHLII *(PLECTRANTHUS BARBATUS):* The forskolin extract increases myocardial contractile strength and peripheral vasodilation and may also reduce cardiac preload and afterload, possibly by activating adenylate cyclase (Baumann, 1990).

CHINESE SALVIA, DAN SHEN *(SALVIA MILTIORRHIZA):* This herb was traditionally used in Chinese herbal combinations; it may decrease vascular resistance (Huang, 2000).

VALERIAN *(VALERIANA OFFICINALIS):* This herb was found to dilate pulmonary vascular smooth muscle in cats, probably through a nonselective γ-aminobutyric acid (GABA)-mediated mechanism (Fields, 2003).

EUCOMMIA *(EUCOMMIA ULMOIDES):* Older studies suggest that this herb may reduce blood pressure. There are anecdotal reports of success with it in early cases of hypertension.

UNCARIA *(UNCARIA RHYNCHOPHYLLA):* This relative of cat's claw (both containing the vasoactive alkaloid rhyncophylline) (Shi, 2003) is known as *gou teng* in Chinese medicine. The herb mediates endothelium-dependent relaxation in spontaneously hypertensive rats in in vitro studies. One extract resulted in peripheral vasodilation in anesthetized dogs (Ozaki, 1990).

Diuretics

Cardioactive herbs were often traditionally classified as diuretics, in many cases because of their effect of increasing renal blood flow secondary to improving ventricular function.

(See the section on urinary system for more information on diuretics.)

DANDELION ***(TARAXACUM OFFICINALE):*** The German Commission E discovered evidence of a diuretic effect. Oral administration of dandelion extracts had a diuretic effect in rats and mice, and in one study, the effect was assessed as equal to that of furosemide and stronger than juniper berry and horsetail (Bisset, 1994).

PARSLEY ***(PETROSELINUM CRISPUM):*** This root and fruit was used historically as a diuretic for patients with dropsy.

Nervines

MOTHERWORT ***(LEONURUS CARDIACA):*** The later Eclectics valued motherwort as a nervine and heart tonic, in addition to its better known effects on women's menstrual functions. It was recommended for "nervous debility" and is used by modern herbalists to treat patients with arrhythmias.

LINDEN ***(TILIA PLATYPHYLLOS):*** This traditional anxiolytic herb is sometimes used in cardiac formulas, although no clinical trials or animal studies have been undertaken. The dose for humans is $^{3}/_{4}$ to 1 teaspoon (3-5 mL) of the tincture three times daily, or 1 cup of tea (1-2 tsp in 1 cup water) three times daily.

VALERIAN ***(VALERIANA OFFICINALIS):*** This is a recognized hypnotic herb. Cropley and colleagues investigated heart rate and blood pressure reactions in a group of people presented with stressful mental tasks. Compared with the placebo group, those treated with valerian demonstrated significantly attenuated heart rate and blood pressure changes (Cropley, 2002).

Angiotensin-converting enzyme inhibitors

TRIBULUS (PUNCTUREVINE) ***(TRIBULUS TERRESTRIS):*** Laboratory animal studies suggest that Tribulus has ACE inhibition activity (Sharifi, 2003b). Heart disease is not a traditional indication for this herb.

DAN SHEN ***(SALVIA MILTIORRHIZA):*** This herb has shown significant ACE inhibition activity in a rat model of hypertension (Kang, 2002), and is a traditional Chinese herb for blood stagnation and chest pain.

Antiarrhythmics

BERBERINE-CONTAINING PLANTS ***(GOLDENSEAL [HYDRASTIS CANADENSIS],*** COPTIS ***[COPTIS CHINENSIS],*** BARBERRY ***[BERBERIS VULGARIS],*** OREGON GRAPE ***[MAHONIA AQUIFOLIUM]):*** These herbs were not used traditionally for heart or cardiovascular disease. King's says that goldenseal "appears to stimulate the respiratory and circulatory apparatus, imparting increased tone and power. Arterial tension is augmented, and blood pressure in the capillaries increased, rendering it valuable, like belladonna and ergot, in overcoming blood stasis. Its action upon the nervous system has been compared [with] that of strychnine (Ellingwood, 1919), [although] less energetic, but more permanent. Thus, the tone imparted to the heart muscle is permanent, rather than intermittent or spasmodic." Animal studies show that berberine decreases heart rate and may act like a Class III antiarrhythmic (Riccioppo, 1993; Huang, 1992). Zeng and associates investigated the effects of 1.2 to 2.0 g berberine given daily to people with congestive heart failure who were experiencing ventricular premature complexes (VPCs) or ventricular tachycardia. Compared with people taking placebo, a significantly greater increase was noted in left ventricular ejection fraction, exercise capacity, and the dyspnea–fatigue index, as was a decrease in the frequency and complexity of VPCs. Over the following 24 months, a significant decrease in mortality was observed in these patients as well (Zeng, 2003). Goldenseal root may consist of 0.5% to 6% berberine, and *Coptis rhizome* may contain 4% to 9% berberine. The barberry plant may contain 1% to 3% berberine.

LILY OF THE VALLEY: This herb is recommended by herbalist David Winston for simple arrhythmias, with or without cardiac hypertrophy.

Other herbs with potential antiarrhythmic activity include Broom, Bugleweed, Motherwort, Ailanthus *(Ailanthus altissima),* Cactus, Dogbane *(Apocynum cannabinum),* Adonis *(Adonis vernalis),* Gelsemium *(Gelsemium sempervirens),* Hawthorn, Lobelia seed *(Lobelia inflata),* Pink root *(Spigelia marilandica),* Pulsatilla *(Anemone patens, A. pulsatilla),* Skullcap *(Scutellaria lateriflora),* Veratrum *(Veratrum verde),* and Valerian according to Winston. Adonis, Ailanthus, Dogbane, Gelsemium, Lobelia, Lily of the Valley, Pink root, Pulsatilla, and Veratrum are potentially toxic herbs. Corydalis, Devil's claw, *Panax ginseng, Panax notoginseng,* and *Stephania tetandra* are also used for their antiarrythmic activity.

Anticoagulants

GARLIC ***(ALLIUM SATIVUM):*** This herb has been shown in many human and animal trials to inhibit platelet aggregation (Rahman, 2000; Ali, 1995; Legnani, 1993; Morris, 1995). Its red blood cell toxicity to cats and dogs in high doses may limit its use to lower doses.

DAN SHEN ***(SALVIA MILTIORRHIZA):*** This herb inhibits platelet activity, has antithrombin III–like activity, and promotes fibrinolysis (Chan, 2001).

REVIEW OF SPECIFIC CARDIOVASCULAR CONDITIONS

Dilated Cardiomyopathy

Therapeutic rationale

- Optimize cardiac output (increase contractility and reduce cardiac afterload).
- Prevent arrhythmias.
- Decrease oxidative stress.

- Rule out metabolic and nutritional abnormalities, such as hypothyroidism, taurine deficiency, and carnitine deficiency.
- Prevent obesity or cardiac cachexia through proper nutritional support.

David Hoffman's formula for mild congestive heart failure in people consists of the following: 3 parts hawthorn, 1 part ginkgo, 1 part linden, 1 part dandelion leaf, 1 part cramp bark, and 1 part valerian (Hoffmann, 2004). Winston recommends a "Hawthorn Compound" that contains hawthorn flower and berry, ginkgo, lemon balm, linden, prickly ash, bugleweed, and cactus (Winston, 2003).

A prescription for dilated cardiomyopathy follows:

Hawthorn	30% (cardiotonic, coronary vasodilator, hypotensive, antioxidant)
Cactus	20%
Terminalia	20% (cardioprotective, hepatoprotective, mild diuretic)
Dan shen	20% (cardioprotective, hypotensive, anticoagulant, antiplatelet, hepatoprotective)

Another prescription used by the author (BF) for cardiac support is:

Hawthorn	40% (cardiotonic, coronary vasodilator, hypotensive, antioxidant)
Dandelion leaf	20% (diuretic, laxative, cholagogue, antirheumatic)
Ginkgo	20% (PAF inhibitor, antioxidant, circulatory stimulant, cognitive enhancer)
Lemon balm	20% (carminative, antispasmodic, sedative)

Heartworm Disease

Therapeutic rationale

- Kill parasites (adults and microfilaria).
- Reduce intimal damage.
- Control secondary heart failure.
- Prevent thromboembolism with cage rest and administration of aspirin.
- Prevent obesity or cardiac cachexia through proper nutritional support.

BLACK WALNUT *(JUGLANS NIGRA)*: This treatment is popular for gastrointestinal parasites, as well as for heartworm disease; no data are available on the latter. Black walnut hull has also been recommended for heartworm prevention at a dosage of approximately 1 capsule of ground herb per day, but long-term safety is unknown. Therapy should be discontinued if diarrhea arises.

GINGER *(ZINGIBER OFFICINALIS)*: A dosage of 100 mg/kg of alcoholic extract of ginger, given subcutaneously by 12 injections to dogs infected with heartworm, caused 98% reduction in microfilarial counts and appeared to have some adulticidal activity (Datta, 1987). How this study relates to oral dosing is uncertain.

The authors do not recommend substituting an unproven herbal formula for effective conventional therapy but recognize that some clients and some situations do not support conventional therapy.

A prescription for general support for patients undergoing treatment or posttreatment follow-up or heartworm disease follows:

Hawthorn	40% (cardiotonic, coronary vasodilator, hypotensive, antioxidant)
Dandelion leaf	20% (diuretic, laxative, cholagogue, antirheumatic)
Ginger	20% (carminative, antispasmodic, anti-inflammatory, antiplatelet)
Dan shen	20% (cardioprotective, hypotensive, anticoagulant, antiplatelet, hepatoprotective)

Hypertension

Therapeutic rationale

- Treat underlying disease, if possible.
- Use pharmacologic therapy to reduce blood pressure.
- Manage obesity, if present.
- Recommend other nutrients with antihypertensive effects, such as omega-3 fatty acids.
- Avoid the use of drugs that promote hypertension.

David Hoffman (2004) recommends a general hypertension formula consisting of the following ingredients:

Hawthorn	40%
Linden	15%
Yarrow	15%
Cramp bark	15%
Valerian	15%

A prescription for renal or cardiac hypertension follows:

Hawthorn	20% (cardiotonic, coronary vasodilator, hypotensive, antioxidant)
Yarrow	20% (antispasmodic, mild vasodilator, hypotensive, bitter)
Astragalus	20% (immune enhancing, tonic, cardiotonic, nephroprotective, diuretic, hypotensive)
Withania	40% (tonic, adaptogen, nervine, sedative, anti-inflammatory)

Hypertrophic Cardiomyopathy

Therapeutic rationale

- Relax the myocardium.
- Enhance ventricular filling.
- Control signs of heart failure, such as pulmonary edema.
- Manage arrhythmias and reduce risks for thromboembolism.
- Rule out hyperthyroidism, systemic hypertension, and acromegaly (rare).
- Prevent obesity or cardiac cachexia through proper nutritional support.

A prescription for hypertrophic cardiomyopathy follows:

Dan shen	20% (cardioprotective, hypotensive, anticoagulant, antiplatelet, hepatoprotective)
Motherwort	20% (sedative, antispasmodic, cardiac tonic)

Ginkgo	20% (PAF inhibitor, antioxidant, circulatory stimulant, cognitive enhancer)
Valerian	20% (sedative, hypnotic, antispasmodic, hypotensive, carminative)
Dandelion	20% (diuretic, laxative, cholagogue, antirheumatic)

David Winston's Melissa/Lycopus compound may be useful for these cats; it consists of Motherwort, Bugleweed, and Lemon balm (Winston, 2003).

DERMATOLOGIC HERBS

General Considerations

Many underlying factors, such as genetics, deficient diet, fleas, allergies (including food), endocrine disorders, and others, contribute to skin disease, as recognized in conventional veterinary medicine. These are generally determined during the processes of history taking and diagnosis, and awareness of them helps the clinician to gain an understanding of the pathogenesis of the skin disorder. However, the treatment of patients with skin disorders in herbal medicine draws on some different traditional concepts.

Skin disorders are considered manifestations of deeper disease processes and therefore indicate metabolic imbalance somewhere in the body. Hence, topical herbs are employed judiciously but represent only a superficial approach. It is important to note that the skin should not be treated in isolation but as a tissue that is intimately connected to and affected by other organ systems. In many cases, a skin lesion is considered a valid attempt by the body to discharge or metabolize toxic agents, so paradoxically, medications that suppress this process (e.g., corticosteroids) are sometimes considered counterproductive over the long term.

Traditional and modern phytotherapeutic concepts that are relevant to chronic skin disease and that help to clarify the issues of "toxicity" include toxemia, leaky gut syndrome, and dysbiosis.

Mechanisms of Interest

Topical vulnerary, astringent, and emollient herbs are discussed under the section "Herbs for Topical Use." From a phytotherapy perspective, topical treatment alleviates skin conditions, but for chronic skin disease, systemic treatment is usually necessary.

Toxemia and chronic skin disease

Traditionally, chronic skin disease was considered a sign of internal toxicity that indicated that the body had failed to eliminate fully. In toxemia, normal elimination through the liver, gut, and kidneys is impaired, allowing the accumulation of toxic metabolites. In the case of chronic dermatitis, the eliminative process most frequently impaired is considered the digestive system. The aim of therapy was always to remove toxins by enhancing and supporting the eliminatory functions of the body. The most useful herbs that have been employed traditionally are the alteratives, also known as depuratives or "blood cleansers." These herbs effect changes in metabolic processes within the body and usually have mild laxative or diuretic actions, among others, so it can be seen that the approach of improving "elimination" has some merit if toxemia is present. Other herbs facilitate the various detoxification mechanisms used by the body and can help restore normal metabolism and immune function.

Although this theory of toxemia is a traditional one, perhaps some scientific support can be provided for it. Incomplete digestion, inflammation, and failure of the local immune response (for systemic tolerance) facilitate gut absorption of macromolecules with high antigenicity (Halliwell, 1995). These can bind to immunoglobulin (Ig)E and precipitate mast cell degranulation or activate the complement cascade via the alternate pathway (thus allowing the subsequent development of food sensitivities and allergies). They can also combine with antibodies to form immune complexes that promote inflammation.

Inflammation of the gut from any cause can make the gut more permeable to macromolecules, causing hyperpermeability, or leaky gut syndrome. Predisposing factors for leaky gut include use of nonsteroidal anti-inflammatory agents or steroids, allergy or intolerance to food, and environmental sensitivities. Similarly, impaired liver function can reduce hepatic detoxification and allow toxins and free radical metabolic intermediates to enter the circulation, thereby contributing to widespread cellular damage (including damage within the epithelium).

Food substances and consequently food allergies and food intolerances are typically associated with chronic dermatitis, alongside exposure to common drugs (especially those that impair liver function or inflame the gut wall) and chemicals that enter the body (through the skin, mouth, or lungs). When subclinical allergy occurs, the potential exists for histamine-releasing foods to become mediators of histamine release, thereby initiating clinical disease (Halliwell, 1995).

Thus, although food allergies (involving an immune reaction) are not considered common in veterinary medicine (less than 10% of atopic dogs are considered to have food allergy [Halliwell, 1995]), food intolerance or adverse reactions to food may go unrecognized. In a study of dogs with allergic dermatoses (excluding flea allergy dermatitis) and not considered to have food intolerance or food allergy, 45.7% improved on a commercial chicken and rice elimination diet. Of the dogs that improved, 68.8% were finally diagnosed with atopic dermatitis (Nagata, 1999). Although the mechanism involved was unclear, this demonstrates the importance of dietary manipulation in the treatment of patients with chronic dermatitis, even when it would not seem obvious in conventional veterinary medicine.

Leaky gut syndrome and chronic skin disease

Another concept employed in herbal medicine is that of "leaky gut syndrome." A major task of the intestine is to form a defensive barrier that prevents absorption of damaging substances from the external environment. In human medicine, inert, nonmetabolized sugars such as mannitol, rhamnose, or lactulose are used to measure the permeability barrier or the degree of leakiness of the intestinal mucosa. Permeability is increased in a number of gastrointestinal tract diseases (such as parasitic infestation, infection, inflammation) and can be increased through trauma, burns, and nonsteroidal anti-inflammatory drugs. The major determinant of the rate of intestinal permeability is the opening or closure of the tight junctions between enterocytes in the paracellular space (Hollander, 1999).

Increasing evidence suggests that a leaky, more permeable bowel wall may lead to translocation of bacteria or endotoxin, which may be an important stimulus for inflammatory cytokine activation (Krack, 2005) and may increase the level of toxic insult to the liver. Leakage of imperfectly digested proteins (peptides) through an incompetent intestinal lining is thought to be the most common cause of environmental sensitivities, acquired food allergies, and an underlying contributing factor to many chronic and degenerative diseases.

Although this syndrome is not yet recognized in veterinary medicine, attention to correcting the "leaky gut" can improve overall health, reduce allergies, and help eliminate one of the major contributing factors to chronic disease.

Dysbiosis theory and chronic skin disease

Related to the theory of the leaky gut syndrome is dysbiosis, which is thought to be a major contributing factor to chronic disease, including skin disorders and food allergies (Fratkin, 1996). It follows the use of antibiotics, other medications, or diets that adversely alter the normal flora, or it may be associated with conditions that allow pathogenic microbes to multiply, producing endotoxins that challenge and deplete the immune system and increase gut permeability (thus predisposing to food allergies and sensitivities). Conditions and symptoms of dysbiosis recognized in human medicine that can be associated with this disturbance include allergies, anxiety, constipation or diarrhea, decreased liver function, decreased pancreatic function, food allergies, muscle pain, pain or swelling in the joints, autoimmune disease, cancer, chemical sensitivities, hyperactivity, chronic hepatitis and pancreatitis, inflammatory bowel disease, malabsorption syndrome, irritable bowel syndrome, and skin conditions such as eczema, psoriasis, urticaria, and acne.

Dysbiosis could be an important unrecognized contributing factor to chronic skin disease, leading to low levels of normal flora (influencing digestion and removal of biodegradable toxins), increased intestinal permeability (toxic overload to liver, lymphatics, interstitial fluids; food sensitivities; autoimmune disease), suppressed immune function, and allergy. Attention to correcting a suspected dysbiosis is worthwhile, and the approach is relatively straightforward.

Therefore, in the treatment of patients with chronic skin disease, whether autoimmune, atopic, infected, or simply chronic, attention must be paid not just to the diagnosis, but to the myriad of contributing factors, such as leaky gut syndrome, dysbiosis, and toxemia, as well as diet, stress levels, drug administration, and so forth. Emphasis is placed on improving systemic health—not just skin health.

When appropriate, herbal interventions may involve the regulation or enhancement of specific body systems, organs, or tissues, or they may require that imbalances be corrected, nutrition optimized, detoxification enhanced, and the energy of the body increased through enhanced vitality (attained with the use of tonics and adaptogens). In chronic disease, an important goal is the stimulation of detoxification, particularly when poor organ function or increased toxic loading is suspected. Detoxification can be achieved by stimulating both the eliminatory organs and the detoxifying processes.

As an informal rule of thumb, chronic skin disease cannot be corrected quickly. The practitioner should allow approximately 3 months' treatment for a condition with duration of 1 year, plus 1 month per each additional year.

Adaptogens

Stress is often a contributing factor to any chronic disease. Adaptogens should be considered if the patient is stressed, anxious, or depressed, in chronic discomfort, and for convalescence. (See Adaptogens in neurology, pain, and behavior section.)

ASHWAGANDHA ***(WITHANIA SOMNIFERA):*** This agent is a tonic, adaptogen, nervine, and anti-inflammatory.

BUPLEURUM ***(BUPLEURUM FALCATUM):*** This is an anti-inflammatory, hepatoprotective, renal protective, and tonic treatment.

LICORICE ***(GLYCYRRHIZA GLABRA):*** This herb is an anti-inflammatory and laxative. It also improves taste.

REHMANNIA ***(REHMANNIA GLUTINOSA):*** This herb is an anti-inflammatory (useful if the patient is on corticosteroids, or when given following their use).

ELEUTHERO ***(ELEUTHEROCOCCUS SENTICOSIS):*** This is an immunomodulatory herb.

GOTU KOLA ***(CENTELLA ASIATICA):*** This herb is a connective tissue regenerator, alterative, nerve tonic, and mild diuretic.

Alteratives/Depuratives

Traditionally, these herbs have been used to detoxify and help eliminatory organs reduce metabolic waste products. Otherwise known as "blood cleansers," they are used to effect a gradual change in chronic disease states, including skin disease. They are said to act by improving the processes of detoxification and elimination, hence they act slowly. A paucity of research data supports their proposed use, but a long tradition of use has been established. Long-term therapy is usually safe and helpful.

BURDOCK ROOT ***(ARTICUM LAPPA):*** This herb is traditionally used as a "tissue cleanser" to eliminate accumulated toxins; it is used for eczema and septic conditions, as a poultice for boils, and in the management of chronic inflammatory states. It contains inulin which acts as a prebiotic and may work as a gentle laxative. It also has demonstrated anti-inflammatory activity in vivo (Lin, 1996a), antioxidant activity in vitro (Duh, 1998), and antimicrobial activity in vitro (Holetz, 2002). Wood (2004) recommends it for dry, red, scaly skin with hair loss and overall dry skin. Felter and Lloyd write in *King's American Disensatory* that Burdock is considered an alterative and a tonic, and they recommend its use in psoriasis and other cutaneous affectations.

OREGON GRAPE ***(MAHONIA AQUIFOLIUM):*** Mahonia is suited to dry, atrophic conditions (rough, dry, scaly skin) when the anabolic function of the liver and the secretory aspect of digestion are compromised. Scudder claimed it "is a blood maker" and a "blood cleanser" that promotes secretion and excretion. It is indicated for dry, scaly, pruritic skin and dandruff (Wood, 2004).

CLEAVERS ***(GALLIUM APARINE):*** This diuretic and lymphatic is used in skin disease. Cleavers has also been used for dry skin eruptions and as a remedy for ulcers and tumors. Wood (2004) recommends it for skin eruptions that have a neurologic association (resembling neurofibrositis). It is considered a valuable diuretic to assist in the treatment of eczema, seborrhea, and psoriasis. It contains iridoid glycosides that are mildly laxative.

RED CLOVER FLOWERS ***(TRIFOLIUM PRATENSE):*** Traditionally, red clover has been used for chronic skin disease, specifically for eczema and psoriasis. No scientific data link specific compounds to distinct dermatologic effects.

YELLOW DOCK ROOT ***(RUMEX CRISPUS):*** Yellow dock is believed to possess gentle purgative and cholagogue properties. Traditionally, it has been used for chronic skin disease, specifically for psoriasis with constipation. Cook, writing in *The Physiomedical Dispensatory* (1869), states that yellow dock is an alterative of the slowly relaxing and stimulating class. It is used in all forms of dry, scaly, itchy, and pustular skin disease.

HEARTSEASE ***(VIOLA TRICOLOR):*** This herb has traditionally been used for the treatment of patients with eczema, psoriasis, and acne. In folk medicine, it is considered a "blood cleanser." Its anti-inflammatory action may in part be due to the presence of both salicylates and rutin (Willuhn, 1994).

BLUE FLAG ***(IRIS VERSICOLOR):*** This herb has traditionally used for skin disease, as a "blood purifier and cleanser of toxins" (Meybe, 1988).

SARSAPARILLA (***SMILAX*** SPP): European physicians considered this an alterative tonic, blood purifier, diuretic, and diaphoretic (Hobbs, 1988). The ability of Smilax to bind with endotoxins and its antibiotic action may explain its effectiveness.

Herbs with activity within the immune system are also regarded as possessing depurative activity.

ECHINACEA ***(ECHINACEA PURPUREA):*** This herb has a long history of medicinal use for a wide variety of conditions, primarily infections such as syphilis and septic wounds; it has also been used as an antitoxin for snakebites and blood poisoning (Hobbs, 1994). Traditionally, Echinacea was known as an anti-infective agent that was indicated in bacterial and viral infections, mild septicemia, furunculosis, and other skin conditions such as boils, carbuncles, and abscesses (Bradley, 1992; British Herbal Pharmacopoeia, 1983).

POKE ROOT ***(PHYTOLACCA DECANDRA):*** King's (Felter, 1898) states that the herb kills scabies mites and is useful for other skin conditions characterized by scaly, vesicular or pustular eruptions, especially those accompanied by lymphatic enlargement. It was recommended for use both locally and systemically in the treatment of patients with skin problems.

Choleretic herbs, such as those listed here, are also considered to have depurative activity:

- Dandelion *(Taraxacum officinale)*
- Fumitory *(Fumaria officinalis)*
- Barberry *(Berberis vulgaris)*
- Globe artichoke *(Cynara scolymus)*

Diuretic herbs that increase detoxification through the urinary tract include the following:

- Dandelion leaf *(Taraxacum officinale)*
- Cleavers *(Gallium aparine)*
- Burdock *(Arctium lappa)*
- Red clover *(Trifolium pratense)*
- Heartease *(Viola tricolor)*

Antiallergy Herbs

The following herbs may help suppress hypersensitivity reactions at any of a number of steps in the process, but their mechanisms of action in vivo are not known. Topical herbs are very useful, but systemic treatment is usually necessary.

NETTLE LEAF ***(URTICA DIOICA FOLIA):*** This herb, also called *stinging nettles,* induces an allergic skin reaction. Herbalists have traditionally prescribed the juice of the nettle as an antidote to rash. One study found that freeze-dried nettles were helpful for symptoms of allergic rhinitis (Mittman, 1990). The mechanism may be partially due to the presence of quercetin; this herb also has anti-inflammatory activity.

ALBIZIA ***(ALBIZIA LEBBECK, ALBIZIA KALKORA):*** This plant, also known as mimosa, is an Ayurvedic herb that is used to treat patients with asthma and dermatitis; it is also a traditional Chinese herb that is used as a sedative. In vivo studies on a bark extract of this plant showed antiallergy activity against anaphylaxis (Tripathi, 1979) and atopic allergy (Tripathi, 1979). Albizia has been shown to stabilize mast cell degranulation, depress levels of antiallergy antibodies, and decrease the overaggressive actions of T and B lymphocytes.

BAICAL SKULLCAP ROOT ***(SCUTELLARIA BAICALENSIS):*** Also called *Huang Qin* in traditional Chinese medicine, this herb has been used traditionally to reduce inflammation and fever. It contains the flavonoids baicalin and wogonin (similar in mechanism of action to quercetin), both of which have antiallergy and free radical scavenging activities (Bochorakova, 2003; Lin, 1996b). Another constituent, baicalein, reduces leukotriene B4 and C4 production by inhibiting lipoxygenase, an action that may lend anti-inflammatory and antiallergy activities (Chang, 1987).

LICORICE ***(GLYCYRRHIZA GLABRA):*** This herb contains glycyrrhizic acid, which is the major bioactive triterpene glycoside of licorice. It possesses a wide range of pharmacologic properties (anti-inflammatory, antiulcer, antiallergic, antidote, antioxidant, antitumor, antiviral, etc.) (Baltina, 2003).

REHMANNIA ***(REHMANNIA GLUTINOSA):*** This herb has demonstrated antiallergic effects on induced allergic reactions in vivo and in vitro. The aqueous extract reduces plasma histamine levels in a dose-dependent manner. It also dose dependently inhibits histamine release from rat peritoneal mast cells (Kim, 1998).

OTHER HERBS: Other antiallergic herbs include achyranthes, alisma, alpinia, apricot seed, arctium, asarum, astragalus, atractylodes, bupleurum, cardamom, ching pi, cinnamon, citrus, cornus, ephedra (ma huang), galanga, ganoderma, gentian, ginger, ginseng, hoelen, licorice, magnolia, moutan, pinnelia, polyporus, pueraria, rehmannia, scute, stephania, tang-kuei, zedoaria, and ziziphus (Tsung, 1987).

Anti-inflammatory Herbs (Systemic Use)

Anti-inflammatory herbs help to control but not suppress symptoms while longer-term alterative strategies take effect.

EVENING PRIMROSE OIL ***(OENOTHERA BIENNIS):*** The actions of evening primrose oil are attributable to the essential fatty acid content of the oil and to the involvement of these compounds in prostaglandin biosynthetic pathways. Evening primrose oil contains 8%-10% gamma linolenic acid (GLA), which displaces and competes with more inflammatory fatty acids in cell membranes. Evening primrose oil had inconsistent benefit, improving a portion of patients tested, in multiple clinical trials in dogs and cats (Harvey, 1993a; Harvey, 1993b; Scarf, 1992; Bond, 1992; Scott, 1992; Bond, 1994).

TURMERIC ***(CURCUMA LONGA):*** This herb has a long history in both Chinese and Ayurvedic medicine as an anti-inflammatory agent. When used orally, curcumin inhibits leukotriene formation, inhibits platelet aggregation, and stabilizes lysosomal membranes, thus inhibiting inflammation at the cellular level (Srimal, 1973). At low levels, curcumin is a prostaglandin inhibitor, and at higher levels, it stimulates the adrenal glands to secrete cortisone (Srivastava, 1985). Powdered turmeric contains 0.6% curcumin (Mukhopadhyay, 1982).

BUPLEURUM ***(BUPLEURUM FALCATUM):*** The anti-inflammatory activity of bupleurum has been demonstrated by in vivo studies (Chang, 1987); the inhibition of arachidonic acid metabolism by saikosaponins is one of the biochemical mechanisms that has been elucidated (Bermejo, 1998). The potency of anti-inflammatory activity of the saikosaponins is similar to that of prednisolone (Chang, 1987).

LICORICE ***(GLYCYRRHIZA GLABRA):*** Glycyrrhizin, a major component of *Glycyrrhiza uralensis* (licorice) root, is a saponin that exhibits a number of pharmacologic effects, including anti-inflammation, antiulcer, antiallergy, and anticarcinogenesis (Hsiang, 2002). It has been shown to inhibit the activity of proinflammatory prostaglandins and leukotrienes and appears to have a cortisone-like effect, accounting for its usefulness as an anti-inflammatory (Okimasu, 1981).

GOTU KOLA ***(CENTELLA ASIATICA):*** This herb is an adaptogen, alterative, and nerve tonic. Triterpenoids are regarded as active principles and are reported to possess wound-healing abilities associated with their stimulating effects on the epidermis and promotion of keratinization. Both asiaticoside and madecassoside are documented to be anti-inflammatory agents (Jacker, 1982). Oral and topical administration of an alcoholic extract of *C. asiatica* for rat dermal wound healing was investigated. The extract increased cellular proliferation and collagen synthesis at the wound site, as evidenced by increased DNA, protein, and collagen content of granulation tissues; wounds treated with the extract were found to epithelialize faster and the rate of wound contraction was higher, as compared with control wounds. Results showed that *C. asiatica* produced different actions in the various phases of wound repair (Suguna, 1996).

OREGON GRAPE ***(BERBERIS AQUIFOLIUM):*** Products of lipoxygenase metabolism are known to play a role in the pathogenesis of human psoriasis. Alkaloids in Oregon grape were tested in vitro and were found to inhibit lipid peroxide substrate accumulation by direct reaction with peroxide, by scavenging, or through lipid-derived radicals (Bezakova, 1996).

NETTLE ***(URTICA DIOICA):*** This traditional herb is used for the treatment of patients with eczema; it is considered to have antiallergic properties and is used to treat itchy skin conditions and insect bites. Nettle leaf extract and caffeic malic acid (the major phenolic component of the extract) were shown to partially inhibit COX- and 5-lipoxygenase (5-LOX)–derived reactions (Obertreis, 1996); also, nettle leaf significantly reduced the release of cytokines in a concentration-dependent manner, and it indirectly decreased PGE_2 synthesis, suggesting an anti-inflammatory effect (Obertreis, 1996).

Antioxidant Herbs

Most herbs have antioxidant activity that is beneficial in reducing oxidative damage associated with inflammation. Herbs that might be useful adjuncts in a formula include Ginger *(Zingiber officinale), Ginkgo biloba,* Grapeseed *(Vitis vinifera),* Green tea *(Camellia sinensis),* Reishi *(Ganoderma lucidum),* Rosemary *(Rosmarinus officinale),* Skullcap *(Scutellaria lateriflora),* Milk thistle *(Silybum marianum),* and Turmeric *(Curcuma longa).*

Antipruritics (Systemic)

CHAMOMILE ***(MATRICARIA RECUTITA):*** The antipruritic effects of diets containing German chamomile on induced scratching in mice have been examined. In mice fed a diet containing 1:2 w/w% of ethyl acetate extract of dried flower of German chamomile for 11 days, scratching behavior was significantly suppressed with no effect on body weight. Inhibitory effects of the dietary intake of German chamomile extract were comparable with those of the antiallergic agent oxatomide (Kobayashi,

2003). The ethyl acetate extract or essential oil of German chamomile showed significant dose-dependent inhibition of induced scratching in mice. The antipruritic effects of the H1 antagonists oxatomide and fexofenadine were only partial in this test. However, the antipruritic effects of these agents were enhanced through combined administration of the ethyl acetate extract of German chamomile (300 mg/kg). Comedication with the ethyl acetate extract, or essential oil of German chamomile, and antihistamines may be more effective for pruritus than either agent alone (Kobayashi, 2005).

TEA ***(CAMELLIA SINENSIS):*** An open study suggests that consumption of oolong tea helps speed the clearance of atopic dermatitis lesions. A total of 118 people continued their usual medications but also drank oolong tea (10 g steeped in 1000 mL water per day, divided into three doses). Beneficial results were observed after 1 to 2 weeks, and 63% of participants showed marked to moderate improvement in lesions after 1 month. After 6 months, 54% still demonstrated a good response (Uehara, 2001).

Immune-Modulating Herbs

HEMIDESMUS ***(HEMIDESMUS INDICUS):*** This root is an Ayurvedic herb (Anant Mool, also known as Krishna powder and Indian Sarsaparilla). It is a depurative and tonic that is used to treat patients with chronic skin disease and other conditions such as cough, genitourinary disease, and rheumatism. Oral administration of an ethanol extract decreased activity in both cell-mediated and humoral components of the immune system in mice (Nadkarni, 1976). Its activity is mild and may benefit patients with autoimmune disease by suppressing the Th-2 cell response.

ASTRAGALUS ***(ASTRAGALUS MEMBRANACEUS):*** This popular herbal medicine is used in Korea, Japan, and China to treat patients with allergic disease. An ethanol extract was tested both in vitro and in vivo to assess murine CD4 T-cell differentiation. Data indicated that astragalus selectively alters Th-1/Th-2 cytokine secretion patterns, which may provide the pharmacologic basis for its clinical applications (Kang, 2004). Astragalus was given to 106 people with herpesvirus keratitis; it changed the state of imbalance of Th-1/Th-2 in these patients and alleviated their immune function disturbance (Mao, 2004).

Nervines

Many animal patients with skin disease display corresponding behavioral signs of anxiety or restlessness. Stress can deplete noradrenaline stores. Adaptogens and nervine herbs may be beneficial. Skullcap *(Scutellaria lateriflora),* Oats *(Avena sativa),* and Saint John's Wort *(Hypericum perforatum)* should be considered.

Effects of Herbal Treatment on Melanin Synthesis

UVA URSI ***(ARCTOSTAPHYLOS UVA URSI):*** This extract may assist in the treatment of patients with hyperpigmentary disorders because arbutin inhibits melanin synthesis in vitro by inhibiting tyrosinase activity (Matsuda, 1992a).

It should be noted that relatively high levels of melatonin are found in Feverfew flowers *(Tanacetum parthenium);* with 2 μg/g, melatonin (dry weight) levels were reduced by about 30% after fresh leaves were oven-dried. Saint John's Wort flowers *(Hypericum perforatum)* contained about 4 μg/g, and the leaves contained about half that level. Baical skullcap leaves *(Scutellaria baicalensis)* consisted of about 7 μg/g melatonin (Murch, 1997). It should be noted that melatonin can cause marked biological effects, even at very low levels.

DONG QUAI ***(ANGELICA SINENSIS):*** This herb promoted melanocytic proliferation and enhanced melanin synthesis and the tryosinase activity of melanocytes, which may be the mechanism for validating its clinical usefulness in the treatment of human patients with skin pigmentation problems (Deng, 2003).

Hair Growth

ASIAN GINSENG: A methanol extract of red ginseng promoted hair growth in mouse vibrissal follicles in organ culture. This suggests that *Panax ginseng* possesses hair growth–promoting activity, and that its bioactive components are partially attributable to the ginseng saponin components (Matsuda, 2003).

REVIEW OF SPECIFIC DERMATOLOGIC CONDITIONS

As a starting point, the following prescriptions are suggested. Selection of herbs will depend on pathophysiology of the disorder, as well as the patient and actions and herbs most suited to the individual.

The importance of the connection between the gut and the skin cannot be underestimated. Even in veterinary medicine in the early part of the 20th century, reference was made to the use of aloes for horses and jalap for dogs for eczema, and to the use of alteratives for urticaria. Barbados aloe, aniseed, ginger, gentian, fenugreek, fennel, and linseed meal were common ingredients in alterative physick balls that were designed to improve such conditions in horses (Leeney, 1921).

Dry Skin and Coat (nonpruritic)

In general, dry skin should prompt the practitioner to evaluate dietary fat content first. Flaxseed and other vegetable oils, as well as increased animal fats, easily reverse this simple problem. When dietary influences have been addressed and the problem persists, herbs may be employed.

A prescription for dry skin and dry or coarse coat, as well as brittle nails follows (dose is 1 ml per 5 kg body weight):

Horsetail	20% (contains minerals, including silica)
Bladderwrack	10% (contains iodine; may be useful in subclinical hypothyroidism)
Red clover	20% (alterative)

Burdock	20% (alterative, mildly laxative; contains linoleic acid)
Rehmannia	30% (adaptogen, blood tonic)

"Condition" powders for horses (adapted from those published in 1920 by the Royal College of Veterinary Surgeons):

Gentian	1 part powdered
Ginger	1 part powdered
Fenugreek	1 part powdered
Licorice	1 part powdered

Atopy and Skin Allergies

Therapeutic rationale

- Reduce exposure to known allergens.
- Consider an elimination diet.
- Modulate immune function.
- Reduce allergic pruritus.
- Inhibit mast cell release of histamine.
- Reduce inflammation.

A study from the University of Minnesota College of Veterinary Medicine investigated three herbs for control of pruritus in atopic dogs. Fifty dogs with atopic dermatitis were assessed by both owners and veterinarians and were given placebo or a combination of Licorice, White peony *(Paeonia lactiflora),* and Rehmannia *(Rehmannia glutinosa).* These herbs were chosen as components of a well-tested human product (not now commercially available) on the basis of company (Phytopharm, United Kingdom) bioassay and palatability. Of dogs receiving herbs, 37.5% improved, compared with 13% in the placebo group, and deterioration scores were worse in the placebo group at the final visit. Although neither result reached statistical significance, researchers were encouraged by the results and suggested further study (Nagle, 2001).

Although the modes of action of alteratives are not clear, they are invaluable in the treatment of patients with chronic allergic skin disease. Concurrent conventional therapy may be required initially, and doses may have to be reduced after 4 to 6 weeks. Herbal therapy should be continued for a minimum of 3 months.

A prescription for allergic dermatitis with dry or moist skin lesions follows:

Burdock	20% (depurative, mild laxative, nutritive)
Red clover	20% (alterative)
Cleavers	20% (diuretic, astringent)
Nettle (leaf)	20% (nutritive, circulatory stimulant, anti-inflammatory, diuretic)
Astragalus	20% (immune modulating, tonic, diuretic)

An alternate prescription for atopic dermatitis is:

Baical skullcap	20% (antiallergy, anti-inflammatory, antibacterial, mild sedative, diuretic, bitter)
Nettles (leaf)	20% (nutritive, circulatory stimulant, anti-inflammatory, diuretic)
Burdock	20% (depurative, mild laxative, nutritive)
Licorice	20% (anti-inflammatory, adaptogen. laxative, taste improver)
Astragalus	20% (immune modulating, tonic, diuretic)

Another prescription for atopic dermatitis is:

Rehmannia	25% (blood tonic, immune modulating)
Licorice	10% (anti-inflammatory, adaptogen. laxative, taste improver)
White peony	25% (anti-inflammatory, antiallergic, immune enhancing)
Sarsaparilla	15% (anti-inflammatory, antiseptic)
Yellow dock or Oregon grape	25% (alterative, cholagogue)

David Hoffman (Hoffmann, 2004) has published this prescription for eczema:

Cleavers	33%
Nettles	33%
Red clover	33%

For acute moist dermatitis (or "hot spots"), black or green tea applied topically (in the moistened tea bag, or as tea on a compress, or as a spray) is very useful for reducing inflammation and pruritus.

Autoimmune Skin Disease*

Therapeutic rationale

- Improve systemic health by improving digestion.
- Eliminate triggers (bacterial, viral, vaccine-related, etc.).
- Reduce stress.
- Regulate immune function.

A prescription for autoimmune skin disease follows:

Bupleurum	20% (anti-inflammatory, hepatoprotective, renal protective, tonic)
Echinacea*	20% (immune modulating, anti-inflammatory, antibacterial, antiviral, vulnerary)
Rehmannia	20% (anti-inflammatory, antiallergy, immune modulating)
Burdock	20% (depurative, mild laxative, nutritive)
Licorice	20% (anti-inflammatory, adaptogen, laxative, taste improver)

Chronic Demodectic Mange

Therapeutic rationale

- Improve immunity.
- Reduce bacterial load.
- Improve systemic health, especially gastrointestinal health.
- Nourish the skin.

A prescription is provided:

Echinacea	20% (immune modulating, anti-inflammatory, antibacterial, antiviral, vulnerary)
Burdock	20% (depurative, mild laxative, nutritive)
Blue flag	20% (cholagogue, laxative, diuretic, alterative, lymphatic)
Baptisia	20% (antimicrobial, antipyretic, antiseptic)
Calendula	20% (lymphatic, anti-inflammatory, astringent, vulnerary, cholagogue)

For other ectoparasitic diseases, see section "Herbs for Topical Use".

*See Author's note on page 320.

Authors' note: The use of immune-enhancing herbs in autoimmune disease is very controversial. The German Commission E monograph recommends that Echinacea not be used in patients with autoimmune disease because of the risk that its immune-stimulating effects could lead to exacerbation of autoimmune illness. Despite several adverse event reports associated with the use of Echinacea in patients with autoimmune disease, the risk has not been adequately studied. The British Herbal Pharmacopoeia (1983) and the British Herbal Compendium offer no contraindications for Echinacea. In fact, it is proposed (Bone, 1997) that molecular mimicry by infectious organisms may be causative in autoimmune disease, and that Echinacea may be benefical in decreasing the chronic presence of microorganisms. Echinacea increases phagocytic activity and increases immune surveillance. This may assist the body in eliminating organisms or neutralizing their imbalancing effects on the immune system, thereby down-regulating an inappropriate immune response.

Chronic or Recurrent Pyoderma

Therapeutic rationale

- Improve systemic health.
- Improve immunity.
- Reduce bacterial load.

A prescription for immune support and lymphatic drainage follows:

Echinacea	20% (immune modulating, anti-inflammatory, antibacterial, antiviral, vulnerary)
Cleavers	20% (diuretic, astringent)
Astragalus	20% (immune modulating, tonic, diuretic)
Blue flag	20% (cholagogue, laxative, diuretic, alterative, lymphatic)
Calendula	15% (lymphatic, anti-inflammatory, astringent, vulnerary, cholagogue)
Poke root	5% (immune enhancing, lymphatic)

A prescription for deep pyoderma (modified from Weiss, 1988) is given here:

Nettle	10%
Dandelion root and herb	15%
Cascara bark	20%
Senna leaf	15%
Anise fruit	20%
Oregon grape root	20%

See also the section on herbs for topical use, especially pertaining to tea tree oil *(Melaleuca alternifolia)*. Tea tree has been shown in human trials to be beneficial in the treatment of acne and Staphylococcus infections (Martin, 2003), as well as in trials in dogs with dermatitis.

ENDOCRINE HERBS

Many herbs can influence the functioning and metabolism of endocrine organs like the thyroid, or endocrine tissue such as the pancreas; however, the therapeutic effects of these herbs may not be an adequate substitute for the efficacy of hormone replacement like insulin and thyroxine. Although conventional drugs target replacement of various hormone compounds, or regulate their production, herbs may be used to reduce drug doses, regulate drug requirements, improve systemic health, and alleviate the secondary effects of systemic disease that result from endocrine changes. The following herbs have activity relating to the endocrine system but can be prescribed alongside herbs for any other system.

Mechanisms of Interest

Adrenal activity

Adaptogens (discussed under the neurologic system) are key herbs for consideration in conditions affecting the adrenal medulla. Nervine tonics also help to reduce anxiety and stress.

CORDYCEPS ***(CORDYCEPS SINENSIS):*** In vitro, a water-soluble extract of *C. sinensis* induced a dose-dependent increase in corticosterone production in rat adrenal cells from 1 hour after the addition of the extract up to 24 hours later. It was concluded that the effect was different from that of adrenocorticotrophic hormone (ACTH) (Wang, 1998).

ASIAN GINSENG ***(PANAX GINSENG):*** Many activities exhibited by *Panax ginseng* have been compared with corticosteroid-like actions, and results of endocrinologic studies have suggested that the ginsenosides may primarily augment adrenal steroidogenesis via an indirect action on the pituitary gland (Ng, 1987). Ginsenosides have increased adrenal cAMP in intact, but not in hypophysectomized, rats, and dexamethasone (which provides positive feedback at the level of the pituitary gland) has blocked the effects of ginsenosides on pituitary corticotropin and adrenal corticosterone secretion (Li, 1987). Ginsenosides may augment adrenocortical steroid production, accounting for its adaptogenic activity (Nocerino, 2000; Rai, 2003b; Kim, 2003). Ginseng saponin was found to act on the hypothalamus or the hypophysis primarily; it stimulated ACTH secretion, which resulted in increased synthesis of corticosterone in the adrenal cortex (Hiai, 1979).

ASHWAGANDHA ***(WITHANIA SOMNIFERA):*** The alcohol extract of ashwagandha (100 mg/kg twice daily on day 1, 4, or 7) attenuated stress-induced increases in blood urea nitrogen, lactic acid, and adrenal hypertrophy but did not affect changes in thymus weight and hyperglycemia in rats (Dadkar, 1987). Ashwagandha reversed stress-induced increases in plasma corticosterone in rats (Archana, 1999). The adaptogenic activity of a standardized extract of ashwagandha root was investigated in a rat model of chronic stress. Stress-induced significant hyperglycemia, glucose intolerance, increased plasma corticosterone levels, gastric ulcerations, male sexual dysfunction, cognitive deficits, immunosuppression, and mental depression. These stress-induced changes were attenuated by ashwagandha (25 and 50 mg/kg given orally) administered before stress induction (Bhattacharya, 2003).

LICORICE ***(GLYCYRRHIZA GLABRA):*** Much has been documented regarding the steroid-type actions of licorice.

Both glycyrrhizin and glycyrrhetinic acid (GA) have been reported to bind to glucocorticoid and mineralocorticoid receptors with moderate affinity, and to estrogen receptors, sex hormone–binding globulin, and corticosteroid-binding globulin with very weak affinity (Tamaya, 1986; Armanini, 1983, 1985). It has been suggested that glycyrrhizin and GA may influence endogenous steroid activity via a receptor mechanism, with displacement of corticosteroids or other endogenous steroids (Tamaya, 1986).

The relatively low affinity of glycyrrhizin and glycyrrhetinic acid for binding to mineralocorticoid receptors, together with the fact that licorice does not exert its mineralocorticoid activity in adrenalectomized animals, indicates that a direct action at the mineralocorticoid receptors is not the predominant mode of action (Stewart, 1987). It has been suggested that glycyrrhizin and GA may exert their mineralocorticoid effects via inhibition of 11β-hydroxysteroid dehydrogenase (11β-OHSD) (Stewart, 1987). 11β-OHSD is a microsomal enzyme complex found predominantly in the liver and kidneys that catalyzes the conversion of cortisol (potent mineralocorticoid activity) to inactive cortisone. Deficiency of 11β-OHSD results in increased concentrations of urinary free cortisol and cortisol metabolites. GA has been shown to inhibit renal 11β-OHSD in rats (Stewart, 1987). It has also been proposed that glycyrrhizin and GA may prevent cortisol from binding to transcortin (Forslund, 1989). One recent case study reports the use of licorice in an Addisonian dog with persistent hyperkalemia. Preliminary results show the dog to be normokalemic after licorice administration (Jarrett, 2005).

ANISEED *(PIMPINELLA ANISUM)*: The pharmacologic effects of aniseed are largely due to the presence of anethole, which is structurally related to the catecholamines adrenaline, noradrenaline, and dopamine. Anethole dimers closely resemble the estrogenic agents stilbene and diethylstilbestrol (Albert-Puleo, 1980).

GINKGO *(GINKGO BILOBA)*: It has been shown that long-term administration of a *Ginkgo biloba* extract inhibits stress-induced corticosterone hypersecretion through a reduction in the number of adrenal peripheral-type benzodiazepine receptors (PBRs). In addition, ginkgo constituents act at the hypothalamic level and are able to reduce corticotrophic releasing hormone expression and secretion (Marcilhac, 1998). Treatment of rats and adrenocortical cells with ginkgolide B reduced mRNA, protein, and ligand binding levels of the adrenal PBR, leading to decreased corticosteroid synthesis. Results of this study demonstrated that ginkgolide B–activated inhibition of glucocorticoid production is due to transcriptional suppression of the adrenal PBR gene and the authors suggest that this might serve as a pharmacologic tool for controlling excess glucocorticoid formation (Amri, 2003).

Androgenic activity

GINGER *(ZINGIBER OFFICINALE)*: An aqueous extract was tested for possible androgenic activity in male rats. It significantly increased the relative weight of the testis, serum testosterone level, testicular cholesterol level, and level of epididymal α-glucosidase activity (Kamtchouing, 2002). Effects on aggression of oral application of 3 mg/day of the ethanolic extracts of ginger were investigated for 6 weeks in intact male mice. The use of ginger showed a dramatic increase in attacks between mice, along with increased spermatozoa count and motility (Homady, 2001).

Antigonadotrophic activity

LYCOPUS *(LYCOPUS EUROPAEUS)*: This herb reduces luteinizing hormone, thyroid-stimulating hormone, and testosterone levels, but not levels of prolactin, in rats administered oral treatment. This reduction was pronounced in spite of reduced thyroxine (T4) and triiodothyronine (T3) levels, suggesting a central point of activity of the plant extract (Winterhoff, 1994). The antigonadotrophic activities of *Lycopus* species can be attributed to their phenolic components. These compounds represent precursors of biologically active products that are formed through an oxidation step. Among the oxidation products of phenolic substances, the corresponding quinones are found. It can be demonstrated that the reaction between quinones and unoxidized diphenols yields products with strong antigonadotrophic activity. This type of reaction—the formation of quinhydrones—is proposed to be involved in the formation of various products with antigonadotrophic activity (Gumbinger, 1981).

Antidiabetic activity

ASIAN GINSENG *(PANAX GINSENG)*: Hypoglycemic activity has been documented for ginseng and has been attributed to both saponin and polysaccharide constituents. In vitro studies using isolated rat pancreatic islets have shown that ginsenosides promote an insulin release that is independent of extracellular calcium and that uses a different mechanism from that of glucose (Guodong, 1987). In addition, in vivo studies in rats have reported that a ginseng extract increases the number of insulin receptors in bone marrow and reduces the number of glucocorticoid receptors in rat brain homogenate (Yushu, 1988). Both of these actions are thought to contribute to the antidiabetic actions of ginseng.

TURMERIC *(CURCUMA LONGA)*: This herb has been used for the treatment of patients with diabetes. One study evaluated turmeric and curcumin in treating rats with induced diabetes. The lower rate of weight gain by diabetic rats, compared with nondiabetic rats, was normalized by oral administration of an aqueous extract of turmeric (1 g/kg) or curcumin (0.08 g/kg) for 21 days. Results revealed a decrease in the cellular leakage of acid phosphatase, alkaline phosphatase, and lactate dehydrogenase into the serum of diabetic animals. Curcumin appeared to be more effective in attenuating diabetes mellitus than turmeric (Arun, 2002).

COMBINATION OF UVA URSI *(ARCTOSTAPHYLOS UVA URSI)*, GOLDENSEAL *(HYDRASTIS CANADENSIS)*, MISTLETOE *(VISCUM ALBUM)*, AND TARRAGON *(ARTEMISIA DRACUNCULUS)*: This combination significantly reduced the hyperphagia and polydipsia associated with streptozotocin–diabetic mice. Treatments were supplied as 6.25% by weight of the diet for 9 days. No effect on insulin or glucose concentrations was observed (Swanston-Flatt, 1989).

CORDYCEPS *(CORDYCEPS SINENSIS):* A study on rats with induced diabetes revealed that the fruiting body—not the carcass of Cordyceps—attenuated diabetes-induced weight loss, polydipsia, and hyperglycemia. This suggested that the fruiting body of Cordyceps has potential as a functional food for patients with diabetes (Lo, 2004). Effects of *C. sinensis* on pancreatic islet B cells of rats with hepatic fibrogenesis were investigated. No change was seen in levels of serum insulin and basal insulin between the test group and the normal group at week 3; however, at week 6 serum insulin and basal insulin were higher in the test group than in the normal group. It was concluded that Cordyceps can increase the basal insulin levels of islets in rats with induced liver fibrosis (Zhang, 2003a).

GINGER *(ZINGIBER OFFICINALE):* The effects of ginger juice (4 mL/kg orally daily, given for 6 weeks) on rats with induced type I diabetes were studied. In normoglycemic rats, 5-HT (1 mg/kg intraperitoneally) produced hyperglycemia and hypoinsulinemia, which were significantly prevented by ginger juice. Treatment with ginger produced a significant increase in insulin levels and a decrease in fasting glucose levels in diabetic rats as well as a decrease in serum cholesterol, serum triglyceride, and blood pressure. The data suggested potential antidiabetic activity of ginger juice in type I diabetic rats, possibly involving 5-HT receptors (Akhani, 2004).

Antihyperglycemic effects

GINSENG *(PANAX GINSENG AND P. QUINQUEFOLIUS):* These herbs have been studied extensively, and data suggest that the antihyperglycemic activity of ginseng may be highly variable. In healthy humans, two batches of American ginseng demonstrated acute postprandial glycemic index lowering efficacy, and a third batch was ineffective, whereas Japanese, Asian red, and Sanchi ginsengs had null effects, and Asian, American wild, and Siberian ginsengs raised glycemia (Sievenpiper, 2004). The dose and the quality of the herb are therefore important, which demonstrates the need for monitoring of patients who are taking herbal medicines.

GYMNEMA *(GYMNEMA SYLVESTRE):* This herb has been found to reduce hyperglycemia in both animal and human studies. Its antidiabetic activity appears to be due to a combination of mechanisms. Animal studies on beryllium nitrate–and streptozotocin–diabetic rats found that Gymnema doubled the number of insulin-secreting β cells in the pancreas and returned blood sugars to almost normal (Prakash, 1986; Shanmugasundaram, 1990). Gymnema increased the activity of enzymes responsible for glucose uptake and utilization (Shanmugasundaram, 1983) and inhibited peripheral utilization of glucose by somatotrophin and corticotrophin (Gupta, 1964). Gymnema has also been found to inhibit epinephrine-induced hyperglycemia (Gupta, 1961).

MADAGASCAR PERIWINKLE LEAF JUICE *(CATHARANTHUS ROSEUS)* AND SEED POWDER OF FENUGREEK *(TRIGONELLA FOENUM-GRAECUM):* These herbs were tested for their hypoglycemic actions when used individually and in combination in normal and alloxan-induced diabetic rabbits. Blood glucose was determined in all groups before and after treatment with *C. roseus* (0.5, 0.75, and 1.0 mL/kg) and fenugreek (50, 100, and 150 mg/kg) throughout a 24-hour period, after fasting for 18 hours. The effects were dose dependent with both treatments. The percentage of blood glucose reduction produced by the combination of periwinkle (0.5 mL/kg) and fenugreek (50 mg/kg) was greater than the sum of the individual percentages of blood glucose reduction in both normal and diabetic rabbits, suggesting that the combination produced a synergistic action (Satyanarayana, 2003).

FENUGREEK *(TRIGONELLA FOENUM-GRAECUM):* This herb and isolated fenugreek fractions have been shown to act as hypoglycemic and hypocholesterolemic agents in both animal and human studies. The dietary fiber composition and high saponin content in fenugreek appear to be responsible for these therapeutic properties (Madar, 2002). Fractions of seeds were given to normal and diabetic dogs for 8 days. Effects on glucose and pancreatic hormones were tested. The lipid fraction of the herb had no effect; the defatted fraction of the herb lowered basal blood glucose, glucagon, and somatostatin and reduced the orally induced hyperglycemia. In diabetic dogs on insulin, the defatted fraction reduced hyperglycemia and glycosuria (Ribes, 1986). In diabetic rats, the inclusion of fenugreek overcame the toxicity of vanadium when given alone. Lower rates of vanadate were needed in combination with fenugreek, and the combined effects were better at restoring the above parameters than was insulin (Dhananjay, 1999).

INULA *(INULA RACEMOSA)* AND GYMNEMA *(GYMNEMA SYLVESTRE):* These (leaf) extracts given alone or in combination were evaluated in the amelioration of corticosteroid-induced hyperglycemia in mice. The extracts in combination were more effective than the individual extracts. The effects were comparable with those of a standard corticosteroid-inhibiting drug, ketoconazole. Because no marked changes in thyroid hormone concentration were observed with the administration of any extracts in corticosteroid-treated animals, it was suggested that these plant extracts may not be effective in thyroid hormone–mediated type II diabetes, but that they would be for steroid-induced diabetes (Gholap, 2003).

BILBERRY *(VACCINIUM MYRTILLUS)* (BILBERRY LEAF TEA): This herb reduced high blood glucose levels in normal and diabetic dogs, even when glucose was concurrently injected intravenously (Allen, 1927). Bilberry extracts are widely used in Europe for the treatment and prevention of secondary eye problems (e.g., diabetic retinopathy cataracts) in people (Murray, 1995); the berry rather than the leaf is most beneficial here. This is a very safe herb that has no known adverse effects.

ALOE *(ALOE VERA):* The dried sap is a traditional remedy for diabetes; it has been reported to reduce blood glucose in patients with type 2 diabetes and in an animal model (Ghannam, 1986). Oral administration of the juice (prepared from the gel) has been reported to reduce fasting blood glucose and triglyceride levels in patients with type 2 diabetes; the amount used was 1 tablespoon taken twice daily (Bunyapraphatsara, 2003; Yongchaiyudha, 1996).

Rehmannia *(Rehmannia glutinosa)*: The hypoglycemic and antidiabetic effects of Rehmannia oligosaccharide in glucose-induced hyperglycemic and alloxan-induced diabetic rats were investigated. It was shown that this herb exerted a significant hypoglycemic effect in normal and alloxan-induced diabetic rats. The regulatory mechanism of glucose metabolism was adrenal dependent and was closely related to the neuroendocrine system (Zhang, 2004).

Dandelion *(Taraxacum officinale)*: In vitro testing of an extract of dandelion revealed insulin secretagogue activity (Hussain, 2004).

Other herbs with hypoglycemic effects

The antihyperglycemic effects of fenugreek *(Trigonella foenum-graceum)*, Damania *(Turnera diffusa)*, and *Euphorbia prostrata* were studied. Each plant was processed in the traditional way and was intragastrically administered to temporarily hyperglycemic rabbits. Results showed that several plants significantly decreased the hyperglycemic peak or the area under the glucose tolerance curve (Alarcon-Aguilara, 1998).

Other herbs with hyperglycemic effects include agrimony, alfalfa, bugleweed, burdock, celery, corn silk, dandelion, elecampane, eucalyptus, garlic, ginger, ginseng, goat's rue, panax, ispaghula, Java tea, juniper marshmallow, myrrh, nettle, sage, senega, siberian ginseng, tansy (Brinker, 1997).

Hyperglycemic activity

Herbs that may increase blood sugar include Elecampane, *Panax ginseng*, Gotu kola, Licorice, Rosemary, and Tea *(Camellia sinensis)*. These herbs may be contraindicated in the treatment of some diabetic patients.

Thyroid-stimulating activity

Ashwagandha *(Withania somnifera)*: A root extract (1.4 g/kg) increased T4 and liver glucose-6-phosphatase in mice and decreased liver lipid peroxidation (Panda, 1999). The same dose rate given for 20 days to mice increased liver superoxide dismutase, glucose-6-phosphatase, and catalase and increased serum 3,3′,5-triiodothyronine (T3) and tetraiodothyronine (T4) (Panda, 1998).

Brahmi *(Bacopa monniera)*: Leaf extracts (200 mg/kg) were investigated in the regulation of thyroid hormone concentrations in male mice. T4 concentration was increased by Bacopa, suggesting a thyroid-stimulating role. Bacopa increased T4 concentration by 41% while decreasing hepatic lipid peroxidation and increasing superoxide dismutase (SOD) and catalase (CAT) activities, thereby showing an antiperoxidative role (Kar, 2002).

Bladderwrack *(Fucus vesiculosus)*: Bladderwrack (kelp) is often touted as a treatment for patients with hypothyroid disease; however, published supporting evidence is distinctly lacking. The charcoal derived from kelp (under the name of *Aethiops vegetabilis*, or vegetable ethiops) was once used in the treatment of patients with goiter and scrofulous swelling. Experiments of Hunt and Seidell in 1910 presented evidence to show that the extract of this plant is a powerful stimulant for the thyroid gland (Remington, 1918). It may be of greatest value in conditions associated with iodine deficiency.

Thyroid-inhibiting activity

Aloe Vera: An extract (125 mg/kg) was investigated for the regulation of thyroid hormone concentrations in male mice. Serum levels of both T3 and T4 were inhibited by *A. vera* (Kar, 2002).

Bugleweed *(Lycopus virginicus)*: This herb decreases levels of several hormones in animal models, particularly thyroid-stimulating hormone (TSH) and the thyroid hormone T4 (Wagner, 1970). In rats, an ethanolic extract of *Lycopus europaeus* caused a long-lasting (for a period longer than 24 h) decrease in T3 levels, presumably as a consequence of reduced peripheral T4 deiodination. Pronounced reductions in T4 and TSH concentrations were observed 24 h after application of the extract by gavage (Winterhoff, 1994). *Lycopus virginicus* and *Lycopus europaeus* have the ability to inhibit many of the effects of exogenous and endogenous TSH on the thyroid gland; they inhibit adenylate cyclase in the thyroid and inhibit cAMP, particularly at high doses (Auf'mkolk. 1984b). Aqueous extracts from *L. virginicus* also inhibit extrathyroidal enzymic T4-5′-deiodination to T3 and T4-5′-deiodination. These effects are dose dependent. Rosmarinic acid, ellagic acid, and luteolin-7 β-glucoside are active inhibitory components (Auf'mkolk, 1984a).

Lemon balm *(Melissa officinalis)*: In vitro investigation showed lemon balm to disrupt thyroid activity by inhibiting TSH-stimulated adenylate cyclase production. It also produced significant inhibition of TSH binding to its receptor and of antibody binding to TSH. Data suggest that lemon balm may block the binding of TSH to its receptor by acting on both the hormone and the receptor itself (Santini, 2003).

REVIEW OF SPECIFIC ENDOCRINOLOGIC CONDITIONS

Hypoadrenocorticism

Therapeutic rationale

- Correct electrolyte abnormalities.
- Improve adrenal and systemic health and alleviate signs of Addison's disease.
- Supply corticosteroid-like action.

A prescription for adrenal support follows here:

Siberian ginseng	20% (adaptogenic, immunomodulatory)
Astragalus	20% (immune modulating, tonic, cardiotonic, diuretic, hypotensive, antitumor)
Licorice	20% (anti-inflammatory, adaptogen, mineralocorticoid and corticoid-like activity)
Ashwagandha	40% (tonic, adaptogen, nervine, anti-inflammatory, antitumor)

Panax ginseng can be substituted for Siberian ginseng in a debilitated or elderly patient.

Hyperadrenocorticism

Therapeutic rationale

- Reduce production of corticosteroids.
- Improve adrenal and systemic health (including the liver) and reduce signs.
- Improve immunity (and reduce secondary infection).

A prescription for hyperadrenocorticism follows:

Ginkgo	20% (antioxidant, circulatory stimulant, cognition enhancer, may reduce corticosteroid production)
Milk thistle	20% (hepatotonic, antioxidant, hepatoprotective)
Dandelion	20% (diuretic, alterative, laxative, cholagogue)
Rehmannia	20% (renal protective, adaptogen)
Astragalus	20% (immune modulating, tonic, cardiotonic, diuretic, hypotensive, antitumor)

Hyperadrenocorticism (Cushing's Disease) in Horses

In an open trial involving 25 horses and ponies diagnosed with Cushing's disease, chaste tree was administered to animals that should have already been shed. Each of the animals was given a daily dose of *Vitex agnus-castus* for 3 months. The study demonstrated the following: reduced hirsutism—with subsequent reduction in hyperhidrosis—improved energy levels and mood; apparent reduction in the incidence of laminitis; reduced polyuria and polydipsia; and decreased abnormal fat deposits. The results encourage further research into therapeutic effects of *Vitex-agnus castus* in horses (Self, 2003). However, another study showed that *Vitex-agnus castus* extract did not have a beneficial effect in horses with pituitary pars intermedia hyperplasia (equine Cushing's syndrome) (Beech, 2002).

Diabetes Mellitus

Therapeutic rationale

- Improve metabolism of food.
- Use hypoglycemic agents (note that careful monitoring is required because insulin adjustments will be needed).
- Prevent long-term complications.
- Improve systemic health and pancreatic health.

Prescription 1 for diabetes mellitus:

Gymnema	30% (hypoglycemic, pancreatic trophorestorative, astringent, mild diuretic)
Panax	30% (adaptogenic, tonic, hypoglycemic, immunostimulant, hepatoprotective, cardioprotective)
Fenugreek	20% (hypoglycemic, laxative, nutritive)
Bilberry	20% (vasoprotective, antioxidant, anti-inflammatory, astringent)

Prescription 2 for diabetes mellitus:

Bilberry	20% (vasoprotective, antioxidant, anti-inflammatory, astringent)
Gymnema	30% (hypoglycemic, pancreatic trophorestorative, astringent, mild diuretic)
Dandelion	20% (diuretic, alterative, laxative, cholagogue)
Rehmannia	30% (hypoglycemic, renal protective, adaptogen)

Prescription for prevention of complications:

Gymnema	30% (hypoglycemic, pancreatic trophorestorative, astringent, mild diuretic)
Bilberry	20% (vasoprotective, antioxidant, anti-inflammatory, astringent)
Globe artichoke	20% (diuretic, hepatoprotective, choleretic, bitter, hepatic trophorestorative)
Astragalus	30% (immune modulating, tonic, cardiotonic, diuretic, hypotensive, antitumor)

Hyperthyroidism

Therapeutic rationale

- Use relaxing nervines and adaptogens to help prevent the adverse effects of the condition.
- Cardiac tonics may be beneficial.
- Herbs can support the work of conventional medications.

Prescription for feline hyperthyroidism with hyperactivity include the following:

Bugleweed	25% (cardioactive diuretic, reduces heart rate, sedative, thyroxine antagonist)
Motherwort	25% (sedative, cardiotonic)
Hawthorn	25% (cardiotonic, hypotensive, antioxidant)
Passionflower	25% (sedative, nervine, antispasmodic)

Prescription for feline hyperthyroidism with renal disease:

Hawthorn	25% (cardiotonic, hypotensive, antioxidant)
Motherwort	25% (sedative, cardiotonic)
Bugleweed	25% (cardioactive diuretic, reduces heart rate, sedative, thyroxine antagonist)
Rehmannia	25% (adaptogen, renal protective)

Note description of herbs for hypertrophic cardiomyopathy in the section on cardiovascular herbs; the formulas above may be modified by adding lemon balm, Oregon grape, ginkgo, valerian, or pharmacological effect of ethanol extract.

Hypothyroidism

Therapeutic rationale

- No herbs contain thyroxine.
- Stimulate the thyroid, if appropriate, although autoimmune herbs may be more strategic.
- Treat associated disorders: bitters, skin emollients, and circulatory stimulants may be helpful; constipation can be alleviated with mild laxative herbs; antidepressant herbs may be beneficial.

A prescription for hypothyroidism is provided here:

Ginger	10% (bitter, carminative, antispasmodic, anti-inflammatory, circulatory stimulant)
Milk thistle	20% (hepatotonic, antioxidant, hepatoprotective)
Bupleurum	30% (anti-inflammatory, hepatoprotective, renal protective, tonic)

Ashwagandha	40% (tonic, adaptogen, nervine, anti-inflammatory, antitumor)

HERBS FOR GASTROINTESTINAL TRACT DISORDERS

General Considerations

"Let your food be your medicine," said Hippocrates. Throughout history, plants have been our medicine; they have a direct effect on digestion attained via absorption, metabolism, and elimination of plant chemicals, and a direct action achieved through tissue contact in the GI tract. The GI tract is central to systemic health, and a recognized fundamental linkage exists between the gut and systemic health in conditions as wide ranging as asthma, atopy, autoimmune disease, and even arthritis. Visceral reflex connections between the gut and other mucous membranes in the body are employed in herbal medicine, so anything that improves digestion will improve tissues elsewhere in the body.

Considering that the gut plays a significant role in immune function, this is no surprise. Therefore, in herbal medicine, significant emphasis is placed on the health of the digestive system; history taking includes nature of bowel movements and any symptoms related to gut function. Clinically, even mild digestive disturbances, such as burping, mild constipation, inconsistent stools, or excessive flatulence, are always considered significant, even if they are not the reason why a patient presents for consultation.

Mechanisms of Interest

Antacids and antiulcer herbs

A number of herbs counteract stomach acidity and have demonstrated a protective effect against the induction of gastric and duodenal ulcers, as well as efficacy in the treatment of patients with ulcers. These herbs are discussed in the following paragraphs.

EXTRACTS FROM LEMON BALM *(MELISSA OFFICINALIS)*, CHAMOMILE *(MATRICARIA RECUTITA)*, PEPPERMINT *(MENTHA X PIPERITA)*, LICORICE *(GLYCYRRHIZA GLABRA)*, ANGELICA ROOT *(ANGELICA ARCHANGELICA)*, MILK THISTLE *(SILYBUM MARIANUM)*, AND GREATER CELANDINE *(CHELIDONIUM MAJUS)*: Singly and combined, these herbs were tested for their potential antiulcerogenic activity against indomethacin-induced gastric ulcer in rats, as well as for their antisecretory and cytoprotective activities. All extracts produced dose-dependent antiulcerogenic activity associated with reduced acid output and increased mucin secretion, increased prostaglandin E_2 release, and leukotrienes that were decreased in the gastric mucosa. The most beneficial effects were observed with combinations and were comparable with the effects of cimetidine. It was concluded that the cytoprotective effects of the extracts could in part be due to their flavonoid content and free radical scavenging properties (Khayyal, 2001).

MEADOWSWEET *(FILIPENDULA ULMARIA)*: This herb is considered to be a normalizer of acidity in the stomach. Its positive effect on the mucosa is paradoxical because it also contains salicylates. When used in an experimental model of ulcers induced by acetylsalicylic acid (aspirin), meadowsweet, given at rates of 0.7 and 1.25 mL/kg, caused reduced numbers of ulcers by 25.4% and 26.2%, respectively. Injection of the infusion at rates of 0.35 to 15.0 mL/kg accelerated the evacuation of gastric contents, providing better protection of the mucous membrane (Gorbacheva, 2002).

TURMERIC *(CURCUMA LONGA)*: Curcuma longa has been commonly used as a traditional remedy for a variety of symptoms such as inflammation, gastritis and gastric ulcer. One study showed that an ethanol extract from *C. longa* specifically inhibits gastric acid secretion by blocking H(2) histamine receptors in a competitive manner (Kim 2005). Intragastric administration of an ethanol extract of turmeric to rats inhibited gastric secretion and protected the gastroduodenal mucosa against chemical, physical, and drug-induced injuries. Turmeric stimulated the production of gastric wall mucus and restored non-protein sulfides in rats (Rafatullah, 1990). The German Commission E monograph is frequently used as an authoritative source for information on herbal medicine. It lists gastric ulcer, hyperacidity, peptic ulcer as contraindications for use of turmeric, however, newer studies suggest that these cautions are unwarranted.

BILBERRY *(VACCINIUM MYRTILLUS)*: Anthocyanins have been shown to have antiulcer activity in various experimental models of acute gastric ulcer and in chronic ulcer induced by acetic acid. The mechanism for this may be potentiation of the defensive barriers of the gastrointestinal tract mucosa, such as the secretion of gastric mucus or the stimulation of cellular regeneration (Magistretti, 1988).

COMFREY *(SYMPHYTUM OFFICINALIS)* AND CALENDULA *(CALENDULA OFFICINALIS)*: This combination was used, alone (137 patients) or in combination with an antacid (33 patients), to treat patients with gastroduodenitis and gastric ulcer. In all, 90% of patients were relieved of pain and the ulcers healed (Chakurski, 1981a). Comfrey is not available in US commercial trade for oral use because of its content of pyrrolizidine alkaloids.

CHAMOMILE *(CHAMOMILLA/MATRICARIA RECUTITA)*: This extract inhibited ethanol-induced ulceration, and antiulcerogenic activity in rats has been reported for α-bisabolol (Mann, 1986; Szelenyi, 1979).

MILK THISTLE *(SILYBUM MARIANUM)*: Administration of this herb to rats prevented gastric ulceration induced by cold stress. Gastric secretion volume and acidity were not affected, but histamine concentration was significantly decreased. It was suggested that the antiulcerogenic effects of silymarin may be related to inhibition of enzymic peroxidation by the lipoxygenase pathway (Alacrin De Le Lastra, 1992). The protective effects of silymarin and its effects on mucosal myeloperoxidase have been compared with those of allopurinol. Mean ulcer indexes of rats treated with 25, 50, and 100 mg/kg silymarin were significantly lower than those in control rats, although allopurinol was considerably more potent (2.3; 100 mg/kg) (Alarcon De La Lastra, 1995).

Dan Shen *(Salvia miltiorrhiza)*: This herb increased gastric mucosal blood flow in normal dogs. In this way, dan shen supported the integrity of the mucosal barrier and improved its defense function. When aspirin was administered, however, dan shen could only delay the onset of mucosal lesions (Yan, 1990).

Fenugreek Seeds *(Trigonella foenum-graecum)*: These have been shown to have significant ulcer protective effects. The cytoprotective effect of the seeds seemed to be due not only to their antisecretory action but also to their effects on mucosal glycoproteins (Pandian, 2002).

Licorice *(Glycyrrhiza glabra)*: This herb is well known for its antiulcer action. One mechanism of antiulcer activity involves acceleration of mucin excretion through increased synthesis of glycoprotein at the gastric mucosa, which prolongs the life of the epithelial cells and lengthens antipepsin activity (Dehpour, 1995). Oral administration of deglycyrrhizinated licorice (380 mg, 3 times daily) to 169 patients with chronic duodenal ulcers was as effective as antacid or cimetidine treatment (Kassir, 1985).

Corydalis *(Corydalis ambigua)*: In humans with stomach or intestinal ulcer or chronic inflammation of the stomach lining, a 90- to 120-mg extract of corydalis per day (equal to 5-10 g crude herb) was found to improve ulcer repair and alleviate symptoms in 76% of patients (Chang, 1986).

Gotu Kola *(Centella asiatica)*: Oral doses of 200 and 600 mg/kg twice daily for 5 days showed significant protection against in a rat model of experimental gastric ulcer; the results were comparable with those elicited by sucralfate. At 600 mg/kg, gotu kola significantly increased gastric juice mucin secretion and increased mucosal cell glycoproteins, signifying increased cellular mucus. It also decreased cell shedding, indicating fortification of the mucosal barrier. Thus, the ulcer protective effect may be due to strengthening of mucosal defensive factors (Sairam, 2001a).

Bacopa *(Bacopa monniera)*: When given as a dose of 10 to 50 mg/kg twice daily to rats for 5 days, this herb showed dose-dependent antiulcerogenic effects on various gastric ulcer models. At 20 mg/kg, it showed no effect on acid–pepsin secretion, and it increased mucin secretion; it also decreased cell shedding with no effect on cell proliferation. Bacopa showed significant antioxidant effect. Thus, its gastric prophylactic and curative effects may be due to its predominant effect on mucosal defensive factors (Sairam, 2001b).

Anti-inflammatory, demulcent, and astringent herbs

Many herbs have demonstrated anti-inflammatory activity in various animal models and traditionally are considered anti-inflammatory for the gastrointestinal tract, although few have been studied specifically for their mechanisms in the gut. Demulcent and astringent herbs are included here because they are used traditionally to relieve inflammation through their physical action.

Anti-Inflammatory Herbs

Boswellia *(Boswellia serrata)*: Extracts of the gum resin possess anti-inflammatory properties. In particular, the boswellic acids inhibit the enzyme 5-lipoxygenase, which is responsible for the production of leukotrienes. Inflammatory bowel disease (IBD) is associated with enhanced leukotriene function, and the benefits of Boswellia in the treatment of patients with chronic colitis (ulcerative colitis) or Crohn's disease have been investigated. A total of 20 patients with chronic colitis received Boswellia gum resin (900 mg/d for 6 wk), and another 10 patients were given sulfasalazine (3 g/d for 6 wk). Of 20 patients treated with Boswellia, 14 went into remission (70%, compared with 40% for sulfasalazine) (Bone, 1999). The safety and efficacy of a Boswellia extract were compared against mesalazine for the treatment of 102 patients with active Crohn's disease in an 8-week, randomized, double-blind study. The authors concluded that the Boswellia extract was as effective as mesalazine (Bone, 2004).

Butterbur *(Petasites hybridus)*: This herb has been used for hundreds of years to treat patients with gastrointestinal tract complaints. Petasines—the main components of butterbur—inhibit the synthesis of leukotrienes and decrease the intracellular concentration of calcium, which explains the anti-inflammatory and spasmolytic properties of extracts of butterbur (Kalin, 2003).

Chamomile *(Matricaria recutita)*: The German Commission E has approved the use of chamomile for gastrointestinal spasms and inflammatory diseases of the gastrointestinal tract (Blumenthal, 1998).

Other herbs

Other herbs traditionally used for their anti-inflammatory activity in gastrointestinal tract conditions include the following:

- Dong quai *(Angelica sinensis)*
- Baical skullcap *(Scutellaria baicalensis)*
- Calendula *(Calendula officinalis)*
- Wild yam *(Dioscorea villosa)*
- Licorice *(Glycyrrhiza glabra)*
- Meadowsweet *(Filipendula ulmaria)*
- Goldenseal *(Hydrastis canadensis)*
- Devil's claw *(Harpagophytum procumbens)*

Demulcents: Demulcents are used to lubricate and protect the alimentary mucous membrane, but the term is usually applied only to those agents that affect the buccal, pharyngeal, esophageal, and gastric mucosa. Demulcents can be used to protect the mucous membranes before or during administration of irritant substances; to allay irritation and inflammation already caused by chemical or bacterial action, or to act as bulking agents for other drugs and herbs.

Mucilage refers to mucilaginous substances in plants that cause demulcency—usually, polysaccharide gels. These substances may protect mucosal surfaces by adhering to the mucosa, and may also act as a prebiotic, reducing epithelial inflammation by normalizing intestinal flora populations.

Polysaccharides from Marshmallow *(Althaea officinalis)*, Ribwort *(Plantago lanceolata)*, *Malva moschata*, or *Tilia cordata* showed only moderate bioadhesion to epithelial tissue, whereas strong adhesive processes were observed with polysaccharides from Bladderwrack *(Fucus vesiculosus)* and Calendula *(Calendula officinalis),* and the adhesive effects were concentration dependent. Histologic studies of membranes revealed the presence of distinct polysaccharide layers on the apical membrane surface (Schmidgall, 2000).

MARSHMALLOW ***(ALTHAEA OFFICINALIS):*** This herb contains mucilage polysaccharides (5%–10%) that consist of galacturono-rhamnans, arabinans, glucans, and arabinogalactans (ESCP, 1999). The German Commission E approved the use of root and leaf for irritation of oral and pharyngeal mucosa and associated dry cough, and root for mild inflammation of the gastric mucosa (Blumenthal, 1998).

SLIPPERY ELM ***(ULMUS FULVA):*** This herb consists of mucilage as a major component and 3% to 6.5% tannin. Traditionally, it has been used for inflammation or ulceration of the stomach or duodenum, convalescence, colitis, and diarrhea. It forms a viscous mucilage with moisture.

LICORICE ***(GLYCYRRHIZA GLABRA):*** Carbenoxolone, an ester derivative of glycyrrhetinic acid, has been used in the treatment of patients with gastric and esophageal ulcers and is thought to exhibit mucosal protective effects by beneficially interfering with gastric prostanoid synthesis, thereby increasing production of mucus and promoting mucosal blood flow (Guslandi, 1985).

BLADDERWRACK ***(FUCUS VESICULOSUS):*** The mucilaginous thallus has been used for a long time to treat patients with irritated and inflamed tissues (Newall, 1996)

COMFREY ***(SYMPHYTUM OFFICINALIS):*** Comfrey is believed to possess vulnerary, cell proliferant, astringent, antihemorrhagic, and demulcent properties. It has been used for colitis, gastric and duodenal ulcers, and hematemesis (Blumenthal, 1998); however, in view of the hepatotoxic properties documented for the pyrrolizidine alkaloid constituents, comfrey should not be taken internally.

FENUGREEK ***(TRIGONELLA FOENUM-GRAECUM):*** This herb is stated to possess mucilaginous demulcent, laxative, and nutritive properties and has been used in the treatment of patients with anorexia, dyspepsia, gastritis, and convalescence (Blumenthal, 1998; Bisset, 1994).

Astringents: An astringent such as tannic acid is a compound that precipitates protein. Similar to mucilages, astringents form a temporary film of clotted protein over the mucosal surface that effectively protects it from caustic agents and dulls the sensory nerve endings that are responsible for any reflex hyperexcitability. The precipitate is relatively impermeable to the passage of fluids in either direction (Daykin, 1960). Tannins belong to two main classes. Condensed tannins (flavanols) include catechins, epicatechins, and epigallocatechin gallate, which is found in teas and red wine; they are considered to be very safe. Hydrolyzable tannins, including tannic acid, typically occur in the bark and fruit of trees, such as oak. These tannins are used in the dying and tanning industries and are not found in teas.

It is usually suggested that astringents be used for a limited time (no longer than about 2 weeks). Herbs that are high in tannins can interact with or limit the absorption of some alkaline drugs.

AGRIMONY ***(AGRIMONIA EUPATORIA):*** This herb contains 3% to 21% condensed tannins and some hydrolyzable tannins (e.g., ellagitannin). The tannin constituents may justify the astringent activity attributed to the herb.

TORMENTIL ***(POTENTILLA TORMENTILLA):*** The roots of this herb contain up to 20% tannins, primarily condensed tannins and essential oils (tormentol). The root was traditionally used to reduce bowel inflammation associated with diarrhea and as an antidote for consumption of poisons; it is strongly astringent and relieves enteritis and episodes of food poisoning (Blumethal, 1998).

BLACKBERRY ***(RUBUS FRUCTOSIS):*** The presence of large amounts of tannins gives blackberry leaves and roots an astringent effect that may be useful for treating patients with diarrhea.

CRANESBILL ***(GERANIUM MACULATUM):*** This herb contains tannins, which hydrolyze to gallic acid, and geranium red (the roots contain 10% to 28% tannins).

OTHER HERBS: Other herbs that contain tannins include Artichoke, Bayberry, Bilberry, Black cohosh, Blue flag, Borage, Cascara, Cassia, Chamomile (German), Cinnamon, Clivers, , Comfrey, Cornsilk, Elder, Ephedra, Eucalyptus, Eyebright, Feverfew, Gentian, Hawthorn, Hops, Horse chestnut, Juniper, Marshmallow, Meadowsweet, Mistletoe, Motherwort, Nettle, Pilewort, Plantain, Poplar, Prickly ash, Raspberry, Rhubarb, Sage, Sassafras, Saw palmetto, Skullcap, Slippery elm, Saint Johns Wort, Tansy, Thyme, Uva ursi, Valerian, Vervain, Willow, Witch hazel, Yarrow, and Yellow dock.

Anthelmintics

In veterinary medicine, before modern anthelmintics became available, Areca *(Areca catechu),* extract of Male fern *(Dryopteris fillix-mas),* kamala, pomegranate (granatum), and santonin (from *Artemisia* spp) were used in different animal species with varying effects. Modern anthelmintics probably pose less of a risk for adverse effects; however, some animal owners prefer to refrain from using drugs and will wish to consider herbal options.

Other issues for consideration include comparative efficacy, safety, risk of zoonoses, resistance, and owner compliance (many protocols involve long-term use). For example, cucurbitine contained in crushed pumpkin seeds is only 55% efficacious against *Taenia saginata* (Pawlowski, 1970), and arecoline hydrobromide, derived from *Areca catechu* (the betel nut palm), is very effective against all kinds of tapeworms; however, emesis and diarrhea are common adverse events. A common procedure was to follow administration of these plant compounds with a purgative, causing diarrhea to expel the affected worms. Because of the difficulty involved in killing intestinal worms without harming the patient, skill was always required in administering these anthelmintics (Mills, 1989).

One of the future directions of herbal anthelmintics involves ethnoveterinary investigation into suitable plants for helminth control in production animals in tropical countries. For example, *Spondias mombin* has been studied in vivo for evaluation of the therapeutic efficacy of water and alcohol extracts administered to sheep naturally infected with gastrointestinal nematodes. The mean percentage of fecal egg reduction on day 12 in sheep drenched with 500 mg/kg *S. mombin* extract was up to 100% against *Haemonchus* species, *Trichostrongylus* species, *Oesophagostomum* species, *Strongyloides* species, and *Trichuris* species, varying with concentration (Ademola, 2005). In Pakistan, plants identified through ethnoveterinary research were screened for their in vitro anthelmintic activity. In vitro results showed that ginger killed all test worms *(Haemonchus contortus)* within 2 hours postexposure. Most worms exposed to control (normal saline) remained alive until 4 hours postexposure; then, 50% died within 6 hours postexposure. It was concluded that all studied plants had some anthelmintic activity (Zafar, 2001). An experiment was carried out to investigate the anthelmintic activity of papaya latex *(Carica papaya)* against natural infection of *Ascaris suum* in pigs. Pigs given 4 or 8 g of papaya latex per kilogram had worm count reductions of 80.1% and 100%, respectively. Some of the pigs receiving the highest dose of latex showed mild diarrhea on the day following treatment. Otherwise, no clinical or pathologic changes were observed in treated animals (Satrija, 1994). Other herbs that have been traditionally used for their anthelmintic activity in humans and animals are discussed in the following paragraphs.

WORMWOOD (*ARTEMISIA* SPP): These herbs, including *Artemisia absinthium,* include bioactive compounds with some anthelmintic activity. The powdered shoots of *Artemisia herba-alba* were investigated in experimental hemonchosis in Nubian goats. Treatment with 2, 10, or 30 g of Artemisia shoots prevented caprine hemonchosis, suppressing egg production and the development of abomasal lesions (Idris, 1982).

GARLIC *(ALLIUM SATIVUM)*: This herb has been used in the treatment of patients with roundworm *(Ascaris strongyloides)* and hookworm *(Ancylostoma caninum* and *Necator americanus).* Allicin appears to be the anthelmintic constituent; diallyl disulphide was not effective (Kempski, 1967, Soh 1960). Allicin is formed through the action of allinase on alliin, which occurs on crushing fresh garlic. Minced garlic has been reported to be successful in reducing parasitism by *Capillaria* species in carp (Peoa, 1988), but it was unsuccessful as an anthelmintic in the treatment of 12 donkeys, when compared with control and fenbendazole treatment groups (Abells, 1999) (note that whole bulbs were used).

ELECAMPANE *(INULA HELENIUM)*: Alantolactone has been used as an anthelmintic in the treatment of patients with roundworm, threadworm, hookworm, and whipworm infection (Reynolds, 1982).

FUMITORY *(FUMARIA PARVIFLORA)*: As an ethanol extract, this agent caused a marked reduction in fecal egg count (100%) and 78.2% and 88.8% reduction in adult *Haemonchus contortus* and *Trichostrongylus colubriformis,* respectively, on day 13 posttreatment in lambs; it was as effective as the reference compound pyrantel tartrate (Hordegen, 2003).

BLACK WALNUT *(JUGLANS NIGRA)*: A decoction has been used to remove worms from people (Felter, 1898); the oil of black walnut *(Juglans nigra)* is often effectual in expelling worms and has even been known to cause ejection of the tapeworm (Cook, 1869). However, toxicity has been reported in dogs ingesting moldy walnuts, and horses exposed to walnut shavings.

GOLDENSEAL *(HYDRASTIS CANADENSIS)*: The effect of hydrastine on the protoscolices of the tapeworm *(Echinococcus granulosus)* has been studied in vitro and in vivo. Hydrastine at 0.3% concentration produced 70% mortality of the larvae in both experiments (Chen, 1991).

OTHER HERBS: Others herbs used historically include the following:

- Tansy *(Tanacetum vulgare)*
- Rue *(Ruta graveolens)*
- Thuja *(Thuja occidentalis)*

Antiemetics

Herbs should not usually be administered orally to animals that are vomiting. They may be administered by enema, if necessary, although conventional injectable medications are probably more appropriate. However, herbs that assist in suppressing emesis include demulcents, which coat, protect, and lubricate the gastric mucosa; local gastric sedatives (antacids and alkaline stomachics), which act through acid neutralization, by coating the gastric mucosa, or by local nerve sedation; and centrally acting antiemetics, which exert their effects by depressing the vomiting center. The aim of antiemetic administration is to suppress the vomiting reflex, thus conserving the animal's strength, preventing loss of nutrients, and preserving the chloride content of the stomach, blood, and tissues. Gastric sedation should not be used to override essential vomition. Once this material has been removed, the reflex can be suppressed (Daykin, 1960). When emesis is centrally initiated, the cause must be diagnosed.

GINSENG *(PANAX GINSENG)*: This herb contains saponins that inhibit the serotonin (5-HT) type 3A receptor, which is known to mediate nausea and vomiting and may have an antagonistic action against them (Min, 2003). Ginseng is included in many traditional Chinese formulas aimed at tonifying digestion, but it is not generally used as an antiemetic alone.

GINGER *(ZINGIBER OFFICINALE)*: This herb is often advocated as beneficial for nausea and vomiting. In a review of evidence from randomized controlled studies, one study was found for each of the following conditions: seasickness, morning sickness, and chemotherapy-induced nausea; these studies collectively favored ginger over placebo (Ernst, 2000a). A later review of antiemetic therapies by the Cochrane Collaboration found 7 trials of ginger for vomiting in early pregnancy (Jewell, 2006). Studies have documented the antiemetic effects of ginger extract in vivo in dogs (Chang, 1986; Sharma, 1997) and frogs (Kawai, 1994). In dogs, acetone and ethanolic extracts of ginger, administered intragastrically at doses of 25, 50, 100, and 200 mg/kg, protected against cisplatin-induced emesis (3 mg/kg administered intravenously 30 minutes before ginger extract), compared with control. However, ginger extracts were less effective in preventing emesis than was the 5-HT_3 receptor antagonist granisetron, and they were ineffective against apomorphine-induced emesis (Sharma, 1997). The emetic action of the peripherally acting agent copper sulfate was inhibited in dogs given an intragastric dose of ginger extract, but emesis in pigeons treated with centrally acting emetics such as apomorphine and digitalis could not be inhibited by a ginger extract (Zhou, 1960). These results suggest that ginger's antiemetic activity is peripheral and does not involve the central nervous system. The antiemetic action of ginger has been attributed to the combined action of zingerones and shogaols (Ghazanfar, 1994).

BLACK HOREHOUND *(BALLOTA NIGRA)*: Black horehound is stated to possess antiemetic, sedative, and mild astringent properties. Traditionally, it has been used for nausea, vomiting, nervous dyspepsia, and specifically for vomiting of central origin (British Herbal Pharmacopoeia, 1983).

OTHER HERBS: Other herbs that can provide symptomatic relief of nausea include the following:

- Chamomile *(Chamomilla recutita)*
- Fringe tree *(Chionanthus virginicus)*
- Peppermint *(Mentha x piperita)*
- Meadowsweet *(Filipendula ulmaris)*
- Lemon balm *(Melissa officinalis)*

Antimicrobials

Many herbs have direct antimicrobial activity in the gastrointestinal tract. Berberine (contained in goldenseal, Oregon grape root, Coptis root, barberry root bark, and Goldthread bark) and hydrastine (contained in goldenseal only) are some of the best studied for gastrointestinal tract infection; however, most herbs have other properties that should be taken into account, depending on the nature of the condition. For example, berberine also inhibits the activity of enterotoxins.

Berberine is reported to be effective against diarrhea caused by enterotoxins such as *Vibrio cholerae* and *Escherichia coli* (Preininger, 1975). In vivo and in vitro studies in hamsters and rats have reported significant activity for berberine against *Entamoeba histolytica* (Pizzorno, 1985). Berberine is stated to have shown significant success in the treatment of patients with acute diarrhea in several clinical studies. It has been found to be effective against diarrhea caused by *Escherichia coli, Shigella dysenteriae, Salmonella paratyphi* B, *Klebsiella, Giardia lamblia,* and *Vibrio cholerae* (Pizzorno, 1985).

CHAMOMILE *(MATRICARIA RECUTITA)*: The oil has been reported to have antifungal activity and antibacterial activity against gram-positive bacteria (ESCP, 1999).

THYME *(THYMUS VULGARIS)*: This herb possesses anthelmintic (especially hookworms), antibacterial, and antifungal properties (Meybe, 1988). The antibacterial activities of thymol and thyme oil have been reviewed. Thymol, carvacrol, and thyme oil have antifungal activity against a range of organisms (Mitchell, 1979).

Antiprotozoals

Antiprotozoal agents include Propolis, *Artemisia annua,* berberine-containing herbs, and Euphorbia *(Euphorbia hirta).* Essential oils may also be effective preventive or curative treatment against several flagellated parasites.

GARLIC *(ALLIUM SATIVUM)*: The essential oils obtained from garlic bulbs were investigated in vitro on *Tetratrichomonas gallinarum* and *Histomonas meleagridis* in poultry, and it appears that these oils may be useful as chemotherapeutic agents against several poultry parasites (Zenner, 2003).

CHAPARRAL *(LARREA MEXICANA)*: Amoebicidal action against *Entamoeba histolytica* has been reported for a chaparral extract (0.01%). This action may be attributable to the lignin constituents, which are documented as both amoebicidal and fungicidal (Fronczek, 1987).

EUPHORBIA *(EUPHORBIA HIRTA)*: In vitro amoebicidal activity versus *Entamoeba histolytica* has been reported for a *Euphorbia hirta* decoction (Basit, 1977).

OTHER HERBS: *Sophora flavescens, Sinomenium acutum, Ulmus macrocarpa, Pulsatilla koreana,* and *Quisqualis indica* were effective against *Eimeria tenella* in broiler chicks (Youn, 2001).

Antiviral herbs

Several herbs (such as *Echinacea* species, *Thuja occidentalis, Uncaria tomentosa, Phyllanthus amarus, Tabebuia avellanedae,* and *Hypericum perforatum*) may have antiviral activity, but few have been investigated for their antiviral activity against gastrointestinal viruses.

TORMENTIL ROOT *(POTENTILLA ERECTA)*: This extract in controlled doses shortened the duration of rotavirus diarrhea and decreased the requirement for rehydration solution in children with rotavirus diarrhea (Subbotina, 2003); it may be useful in rotaviral infection in animals.

Bitters, sialagogues, and stomachics

Bitters, sialogogues, and stomachics refer to herbs that improve a patient's digestion and appetite by increasing saliva production (sialogogue) or increasing gastric secretion (stomachics); they frequently are bitter tasting (hence, "bitters"). A stomachic is an herb that stimulates gastric function, gastric secretion, and gastric motility; the term refers to many of the bitters. In low doses, they act as "stomach tonics" to improve appetite and upper digestive function.

The taste of bitterness is an extremely common feature of many herbs; it has a major pharmacologic action, which is to stimulate the bitter receptors inside the mouth. These, in turn, send signals via the gustatory nerve (Mills, 1997) to promote the release of gastrointestinal hormones; they also have effects on other physiologic functions. Work published in 1915 by Moorhead revealed that a tincture of the herb Gentian *(Gentiana lutea)* given by mouth or directly into the stomach of cachectic dogs caused a marked increase in appetite. Only when gentian was given by mouth (i.e., tasted) did it cause a marked increase in gastric secretion of acid and pepsin content, and this effect occurred only after normal feeding. These effects provide rational explanations for the traditional use of bitters for liver and digestive complaints, poor appetite, debility, and a wide range of other conditions. It has been postulated that bitters applied to the mouth before a meal have a priming effect on upper digestive function, which is most marked in states in which digestion is below optimum. The increase in digestive function is probably mediated by a nerve reflex caused by the bitter taste buds and involves an increase in vagal stimulation (ACP, 1999). Vagal stimulation causes an increase in gastric acid secretion, a transient rise in gastrin, an increase in pepsin secretion, a slight increase in gallbladder motility, and priming of the pancreas.

Bitters can be used to (1) stimulate the appetite (anorexia or poor appetite), (2) increase the flow of digestive juices, (3) reduce the risk of enteric infection and improve the microenvironment of the gut, (4) promote bile flow, (5) regulate the secretion of insulin and glucagons, and (6) stimulate repair of the gut wall lining; bitters are not necessarily contraindicated in ulcer or other erosive conditions. In short, the action of bitters can be seen to enhance the whole upper digestive function and to improve assimilation of nutrients into the system.

In traditional medicine, this property was highly regarded as leading to a real tonic improvement in health. Bitters were seen as "cooling," that is, reducing fever by switching blood flow to the breakdown of food and reducing toxin resorption in such conditions, but in a more general way, improving nourishment at the expense of "circulatory heat." Bitters were therefore prescribed in "hot" conditions—those in which the patient feels the heat; the patient experiences thirst; the tongue is dry and red; and nervous agitation, restlessness, and tension are observed. The bitter option is one of the most central choices facing the herbalist (Mills, 1989).

Because they act locally on the taste buds, bitters must be administered in the form of a tea, powder, or tincture. Tablets, pills, and capsules bypass the taste buds. They should be administered 5 to 15 minutes before feeding, or should actually be mixed in with food. Dogs and cats usually object to the taste, and meat or meat extracts are probably more useful as salivary or gastric stimulants. In convalescing cattle and horses, gentian can be mixed with bran mashes (Daykin, 1960).

The two most famous bitters are Gentian and Wormwood *(Artemisia absinthium),* the latter of which is the central ingredient in Angostura bitters.

GENTIAN *(GENTIANA LUTEA)*: Elevation of gastric secretion by up to 30% has been reported following the administration of gentian tincture to dogs. An infusion given orally to sheep as a single daily dose (5 g) stimulated enzyme secretion in the small intestine. A root extract (12 mg/kg/d) applied by gavage to rats for 3 days elevated bronchosecretion. A standardized extract perfused into the stomachs of anesthetized rats increased gastric secretion in a dose-dependent manner. Lower doses caused no changes in gastric pH, whereas higher doses increased pH from 4.25 to 4.85. A dose of 0.5 mL/kg did not affect the incidence of gastric ulceration in rats (EMEA, 2002). In an open, uncontrolled study, a single dose of an alcoholic extract of gentian (equivalent to 0.2 g) given to 10 healthy volunteers was reported to result in stimulation of gastric juice secretion (Glatzel, 1967). Gallbladder emptying was increased and prolonged while protein and fat digestion was enhanced. A total of 19 patients with inflammatory conditions of the gastrointestinal tract (e.g., colitis, Crohn's disease, nonspecific inflammation) and elevated secretory immunoglobulin A (IgA) concentrations and 8 healthy individuals were treated with gentian tincture (3 × 20 drops/d) for 8 days. IgA concentrations decreased in both groups (ESCP, 1999).

OTHER HERBS: Other herbs that can be used for their "bitterness" include the following:

- Oregon grape *(Berberis aquifolium)*
- Barberry *(Berberis vulgaris)*
- Bupleurum *(Bupleurum falcatum)*
- Burdock *(Arctium lappa)*
- Forskohlii *(Plectranthus forskholi)*
- Wild yam *(Dioscorea villosa)*
- Echinacea species
- Fringe tree *(Chionanthus virginicus)*
- Fumitory *(Fumaria officinalis)*
- Goldenseal *(Hydrastis canadensis)*
- Chamomile *(Matricaria recutita)*
- Picrorrhiza *(Picrorrhiza kurroa)*
- Baical skullcap *(Scutellaria baicalensis)*
- Dandelion (*Taraxacum officinale folia* and *radix*)
- Thyme *(Thymus vulgaris)*
- Prickly ash *(Zanthoxylum clava-herculis)*
- Ginger *(Zingiber officinale)*
- Yellow dock *(Rumex crispus)*

Carminatives and spasmolytics

Carminatives cause the expulsion of gases from the stomach via eructation and have also been used in flatulent colic to assist in the evacuation of gases from the large intestine. These compounds cause mild irritation of the gastrointestinal tract mucosa, which results in vasodilation. This is probably responsible for the well-known "warm feeling" that follows the swallowing of these compounds. Other actions that result are the relaxation of the gastrointestinal tract musculature, but particularly the cardiac sphincter, for a period of up to 30 minutes, which probably plays a large part in releasing gases from the stomach. The antispasmodic action of some of these, especially ginger, is due to the same factors, which give the carminative effect. The rhythm and tone of peristalsis may be initially increased, but this is often followed by a decrease in movement, which helps in relaxing colic spasms (Daykin, 1960).

ANISEED OIL *(PIMPINELLA ANISUM)*: This herb (200 mg/L) was shown to antagonize carbachol-induced spasms in a guinea pig tracheal muscle preparation.

CHAMOMILE *(MATRICARIA RECUTITA)*: The spasmolytic activity of chamomile has been attributed to apigenin, apigenin-7-O-glucoside, and α-bisabolol, all of which have activity similar to that of papaverine (Bruneton, 1995).

CARDAMOM OIL: The antispasmodic activity of this herb was determined from a rabbit intestine preparation, using acetylcholine as agonist. Results proved that cardamom oil exerts its antispasmodic action through muscarinic receptor blockage (al-Zuhair, 1996).

FENNEL SEED OIL *(FOENICULUM VULGARE)*: This herb has been shown to reduce intestinal spasms and enhance motility of the small intestine. In a randomized, placebo-controlled trial fennel seed oil emulsion was compared with placebo in infantile colic. One study suggested that fennel seed oil emulsion is superior to placebo in decreasing the intensity of infantile colic (Alexandrovich, 2003).

LAVENDER *(LAVANDULA ANGUSTIFOLIA)*: This herb is said to have carminative, antiflatulence, and anticolic properties. Lavender also exhibits spasmolytic activity on guinea pig ileum and rat uterus in vitro, which is most likely to be mediated through cAMP—not through cyclic guanosine monophosphate (Lis-Balchin, 1999).

THYME *(THYMUS VULGARIS)*: In vitro antispasmodic activity of thyme and related herbs has been associated with the phenolic components of the volatile oil and with the flavonoid constituents; their mode of action is thought to involve calcium channel blockage (Cruz, 1989).

PEPPERMINT *(MENTH X PIPERITA)*: Peppermint oil is used to relieve the symptoms of irritable bowel syndrome, relaxing intestinal smooth muscle by reducing the availability of calcium (Beesley, 1996). In a trial of 50 children with irritable bowel syndrome, patients received 187-374 mg daily of a pH-dependant, enteric coated peppermint oil preparation, or placebo. Seventy one percent of those receiving peppermint oil experienced improvement in abdominal pain, as opposed to 43% of those administered placebo ($p < 0.002$) (Kline, 2001). Grigoleit et al (2005) monitored the gastrointestinal effects of peppermint oil in 269 people. Peppermint administration resulted in a substantial spasmolytic effect (Grigoleit, 2005). Menthol in peppermint oil is thought to have the strongest effect in suppressing smooth muscle contraction (Grigoleit, 2005b).

LEMON BALM *(MELISSA OFFICINALIS)*: An ethanol extract of lemon balm leaves inhibited histamine- and barium-induced contractions of guinea pig ileum in vitro (200 mg/mL); an aqueous extract was inactive (Itokawa, 1983).

LICORICE *(GLYCYRRHIZA GLABRA)*: The spasmolytic activity of licorice has been demonstrated in vivo (guinea pig, rabbit, and dog) and appears to be due to the flavonoids liquiritigenin and isoliquiritigenin (Chandler, 1985).

OTHER HERBS: Other carminatives and spasmolytics are listed here:

- Ginger *(Zingiber officinale)*
- Rosemary *(Rosmarinus officinalis)*
- Cinnamon *(Cinnamomum zeylanicum)*
- Catnip *(Nepeta cataria)*
- Cramp bark *(Viburnum opulus)*

Cholagogues and choleretics

Cholagogues stimulate release of bile already formed in the liver and possibly stimulate contraction of the gallbladder. Cholagogue activity is generally a characteristic of bitters but can be attributed to other plant constituents as well. Cholagogues are traditionally prescribed for "cleansing of the liver" and may aid bile movement into the gastrointestinal tract. They are often combined with laxatives (and formerly emetics) and make up an important part of the eliminative regimen; they are useful in the treatment of liver disease and wider liver dysfunction (Mills, 1989).

Choleretics stimulate bile production by hepatocytes, and most have effective cholagogue properties as well. Contraindications for choleretics and cholagogues include obstructed bile ducts (e.g., cancer of the bile duct or pancreas), jaundice following hemolytic disease, and acute or severe hepatocellular disease (e.g., viral hepatitis, septic cholecystitis, intestinal spasm, or ileus or liver cancer). Strongly choleretic herbs include Goldenseal *(Hydrastis canadensis)*, Barberry *(Berberis vulgaris)*, and Greater celandine *(Chelidonium majus)*. It should be noted that bitter herbs can cause nausea in patients with liver damage, so they should be avoided until after hepatic restoratives have been used.

ANDROGRAPHIS *(ANDROGRAPHIS PANICULATA)*: Andrographolide produces a significant dose-dependent (1.5-12 mg/kg) choleretic effect (4.8%-73%), as evidenced by increases in bile flow, bile salt, and bile acids in conscious rats and anesthetized guinea pigs. Paracetamol-induced decreases in volume and contents of bile were prevented significantly by andrographolide pretreatment. It was found to be more potent than silymarin, a clinically used hepatoprotective agent (Shukla, 1992).

CHAMOMILE *(MATRICARIA RECUTITA)*: This oil has been reported to increase bile secretion and concentration of cholesterol in the bile following the administration of 0.1 mL/kg by mouth to cats and dogs (Ikram, 1980).

OREGON GRAPE *(MAHONIA AQUIFOLIUM)*, GOLDENSEAL *(HYDRASTIS CANADENSIS)*, BARBERRY *(BERBERIS VULGARIS)*: Clinical studies have shown berberine to stimulate bile and bilirubin secretion (Pizzorno, 1985).

DANDELION *(TARAXACUM OFFICINALE)*: Bile secretion was doubled in dogs by a decoction of fresh root (equivalent to 5 g dried plant); similar activity has been observed for rats (ESCP, 1999).

GLOBE ARTICHOKE *(CYNARA SCOLYMUS)*: Globe artichoke leaf extract not only increases choleresis and, therefore, cholesterol elimination, but it has also been shown to inhibit cholesterol biosynthesis (Kraft, 1997b).

OTHER HERBS: Other herbs include Greater celadine *(Chelidonium majus)*, Turmeric *(Curcuma longa)*, Agrimony *(Agrimonia eupatoria)*, Calendula *(Calendula officinalis)*, Fringe tree *(Chionanthus virginicus)*, *Picrorrhiza kurroa*, Gentian *(Gentiana lutea)*, Yellow dock *(Rumex crispus)*, Milk thistle *(Silybum marianum)*, Wormwood *(Artemisia absinthium)*, Licorice *(Glycyrrhiza glabra)*, Peppermint *(Mentha x piperita)*, and Ginger *(Zingiber officinale)*.

Hypolipidemic and hypocholesterolemic activity

A few herbs have been well studied for their lipid- and cholesterol-lowering effects and may have some application in veterinary treatment.

Garlic *(Allium sativum)*: The cholesterol- and lipid–lowering effects of garlic and its constituents have been documented in several animal models (e.g., rabbits, rats, chickens, pigs) of atherosclerosis, hypercholesterolemia, and hyperlipidemia (Koch, 1996). The cholesterol-lowering effect of garlic is thought to be dose related; proposed mechanisms of action include inhibition of lipid synthesis and increased excretion of neutral and acidic sterols (Lau, 1983; Fulder, 1989). The potential for causing Heinz body anemia in dogs and cats may limit the dose size and duration of treatment in these species.

Globe Artichoke *(Cynara scolymus)*: Hypolipidemic, hypocholesterolemic, and choleretic activities are well documented for globe artichoke leaf extract. Luteolin was considered to be one of the most important constituents for this effect, and it was suggested that a possible mechanism of action might be indirect inhibition of hydroxymethylglutaryl-CoA reductase (HMG-CoA) (Gebhardt, 1998). Several other experimental studies have documented lipid-lowering effects for globe artichoke leaf extract and cynarin in vivo (Kraft, 1997b; Fintelmann, 1996) and have shown benefit in human clinical patients (Thompson, 2003; Lupatelli, 2004).

Fenugreek *(Trigonella foenum-graecum)*: Hypocholesterolemic activity has been reported for fenugreek in rats (Sharma, 1986) and alloxan-diabetic dogs (Ribes, 1984). Activity has been attributed to the fiber and saponin fractions, with reduction in cholesterol but not in triglyceride concentrations (Ribes, 1984).

Other herbs: Other herbs with hypolipidemic activity include Myrrh and Senega (both hypolipidemic in vivo). Other herbs with hypocholesterolemic activity include alfalfa, bilberry, capsicum, black cohosh, ginger, ispaghula, milk thistle, plantain, tansy, and skullcap. It should also be noted that Gotu kola has shown hypercholesterolemic activity.

Hepatoprotective and hepatorestorative herbs

A number of herbs have demonstrated hepatoprotective and hepatorestorative (restore liver parenchyma) activity.

Milk Thistle *(Silybum marianum)*: After poisoning with *Amanita phalloides* in beagles, silibinin administration (50 mg/kg) 5 and 24 hours after intoxication markedly reduced hemorrhagic necrosis induced in the liver and more effectively prevented death in all of the silibinin-treated dogs compared with controls (Vogel, 1984). The active principle silymarin protects when given 60 minutes before intoxication with phalloidine, or 10 minutes after intoxication. However, as the time span between administration of the toxic substance and the start of treatment increases, so the efficacy of silymarin decreases; after 30 minutes, its curative effect is negligible (Desplaces, 1975). Silymarin was tested in dogs that were subjected to carbon tetrachloride (CCl_4) intoxication, which leads to damage of the liver. The protective effects of silymarin were manifested by the significantly lower aspartate aminotransferase (AST) and alanine aminotransferase (ALT) activities and by the insignificantly reduced extent of lesions in the liver parenchyma, compared with the control CCl_4-intoxicated group (Paulova, 1990). In another study, beagles were divided into 5 groups, and given 85 mg/kg Amanita phalloides lyophilizate orally. The 5 groups, after receiving Amanita extract, were then administered either no treatment (as a control group), prednisolone 30 mg/kg iv at 5 and 24 hours, cytochrome C 50 mg/kg iv at 5 and 24 hours, penicillin G 1000 mg/kg iv at 5 hours, or silymarin 50 mg/kg iv at 5 hours and 30 mg/kg iv at 24 hours. Blood was sampled at 5, 24, 48, 96 and 192 hours and changes in liver enzymes were monitored. At 24 hours post Amanita administration, GPT and GOT levels of the control group averaged over 4000 U/l while those of the silymarin group remained under 60 U/l, slightly lower than the penicillin group and significantly lower than those dogs administered prednisone or cytochrome C. At 48 hours, the control groups' values had returned to near normal with the exception of GPT, which averaged 2250 U/l. The prednisone group transaminase values continued to climb rather than resolve, and the other groups, including the silymarin group, remained in normal ranges (Floersheim, 1978). Studies were conducted on the effects of silybin on the biological activities of Kupffer cells in regenerating livers of rats subjected to partial hepatectomy; results showed that silybin increased the mitotic activity of Kupffer cells (Magliulo, 1979).

Globe Artichoke *(Cynara scolymus)*: In vivo hepatoprotectivity against tetrachloromethane–induced hepatitis has been documented for globe artichoke leaf extract (500 mg/kg) administered orally to rats 48 hours, 24 hours, and 1 hour before intoxication (Adzet, 1987). A hepatoregenerating effect has also been described for an aqueous extract of globe artichoke leaf administered orally to rats for 3 weeks following partial hepatectomy (Maros, 1966). Regeneration was determined in globe artichoke–treated rats, compared with controls, by stimulation of mitosis and increased weight in the residual liver when animals were sacrificed.

Dan Shen *(Salvia miltiorrhiza)*: This herb has been traditionally used in chronic hepatitis and hepatic fibrosis. It protects rat hepatocytes against CCl_4-induced necrosis (Hase, 1997).

Schisandra *(Schisandra chinensis)*: This herb is effective in protecting the liver from harmful toxins, and it may stimulate liver repair (Shiota, 1996; Ohtaki, 1996).

Andrographis *(Andrographis paniculata)*: Hepatoprotective effect was studied on acute hepatitis induced in rats. Treatment of rats before galactosamine administration or after paracetamol challenge leads to complete normalization of toxin-induced increase in the levels of hepatic biochemical parameters, and significantly ameliorates toxin-induced histopathologic changes in the livers of experimental rats (Handa, 1990).

Asian Ginseng *(Panax ginseng)*: Oral administration (250-500 mg/kg) accelerated liver regeneration and

ameliorated liver injury after hepatectomy in dogs (Kwon, 2003).

ANISEED OIL *(PIMPINELLA ANISUM)*: When given to rats (100 mg/kg given subcutaneously), this herb stimulated liver regeneration after partial hepatectomy (ESCP, 1999).

CHAMOMILE *(MATRIACRAIA RECUTITA)*: The ability of the volatile oil of Chamomile to regenerate liver tissue in partially hepatectomized rats has been attributed to the azulene constituents (Mann, 1986).

OTHER HERBS: Other hepatoprotective and hepatorestorative herbs include the following:

- Phyllanthus *(Phyllanthus amarus)*
- Picrorrhiza *(Picrorrhiza kurroa)*
- Dandelion root *(Taraxacum officinale)*
- Burdock *(Articum lappa)*
- Bupleurum *(Bupleurum falcatum)*
- Turmeric *(Curcuma longa)*

Liver tonics, hepatotonics

Liver tonics include those with choleretic, cholagogue, hepatoprotective, or hepatorestorative properties, as described previously.

Laxatives and aperients

Aperient: *Aperient* is the traditional term for a mild laxative that increases stool moisture to promote bowel movements. These plants often contain soluble fibers and oligosaccharides such as inulin and are mild in their effect. They are used traditionally to aid digestion and assimilation and are frequently cholagogue or choleretic in their action. They include the following:

- Fringe tree *(Chionanthus virginicus)*
- Fumitory *(Fumaria officinalis)*
- Licorice *(Glycyrrhiza glabra)*
- Dandelion root *(Taraxacum officinale)*
- Fenugreek *(Trigonella foenum-graecum)*
- Burdock *(Articum lappa)*
- Oregon grape *(Berberis aquifolium)*
- Barberry *(Berberis vulgaris)*
- Rehmannia *(Rehmannia glutinosa)*

Laxatives include mechanical stimulants, bulk purgatives, irritant purgatives, and neuromuscular purgatives. Mechanical stimulants like paraffin oil may hinder absorption of nutrients by coating the mucosa. Chronic constipation or impaction will not benefit and may be aggravated; in small animals, liquid paraffin may actively encourage the continued existence of fecoliths because the oil facilitates the passage of soft feces past solid masses.

Bulk laxatives increase the volume of intestinal contents, causing distention of the intestines, which induces a reflex that initiates contraction of the musculature and an increase in the power and speed of peristalsis. Wheat bran, plantain seeds (psyllium), and seaweeds fall into this group. The swelling properties of mucilage in herbs also enable it to absorb water in the gastrointestinal tract, thereby increasing the volume of the feces and promoting peristalsis. These laxatives have only mild stimulant effects and are particularly useful when sharp foreign bodies (e.g., needles, sharp bones, stones) have been swallowed. Bulk laxatives lower transit time through the gastrointestinal tract and therefore may delay the absorption of other drugs.

Vegetable oils are probably the most efficient and safe of the direct irritant purgatives. As a group, they act by combining in a saponification process with alkaline bile salts of the small intestine. This process produces monobasic, dibasic, and tribasic soaps that exert irritant effects. Glycerol is a by-product of this process and is useful in lubricating and breaking up fecal masses; it also assists in defecation by exerting strong osmotic pressure to retain fluid within and possibly attract fluid into the intestinal lumen. The soaps produced by these oils differ in their irritant properties, so olive oil produces oliveic acid, castor oil ricinoleates, and linseed oil linoleates and linolenates—all of which are relatively strong irritants. Small quantities of stearates and palmitates are also produced (Daykin, 1960).

The effect is seen within 4 to 8 hours in smaller species and in 12 to 18 hours in the horse. An almost complete clearance of the intestines results when these oils are used. Defecation is temporarily suspended until sufficient bulk reaches the colon again; therefore, oleaginous purgatives are not recommended for chronic constipation.

Indirect irritant purgatives contain precursors that are broken down to anthrones and anthraquinones, which themselves pass unchanged through the colon; there, they exert an irritant action and stimulate intestinal movement. Systemic absorption is limited, especially in the case of whole anthraquinone glycosides. Their main effects probably involve stimulation of active chloride secretion, which is electrochemically and osmotically balanced by an increase in sodium and water secretion—an effect that is counteracted by morphine, with 5-HT as a likely mediator.

Neuromuscular Purgatives: A separate effect of anthraquinones is observed in increasing gut motility of the bowel musculature—a response that may be more sensitive than changes in secretion. Bowel flora metabolism has been firmly implicated in the action of sennosides in the gut (Mills, 1997). The primary members of this group are aloes, cascara, Senna *(Cassia angustifolia)*, and rhubarb (rhizome).

ALOE *(ALOE BARBADENSIS)*: This was the most widely used anthracene purgative until synthetic anthraquinones were introduced into veterinary medicine. The emodins (anthraquinones) of Aloes are excreted in the large intestine and are of greatest value in those animals that suffer from impaction of the large intestine. The horse with its numerous colon flexures and its decrease in diameter at the pelvic flexure benefits from this type of purgative. Purgation in the horse is delayed for at least 18 hours. In other animals, the action is far more rapid (Daykin, 1960). The glycosides are metabolized by glycosidases in the intestinal flora to form active anthrones. The laxative action is due to increased motility of the large intestine attained by inhibition of the Na^+/K^+ pump and chloride ion channels; enhanced fluid secretion occurs because of stimulation of secretion of mucus and chloride ion (ESCP, 1997).

Senna Pod *(Cassia angustifolia):* At very small doses, this herb produces sublaxative effects, whereby bowel motions are made comfortable, normal, and soft. At larger doses, it produces a laxative or purgative effect. The effects of sennosides on colonic motility were investigated in eight conscious dogs. Oral sennosides (30 mg/kg) inhibited colonic motility for 12 to 18 hours after a 3- to 6-hour delay and were associated with giant contractions and diarrhea. The minimal oral dose of sennosides needed to produce such changes varied from 5 to 15 mg/kg. Intracolonic sennosides at the minimal effective dose and at 30 mg/kg reproduced the effects of oral sennosides, but with a shorter latency (0.5-1.5 h). This study suggested that colonic motor actions of sennosides are mediated through local prostaglandin synthesis because they were blocked by cyclooxygenase inhibitor and reproduced by PGE_2 (Staumont, 1988).

Parsley *(Petroselinum crispum):* The mechanism of action for the purported laxative effects of parsley has been investigated. In rat colon, an aqueous extract of parsley seeds significantly reduced net water absorption from the colon, as compared with controls. Results suggest that parsley acts by inhibiting sodium and consequently water absorption through inhibition of the Na^+/K^+ pump, by stimulating the NaKCl transporter, and by increasing electrolyte and water secretions (Kreydiyyeh, 2002).

Rhubarb *(Rheum officinale):* The laxative action of anthraquinone derivatives is well recognized. Rhubarb also contains tannins, which exert an astringent action. At low doses, rhubarb is stated to act as an antidiarrheal because of its tannin components, whereas at higher doses, it exerts a cathartic action (Meybe, 1988).

Psyllium (Ispaghula/Metamucil) *(Plantago ovata):* In addition to its stool bulking effects, psyllium exhibits cholinergic activity. Mild laxative action has also been reported in mice administered iridoid glycosides, including aucubin (Inouye, 1974). Four-week supplementation of a fiber-free diet with ispaghula seeds (100 or 200 g/kg) was compared with that of husks and wheat bran in rats (Leng-Peschlow, 1991). The seeds increased fecal fresh weight by up to 100% and fecal dry weight by up to 50%. Total fecal bile acid secretion was stimulated, and β-glucuronidase activity reduced, by ispaghula. The study concluded that ispaghula acts as a partly fermentable dietary fiber supplement that increases stool bulk, and that it probably has metabolic and mucosaprotective effects.

Other herbs: Other laxative herbs include the following:

Cascara *(Rhamnus purshiana)*	Hydroxyanthracene constituents
Eyebright *(Euphrasia officinalis)*	Iridoids
Plantain *(Plantago major)*	Iridoids (much less than senna)
Yellow dock *(Rumex crispus)*	Hydroxyanthracene constituents
Buckthorn *(Rhamnus frangulara)*	Hydroxyanthracene constituents
Butternut *(Juglans cinerea)*	Hydroxyanthracene constituents

Pancreatic protectives and trophorestoratives

These herbs have some affinity for pancreatic tissue and aid chronic and acute pancreatic conditions.

Fringe Tree *(Chionanthus virginicus):* This traditional herb is advocated for pancreatic disease, inflammatory or otherwise, and for diabetes (Felter, 1898)

Aloe *(Aloe vera):* The constituent emodin (also found in other herbs) is a potent agent in the management of clinical and experimental acute pancreatitis. In induced pancreatitis in rats, the serum amylase level was decreased significantly in the emodin-treated group compared with controls. It was concluded that emodin might upregulate gene expression, which subsequently increases DNA synthesis and protein content and thus accelerates pancreatic repair and regeneration (Gong, 2002). Emodin in combination with baicalein has significant therapeutic benefit in severe acute pancreatitis in rats (Zhang, 2005).

Dandelion *(Taraxacum officinale):* This herb (10 mg/kg orally) reduced IL-6, a principal mediator of acute phase response and TNF-α production during cholecystokinin-induced acute pancreatitis in rats (Seo, 2001).

REVIEW OF SPECIFIC GASTROINTESTINAL TRACT CONDITIONS

In the following symptoms or conditions, the underlying pathophysiology is assumed to be known. However, it is not uncommon for the veterinary clinician to be presented with a case in which a definitive diagnosis is not made. These are ideal cases for herbal medicine, which can be used to treat the presenting signs. For this reason, both signs and disease conditions of the gastrointestinal tract are listed.

One of the primary considerations in gastrointestinal tract disease is how to avoid aggravating the condition by giving something orally. However, in the authors' experience, the oral route is the main route of administration, with only a handful of adverse events recorded. Many herbs can be given as teas rectally, particularly when vomiting is a major issue.

In human medicine, increasing attention is being paid to physiological, emotional, cognitive and behavioral components of chronic GI disease (Mulak, 2004); stress may similarly impact GI problems in animals and can be addressed with nervines and adaptogens. Attention to diet, probiotics, and contributing or perpetuating factors is essential, as is consideration of conventional treatment.

Colic

Therapeutic rationale

- Identify the cause and relieve obstructions, if applicable.
- Relieve pain.
- Reduce spasm.
- Relieve gas.

The main herbal agents for consideration are spasmolytics, carminatives, nervines, and analgesics (see neurologic section). Fennel *(Foeniculum vulgare),* Chamomile *(Matricaria recutita),* Peppermint *(Mentha x piperita),* Cramp bark *(Viburnum opulus),* and Ginger *(Zingiber officinale)* are well indicated and usually work best when incorporated in a formula (tincture or tea), although a tea of one or two herbs may be sufficient for mild cases.

For example, colic in infants is a common problem in human medicine. For 1 week, 33 healthy infants 2 to 8 weeks of age with colic were given an herbal tea that contained extracts of chamomile, vervain, licorice, fennel, and balm mint; 35 infants were given a placebo drink that included no herbs. At the end of treatment, the colic improvement score was significantly better with herbal tea. Colic was eliminated in 19 infants given herbal tea and in 9 given placebo. No adverse events were reported in either group (Weizman, 1993).

David Hoffmann recommends dill, fennel, chamomile, lemon balm, peppermint, catnip, linden, and red clover for colic. For mild colic in cats or dogs, one should consider using chamomile tea, 1 teaspoon to 1 tablespoon every half-hour. In the author's experience, this is a gentle, readily available herb that provides anti-inflammatory, antispasmodic, carminative, antimicrobial, and bitter actions. It is very useful when stress is a feature of the history, and it is especially useful in German shepherds with stress-induced diarrhea.

For mild colic in veterinary staff, peppermint or chamomile tea, 1 cup sipped every 2 to 3 hours, should be prescribed.

A prescription for recurrent colic signs in small animals that should be given twice daily over 2 to 3 weeks might include the following:

Chamomile	40% (carminative, anti-inflammatory, bitter, spasmolytic, mild sedative)
Fennel	20% (carminative, antimicrobial, anti-inflammatory)
Cramp Bark	20% (bitter, antispasmodic, sedative, astringent)
Licorice	20% (adaptogen, antispasmodic, mild laxative, antiulcerogenic, taste improver)

For mild colic in horses, one historical formula follows:

Aloe	33% (1 oz)
Buckthorn	33% (1 oz)
Ginger	33% (1 oz)

This should be prepared as powders dissolved in a pint of water and given as a drench (Manning, 1883).

Colitis

(See also "Inflammatory Bowel Disease.")

Therapeutic rationale

- Eliminate parasites.
- Reduce inflammation and infection.
- Rule out food allergy—consider an elimination diet.
- Manage stress.

The primary actions that should be considered involve anti-inflammatory, spasmolytic, and nervine herbs. Astringents may be necessary when bleeding is a sign; demulcents and mucilages can reduce mucosal irritation, and vulnerary herbs enhance healing. Immune system support and antimicrobial herbs may be needed when infection is present.

When pain is evident controlling spasm is probably more important than correcting epithelial defects, so peppermint oil is among the most important herbs for consideration. Two drops per 2 oz can be added easily to a tincture.

Herbs to be considered include agrimony, wild yam, angelica, calamus, ginger, licorice, chamomile, lavender, bayberry, turmeric, and fiber-containing herbs such as psyllium, flaxseed, or slippery elm.

Weiss (1988) recommends chamomile, tormentil, and senna in equal parts but also notes that local topical treatments may be most valuable. Herbs used as retention enemas include chamomile, tormentil, and a stimulant "tonic" herb that would enhance secretory activity, such as calamus or red clover. Saint John's Wort can also be used as a vulnerary, and licorice can be used as an anti-inflammatory.

A prescription for colitis follows:

Cramp bark	20% (bitter, antispasmodic, sedative, astringent)
Chamomile	20% (carminative, anti-inflammatory, bitter, spasmolytic, mild sedative)
Marshmallow	20% (demulcent, vulnerary)
Licorice	20% (adaptogen, antispasmodic, mild laxative, antiulcerogenic, taste improver)
Calendula	20% (antimicrobial, anti-inflammatory, astringent, spasmolytic, vulnerary, cholagogue)

Peppermint oil, 1 drop per 25 mL of formula (antispasmodic, carminative, antiemetic)

If stress is involved, one should consider the use of nervines such as skullcap, valerian, or lime blossom and adaptogens such as Eleuthero or *Withania somnifera.*

In an open trial, 24 patients with chronic nonspecific colitis were treated with an herbal combination of *Taraxacum officinale, Hypericum perforatum, Melissa officinalis, Calendula officinalis,* and *Foeniculum vulgare.* As a result of treatment, spontaneous and palpable pains along the large intestine disappeared in over 95% of patients by the 15th day of treatment. Defecation occurred daily in patients with obstipation syndrome, but a combination of *Rhamnus frangula, Citrus aurantium,* and *Carum carvi* was added to the herbal combination already described. Defecation was normalized in patients with diarrhea syndrome. The pathologic admixtures in feces disappeared (Chakurski, 1981b). The inclusion of nervine herbs in this formula should be noted.

A double-blind, randomized, placebo-controlled trial of the efficacy and safety of aloe vera gel for the treatment of patients with mildly to moderately active ulcerative colitis was undertaken in 44 patients given oral aloe vera gel 100 mL twice daily for 4 weeks (2:1), or placebo. Aloe produced a clinical response more often than placebo; it also reduced histologic disease activity and appeared to be safe (Langmead, 2004a).

An open-label, parallel-group, multicenter, randomized clinical trial to assess the efficacy and safety of *Plantago ovata* (psyllium) seeds as compared with mesalamine in maintaining remission was conducted in patients with ulcerative colitis. A total of 105 patients with ulcerative colitis who were in remission were randomized into groups to receive treatment with *P. ovata* seeds (10 g twice daily), mesalamine (500 mg three times daily), and *P. ovata* seeds plus mesalamine at the same doses. The primary outcome was maintenance of remission for 12 months. After 12 months, the treatment failure rate was 40% in the *P. ovata* seed group, 35% in the mesalamine group, and 30% in the *P. ovata* plus mesalamine group. A significant increase in fecal butyrate levels was observed after *P. ovata* seed administration. It was concluded that *P. ovata* seeds may be as effective as mesalamine in maintaining remission in patients with ulcerative colitis (Fernandez-Banares, 1999).

The use of wheat grass *(Triticum aestivum)* in the treatment of patients with ulcerative colitis has been investigated in a randomized, double-blind, placebo-controlled study. A total of 23 patients with active distal ulcerative colitis were randomly allocated to receive 100 mL of wheat grass juice or a matching placebo daily for 1 month. Treatment with wheat grass juice was associated with significant reductions in overall disease activity; treatment appeared effective and safe when given as a single or adjuvant treatment for distal ulcerative colitis (Ben-Arye, 2002).

Constipation

Therapeutic rationale

- Increase systemic hydration and exercise.
- Increase stool bulk (if appropriate, pelvic narrowing would be a contraindication).
- Increase gastrointestinal tract lubrication.
- Use gentle aperients to stimulate peristalsis.
- Suppress spasm when appropriate.
- Improve liver function.

If laxative herbs are needed, initial treatment with bulk-forming (mucilage-containing) herbs such as flax seed or psyllium seed is usually appropriate. Attention to systemic hydration is important in the use of these herbs because they lead to water reabsorption into the intestine. Use of anthraquinone-containing herbal laxatives is generally safe and effective. However, they are best used as a last resort after obvious factors, such as hydration status, diet, and exercise, have been addressed. These herbs have a tendency to cause flatus and can aggravate discomfort. Because they cause emptying of the bowel, it is not uncommon for the client to believe that the animal is still constipated if it does not have a bowel movement for a day or two after use. If needed, modest doses of Senna, Butternut, and Cascara may be used.

A prescription for constipation is provided here:

Licorice	30% (adaptogen, antispasmodic, mild laxative, antiulcerogenic, taste improver)
Marshmallow	20% (demulcent, vulnerary)
Cascara	40% (mild purgative)
Yellow dock	10% (gentle purgative, cholagogue)

Tincture: Give 1 mL per 10 lb twice daily in food for 3 weeks.
Tea: Give 1 dessert spoonful twice daily in food for 3 weeks. Repeat, if necessary.

Megacolon in cats: Marsden in (Wynn, 2003) recommends the following formula for megacolon in cats (proportions are modified):

Cascara	60%
Ginger	10%
Licorice	30%

0.2 mL per 5 kg twice daily

Manning (1883) published the following recipes for constipation in cattle:

Laxative clyster (for obstinate constipation):

- 3-4 quarts warm water
- 8 oz linseed oil
- 1 tablespoon common salt

Stimulating clyster (for inactive rectum and small intestine with gas or loaded with feces):

- 3 quarts thin mucilage of slippery elm bark or linseed tea
- 1 teaspoonful pure cayenne

or

- $^1/_2$ tablespoon powdered ginger
- 3 quarts boiling water

Diarrhea

Therapeutic rationale

- Maintain hydration.
- Normalize intestinal motility.
- Reduce mucosal inflammation.
- Eliminate parasites.
- Rule out food allergies.
- Restore bowel flora.

Depending on the cause of diarrhea, herbs to be considered may have demulcent properties or anti-inflammatory, spasmolytic, astringent, or antimicrobial activity.

For simple, mild diarrhea of nonspecific origin, one should consider *Hydrastis canadensis* (goldenseal). It inhibits enterotoxins and is most useful for gastrointestinal tract infection and giardiasis. *Geranium maculatum* (cranesbill) contains tannin and is a gentle astringent and almost a specific for mild diarrhea. *Hamamelis virginiana* (witch hazel) is an astringent and anti-inflammatory for nonspecific diarrhea. *Harpagophytum procumbens* (devil's claw) has a traditional use in nonspecific diarrhea as a bitter tonic and anti-inflammatory herb.

Matricaria recutita (chamomile) is ideal for inflammation or spasm of the digestive tract, especially with nervous diarrhea, travel sickness, and anxiety. *Filipendula ulmaria* (meadowsweet) has astringent properties and, according to Grieves (1931), is almost a specific for children's diarrhea. King's Dispensatory (Felter, 1898) reports that it is effective in debility and convalescence from diarrhea. *Chelidonium major* (greater celadine) is used in China to treat patients with enteritis and abdominal pain.

In a prospective, double-blind, randomized, multicenter, parallel-group study, children (6 months to 5.5 years of age) with acute, uncomplicated diarrhea received apple pectin and chamomile extract (n = 39) or placebo (n =

40), in addition to rehydration and realimentation diet. After 3 days, the diarrhea had ended significantly more frequently in the pectin/chamomile group than in the placebo group, and pectin/chamomile reduced the duration of diarrhea significantly by at least 5.2 hours. Parents expressed their contentment more frequently (82%) with pectin/chamomile than with placebo (60%) (de la Motte, 1997).

Many cats and dogs with simple diarrhea respond to a combination of probiotics and slippery elm powder (1/4 teaspoon per 10 lb, or 5 kg twice daily) administered with water or fresh food.

Preweaning diarrhea is a very common disease in piglets. Oral administration of 0.5 g of Ko-ken-huang-lien-huang-chin-tang (pueraria, coptis, scute, and licorice combination) to piglets at 1 day of age was effective in reducing the incidence of gastrointestinal tract infection and increasing body weight gain during the first 10 days of life (Lin, 1988).

A prescription for nonspecific diarrhea in animals is provided here:

Goldenseal	20% (antimicrobial, mucous membrane tonic, stomachic)
Marshmallow	20% (demulcent, vulnerary)
Cramp bark	20% (bitter, antispasmodic, sedative, astringent)
Chamomile	20% (carminative, anti-inflammatory, bitter, spasmolytic, mild sedative)
Agrimony	20% (astringent, bitter tonic)

Tincture: Give 1 mL per 10 lb twice daily in food for 3 weeks.

A historical recipe for an astringent enema for scours in cattle is as follows:

1 tablespoon bayberry bark
3 quarts boiling water

Digestive Weakness

Veterinarians are sometimes presented with a general picture of intestinal disturbance. Bloating, flatulence, mild diarrhea, mild constipation, mild abdominal pain, mucus in the stool, and anorexia or fussy eating habits, as well as borborygmus and pica, can all be evidence of inherent "digestive weakness" and dysbiosis (an alteration in normal bowel flora, leading to bowel function changes). Poor digestion in animals may also be largely nonclinical but can contribute to other conditions, such as food intolerance or allergies, constipation, dysbiosis, and nutrient deficiencies (and skin problems). Herbalists suspect that many chronic diseases begin with subclinical poor digestive function. Herbs that improve upper digestive function include bitters, carminatives, pungent herbs to stimulate gastric secretions, choleretics, and cholagogues.

A prescription for digestive weakness is provided:

Barberry	20% (alterative, mild laxative, cholagogue, liver and digestive tonic antiseptic)
Ginger	10% (carminative, antispasmodic, anti-inflammatory)
Dandelion	20% (laxative, cholagogue, bitter)
Licorice	20% (adaptogen, antispasmodic, mild laxative, antiulcerogenic, taste improver)
Eleuthero	30% (adaptogen, immune modulatory)

Use alcohol or glycerin tinctures for best results; alternatively, use teas.

Tincture: Give 1 mL per 10 lb twice daily in food for 3 weeks.

Emaciation

If emaciation is due to anorexia, one should consider using gentian or some of the bitters and stomachics. Also, consideration should be given to adaptogens and nutritive herbs like ashwagandha, alfalfa, nettle, and others. Of course, the predisposing cause of emaciation must be identified and addressed.

Flatulence

Therapeutic rationale

- Identify food intolerances and hypersensitivities.
- Improve digestibility.
- Rule out dysbiosis, bacterial overgrowth, and pancreatic insufficiency.

Carminative herbs are used to relieve gas and gas pain. These include anise seed, fennel, cardamom, peppermint, cilantro, bergamot, lavender, hyssop, and chamomile. Spasmolytic herbs such as wild yam and cramp bark may also be useful.

Perianal Fistula

An association may be found between colitis and perianal fistula; food sensitivities and allergies should be ruled out. One should consider using immune-modulating herbs, astringent, and vulnerary herbs. Two herbs used in human furunculosis are *Baptisia tinctoria* (wild indigo) and *Potentilla erecta* (tormentil).

Prescription for perianal fistula:

Barberry	30% (alterative, anti-inflammatory, mild laxative, liver tonic, digestive tonic, antiseptic)
Echinacea	20% (immunostimulant, anti-inflammatory, antibacterial, vulnerary)
Marshmallow	20% (demulcent, vulnerary)
Licorice	10% (anti-inflammatory, adaptogen, taste improver, antiulcerogenic)
Astragalus	20% (immune enhancing, tonic)

Gallbladder Disorders

Therapeutic rationale

- Use mild bitter herbs to improve digestion and gallbladder function.
- Spasmolytic and carminative herbs can be used to relieve pain.
- Regulate bowel function simultaneously.

Agents of value include anti-inflammatories, hepatic tonics, antispasmodics, and antimicrobial herbs. Caution should be used with choleretic herbs that improve bile flow and cholagogue herbs that stimulate gallbladder motility; these may increase peristalsis and therefore worsen discomfort. Only mild choleretics and cholagogues should be used.

Weiss (1988) suggests that, in treating gallbladder disease, a therapeutic triad to guide the prescription should involve a specific biliary remedy that includes a carminative and an antispasmodic, as well as a supporting laxative. His example formula is as follows:

Peppermint (as a cholagogue)	50%
Melissa (sedative adjuvant)	20%
Fennel seed (carminative)	20%
Buckthorn bark (laxative)	10%

Another example given by Weiss (1988) is composed of 10% caraway seed, 10% fennel seed, 30% peppermint, 20% yarrow, 20% everlasting flower, and 15% senna. Other herbs that are included in his formulas are wormwood, milk thistle, blessed thistle, and dandelion.

A prescription for cholecystitis is provided:

Barberry	20% (alterative, mild laxative, liver and digestive tonic, antiseptic)
Globe artichoke	10% (bitter tonic, choleretic, cholagogue, hepatic tonic)
Wild yam	20% (spasmolytic, anti-inflammatory, cholagogue)
Milk thistle	20% (hepatotonic, antioxidant)
Dandelion	30% (laxative, cholagogue)

Gastritis

Therapeutic rationale

- Reduce inflammation.
- Identify and remove the cause.
- Control nausea and vomiting.
- Rule out bacterial infection.

A number of herbs have demonstrated therapeutic effects on the stomach and may be particularly useful in the prevention of gastritis or gastric ulcers associated with some conventional medicines. Herbs to consider include Licorice, Chamomile, Dan shen, Fenugreek, Goldenseal, Thyme, and Cat's claw. If bacterial infection (such as *Helicobacter*) is suspected, Goldenseal, Barberry, and Grapeseed extract may be added. Garlic, on the other hand, may exacerbate gastritis and worsen gastric ulceration (see Garlic monograph in Chapter 24).

One formula advocated for gastritis by Hoffmann (1992) is provided here (proportions slightly modified):

Comfrey root	30%
Marshmallow root	30%
Meadowsweet	30%
Goldenseal	10%

Administer as a tea.

Prescription for simple gastritis:

Chamomile flowers 50.0g, 1 teaspoon to 1 cup boiling water, or

Chamomile tincture, 10 to 20 drops in $^1/_2$-glass lukewarm water.

Chamomile is easily accepted by small animals with gastritis as a tea or a diluted tincture.

Prescription for chronic gastritis:

Meadowseet	40% (antiulcerogenic, antacid, anti-inflammatory, astringent)
Marshmallow	30% (demulcent, vulnerary)
Chamomile	30% (carminative, spasmolytic, anti-inflammatory, cholagogue, antiallergic, mild sedative, and vulnerary)

Or, a simple infusion can be prepared of equal parts fennel seeds, peppermint leaves, melissa leaves, and calamus (sweet flag); 1 teaspoon to 1 cup in boiling water should be given.

Gastroenteritis

Therapeutic rationale

- Treat infection (viral, bacterial, protozoal, etc.).
- Reduce inflammation.
- Control nausea and vomiting.

The prescription should include astringent herbs if the problem is acute, as well as anti-inflammatory and antimicrobial herbs. If the patient is vomiting, one should consider delivery of herbal teas via enema.

Prescription for gastroenteritis, given as tea or tincture (no vomiting):

Marshmallow	20% (demulcent, vulnerary)
Meadowsweet	30% (antiulcerogenic, antacid, anti-inflammatory, astringent)
Goldenseal	20% (antimicrobial, mucous membrane tonic, stomachic)
Angelica root	20% (warming, bitter, carminative, spasmolytic)
Agrimony	10% (astringent, bitter, cholagogue)

Gastric Dilation

The gastric dilation–volvulus (GDV) syndrome in the dog is considered to be multifactorial; however, an association between GDV and inflammatory bowel disease has been raised as a possibility, on the basis of an evaluation of the correlation between GDV and preexisting gastrointestinal tract disease (Braun, 1996). Prevention in large-breed dogs is desirable, and prevention of recurrence post-GVD may be aided by herbal medicine, along with appropriate diet and lifestyle changes. The most important herbs to be included are the carminatives, stomachics, bitters, and anti-inflammatories. Along with dietary and lifestyle management, the following formula should be considered.

A preventative prescription for GDV:

Fennel	25% (carminative, antimicrobial, anti-inflammatory)
Peppermint	25% (antispasmodic, carminative, antiemetic)
Chamomile	25% (carminative, spasmolytic, anti-inflammatory, cholagogue, antiallergic, mild sedative, and vulnerary
Dandelion	25% (laxative, cholagogue)

One should give 1 mL per 5 kg to large-breed dogs in divided doses in food; for long-term use, 3 weeks on and 1 week off the formula is recommended, with chamomile tea during the rest week given at a half-cup twice daily with food.

Giardia

Numerous medicinal herbs, including Berberine-containing herbs (Coptis, Goldenseal, Oregon grape, Barberry), show promise. For example, a group of 42 human patients with giardia received 10mg/kg/d of berberine orally for 10 days. A total of 90% had negative stool specimens after treatment, although a small number relapsed 1 month later. Results compared favorably with those of the other three antigiardial drugs that were investigated (Gupte, 1975). Others, such as Indian Long Pepper *(Piper longum)*, the Ayurvedic formulation consisting of Indian Long Pepper and Palash *(Butea monosperma)*, and propolis, also showed antigiardial activity (Hawrelak, 2003). Flavonoid-containing herbs, including Oregano *(Origanum vulgare)*, Guava leaves *(Psidium gujava)*, Mango leaves *(Mangifera indica)*, and plantain leaves *(Plantago major)*, demonstrated antigiardial activity equal to tinidazole (Ponce-Macotela, 1994). Probiotics are well indicated, as is a low-fat diet (Giardia trophozoites depend on bile acids for survival). Wheat germ may also be therapeutic (human dose 2g, or 1tsp three times daily).

Prescription for chronic or recurrent giardiasis:

Goldenseal	20% (antimicrobial, mucous membrane tonic, stomachic)
Meadowsweet	20% (antiulcerogenic, antacid, anti-inflammatory, astringent)
Cramp bark	20% (bitter, antispasmodic, sedative, astringent)
Echinacea	20% (immunostimulant, anti-inflammatory, vulnerary)
Marshmallow	20% (demulcent and vulnerary)

Although conventional medicines (e.g., metronidazole) may be effective, herbal medicine may help to alleviate the signs and duration of infection.

Gingivitis/Periodontal Disease

Therapeutic rationale

- Identify the cause.
- Treat accompanying dental or periodontal disease.
- Reduce inflammation.
- Treat infection and inflammation.

Herbs with potential use in the treatment of patients with periodontal disease include antimicrobials, vulnerary herbs, and anti-inflammatory herbs. Astringents may help reduce bleeding, and circulatory stimulants might improve circulation of blood to the gums. Immune system support should be considered, given the potential for systemic effects caused by bacteremia. Traditionally, propolis, marshmallow, aloe, calendula, Echinacea, witch hazel, goldenseal, myrrh, balm of gilead, coptis, spilanthes, and other herbs have been used.

One study investigated the treatment of patients with chronic catarrhal gingivitis with polysorb-immobilized calendula. The results of this use for periodontal disease in clinic cases showed the greatest effect of calendula after treatment (Krazhan, 2001). Epigallocatechin gallate (EGCG), the main constituent of green tea polyphenols, has been reported to have inhibitory effects on the activity and expression of matrix metalloproteinases (MMPs) that are involved in alveolar bone resorption in periodontal disease (Yun, 2004). Likewise, baicalin inhibits metalloproteinases, which suggests that baicalin and plants that contain high levels of it may play an important role in preventing and treating periodontal disease (Li, 2004).

Centella asiatica and *Punica granatum* have been investigated for periodontal healing following scaling and root planing in adult human patients with periodontitis. Study results showed significant improvement in pocket depth and attachment level in test sites when compared with placebo sites at 3 months, and with placebo and control sites at 6 months. Results indicate that local delivery with *C. asiatica* and *P. granatum* extracts plus scaling and root planing significantly reduced the clinical signs of chronic periodontitis (Sastravaha, 2003).

Methanol extracts of *Hamamelis virginiana* and *Arnica montana* and, to a lesser extent, *Althaea officinalis* were shown to possess antimicrobial activity and may be useful as topical medications in periodontal prophylaxis (Iauk, 2003). Similarly, a perilla seed *(Perilla frutescens)* extract was examined for its antimicrobial activity against oral cariogenic bacteria. Luteolin, one of the components of perilla seed, showed the strongest antimicrobial effect among the phenolic compounds; therefore, perilla seed may be used to prevent dental caries and periodontal disease (Yamamoto, 2002).

Prescription for periodontal disease/gingivitis for internal use:

Echinacea	30% (immunostimulant, anti-inflammatory, vulnerary)
Baptisia	20% (antimicrobial, antiseptic)
Baical skullcap	30% (anti-inflammatory, antibacterial, antiallergic)
Devil's claw	20% (anti-inflammatory, analgesic, bitter tonic)

For topical use: For small animals, consider a flush with fresh, cooled green tea twice daily, and add the remaining tea to food.

Halitosis

Halitosis may have three main causes: dental or periodontal disease, gastric disease, or rhinitis/sinusitis. If it is due to poor digestion, one should consider starting treatment with bitters like *Gentiana lutea* (gentian) or stomachics.

Inflammatory Bowel Disease

(See also "Colitis.")

Therapeutic rationale

- Rule out parasites.
- Reduce inflammation.
- Address food allergy and food intolerance.
- Identify and remove behavioral or stress triggers.

The cause or causes of inflammatory bowel disease (IBD) remain obscure. Food allergy or intolerance contributes in many dogs and in up to 66% of cats. Antigens that have been implicated include parasites, dietary proteins, and bacteria, including commensal species. In cats with chronic IBD, triaditis (an associated inflammation of liver and pancreas) may also develop. Herbal agents indicated include astringents, demulcents, vulneries, carminatives, antispasmodics, and nervines, as well as immune system support (antiallergy herbs should be considered). Herbs frequently recommended for human patients with IBD include catnip, chamomile, sarsaparilla, belladonna, bayberry, turmeric, wild yam, and agrimony.

It has been suggested that reactive oxygen metabolites produced by inflamed colonic mucosa may contribute to the pathogenesis of the disease. In one in vitro study, slippery elm, devil's claw, Mexican yam, tormentil, and wei tong ning (a traditional Chinese medicine) scavenged superoxide dose dependently, so they may deserve a role in treatment of IBD (Langmead, 2002). In another in vitro study, the inflammatory action of aloe vera gel provided support for the proposal that it may have a therapeutic effect in IBD (Langmead, 2004b).

A formula consisting of Bilwa *(Aegle marmelos)*, Dhanyak *(Coriandrum sativum)*, Musta *(Cyperus rotundus)*, and Vala *(Vetiveria zizanioides)* was evaluated for its activity against IBD. The formulation showed significant inhibitory activity against IBD induced in rat models; the activity was comparable with that of prednisolone (Jagtap, 2004).

A prescription for IBD follows:

Chamomile	20% (carminative, anti-inflammatory, vulnerary, bitter, spasmolytic, antiallergic, cholagogue, mild sedative)
Calendula	20% (antiseptic, anti-inflammatory, astringent, spasmolytic, vulnerary, cholagogue)
Meadowsweet	20% (antiulcerogenic, antacid, anti-inflammatory, astringent)
Astragalus	20% (immunomodulatory)
Baical skullcap	20% (anti-inflammatory, antibacterial, antiallergic)

One should give 1 mL per 5 kg for large-breed dogs in divided doses in food.

An emollient clyster published by Manning (1883) for cattle was:

2 oz slippery elm bark
2 quarts boiling water

Irritable Bowel Syndrome

Therapeutic rationale

- Rule out food allergy.
- Manage stress/behavioral triggers.

It is estimated that 10% to 15 % of dogs with chronic large bowel diarrhea have irritable bowel syndrome (IBS). IBS has an unclear cause and, in humans, stress, anxiety, and psychological issues are common triggers, along with possible food intolerance. In animals, stressful episodes such as boarding or shows can be linked to onset of clinical signs. Food intolerance may also contribute, and leaky gut and poor liver function should be ruled out. Signs may include constipation or diarrhea, or alternating between these two. The colon is generally more sensitive than normal, so key signs include urgency to defecate, cramping, and diarrhea.

Spasmolytic herbs, including chamomile, cramp bark, peppermint, and bayberry, and nervine herbs, especially chamomile, should be used for nervous dogs with stress-related diarrhea. The presence of mucus implies inflammation, and gastrointestinal anti-inflammatory and astringent herbs, like meadowsweet, might be considered. Other herb classes for consideration when appropriate include hepatic, choleretic, antimicrobial, and demulcent herbs.

A modern Chinese herbal formula significantly improved symptoms of irritable bowel syndrome in a randomized controlled trial in human patients (Bensoussan, 1998). This trial compared patients given placebo, individualized Chinese herbal prescriptions, and standard formula. Initially, both treatment groups improved significantly compared to the placebo group; at follow-up 14 weeks later, only those receiving individualized prescriptions maintained improvement.

Standard Chinese herbal formula in Bensoussan trial

Dang Shen	*Codonopsis pilosulae*	7 gm
Huo Xiang	*Agastaches seu pogostemi*	4.5 gm
Fang Feng	*Ledebouriella sesiloidis*	3 gm
Yi Yi Ren	*Coicis lacryma-jobi*	7 gm
Chai Hu	*Bupleurum Chinense*	4.5 gm
Yin Chen	*Artemisia capillaris*	13 gm
Bai zhu	*Atractylodes macrocephalae*	9 gm
Hou Po	*Magnolia officinalis*	4.5 gm
Chen Pi	*Citrus reticulata*	3 gm
Pao Jiang	*Zingiber officinalis*	4.5 gm
Qin Pi	*Fraxinus rhynchophylla*	4.5 gm
Fu Ling	*Poria cocos*	4.5 gm
Bai Zhi	*Angelica daihurica*	2 gm
Che Qian Zi	*Plantago asiatica*	4.5 gm
Huang Bai	*Phellodendron amurense*	4.5 gm
Zhi Gan Cao	*Glycyrrhiza uralensis*	4.5 gm
Bai Shao	*Paeonia lactiflora*	3 gm
Mu Xiang	*Aucklandia lappa*	3 gm
Huang Lian	*Coptis sinensis*	3 gm
Wu Wei Zi	*Schisandra chinensis*	7 gm

Hoffmann suggests the following formula for IBS (proportions modified):

Bayberry	25%
Mugwort *(Artemisia vulgaris)*	15%
Chamomile	15%
Peppermint	15%
Wild yam	15%
Valerian	15%

A simplified prescription for IBS:

Chamomile	25% (carminative, anti-inflammatory, vulnerary, bitter, spasmolytic, antiallergic, cholagogue, mild sedative)
Passionflower	25% (sedative, antispasmodic, anodyne)
Calendula	25% (antiseptic, anti-inflammatory, astringent, spasmolytic, vulnerary, cholagogue)
Marshmallow	25% (vulnerary and demulcent)

Liver Hypofunction

Phytotherapeutic and naturopathic thinking recognizes a condition wherein the liver functions below optimum, even when no clinical evidence of liver disease or damage is apparent. Because the liver plays an important role in detoxification and many other metabolic processes, a poorly functioning liver can broadly affect health.

Signs of a poorly functioning liver might include food or drug intolerance, chronic constipation, fat intolerance, and poor digestion; poor liver functioning may contribute to chronic skin disease, autoimmune disease, allergies, IBD, and cancer.

Depending on severity and signs, treatment of patients with subclinical liver dysfunction should include hepatoprotective and hepatorestorative herbs, especially if a history of liver damage or exposure to liver toxins or drug toxicity is reported. Choleretic herbs, such as artichoke and dandelion, are also included to improve liver function, especially if digestion is compromised. Choleretics aid detoxification and may be useful in chronic skin disease and cancer, as may long-term prednisolone therapy. Depuratives such as burdock and yellow dock may also be considered.

A prescription to aid liver function:

Schisandra	20% (hepatoprotective, nervine tonic, adaptogen)
Dandelion root	20% (laxative, cholagogue)
Milk thistle	20% (hepatotonic, hepatoprotective, antioxidant)
Panax ginseng	20% (adaptogen, anti-inflammatory, antiallergic, immune enhancing)
Burdock	20% (alterative, bitter, mild laxative)

Another simple liver formula might consist of equal parts milk thistle, turmeric, artichoke, and schisandra.

An initial recommended dosage is 1 mL per 5 kg, given daily to twice daily.

Hepatitis

Therapeutic rationale

- Identify precipitating cause.
- Suppress inflammation to reduce fibrosis.

Knowledge of the underlying pathophysiology of particular hepatic disorders is important if treatment will be tailored for the individual case. Primary herbs for consideration in liver disease include barberry, milk thistle, dandelion, Oregon grape, bupleurum, fringe tree, artichoke, phyllanthus, turmeric, and schisandra. Antimicrobial, antiviral, and immune-enhancing herbs may be necessary. When fibrosis is a concern, hepatotrophorestorative herbs are an important part of strategic treatment. Hepatoprotective herbs given to minimize liver damage may include bupleurum, dandelion root, globe artichoke, and milk thistle. One should consider using milk thistle and schisandra in more concentrated forms, perhaps by giving tablet forms in addition to a formula. Because of the high prevalence of viral hepatitis, the human herbal literature lists antiviral herbs such as picrorrhiza, but these syndromes have not been documented in veterinary medicine at this writing. Immune-enhancing herbs such as *Astragalus membranaceus* (astragalus) and antimicrobial herbs such as *Echinacea* may still be appropriate for acute or chronic infection. For toxic insults to the liver, Schisandra and milk thistle should be considered.

The general liver health formula of herbalist Christopher Hobbs consists of milk thistle, artichoke, dandelion root, turmeric, skullcap, and California coast sage. David Winston's thistle compound for liver problems (Winston, 2003) contains dandelion root, watercress, blessed thistle, milk thistle, turmeric, and Oregon grape.

Hoffmann's chronic hepatitis formula (Hoffmann, 2004) consists of the following (proportions slightly modified):

Dandelion root	25%
Milk thistle	25%
Echinacea	20%
Mugwort	15%
Fringe tree	15%

A veterinary prescription for hepatitis :

Bupleurum	20% (hepatoprotective, anti-inflammatory, tonic)
Schisandra	20% (hepatoprotective, nervine tonic, adaptogen)
Milk thistle	20% (hepatotonic, hepatoprotective, antioxidant)
Panax ginseng	20% (adaptogen, anti-inflammatory, antiallergic, immune enhancing)
Astragalus	20% (immunomodulatory)

Another prescription is:

Milk thistle	20%
Artichoke	20%
Oregon grape	30%
Echinacea	30%

The recommended dosage is 1 mL per 5 kg, given daily to twice daily.

Megacolon

See "Constipation."

Parvovirus

Therapeutic rationale

- Maintain hydration.
- Control systemic bacterial infection via translocation from compromised gut.
- Maintain nutritional support.

Dogs with parvoviral enteritis may benefit from antiviral herbs, astringent herbs, and mucosal support provided by mucilaginous herbs. Herbs should be delivered via enema if administered to vomiting dogs. African plants *Bauhinia thonningii, Boswelia dalzielii, Detarium senegalensis*, and *Dichrostachys glomerata* inhibited replication of canine parvovirus in vitro (Kudi, 1999).

Stomatitis

Therapeutic rationale

- Control plaque.
- Identify other inciting causes, where possible.
- Control inflammation and bleeding.
- Control pain.

Classic herbs for gum disease include myrrh, goldenseal, sage, coptis, propolis, and calendula. For bleeding gums, astringent herbs (tormentil, agrimony) or yunnan pai yao can be used as needed. Echinacea is an antimicrobial herb, but it also acts as a local anesthetic. Weiss (1988) provides formulas that contain tormentil, sage, and arnica, and also recommends that lidocaine be added to one formula for pain.

One suggested formula follows:

Tormentil	30%
Echinacea	20%
Propolis	20%
Sage	20%
Myrrh	10%

Marsden has recommended Hoxsey formula for animals that present with an energetically "hot" constitution (Wynn, 2003), along with other formulas:

Agrimony	6 parts
Yellow dock	2 parts

Administer 0.2 mL/5 kg twice daily.

Or

Sarsaparilla	2 parts
Burdock	2 parts
Agrimony	3 parts
Yellow dock	1 part

Give 0.2 mL/5 kg twice daily.

Vomiting and Nausea

Therapeutic rationale

- Identify cause.
- Provide gastrointestinal tract rest in acute cases.
- Allow vomiting to remove offending material, if the cause is believed to be local.

Herbs traditionally used for symptomatic treatment of nausea in human medicine include ginger, gentian, goldenseal, peppermint, licorice, lavender, catnip, chamomile, and wild yam. Peppermint and ginger are probably the most effective.

Ulcers, Gastric or Intestinal

Therapeutic rationale

- Identify cause.
- Reduce formation of hydrogen ions.
- Protect ulcerated tissue.

The primary herbs used traditionally for gastrointestinal tract ulceration are chamomile and gotu kola, which appear to enhance healing of the ulcers and should be given on an empty stomach. Astringent herbs such as meadowsweet can be used but are of secondary importance. Mucilaginous herbs such as marshmallow or slippery elm may help protect ulcerated surfaces and, if used, should follow the vulnerary chamomile or gotu kola. See "Antiulcer Herbs."

HERBS FOR MUSCULOSKELETAL DISORDERS

General Notes

Musculoskeletal disorders result in loss of function and pain. This is generally associated with joint irregularities (hypermobility, instability, arthrosis, bony proliferation, ligamentous thickening) and muscle changes (spasms, both acute and chronic; atrophy). Goals of therapy include normalizing joint and muscle function and controlling pain. Joint instability itself may require surgical intervention; however, herbal analgesics and anti-inflammatory herbs may be useful in acute situations. In chronic situations, chondroprotectives, anti-inflammatories, alteratives, and analgesics are required. In older patients and those with chronic joint disease, muscle spasm is a dramatic but rarely recognized clinical finding. Deep palpation of thoracic, lumbar, and upper limb muscles reveals sensitivity that indicates massage therapy and antispasmodic herbs. Other useful therapies include physiotherapy, as well as chiropractic treatment and acupuncture.

In earlier times, arthritis was sometimes viewed as resulting from abnormal accumulations of metabolic toxins, which could be cleared with dietary changes, diuretics, and hepatics. There may be reason to connect toxin accumulation with pain and inflammation, and the more modern concept of "leaky gut" can explain why herbalists generally direct some efforts toward normalizing gut function, as well as directly addressing joint and muscle pain and inflammation. Leaky gut occurs in animals that may be older and stressed because of chronic pain or disease, especially when steroids and nonsteroidal anti-inflammatory drugs (which may often lead to mucosal inflammation) change normal gut permeability. When the gut mucosa is altered in this way, large proteins such as food as well as bacterial, and self antigens may gain access to the submucosa and possibly even the portal circulation. The normal gut is responsible for making primary immune responses, but it also makes significant neuroendocrine responses, including the production of serotonin, benzodiazepines, glutamate, enkephalins, nitric oxide, and dopamine. The end clinical response is increased immune responsiveness, systemic inflammation and perhaps altered behavior (Figure 20-2).

Mechanisms of Interest

Antirheumatics

Veterinarians are not prone to use the term *rheumatism,* and most are not searching for it in the clinic. Chronically arthritic animals use other body regions to compensate for pain and suboptimal function. In the case of hip dysplasia, for instance, most animals exhibit sensitivity on palpation of thoracic and lumbar muscles. Treatment of the primary problem may or may not resolve the

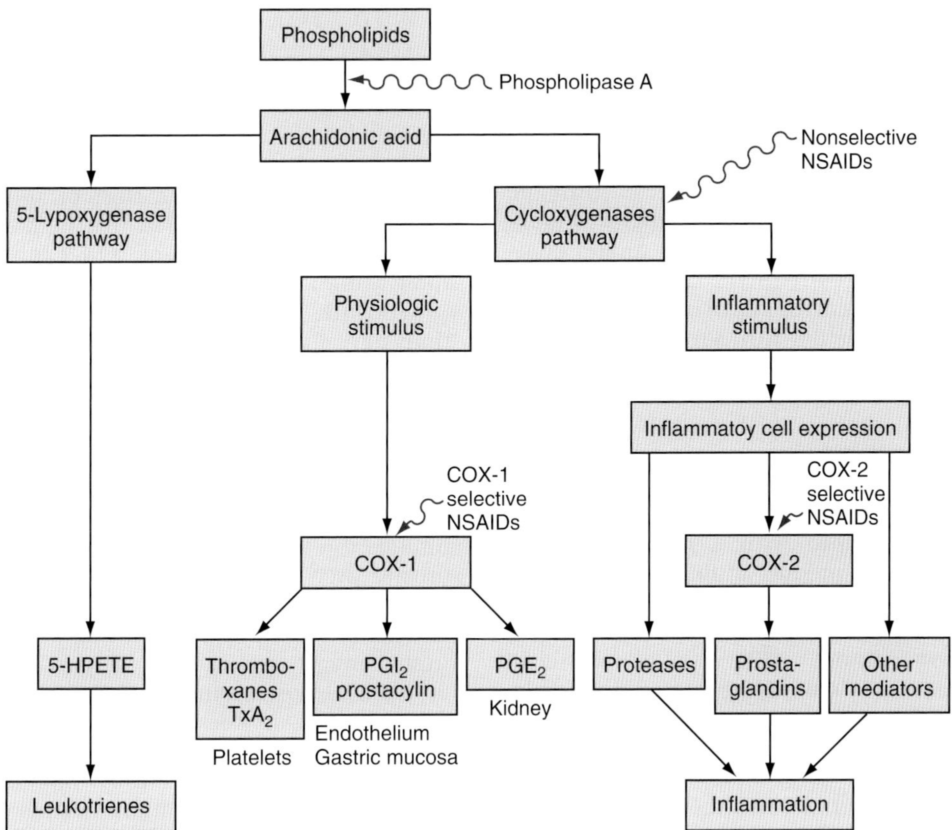

Figure 20-2 Inflammatory pathways and sites for herb interventions.

painful muscle spasms that limit mobility in these animals. Massage and other physical therapies can be very helpful, but herbs can provide a variety of therapeutic actions, including antispasmodic, anti-inflammatory, and circulatory enhancement to these areas. Most of the herbs that are useful in treating "rheumatic" animals are discussed below by putative mechanism, but the entire list given by Hoffmann (2004) is long and includes the following: yarrow, angelica, celery seed, burdock, uva ursi, arnica, horseradish, wormwood *(Artemisia absinthium),* mugwort, birch, brassica, cayenne, blue cohosh, black cohosh, wild yam, boneset, gravelroot, meadowsweet, bladderwrack, wintergreen, guaiacum, devil's claw, blue flag, juniper, Oregon grape, bogbean, bayberry, parsley, poke, aspen, rosemary, yellow dock, willow, sarsaparilla, feverfew, dandelion, nettle, cramp bark, prickly ash, and ginger.

Anti-inflammatory agents

These herbs appear to inhibit the inflammatory processes that accompany degenerative processes, immune-mediated events, and other inflammatory and traumatic conditions.

DEVIL'S CLAW *(HARPAGOPHYTUM PROCUMBENS)*: This plant is used in traditional African medicine for arthritis. Studies suggest that devil's claw may suppress prostaglandin E_2 (PGE_2) synthesis and nitric oxide production by inhibiting lipopolysaccharide-stimulated enhancement of cyclooxygenase (COX)-2 and inducible nitric oxide synthase mRNA expression. Human clinical trials show that it is clearly effective in the treatment of low back pain.

MEADOWSWEET *(FILIPENDULA ULMARIA)*: This was the first source identified for commercial production of salicin, a nonselective COX-1 and COX-2 inhibitor.

WILLOW BARK (*SALIX ALBA* AND OTHER SALIX SPECIES): Willow contains high levels of salicin, a nonselective COX-1 and COX-2 inhibitor. *Betula* (Birch) species are also recognized as having significant salicin levels in their barks.

FEVERFEW *(TANACETUM PARTHENIUM)*: Clinical trial evidence for use of feverfew in osteoarthritis is not yet convincing (Ernst, 2000b). A well-studied constituent, parthenolide, specifically binds to and inhibits IKK-beta, which is involved in cytokine-mediated signaling. Parthenolide and other constituents also apparently inhibit COX expression and have various other effects on a variety of eicosanoids. Feverfew powder (more so than its extracts) has antiserotonergic activity (Mittra, 2000).

NETTLE *(URTICA DIOICA)*: In his review, Ernst (2000) describes unpublished data from a randomized controlled trial in which a stew of aerial parts of the plant was effective for pain, but a concentrated juice containing 10 times more of the presumed active ingredient (lipoxygenase inhibitor caffeoyl malic acid) was not. Nettle inhibits the activity of NF-kappa-B (Riehemann, 1999), and proprietary extracts of nettle were found to suppress the activity matrix metalloproteinases, which enhance degradation of extracellular matrix in joint cartilage (Schulze-Tanzil, 2002).

GINGER ***(ZINGIBER OFFICINALIS):*** This has been recommended for anti-inflammatory effects through eicosanoid modulation, as it inhibits the activity of both cyclooxygenase and lipoxygenase. The few studies done may suggest some such activity (Bliddal, 2000).

BOSWELLIA ***(BOSWELLIA SERRATA):*** Boswellia may reduce pain and inflammation through its activity as a lipoxygenase inhibitor. In bovine serum albumin-induced arthritis, boswellic acids reduced inflammatory cell infiltrates (Sharma, 1989). One study showed that boswellic acids have activity against 5-lipoxygenase, but that they did not affect 12-lipoxygenase or cyclooxygenase (Ammon, 1993). An open, multicenter (10 veterinarians) clinical trial was performed with a resin extract of *Boswellia serrata* (BSB108, product of Bogar AG). A total of 29 dogs with signs of chronic joint and spinal disease were enrolled; 25 had radiologic signs of osteoarthritis and "degenerative conditions." BSB108 was administered in the diet at a dose of 400 mg/10 kg body weight daily for 6 weeks. Of 24 eligible dogs, the investigators believed that 71% of them showed improvement. A statistically significant reduction in severity and resolution of typical clinical signs, such as intermittent lameness, local pain, and stiff gait reported after 6 weeks, were observed in individual animals; however, no control group was included. Adverse effects were rare and mild, consisting only of brief episodes of diarrhea and flatulence (Reichling, 2004).

TURMERIC ***(CURCUMA LONGA):*** This has been used in Ayurvedic medicine for arthritis and other types of pain, and in Chinese medicine for abdominal pain, and is often found in formulas with Boswellia. Human clinical trials have demonstrated some anti-inflammatory activity (Chainani-Wu, 2003). A clinical trial using similar species of turmeric—Indian turmeric *(C. domestica)* and Javanese turmeric *(C. xanthorrhiza)*—was conducted with 61 client-owned dogs with arthritis. The dogs were evaluated by veterinarians and owners, then were administered a placebo or a standardized extract containing 20 mg curcuminoids, 50 mg *C. xanthorrhiza* volatile oil, and 150 mg *C. domestica* essential oil. The dose used was 2 capsules per 10 kg body weight twice daily. Veterinary evaluations were statistically significantly in favor of the turmeric preparation over placebo, but force plate analysis and owner evaluations were not. Investigators noted that minor adverse effects occurred in the turmeric group, including a peculiar smell that may have compromised the blinding of the clinical evaluators (Innes, 2003).

YUCCA ***(YUCCA SCHIDIGERA):*** This herb is popular but not well studied. One proposed mechanism of action involves the suppression of gut bacterial endotoxin production by saponins, which thus removes a supposed suppressor of proteoglycan synthesis. One study suggested that a single constituent, Yuccaol C, reduced inducible nitric oxide synthase expression via the transcription factor NF-kappa-B (Marzocco, 2004).

WILD YAM, OR MEXICAN YAM ***(DIOSCOREA VILLOSA):*** This herb has traditionally been used for pain control. It contains diosgenin, which has been used as a precursor in the manufacture of commercial corticosteroids. Diosgenin does not appear to be converted to glucocorticoid by mammalian systems, so plant sterols may have effects that are like or unlike mammalian steroids. One study showed that extracts of a Japanese yam inhibited production of COX-2 and nitric oxide synthase (Kim, 2004).

GUGGUL ***(COMMIPHORA MUKUL):*** Clinical investigations have shown that guggul reduced pain and stiffness and improved function in older patients with osteoarthritis of the knee. Guggul was administered in capsule form (500 mg concentrated exact delivered three times daily) along with food. No adverse effects were reported during the trial (Singh, 2003b).

ARNICA ***(ARNICA MONTANA):*** This strong herb inhibits the activation of NF-kappa-B (Klaas, 2002). It is usually used only topically, or orally in homeopathic doses. An open multicenter clinical trial was conducted to determine the safety and efficacy of an *Arnica montana* fresh plant gel, applied twice daily, in 79 people with mild to moderate osteoarthritis of the knee. After 3 and 6 weeks, significant decreases in scores for pain, stiffness, and function scales showed significant reductions at these time points, with only one allergic reaction. (Knuesel, 2002). A preparation like this may be useful in horses, but dogs would have to be prevented from licking the gel because of its oral toxicity. Arnica was also investigated in a double-blind trial with 37 humans undergoing bilateral endoscopic carpal tunnel release surgery. Patients were administered homeopathic Arnica orally and arnica gel topically. A significant reduction in pain was noted after 2 weeks in the Arnica-treated group (Jeffrey, 2002).

GUAIACUM ***(GUAIACUM OFFICINALE):*** This herb has been listed as a traditional analgesic, but one study suggested that it has anti-inflammatory activity (Duwiejua, 1994).

BOGBEAN ***(MENYANTHES TRIFOLIATA):*** This plant contains unusually high levels of betulinic acid, a potent anti-inflammatory agent (Patočka, 2003).

OTHER HERBS: Other anti-inflammatory agents suggested in traditional herbal texts include Angelica *(Angelica archangelica),* Celery *(Apium graveolens),* Blue cohosh *(Caulophyllum thalictroides),* Black cohosh *(Actea racemosa),* Wintergreen *(Gaultheria procumbens),* and Quaking aspen *(Populus tremuloides).*

Analgesics

Analgesics alleviate pain without causing loss of consciousness, although they may also have central nervous system effects that affect awareness. (Analgesic herbs are discussed further under neurologic and behavioral herbs.)

CORYDALIS ***(CORYDALIS YANHUSUO, C. TURTSCHANINOVII, C. TECUMBENS, AND C. INCISA):*** These herbs account for part of traditional Chinese herbal combinations for pain. Although a specific mechanism of action has not been well described, authorities state that continued use leads to tolerance and to cross-tolerance with opioids.

Jamaican Dogwood *(Piscidea erythrina)*: This herb is not well studied, but early laboratory animal studies suggested some spasmolytic and possible sedative effects. *King's American Dispensatory* opined that it had a central pain-relieving action.

Saint John's Wort *(Hypericum perforatum)*: Although it is better known as an antidepressant, this herb has exhibited analgesic and anti-inflammatory activities in laboratory animals; two other *Hypericum* species *(H. cordatum* and *H. caprifoliatum)* have shown antinociceptive activity, possibly via opioid systems, in laboratory animal pain models (Viana, 2003). Antidepressants are recognized elements of pain control in human medicine, and they may act through a number of pharmacologic actions; for example, by blocking reuptake of noradrenaline and 5-hydroxytryptamine through direct and indirect actions on opioid receptors; inhibiting histamine, cholinergic, 5-hydroxytryptamine and *N*-methyl-D-aspartate receptors; inhibiting ion channel activity; and blocking adenosine uptake (Sawynok, 2001).

California Poppy *(Eschscholtzia californica)*: This plant has not been well investigated for analgesic properties, but the U.S. Dispensatory of 1918 claimed it to be a powerful but safe soporific and analgesic, containing small amounts of morphine and other alkaloids. Rolland et al (2001) showed analgesic effects in mice.

Indian Pipe *(Monotropa uniflora)*: This has also been used for pain control and is said to have mild dissociative effects.

Spasmolytic agents

Although spasmolytic agents are generally thought to apply more to smooth muscle (such as in the gastrointestinal, reproductive, respiratory, and urinary tracts), skeletal muscle may also be relieved of spasm, probably because of central effects.

Black Cohosh *(Actaea racemosa)*: The single constituent, cimicifugoside, was recently shown to selectively inhibit N-acetylcholine receptor–mediated responses in bovine chromaffin cells (Woo, 2004). No other studies related to pain or spasm could be located.

Valerian *(Valeriana officinalis)*: Older German studies indicate that valerenic acid is spasmolytic and relaxes muscles (Wagner, 1979; Bisset, 1994).

Cramp Bark *(Viburnum opulus)*: This herb and other *Viburnum* species have shown the ability to reduce smooth muscle spasm in a number of in vitro studies (Cometa, 1998; Calle, 1999; Nicholson, 1972). Whether they also have skeletal muscle effects has not been investigated.

Other herbs: Other herbs used for their spasmolytic effects include Black haw, Skunk cabbage, Lobelia, Myrrh, Skullcap, and Kava kava.

Alteratives

Alterative herbs cause a change in a chronic condition, or tend to restore to health ["without sensible evacuations," according to *Webster's Dictionary*]. Traditional lore had it that these herbs were blood purifiers that supported toxin elimination. Modern medical science may also conceive of these herbs as supplying nutritional elements or acting as immune modulators, enhancing liver detoxification activity, antioxidants, anti-inflammatories, or normalizing gut function or gut bacterial populations.

Burdock *(Arctium lappa)*: This herb has shown antioxidant and anti-inflammatory activities in laboratory animal studies (Lin, 1996a). The root is also high in starch (especially inulin), which accounts for its mild laxative effect, and may improve gut bacterial populations.

Blue Flag *(Iris versicolor)*: This herb is usually used for liver disease (chronic skin and musculoskeletal diseases are often treated with the same alteratives for many of the same reasons). The herb is traditionally considered to be hepatic, cholagogue, diuretic, laxative, and anti-inflammatory.

Oregon Grape *(Mahonia aquifolium)*: The components jatrorrhizine and magnoflorine are powerful antioxidants (Rackova, 2004). The aporphine alkaloids isothebaine and isocorydine showed relaxant properties in the rat aorta (Sotnikova, 1997). This herb is a traditional hepatic, laxative, and cholagogue.

Yellow Dock or Curly Dock *(Rumex crispus)*: This herb is a traditional hepatic, cholagogue, and mild laxative. Studies on other species of Rumex *(R. maritima, R. patientia,* and *R. saggitatus)* show anti-inflammatory activity in laboratory animal and in in vitro studies (Islam, 2003; Suleyman, 2001; Jager, 1996).

Sarsaparilla (*Smilax* spp): Various species of *Smilax* have shown immune modulatory and anti-inflammatory activities in laboratory animal studies of chronic inflammation (Lu, 2003; Jiang, 2003; Ageel, 1989).

Pokeweed *(Phytolacca americana)*: This strong plant is not used often for patients with arthritis but may be a powerful immune modulant or anti-inflammatory agent. It was an important plant for rheumatism in American folk medicine

Circulatory stimulants

Traditional circulatory stimulants are generally warming and pungent herbs, the peripheral effects of which can sometimes be seen in nearly immediate sweating. Practically speaking, these herbs probably have anti-inflammatory AND analgesic effects.

Capsicum *(Capsicum annuum)*: This herb has been used orally as a traditional circulatory stimulant. Capsaicin is the best known analgesic compound in this pepper, and it is the parent compound of a group of vanillyl fatty acid amides. It acts specifically by depleting stores of substance P from sensory neurons; it has been used successfully in the treatment of rheumatoid arthritis, osteoarthritis, peripheral neuropathies, and fibromyalgia, and is applied topically. Capsicum oleoresin, however, contains more than 100 volatile compounds and may have a variety of other actions. Other capsaicinoids have anti-inflammatory activity, inhibiting activation of NF-kappa-B and certain events in T-cell activation (Sancho, 2002).

PRICKLY ASH *(ZANTHOXYLUM AMERICANUM)*: This traditional circulatory stimulant has not been examined for activity in musculoskeletal pain. The Eclectics used it primarily for muscular rheumatism and neuromuscular problems. Other species of *Zanthoxylum* have shown antinociceptive and antispasmodic activities in laboratory animals and in in vitro studies (de Moura, 2002; Rahman, 2002).

OTHER HERBS: Ginger has been reviewed in the anti-inflammatory herb section.

Diuretics

Diuretics have traditionally been considered important to help eliminate end products of metabolism and inflammatory by-products. Although the plants discussed in this section have diuretic activity, it is unclear that this is a primary mechanism for consideration in patients with musculoskeletal disease, because they also appear to work via other mechanisms.

YARROW *(ACHILLEA MILLEFOLIUM)*: This herb and other species of yarrow contain anti-inflammatory principles, including sterols, flavonoids, and sesquiterpenes.

CELERY *(APIUM GRAVEOLENS)*: This traditional remedy is used for gout, a type of inflammatory arthritis that develops in people with accumulation of uric acid in the joints. Celery seed has a reputation for increasing urinary uric acid excretion, but studies have not confirmed this. One group did identify multiple compounds in celery seed that inhibited both COX-1 and COX-2 activity, as well as compounds that had antioxidant activity (Momin, 2002).

BONESET *(EUPATORIUM PERFOLIATUM)*: A component of Joe Pye Weed *(E. purpureum)* has been shown to have anti-inflammatory activity (Habtemariam, 2001). Other species of *Eupatorium* have shown antinociceptive activity that is not related to opioids (Clavin, 2000). No relevant studies were found for use of boneset.

Nervines

See the neurologic and behavioral herb section.

Nervines may be effective in reducing the stress associated with chronic pain. The herbs listed here have other actions that have been described previously.

- Celery *(Apium graveolens)*
- Jamaica dogwood *(Piscidia erythrina)*
- Valerian *(Valeriana officinalis)*

Other herbs

Other herbs that have been used for their effects on the musculoskeletal system include Blue vervain, Butterbur, Chamomile, Hops, Skunk cabbage, Valerian, Willow bark, and Wood Betony.

Review of Specific Musculoskeletal Conditions

Musculoskeletal pain and inflammation

The formulas given here are simply starting points and should be customized (in content and dose) for the patient's condition. These formulas may be dosed at approximately 0.25-1.0 mL per 10 lb two to three times daily.

A prescription for early osteoarthritis or presurgical patients with anti-inflammatory and analgesic activity follows:

Devil's claw	25%
Meadowsweet	25%
Ginger	25%
Ashwagandha	25%

A stronger formula, used only after chondroprotectives, massage, exercise, and milder formulas have failed, is provided here:

Devil's claw	30%
Corydalis	30%
Prickly ash	30%
Sarsaparilla	10%

Formulas similar to those above can be considered for the following conditions.

Cranial cruciate ligament rupture

Complete rupture of the ligament will probably require surgery for best results, but partial tears may be managed with anti-inflammatory herbs and physical therapy. Analgesics or acupuncture may be necessary for animals undergoing physical therapy.

Luxating patella

Anti-inflammatory herbs are useful if the condition is of low grade and surgery is not required. Severe arthritis of the stifle may require more integrated therapy with anti-inflammatory, antispasmodic, analgesic, and alterative herbs, as well as acupuncture and physical therapy.

Myopathy

Owners of animals with diseases such as feline congenital myotonia, Devon Rex myopathy, Scotty cramp, German shepherd fibrotic myopathy, Labrador stress syndrome, and other unusual muscle diseases frequently seek herbal and other therapies when conventional medicine fails their pets. These animals may benefit from spasmolytic and nervine herbs. Cramp bark, black haw, valerian, Jamaica dogwood, wild yam, and prickly ash might be candidates for these patients.

Osteoarthritis

Anti-inflammatory herbs are frequently used for osteoarthritis. The most popular are Boswellia, Ginger, Devil's claw, Meadowsweet, and Yucca. For chronic arthritis, analgesic, spasmolytic, nervine, and alterative herbs may be used.

One Chinese herbal combination tested in dogs appeared effective (Bonnett, 1996). In a study of 143 clinical canine patients in four groups, a proprietary Chinese herbal combination was compared with Devil's claw combination, aspirin, and placebo. The Chinese herbal prescription contained White peony, Licorice, Epimedium, Oyster shell, Reishi mushroom, Isatidis, and Corydalis. The Chinese herbal combination and aspirin groups experienced significant improvement according to owner and veterinary evaluation, whereas the response to Devil's claw combination was equivalent to the placebo response (Bonnett, 1996). The specific formula used in this study is not commercially available, but similar combinations can be formulated on request by reputable Chinese pharmacies.

A prescription for relief from osteoarthritis:

Devil's claw	20%
Corydalis	20%
Saint John's Wort	20%
Ashwagandha	40%

Osteochondrosis

Acute osteochondrosis requires surgery, but the consequence of this disease is osteoarthritis. See the section on osteoarthritis for suggested herbs.

Panosteitis

Analgesic herbs may be helpful in this condition. Boneset has a reputation for relieving deep bone pain. Boneset has a specific indication for deep "bone" pain and may be useful in a formula as well. *King's American Dispensatory* describes the indications for boneset in this way: "Its popular name, "boneset," is derived from its well-known property of relieving the deep-seated pains in the limbs which accompany [influenza], and colds and rheumatism. Often, this pain is periosteal, and if neuralgic in character, or due to a febrile condition, eupatorium will relieve it. But it is not a remedy for periosteal pain due to inflammation or to organic changes in the periosteum."

Muscular rheumatism (old age stiffness)

Merriam Webster Online defines rheumatism as, "any of various conditions characterized by inflammation or pain in muscles, joints, or fibrous tissue." Herbs that may be helpful for this kind of pain include prickly ash, valerian, and the viburnums (Black haw and Cramp bark).

Rheumatoid arthritis

Patients with rheumatoid arthritis may benefit from immune modulators, alteratives, and anti-inflammatory herbs. One plant that has been shown to have activity in rheumatoid arthritis patients is *Tripterygium wilfordii* (Tao, 2000); however, the adverse effects have led researchers to try to isolate a safer single constituent (triptolide). Other herbs for consideration are those with anti-inflammatory and analgesic activities.

These may include bogbean, meadowsweet, wild yam, guaiacum, valerian, celery seed, angelica, and Saint John's wort.

Spondylosis deformans

Although many still consider this a nonpainful condition, we disagree. Anti-inflammatory herbs may be useful, but circulatory stimulants and analgesics may be more useful. These might include capsicum, prickly ash, valerian, boswellia, peony, and yucca.

Trauma

Arnica is a specific remedy for trauma. It is a very strong herb and, if used orally, is generally administered in homeopathic (or low-dose) form. Arnica ointments are available for topical use but may be toxic if the animal licks the area.

Rabbits with induced impacted vertebrae and spinal cord injury that were treated with dan shen *(Salvia miltiorrhiza),* compared with controls, demonstrated less serious damage histologically. It was concluded that dan shen injection has some protective effect on spinal cord injury in its early stage (Ni, 2002).

Fracture repair

In addition to conventional treatment, one may consider using dan shen *(Salvia miltiorrhiza)*. Dan shen was used in an experimental group of rabbits with induced bone defects. It increased osteoblast activity to a greater extent than did controls, and it stimulated synthesis of protein in fibroblasts. Dan shen caused early formation of dense callus, and microscopic examination revealed increased activity of osteoblasts. It was concluded that dan shen could improve mandibular bone fracture healing (Lin, 1992).

HERBS FOR PAIN AND NEUROLOGIC AND BEHAVIORAL DISORDERS

General Considerations

In no other system is it so obvious that plants and animals coevolved to use each other for conducting the business of life—beyond mere nutrition. Plant and animal physiologic master plans developed in concert, sometimes during battles (as plants developed defenses against herbivores) but seemingly to everyone's benefit in the end. Plants learned to use animals for reproduction (for a surprising read, *The Botany of Desire* is highly recommended). Animals have receptors for plant chemicals—opioid receptors, named for the opium poppy, as well as cannabinoid receptors, benzodiazepine receptors, and vanilloid receptors (for cayenne's constituent, capsaicin). Many plants can have an effect on animal consciousness and pain perception. Veterinarians have learned many of these in poisonous plant lists. For herbalists, these plants may provide additional tools with which to treat patients with abnormal behavior, seizures, neuromuscular disease, and pain.

In traditional herbal medicine, any plant that affects the nervous system is called a *nervine*. A nervine can therefore encompass several kinds of therapeutic activity. For example, an herbalist might prescribe a nervine to calm and sedate a patient who exhibits hyperactivity or anxiety, or a nervine may be prescribed for a depressed patient, to restore a sense of well-being. In veterinary neurology, one of the most important contributions that herbal medicine can make is in "strengthening" the nervous system. Nervines can be broadly classified into three main groups, although many nervine herbs have overlapping activity.

1. Nervine relaxants have sedating, hypnotic, or calming and anxiolytic activity, and many have antispasmodic activity. Relaxant nervines are prescribed for anxiety, hyperactivity, and sleeplessness and restlessness. They

include herbs such as valerian, lavender, hops, passionflower, and lemon balm. Nervine relaxants include antispasmodic nervines that are prescribed for muscle cramping or twitches, such as smooth muscle spasm of the colon, bronchi, stomach, bladder, and so forth. An example is chamomile, which is used for painful spasm of the gastrointestinal tract.

2. Nervine stimulants may be beneficial in a depressed or hypoactive nervous system. Rarely needed in veterinary medicine, these herbs are widely used by people and include coffee, tea, cola (kola nut), and guarana; all can induce anxiety and tension. Stimulating nervines are prescribed for low-energy states, lethargy, and depression. Saint John's wort can be useful for mild depression; also, this group may include the cognition-enhancing herbs outlined later.
3. Nervine tonics can restore tissues directly (see later) by contributing to tissue repair, or they may help reduce the effects of undue stress on the body; these include adaptogens, nervine trophorestoratives, and most herbs that reduce anxiety and stress. One example is *Ginkgo biloba,* which appears to work by promoting vasodilation in the brain, thus improving oxygenation to brain tissue. Others include Saint John's wort and Oats.

Although these classifications may appear paradoxical, in all cases of neurologic or behavioral imbalance, the goals of herbal medicine are fundamentally the same: to nourish the nervous system and restore and balance activity. The following herbs may give veterinary herbalists additional tools for use in treating patients with abnormal behavior, seizures, neuromuscular disease, and pain; their mechanisms of action are presented.

Mechanisms of Interest

Nervine relaxants

BLACK COHOSH *(ACTAEA RACEMOSA):* Most Eclectic uses of black cohosh as a nervine were associated with menstrual or menopausal disorders in women, and it is difficult to separate the antispasmodic and analgesic effects within traditional literature. King's (Felter 1898) has this to say of Black cohosh: "exerts a powerful influence over the nervous system, and has long been favorably known as a remedy for chorea. It may be used alone or with specific valerian, equal parts. Its action is slow, but its effects are permanent. It has been used successfully as an antispasmodic in hysteria, epilepsy when due to menstrual failures, asthma and kindred affections, periodical convulsions, nervous excitability, pertussis, delirium tremens, and many other spasmodic affections."

HOPS *(HUMULUS LUPULUS):* This traditional sedative is used for neuralgia, insomnia, excitability, priapism, mucous colitis, and, specifically, for restlessness associated with nervous tension headache or indigestion. The German Commission E approved its use for mood disturbances such as restlessness and anxiety, as well as for sleep disturbances (Blumenthal, 1998). King's describes hops this way: "They are principally used for their sedative or hypnotic action—producing sleep, removing restlessness, and abating pain, but which they often fail to accomplish." Whole extracts of hops were generally administered for this purpose in the form of ale or porter. The Eclectics preferred a powdered extract called *lupulin,* and found it much more reliable. Early laboratory animal and human clinical studies showed no sedative effects (Hansel, 1967; Stocker, 1967). Later studies showed that one auto-oxidation product had strong sedative properties in animals (Wohlfart, 1983; Hänsel, 1980; Wohlfart, 1982). This is an aromatic principle, and the authors warned that it may be present in traditional hops pillows, but not in many herb extracts. However, it has also been suggested that isovaleric acid residues present in hops may contribute to its sedative action in mice. Hops extract administered intraperitoneally 30 minutes before a series of behavioral tests resulted in dose-dependent suppression of spontaneous locomotion at a dose of 250 mg/kg for up to 1 hour (Lee, 1993).

ASHWAGANDHA *(WITHANIA SOMNIFERA):* The alkaloid root extract (ashwagandholine) exhibited a taming effect and had a mild depressant (tranquilizer) effect on the central nervous system of monkeys, cats, dogs, rats, and mice (Malhotra, 1965). Glycowithanolides of withania (10 and 20 mg/kg/day, intraperitoneally, for 21 days) induced a dose-related increase in superoxide dismutase, catalase, and glutathione peroxidase activity in rat brain; this effect was comparable to the benefit of deprenyl (Bhattacharya, 1997). Sitoindosides VII through X and withaferin-A were studied on brain cholinergic, glutamatergic, and gamma-aminobutyric acid (GABA)ergic receptors in rats. Results suggested that the compounds preferentially affect events in the cortical and basal forebrain cholinergic signal transduction cascade. The drug-induced increase in cortical muscarinic acetylcholine receptor capacity might explain in part the cognition-enhancing and memory-improving effects of extracts from *Withania somnifera* observed in animals and humans (Schliebs, 1997). GABA binding was inhibited by 20% with 5 µg Withania root extract and completely by 1 mg. This extract increased Cl influx, which was blocked by bicuculline and picrotoxin and was enhanced by diazepam. These results suggest that the *W. somnifera* extract contains an ingredient that has a GABA-mimetic activity (Mehta, 1991). Withania has been used to stabilize mood in patients with behavioral disturbances.

ZIZYPHUS SEED *(ZIZYPHUS SPINOSA):* The flavonoids and saponins were tested for sedative activity. All compounds tested potentiated hexobarbital-induced hypnosis and reduced ladder climbing and caffeine-induced hyperactivity. It was found that these compounds produced sleep but were not anticonvulsants or muscle relaxants (Shin, 1981). Jujuboside A (JuA), a major constituent of the seed, has inhibitory effects on the glutamate-mediated excitatory signal pathway in the hippocampus and probably acts through its anticalmodulin action (Zhang, 2003b).

MOTHERWORT *(LEONURUS CARDIACA):* This herb has not been investigated for its nervine qualities. King's describes its indications as "nervous excitability, all chronic diseases attended with restlessness, wakefulness, disturbed sleep. . . . It is adapted to cases of nervous debility with irritation, nervous unrest, tendency to choreic or spasmodic movements."

CHAMOMILE *(MATRICARIA RECUTITA)***:** The dried flower heads of chamomile are used in folk medicine to prepare a spasmolytic and sedative tea. Laboratory animal studies suggest that this plant has some sedative activity (Della Loggia, 1981). The essential oil of chamomile improved mood in a human clinical trial (Roberts, 1992). King's describes the indications as "nervous irritability, with peevishness, fretfulness, discontent, and impatience; sudden fits of temper during the catamenial period; muscular twitching; morbid sensitiveness to pain." This herb was considered most important for children and for those who exhibited signs that were out of proportion to the actual pain that was experienced. The text also notes that the nervine effects of Chamomile are more marked at low (drop) doses than at typical herb doses.

LEMON BALM *(MELISSA OFFICINALIS)***:** Laboratory animal studies have shown that Lemon balm has sedative activity (Bisset, 1994). Two randomized, placebo-controlled, double-blind, balanced-crossover studies investigated the effects of a standardized extract in healthy people who received single doses of 300, 600, 900, 1000, or 1600 mg or a placebo at 7-day intervals. Cognitive performance was assessed immediately before dosing and at 1, 2.5, 4, and 6 hours thereafter. Calmness (self-assessed) was increased after the lowest doses, and alertness was decreased following the higher doses. Higher doses improved memory performance, however (Kennedy, 2002; Kennedy, 2003b). In a subsequent study, this group showed that in healthy humans, 300 mg or 600 mg of standardized extract increased calmness and decreased alertness in the face of stress, but the speed of mathematical processing was increased at the lower dose (Kennedy, 2004). Patients with agitation due to severe dementia were administered a lotion with essential oil of Melissa or a placebo aromatherapy lotion. In this study, there was significant improvement in agitation and quality of life indices for those being treated with Lemon balm (Ballard, 2002). The Eclectics considered the plant stimulant and diaphoretic.

CATNIP *(NEPETA CATARIA)***:** This herb was used by the Eclectics for headaches and nervous irritability. It was also used as an antispasmodic, and Cook's *Physiomedical Dispensatory* (1869) calls it a "diffuse nervine and antispasmodic of much service." Laboratory animal studies have produced somewhat conflicting results regarding sleep time and activity. Two studies suggest that components of catnip have some sedative activity. Catnip oil (500 mg/kg) and nepetalic acid (62.5 mg/kg) were found to significantly increase sleep time in mice. Rats showed a significant decrease in performance in avoidance studies after intraperitoneal injections of catnip oil (500-750 mg/kg), nepetalic acid (125-250 mg/kg), and the nepetalactone-enriched fraction (500-750 mg/kg) (Harney, 1978). The alcohol extract of catnip showed a biphasic effect on the behavior of young chicks, increasing the number of chicks who slept at low and moderate doses (25-1800 mg/kg), while high dose levels (i.e., above 2 g/kg) led fewer chicks to sleep (Sherry, 1979). On the other hand, Massoco and colleagues (1995) fed mice catnip at 10% of their dietary intake and discovered amphetamine-like activity. A case report described a single child who ate a large amount of catnip and was obtunded (Osterhoudt, 1997). Aydin (1998) determined that nepetalactone (a component of *Nepeta cataria* and other species of *Nepeta*) had specific activity at some opioid receptor subtypes. Unique behavioral reactions of cats have been observed in the presence of catnip. The chemosensory stimulus evoking the catnip reaction is undoubtedly mediated through the main olfactory system. These behaviors, include sniffing and chewing as associated with oral appetitive behavior, rolling and rubbing characteristic of female sexual behavior, batting the catnip source characteristic of play behavior, and a type of kicking associated with predatory behavior. These behavioral reactions occur randomly and intermittently (Hart, 1985).

PASSIONFLOWER *(PASSIFLORA INCARNATA)***:** The methanol leaf extract was evaluated for various central nervous system (CNS) effects in experimental animals. This extract exhibited significant sedative, anticonvulsant, and CNS-depressant activities at a dose of 200 mg/kg in mice. The extract also exhibited analgesic and anti-inflammatory activities against induced pain and induced edema, respectively, in experimental animals (Kamaldeep, 2003).

JAMAICA DOGWOOD *(PISCIDIA PISCIPULA,* FORMERLY *PISCIDEA ERYTHRINA)***:** Ellingwood's *Materia Medica* (1919) describes this herb's indications as follows: "In susceptible patients, it will control pain and relieve general distress. It is distinctly a nerve sedative, and overcomes nervous excitability and also reflex irritability. It is an antispasmodic of much power in mild cases." It is also known for its ability to induce deep, restful sleep. Laboratory animal studies suggest that this plant has some sedative activity (Della Loggia, 1981). The herb is toxic in high doses (producing seizures and cardiorespiratory arrest) and probably is not appropriate for long-term use. The human dose of the fluid extract recommended by King's (Felter, 1898) is 10 drops to 2 fluid drachm (approximately 7 mL) daily, but doses recommended by the *British Herbal Compendium* are higher: 2 to 4 g of dried root bark, 5 to 15 mL of the tincture (1:5 in 45%), or 2 to 8 mL of the liquid extract (1:1 in 60%) three times daily (Bradley 1992).

PULSATILLA *(PULSATILLA VULGARIS,* FORMERLY *ANEMONE PULSATILLA)***:** This herb is also called European pasqueflower, Meadow anemone, and Windflower. The 1918 US Dispensatory summarizes the available anecdotes and literature on this herb, saying that it leads to progressive paralysis and that there is contradictory information on any effect on the heart; it does not list nervousness or anxiety as an indication. On the other hand, King's describes the specific indications for Pulsatilla to include "nervousness and despondency, sadness, unnatural fear, tendency to weep, morbid mental excitement, marked depression of spirits, pain, with debility, nervousness . . ." The US Dispensatory related the fatal dose for the rabbit as 200 mg/kg and for the guinea pig as 0.16 g/kg. This reference provided a dose for humans of from $^5/_6$ to $1^1/_2$ grains (0.05-0.096 g) divided daily.

SKULLCAP *(SCUTELLARIA LATERIFLORA)*: King's lists the specific indications for Skullcap as "Nervousness, attending or following acute or chronic diseases, or from mental or physical exhaustion, teething, etc.; nervousness manifesting itself in muscular action; tremors, subsultus, etc.; hysteria, with inability to control the voluntary muscles; functional cardiac disorders of a purely nervous type, with intermittent pulse." The 1918 US Dispensatory proclaimed it devoid of medicinal effects, but evidence is accumulating that it may indeed act as a mild nervine. Scutellarin and ikonnikoside bind a 5-HT receptor subtype (Gafner, 2003). The plant contains baicalin and baicalein, which bind the benzodiazepine site of the GABA A receptor (Awad, 2003).

LINDEN *(TILIA PLATYPHYLLOS)*: This is a mild traditional nervine that was more popular in Europe than in the United States. The Eclectics considered the flowers a stimulant and nervine, as well as a remedy for mild hysteria. No studies were found on the putative medicinal effects of Linden.

VALERIAN *(VALERIANA OFFICINALIS)*: The 1918 US Dispensatory discusses valerian as follows: "Valerian is used as a sedative to the higher nerve centers in conditions of nervous unrest, hysteria, hypochondriasis, neuralgic pains, and the like." There is fairly good evidence for valerian as a hypnotic; clinical trials have shown that it can decrease sleep latency and nocturnal awakenings and improve subjective sleep quality (Beaubrun, 2000), but the evidence for a sedative effect is less strong. In laboratory animal studies, valerian extracts appear to influence GABAergic neurons, including increased release of GABA, decreased GABA reuptake, and decreased GABA degradation. Studies in rats and mice have shown sedative and anticonvulsant activities for whole plant extracts, as well as for valerenic acids, valepotriates, and the volatile oil (Schulz, 2001). Cats given 10 mg of valepotriates by stomach tube showed decreased restlessness, fear, and aggressive behaviors (Eickstedt, 1969).

MISTLETOE, EUROPEAN *(VISCUM ALBUM)*: This herb is classed as a nervine by some herbalists. The Eclectic literature evolved from originally calling the herb a *narcotic,* used for calming seizures (in King's 1898), to calling it *toxic* and possibly indicated most often for heart disorders (Felter, 1922). Modern studies concentrate on its immune modulating and antineoplastic effects. It cannot be recommended as a nervine for animals without additional studies or experience.

GOTU KOLA *(CENTELLA ASIATICA)*: In vivo studies in mice and rats using brahmoside and brahminoside, given by intraperitoneal injection, have shown a CNS-depressant effect. These compounds were found to decrease motor activity, increase hexobarbitone sleeping time, and slightly decrease body temperature; they were thought to act via a cholinergic mechanism (Ramaswamy, 1970).

Herbs with anxiolytic activity

CALIFORNIA POPPY *(ESCHSCHOLZIA CALIFORNICA)*: Rolland and associates investigated the anxiolytic effects of an aqueous extract in mice. Doses of 25 mg/kg were anxiolytic when measured by standard anticonflict tests. Additional behavioral effects were noted at doses of 100 mg/kg and 200 mg/kg, and no adverse effects were noted when the herb was administered intraperitoneally and orally (Rolland, 1991). This extract was evaluated for benzodiazepine, neuroleptic, antidepressant, antihistamine, and analgesic properties. Investigators concluded that the extract had an affinity for benzodiazepine receptors, and that it had peripheral analgesic effects (Rolland, 2001).

SAINT JOHN'S WORT *(HYPERICUM PERFORATUM)*: Saint John's wort extracts have been shown in multiple laboratory animal studies to bind at GABA A and GABA B receptors, to inhibit GABA reuptake, to evoke GABA release, and to exert anxiolytic-like effects that are blocked by the benzodiazepine antagonist flumazenil (Skalisz, 2004; Beijamini, 2003a; Beijamini, 2003b; Zanoli, 2002; Perfumi, 2002; Flausino, 2002). The Eclectics mentioned that it had sedative properties but did not make much use of the plant for this purpose. A modern application may be its use in the treatment of obsessive-compulsive disorder. The mechanism of action of Saint John's wort is postulated to be inhibition of the synaptosomal uptake of serotonin. Twelve subjects were evaluated with a primary diagnosis of obsessive-compulsive disorder of at least 12 months' duration. Treatment lasted for 12 weeks, with a dose of 450 mg of 0.3% hypericin twice daily. Weekly and monthly evaluations were conducted. A significant change from baseline to endpoint was found, which occurred at 1 week and continued to increase throughout the trial. At endpoint, 5 of 12 were rated much or very much improved, 6 were minimally improved, and 1 had no change (Taylor, 2000). Saint John's Wort induces CYP3A4 and P-glycoprotein, and has been shown to reduce blood levels of alprazolam (Madabushi, 2006).

LAVENDER (*LAVANDULA* SPP): This herb is listed as a calming agent in some herbal texts, but the Eclectic *Materia Medicas* all describe it as a stimulant. A clinical trial examining the effects of inhaled lavender oil suggests that it increases arousal but decreases stress (Motomura, 2001). A study of plant-derived essential oils that possess an anticonflict effect in mice showed that the anxiolytic diazepam, as well as lavender essential oil, increased response rate during the alarm period and demonstrated an anticonflict effect in the same manner (Umezu, 2000).

WITHANIA *(WITHANIA SOMNIFERA)*: One study investigated the anxiolytic and antidepressant actions of the glycowithanolides (WSG), isolated from withania roots, in rats. WSG (20 and 50 mg/kg) was administered orally once daily for 5 days, and the results were compared with those elicited by the benzodiazepine lorazepam (0.5 mg/kg, intraperitoneally) for anxiolytic studies, and by the tricyclic antidepressant imipramine (10 mg/kg, intraperitoneally), for antidepressant investigations. WSG induced an anxiolytic effect, comparable with that produced by lorazepam, and both WSG and lorazepam reduced rat brain levels of tribulin, a marker of clinical anxiety, when the levels were increased following administration of the anxiogenic agent, pentylenetetrazol. WSG also exhibited an antidepressant effect, comparable with that induced by imipramine (Bhattacharya, 2000).

CHAMOMILE ***(MATRICARIA RECUTITA):*** Study of the aqueous extract detected several fractions with significant affinity for the central benzodiazepine receptor and isolated apigenin in one fraction. Apigenin showed anxiolytic activity in mice without sedation and muscle relaxant effects or anticonvulsant action. A 10-fold increase in dosage produced a mild sedative effect (Viola, 1995). Individual flavonoids contained in chamomile have also been shown to have anxiolytic and antispasmodic activities (Paladini, 1999; Bisset, 1994).

PASSIONFLOWER ***(PASSIFLORA INCARNATA):*** Laboratory animal (Bisset, 1994) and human clinical trial evidence indicates that Passionflower has anxiolytic activity. Various extracts, including methanol and water extracts of Passionflower whole plant and plant parts, have been evaluated for their anxiolytic activity in mice. The methanol extracts of leaves, stems, flowers, and whole plant exhibited anxiolytic effects at 100, 125, 200, and 300 mg/kg, respectively. The roots were practically devoid of anxiolytic effects (Dhawan, 2001). A double-blind randomized trial in 36 patients compared the efficacy of Passionflower extract with that of oxazepam in the treatment of patients with generalized anxiety disorder. Patients were allocated in a random fashion for a 4-week trial: 18 to the Passionflower 45 drops/day plus placebo tablet group, and 18 to the oxazepam 30 mg/day plus placebo drops group. Both were effective in the treatment of patients with generalized anxiety disorder with no significant difference between the two protocols. Oxazepam showed a rapid onset of action but significantly more problems related to impairment of job performance. The results suggested that Passionflower is an effective drug for the management of generalized anxiety disorder with a low incidence of impaired job performance (Akhondzadeh, 2001b). Dhawan and colleagues (2003, 2004) have investigated a benzoflavone of Passionflower with particularly potent CNS depressant activity.

KAVA KAVA ***(PIPER METHYSTICUM):*** Good evidence suggests that Kava is anxiolytic (Pittler, 2003; Basch, 2005), and it is generally agreed that the risk/benefit ratio (despite recent reports of hepatotoxicity) is good compared with that of anxiolytic drugs (Clouatre, 2004). The mechanisms thought to be operative include blockade of voltage-gated sodium channels, enhanced GABA A receptor binding, diminished excitatory neurotransmitter release due to calcium channel blockade, reduced neuronal reuptake of norepinephrine, monoamine oxidase (MAO)-B inhibition, and thromboxane A2 synthesis suppression, the latter of which antagonizes GABA A receptor function (Singh, 2002). The Eclectics did not seem to recognize this herb as anxiolytic but did note pain-relieving properties and diuresis. Felter listed the specific indications as "irritation, inflammation, or debility of the urinary passages; chronic catarrhal inflammations; vesical irritation and inflammation; vesical atony; painful micturition, strangury, and dysuria." With consideration of its accepted anxiolytic properties and traditional indications for diuresis, urinary tract pain, and inflammation, kava seems particularly appropriate for cases of feline interstitial cystitis, in addition to short-term use for other conditions in which anxiety is present.

SKULLCAP ***(SCUTELLARIA LATERIFLORA):*** One animal and one human clinical trial have suggested that the plant has anxiolytic effects (Awad, 2003; Wolfson, 2003).

BAICAL SKULLCAP ***(SCUTELLARIA BAICALENSIS):*** The constituent wogonin was investigated. Oral wogonin (7.5-30 mg/kg) elicited an anxiolytic response, similar to diazepam. However, the anxiolytic effects of wogonin were not accompanied by the sedative and muscle relaxant adverse effects that are typical of benzodiazepines (Hui, 2002).

BACOPA ***(BACOPA MONNIERI):*** One study investigated the anxiolytic activity of a standardized extract (bacoside A content 25.5% ± 0.8%) of Bacopa at doses of 5, 10, and 20 mg/kg, given orally in rats, and results were compared with those elicited by lorazepam at 0.5 mg/kg, given intraperitoneally. In all test parameters, Bacopa produced dose-related anxiolytic activity that was qualitatively comparable with that of lorazepam. Significant results were attained, usually at 10 and 20 mg/kg. Bacopa did not produce any significant motor deficit (Bhattacharya, 1998).

GINGER ***(ZINGIBER OFFICINALIS)*** AND GINKGO ***(GINKGO BILOBA):*** The anxiolytic effects of a range of doses (0.01-10 mg/kg) of combination preparations containing different mixture ratios of standardized extracts of ginkgo leaf and ginger root have been tested in rats by means of a maze test. Compared with controls, rats treated with the combination preparation (mixture ratio of ginger extract to ginkgo extract, 2.5 : 1; 1 mg/kg, intragastrically) spent increased amounts of time in the open arms of the maze, whereas the behavior of rats treated with preparations of mixture ratios of 1 : 1 and 1 : 2.5 did not change (Hasenöhrl, 1998). Zingicomb, a preparation consisting of ginger and *Ginkgo biloba* extracts, administered intragastrically has anxiolytic-like properties. A study assessed the effects of acute treatment with this preparation on inhibitory avoidance learning. The influence of zingicomb on avoidance conditioning was investigated in rats treated intragastrically with vehicle or 0.5, 1, 10, or 100 mg/kg zingicomb 60 minutes before the trial. When tested 24 hours after training, rats that had received 10 mg/kg zingicomb exhibited significantly longer step-through latencies than did vehicle-treated animals. In contrast to conventional anxiolytic drugs, which tend to have amnesic properties, zingicomb is a potent anxiolytic agent that may facilitate performance on a learning task (Topic, 2002).

ASIAN GINSENG ***(PANAX GINSENG):*** The anxiolytic activities of the white and red varieties of ginseng were investigated in rats and mice and compared with those of diazepam. Pilot studies indicated that single-dose ginseng had little to no acute behavioral effects; so, the two varieties of ginseng were administered orally at two dose levels twice daily for 5 days, and diazepam (1 mg/kg intraperitoneally) was administered acutely. White and red varieties of ginseng (20 and 50 mg/kg) showed positive results when tested against several paradigms of experimental anxiety. Both were effective in maze tests, and they reduced conflict behavior in thirsty rats and during footshock-induced fighting in paired mice. Ginseng also attenuated pentylenetetrazol-induced decrease in rat brain MAO activity, confirming its anxiolytic activity. The effects of white and red ginseng (50 mg/kg × 5 days) were comparable with those of diazepam (Bhattacharya, 1991).

Hypnotics

Insomnia is an occasional complaint that is usually reported in elderly animals. These animals may well be experiencing "sundowner syndrome"—increasing agitation and confusion in the evening, seen in patients with Alzheimer's disease. Medical problems such as hypertension, hyperthyroidism, pain, and other disorders also must be considered. Traditional hypnotics do not always have a chemical sleep-inducing effect; in some cases, these plants are anxiolytic and help calm people, leading to better sleep. It is unknown whether this is applicable to animals.

California Poppy *(Eschscholzia californica):* The US Dispensatory of 1918 describes it as "a powerful soporific and analgesic, which is free from the disadvantages of opium," and laboratory animal studies (described earlier, in the section on relaxants) suggest that it does have anxiolytic properties. In one study (Rolland, 1991), investigators found that the extract induced sleep at doses above 100 mg/kg. It may act via benzodiazepine receptors (Rolland, 2001).

Hops *(Humulus lupulus):* The aromatic principles in hops may have sedative activity, thus enhancing sleep. (See discussion of hops in the section on nervine relaxants.)

Wild Lettuce *(Lactuca virosa):* King's claims that 20 to 30 grains (1.3-1.9 g) of the dried sap of wild lettuce "will cause a dog to sleep." It was said to be insufficiently investigated but used primarily as a calmative and hypnotic. The human dose for the tincture was 30 to 60 drops. No supporting studies could be found.

Passionflower *(Passiflora incarnata):* The Eclectics found Passionflower useful for inducing sleep from mental overwork; this reflects the anxiolytic effect better than a specific hypnotic effect, for which no data can be found.

Kava Kava *(Piper methysticum):* This herb has been shown to assist people with anxiety in falling to sleep (Lehrl, 2004). A total of 61 patients were administered 200 mg of the standardized extract WS 1490 or a placebo in a multicenter, randomized, double-blind, placebo-controlled trial. According to sleep and anxiety questionnaires, 4 weeks of treatment resulted in statistically significant improvement.

Jamaica dogwood *(Piscidia piscipula):* This herb had a reputation for inducing deep and restful sleep. (Also see the section on anxiety.)

Valeria *(Valeriana officinalis):* Fairly good evidence has been found that indicates that valerian is a hypnotic. Clinical trials have shown that it can decrease sleep latency and nocturnal awakenings and improve subjective sleep quality (Beaubrun, 2000); however, the evidence for a sedative effect is less strong. In laboratory animal studies, valerian extracts appear to influence GABAergic neurons, including increased release of GABA, decreased GABA reuptake, and decreased GABA degradation.

Chamomile *(Matricaria chamomilla):* Intraperitoneal administration to mice of a lyophilized infusion of chamomile decreased basal motility and exploratory and motor activities and potentiated hexobarbital-induced sleep. These results demonstrated that in mice, chamomile depresses the central nervous system (Della Loggia, 1982).

Anesthetics

Clove Oil *(Syzygium aromaticum):* This was tested for anesthesia induction, recovery time, hematology, and stress indicators in gilthead sea bream and rainbow trout and was compared with 2-phenoxyethanol. Results showed only slight differences in anesthetic efficiency and physiologic effects, and suggested that clove oil does not block cortisol response to stress in fish, as do other anesthetics (Tort, 2002; Vykusova, 2003). In a similar study, clove oil (85%–95% eugenol) was only slightly less effective than quinaldine and more effective than benzocaine, MS-222, and 2-phenoxyethanol. Clove oil had a much calmer induction to anesthesia than did quinaldine, along with a recovery time that was 2 to 3 times longer (Munday, 1997). The anesthetic effects of clove oil–derived eugenol were studied in juvenile rainbow trout. Times to induction and recovery from anesthesia were measured and compared with those of MS-222. Eugenol induced anesthesia faster and at lower concentrations than did MS-222, and recovery times for eugenol were 6 to 10 times longer. Clove oil eugenol was determined to be an acceptable anesthetic for use in aquaculture and aquatic research. It was found that 40 to 60 ppm eugenol induced rapid anesthesia, with a relatively short time for recovery in juvenile trout (Keene, 1998). Juvenile rabbitfish were anesthetized and their length and weight recorded on three separate occasions. Fish were fed shortly afterward, and no mortality was observed. Clove oil appeared to be highly effective as a fish anesthetic with potentially few or no adverse effects (Soto, 1995).

Lavender *(Lavandula officinalis):* The local anesthetic activity of the essential oil of lavender was investigated and compared with that of the essential oils of *Citrus reticulata* and *C. limon*. Tests were also performed on the components of lavender essential oil, linalool, and linalyl acetate. The essential oil of lavender, linalyl acetate, and linalool (0.01-10 μg/mL)—but not the Citrus essential oils—reduced electrically evoked contractions of rat phrenic hemidiaphragm. In the rabbit, conjunctival reflex test treatment with a solution of essential oil of lavender, as well as linalyl acetate and linalool, confirmed the local anesthetic activity that had been observed in vitro (Ghelardini, 1999).

Kava *(Piper methysticum):* This herb has been reported to have analgesic activity (Jamieson, 1990) and was used by the Eclectics as a local anesthetic.

Antispasmodics

Antispasmodic herbs are listed in neurologic *Materia medicas* for their ability to relax skeletal muscle tension and reduce the consequences of stress, such as asthmatic bronchiolar constriction and intestinal/colonic spasm. Anxiolytics can be employed, but some herbs have specific activity on smooth and skeletal muscle.

KAVA KAVA *(PIPER METHYSTICUM):* The kavapyrone, kavain, has been shown in vitro to inhibit contraction (and relax precontracted muscle) in vascular and gastrointestinal smooth muscle, possibly by interfering with Ca^{2+} channels (Martin, 2002; Seitz, 1997).

BAICAL SKULLCAP *(SCUTELLARIA BAICALENSIS):* This agent has shown smooth muscle relaxant properties (Usow, 1958). Recent in vitro studies in vascular and respiratory smooth muscle suggest a different effect, depending on the dose of the flavonoid baicalein (Ajay, 2003; Miyamoto, 1997).

VALERIAN *(VALERIANA OFFICINALIS)*: This is a potent smooth muscle relaxant in feline pulmonary vasculature, probably via GABA-mediated mechanisms (Fields, 2003). Isovaltrate, valtrate, and valeranone caused suppression of peristaltic contractions in guinea pig ileum in vivo (Hazelhoff, 1982).

CRAMP BARK *(VIBURNUM OPULUS)* AND BLACK HAW *(VIBURNUM PRUNIFOLIUM):* These herbs probably have similar properties in that both are used as antispasmodics for uterine cramps. King's says that Cramp bark is useful in asthma, spasms, and cramps of the limbs as well. Tests in guinea pigs, rats, and human uteri suggest that Black haw has smooth muscle relaxant properties (Horhammer, 1965; Horhammer, 1966).

JAMAICA DOGWOOD *(PISCIDIA PISCIPULA):* Ellingwood (1919) recommended the plant for gallstone, renal, and intestinal colic. Some studies have shown spasmolytic activity (Della Loggia, 1988; Costello, 1948).

OTHER HERBS: Others include California poppy, Motherwort, Lobelia, Lemon balm, Peppermint, Catnip, Aniseed, Rosemary, Sage, Bloodroot, Tilia, Licorice, Peony, Passionflower, Parsley, Thyme, Verbena, and Ginger.

Adaptogens

The original definition of adaptogen was as follows (Panossian, 1999):

1. The adaptogenic effect is nonspecific in that the adaptogen increases resistance to a very broad spectrum of harmful factors ("stressors") of different physical, chemical, and biological natures;
2. An adaptogen is said to have a normalizing effect, that is, it counteracts or prevents disturbances brought about by stressors; and
3. An adaptogen must be innocuous to have a broad range of therapeutic effects without causing any disturbance (other than very marginally) to the normal functioning of the organism.

More recently, a theory has been advanced to explain that changing levels of mediators such as nitric oxide (NO), platelet-activating factor (PAF), catecholamines, cortisol, and PGE_2 are held in tighter homeostatic control, unlike the wide swings that a normal stress response brings with it (Panossian, 1999).

Herbalists believe, in addition, that adaptogens must work through the hypothalamic-pituitary-adrenal axis, differentiating them from other function regulators, such as immune stimulants. Adaptogenic herbs are especially useful for mitigating the effects of stress in overworked horses and dogs, run-down production animals such as dairy cows, and perhaps chronically stressed dogs and cats that exhibit anxiety-related behaviors, or for elderly or chronically ill animals to help counteract lethargy and weakness. These herbs have been investigated for use in enhancing performance in healthy athletes—early clinical trials in humans suggested the effect, but more recent high-quality studies do not support this use.

ELEUTHERO, SIBERIAN GINSENG *(ELEUTHEROCOCCUS SENTICOSIS):* Animal studies showed a "protein anabolic" effect (Kaemmerer, 1980). One study of mice that ingested different ginseng infusions in comparison with water showed no increase in stamina or longevity, and no difference in survival, under major environmental stress (Lewis, 1983). Another showed that various extracts increased swimming time and attenuated the rise in blood corticosterone (Kimura, 2004). Mouse studies also suggest that Eleuthero can enhance cellular and humoral immunity (Rogala, 2003). Elderly human patients given Eleuthero experienced temporary improvements in social functioning that were measured at 4 weeks but did not last to 8 weeks of the trial (Cicero, 2004). Hartz and associates examined 96 people with chronic fatigue who had been given Eleuthero or placebo and found no statistically significant differences between groups (Hartz, 2004). Some animal studies and one human study in athletes (Gaffney, 2001) showed that Eleuthero actually increased hormonal indices of stress. In a controlled study of 1000 Siberian factory workers, a 50% reduction in illness and a 40% reduction in lost workdays were noted over 1 year (Bone, 2003).

ASIAN GINSENG *(PANAX GINSENG):* Oriental, Red, or Asian ginseng is one of the most studied of herbs. Some of the established effects include antioxidant activity, improved immune function, improved cognition and memory, modification of vasomotor function, reduced platelet adhesion, an influence on ion channels, modulation of autonomic neurotransmitter release, improved lipid profiles, and improved glucose metabolism and glycemic control (Zhou, 2004; Kiefer, 2003; Kennedy, 2003a). Animal studies have shown that ginseng increases resistance to irradiation, temperature stress, hyperbaric stress, physical exercise, and viral and tumor load (Nocerino, 2000). The mechanism is still under investigation, but it is possible that ginsenosides may augment adrenocortical steroid production (Nocerino, 2000; Rai, 2003b; Kim, 2003).

AMERICAN GINSENG *(PANAX QUINQUEFOLIUS):* Although the energetic characteristics and traditional Chinese uses of American and Asian ginseng are different, the constituents and clinical studies suggest that they have similar broad uses as adaptogens. Few clinical trials have specifically addressed the effects of *P. quinquefolius* on stress.

SCHISANDRA *(SCHISANDRA CHINENSIS)*: A clinical trial in athletes undergoing heavy exercise indicated that administration of Schisandra attenuated the rise in salivary nitric oxide that is usually seen after physical stress (Panossian, 1999b). Russian studies examining job-related stress suggested that Schisandra decreased illness, increased stamina, and prevented some stress-induced physiologic changes in people (Bone, 2003).

ASHWAGANDHA *(WITHANIA SOMNIFERA)*: A variety of animal models of stress have shown an adaptogenic effect for this plant. In chronically stressed rats, ashwagandha administered at 25 to 50 mg/kg attenuated stress-related hyperglycemia, gastric ulcers, cognitive deficits, male sexual dysfunction, mental depression, and immune suppression (Bhattacharya, 2003). A withanolide-free extract also showed antistress effects in rats and mice (Singh, 2003a; Singh, 2001). Withania extract increased corticoid levels in stressed mice (Singh, 2000).

OTHER HERBS: Others include *Andrographis paniculata,* Gotu kola *(Centella asiatica),* and Licorice *(Glycyrrhiza glabra).*

Herbs with antistress activity

SIBERIAN GINSENG *(ELEUTHEROCOCCUS SENTICOSIS)*: This plant is known to have protective effects on stress-induced disturbance of mental status. One study evaluated whether administration of Siberian ginseng (500 mg/kg) can affect concentrations of noradrenaline (NA), dopamine (DA), and their metabolites in the normal rat brain. Even a single oral administration of Siberian ginseng elevated NA and DA levels in the brain in a dose-dependent manner. Results suggested that Siberian ginseng may act by regulating NA and DA levels in specific brain regions related to stress response and Parkinson's disease (Fujikawa, 2002).

SAINT JOHN'S WORT *(HYPERICUM PERFORATUM)*: The antistress activity of an ethanolic extract was investigated on 14-day foot-shock stress (FSS)-induced behavior in albino rats. Gastric ulceration and adrenal gland and spleen weight were used as the stress indices. *Panax ginseng* (PG) was used as the standard adaptogenic agent for comparison. FSS induced marked gastric ulceration and a significant increase in adrenal gland weight with a concomitant decrease in spleen weight. Chronic stress also suppressed male sexual behavior and induced behavioral depression and cognitive dysfunction. All FSS-induced perturbations were attenuated dose dependently by Saint John's wort (100 and 200 mg/kg orally) and PG (100 mg/kg orally) (Vikas, 2001).

Antidepressants

Antidepressants such as tricyclic antidepressants and selective serotonin reuptake inhibitors (SSRIs) are used in veterinary medicine for a variety of behavior problems, including anxiety-related behaviors such as house soiling and phobias, aggression, compulsive behaviors, and, recently, for chronic pain and "behavioral dermatoses." These uses are based on specific receptor pharmacology and not necessarily on the clinical effects noted with traditional herbal antidepressants such as Mugwort *(Artemisia vulgaris),* Milky oat *(Avena sativa),* and Damiana *(Turnera diffusa).*

SAINT JOHN'S WORT *(HYPERICUM PERFORATUM)*: This is a well-recognized and effective treatment for patients with mild to moderate depression. It has multiple constituents that may be active in the treatment of depression, including weak MAO-A and MAO-B inhibition; glutamate, GABA-A, and GABA-B affinity; downregulation of beta-adrenergic receptors and upregulation of 5-HT_2 receptors; and regulation of genes involved in the hypothalamic-pituitary-adrenal axis (Butterweck, 2003). The range of compounds at work include hypericin, hyperforin, and a number of flavonoids such as amentoflavone, quercetin, and a form of apigenin.

LAVENDER *(LAVANDULA OFFICINALIS)*: Akhondzadeh (2003a) investigated the use of lavender in the treatment of patients with mild to moderate depression. In a 4-week, double-blind, randomized trial, 45 adults with depression received lavender tincture (1:5 in 50% alcohol, 60 drops/day, plus placebo tablet; imipramine alone; or lavender tincture plus imipramine). The combination of lavender and imipramine was more effective than either treatment alone. In cancer hospice patients, lavender administered by aromatherapy was compared with simple water humidification, and vital signs, depression, sense of well-being, pain, and anxiety were monitored. Lavender was superior to water humidification in pain and anxiety levels (Louis, 2002).

BACOPA *(BACOPA MONNIERI)*: A standardized methanolic extract of Bacopa (bacoside A 38.0 ± 0.9) was investigated for potential antidepressant activity in rodent models of depression. The effect was compared with that of the standard antidepressant drug imipramine (15 mg/kg, intraperitoneally). The extract, when given at 20 and 40 mg/kg orally once daily for 5 days, was found to have significant antidepressant activity in models of depression that was comparable with that of imipramine (Sairam, 2002).

Analgesics

Before the advent of ether and subsequent improvements in anesthesia drugs, surgery and other painful procedures were accomplished under the influence of alcohol and toxic plants. These plants included datura *(Datura stramonium),* gelsemium *(Gelsemium sempervirens),* henbane *(Hyoscyamus niger),* poison hemlock *(Conium maculatum),* and opium poppy *(Papaver somniferum).* With the exception of gelsemium, most of the plants discussed in this section are less dramatic in their activity and can be used in formulas given over the long term.

CORYDALIS (*CORYDALIS YANHUSUO* AND OTHER SPECIES): This herb inhibits the reticular activating system (RAS) of the brain stem, and long-term use may result in tolerance and cross-tolerance with morphine (Huang, 2000). The herb was shown to reduce pain from inflammation in a rat model (Wei, 1999). A clinical trial in people administered pain via a cold-pressor test showed that corydalis had a significant ($P < .01$) dose-related analgesic effect (Yuan, 2004).

LAVENDER *(LAVANDULA OFFICINALIS):* A hydroalcoholic extract, polyphenolic fraction, and essential oil of lavender leaves were prepared and their analgesic effects and anti-inflammatory activities were studied in mice. Results of the study confirmed the traditional use of lavender for the treatment of patients with painful and inflammatory conditions (Hajhashemi, 2003).

WILD YAM *(DIOSCOREA VILLOSA):* Although research support has not been found for an analgesic or spasmolytic effect for this herb, traditional use centers primarily on abdominal pain and spasm. The US Dispensatory of 1918 claims that an indication for the pain of rheumatism was a Southern regional use. Interestingly the root of a species Dioscorea *(Dioscorea opposita)* has been used for the treatment of arthritis, muscular pain and urinary diseases in oriental medicine. A methanol extract of Dioscorea root down regulated the expression of cyclooxygenase-2 (COX-2) and inducible nitric oxide synthase and reduced the level of reactive oxygen species in vitro (Kim, 2005b).

CALIFORNIA POPPY *(ESCHSCHOLZIA CALIFORNICA):* Rolland (1991, 2001) found that this extract had peripheral analgesic effects in laboratory animal studies. The US Dispensatory of 1918 describes it as "a powerful soporific and analgesic, which is free from the disadvantages of opium. . . . The narcotic power of the drug seems to be very weak, since . . . three drachms (5.3 g) were necessary to kill a rabbit . . . the alcoholic extract acts as a respiratory depressant and narcotic, affecting in toxic dose also the spinal cord . . . the extract [was used] in commencing doses of twelve grains (0.78 g) increasing to one hundred and eighty-five grains (12 g) a day . . ."

GELSEMIUM *(GELSEMIUM SEMPERVIRENS):* The 1918 US Dispensatory advocated this root mostly in "the treatment of neuralgias, especially those involving the facial nerves. The mode of its action in these cases is obscure, but there is considerable clinical evidence of its utility." It was also used for headache and toothache. This is a toxic herb that may cause extreme weakness, seizures, and respiratory arrest. It is not in popular use in veterinary herbal medicine, and should be used with care, as part of pain formulas, if at all.

JAMAICA DOGWOOD *(PISCIDIA PISCIPULA):* Ellingwood listed indications related to pain as gallstone colic, renal colic, intestinal colic, neuralgias, and as an anodyne for toothache and developing abscesses. No supporting studies can be found for an analgesic effect.

SAINT JOHN'S WORT *(HYPERICUM PERFORATUM):* King's relates that *Hypericum* was used for the pain of spinal injuries, spinal irritation, and wounds. Multiple species of *Hypericum* have shown analgesic effects in laboratory animal studies, including *H. perforatum, H. brasiliense, H. cordatum,* and *H. empetrifolium* (Viana, 2003; Rieli, 2002; Kumar, 2001; Trovato, 2001). A human clinical trial using Saint John's wort for painful polyneuropathy showed no statistical significance from placebo, but a trend existed showing some pain relief for the extract—nine patients on Saint John's wort had complete, good, or moderate pain relief, and only two of those on placebo had the same benefit (Sindrup, 2001). No description of a possible analgesic mechanism was found.

OTHER HERBS: Anti-inflammatory herbs, such as Willow *(Salix alba),* Devil's claw *(Harpagophytum procumbens),* Boswellia *(Boswellia serrata),* Prickly ash *(Zanthoxylum* spp*),* Ginger *(Zingiber officinalis),* and others, are useful in controlling the pain of inflammation.

Anticonvulsants

SAINT JOHN'S WORT *(HYPERICUM PERFORATUM):* Effects of different extracts of Saint John's wort on kindling epileptic discharges were analyzed in rabbits with chronically implanted electrodes in cortical structures and the hippocampus. Results showed that the effect depends on the constituents present; in particular, fractions and repression of epileptic activity correlated with polarity of plant constituents. Most polar constituents in the water fraction exerted the highest antiepileptic activity in 100% of animals tested. Substances present in the butanol fraction repressed the epileptic manifestations in 40% of animals with kindling epilepsy, whereas lipid-soluble constituents in the ether fraction potentiated epileptic activity (Ivetic, 2002).

SKULLCAP *(SCUTELLARIA LATERIFOLIA):* In rats given lithium and pilocarpine to induce status epilepticus, seizures resolved completely when skullcap was given in the water, but they returned when the herb was discontinued (Peredery, 2004). It contains the active constituents baicalin and baicalein, also found in Baical skullcap.

BAICAL SKULLCAP *(SCUTELLARIA BAICALENSIS):* Research suggests that the active component baicalein is a major contributor to the antiepileptic and neuronal protective effects of a traditional formula, and that the mechanism of its pharmacologic action is based on radical quenching and antioxidative effects (Hamada, 1993).

KAVA *(PIPER METHYSTICUM):* Studies described in the older literature have documented anticonvulsant effects for kavalactones in several experimental models (Gleitz, 1996a, b, c). The anticonvulsant properties of methysticin in vitro may arise from direct membrane action on the excitability of neurons, and in vitro assays have shown that methysticin, kavain, and the synthetics kavalactone and kavain appear to interact with voltage-dependent sodium channels, and that kavain also interacts with voltage-dependent calcium channels (Magura, 1997; Gleitz, 1996a,b,c; Schirrmacher, 1999). Substances that reduce extracellular glutamate concentrations are of interest for their potential as anticonvulsant agents. Reduction in veratridine-induced glutamate release following kavain administration has been reported both in vitro and in vivo in freely moving rats (Gleitz, 1996c; Ferger, 1998).

GELSEMIUM *(GELSEMIUM SEMPERVIRENS):* In rats given lithium and pilocarpine to induce status epilepticus, seizures resolved completely when gelsemium was given in the water but returned when the herb was discontinued (Peredery, 2004).

GASTRODIA *(GASTRODIA ELATA)*: This Chinese herb is contained in many traditional formulas for seizures, often in combination with *Uncaria rhynchophylla*. In a study of rats with seizures induced by kainic acid, administration of Gastrodia extract 0.5 to 1 g/kg reduced lipid peroxidation in brain tissue, as well as seizure activity (Hsieh, 2001).

UNCARIA *(UNCARIA RHYNCHOPHYLLA)*: In a study of rats with seizures induced by kainic acid, Uncaria 1 g/kg alone or Uncaria 1 g/kg plus Gastrodia 1 g/kg was administered to rats with induced epileptic seizures. Results showed that Uncaria alone reduced induced lipid peroxide levels in vitro. It was concluded that Uncaria has anticonvulsive and free radical scavenging activities, and effects appeared synergistic with those of Gastrodia (Hsieh, 1999).

BACOPA *(BACOPA MONNIERI)*: This plant has been used for epilepsy in animals in traditional Indian medicine, although no supporting studies have been found.

CORYDALIS *(CORYDALIS YANHUSUO)*: The influence of the constituent tetrahydropalmatine (THP), isolated from corydalis, was tested on the development of electrically kindled amygdala. Intraperitoneal injection of THP before application of the stimulus prevented development of the kindling process. The behavioral seizure score and motion responses that normally develop during electrical kindling were reduced to below initial values. Results suggest that THP may have antiepileptogenic and anticonvulsant activity (Lin, 2002). Administration of picrotoxin increases locomotion, elevation of turning, and inhibition of postural freezing in rats; it also increases amygdaloidal release of dopamine in anesthetized rats. All these activity measures induced by picrotoxin were suppressed following THP treatment. Results indicate that THP may act through inhibition of amygdaloid dopamine release to inhibit seizures (Chang, 2001).

OTHER HERBS: Chinese herbal combinations have been investigated more thoroughly and may be more effective than any single herb. Uncontrolled trials in humans suggest that the combination Sho saiko to and similar formulas (Xiao Chai Hu Tang, Minor Bupleurum formula) can help reduce seizure severity and frequency in people who are unresponsive to normal seizure medications. Combinations of the two herbs *Uncaria rhynchophylla* and *Gastrodia elata* have shown anticonvulsant activity in laboratory animals.

Nervine stimulants *(cognitive enhancers)*

GINKGO *(GINKGO BILOBA)*: It is now clear that ginkgo is effective in the treatment of people with dementia and cognitive decline. A Cochrane meta-analysis showed some methodologic problems with earlier trials, but in general, ginkgo benefits cognition, activities of daily living, mood, and emotional function in people, with no difference from placebo in adverse effects (Birks, 2002).

LEMON BALM *(MELISSA OFFICINALIS)*: This herb has been examined in two different forms for the treatment of patients with Alzheimer's disease. Akhondzadeh (2003b) administered 60 drops/day of an extract for 4 months to patients with mild to moderate Alzheimer's disease. The Melissa extract had a significantly better outcome for cognitive function than did placebo. In another human clinical trial, patients with Alzheimer's with severe dementia and agitation were treated with lemon balm oil via massage, and the placebo group was massaged with sunflower oil only. Agitation score was 30% improved in 60% of the Melissa group, but in only 14% of the placebo group. Quality of life improved significantly more in people receiving lemon balm than in those receiving placebo. It was concluded that lemon balm extract is of value in Alzheimer's disease and that it mitigates agitation (Akhondzadeh, 2003b).

SAINT JOHN'S WORT *(HYPERICUM PERFORATUM)*: A standardized 50% ethanolic extract of Saint John's wort was investigated in various experimental paradigms of learning and memory in rats. A dosage of 100 or 200 mg/kg was administered orally once daily for 3 days; piracetam (500 mg/kg intraperitoneally), was administered to rats as the standard drug control. Saint John's wort at both doses and piracetam facilitated acquisition and retention of active avoidance; the Saint John's wort effects were dose dependent. Results indicated a possible nootropic action of Saint John's wort that was qualitatively comparable with piracetam (Vikas, 2000). Another study investigated the effects of long-term Saint John's wort treatment on spatial learning and memory in rats. Saint John's wort standardized to 0.3% hypericin content was administered for 9 weeks in doses of 4.3 and 13 μg/kg, corresponding to therapeutic dosages in humans of 0.3 and 0.9 mg of total hypericins daily. Findings showed that the long-term administration of Saint John's wort can improve learning and spatial memory, with significant changes in the content of monoamines in several brain regions (Widy-Tyszkiewicz, 2002).

BACOPA *(BACOPA MONNIERI)*: This herb has been shown to exert cognition-enhancing effects in animals. A human, double-blind, placebo-controlled trial found that *Bacopa monnieri* (300 mg; n = 18) or placebo (n = 20) had no acute effects on cognitive functioning in normal healthy subjects (Nathan, 2001). However, in a double-blind, randomized, placebo-controlled study in which various memory functions were tested and levels of anxiety measured in people, results showed a significant effect of Bacopa on a test for retention of new information. Follow-up tests showed that the rate of learning was unaffected, suggesting that Bacopa slows the rate at which people forget new information (Roodenrys, 2002).

KOREAN GINSENG *(PANAX GINSENG)*: Studies have demonstrated that two ginsenosides—Rb(1) and Rg(1)—improve performance in a passive avoidance-learning paradigm and enhance cholinergic metabolism. One study examined the cellular neurotrophic and neuroprotective actions of these ginsenosides in two model systems. Results suggested that Rb(1) and Rg(1) have neurotrophic and selective neuroprotective actions that may contribute to the purported enhancement of cognitive function (Rudakewich, 2001).

Herbs with stimulant activity

Rosemary (*Rosmarinus officinalis*): An increase in locomotor activity has been observed in mice following inhalation or oral administration of rosemary oil. The increase in activity paralleled a dose-related increase in serum 1,8-cineole level (Kovar, 1987).

Cola (*Cola nitida*): The xanthine constituents, caffeine and theobromine, are the active principles in cola. The pharmacologic properties of caffeine are well documented and include stimulation of the CNS, respiratory system, and skeletal muscle, as well as cardiac stimulation, coronary dilatation, smooth muscle relaxation, and diuresis (Leung, 1980).

Asian Ginseng (*Panax ginseng*): A double-blind, placebo-controlled clinical study assessed the effect of standardized ginseng (100 mg twice daily for 12 weeks) on psychomotor performance in 16 healthy individuals. Tests of psychomotor performance found favorable effects on attention, processing, integrated sensory motor function, and auditory reaction time. This study concluded that ginseng was superior to placebo in improving certain psychomotor functions in healthy subjects (D'Angelo, 1986).

Dong Quai (*Angelica sinensis*): Hot aqueous extracts of dong quai stimulated smooth muscle contractions of the bladder, intestine, and uterus when administered intravenously to dogs (10 g/kg body weight) (Schmidt, 1924). Intravenous administration of an aqueous or 95% ethanol extract dong quai to cats, rats, and rabbits increased the strength of the contractions and the tone of uterine smooth muscles (Zhu, 1987).

Nux Vomica Seed (*Strychnos nux vomica*): This spinal stimulant is the source of strychnine. Veterinarians are more familiar with the signs of overdose of strychnine than they are with its historical use as a spinal stimulant. Gresswell's *Veterinary Pharmacopeia, Materia Medica, and Therapeutics* (1887) describes the official preparation as the liquid extract that contains 15% alkaloids, or the tincture that contains 1 grain (65 mg) of alkaloids per fluid ounce. The dose for dogs was 0.5 to 2 grains (30-130 mg); for horses, 20 grains to 1 drachm (1.3-1.8 g). By 1949, Milks describes the official preparations as follows:

1. Fluid extract, containing 1.15% strychnine and 25% alkaloids. The dose of this form was 0.5 to 2 dram (1.8-7.1 mL) for horses, and 0.5 to 2 minims (0.03-0.12 mL) for dogs.
2. Extract, containing 7% to 7.5% strychnine. Horse dose was 7 to 15 grains (0.45-0.97 g), and dog dose was 1/8 to 1/4 grain (8.1-16.2 mg)
3. Tincture, containing 0.1% strychnine and 0.25% alkaloids. Horse dose was 3 dram to 2.5 oz (10.7-74 mL), and dog dose was 5 to 20 minims (0.3-1.2 mL).

The author (SW) has used Chinese formulas containing this herb with some success in the treatment of degenerative myelopathy.

Herbs with aphrodisiac activity

Clove (*Syzygium aromaticum*): Spices can be considered sexual invigorators. Ethanol extracts of nutmeg and clove were found to stimulate the mounting behavior of normal male mice and to significantly increase their mating performance (Tajuddin, 2003).

Passionflower (*Passiflora incarnata*): The aphrodisiac properties of the methanol extract of Passionflower leaves were evaluated in mice by observing mounting behavior. The methanol extract exhibited significant aphrodisiac behavior in male mice at all doses (i.e., 75, 100, and 150 mg/kg). Among these, the highest level of activity was observed with the 100 mg/kg dose when the mountings were calculated about 95 minutes after the administration of the test extracts (Dhawan, 2003).

Tribulus (*Tribulus terrestris*): The puncturevine plant has long been considered an energizer and vitalizer in traditional medicine. Weight gain and improvement in sexual behavior parameters observed in rats, as well as the increase in intracavernous pressure, which confirms the proerectile aphrodisiac property, could be the result of an increase in androgen (Gauthaman, 2003). An experiment was carried out to define the stimulating effects of Tribestan on rams that were intended for breeding, as well as on rams that exhibited sexual impotence and deteriorated semen qualities. Treatment led to an extended period of sexual activity and improvement of semen production in rams over the service period. Results of Tribestan therapy with rams with reduced libido showed that the animals could recover with no morphologic changes in the structure of the testes and epididymides. The use of this preparation raised the testosterone level and normalized the sexual activity of rams affected by impotence (Dimitrov, 1987). Tribestan increased testosterone levels and accelerated sexual development in rams and male lambs, respectively (Georgiev, 1988). Libido and sexual reflexes were restored in boars with long-term sexual impotence (Zarkova, 1984).

Nervine tonics *(neurologic trophorestoratives)*

Eleuthero, Siberian Ginseng (*Eleutherococcus senticosis*): This was found to reduce the pathologic effects of cerebral lesions in mice (Kaplan, 1965). A study conducted over several years examined the therapeutic value of Siberian ginseng in human brain injury. Most of the 124 patients were severely affected. The test group received Siberian ginseng extract 1/2 hour before meals, and the control group received a placebo. Siberian ginseng administration resulted in a normalizing effect on brain activity and a higher functional level of recovery. Alleviation of neurodynamic disturbances in the vestibular apparatus and normalizing of effects on cerebral hemodynamics, cortical neurodynamics, unconditioned reflex vascular motor reactions, and leukocyte counts were found (Sandler, 1972).

Baical Skullcap (*Scutellaria baicalensis*): Clinical investigation of scutellarin involving 634 cases of cerebral thrombosis, cerebral embolism, and paralysis caused by stroke has been undertaken. An overall positive effect rate higher than 88% was reported following intramuscular, intravenous, or oral administration (Peigen, 1987).

Kava (*Piper methysticum*): A neuroprotective effect against ischemic brain damage in mice and rats has been demonstrated for kava extract (WS-1490 containing 70% kavalactones) and the individual kavalactones methysticin and dihydromethysticin. Kava extract 150 mg/kg given orally 1 hour before experimentally induced ischemia, and methysticin and dihydromethysticin (both 10 and 30 mg/kg intraperitoneally 15 minutes before induction of ischemia) significantly reduced the size of the infarct area in mice brains. In rats, kava extract administered according to the same regimen as that used in mice significantly reduced infarct volume compared with control findings (Backhauss, 1992).

GINKGO *(GINKGO BILOBA)*: Several studies have reported that treatment with standardized extract of ginkgo leaf (EGb 761) aids recovery of function following brain injury, as demonstrated by behavioral tests in rats who had undergone bilateral frontal lobotomy or septohippocampal deafferentation, and in rat models of cortical hemiplegia. It has been suggested that the effects of EGb 761 in the experimental animal models described previously may involve aspects of neuronal plasticity (e.g., neuronal regeneration) (DeFeudis, 1998). Ischemia-induced lipid peroxidation is one of the most important causes of tissue damage in spinal cord injury. In one study, the protective effects of *Ginkgo biloba*, thyroid-releasing hormone (TRH), and methylprednisolone on compression injury of the rat spinal cord were investigated. *Ginkgo biloba* treatments significantly decreased malondialdehyde levels, which suggests that methylprednisolone and *Ginkgo biloba* may provide protection against ischemic spinal cord injury through the antioxidant effect (Koc, 1995). In another study, when pretreatment with a ginkgo extract was given 7 days before induced ischemia, followed by reperfusion, treated rabbits had only a slight tremor in the hind limbs compared with completely paraplegic controls. This study indicated that the ginkgo extract can scavenge free radicals produced during ischemia/reperfusion and may reduce reperfusion damage (Mechirova, 2002).

AMERICAN GINSENG *(PANAX QUINQUEFOLIUS* [GINKGO *(GINKGO BILOBA)* EXTRACT AND SAINT JOHN'S WORT *(HYPERICUM PERFORATUM)* EXTRACT]): The effects of this combination on the survival and regeneration of transected axotomized retinal ganglion cells was studied in an optic nerve transection model in adult hamsters. Animals that had undergone surgery received daily oral administration of vehicle or herbal extracts, alone or in combination, for 7 and 21 days, respectively. Treatment with American ginseng, ginkgo extract, or Saint John's wort alone failed to offer neuroprotection to injured retinal ganglion cells. However, treatment with a mixture of American ginseng, ginkgo extract, or Saint John's wort significantly augmented retinal ganglion cells survival 7 days postaxotomy. Treatment with the combination also induced a significant increase in the number of regenerating RGCs 21 days after optic nerve transection. This study suggests that herbs can act as potential neuroprotective agents for damaged retinal ganglion cells and that the therapeutic value of herbal remedies may be maximized through the use of mixtures of appropriate herbs (Cheung, 2002).

WITHANIA *(WITHANIA SOMNIFERA)*: Extensions of dendrites and axons in neurons may compensate for and repair damaged neuronal circuits in the brain. One study investigated the effects of activating neurite outgrowth and regenerating the neuronal network. A methanol extract of Ashwagandha significantly increased the percentage of cells with neurites in human neuroblastoma cells. The effects of the extract were dose and time dependent (Tohda, 2000).

Review of Specific Pain, Neurologic, and Behavioral Disorders

Anxiety

Anxiety is the root of many major complaints presented to veterinarians; it is also a leading reason for surrender of pets to shelters. Owner education about inappropriate interactions and behavior modification techniques is critical, but herbs may help the animal to focus on training and ignore distractions. All of the herbs in the "nervine relaxant" sedating, anxiolytic, antistress activity, and "antidepressant" sections should be considered.

The effects of supplementing tryptophan, vitamin E, or an herbal product with passionflower and valerian were investigated in terms of the effects on stress response in pigs during transport simulation. Pigs supplemented with tryptophan tended to spend more time lying down during the second hour of vibration. Vitamin E decreased peak heart rate, ventricular ectopic beats, and ST elevation. The herbal supplement caused smaller increases in heart variables (i.e., minimum heart rate, ventricular ectopic beats, ST elevation) during and after stress evocation compared with the control group. Tryptophan had a positive behavioral effect in this experiment, and vitamin E and the herbal supplement mediated an increase in some heart variables, suggesting sedative and antianxiety effects (Peeters, 2004).

Various combinations of kava, skullcap, valerian, lemon balm, Saint John's wort, Jamaica dogwood, and hops may be used. Formulas recommended by herbalists and marketed by herbal pharmacies contain variously skullcap, oat seed, hops, passionflower, valerian, California poppy, Eleuthero, chamomile, motherwort, and linden.

Because the mechanisms of action for most anxiolytic herbs are not well defined, it is recommended that herbs be used instead of anxiolytic drugs only if the owner gives informed consent. Herb–drug interactions in this area are not yet well defined.

Adaptogenic herbs may also be considered for chronically stressed animals.

A prescription for mild anxiety follows:

Chamomile	100% (carminative, bitter, spasmolytic, mild sedative, anxiolytic, cholagogue)

Chamomile tea can be added to food, 1 mL per kg once to twice daily.

A prescription for moderate (separation) anxiety is provided here:

Passionflower	20% (sedative, hypnotic, antispasmodic, anxiolytic)

Saint John's Wort	20% (antidepressant, nervine tonic, anti-inflammatory, anxiolytic)
Withania	40% (tonic, adaptogen, nervine, sedative, anxiolytic, anti-inflammatory, antitumor)
Chamomile	20% (carminative, bitter, spasmolytic, mild sedative, anxiolytic, cholagogue)

Give 1 mL per 5 kg.

An alternative prescription for moderate to severe anxiety is:

Kava kava	40%
Eleuthero	20%
Passionflower or California Poppy	40%

Give 1 ml per 5 kg BID-TID

A prescription for separation anxiety with stress-related gastrointestinal symptoms is given below:

Saint John's Wort	30% (antidepressant, nervine tonic, anti-inflammatory, anxiolytic)
Withania	40% (tonic, adaptogen, nervine, sedative, anxiolytic, anti-inflammatory, antitumor)
Chamomile	30% (carminative, bitter, spasmolytic, mild sedative, anxiolytic, cholagogue)

Administer 1 mL per 5 kg.

Cognitive dysfunction

Therapeutic Rationale

- Improve cognitive function and antioxidant status.

Ginkgo and lemon balm may be combined with other herbs appropriate to the patient in terms of concomitant signs and energetic presentation. Commercial formulas for Alzheimer's disease and other human cognitive disorders may contain gotu kola, rosemary schisandra, ginkgo, and lemon balm. A foundation formula for dogs may contain the following:

Lemon balm	50%
Gotu kola	25%
Bacopa	25%

An alternative prescription for cognitive disorder is as follows:

Ginkgo	40% (antioxidant, circulatory stimulant, cognition enhancer, neurorestorative)
Bacopa	20% (nervine tonic, spasmolytic, mild sedative, mental tonic, cognitive enhancer)
Withania	20% (tonic, adaptogen, nervine, sedative, anxiolytic, anti-inflammatory, antitumor)
Gotu kola	20% (adaptogen, alterative, nerve tonic, mild diuretic)

The recommended dose is 1 mL per 5 kg.

Degenerative myelopathy

Therapeutic Rationale: Because the cause of degenerative myelopathy (DM) is unknown, different therapeutic regimens have been suggested on the basis of the possibility of autoimmune disorder, vitamin E deficiency, vitamin B deficiency, or simple degenerative disorder.

- Maintain neurologic integrity and muscular function through exercise.
- In the absence of a known mechanism to be targeted with herbal therapy, formulas may be directed toward reducing inflammation, alleviating stress, and possibly stimulating spinal cord and muscle function.

A prescription for degenerative myleopathy is given here:

Prickly ash	40% (circulatory stimulant, carminative, diaphoretic, antirheumatic)
Capsicum	20% (circulatory stimulant, diaphoretic, digestive, carminative, metabolic stimulant)
Eleuthero	10% (adaptogen, nervine stimulant)
Panax ginseng	10% (adaptogen, anxiolytic, stimulant, tonic, immune stimulant, hepatoprotective, cardioprotective)
Schisandra	20% (hepatoprotective, nervine tonic, adaptogenic)

Another prescription for degenerative myelopathy follows:

Turmeric	20% (anti-inflammatory, antioxidant, antiplatelet, cholagogue, hepatoprotective, anticancer)
Bacopa	20% (nervine tonic, spasmolytic, mild sedative, mental tonic, cognitive enhancer)
Siberian ginseng	20% (adaptogenic, immune modulating, neurologic trophorestorative)
Ginkgo	20% (antioxidant, circulatory stimulant, cognition enhancer, neurotrophorestorative)
Bilberry	20% (vasoprotective, antiedema, antioxidant, anti-inflammatory)

NOTE: Nux vomica is available in tincture form in the U.S. and should be used only by experienced herbalists at very low doses. It is contained in some traditional Chinese veterinary herbal products.

Depression

Therapeutic Rationale

- Rule out physical disorders.

A prescription for mild depression is provided:

Saint John's Wort	30% (antidepressant, nervine tonic, vulnerary, anti-inflammatory)
Siberian ginseng	30% (adaptogenic, antistress, immune modulating, neurologic trophorestorative)
Bacopa	20% (nervine tonic, antidepressant, spasmolytic, mild sedative, mental tonic, cognitive enhancer)
Lavender	10% (carminative, spasmolytic, antidepressant, antirheumatic)

Oats *(Avena sativa)* can be given in the diet as porridge for use as a nourishing nervine.

Lavender is particularly indicated when disturbances in gastrointestinal function are apparent as well.

Epilepsy

See the general section on seizures later.

Facial paralysis

Therapeutic Rationale

- Identify treatable causes, which include otitis media or interna, hypothyroidism, neoplasia, encephalitis, polyneuropathy, and facial neuritis.

Although we would recommend primarily acupuncture and massage for this condition, an herbal adjunct might consist of the following.

A prescription for facial paralysis is provided:

Gelsemium	5% (analgesic, sedative, hypotensive)
Prickly ash or capsicum	25% (circulatory stimulant, carminative, diaphoretic, antirheumatic)
Ginkgo	25% (antioxidant, circulatory stimulant, cognition enhancer, neurotrophorestorative)
Ashwagandha	45% (tonic, adaptogen, nervine, sedative, anxiolytic, anti-inflammatory, antitumor)

Feline hyperesthesia syndrome

Therapeutic Rationale

- Control seizures.
- Reduce allergies, skin irritation and panniculitis.
- Rule out other musculoskeletal and central nervous system (CNS) disorders and abscessation of the tail head.

Hyperesthesia in cats is a sign, rather than a diagnosis. Underlying diseases that lead to the biting, licking, scratching, and even seizure activity are many, and any cause of pain or irritation should be ruled out. These include flea allergy, spinal or muscular pain (including a specific inclusion body myositis that has been identified in these cats), cystitis and dermatitis. True seizure or behavioral disorders are probably rare. Environmental stress can worsen the condition.

A formula for cats that have been treated for any skin disease after thorough orthopedic and chiropractic examination might include the following:

Saint John's Wort	50% (antidepressant, nervine tonic, anti-inflammatory, anxiolytic)
Valerian	10% (sedative, hypnotic, antispasmodic, carminative)
Bacopa or skullcap	20% (anxiolytic, nervine relaxant)
California poppy	20% (sedative, hypnotic, antispasmodic, analgesic)

Also, see the section on neuropathy, later.

Fly-biting seizures

See the general section on seizures later in the chapter.

Hyperactivity

Therapeutic Rationale

- Determine underlying cause.
- Counsel owner to provide high levels of exercise.
- Rule out owner lack of leadership.
- Rule out anxiety.
- Rule out possible dietary manifestation or hypersensitivity. Consider an elimination diet.
- Provide sedative and anxiolytic herbs.

A mild prescription for hyperactivity is given here:

Ashwagandha	40% (tonic, adaptogen, nervine, sedative, anxiolytic, anti-inflammatory, antitumor)
Motherwort	20% (sedative, antispasmodic, cardiac tonic)
Lemon balm	20% (carminative, spasmolytic, sedative)
Chamomile	20% (carminative, bitter, spasmolytic, mild sedative, anxiolytic, cholagogue)

Insomnia/Nocturnal restlessness

Therapeutic Rationale

- Rule out cognitive dysfunction, hyperthyroidism, hypertension and so forth.
- Provide sedating, anxiolytic, and relaxing herbs.

A prescription for insomnia or restlessness at night follows:

Ashwagandha	40% (tonic, adaptogen, nervine, sedative, anxiolytic, anti-inflammatory, antitumor)
Chamomile	20% (carminative, bitter, spasmolytic, mild sedative, anxiolytic, cholagogue)
Skullcap	20% (sedative, nervine relaxant)
Chaste tree	20% (enhances melatonin production)
Ginkgo	20% (antioxidant, circulatory stimulant, cognition enhancer, neurotrophorestorative)

Alternatively, valerian alone can be used.

Intervertebral disk disease *(cervical and thoracolumbar)*

Therapeutic Rationale

- Minimize spinal movement in acute stages.
- Reduce pain and inflammation.
- Maintain muscular strength throughout recovery.
- Give bladder care.
- Reduce pain.
- Reduce risk of trauma.

Formulas for this disorder should seek to relieve pain from spinal impingement, inflammation, and muscle spasm. A suggested foundation for formula building is provided here:

Corydalis	30% (analgesic, sedative, cardioprotective)
Kava kava or cramp bark	15%
Meadowsweet	20% (anti-inflammatory, possible diuretic)
Ashwagandha	10% (tonic, adaptogen, nervine, sedative, anxiolytic, anti-inflammatory, antitumor)
Prickly ash or capsicum	20% (circulatory stimulant, carminative, diaphoretic, antirheumatic)

Kirk (1948) indicated that nux vomica and belladonna are "two sovereign remedies" for lack of tone in the bladder.

Meningitis and encephalitis

Therapeutic Rationale

- Identify predisposing or associated injury, infection, or immune compromise.
- Control seizures.
- Improve circulation.

Cases of intractable meningitis (such as granulomatous meningitis, beagle meningitis, etc.) are frequently presented after other treatments have been ineffective.

A foundation formula in this case might be as follows:

Prickly ash or capsicum	20% (circulatory stimulant, carminative, diaphoretic, antirheumatic)
Kava kava or cramp bark	35%
Black cohosh	25% (relaxing nervine, sedative, antirheumatic)
California poppy or Jamaica dogwood	15%
Gelsemium	5% (analgesic, sedative, hypotensive)

Pain

Corydalis: Add to system-based formula, 20% to 50%.

Obsessive-compulsive disorder

Therapeutic Rationale

- Reduce stress.
- Provide adaptogens and anxiolytics.

A mild prescription for obsessive-compulsive disorder is provided:

Saint John's Wort	20%
Chaste tree	20%
Siberian ginseng	20%
Ashwagandha	40%

Peripheral neuropathy

Therapeutic Rationale

- Identify cause, if possible.
- Control immune-mediated damage, if present.
- Provide physical therapy.

A formula for oral use in animals that experience neuralgic pain might contain Saint John's Wort, corydalis, and prickly ash. If the animal can be prevented from licking the area, a local application of capsicum may be of benefit. For paralysis, the authors would prefer acupuncture and physical therapy, but herbal support with circulatory stimulants (such as prickly ash) may also be warranted.

Professional herbalists for humans include herbs such as Saint John's Wort, skullcap, oat seed, and Eleuthero. Peppermint oil may be used as a topical analgesic.

A prescription for neuralgia is offered:

Saint John's Wort	20%
Passionflower	20%
Ashwagandha	20%
Bacopa	20%
Lemon balm	20%

Nerve restorative and protective herbs should be used when nerve damage is suspected. Antioxidant status should be attended to as well.

A general foundation formula to build on for nerve damage is given here:

Ashwagandha	20%
Bacopa	20%
Gingko	20%
Bilberry	20%
Saint John's Wort	20%

Seizures, general

Therapeutic Rationale: The diagnosis of "epilepsy" is oversimplified in that a number of syndromes may cause recurrent seizures. The alternative therapies described in this section may help in a percentage of cases depending on the cause, but at this point, mechanisms are largely unknown and treatment must be provided on a trial-and-error basis.

The practitioner should first attempt to control seizures with conventional drugs because seizures usually become more frequent if untreated, and veterinary herbalists have not found consensus on the most useful herbal anticonvulsants.

Historical texts, both human and veterinary, seem to lament the fact that no cures have been found for this disease, and they point to bromide salts, amyl nitrate, and, later, phenobarbital. The herbs that are most often recommended include gelsemium, passionflower, verbena, and valerian. Kirk (1948) also recommends belladonna if bromide has had no effect on the condition in dogs.

A foundation formula for dogs that do not respond to dietary changes or administration of conventional drugs might consist of these ingredients:

Skullcap	45% (anticonvulsive, sedative)
Gelsemium	5% (analgesic, sedative, hypotensive)
Valerian	20% (sedative, hypnotic, antispasmodic, hypotensive)
Passionflower	30% (sedative, hypnotic, antispasmodic)

A prescription for epilepsy support (assuming conventional medicine is being given concurrently):

Bacopa	20% (nervine tonic, spasmolytic, mild sedative, mental tonic)
Milk thistle	40% (hepatotonic, hepatoprotective, antioxidant)
Baical skullcap	20% (anticonvulsive, anti-inflammatory, antiallergic, mild sedative, hypotensive, diuretic, bitter)
Ginkgo	20% (antioxidant, circulatory stimulant, cognitive enhancer)

Stress

Stress occurs commonly in domestic animals, but aside from behavior counseling and modification, it is not a focus for treatment. The effects of chronic stress in people are well documented.

Stress occurs in large animals such as horses and food animals during shipping and in feedlots. Small animals that have maladapted to their environments are also stressed—these might include cats in crowded environments, high-energy dogs not given enough exercise, and interdog/intercat aggression circumstances.

A study in horses examined changes in cortisol, white blood cell count, and lymphocyte subpopulations in horses following 24 hours of transport. These horses were given an adaptogenic combination proprietary supplement, consisting of eleuthero, schisandra, rhodiola, and Asian devil's club *(Echinopanax elatus),* 8 mL once daily, or placebo. No differences were observed between treatment and placebo groups. In the horses housed in stalls and not exposed to transport stress, differences in lymphocyte subpopulation counts were noted, but no differences in cortisol, weight, white blood cell count, or lymphocyte responsiveness were reported. This supplement has documented effects in people, so it is possible that the supplement does not work in horses; that the level of stress intensity is different from that tested in humans, or that the dose was inadequate (Stull, 2004).

Stroke *(cerebrovascular accident)*

Therapeutic Rationale

- Improve circulation.
- Improve antioxidant status.
- Provide nerve restoratives.

A prescription to be given following stroke or suspected stroke is given:

Ginkgo	30% (antioxidant, circulatory stimulant, cognition enhancer, neurorestorative)
Lesser periwinkle *(Vinca minor)*	20% (circulatory stimulant [cerebral blood flow], increases cerebral oxygen uptake and glucose absorption, sedative, hemostatic)
Bacopa	20% (nervine tonic, spasmolytic, mild sedative, mental tonic, cognitive enhancer)
Withania	30% (tonic, adaptogen, nervine, sedative, anxiolytic, anti-inflammatory, antitumor)

Vestibular disease

Therapeutic Rationale

- Improve cerebral blood flow.
- Control nausea.

The recommended prescription is as follows:

Ginkgo	15% (antioxidant, circulatory stimulant, cognition enhancer, neurorestorative)
Lesser periwinkle *(Vinca minor)*	25% (circulatory stimulant [cerebral blood flow], increases cerebral oxygen uptake and glucose absorption, sedative, hemostatic)
Skullcap	15% (anticonvulsive, sedative)
Ginger	20%
Saint John's Wort	25% (antidepressant, nervine tonic, anti-inflammatory, anxiolytic)

HERBS FOR REPRODUCTIVE DISORDERS

General Considerations

Herbal medicine is commonly employed to assist men and women with reproductive disorders. It is curious that veterinary herbalists have much less experience in targeting herbs toward animal reproductive diseases, even though infertility and false pregnancy are common reasons for clients to seek herbal medicine treatment. Differences in female reproductive cycle types are likely one factor. In addition, our inability to evaluate sensations that go along with the physiologic processes of ovulation, gestation, and ejaculation, or clinical signs such as uterine bleeding or lack of libido in animals, undoubtedly contribute to this deficiency in herbal tools. This brief section attempts to pull together some clinical targets in human medicine and suggests possible strategies for the future in veterinary reproductive medicine.

Mechanisms of Interest

Emmenagogues

This traditional term refers to any plant that stimulates the menstrual process in women; it may apply to stimulation of menstrual bleeding or to normalization of the menstrual cycle in general. In veterinary medicine, emmenagogues may or may not normalize estrus cycles, but a few herbs with their potential mechanisms of action are given in the female endocrine modulators section that follows. Others include those listed here:

- Partridgeberry *(Mitchella repens)*
- Parsley *(Petroselinum crispum)*
- Rue *(Ruta graveolens)*
- Mugwort *(Artemisia vulgaris)*

Endocrine modulators

Female

VITEX (CHASTE TREE BERRY) ***(VITEX AGNUS-CASTUS):*** This herb is dopaminergic. The berries of this plant are used primarily in women for complaints of premenstrual syndrome. Animal studies have shown that vitex inhibits prolactin and appears to selectively stimulate D_2-type dopamine receptors. A randomized, placebo-controlled trial in men showed no dose-dependent changes in serum prolactin, but studies in women with mastodynia showed that treatment with vitex reduced serum prolactin levels. Vitex has also been shown to reduce the symptoms of premenstrual syndrome and mastalgia in women (Schulz, 2001; Wuttke, 2003). Prolactin may inhibit estrus; vitex may be helpful in suppressing prolactin in animals and may have utility in the treatment of false heat in dogs. It should not be used in pregnant or lactating animals.

BLACK COHOSH ***(CIMICIFUGA RACEMOSA):*** This plant is antiestrogenic. The root of the plant is used primarily in women for menopausal symptoms. Experiments have demonstrated that black cohosh contains compounds with antiestrogenic properties, and that the herb reduces levels of luteinizing hormone (which induces ovulation), with no changes in follicle-stimulating hormone. The triterpene glycosides also affect the hypothalamic-pituitary axis, potentially leading to a variety of secondary effects on the reproductive, nervous, and circulatory systems. Traditionally, black cohosh is considered a uterine tonic and nervine as well. To our knowledge, the herb is not recommended in historic veterinary texts for reproductive or hormonal disorders, and any clear indication for its use in animals is unknown.

FENNEL ***(FOENICULUM VULGARE):*** Fennel extracts have been shown in mice to trigger a mating response, induce estrus, and increase the size of mammary glands, cervix, vagina, endometrium, and myometrium. On the other hand, an aqueous extract of the seed has been shown to reduce female fertility (Mills, 2000).

SZECHUAN LOVAGE ROOT ***(LIGUSTICUM WALLICHII):*** This herb is a luteal phase normalizer that is traditionally prescribed for menstrual disorders caused by blood stasis.

Effects of ligusticum on the endocrine function of the ovary/uterus were studied in rats. Ligusticum had no influence on immature rats, except that it decreased prostaglandin E2 content in the ovary; in pseudopregnant rats, it inhibited the function of the corpus luteum, decreased the level of progesterone in the plasma, and reduced the hCG/luteinizing hormone receptor binding capacity of the ovary, compared with controls (Li, 1992).

DAN SHEN *(SALVIA MILTIORRHIZA)*: This herb was investigated in terms of the endocrine function of the ovary and the uterus. In immature Wistar rats, it increased the level of estradiol in plasma, the weight of the uterus, and the ovarian prostaglandin F2 alpha content, but the ovarian prostaglandin E_2 content was reduced when compared with that in the control group. It stimulated ovulation in immature mice pretreated with PMSG. In pseudopregnant rats, it also inhibited the function of the corpus luteum, decreased the level of progesterone in the plasma, and reduced the hCG/luteinizing hormone receptor binding capacity of the ovary (Li, 1992).

OTHER HERBS: Herbs with estrogen-like activity include ladies' mantle *(Alchemilla vulgaris)*, false unicorn root *(Chamaelirium luteum)*, wild yam *(Dioscorea villosa)*, fennel *(Foeniculum vulgare)*, licorice *(Glycyrrhiza glabra)*, white peony *(Paeonia lactiflora)*, *Panax ginseng*, trillium *(Trillium erectum)*, and vervain *(Verbena officinalis)*.

Male

SAW PALMETTO *(SERENOA REPENS)*: This herb may have numerous mechanisms of action, including an antiandrogenic action, an anti-inflammatory effect, and an antiproliferative influence attained through the inhibition of growth factors. It is effective in reducing symptoms in human benign prostatic hypertrophy (BPH) in men. The most intensively investigated form is the n-hexane lipidosterolic extract known as *Permixon* (Pierre Fabre Medicament, Boulogne, France) (Buck, 2004). It has been tested in dogs and was not effective in correcting measurements of BPH; however, these dogs were asymptomatic (Barsanti, 2000), so a true parallel to the demonstrated efficacy in human BPH has not yet been investigated.

NETTLE *(URTICA DIOICA)*: This plant may be mildly effective in human males with BPH. Nettle is commonly used in combination with other herbs. Only the root is considered to have activity in BPH. Clinical observations of men after long-term treatment with an alcoholic extract of nettle root reported an improvement in bladder outlet obstruction symptoms and a decrease in postvoiding residual urine (Bruneton, 1995).

PYGEUM *(PYGEUM AFRICANUS)*: This herb has been shown in clinical trials to reduce symptoms associated with BPH in men (Ishani, 2000). The mechanism by which it works is unknown, and pygeum use has not been popular for use in dogs to date.

PUMPKIN SEED *(CUCURBITA PEPO)*: These contain sterols, similar to the herbs listed above, and have also been used for the treatment of BPH in men.

TRIBULUS *(TRIBULUS TERRISTIS)*: In male rats, tribulus showed considerable stimulation of sperm production. Sperm cells were more viable, suggesting improved fertility (Zarkova, 1984). An experiment was carried out to define the stimulating effect of Tribestan, a proprietary extract on rams that were intended for breeding, as well as on rams that exhibited sexual impotence and deteriorated semen qualities. Treatment led to an extended period of sexual activity and to improved semen production in rams over the service period. Rams with reduced libido recovered by the seventh or eighth day with no morphologic changes in the structure of both testes and epididymides. The use of this preparation led to changes in the endocrine activity of the testis, raising the testosterone level and normalizing the sexual activity of rams affected with coital impotence (Dimitrov, 1987). Tribestan increased testosterone levels and accelerated sexual development in rams and male lambs, respectively (Georgiev, 1988). Libido and sexual reflexes were restored in boars with long-term sexual impotence (Zarkova, 1984).

Galactagogues

FENNEL *(FOENICULUM VULGARE)* OIL: This was shown to increase milk production and fat content in goats (Mills, 2000). Fennel has been used since at least the time of Dioscorides for this purpose.

GUAN MU TONG *(ARISTOLOCHIA FANGCHI OR A. MANSHURIENSIS)*: This herb was administered in drinking water to lactating mice. A 5% solution suppressed lactation and was associated with decreased mammary RNA levels; a 0.05% solution improved lactation (Wu, 1995). This herb is carcinogenic with long-term use, and it has been removed from the market in some countries.

GOAT'S RUE *(GALEGA OFFICINALIS)*: "In 1873, Gillet-Damitte, in a communication to the French Academy, stated that this plant when fed to cows would increase the secretion of milk from 35 to 50 per cent. Others have affirmed that goat's rue is a powerful galactagogue. The best preparation appears to be an aqueous extract prepared from the fresh plant" (Remington, 1918).

CHASTE TREE *(VITEX AGNUS-CASTUS)*: This herb is used traditionally as a galactagogue, though no supporting evidence could be found; in fact, clinical trial evidence suggests that Vitex reduces serum prolactin levels (Wuttke, 2003), which would theoretically suppress milk production.

Uterine astringents

Astringents are used to suppress excessive bleeding—in women, they are used primarily for metrorrhagia (bleeding between periods), menorrhagia (heavy periods), or fibroids. Their use for this purpose is questionable in veterinary medicine.

- Ladies' mantle *(Alchemilla vulgaris)*
- Shepherd's purse *(Capsella bursa-pastoris)*
- Cranesbill *(Geranium maculatum)*

Uterine tonics

These plants are used traditionally to prepare the uterus for normal functions, including birth and involution, and may improve circulation or normalize hormonal influence on the uterus.

DONG QUAI *(ANGELICA SINENSIS):* Hot aqueous extracts of dong quai stimulated smooth muscle contractions of the bladder, intestine, and uterus when administered intravenously to dogs (10 g/kg body weight) (Schmidt, 1924). Intravenous administration of an aqueous or 95% ethanol extract of dong quai to cats, rats, and rabbits increased the strength of the contractions and improved the tone of uterine smooth muscle (Zhu, 1987). In vitro assays demonstrated that a decoction of dong quai stimulated the H1 receptor of the mouse uterus (Shi, 1995). It had varied actions on the uterus that were not related to estrogenic activity, and it promoted relaxation and uterine contractility and uterine hyperplasia (Belford-Courtney, 1994).

BLUE COHOSH *(CAULOPHYLLUM THALICTROIDES):* This plant was used by American natives to assist labor and delivery and is described in King's this way: "There is no doubt but that caulophyllum has a decided action upon the gravid uterus. During labor, it relieves *false pains* and coordinates muscular contractions, at the same time increasing their power. When used by delicate women, or those who experience prolonged and painful labors, for several weeks previous to confinement, it gives tone and vigor to all the parts engaged in the accouchement, facilitating its progress and relieving much suffering . . . Chronic corporeal or cervical endometritis, metritis, ovaritis, ovarialgia, uterine leucorrhoea, amenorrhoea, and dysmenorrhoea are conditions in which it has been most successfully employed." This herb has been associated with acute onset of labor and myocardial infarction in a woman, and a review by Paul Bergner notes that it was used in excess of traditional doses, and that it was not traditionally used alone (Bergner, 2001).

BLACK COHOSH *(ACTAEA RACEMOSA):* King's designates this plant as a remedy for "atony of the reproductive tract" and an "excellent *'partus praeparator.'*" No studies were found to support this use.

PARTRIDGEBERRY *(MITCHELLA REPENS):* This herb had similar uses as blue cohosh and black cohosh; it was taken a few weeks before birth to "tone" the uterus.

FALSE UNICORN ROOT *(CHAMAELIRIUM LUTEUM):* King's describes the value of false unicorn root in diseases of the reproductive organs of females. "Especially of the uterus, it is one of our most valuable agents, acting as a uterine tonic, and gradually removing abnormal conditions, while at the same time, it imparts tone and vigor to the reproductive organs. Hence, it is much used in leucorrhoea, amenorrhoea, dysmenorrhoea, and to remove the tendency to repeated and successive *miscarriages*. A particular phase removed by it is the irritability and despondency that often attends uterine troubles."

RASPBERRY *(RUBUS IDAEUS):* This plant is commonly used by breeders to ease parturition in dogs and cats. This use is somewhat mysterious, as it is not a traditional indication in the older literature. No studies can be found to support its use.

OTHER HERBS: Infusions of some medicinal plants were studied for their activity in enhancing uterine tone in in vitro experiments performed on isolated rabbit and guinea pig uterine smooth muscle. In concentrations of 1 to 2 mg crude herb per ml, the plants were ranked in descending order with regard to their tone-enhancing effects on the uterus: chamomile *(Matricaria chamomilla)*, calendula *(Calendula officinalis)*, cockscomb *(Celosia cristata)*, plantain *(Plantago lanceolata)*, comfrey *(Symphytum officinale)*, shepherd's purse *(Capsella bursa-pastoris)*, and Saint John's Wort *(Hypericum perforatum* L.*)*. No effect resulted from infusions of flaxseeds *(Linum usitatissimum* L.*)* and bearberry leaves *(Arctostaphylos uva ursi* L.*)* (Shipochliev, 1981).

Uterine relaxants

These may be useful in threatened miscarriage and false labor.

CRAMP BARK *(VIBURNUM OPULUS):* Cooks (1869) describes the bark as a "slowly acting relaxant, with gentle (mild) tonic properties that chiefly influences the nervous system. Because of its antispasmodic action, it is chiefly employed in hysteria, painful menstruation, neuralgia and rheumatism of the womb, and the uterine cramping incident to pregnancy (and is usually combined with *Mitchella*)."

OTHER HERBS: Others include *Ligusticum wallichii*, black haw *(Virburnum prunifolium)*, and blue cohosh *(Caulophyllum thalictroides)*.

Nervines and antispasmodics

Breeders frequently report signs of irritability, depression, and possibly pain in mares and bitches. Whatever the causes of the clinical signs, the herbs below have been used in women for the pain and emotional/behavioral symptoms of premenstrual syndrome and may have use if the breeder elects to experiment with them.

BLACK COHOSH *(ACTAEA RACEMOSA):* Most Eclectic uses of black cohosh as a nervine were associated with menstrual or menopausal disorders in women, and it is difficult to separate the antispasmodic and analgesic effects from any nervine effect in traditional herbal literature.

BLACK HAW *(VIBURNUM PRUNIFOLIUM)* AND CRAMP BARK *(VIBURNUM OPULUS):* Cramp bark and other *Viburnum* species have shown ability to reduce smooth muscle spasm in a number of in vitro studies (Cometa, 1998; Calle, 1999; Nicholson, 1972).

Anti-inflammatories *(female reproductive system)*

- Dong quai *(Angelica sinensis)*
- Wild yam *(Dioscorea villosa)*
- White peony *(Paeonia lactiflora)*

REVIEW OF SPECIFIC REPRODUCTIVE SYSTEM CONDITIONS

Abortion

Therapeutic rationale

- Determine infectious, toxic, or hormonal influences.

Antispasmodic herbs such as wild yam, black haw, and cramp bark and uterine relaxants have been suggested for impending miscarriage in women. For repeated miscarriage, false unicorn root can be incorporated into any formula. Peterson (1905) described the action of caulophyllum in pregnancy by saying that it is used "to prolong gestation to the normal period. In labor, it is of value when the pains are feeble from atony of the uterus, patient weak, nervous."

Many, many herbs have been implicated as abortifacients. Although it is better to be safe than sorry, the reader should remember that many of the herbs discussed in the following section have only theoretical contraindications. With an abundance of caution, we have listed all herbs mentioned in our search of the literature. Types of herbs to be avoided include the following:

- Emmenagogues
- Herbs that may stimulate uterine contractions
- Herbs that are high in alkaloids (which may stimulate the uterus)
- Herbs that are high in volatile oils (which may stimulate or irritate the uterus)
- Herbs that affect hormonal function
- Harsh laxatives
- Strong diuretics

Specific Herbs to be Avoided in Pregnant Animals

Potentially toxic herbs should generally be avoided; however, some are used in low doses or during the last weeks of pregnancy (see individual monographs, where applicable, for more information) (Box 20-1).

Agalactia

Therapeutic Rationale

- Normalize hormonal control of milk production (prolactin and oxytocin).
- Evaluate for systemic illness, excessive epinephrine production (stress or pain induced), debility, or malnutrition.

Herbs with galactagogue activity are used in this condition. Fennel may be employed to increase milk production. Mouse studies suggest that the taste does cross into the milk.

Benign prostatic hyperplasia

Therapeutic Rationale

- Rule out infection.
- Normalize hormonal influences, if possible (although BPH in men and in dogs occurs through different processes).

In men, saw palmetto is well studied and apparently effective. The single trial that investigated saw palmetto in dogs reported a lack of effect for saw palmetto extract on prostatic weight, prostatic volume, prostatic histologic scores, prostatic ultrasonographs, and serum testosterone concentrations (Barsanti, 2000). Dogs included in this

BOX 20-1

Herbs and Poisonous Plants to Be Avoided During Pregnancy*

Achillea millefolium
Aconitum species
Acorus calamus
Adhatoda vasica
Aesculus hippocastanum
Agathosma betulina
Aloe vera (latex)
Ammi visnaga
Andrographis paniculata
Anemone pulsatilla
*Angelica sinensis***
Angelica archangelica
Anthemis nobilis
Apium graveolens
Arctostaphylos uva ursi
Aristolochia (all or any species)
Arnica (all or any species)
Artemisia species
Asarum canadense
Asclepias tuberosa
Atropa belladonna
Baptisia tinctoria
Berberis vulgaris
Borago officinalis
Brassica nigra
Brugmansia spp.
Brunfelsia uniflora
Calotropis procera, C. gigantea
Capsella bursa-pastoris
Cassia senna
Catha edulis
Caulophyllum thalictroides
Cephalis ipecacuanha
Chelidonium majus
Chenopodium ambrosioides
Cicuta virosa
Cimicifuga (Actea) racemosa
Cinchona spp
Cinnamomum species
Cnicus benedictus
Colchicum autumnale
Commiphora spp.
Convallaria majalis
Coptis teeta
Coronilla varia
Corydalis ambigua
Crocus sativus
Crotalaria (all or any species)
Croton (all or any species)
Cynoglossum officinale
Cystis scoparius
Daphne mezereum

BOX 20-1

Herbs and Poisonous Plants to Be Avoided During Pregnancy*—cont'd

Datura stramonium
Dauca carota (seed only)
Digitalis purpurea
Dryopteris fillix-mas
Duboisia myoporoides
Echium vulgare
Embelia ribes
Ephedra sinica
Erysimum cheiranthoides
Euonymus europaeus
Galanthus nivalis
Gelsemium sempervirens
Glycyrrhiza glabra
Gossypium herbaceum
Harpagophytum procumbens
Hedeoma pulegoides
Heliotropium (all or any species)
Helleborus (all or any species)
Hydrastis canadensis
Hyoscyamus niger
Hyssopus officinalis
Iris versicolor
Juniperus communis
Lantana camara
Larrea divaricata
Lathyrus sativus, other than the cooked seed
Leonurus cardiaca
Ligusticum chuanxiong
Ligusticum porterii
Lithospermum (any species)
*Lobelia inflata***
Lomatium dissectum
Lycopus species
Mahonia spp
Mandragora
*Marrubium nigrum***
Menispermum canadense
Momordica charantia
Myristica fragrans
Nerium oleander
Nicotiana tabacum
Opuntia cylindrica
Panax notoginseng
Panax pseudoginseng
Papaver somniferum
Paullinia cupana
Pausinystalia yohimbe
Peganum harmala
Petasites frigida
Petroselinum crispum root or seed
Peumus boldus
Phytolacca americana
Picrasma excelsa
Picrorrhiza kurroa
*Piper methysticum***
Piscidia erythrina
Podophyllum peltatum
Prunus africanum
Prunus serotina
Pteridium aquilinum
Pulsatilla vulgaris
Rauwolfia serpentina
Rhamnus cathartica
Rhamnus purshiana
Rheum palmatum
Ricinus communis
Robinia pseudoacacia, other than the leaf
Ruta graveolens
Salvia miltiorrhiza
Salvia officinalis
Sanguinaria canadensis
Santalum album
Schisandra chinensis, except in last 6 weeks to assist with birth
Schoenocaulon officinale (Sabadilla officinarum, Veratrum officinale)
Scopolia carniolica
Semecarpus anacardium (Anacardium orientale), other than the seed
Senecio aureus
Solanum (all or any species) except stems of *Solanum dulcamara* (Bittersweet) and potatoes
Sophora secundiflora
Spigelia marilandica
Strophanthus spp
Strychnos nux-vomica
Strychnos gaultheria
Strychnos ignatii (Ignatia amara)
Symphytum officinale
Tamus communis fruit and root
Tanacetum parthenium
Tanacetum vulgare
Teucrium (all or any species)
Thuja occidentalis
Thymus vulgaris
Toxicodendron radicans (Rhus toxicodendron)
Tribulus terrestris
Trigonella foenum-graecum
Trillium erectum
Tussilago farfara
Tylophora indica
Uncaria tomentosa
Urginea spp
Verbena hastate
Veronicastrum virginiana
Vinca rosea
Virola sebifera
Viscum album
*Vitex agnus-castus***
Xanthorrhiza simplicissima
*Zanthoxylum americanum***

*This list is compiled from multiple sources with an eye to conservatism
**These herbs may be used by experienced herbalists during pregnancy

study did not have the clinical signs of BPH (i.e., decreased urinary flow and residual urine volume) that often occur in men with BPH. Dogs did not appear to be randomly assigned to treatment, and mean prostatic volume in the control group was higher than that in the active treatment groups before treatment.

Crataeva may also be beneficial in animals with concurrent infection or bleeding from the penis, or when bladder tone may be compromised (see section on urinary tract herbs). Formulas for men are available over the counter and may contain saw palmetto, pygeum root, nettle root, and other herbs.

Herbalists tend to use formulas that contain saw palmetto berry, hydrangea, pygeum, sarsaparilla, white sage *(Salvia apiana)*, collinsonia *(Collinsonia canadensis)*, corn silk, and nettle root.

Infertility, female

Therapeutic Rationale

- Determine whether anatomic abnormalities prevent insemination.
- Identify potential ovarian or ovum dysfunction (due to toxins, systemic diseases, or congenital or hereditary problems).
- Identify potential hormonal imbalances that may prevent normal cycling, ovum production, maturation, implantation, and so forth.
- Determine whether uterine infection may be present.

Herbal treatment of female infertility should be attempted only after physical problems such as anatomic abnormalities and problems with the male have been ruled out. These may include hormone balancers such as vitex and tonics such as dong quai. Chinese medicine offers many formulas that may be appropriate; these may contain herbs such as white peony, rehmannia, ligusticum, cyperus, and others. It is good to remember that dogs are sensitive to estrogenic compounds and may exhibit bone marrow suppression when given high doses of pharmacologic estrogen compounds. How this relates to herbal estrogenic compounds is unknown.

Infertility, male

Therapeutic Rationale

- Determine whether anatomic abnormalities are present (e.g., testicular hypoplasia, persistent penile frenulum, hypospadia).
- Identify causes of low libido (e.g., behavioral problem, pain, neurologic disorder).
- Determine causes of abnormal or dysfunctional sperm.
- Determine whether genetic disorders are present (e.g., Klinefelter's syndrome, XX male syndrome).
- Identify infection, injury, or tumors that may cause testicular degeneration.

Ginsenosides from *Panax ginseng* may facilitate penile erection by directly inducing the vasodilation and relaxation of penile corpus cavernosum. These effects may be mediated by modification of nitric oxide release from endothelial cells and perivascular nerves. American ginseng *(P. quinquefolius)* has also been shown to enhance male copulatory behavior and lower prolactin levels in male rats (Murphy, 2002). Damiana may also be included in a formula for impotence.

Astragalus may improve sperm motility. In a study on how herbs influence human spermatozoal motility, *Astragalus,* as well as *Acanthopanax senticosus,* significantly enhanced percent viability, number of progressive motile spermatozoa, curvilinear velocity, average path velocity, and amplitude of lateral head displacement (as compared with other herbs in the study, which were ineffective) (Liu, 2004).

Mastitis

Therapeutic Rationale

- Make sure the environment is clean.
- Treat infection with appropriate antibiotics.
- Reduce inflammation to relieve pain.
- Protect infants from nursing abscessed or gangrenous teats.

Most herbalists recommend poultices or compresses, as well as systemic treatments. (See section on immune system and infections.) External applications of chamomile and calendula may have anti-inflammatory activity. Poke root is a stronger herb with a tradition of use in mastitis; King's says, "No other remedy equals phytolacca in acute mastitis." Safety for nursing infants is unknown, and they should not be allowed to nurse if this herb is in use.

Topical applications of Comfrey *(Symphytum offinale)* extract (in propylene glycol base with allantoin, ascorbic acid, and chlorophyll or carotene) to the teats of dairy cows and infusion of the extract into the udder cured acute mastitis after two applications (Noorlander, 1987). Chronically infected cows did not respond as well. Seven cows with teat ends that were ruptured and cracked received topical application of this extract, which healed the tissue. Similar success rates were observed in another herd—cows with chapped teats and skin lesions healed in less than 3 days, and the tissue became soft and smooth. A deep cut on the surface of one teat of one cow healed in less than 5 days after treatment was provided (Noorlander, 1987).

Tea leaves *(Camellia sinensis)* as a poultice were recommended by Sheldon (1880) in a treatise on treatment of mastitis in dairy cows.

Aloe *(Aloe vera)* for the treatment of cows with mastitis was described by Coats in 1985. Therapy was provided through injection of 20 to 60 mL of aloes (in gel or juice form) into the infected quarter at least once a day. It was claimed that aloe helps to drain the infection, has anti-inflammatory properties, and is a coagulant. It has a diuretic property also, which serves to soften the hardened udder.

Chamomile *(Matricaria recutita)* has a traditional use in external application for mastitis and mammary abscesses, as does cabbage, made into a poultice.

Panax ginseng: Cows with subclinical mastitis caused by *Staphylococcus aureus* were subjected to subcutaneous injection with an extract from the root of *Panax ginseng* at a dose of 8 mg/kg body weight per day for 6 days. After the end of treatment, the numbers of *S. aureus*–infected quarters and milk and somatic cell count tended to decrease in ginseng-treated cows, but not in the control group. Findings indicated that ginseng treatment may activate the innate immunity of cows and may contribute to the cow's recovery from mastitis (Hu, 2001).

KELP *(ASCOPHYLLUM NODOSUM):* This herb has been used to prevent mastitis (Vacca, 1954). In a 7-year experiment with twin cows, in which one was given kelp in its ration and the other was not, the incidence of mastitis was greatly reduced in the cows who received kelp. The original research is difficult to trace. Another study (Jensen, 1968) found the total milk yield to be around 6% higher in dairy cows fed 3% *Ascophyllum nodosum* in a fortified seaweed meal, over a 7-year period in Norway, than in controls. The test concluded that the fortified seaweed meal was superior to the standard mineral mixtures for milk production. In the seaweed group, the incidence of mastitis was markedly reduced (90% in the control group); the number of services needed per conception was decreased and the number of no returns was increased; and a marked increase was seen in the iodine content of milk. Trials at the Institute of Animal Husbandry at the University of Giessen, West Germany, affected an increase in number and "much greater" durability of live semen in bulls (Stephenson, 1974).

CALENDULA *(CALENDULA OFFICINALIS):* This herb is used in bioorganic farming as a mastitis salve (Jost, 1984).

PERSICARIA SENEGALENSE: This plant was studied through the use of in vitro and in vivo antimicrobial tests, with crude extracts and the leaf in different forms. The in vitro test showed that isolates of *Staphylococcus aureus, Candida albicans,* and *Corynebacterium bovis* from subclinical cases and an isolate of *Pseudomonas aeruginosa* from a clinical case of mastitis were all inhibited by the three crude extracts at an 820-μg concentration. A trial feeding of 1.5 kg of the cooked leaf per day for 5 days did not yield a significant cure rate, whereas a second trial in which 0.77 kg of leaf powder (equivalent to 3 kg of wet leaf) was fed per day for 5 days resulted in an apparent cure rate of 92.8% (52.8% actual); a 40% spontaneous cure rate was seen in the negative control group, in contrast to 80% (40% actual) in the positive control group that had been treated with an intramammary antibiotic preparation. The difference in cure rate between the negative control group and the experimental group given 0.77 kg leaf powder was significant ($P = .008$) (Abaineh, 2001).

HOUTTUYNIA CORDATA: An aqueous intramammary solution obtained from *Houttuynia* was made for the treatment of bovine clinical mastitis. A total of 104 acute and subacute mastitis cases were randomly assigned into two groups (with 52 cases in each group)—a treatment group and a control group (in which intramammary administration of 800,000 IU penicillin G in combination with 1 g streptomycin was conducted). No statistically significant difference was found between the treatment group and control groups in the treatment of acute and subacute mastitis. In addition, an inhibitory effect was seen on the growth of lactic streptococcus in the milk collected within 48 hours of intramammary treatment with penicillin G in combination with streptomycin. However, for the herbal preparation, a mild inhibitory effect on lactic streptococci was detected in the milk within 12 hours of treatment (Hu, 1997).

Metritis

Therapeutic Rationale

- Identify and treat infection.

Herbs such as blue cohosh, white dead nettle *(Lamium album),* and goldenseal have been recommended for women with endometritis. Echinacea and baptisia may be added for infection. Herbalists often recommend making these herbs into a vaginal suppository to be inserted at bedtime, whereas veterinarians may choose to use infusions. In small animals, however, vaginal douching or uterine infusions are not typically used, as an increase in inflammation usually results. The exception would be a case of vaginitis in which a large amount of pus has pooled (as with a foreign body).

A comfrey extract has also been used in the treatment of metritis of dairy cows. Treatment consisted of 90 mL of extract infused into the uterus every day for 3 days. No visible irritation to the mucous membrane or epithelial tissue was noted; however, a beneficial effect on the endometrium was observed (Noorlander, 1987).

Pseudocyesis (false pregnancy)

Therapeutic Rationale

- Lower prolactin levels.
- Evaluate for hormonal influences, such as hypothyroidism.

Chaste tree *(Vitex angus castus)* is the premier herb for consideration in lowering prolactin levels for these animals.

Pyometra

See the section on metritis. Surgery or luteolytic drugs are recommended for pyometra. As with any potentially life-threatening condition, open pyometra should be managed with extreme caution and diligent follow-up, if unproven alternative medical treatments are used. Herbal medicine is ideal for assisting in the recuperative stage following surgery or as a complementary approach, alongside antibiotics, in open pyometra. Uterine tonics and immune-supporting herbs should be used, as well as adaptogens.

Vaginitis

Therapeutic Rationale

- Address underlying causes (e.g., anatomic abnormalities, subclinical urinary incontinence, obesity-induced fat folds over vulva).
- Identify and suppress pathogenic bacteria.
- Reduce inflammation.

In addition to probiotics, quite a few herbs have been recommended for women with this problem, usually as a douche (see previous note) or sitz bath. These herbs include marshmallow, yerba mansa, black cohosh, myrrh, coptis, echinacea, gossypium, goldenseal, calendula, grindelia, and comfrey leaf.

A classic formula for vaginal discharge consisted of equal parts cranesbill *(Geranium maculatum),* bethroot

(Trillium erectum), marshmallow *(Althaea officinalis)*, and agrimony *(Agrimonia eupatoria)*.

The author (BF) has successfully treated a chronic case of lymphocytic plasmacytic vulvitis/vaginitis in a dog with Chinese formula Rehmannia 6.

HERBS FOR RESPIRATORY DISORDERS

Practitioners rely heavily on the traditional uses of respiratory herbs because these herbs have been less well researched than those used in other areas of herbal medicine. Similar to conventional medicine, symptomatic management is the mainstay of treatment, and a diagnosis assists herbalists in treating the underlying pathophysiology.

One of the first signs of respiratory disease is coughing, which in itself may be beneficial. Generally, coughs should be treated when they are unproductive, or when they keep the owner awake at night. Herbal treatment for respiratory disease may include tinctures, but steam inhalation and cough syrups are also useful. Herbs are commonly found in many cough syrups used in conventional medicine. Some of the actions we look for in treating respiratory disease include expectorants, which help remove excess mucus; demulcents, which reduce irritation;. antitussives, to prevent or reduce the severity of coughing; suppressants, which inhibit the coughing reflex; antimicrobials, to reduce infection; and, more recently, herbal antihistamines and immune modulators, to treat allergic respiratory disease.

Mechanisms of Interest

Antitussive herbs

Coughing is a complex reflex that originates in peripheral cough receptors, which are most concentrated in the epithelium of the upper and lower respiratory tracts but are also found in the external auditory meatus, tympanic membrane, esophagus, stomach, pericardium, and diaphragm. Vagal afferent nerves carry signals from irritants and mechanoreceptors to the central medullary cough center (or centers), and efferent signals reach bronchial smooth muscle through the vagal, phrenic, and spinal motor nerves. Stimulation at any point in this reflex arc may lead to a cough.

Antitussives work through central or peripheral means. Central-acting antitussives act on the central cough center. Conventional drugs with central antitussive activity include opioid agonists; however, few herbs with demonstrated opioid activity are also used as antitussives. One source (Mills, 2000) claims that cyanogenic glycosides have central antitussive activity—the premier herb in this case is wild cherry bark. Peripheral antitussives may have bronchodilator, expectorant, demulcent, or anti-inflammatory activity; these are discussed in their respective sections.

Swallowing itself helps to suppress coughing. In humans, cough lozenges include ingredients that work via several modes of action, but it should be noted that even the sugar in these lozenges may suppress cough by stimulating salivation and subsequent swallowing.

Wild Cherry Bark *(Prunus serotina)*: Studies to support the antitussive activity of wild cherry bark could not be found. Wild cherry was often confused with *P. virginiana*, which is actually choke cherry, but for the reader's own information, it is useful to note that the Eclectic writers and the early US Dispensatory may have considered them synonymous. Ellingwood (1919) describes the indications as follows: "a common remedy in the treatment of chronic coughs, especially those accompanied with excessive expectoration . . . The syrup is used as a menstruum for the administration of other remedies in this disease. It is excellent also in reflex cough—the cough of nervous patients without apparent cause." The US Dispensatory (Remington, 1918) stated that hydrocyanic acid was believed to be the active principle, but wild cherry bark was not believed to be very effective. The dose recommended for people was 30 to 60 grains (1.9-3.8 g). Winslow states that the official products (fluid extract and syrup) were often used in cough mixtures for dogs, but that the official hydrocyanic acid was more reliable. Milks (1949) recommends doses of 2 mL of the fluid extract for dogs, or 4 mL of the syrup.

Licorice *(Glycyrrhiza glabra)*: Constituents may have some direct central effects on the cough reflex. Laboratory animal studies have suggested that the effect was comparable with that of codeine (Anderson, 1961), and that one component—liquiritin apioside—had antitussive effects that were dependent on both peripheral and central mechanisms (Kamei, 2003). The herb is considered both demulcent and expectorant and is used to decrease inflammation in the respiratory tract, and often as a stabilizing and flavoring base for troches or pills that included other antitussives.

Burdock *(Arctium lappa)*: A constituent (fructofuranan—a type of inulin), has been tested for antitussive activity in cats. It was found to be equally as active as some nonnarcotic, synthetic preparations used in clinical practice to treat patients with cough; in mitogenic and comitogenic tests, its biological response was comparable with that of the commercial zymosan immune modulator (Kardosova, 2003).

Other herbs: Other antitussive herbs include the following:

- Neem *(Azadirachta indica)*
- Bupleurum *(Bupleurum falcatum)*
- Black cohosh *(Cimicifuga racemosa)*
- Pinellia *(Pinellia ternata)*
- Elecampane *(Inula helenium)*
- Thyme *(Thymus vulgaris)*
- Marshmallow *(Althaea officinalis)*
- Irish moss *(Chondrus crispus)*

Anti-inflammatory and antiallergic herbs

These herbs may stabilize mast cells, reduce leukotriene production, or have other effects that suppress acute allergic responses that lead to bronchoconstriction, inflammation, and mucous production.

Perilla Seed *(Perilla frutescens)*: This is a traditional Oriental remedy for asthma. This treatment is frequently used in cats; they tolerate it well because of the neutral taste.

Boswellia *(Boswellia serrata)*: In a controlled study, 40 human patients with asthma were treated with boswellia gum resin (300 mg three times daily for 6 weeks). In all, 70% of patients showed improvement in physical symptoms such as dyspnea, rhonchi, and frequency. Only 27% of control patients treated with lactose showed improvement (Gupta, 1998).

Nettle Leaf *(Urtica dioica)*: A double-blind, randomized trial examined the effects of freeze-dried nettle on 69 people with allergic rhinitis. Nettle was rated higher or slightly higher by physician assessment and patient diary entries, respectively (Mittman, 1990).

Licorice Root *(Glycyrrhiza glabra)*: King's (Felter, 1898) suggests that licorice is useful in "old bronchial affections." Because the herb inhibits 11-hydroxysteroid dehydrogenase, endogenous steroid levels may be elevated, which may also suppress allergic responses. Licorice is most often used as part of a formula because of concerns about mineralocorticoid-like adverse effects when it is used over the long term.

Butterbur Rhizome *(Petasites hybridus)*: Extracts of butterbur have been shown to bind the H1 histamine receptor (petasin), inhibit cyteinyl-leukotriene synthesis, and selectively inhibit cyclooxygenase (COX)-2 in vitro (Fiebich, 2005). The Asthma & Allergy Research Group at the University of Dundee has completed multiple human clinical trials undertaken to investigate the effects of butterbur extracts in allergic respiratory disease. Using the patented butterbur extract Petaforce® (50 mg twice daily), they compared the extract with placebo in patients challenged with adenosine monophosphate. In two randomized, double blind, crossover trials, butterbur effectively suppressed the signs of allergic rhinitis (Lee, 2004b; Lee, 2003); in another trial, it was ineffective (Gray, 2004). Tesalin® was used by another group and was compared with cetirizine in a double-blind, parallel-group trial. Tesalin contains the equivalent of 8 mg petasins per tablet. Similar improvements were noted in the two groups, and although butterbur use was not associated with adverse effects, the cetirizine group reported sedation as a common adverse effect (Schapowal, 2002). Petaforce® was also investigated for use in atopic asthmatic human patients who were already being treated with corticosteroid inhalers; it was found to be significantly beneficial as a complement to steroid use in a double-blind, crossover trial (Lee, 2004a). The proprietary product Petadolex® was administered to 80 asthmatic patients for 2 months in an open trial, and the number of asthmatic attacks, peak flow, and forced expiratory volume were measured. All symptoms improved during therapy, and more than 40% of patients were able to reduce their intake of other asthma medications (Danesch, 2004). Butterbur had no effect on skin test reactions to histamine (Jackson, 2004). Butterbur contains pyrrolizidine alkaloids and should not be used as crude herb or crude extract. The products mentioned here have been processed to remove the pyrrolizidine alkaloids, according to the manufacturers. Doses recommended for adult humans are as follows: Petaforce® (25-50 mg twice daily to three times daily), Petadolex® (25-75 mg twice daily to three times daily, maximum 150 mg/day), and Tesalin® (Ze 339; 1-2 tablets twice daily to three times daily).

Ginkgo *(Ginkgo biloba)*: This plant was shown in one trial in asthmatic humans to improve forced expiratory volume significantly over placebo. A dose of 15 g of a concentrated extract was administered three times daily (Li, 1997). A protective effect is exerted by ginkgolides on platelet-activating factor (PAF)-induced bronchoconstriction and airway hyperactivity. Oral or intravenous injection of ginkgolide B antagonizes cardiovascular impairments and bronchoconstriction induced by PAF. Ginkgolide B does not appear to interfere with cyclooxygenase, but it does have an effect in an earlier step involving PAF receptors and phospholipase activation. Eosinophil infiltration occurs in asthma and in allergic reactions, the number of eosinophils increasing during late phase. Because PAF is a potent activator of eosinophil function, it has been argued that ginkgolide B may interfere with the late-phase response (Hosford, 1988). A randomized, double-blind, crossover study involved patients with atopic asthma who were challenged with a specific dust or pollen antigen. After 6.5 hours, participants were subjected to a provocation test with acetylcholine. Mixed ginkgolide standardized extract, 40 mg three times daily, or placebo was given during the 3 days before the test, and a final single dose of 120 mg of extract was given 2 hours before the challenge. Results suggested that ginkgolides were effective in both the early phase and the late phase of airway hyperactivity (Braquet, 1987).

Tylophora *(Tylophora indica/asthmatica)*: This traditional Ayurvedic herb is used for asthma. In vitro studies suggest that constituents from the plant are anti-inflammatory and may suppress mast cell activation. Clinical trial results, however, have been mixed. The human dose is 200 to 400 mg of dried leaf, or 1 to 2 mL of tincture, divided daily. Reported adverse effects include nausea, vomiting, and mouth soreness (Shivpuri, 1969; Shivpuri, 1972; Thiruvengadam, 1978; Gupta, 1979).

Expectorant herbs

Traditional practitioners from many cultures have noted a connection between the secretory functions of the respiratory and digestive tracts. A simple observation has been made that vomiting is preceded by salivation and nausea—but also by respiratory secretions. Ancient medical strategies to reduce phlegm in the respiratory tract concentrate on abnormalities in digestive function. This related reflex is not surprising when one considers the common embryologic origin of the bronchial and alimentary epithelium, as well as the shared vagal innervation. Herbs that cause expectoration do so by one of two mechanisms. Reflex expectorants irritate gastric mucosa, and some (like ipecac, *Cephaelis)* are used most often as emetics. Herbs that contain saponins (mullein, licorice, ivy, cowslip, senega snakeroot, and soap bark) probably stimulate the gastric mucosa. Mucolytic herbs increase the water content of respiratory mucus.

Stimulating expectorants

Lobelia *(Lobelia inflata)*: This herb has not been investigated in controlled trials for its effects on the respiratory system. King's (Felter, 1898) describes the expectorant characteristics of the herb as follows: "It improves innervation and the circulation, and is one of the best remedies to employ in congestive conditions. It is frequently indicated in pleurisy and pleuropneumonia.... Acute pneumonia, with tendency to congestion, the breathing being oppressed, is quickly relieved by lobelia. Chronic pneumonia, bronchitis, and laryngitis are all conditions in which lobelia will be of great service... It is a remedy of great value in chronic catarrh, dry, hard, or barking coughs, colds, and all forms of irritation of the respiratory tract, with oppression. It relaxes the tissues, favors expectoration when a large quantity of mucus is secreted and there is want of power to remove it. The indications for this drug are... difficult respiration, oppression anywhere in the chest, with accumulation of the bronchial secretions, cough with loud mucous rates within the chest..." Milks (1949) lists the following doses: Horses—4 to 30 mL of fluid extract and 30 to 60 mL of tincture; dogs—0.03 to 1.3 mL of fluid extract and 0.2 to 2 mL of tincture.

BLOODROOT *(SANGUINARIA CANADENSIS):* This plant has not been scientifically investigated for possible usefulness in respiratory disease. King's (Felter, 1898) describes its use in this way: "Its action upon the pulmonary organs is somewhat similar to that of lobelia. It is important as a stimulating expectorant, to be used after active inflammation has been subdued... It restores the bronchial secretions when scanty, and checks them when profuse... when... the secretions are checked, it restores them, and removes the dry, harsh cough. It is useful in both acute and chronic bronchitis, laryngitis, sore throat, and acute or chronic nasal catarrh. It acts as a sedative to the irritable mucous surfaces, promotes expectoration, and stimulates their functions... Pharyngitis, with red and irritable mucous membranes, and burning, smarting, or tickling, is cured by it... In pneumonia, after the inflammatory stage has passed, it may be given in 1- or 2-drop doses, frequently repeated, or it may be combined with wild cherry, lycopus, or eucalyptus." Bloodroot does not make an appearance in the old veterinary pharmacopoeias. The human dose recommended by the US Dispensatory (1918) is 0.13 g. This herb is more safely used as part of a formula.

SQUILL *(URGINEA MARITIMA):* This herb was formerly used as a stimulating expectorant, but it contains cardiac glycosides and was said to be a stimulating irritant to the kidney. This plant has more powerful gastrointestinal adverse effects than digitalis. Winslow (1908) recommended it for ascites from heart disease but also said it was indicated in bronchitis with "scanty secretion, or when exudation is excessive, to improve the tone of the bronchial mucous membrane." Milks said that it was a powerful and commonly employed expectorant. The dose given in Milks is as follows: Horses—fluid extract 4 to 8 mL, tincture 15 to 30 mL, syrup 15 mL; dogs—0.06 to 0.3 mL, tincture 0.3 to 2 mL, and syrup 2 to 4 mL. No studies can be found to support its use. Considering the toxic cardiac and kidney effects, this herb should probably be avoided.

IVY LEAF *(HEDERA HELIX):* This herb contains saponins, which are thought to confer expectorant activity. A meta-analysis in 2003 examined five randomized, controlled trials that used ivy extract for the treatment of chronic bronchitis. Only one trial included a control, and three met the inclusion criteria. Analysis showed that ivy leaf extract improved respiratory function in children with bronchial asthma, but more trials were recommended (Hofmann, 2003). The preparation used in the placebo-controlled trial of children aged 4 to 12 years was a hydroethanolic extract, given at 35 mg/dose, equivalent to 210 mg of crude herb. The dose used for trials in adults was 60 mg of the extract, equivalent to 400 mg of crude herb.

MULLEIN *(VERBASCUM THAPSUS, V. DENSIFLORUM):* This is an expectorant and demulcent, but its primary action is thought to be as an expectorant because of its content of saponins (such as verbascosaponin). It is traditionally recommended for bronchitis, tracheitis, laryngitis, asthma, dry cough, and catarrh (1-4 mL three times daily to four times daily; dried herb $^{1}/_{2}$-$^{3}/_{4}$ teaspoon [3-4 g] three times daily).

PRIMULA ROOT *(PRIMULA VERIS, P. ELATIOR):* This is used occasionally as an expectorant, although this does not seem to be a primary traditional use for the plant. It contains saponins. The dose for adult humans is about 1 g of crude herb divided daily. The only scientific studies found on primula used a proprietary formula of thyme and primula, with beneficial results seen in people and horses (van den Hoven, 2003). See section on equine COPD.

SOAP BARK *(QUILLAJA SAPONARIA):* This herb contains saponins and is said to be similar in constituents and activity to senega (see next paragraph). No recent scientific studies have been found to support the use of soap bark. King's recommends $^{1}/_{2}$ to 1 oz of infusion for adult humans.

SENEGA SNAKEROOT *(POLYGALA SENEGA):* No recent scientific studies have been found to support the use of senega. King's describes the use of senega as follows: "Its expectorant properties render it very useful in chronic catarrh, ... bronchorrhoea, chronic bronchitis, with profuse secretion, humoral asthma... In active inflammation, its use is contraindicated."

GRINDELIA (*GRINDELIA SQUARROSA* AND OTHER SPECIES): This plant contains saponins, as well as a volatile oil. No recent scientific studies have been found to support its use. King's recommends it as "especially efficient in asthma, giving prompt relief, and effecting cures in cases previously rebellious to medication. . It has likewise been found efficient in bronchial affections..." The dose for adult humans is as follows: fluid extract, from 15 minims to 1 fluid drachm (0.9-3.7 mL), repeated every 3 or 4 hours; [tincture], 5 to 40 drops.

LICORICE *(GLYCYRRHIZA GLABRA):* This plant contains a saponin (glycyrrhizin), but some authors believe it exerts expectorant activity primarily by other, unexplored, means. Veterinary doses vary, as most authors consider the herb harmless. See monograph on licorice for a discussion of whole versus deglycyrrhizinated DGL form.

Mucolytic expectorants

AROMATIC HERBS, SUCH AS CINNAMON, GINGER, FENNEL, ANISEED, CLOVE, SPRUCE NEEDLE, CAJEPUT, NIAOULI, AND TURPENTINE: Volatile oils have "bronchomucotropic" activity. They are well absorbed orally and are partially excreted through the lungs, acting on bronchial mucous glands as they pass through the bronchial tree. (Schulz, 2001). A typical terpene product called "Ozothin" was studied for its effects on the bronchial glands. In this study, the aromatic compound selectively stimulated serous glands while depressing the function of mucous glands, resulting in a net liquefaction of bronchial secretions (Lorenz, 1985).

PUNGENT HERBS, SUCH AS HORSERADISH, GARLIC, MUSTARD, AND CAYENNE: These may increase blood flow to the lower respiratory tract, stimulated by an increase in blood flow to the upper gastrointestinal mucosa, which occurs after these spicy herbs are ingested. Horseradish and mustard contain sulphoraphanes that may interact with sulfide linkages in mucus as well.

Demulcent herbs

The pharynx, larynx, and trachea contain mechanoreceptors that are sensitive to irritation; the demulcent herbs coat irritated pharyngeal tissue on a short-term basis. Some herbalists speculate that the systemic effect on the lower respiratory tract is mediated via the effect of mucilage on the gastrointestinal tract.

MARSHMALLOW ***(ALTHAEA OFFICINALIS):*** Intragastric administration to cats of an extract of marshmallow root, or the polysaccharide fraction, demonstrated significant antitussive activity, depressing the cough that resulted from irritation of laryngopharyngeal and tracheobronchial mucosa. The isolated polysaccharide, administered at 50 mg/kg, was as effective as marshmallow syrup administered at 1 g/kg and was more effective than the whole extract, administered at 100 mg/kg (Nosal'ova, 1992).

SLIPPERY ELM ***(ULMUS FULVA):*** This demulcent was thought to have expectorant qualities as well by traditional practitioners. King's says that, "for mucous inflammations of the lungs . . . used freely in the form of a mucilaginous drink (1 ounce of the powdered bark to 1 pint of water), it is highly beneficial, as well as in diarrhoea, dysentery, coughs, pleurisy, strangury, and sore throat, in all of which it tends powerfully to allay the inflammation."

ENGLISH PLANTAIN ***(PLANTAGO MAJOR):*** Two observational studies have suggested that plantain has mild antitussive activity, with miminal adverse effects (Matev, 1982; Kraft, 1997a).

ICELAND MOSS ***(CETRARIA ISLANDICA):*** This lichen contains unique depsidones (lichenic acids), although the polysaccharides are considered most important in its demulcent effects. Results of a randomized trial suggested that Iceland moss can prevent dryness and inflammation of the oral cavity in patients who had undergone surgery of the nasal septum who were forced to undergo prolonged mouth breathing. Emollient effects were found with the daily use of 0.48 mg Iceland moss lozenges (Kempe, 1997). The human dose is 4 to 6 g/day of cut herb powdered or made into an infusion, 4 to 6 mL of the fluid extract (1:1), or 20 to 30 mL of the tincture (1:5).

IRISH MOSS ***(CHONDRUS CRISPUS):*** This herb, also called carrageen, is a common ingredient in cough mixtures available in most drug stores. Cook (1869) describes its use as follows: "for its demulcent influence in bronchial and pulmonary irritation, diarrhea and dysentery, and irritability of the kidneys and bladder. It is most available in recent colds and coughs, where it may be used freely in warm decoction. Its mucilaginous, demulcent properties are used traditionally to reduce coughing."

COLTSFOOT ***(TUSSILAGO FARFARA):*** This plant contains 6% to 10% mucilage and inulin, but some specimens also contain pyrrolizidine alkaloids. King's recommended the plant as "useful in coughs, asthma, whooping-cough, laryngitis, pharyngitis, bronchitis, and other pulmonary affections . . ." A sesquiterpene, tussilagone, was shown to produce a pressor effect in anesthetized dogs (0.02-0.3 mg/kg), cats (0.02-0.5 mg/kg), and rats (0.4-4 mg/kg) when administered intravenously (Li, 1988). Tussilagone also stimulated respiration in anesthetized animals. The herb is approved by Commission E for acute catarrhal or inflammatory conditions of the respiratory tract; it is noted that although coltsfoot should not be used on a long-term basis because of its possible pyrrolizidine content, it is safe for acute use. The human dose is 2 to 4 mL of the tincture (1:5), or 1 to 2 tsp of the dried flower and leaf (dry or in infusion), three times daily.

COMFREY ***(SYMPHYTUM OFFICINALE):*** This demulcent herb has traditionally been used for coughing and bronchial irritation. Unfortunately, internal use of the herb has been associated with at least four human deaths, and in laboratory animal studies, it is carcinogenic. It is banned in Australia and Europe. It consistently contains pyrrolizidine alkaloids, and recent studies point to an additional quinoid toxin. Commission E recommends it for external use only; however, some traditional herbalists still use it for **short** periods.

MULLEIN ***(VERBASCUM THASPUS):*** This plant contains only 3% mucilage, and although it is usually listed as a demulcent antitussive, most of its action is probably expectorant, which is caused by saponins.

FENUGREEK ***(TRIGONELLA FOENUM-GRAECUM):*** According to King's, the "only property worth mentioning is its emolliency. It has been used to allay irritation of the throat and breathing passages. Respiratory irritation is thought to be relieved by its internal use."

Spasmolytic herbs

Bronchodilating herbs may suppress cough simply by relaxing bronchoconstriction, which is thought to stimulate some types of cough receptors. Bronchodilating herbs such as ephedra also tend to dry mucosal secretions.

Mechanisms by which bronchial tone is mediated include the following:

1. Parasympathetic system maintains mild bronchoconstriction.
2. Sympathetic system causes constriction via α_1 receptors, and dilation via β_2 receptors.

3. Vasoactive peptides mediate bronchodilation through nonadrenergic, noncholinergic neuroendocrine mechanisms.

LOBELIA ***(LOBELIA INFLATA):*** King's says this about the herb: "It is for its antispasmodic effects that it is given in asthmatic paroxysms, spasmodic croup, and whooping-cough. . . . It has come to be the first of remedies for spasmodic asthma." Lobeline is a nicotinic acid receptor agonist (mimics actions of acetylcholine at nicotinic sites) similar to but weaker than nicotine. Experimentally, it stimulates respiration and induces coughing. However, some trials suggest that lobeline may improve lung function, possibly by suppressing bronchial constriction and thinning mucus (Pocta, 1970). Lobelia is a low-dose herb.

EPHEDRA ***(EPHEDRA SINICA):*** This plant contains sympathomimetic alkaloids (ephedrine, pseudoephedrine, and others) that have bronchodilatory, decongestant, and cardiac stimulant effects. The herb is not now commercially available in many countries, although US Food and Drug Administration (FDA) language leaves the door open for professional herbalists to use it, and current civil cases in the United States (as of 2005) may make it available again to consumers in low doses. The herb was used most commonly in the context of traditional Chinese formulas.

GRINDELIA ***(GRINDELIA CAMPORUM, G. ROBUSTA, G. HIRSUTA, G. HUMILIS, G. SQUARROSA):*** The volatile oil and resin from these herbs have slight antispasmodic activity. Supporting data could not be found, but King's describes the use of grindelia as "especially efficient in *asthma,* giving prompt relief, and effecting cures in cases previously rebellious to medication. . . . It has likewise been found efficient in bronchial affections . . ."

YERBA SANTA ***(ERIODICTYON CALIFORNICUM):*** This herb is described in Ellingwood (1919) this way: "It is of value in chronic bronchitis, chronic pneumonitis and in phthisis pulmonalis, in allaying the cough which seems to increase the patient's feebleness and advance the development of the disease. It is an excellent remedy combined with Grindelia robusta. It acts well in all forms of cough where there is dryness of the mucous membranes, in conjunction with other directly indicated remedies. It is prepared in the form of a syrup . . ."

HYSSOP ***(HYSSOPUS OFFICINALIS):*** This is traditionally used as a mild antispasmodic and expectorant, because of its volatile oil content. It is not well studied.

RED ROOT ***(CEANOTHUS AMERICANUS):*** This is stated in King's to be antispasmodic and expectorant, and to be of value in chronic bronchitis, asthma, whooping cough, and other "pulmonary affections."

THYME ***(THYMUS VULGARIS):*** This herb contains volatile oils and flavonoids that suppress bronchospasm and are mucolytic; the herb also has antibacterial activity (Bisset, 1994; Van Den Broucke, 1983; Muller-Limmroth, 1980). It was not used much by the Eclectic medical doctors, but Lloyd's *History of the Vegetable Drugs of the U.S.P.* (1911) states that it was used in veterinary medicine as oil of origanum or oil of thyme.

CHUAN XIONG ***(LIGUSTICUM WALLICHII):*** This plant was shown in one human clinical trial to improve forced expiratory volume when compared with placebo treatment. A parallel study in guinea pigs suggested that the mechanism of action involved tracheal smooth muscle relaxation and suppression of thromboxane B2. The dose used was 10 mL three times daily, presumably of the decoction (Shao, 1994).

Anticatarrhal herbs

Catarrh is inflammation (and usually subsequent discharge from) mucous membranes, especially in the respiratory tract. Catarrh is a feature of allergic rhinitis and sinusitis, and is also a feature of infections, such as viral upper respiratory infections.

PLEURISY ROOT ***(ASCLEPIAS TUBEROSA):*** This was considered in King's to be one of the best anticatarrhal herbs for the respiratory tract—primarily the upper respiratory tract. It is not a well-studied herb and it contains cardiac glycosides, so high doses should be avoided.

EYEBRIGHT ***(EUPHRASIA OFFICINALIS):*** This plant has been used for acute, watery rhinitis. It is not well studied.

GOLDENSEAL ***(HYDRASTIS CANADENSIS):*** This plant has not been studied for catarrhal respiratory disorders. King's describes its use in this way: "For that disagreeable state accompanying nasal and pharyngeal catarrh, in which the mucus forms in gelatinous masses and drops into the throat, hydrastis is probably without an equal. It should be applied locally and also administered internally."

ELDER FLOWER ***(SAMBUCUS NIGRA):*** This is considered a diaphoretic; it has been suggested in a human clinical trial to hasten recovery from influenza.

OTHER HERBS: Other anticatarrhals, especially for the lower respiratory tract: Bryony, Polygala, Sage, Mullein.

Other anticatarrhals, especially for the upper respiratory tract include: garlic, Indian barberry, eyebright, elder flower, and goldenrod.

Decongestant herbs

Drug decongestants are sympathomimetics or H1 blockers. Ephedra is the only herb of assistance in this category.

Diaphoretic herbs

These herbs cause sweating, sometimes because of inherent qualities in the herb, and sometimes because they were administered as hot teas. Traditionally, these herbs were administered to help the body release "toxins" through the skin by stimulating sweating; they were thought to lower fevers. It is also possible that some of them raise body temperature slightly and transiently, hastening resolution of viral or bacterial infection. The relevance of diaphoretic herb therapy in small animals without the ability to sweat is unknown. Horses and other species that sweat may benefit from their use. The best known diaphoretic herbs are yarrow, elder flower, ginger, cayenne, garlic, boneset, lemon balm, peppermint, linden, and hyssop.

Pectorals

This is an old term that included herbs used in the treatment of diseases of the chest, more often respiratory remedies. The term is too vague to be of much modern use.

Other herbs that have been used for respiratory conditions include astragalus root *(Astragalus membranaceus),* black cohosh, ground ivy *(Glechoma),* lomatium *(Lomatium dissectum),* osha *(Ligusticum porteri),* stillingia *(Stillingia sylvatica),* thyme *(Thymus vulgaris),* usnea *(Usnea barbata), Picrorrhiza kurroa, Solanum xanthocarpum/trilobatum,* Boswellia *(Boswellia serrata),* and sundew *(Drosera rotundifolia).*

Review of Specific Respiratory Conditions

Allergic bronchitis *(feline asthma, canine chronic bronchitis)*

Therapeutic Rationale

- Manage underlying disorders, including lung parasites and infection.
- Manage immune reactivity and inflammation.
- Control bronchoconstriction.
- Loosen airway mucus.

Formulas for allergic bronchitis should include expectorants (mucolytic and stimulating), antispasmodics, antiallergics, immune-modulating herbs, demulcents, and perhaps antimicrobials and adaptogens.

A prescription for allergic bronchitis follows:

Elecampane, mullein, or ivy	25% (stimulating expectorants)
Fennel or ginger	25% (mucolytic expectorants)
Lobelia for acute exacerbation, khella *(Ammi visnaga)* for long-term use	15% (antispasmodics)
Iceland moss or marshmallow	20% (demulcents)
Pyrrolizidine alkaloid (PA)–ree butterbur or licorice	15% (antiallergics)

Human herbalists have recommended various recipes for the treatment of asthma. These may include Reishi, ephedra, anise, *Euphorbia pilufera,* Ginkgo leaf, Khella, Lobelia, grindelia, wild cherry, motherwort and Licorice. Chinese formulas for asthma may include coltsfoot flower, ephedra, licorice, and apricot seed.

Weiss (1988) provides formulas that contain Primula tincture, Ephedra tincture, Anise tincture, and thyme syrup or fluid extract.

For cats that become stressed by administration, marshmallow glycetracts mixed with food or perilla seeds added to food may be used.

Equine chronic obstructive pulmonary disease or heaves

Therapeutic Rationale

- Manage underlying disorders, including lung parasites and infection.
- Manage immune reactivity and inflammation.
- Control bronchoconstriction.
- Loosen airway mucus.

Herbs listed in the allergic bronchitis section (earlier) may also be used for horses with heaves.

Bronchipret®, with extracts of *Thymus vulgaris* and *Primula veris,* is a proprietary remedy for the treatment of human bronchitis. The formula was tested in five warmblood horses with confirmed recurrent airway obstruction by van den Hoven and associates (2003). The horses were administered 2400 mg of Thyme extract and 900 mg of Primula root extract twice daily. Lung compliance, pulmonary pressure, and airway resistance were all significantly improved after 1 month of treatment, but the severity of clinical signs and arterial oxygen partial pressure did not improve.

Titus (1865) recommended that horses be fed no hay, and that 1 tablespoonful of ginger be added to each meal. He thought the best fodder for heavy horses was "good, bright cornstalks." In addition, doses of the following were given:

Tincture of aromatic sulphur acid 1 drachm
1 pint of water

To be followed by an alterative formula, which consisted of these ingredients:

Powdered ginger	2 oz
Powdered gentian	2 oz
Salt	3 oz
Cream of tartar	2 oz
Powdered licorice	2 oz
Powdered elecampane	1 oz
Powdered caraway seed	2 oz
Powdered balm of gilead buds	2 oz

This powder, 1 oz, was given twice daily in food.

Another "cure for heaves" given by Titus was:

Sumach bobs (the flowering head of sumac)	3 pounds
Ginger	1 pound
Mustard seed	1 pound
Rosin (pine resin)	1 pound
Air-slaked lime	1 pound
Cream of tartar	6 oz

This was mixed and divided into 30 doses, given once daily in the morning.

Titus gives a recipe for a strong expectorant powder that contains 2 oz powdered ipecac, 2 oz powdered lobelia, 2 oz powdered bloodroot, and 4 oz powdered licorice.

For a cough in horses, Titus recommended cutting the "boughs of cedar or white pine" finely, and adding it to the grain.

Titus prepared two recipes for cough balsams for horses—one of which contained the active ingredient paregoric. The one containing only herbs is provided here:

Cough balsam No. 1 (the ingredients below are mixed and the dose is $^1/_2$ oz)

Molasses	1 pint
Tincture lobelia	4 oz
Essence peppermint	1 oz
Essence anise	1 oz

More modern approaches to the treatment of heaves may be found in Chapter 21, Herbal medicine in equine practice.

Feline viral upper respiratory disease *(especially herpesvirus)*

Therapeutic Rationale

- Provide nutritional and fluid support.
- Control secondary bacterial infections.

Formulas for viral upper respiratory infection may include antiviral herbs, antibacterial herbs, expectorants, and immune support.

A prescription for viral respiratory disease follows:

Echinacea (immune stimulant, possibly antimicrobial)	50%
Ginger or fennel (mucolytic expectorant)	25%
Goldenseal (anticatarrhal)	25%

In vitro, quite a number of herbs have been shown to have antiviral activity, at least against herpesvirus. Lemon balm has been the subject of more investigations than many other herbs and may be worth including.

Human herbalists may recommend any of the following for "the common cold": Yarrow, Garlic or Onion, Horseradish, Mustard, Cayenne, Boneset, Chamomile, Peppermint, Elder, and Linden.

Another strategy for chronic cat flu is to provide concentrated mushroom extracts, which can be given in small doses mixed with food. The author's cat (SW) loves fresh mushrooms.

Rhinitis/sinusitis

Therapeutic Rationale

- Depends on cause, which may be infectious, neoplastic, allergic, or traumatic, or may be related to a foreign body.

For allergic rhinitis/sinusitis, a typical formula might contain these ingredients:

- Nettle or butterbur (antiallergic)
- Goldenseal, Pleurisy root, Ephedra, or Euphrasia (anticatarrhal)

One prescription for idiopathic sinusitis/rhinitis is provided:

Echinacea	20% (immune enhancing, anti-inflammatory, antibacterial, antiviral, vulnerary)
Nettle	20% (astringent, circulatory stimulant, nutritive, hemostatic)
Eyebright	20% (anticatarrhal, astringent, anti-inflammatory)
Elder flowers	20% (anticatarrhal, diaphoretic)
Marshmallow	20% (demulcent, vulnerary)

Pneumonia; lower respiratory infection

Therapeutic Rationale

- Address cause of infection through culture and sensitivity testing.
- Move airway mucus.
- Provide immune support.

Although antibiotics are necessary for life-threatening infection, herbs may provide support that is particularly helpful for chronic cases. A basic recipe on which to build would include:

Echinacea (immune stimulating, antimicrobial)	35%
Astragalus (immune stimulating)	15%
Fennel or thyme (mucolytic expectorant)	25%
Garlic or elecampane (stimulating expectorant)	25%

Historical recipes for large animals featured stimulating expectorants prominently, along with demulcents. Titus gives a recipe for an expectorant powder that contains 2 oz powdered ipecac, 2 oz powdered lobelia, 2 oz powdered bloodroot, and 4 oz powdered licorice.

For cough in cattle, Titus recommended the following recipe, mixed and divided into 6 parts, with 1 part being administered every 6 hours in linseed tea, or as a ball in syrup:

Powdered elecampane	2 oz
Powdered licorice root	2 oz
Powdered anise seed	2 oz
Powdered honey	4 oz

For cough in sheep, Titus recommended the following, mixed and given as 1 gill every 6 hours:

Lobelia *root*	1 drachm
Licorice root	4 drachm
Bloodroot	2 drachm
Mandrake root	2 drachm
Boiling water	1 quart

After this formula began to "work on the bowels," he recommended administering a teaspoonful of the following combination three times daily:

Powdered licorice root	2 oz
Powdered ipecac	2 drachm

For pneumonia in swine, the recipe was as follows:

Lobelia herb	4 oz
Licorice	2 oz
Boiling water	4 quarts

The tea was administered 1 gill at a time, every 15 to 20 minutes, until symptoms abated; then, the following mixture was administered:

Mandrake root	1 oz
Cream of tartar	2 oz

This was to be divided into 6 doses and given every 6 hours until signs improved.

HERBS FOR URINARY TRACT CONDITIONS

General Considerations

In the urinary system, the emphasis is on supporting the normal functioning of the kidneys and bladder, which is to excrete metabolic wastes in urine. It is no surprise that traditional herbal medicine "diuretics" played an important role in the treatment of urinary tract disorders. However, the term *diuretic* in herbal medicine is not the same as that in conventional medicine; it can be used in a number of other ways. Traditionally, herbs were given as a decoction or infusion for urinary conditions, and the additional water consumption would have produced an observable diuresis. Hence, many herbs were classified as diuretics, whether they had genuine diuretic action or not. The "flushing" of the bladder naturally assisted in the treatment of cystitis. This strategy can also be employed in treating animals. Simply encouraging animals to drink more water or broth may accomplish the same end. Nonetheless, in many traditional herbal writings, diuretics were herbs that were considered to enhance excretion of waste through the kidneys (perhaps better classed as "diuretic depuratives"); they included herbs like Dandelion leaf *(Taraxacum officinale),* Cleavers *(Gallium aparine),* Burdock *(Arctium lappa),* Red clover *(Trifolium pretense),* Heartsease *(Viola tricolor),* and Celery *(Apium graveolens).* Improving elimination through other systems of the body with the use of these alteratives and diuretics was another important strategy that aided one of the most important elimination systems—the urinary tract.

Mechanisms of Interest

Diuretics

Although diuretics might not be the most important agents needed in the treatment of urinary tract disorders, many of the herbs outlined in the following section have diuretic activity that might be useful. Herbal diuretics may also be useful in cases of edema or fluid retention and tissue congestion, and in their role as gentle "blood cleaners," when an excess of metabolic waste is being filtered through the kidneys.

In Europe, phytotherapists have proposed the term *Aquaretic* to describe those herbs that create actual diuresis. It is suggested that these herbs act directly on the glomerulus to increase water excretion, but their impact on electrolytes is neutral (Werk, 1994). In other words, aquaretics work by promoting the formation of urine. Diuretic activity may also be due to the mineral (electrolyte) content of herbs. In decoctions of herbs traditionally regarded as diuretics, the ratio of potassium to sodium was found to be higher compared with other herbs (Szentmihályi, 1998).

Herbs with diuretic or aquaretic activity are discussed here.

NETTLE ***(URTICA DIOICA):*** In an open, uncontrolled study, 32 patients with myocardial or chronic venous insufficiency were treated with 15 mL of nettle juice three times daily for 2 weeks (ESCP, 1999). A significant increase in daily volume of urine was observed throughout the study, and it has been proposed that the diuretic activity of aqueous extracts of nettle may be attributed to the high potassium content (Szentmihályi, 1998).

PARSLEY ***(PETROSELINUM CRISPUM):*** Edema and dropsy have been treated with parsley traditionally in Europe. Galen said, "It provoketh the urine mightily." In France, it was used to treat kidney stones. One experimental study provides evidence for the advocated diuretic effect. Rats offered an aqueous parsley seed extract to drink eliminated a significantly larger volume of urine per 24 hours as compared with when they were drinking water. The mechanism of action of parsley seems to be mediated through an inhibition of the Na^+-K^+ pump that would lead to a reduction in Na^+ and K^+ reabsorption, leading thus to an osmotic water flow into the lumen, and diuresis (Kreydiyyeh, 2002).

CORN SILK ***(ZEA MAYS):*** This herb is stated to possess diuretic and stone-reducing properties. It has been used for cystitis, urethritis, nocturnal enuresis, prostatitis, and, specifically, acute or chronic inflammation of the urinary system (Wren, 1988). The diuretic action confirmed in animals may be due to the high concentration of potassium (2.7%) (Bradley, 1992). Maizenic acid is also claimed to be active; it acts as a cardiac tonic, thus stimulating diuretic action (Willard, 1991). However, no influence of corn silk was recorded for 12- and 24-hour urine output, or sodium excretion, in people tested under standardized conditions in a placebo-controlled, double-blind, crossover model (Doan, 1992).

BUCHU ***(AGATHOSMA BETULINA):*** This is stated to possess urinary antiseptic and diuretic properties. It has been used for cystitis, urethritis, prostatitis, and, specifically, acute catarrhal cystitis (Wren, 1988).

CELERY ***(APIUM GRAVEOLENS):*** This herb is stated to possess mild diuretic and urinary antiseptic properties. It has been used for urinary tract inflammation (Wren, 1988).

COUCH GRASS ***(AGROPYRON REPENS):*** This plant is stated to possess diuretic properties. It has been used for cystitis, urethritis, prostatitis, benign prostatic hypertrophy, renal calculus, lithuria, and, specifically, cystitis with irritation or inflammation of the urinary tract (Wren, 1988). It contains mannitol as a constituent, which is an osmotic diuretic that in small quantities may confer a mild diuretic effect.

LAVENDER ***(LAVANDULA OFFICINALIS):*** The aqueous extract of lavender was compared with acetazolamide. It accelerated elimination of fluid and, at the peak of diuretic response, urinary osmolarity was significantly less than controls; sodium excretion was moderate compared with a synthetic diuretic acetazolamide. The stability of aldosterone and the absence of correlation with plasma sodium concentrations, coupled with the observed clearance of free water, show that the increase in diuresis is of tubular origin (Elhajili, 2001).

DANDELION ***(TARAXACUM OFFICINALIS):*** A diuretic effect in rats and mice was documented in early studies for dandelion extracts, following oral administration (Rácz-Kotilla, 1974). Herb extracts were found to produce greater diuresis than root extracts; a dose of 50 mL (equivalent to 2 g dried herb/kg body weight) produced an effect comparable with that of furosemide, at 80 mg/kg. By contrast, no significant increases in urine volume or sodium excretion were observed in mice following oral administration of leaf or root extracts, or of purified fractions (Hook, 1993). Similarly, oral and intravenous administration of an ethanolic extract of dandelion root failed to produce a diuretic effect in laboratory animals (Tita, 1993).

JUNIPER ***(JUNIPERUS COMMUNIS):*** According to some sources, juniper increases urine volume without loss of electrolytes such as potassium (Blumenthal, 2000). The diuretic activity of juniper berries is attributed to the volatile oil terpinen-4-ol and to hydrophilic constituents that are reported to increase the glomerular filtration rate (Tyler, 1993). Terpenin-4-ol is also stated to be an irritant to the kidneys, although in a later review by the same author, no such statement was made, and the oil was stated to represent no hazards (Tisserand, 1995).

BEARBERRY (*ARCTOSTAPHYLOS UVA URSI*): An aqueous extract was tested for diuretic activity in rats; pharmacologic evaluation revealed that it led to an increase in urine flow (Beaux, 1999).

TRIBULUS (*TRIBULUS TERRESTRIS*): In rats, the aqueous extract of *T. terrestris,* in an oral dose of 5 g/kg, elicited a positive diuresis, which was slightly greater than that of furosemide. Na^+, K^+, and Cl^- concentrations in the urine had also increased greatly (Al Ali, 2003).

OTHER HERBS: A total of 23 herbs traditionally used as diuretics were examined for their effects on horse kidney (Na^+ + K^+)–adenosine triphosphatase (ATPase). Among these Atractylodes *(Atractylodes lanceae* and *A. japonica), Plantago asiatica herb and seed,* and Alisma *(Alisma orientalis)* were shown to have strong inhibitory effects on kidney (Na^+ + K^+)-ATPase activity (Satoh, 1991).

Anti-inflammatory herbs

KAVA (*PIPER METHYSTICUM*): Traditional uses listed for kava rhizome in standard herbal and pharmaceutical reference texts include cystitis, urethritis, infection or inflammation of the genitourinary tract, and rheumatism (British Herbal Medicine Association, 2003).

Antilithics

Antilithic herbs are used to dissolve urinary stones and reduce their formation; they may also help a patient to expel stones. Possible mechanisms of action are discussed in the following paragraphs.

Seven plants with suspected application to prevent and treat kidney stone formation were studied. Changes in urolithiasis risk factors (i.e., citraturia, calciuria, phosphaturia, pH, and diuresis) were evaluated. The herb infusions were believed by the author to cause change primarily due to disinfectant action and because of saponin content. Some solvent action was postulated due to alkalinizing capacity of some of these infusions (Grases, 1994). These include Vervain *(Verbena officinalis),* Lithospermum *(Lithospermum officinale),* Dandelion *(Taraxacum officinale),* Horsetail *(Equisetum arvense),* Bearberry *(Arctostaphylos uva ursi),* Burdock *(Arctium lappa),* and Tufted catchfly *(Silene saxifraga).*

CORN SILK (*ZEA MAYS*): In rats, corn silk was investigated in terms of risk factors for kidney stones; however, an extract did not influence citraturia, calciuria, or urinary pH (Grases, 1994).

FENUGREEK SEEDS (*TRIGONELLA FOENUM-GRAECUM*): Another study investigated the effect of fenugreek seed on experimentally induced kidney stones. Oxalate urolithiasis in male rats was produced by 3% glycolic acid in the diet. Daily treatment with fenugreek significantly decreased the quantity of calcium oxalate deposited in the kidneys. These results supported the similar use of fenugreek in Saudi folk medicine (Ahsan, 1989).

COUCH GRASS (*AGROPYRON REPENS*): This plant did not appear to have any effect on the main urolithiasis risk factors in calcium oxalate urolithiais in rats (Grases, 1995).

STONEROOT (*COLLINSONIA CANADENSIS*): This is stated to possess antilithic, litholytic, mild diaphoretic, and diuretic properties. Traditionally, it has been used for renal calculus, lithuria, and, specifically, urinary calculus (British Herbal Pharmacopoeia, 1983; Wren, 1988).

GRAVELROOT (*EUPATORIUM PURPUREUM*): This herb is stated to possess antilithic, diuretic, antiinflammatory and antirheumatic properties. Traditionally, it has been used for urinary calculus, cystitis, dysuria, urethritis, prostatitis, rheumatism, gout, and, specifically, renal or vesicular calculi (British Herbal Pharmacopoeia, 1983; Wren, 1988, Habtemariam 2001).

HYDRANGEA (*HYDRANGEA ARBORESCENS*): This is stated to possess diuretic and antilithic properties. Traditionally, it has been used for cystitis, urethritis, urinary calculi, prostatitis, enlarged prostate gland, and, specifically, urinary calculi with gravel and cystitis (British Herbal Pharmacopoeia, 1983; Wren, 1988).

CRANBERRY (*VACCINIUM MACROCARPON*): In a study undertaken to investigate the potential influence of cranberry juice on urinary biochemical and physicochemical risk factors associated with the formation of calcium oxalate kidney stones, the ingestion of cranberry juice significantly altered three key urinary risk factors. Oxalate and phosphate excretion decreased, and citrate excretion increased. In addition, a decrease was noted in the relative supersaturation of calcium oxalate, which tended to be significantly lower than that induced by water alone. It was concluded that cranberry juice has antilithogenic properties (McHarg, 2003). However, cranberry juice has a moderately high concentration of oxalate, a common component of kidney stones in humans. In five healthy volunteers, urinary oxalate levels in volunteers significantly increased by an average of 43.4% while they were receiving cranberry tablets. The excretion of potential lithogenic ions calcium, phosphate, and sodium also increased. However, inhibitors of stone formation—magnesium and potassium—rose as well (Terris, 2001).

CRATAEVA (*CRATAEVA NURVALA*): This herb significantly inhibited bladder stone formation in an experimental model in rats. The bladders of treated animals showed less edema, ulceration, and cellular infiltration when compared with those of controls (Deshpande, 1982). A crude extract at 100 mg/kg given orally to rats significantly reduced stone formation (81%) (Prabhakar, 1997). The effects of oral administration of *Crataeva nurvala* bark decoction on calcium oxalate lithiasis have been studied in rats. Crataeva reduced the oxalate-synthesizing liver enzyme, glycolate oxidase, which is produced by the feeding of glycolic acid; this caused a regulatory action on endogenous oxalate synthesis. Increased deposition of stone-forming constituents in the kidneys of calculogenic rats was lowered with decoction administration. Increased urinary excretion of the crystalline constituents, along with lowered magnesium excretion, in stone-forming rats was partially reversed by decoction treatment (Varalakshmi, 1990). Among 46 human patients with calcium oxalate stones that used 50 mL decoction twice daily for between 1 and 47 weeks, 28 passed the stone and 18 experienced symptomatic relief. This is thought to be due to the tonic contractile action of the drug on smooth muscle (Deshpande, 1982). Stem bark decoction was used in patients with calcium oxalate stones. After 12 weeks, a significant reduction in pain and dysuria was observed, along with some reduction in the size of stones (Singh, 1991).

TRIBULUS ***(TRIBULUS TERRESTRIS):*** An ethanolic extract of tribulus fruits showed significant dose-dependent protection against induced uroliths in rats. It protected against deposition of calculogenic material around a glass bead, and it also protected leukocytosis and elevation in serum urea levels (Anand, 1994). In addition to its diuretic activity, *T. terrestris* evoked contractile activity on guinea pig ileum. The diuretic and contractile effects of *T. terrestris* suggest that it may have the potential to propel urinary stones (Al Ali, 2003).

Bladder tonics

Bladder tonics are used to improve the tone of the bladder smooth muscle and are ideal for neurologic conditions of the bladder. They can also be used for more efficient voiding of urine in cystitis, when residual urine increases the risk of bacterial infection, so they may be useful with recurrent cystitis. The most useful tonic is Crataeva.

CRATAEVA ***(CRATAEVA NURVALA):*** In human studies, 50 mL decoction given twice daily for 3 months significantly improved incontinence, pain, and retention in prostatic hypertrophy with hypotonic bladder (Deshpande, 1982). After 4 weeks of treatment, 68% had symptomatic relief of chronic urinary tract infection, and 17% were devoid of microorganisms and neutrophils (Deshpande, 1982). Water extract of the stem bark improved smooth muscle tone (intestine and ureters) of guinea pigs, dogs, and humans, as well as skeletal muscle, in vitro (Das, 1974). After oral treatment with Crataeva for 40 days, a significant increase in bladder tone was noted in dogs (Deshpande, 1982).

Renal protective agents/kidney tonics

Traditionally, kidney tonics (in Western herbal medicine) have been used in conjunction with diuretic depuratives to improve kidney function; they may also provide a protective effect.

ASTRAGALUS ***(ASTRAGALUS MEMBRANACEUS):*** Proteinuria is regarded as a marker for significant renal injury and as a contributor to renal pathology. Astragalus can increase albumin level in plasma, decrease the output of urinary protein, and increase muscle protein. These actions may help prevent glomerular sclerosis (Zhou, 1999). Oral doses improve renal function in rats with experimental nephritis, and large doses are traditionally used in the treatment of chronic nephritis (Chang, 1987). A total of 30 human patients with chronic glomerulonephritis were enrolled in an open study. After injection of 40 mg/day for 3 weeks, proteinuria dropped dramatically—by more than half (Shi, 2002). Two other studies in 106 patients with chronic glomerulonephritis and in animal models that included immune complex nephritis have also demonstrated the ability of Astragalus to significantly reduce proteinuria (Peng, 2005). Thus, the effects of Astragalus on reduction of proteinuria may have benefit in slowing the progression of renal disease. In another study, serum creatinine was significantly reduced and creatinine clearance increased in patients treated with 32 g of Astragalus per day, compared with controls, in whom no significant change was observed (Zhao, 2000).

CHAMOMILE ***(MATRICARIA RECUTITA):*** This volatile oil has been documented to reduce the serum concentration of urea in rabbits with experimentally induced uremic conditions (Grochulski, 1972).

EVENING PRIMROSE ***(OENOTHERA BIENNIS):*** Prostaglandins of the E series are believed to be important in maintaining adequate renal blood flow. Administration of Evening primrose to animals has been reported to prevent or attenuate renal damage. Effects of orally administered *Oenothera biennis* on chronic renal failure were studied in partially nephrectomized rats. Compared with control groups, the group treated with Oenothera showed that urine protein excretion was reduced, serum cholesterol was decreased, levels of PGE_1 and PGE_2 were increased in renal cortex and medulla, 6-keto PGF_1-alpha was increased in cortex, and thromboxane 2 production was increased at only 4 weeks after nephrectomy. Glomerular lesions were more severe in the control group (Bi, 1992). A single, placebo-controlled trial involving human patients postrenal transplantation demonstrated a better graft survival rate for the group receiving evening primrose oil (45 patients) compared with the placebo group (44 patients) (Horrobin, 1990).

CORDYCEPS ***(CORDYCEPS SINENSIS):*** Cordyceps is regarded in Traditional Chinese Medicine as a premier "kidney tonic" that may prevent gentamicin-induced nephrotoxicity in animals. Cordyceps ameliorated deterioration of tubule metabolism and ion transport (Tian, 1991a), promoted DNA synthesis of kidney cells, lessened urinary β-N-acetylglucosaminidase and lysozyme levels, and delayed proteinuria (Tian, 1991b, 1991c). A comparative clinical study of Cordyceps (3-5 g/day) was conducted in 51 patients with chronic renal failure. In all, 28 received Cordyceps and showed a significant increase in renal function and T-lymphocyte subsets, including the T helper cell ratio, compared with the control group (Guan, 1992).

LICORICE ***(GLYCYRRHIZA GLABRA):*** This herb and two constituents—glycyrrhizin and 3-glycyrrhetinic monodesmoside—significantly suppressed lactate dehydrogenase leakage and malondialdehyde release from renal cells subjected to hypoxia–reoxygenation, whereas glycyrrhetinic acid had no effect. However, in rats subjected to ischemia–reperfusion, activities of endogenous antioxidant enzymes, including catalase and glutathione peroxidase, showed recovery, whereas levels of urea nitrogen and creatinine in serum were reduced by oral administration of glycyrrhizin (2.5 or 10 mg/kg daily) for 30 days before ischemia–reperfusion. Results indicated that licorice may be promising for amelioration of hypoxia–reoxygenation injury and for improvement of renal function in that it acts directly or indirectly as an antioxidant and an oxygen radical scavenging agent (Yokozawa, 2000).

ASTRAGALUS *(ASTRAGALUS MONGHOLICUS)* AND DONG QUAI *(ANGELICA SINENSIS)*: These plants have been used in China to treat patients with nephrotic syndrome. Rats with chronic induced nephrosis were treated with astragalus and dong quai or enalapril and were compared with control rats. Astragalus and dong quai significantly reduced deterioration of renal function and histologic damage. This combination of herbs slowed the progression of renal fibrosis and the deterioration of renal function with effects comparable to enalapril (Wang, 2004). The primary cause of anemia of chronic renal failure (CRF) is insufficient production of erythropoietin by diseased kidneys. *Angelica sinensis* improved red blood cell parameters in a person who was nonresponsive to erythropoietin administration (Bradley, 1999).

NETTLE SEED *(URTICA DIOICA)*: This was first suggested by North American herbalist David Winston for the treatment of renal disease. Treasure (2003) reported two cases of humans with persistently elevated serum creatinine that required them to undergo chronic dialysis. A hydroethanolic (1:5) tincture of nettle seed (5 mL given three times daily) led to reductions in serum creatinine in both patients. In one patient, discontinuing the nettle seed was associated with a subsequent rise in creatinine, and when the herb was started again, the creatinine fell once more.

PERILLA LEAVES *(PERILLA FRUTESCENS)*: A decoction of perilla leaves had suppressive effects on the progression of glomerulonephritis in an animal model of spontaneous immunoglobulin (Ig)A nephropathy. The active constituent rosmarinic acid was identified as causing the in vitro antiproliferative effects of perilla decoction (Makino, 2001).

TRIPTERYGIUM WILFORDII: This plant reduced proteinuria, and remission was gained, in 83% of human patients with nephritic syndrome at 2 mg/kg/day for at least 4 weeks (Peng, 2005).

CHUAN XIONG *(LIGUSTICUM WALLICHII)*: This herb has been evaluated in many clinical studies for its effects in reducing serum creatinine, increasing creatinine clearance, and reducing proteinuria. Studies on the phenolic constituent sodium ferulate suggest that it corrects abnormal endothelial gene expression, and that the reduction in proteinuria or improvement in renal functional deterioration associated with the correction of an endothelial disorder (Peng, 2005).

Spasmolytics

Many spasmolytic herbs have been discovered. Some that should be considered for urinary disorders, such as the pain of interstitial cystitis or passing a kidney stone, are discussed here.

CRAMP BARK *(VIBURNUM OPULUS)*: According to King's (Felter, 1898), this herb has been used for spasmodic contraction of the bladder, as well as for spasmodic stricture.

PUMPKIN SEED *(CUCURBITA PEPO)*: The expressed oil of pumpkin seeds, in doses of 6 to 12 drops given several times a day, is said to be an efficient diuretic that provides relief in "scalding of urine, spasmodic affections of the urinary passages" (Felter, 1898).

OTHER HERBS: A combination of uva ursi, hops, and peppermint has been used to treat patients with compulsive strangury, enuresis, and painful micturition. Of 915 patients treated for 6 weeks, success was reported in about 70% (Lenau, 1984).

Urinary tract demulcents

The mucopolysaccharide layer produced by the transitional cells that coat the bladder plays an important role as a defense mechanism of the lower urinary tract. Traditionally, demulcents have been thought to soothe the mucous membrane lining of the urinary tract; therefore, they have been used in inflammatory conditions such as cystitis. It is probable that some of these herbs may work to improve the integrity of this layer through their influence on the mucous membrane, but a paucity of data supports this. For example, carbenoxolone, derived from licorice, was shown to provide a protective effect in laboratory-induced lower urinary tract infection in the rabbit model; in the same way, it is used to treat peptic ulcers in people (Mooreville, 1983).

MARSHMALLOW *(ALTHAEA OFFICINALIS)*: Mucilage content ranges from 10% to 20%, and this herb may work through a reflex effect.

COUCH GRASS *(AGROPYRON REPENS)*: This plant contains both triticum 3% to 8%—a polysaccharide related to inulin—and 8% to 10% mucilage.

CORN SILK *(ZEA MAYS)*: This plant contains allantoin, which is a vulnerary.

LICORICE *(GLYCYRRHIZA GLABRA)*: This herb may provide reflex demulcency.

Urinary antiseptics/antimicrobials

These herbs produce metabolites that are excreted in urine, and they exert their antiseptic effects there. Compared with antibiotics, this effect is expected to be mild; however, these agents may have a role in chronic or recurrent urinary tract infection. Herbs with antiseptic activity include the following.

CRANBERRY *(VACCINIUM MACROCARPA)*: Cranberry juice and crushed cranberries have a long history of use in the treatment and prevention of urinary tract infection (Kingwatanakul, 1996). Initially, it was thought that the antibacterial effect of cranberry juice was a result of its ability to acidify urine and, therefore, to inhibit bacterial growth. However, recent work has focused on the effects of cranberry in inhibiting bacterial adherence and on the effects of antiadhesion agents in cranberry juice. Bacterial adherence to mucosal surfaces is considered to be an important step in the development of urinary tract infection (Reid, 1987). It is facilitated by fimbriae on the bacterial cell wall, which produce adhesins that attach to specific receptors on uroepithelial cells (Beachey, 1981). Proanthocyanidins extracted from cranberries have been shown to inhibit the adherence of P-fimbriated *Escherichia coli* to uroepithelial cell surfaces, suggesting that proanthocyanidins may be important for the stated effects of cranberry in urinary tract infection (Howell,

1998). Cranberry juice cocktail provided antiadherence activity directed toward gram-negative rods, including *Klebsiella, Enterobacter, Pseudomonas,* and *Proteus* species (Schmidt, 1988). In a review of two randomized controlled trials, it was found that cranberry (as juice or capsule) significantly reduced the incidence of urinary tract infection in women. Evidence supports the use of cranberry to prevent urinary tract infection in some populations, but none to support its use as a treatment (Griffiths, 2003).

BUCHU *(AGATHOSMA BETULINA):* In 1821, it was introduced from Africa into Great Britain as an official medicine for treating cystitis, urethritis, nephritis, and catarrh of the bladder (Grieve, 1931). Urinary tract antiseptic actions of buchu are thought to be due to the volatile oils. The primary volatile oil component thought to have antibacterial action is the monoterpene disophenol. However, one test tube study of buchu oil found no significant antibacterial effect (Didry, 1982). Very low activity was observed against *Escherichia coli, Saccharomyces cerevisiae,* and *Staphylococcus aureus,* suggesting little potential for use as an antimicrobial agent (Lis-Balchin, 2001).

UVA URSI *(ARCTOSTAPHYLOS UVA URSI):* Uva ursi is stated to possess diuretic, antiseptic, and astringent properties. Traditionally, it has been used for cystitis, urethritis, dysuria, pyelitis, lithuria, and, specifically, acute catarrhal cystitis with dysuria and highly acidic urine (British Herbal Pharmacopoeia, 1983; Wren, 1988). The antiseptic and diuretic properties claimed for uva ursi can be attributed to its hydroquinone derivatives, especially the constituent arbutin. Arbutin is absorbed intact from the gastrointestinal tract and during renal excretion is hydrolyzed to yield the active principle, hydroquinone, which exerts antiseptic and astringent actions on the urinary mucous membranes (Matsuda, 1992b). In a double-blind, placebo-controlled, randomized clinical trial, 57 women with more than three episodes of cystitis in the previous year received herbal extract or placebo. The herbal medicine consisted of bearberry and dandelion root and leaf. Treatment for 1 month significantly reduced the recurrence of cystitis during the 1-year follow-up, with no cystitis in the treated group and 23% recurrence in the placebo group. No adverse effects were reported (Larsson, 1993). It should be noted that alkaline urine is necessary for arbutin to work. Urinary acidifiers inhibit the conversion of arbutin to an active hydroquinone, making uva ursi less effective (De Smet, 1993).

COUCH GRASS *(AGROPYRON REPENS):* Broad antibiotic activity has been documented for agropyrene and its oxidation products (Leung, 1980).

GOLDENROD *(SOLIDAGO VIRGAUREA):* Fresh Solidago tincture was evaluated in a double-blind, placebo-controlled trial of patients with urinary tract infection. A significant rise (30%) in the amount of secreted urine was observed after a single dose of 100 drops (4-5 mL). A subsequent open trial showed that 70% of patients experienced improvement in symptoms such as dysuria, frequency, and tenesmus (Bruhwiler, 1992).

SAW PALMETTO *(SERENOA REPENS):* This herb is stated to possess diuretic, urinary antiseptic, endocrinologic, and anabolic properties. Traditionally, it has been used for chronic or subacute cystitis, catarrh of the genitourinary tract, testicular atrophy, sex hormone disorders, and, specifically, prostatic enlargement (British Herbal Pharmacopoeia, 1983; Wren, 1988).

Urinary tract astringents

PLANTAIN *(PLANTAGO MAJOR):* This plant is stated to possess diuretic and antihemorrhagic properties. Traditionally, it has been used for cystitis with hematuria and for hemorrhoids with bleeding and irritation (British Herbal Pharmacopoeia, 1983; Wren, 1988).

HORSETAIL *(EQUISETUM ARVENSE):* This has traditionally been used for gravel ulcerations in the urinary tract and for kidney affectations generally. It can be used for irrigation therapy for bacterial and inflammatory diseases of the lower urinary tract and renal gravel (American Botanical Council, 1998). Its hemostyptic effect may be due to silicic acid or flavonoids.

Alkalinizing agents

Cranberry juice has the ability to lower urinary pH (Jackson, 1997). In patients with urostomy, peristomal skin problems are common and may stem from alkaline urine. In a study on patients with human urostomy, drinking cranberry juice did not appear to acidify the urine, as expected; however, improvements were seen in the skin conditions of study participants, suggesting that drinking cranberry juice does positively affect the incidence of skin complications among these patients (Tsukada, 1994).

Review of Specific Urinary Tract Conditions

Cystitis

Therapeutic Rationale

- Evaluate for predisposing causes, such as infection, environmental and food allergies, impaired immune function, and chronic constipation.
- Encourage diuresis by providing broths and soups.
- Provide a source of glycosaminoglycans.

Prescription 1 for cystitis: For recurrent cystitis, rotate between prescriptions. Use alcohol or glycetract tinctures for best results; alternatively, use teas.

Crataeva	20% (antilithic, bladder tonic, anti-inflammatory)
Licorice	20% (anti-inflammatory, adaptogen, antispasmodic, taste improver, demulcent)
Corn silk	20% (diuretic, demulcent, antilithic)
Marshmallow	20% (demulcent, vulnerary, diuretic)
Horsetail	20% (genitourinary astringent, antihemorrhagic)

Prescription 2 for cystitis: Use alcohol or glycetract tinctures for best results; alternatively, use teas.

Goldenrod	20% (anti-inflammatory, antiseptic, diuretic, carminative)
Buchu	20% (diuretic, antiseptic)
Uva ursi	20% (urinary antiseptic, astringent)
Corn silk	20% (diuretic, demulcent, antilithic)
Bilberry	20% (antioxidant, astringent, anti-inflammatory)

Bladder stones—urolithiasis

Therapeutic Rationale

- Enhance diuresis.
- Reduce mucosal inflammation.
- Reduce smooth muscle spasm.
- Control infection, where appropriate.
- Initiate stone dissolution, if possible.
- Restore mucosal polysaccharide layer.
- Avoid using high doses of vitamin C, where appropriate.

A prescription for bladder stones is given here:

Use alcohol or glycetract tinctures for best results; alternatively, use teas.

Crataeva	20% (antilithic, bladder tonic, anti-inflammatory)
Hydrangea	20% (diuretic, antilithic, antihyperprostatic)
Marshmallow	20% (demulcent, vulnerary, diuretic)
Gravelroot	20% (antilithic, diuretic)
Licorice	20% (anti-inflammatory, adaptogen. laxative, taste improver)

Incontinence

Therapeutic Rationale

- Improve sphincter tone.
- Improve bladder tone.
- Reduce odor.
- Prevent infection from residual urine.

Cranberry will help reduce odor of urine; use capsules or powder and add to food.

A prescription for incontinence support follows:

Crataeva	40% (antilithic, bladder tonic, anti-inflammatory)
Uva ursi	20% (urinary antiseptic, astringent)
Marshmallow	20% (demulcent, vulnerary, diuretic)
Add Chaste tree	20% for females (or Saw palmetto 20% for males).

Alternate uva ursi with couch grass or bilberry or horsetail over time.

Interstitial cystitis and feline lower urinary tract disease

Therapeutic Rationale

- Reduce inflammation.
- Reduce pain.
- Relieve stress.
- Improve integrity of bladder wall.
- Reduce risk of uroliths.
- Consider a source of glycosaminoglycans.

Consider Horsetail for irrigation therapy for FLUTD as a tea or diluted tincture, for its astringent, antihemorrhagic, anti-inflammatory, and diuretic properties.

A prescription for feline cystitis is provided:

Crataeva	20% (antilithic, bladder tonic, anti-inflammatory)
Marshmallow	40% (demulcent, vulnerary, diuretic)
Saint John's Wort	20% (antidepressant, nervine tonic, vulnerary, anti-inflammatory)
Horsetail	20% (genitourinary astringent, antihemorrhagic)

Another prescription for interstitial cystitis is:

Kava kava	40% (anxiolytic, anti-inflammatory)
Saint John's Wort	30% (anxiolytic, analgesic)
Marshmallow	30% (demulcent)

A traditional Kampo formula, Choreito, has been investigated in the treatment of lower urinary tract disease in cats. Choreito (Zhu Ling San) has been shown to decrease struvite crystalluria and hematuria in cats (Buffington, 1994, 1997a, 1997b).

Kidney disease

Kidney fibrosis is a common sequel of chronic kidney disease. Standard treatment includes dietary phosphorus restriction, maintenance of proper hydration, blood pressure control, use of angiotensin-converting enzyme inhibitors and aspirin for proteinuria, and so forth. Evidence suggests that there is value in using herbal medicine, including nephroprotective herbs. Many Chinese herbs have been investigated, including Astragalus, Angelica, Ligusticum, Tripolide, and Rhubarb, and some have been shown to slow the progression of chronic kidney disease. On the other hand, some herbs can be nephrotoxic or hazardous to patients with renal disease, so caution is required (Peng, 2005).

A prescription for chronic renal disease is given here:

Marshmallow	20% (demulcent, vulnerary, diuretic)
Rehmannia	20% (anti-inflammatory, antihemorrhagic, antipyretic)
Astragalus	40% (immune modulating, tonic, hypotensive, renal protective)
Siberian ginseng	20% (adaptogenic, immune modulating)

A second prescription is provided:

Rehmannia	25% (anti-inflammatory, antihemorrhagic, antipyretic)
Cordyceps	25% (nephroprotective, immune modulating)
Astragalus	25% (immune modulating, tonic, hypotensive, renal protective)
Nettle seed	25% (reduces creatinine)

Many herbalists use the traditional Chinese formula (Jin Gui Shen Qi Wan or Ba Wei Wan) (Rehmannia, 8) to successfully slow the progression of chronic kidney disease.

HERBS FOR TOPICAL USE

This section presents well-known and less-recognized herbs that are used topically to enhance wound healing, reduce inflammation, and shrink or cause necrosis of tumors. Information on traditional uses comes from the popular herb literature, most of it (and wherever quotes are found below) from *King's American Dispensatory,* 1898 version, by Felter and Lloyd. Scientific literature searches were done on Medline, Google, and the websites of the Southwest School of Botanical Medicine and HealthNotes online. Search terms were generally of two types: (1) the word "herbal" plus the mechanism of action, and (2) the individual herb name, sometimes narrowed with the descriptor "topical" or "topically."

Definitions (from Merriam-Webster Online and Traditional Sources)

Fomentation
The application of hot, moist substances to the body to ease pain, or (as a noun) the material so applied.

Plaster
A medicated or protective dressing that consists of a cloth or plastic film spread with a medicated substance.

Poultice
A soft, usually heated medicated mass spread on cloth and applied to cutaneous lesions.

Compress
A folded cloth or pad applied so as to press upon a body part.

Ointment
A salve or unguent for application to the skin.

Salve
An unctuous adhesive substance for application to wounds or sores.

Cataplasm
Synonymous with plaster or poultice.

Anodyne
An agent that relieves pain via topical application.

Astringent
A substance that contracts and firms tissues and organs; a styptic; an agent that decreases secretions.

Counterirritant
A substance that is externally applied to relieve deep-seated pain by way of causing hyperemia or local irritation.

Demulcent
A substance that soothes, protects, and restores mucous membranes and relieves irritation of inflamed or abraded surfaces, usually through mucilage content.

Embrocation
A liquid or wash applied to a diseased or painful part, usually by rubbing; liniment.

Escharotic
A caustic or corrosive that is capable of producing a slough or eschar (scab).

Hemostatic
A substance that stops the flow of blood.

Rubefacient
Something that reddens the skin by causing capillary dilation from external application.

Scrofula
Tuberculosis or other swellings of the lymph nodes, especially of the neck

Styptic
Something that contracts or binds to prevent bleeding; it stops blood flow by constricting blood vessels.

Vesicant
A substance that causes blistering.

Vulnerary
An agent that aids in wound and skin healing.

TYPES OF TOPICAL APPLICATIONS USED IN VETERINARY PATIENTS

Herbs may be applied to the eyes in the form of infusions, usually water infusions. Stomatitis may be treated with the use of infusions or decoctions (well filtered) administered from a spray bottle. Prescribers should remember that many herbs taste bad, and animals may not accept treatment unless the herb is diluted with a sweet liquid such as juice. Ear treatments may consist of water or oil infusions or decoctions applied as ear drops. Tinctures are usually diluted with an active or inactive vehicle to prevent alcohol from causing pain in inflamed or ulcerated ear canals. Wounds may be best managed with wet or wet-dry dressings, with the use of infusions or decoctions of the herb. Oil infusions or ointments may provide a protective coating for open wounds, chronic ulcers, and so forth.

Cautions

Many of the herbs listed are toxic (e.g., Chinaberry, Henbane, Hellebore, Mayapple) or caustic (e.g., Bloodroot, Chelidonium), if ingested. Readers should refer to individual herb monographs for further information on toxicity.

Mechanisms of Interest

Ectoparasiticidal herbs

Fleas: Fleas are a constant problem in warm climates. Commercial flea sprays and powders are available, mostly based on Neem and various aromatic herbs (e.g., cedar, rosemary). These have not been evaluated critically, to our knowledge.

Flies: Herbal sprays are available to horsekeepers; they generally contain combinations of aromatic herbs and Neem. These must be applied frequently if they are to be effective, especially if the horses sweat a lot. These have not been evaluated critically, to our knowledge.

PYRETHRUM ***(TANACETUM CINERARIIFOLIUM* OR *CHRYSANTHEMUM CINERARIIFOLIUM):*** This agent is the source of pyrethrins used in commercial natural flea products.

CHASTE TREE *(VITEX ANGUS-CASTUS)*: A study suggests that a CO_2 extract of the seeds of the Mediterranean plant Vitex agnus castus (monk's pepper) can be used as a spray to repel especially Ixodes ricinus and Rhipicephalus sanguineus ticks from animals and humans for at least 6 hours. In addition mosquitoes, biting flies and fleas were also repelled for about 6 hours (Mehlhorn 2005).

LOUSEWORT *(DELPHINIUM STAPHISAGRIA LINN)*: A traditional flea remedy, found in veterinary school notes from the early 1900s, was based on Stavesacre or Lousewort seed. Instructions were given as follows: "Crush 1 oz Stavesacre seed well, and boil for 2 hours in 20 to 30 oz of water, making up the original quantity used, and use as a wash."

NEEM *(AZADIRACHTA INDICA)*: This herb may be potentially useful for managing flea and tick infestation in dogs and cats. Azadirachtin and other constituents in various parts of this tree possess more than one mode of action against insects. These include antifeedancy, growth regulation, fecundity suppression and sterilization, oviposition repellency or attractancy, changes in biological fitness, and blockage of the development of vector-borne pathogens. Some of these activities have been studied in mosquitoes, flies, cockroaches, fleas, lice, and other parasites of veterinary importance (Mulla, 1999). In a study in which topical Neem extract was used on both dogs and cats, 1000 to 2400 ppm azadirachtin reduced fleas on Greyhounds and cats by 53% to 93% in a dose-dependent manner for 19 days (Guerrini, 1998). Clinical experience suggests that Neem spray should be applied every few days.

FLEABANE *(ERIGERON CANADENSE)*: This herb has been used for many centuries (Aristotle mentions it). The traditional recommendation is to repel fleas by burning the herb, but some sources recommend rubbing the herb on clothing (or the fur for animals) or applying extracts topically. No data are available to support the use of fleabane for fleas.

LABRADOR TEA *(LEDUM GLANDULOSUM* OR *LEDUM LATIFOLIUM)*: King's claims that the plant was strewn among clothes to prevent moth damage, and that a strong decoction used externally was effective against lice and other insects.

AZEDARACH *(MELIA AZEDARACH)*: The "pulp" of this tree has been used in traditional medicine for destroying human ectoparasites. Azedarach extracts were shown to kill *Boophilus microplus* tick larvae (Borges, 2003). Sixteen of 17 species of parasitic insects consumed significantly less food when treated with an extract of the fruit (Carpinella, 2003). Poisoning caused by eating the berries has been reported in a number of mammalian species.

CHAULMOOGRA, GYNOCARDIA *(GYNOCARDIA ODORATA)*: This herb had a reputation among the Eclectics for destroying lice and scabies mites.

PARSLEY *(PETROSELINUM SATIVUM)*: When an ointment was prepared with the use of seeds and leaves, or when the seeds and leaves were powdered, this was said to be effective in destroying "vermin."

IVY *(HEDERA HELIX)*: This was said to kill "vermin in the hair, which, it is stated, is stained black by the application."

PERU BALSAM TREE *(MYROXYLON PEREIRAE)*: This was used for the treatment of scabies. It was administered as the balsam, 40 drops over the whole body (of a human) for 2 days. It has been known to lead to contact hypersensitivity.

WHITE HELLEBORE *(VERATRUM ALBUM)*: This was used as a decoction or ointment to kill lice and scabies; however, the plant is highly toxic and teratogenic and should be avoided because animals often lick topical applications.

Astringent herbs

TEA *(CAMELLIA SINENSIS)*: This has been used for burns and excoriations. In veterinary medicine, a particularly useful application is for moist dermatitis and traumatic dermatitis, or "hot spots." Tea catechins, when applied percutaneously in the ears of mice and given orally, inhibited signs of oxazolone-induced type IV allergy (Suzuki, 2000). The saponins also reduce allergy mediator release in in vitro studies (Akagi, 1997). The tannins are astringent and may coagulate serum proteins in oozing lesions.

WITCH HAZEL *(HAMAMELIS VIRGINIANA)*: Witch hazel bark contains catechins and has barrier-stabilizing, antimicrobial, and anti-inflammatory activities (Gloor, 2002; Hughes-Formella, 2002; Erdelmeier, 1996; Duwiejua, 1994). The Eclectics used it in poultice form for painful swellings, tumors, and external inflammation. It was also popular, in decoction form, for treating mouth inflammation and ulcers. Typical over-the-counter witch hazel products are preserved with alcohol and may cause irritation.

GERANIUM, CRANESBILL *(GERANIUM MACULATUM)*: This herb has a variety of uses because of its astringency, including ulcers. It may also be used for hot spots and excoriations.

GNAPHALIUM, WHITE BALSAM *(GNAPHALIUM POLYCEPHALUM)*: This was used in fomentation form for bruises, tumors, and other focal cutaneous problems.

HEUCHERA, ALUM ROOT *(HEUCHERA AMERICANA)*: This is considered a very strong astringent and was used for all kinds of mucosal hemorrhage (e.g., epistaxis, wounds, nonhealing ulcers).

MOUNTAIN ASH FRUIT, SORBUS FRUIT *(PYRUS AUCUPARIA, SORBUS AUCUPARIA)*: These were used primarily in poultice form.

BLACK OR WHITE ASH TREE BARK *(FRAXINUS SAMBUCIFOLIA, FRAXINUS AMERICANA)*: This was used in plaster form and was considered tonic as well as astringent.

STATICE, MARSH ROSEMARY *(STATICE CAROLINIANA)*: This was used as a gargle or mouthwash for sore throat and mouth ulcers, and as a decoction for eye inflammation. The powdered root was applied directly to nonhealing ulcers or was mixed into an ointment.

NETTLE, STINGING NETTLE *(URTICA DIOICA)*: This powdered leaf or infusion can be used as a styptic for bleeding surfaces such as abrasions or hot spots.

Antibacterial herbs

ECHINACEA *(ECHINACEA PURPUREA, E. ANGUSTIFOLIA)*: One of the most important traditional uses for this plant was as a wash or dressing for snake and spider bites, or "other envenomations that lead to necrosis; crush injuries leading to necrosis and infection.... [Think of Echinacea for] swelling when extensive, tense, and of a purplish-red hue...." Echinacoside and the polyacetylene constituents have antibacterial activity, and the polyacetylenes have antifungal activity (Bisset, 1994); however, Echinacea demonstrated a propensity for increasing bacterial resistance in vitro by greatly increasing the minimum inhibitory concentration of ampicillin against *E. coli* (Ward, 2002). Nonetheless, it is potentially indicated when given as simultaneous oral medication and topical dressing for serious and infected wounds, snake and brown recluse spider bites, and cat abscesses. An interesting ancillary effect is that Echinacea acts as a mild anodyne.

TEA TREE ***(MELALEUCA ALTERNIFOLIA):*** This herb was used by the Eclectics as mild anodyne for neuralgic pain, but also for various cutaneous problems and to relieve the pain of toothache. Tea tree oil has shown activity in vitro against Malassezia yeast (Weseler 2002; Hammer 2000), and Staphylococcus aureus (including resistant strains)(Halcon 2004), in addition to other skin pathogens. In a clinical case series of dogs treated with a 10% preparation of tea tree for dermatitis, the authors suggested that tea tree oil was effective in reducing the signs of dermatitis (Fitzi 2002). Tea tree has potential as a diluted wound dressing, and in diluted form for other infections such as otitis. Undiluted tea tree oil is highly toxic to cats and potentially toxic to small dogs as well. This author (SW) uses 10% as the highest concentration, but adverse events may still occur.

BASIL ***(OCIMUM GRATISSIMUM):*** This agent is not used traditionally as a topical antimicrobial, but it has potential. In one trial, Ocimum gratissimum oil was found to be equivalent to conventional treatments for acne (Ernst, 2003). Thyme *(Thymus vulgaris)* and various species of Sage (*Salvia* species, especially *S. apiana*) are also used as antibacterial herbs.

Demulcent herbs

QUINCE SEED ***(CYDONIA VULGARIS):*** This herb was used by the Eclectics as a mucilage to soothe oral lesions such as aphthous ulcers and excoriations, as well as for conjunctivitis.

OKRA ***(HIBISCUS ESCULENTUS):*** Seed pods and leaves both contain mucilage and can be used as wound dressing in the form of a cataplasm.

PSYLLIUM ***(PLANTAGO MAJOR):*** This seed contains large amounts of mucilage; one study showed that the capillary action that draws water away from wounds inhibits bacterial growth (Westerhof, 2001). This herb has been used since the time of Gerard, who wrote, "The seed stamped, and boyled in water to the forme of a plaister, and applied, taketh away all swelling of the joynts, especially if you boyle the same with vinegar and oyle of Roses, and apply it as aforesaid... unto any burning heate... or any hot and violent impostume [abscess], asswageth the same...."

MULLEIN ***(VERBASCUM THAPSUS):*** These leaves have been used as a fomentation for inflamed hemorrhoids and ulcers.

FENUGREEK ***(TRIGONELLA FOENUM-GRAECUM):*** This herb, prepared as a poultice or decoction (1 oz of seeds in 1 pint of water) of the seeds, has been used on inflamed mucous membranes, for instance, for throat, rectal, and vaginal irritation.

Hemostatic herbs

YUNNAN PAI YAO: This proprietary Chinese formula is said to be composed of *Panax notoginseng,* San Yu Cao *(Ajuga patantha), Dioscorea opposita,* Chuan Shan Long *(Dioscorea nipponica),* Lao Guan Cao *(Erodium stephanianum), Alpinia officinarum,* Bai Niu Dan, and *Dryobalanops aromatica* (or *Blumea balsamifera*) (package label, 2005). Alternatively, some formulas contain *(Panax pseudoginseng or Radix notoginseng),* and variously Chinese yam *(Dioscorea opposita),* yam rhizome *(Dioscorea hypolglauca),* sweet geranium *(Erodium stephanianum),* and galangal rhizome *(Alpinia officinarum)* (Polesuk 1973). It is used orally and locally to stop bleeding. Studies show decreased bleeding times in an animal model and possible effects on blood platelets (Ogle, 1977; Ogle, 1976).

NETTLE, STINGING NETTLES ***(URTICA DIOICA):*** This is traditionally used as a styptic for bleeding.

ZONAL GERANIUM ***(PELARGONIUM ZONALE):*** This species forms the basis for decorative pot geraniums. The juice has been applied to staunch bleeding, and one study in a rat model confirmed its efficacy (Paez, 2003).

RHATANY, KRAMERIA ***(KRAMERIA TRIANDRA):*** This herb contains tannins and is high in proanthocyanidins. It has been used in epistaxis, bleeding from tooth extraction sites, wounds, anal fissures, and bleeding gums. One traditional preparation used tinctures of rhatany and myrrh mixed with chalk. Contact hypersensitivity has been reported with this herb.

MATICA ***(PIPER ANGUSTIFOLIUM):*** This leaf has been used to stop hemorrhage from wounds and leech bites.

Escharotic herbs

CHELIDONIUM ***(CHELIDONIUM MAJUS):*** A patented extract, Ukrain, has documented cytostatic and cytotoxic effects against a number of cancer cell lines and has immunemodulatory activity as well. Preclinical studies in humans with cancer have been promising (Ernst 2005; Uglyanitsa 2000). This herb was used traditionally as a caustic to remove warts and stimulate healing of indolent ulcers and ringworm. It was also used on the cornea for removal of opacities. It is said to cause inflammation and vesication when applied to normal skin. Contact dermatitis and hepatotoxicity after oral ingestion have been reported.

BLOODROOT ***(SANGUINARIA CANADENSIS):*** This herb is part of the most popular escharotic salves (or black salves) available today, which also include zinc chloride and perhaps other herbs such as galangal root. Clinical experience among multiple veterinarians has been good for small cutaneous tumors. Tumor removal was not an indication for this plant in Eclectic medicine. An extract, sanguinarine, initiates apoptosis in certain tumor cells (Ahmad, 2000). In a clinical series, escharotic ointments that contained bloodroot were effective in removing tumors locally but did not prevent metastasis (McDaniel,

2002). Animals must be prevented from licking the salve. Long-term use of sanguinarine in toothpaste in humans is suspected to be a cause of leukoplakia. Long-term oral ingestion of sanguinarine has led to "epidemic dropsy."

PRICKLY POPPY ***(ARGEMONE MEXICANA):*** This herb was used topically for warts, chancres, and ulcers. It contains sanguinarine, which may in part account for an escharotic-like effect. Oral ingestion causes "epidemic dropsy," a generalized vasculitis that may lead to respiratory impairment, renal tubular necrosis, generalized edema, and death.

Herbs for warts, corns

In small animal practice, clients complain that their dogs develop warts, which are usually sebaceous gland adenomas or other benign tumors. One experimental treatment that is being explored by herbalists at the time of this writing is black salve (see the section on tumors, later).

DROSERA ***(DROSERA ROTUNDIFOLIA):*** This has been used for corns and warts; however, the plant is highly endangered in the wild and should not be used.

HAWKWEED ***(HIERACIUM VENOSUM):*** Fresh juice from the leaves has been recommended to remove warts.

MOSSY STONECROP (*SEDUM* SPP): This is said to be a topical vesicant if the leaves are pounded and applied fresh to warts, corns, and other small growths.

CASHEW NUT RIND JUICE ***(ANACARDIUM OCCIDENTALE):*** This herb is an irritant in the poison ivy family; it has been used to stimulate indolent ulcers, as well as to remove warts and corns.

NETTLE, STINGING NETTLES ***(URTICA DIOICA):*** In King's, this herb is said to make warts disappear with no pain, if they are rubbed with fresh nettle juice 3 to 4 times daily for 10 to 12 days.

THUJA ***(THUJA OCCIDENTALIS):*** This herb is popular today for removal of warts and similar growths, such as sebaceous adenomas. It can be used in ointment or tincture form (although the tincture may be more effective). King's claimed that it was effective on most warts, except for rapidly growing venereal warts.

MAYAPPLE ***(PODOPHYLLUM PELTATUM)*** (GREEN OR DRIED ROOT): This was said to cause irritation and suppuration when applied continuously to warts. Podophyllin, an extract of *Podophyllum peltatum,* is effective in the treatment of human warts (Miller, 1996; White, 1997).

Counterirritants

Capsaicin is a modern example of a counterirritant, which can be used to relieve deep-seated local painful conditions, such as arthritis and shingles. Counterirritants relieve pain locally, possibly via substance P–mediated mechanisms.

MUSTARD ***(SINAPISA ALBA, S. NIGRA):*** Applied topically, this herb causes inflammation, stinging pain, scaling, and, if left long enough, ulceration. The goal was to cause reddening of the skin, but not vesication or ulceration. "Sinapisms" were applied to the abdomen and spine to relieve discomfort or signs of gastrointestinal inflammation, such as vomiting, pain, or even constipation; on the chest for painful chest disorders such as pleurisy; or on the head for headaches. It was also applied to other areas as a rubefacient to relieve local pain caused by joint inflammation. It was applied as a plaster using equal parts wheat or rye flour and lukewarm water with $^{1}/_{12}$ to 2 drops of mustard oil dissolved in a mucilaginous herb, or as a liniment composed of 1 part oil in 16 parts alcohol or 10 parts carrier oil.

AMMONIAC ***(DOREMA AMMONIACUM):*** This is a similar irritant and was formerly used for buboes, joint tumors, enlarged glands, and "other indolent swellings."

OTHER HERBS: Various species of *Clematis* contain triterpenoid saponins. One, *C. hirsutissima,* is a known blistering agent and was used by Native Americans as a "horse stimulant."

Herbs for Eyes

Herbs can be used in infusion form in the eyes, but irritating forms such as alcohol extracts must be avoided. Sterility is a concern, and if teas are made fresh, they must be cooled while covered, and made fresh every day.

EUPHRASIA ***(EUPHRASIA OFFICINALIS):*** This herb is used for conditions that produce serous or mucoid discharges of the eye. An uncontrolled case series that used *Euphrasia rostkoviana* for catarrhal conjunctivitis resulted in resolution or improvement in 98.5% of treated patients (Stoss, 2000). It is most often used for allergic or irritant conjunctivitis.

GOLDENSEAL ***(HYDRASTIS CANADENSIS):*** This is a fairly common prescription for conjunctival inflammation, superficial corneal ulcers, and blepharitis.

DUSTY MILLER, SILVER RAGWORT ***(SENECIO MARITIMA):*** This has been used, especially as a topical homeopathic preparation, for cataracts, on the basis of early laboratory animal studies. The herb is irritating and must be used in very diluted form.

RED ROSE ***(ROSA GALLICA):*** This was used as a poultice, sometimes in infusion form with the pith of sassafras, for acute conjunctivitis.

PRICKLY POPPY ***(ARGEMONE MEXICANA):*** This herb is an irritant that was formerly used for corneal opacities and some forms of chronic conjunctivitis.

LOOSESTRIFE, LYTHRUM ***(LYTHRUM SALICARIA):*** This herb has been used for chronic conjunctivitis and keratitis, as well as for corneal ulcers.

BLACK HAW ***(VIBURNUM PRUNIFOLIUM):*** This was used for "various ophthalmic disorders."

OTHER HERBS: Sunflower (Helianthus annuus), Galbanum (Ferula galbaniflua), Tall Ambrosia, Great Ragweed (Ambrosia trifida), Wild Cherry Bark (Prunus serotina), and Chamomile (Matricaria recutita) were also used for conjunctivitis (called "ophthalmia" in older texts). The pith mucilage of Pitcher plant *(Sarracenia purpurea)* was also used—2 drachms to 1 pint of water.

Herbs for Ears

GOLDENSEAL ***(HYDRASTIS CANADENSIS):*** This was said to be specifically indicated for purulent otitis media, both acute and chronic, otitis externa, and "irritation due to inspissated cerumen." King's recommended about 10 drops of a 1:1 up to a 1:8 solution dropped into the ear, or it could be mixed with a preparation of witch hazel. Berberine has antibacterial activity against *Staphylococcus* and other bacteria, and topical use is most likely to repeat the success demonstrated in in vitro studies.

PRIVET LEAVES *(LIGUSTRUM VULGARE)*: Infusion was said to be indicated for ulcerated ears.

WITCH HAZEL *(HAMAMELIS VIRGINICA)*: This herb was often used with glycerin, or with an equal measure of goldenseal, for otitis externa.

MULLEIN *(VERBASCUM THAPSUS)*: Flowers infused in oil were used primarily for deafness, to normalize cerumen production, and for some possible benefit to an inflamed tympanic membrane.

Base formula for yeast or bacterial otitis (not to be used in place of the appropriate antibiotic for bacterial infections):

Aloe vera gel	40%-50%
Goldenseal	30%-40%
Thyme or white sage (as an antibacterial)	10%-15%
Tea tree (dogs only)	5%-10%

Herbs for Stomatitis

It is important to note that human patients can be instructed to use herbs as a gargle or mouthwash without swallowing the herbs. If these herbs are used in animals, it may be advisable to use a lower dose in the form of a spray. If an herb is nontoxic or is not contraindicated for concurrent medical disorders, herbs may be mixed in liquefied food (such as baby food) for increased contact time with the oral mucosa. Most of the herbs below (except for the astringents) are strongly bitter, and creative flavoring should be attempted to gain the animal's cooperation for more than one treatment!

BAPTISIA *(BAPTISIA TINCTORIA)*: This herb is specifically indicated for severe, painful oral ulceration.

MYRRH *(COMMIPHORA MYRRHA)*: This has been used for oral ulcerations, pharyngitis, and dental caries. Extracts of myrrh have antibacterial and analgesic activities (Dolara, 2000).

BLOODROOT *(SANGUINARIA CANADENSIS)*: Multiple studies suggest efficacy against gingivitis/periodontal disease and plaque build-up; however, the possibility exists that sanguinarine-containing products are associated with a preneoplastic lesion known as leukoplakia. This is a strong plant, and animals should be prevented from ingesting it chronically.

GOLDENSEAL *(HYDRASTIS CANADENSIS)*: This herb was thought by the Eclectics to be indicated specifically for subacute or chronic stomatitis. Berberine and two other extracts of goldenseal root showed antibacterial activity against oral pathogens *Streptococcus mutans* and *Fusobacterium nucleatum* (Hwang, 2003). Other plants containing berberine that have been recommended for stomatitis are Goldthread *(Coptis trifolia)* and Barberry *(Berberis vulgaris)*.

OTHER HERBS: Agrimony (Agrimonia eupatoria), Heuchera, Alum Root (Heuchera americana), and Cranesbill (Geranium maculatum) have been used as astringent gargles for mouth and throat ulceration.

Other herbs that have been used for mouth and throat ulceration or inflammation include Amaranth, Tall ambrosia or Great ragweed *(Ambrosia trifida)*, Red root or New Jersey tea *(Ceanothus americanus)*, Persimmon, Diospyros *(Diospyros virginiana)*, Epilobium or Willow herb *(Epilobium angustifolium, E. palustre)*, Rockbrake or Common brake *(Pteris atropurpurea,* other species), Gnaphalium or White balsam *(Gnaphalium polycephalum)*, Twinleaf or Jeffersonia *(Jeffersonia diphylla)*, Privet leaves *(Ligustrum vulgare)*, Statice or Marsh rosemary *(Statice caroliniana)*, Bellwort *(Uvularia perfoliata)*, Blue whortleberry *(Vaccinium frondosum)*, Pokeweed *(Phytolacca decandra, P. dodecandra, P. americana)*, Kino *(Pterocarpus marsupium)*, Helenium or Frostwort *(Helianthemum canadense)*, Oak gall *(Quercus lusitanica)*, and Bayberry *(Myrica cerifera)*.

Antipruritics

BLACK OR GREEN TEA *(CAMELLIA SINENSIS)*: Tea catechins, when applied percutaneously in the ears of mice and given orally, inhibited signs of oxazolone-induced type IV allergy (Suzuki, 2000). The saponins also reduce allergy mediator release in in vitro studies (Akagi, 1997). The tannins are astringent and may coagulate serum proteins in oozing lesions, such as in acute traumatic dermatitis or hot spots.

GELSEMIUM *(GELSEMIUM SEMPERVIRENS)*: This herb appears to act as an anodyne, which is possibly the reason for traditional use for focal pruritus. This is a potentially toxic herb, and animals should not be allowed to lick any topical preparation of gelsemium.

CAYENNE *(CAPSICUM FRUTESCENS)*: An extract of capsicum, capsaicin is well accepted as a topical analgesic in human medicine. In a trial of capsaicin to suppress pruritus in dogs, owners found it to be effective; investigators did not (Marsella, 2002).

Anodyne

CAYENNE *(CAPSICUM FRUTESCENS)*: This herb was formerly used more as a counterirritant than as an anodyne. The isolated constituent capsaicin has been well investigated as an anodyne and is in commercial trade as Capsaizin. If the animal can be prevented from licking the area, it should be effective for local pain of osteoarthritis or neuritis. The taste itself may act as a deterrent to licking!

NETTLE, STINGING NETTLES *(URTICA DIOICA)*: In a controlled trial that examined "base of thumb pain" in humans, fresh nettle leaf applied to the area was significantly more effective in reducing pain than was placebo (Randall, 2000).

ECHINACEA ROOT *(ECHINACEA ANGUSTIFOLIA)*: This herb has mild anodyne properties.

CONIUM, POISON HEMLOCK *(CICUTA MACULATA):* This extract, combined with petrolatum, was traditionally used as a poultice for painful tumors, ulcers, neuralgia, and so forth. This is a highly toxic herb and should not be used at all.

JIMSON WEED (ALSO KNOWN AS THORNAPPLE OR STRAMONIUM) *(DATURA STRAMONIUM),* BELLADONNA *(ATROPA BELLADONNA),* HENBANE *(HYOSCYAMUS NIGER):* These are other very poisonous plants that should be used only by experienced herbalists, if at all. They were used in ointment form or as fomentations for many local painful disorders such as painful ulcers, tumors, orchitis, and mastitis, but they should not be used in animals because they will lick the applications.

CHELONE *(CHELONE GLABRA):* This herb was used as an ointment for painful ulcers, tumors, mastitis, and hemorrhoids.

MIMULUS, MONKEY FLOWER *(MIMULUS PILOSUS):* This was used by bruising the leaves or as a hot infusion, as a cataplasm.

CYNOGLOSSUM *(CYNOGLOSSUM OFFICINALE):* This herb was particularly used for bruising or chapping, and an interesting indication was for "excoriation of the feet from much traveling."

OTHER HERBS: Lavender (Lavandula vera, L. officinalis, L. angustifolia), Meadow Lily (Lilium candidum) Flowers, Horsemint (Monarda punctata), and Spearmint (Mentha viridis) were used occasionally in fomentation or oil form for local pain. The plants are high in essential oils. Some Lily spp are toxic to cats.

Herbs for Snakebite

Many plants in many cultures have been identified as beneficial in the treatment of snake bites. Mors and colleagues (2000) reviewed these plants and tested some of the plant constituents in a murine snakebite model. The mice were given 100 mg/kg of a specific phytochemical orally 1 hour before subcutaneous injection with the venom of the jararaca snake *(Bothrops jararaca).* The capacity for these phytochemicals to prevent death from envenomation was expressed as percentage of surviving animals in each group. Beta-sitosterol administration resulted in 70% protection; this is a common plant sterol contained in Yarrow *(Achillea millefolium),* Calendula *(Calendula officinalis), Cynanchum paniculatum, Eclipta prostrata, Ocimum basilicum,* Saw palmetto *(Serenoa repens),* Dandelion *(Taraxacum officinale),* and many other herbs. Hydroxybenzoic acids and their methyl esters gave up to 83% protection. Plants that contain these acids include Bistort *(Polygonum bistorta),* Gentian *(Gentiana lutea),* and *Perilla ternata.* Coumarins gave 40% protection, and many flavonoids provided 40% to 80% survival. Secondary metabolites of plants appear to interact with snake venom proteins, either by blocking receptors, chelating enzymes, or inhibiting enzymes in other ways.

This review contains an extensive listing of plants with ethnobotanical data for use in snakebites. Some of the better known plants include *Acacia catechu, Achyranthes aspera, Agrimonia eupatoria, Allium cepa, Arctium lappa, Argemone mexicana, Belamcanda chinensis, Brunfelsia grandiflora, Buddleia brasiliensis, Chenopodium ambrosioides, Cimicifuga racemosa, Coffea arabica, Curcuma longa, Daphne mezereum, Echinacea anugustifolia, Foeniculum vulgare, Gymnema sylvestre, Impatiens balsamina, Impatiens capensis, Morus alba, Nerium oleander, Perilla frutescens, Phyllanthus amarus, Pinellia ternata, Plantago major, Pinus sylvestris, Polygala senega, Ruta graveolens, Strychnos nux-vomica, Thymus vulgaris, and Verbascum thapsus* (Mors, 2000).

LIATRIS SPECIES: Roots were bruised and applied directly to the bite, while the root was also decocted and mixed with milk to be administered orally.

ECHINACEA *(E. ANGUSTIFOLIA):* This herb was used by Native Americans for bites, and this was a primary indication for its use for many years.

LION'S FOOT, NABALUS *(NABALUS ALBUS):* This was used as the root decoction.

BELLWORT *(UVULARIA PERFOLIATA):* This herb was boiled in milk to be administered orally, and the root was applied as a poultice simultaneously.

Herb for Anal Fistula

SWEET GUM *(LIQUIDAMBAR STYRACIFOLIUM):* Resin was melted with equal parts of lard or tallow; this was used as an ointment for anal fistula in people.

Poison Ivy, Poison Oak Herbal Treatment

LOBELIA *(LOBELIA INFLATA):* This herb was used in infusion form on wet cloths that were applied frequently to affected areas.

PUSSY WILLOW, BLACK WILLOW *(SALIX NIGRA):* This was said to be very effective for this condition and was prepared by simmering powdered bark in cream.

JEWELWEED *(IMPATIENS BALSAMIFERA):* This well-known traditional remedy was used for poison ivy, and teachers often point out that it grows near poison ivy. One study demonstrated that an extract of jewelweed was ineffective in the treatment of poison ivy contact dermatitis (Long, 1997)

GRINDELIA *(GRINDELIA SQUARROSA),* DIERVILLA, BUSH HONEYSUCKLE *(DIERVILLA TRIFIDA):* These were also used for poison ivy.

Vulnerary Herbs

Many, many herbs have been used to enhance wound healing. The list that follows was derived from the complete list of herbs in *King's American Dispensatory.* Clearly, some are more effective than others, but the large list below is provided because herbalists often find that they must use the herbs they have if the "best" choice is not available.

ALOE *(ALOE VERA):* This herb has been shown to enhance healing in surgically induced wounds in dogs (Swaim, 1992). Aloe also may have anti-inflammatory and angiogenic properties, and it contains a glycoprotein that stimulates cell proliferation and migration (Vazquez, 1996; Moon, 1999; Choi, 2001).

PLANTAIN *(PLANTAGO LANCEOLATA, P. MAJOR):* The leaves contain constituents with antibacterial, antihistamine, neutrophil-chemotactic, antifungal, analgesic, and anti-inflammatory properties (Samuelsen, 2000). They have been used for all types of skin lesions and wounds since at least the time of Dioscorides and are favorite choices of herbalists worldwide because they grow nearly everywhere.

CALENDULA *(CALENDULA OFFICINALIS):* The petals for the basis for one of the most popular vulnerary herbs in trade. The herb may enhance epithelialization of wounds and may have mild anti-inflammatory properties (Klouchek-Popova, 1982). It was strongly recommended by the Eclectics and used for "cancerous and other ulcers . . . lacerated wounds . . . [enhances] wound healing by replacement or first intention. . . . It is to be made into a saturated tincture with whiskey diluted with one-third its quantity of water; lint is saturated with this, applied to the parts, and renewed as often as it becomes dry . . . to wash abscess cavities, to prevent cicatrization from burns and scalds, in eczematous and ulcerative skin diseases, vaginitis (wash or tampon) . . . calendula has received strong endorsement . . . applied diluted to inflamed conjunctival and aural tissues, and to traumatic injuries of the eye and ear."

GOTU KOLA *(CENTELLA ASIATICA):* This has been used for ulcers, chronic eczema, and other cutaneous disorders. Gotu kola is well documented to enhance wound healing. Mechanisms may include increase of extracellular matrix, angiogenesis, and various growth factors (Maquart, 1999; Coldren, 2003).

CHELIDONIUM *(CHELIDONIUM MAJUS):* This herb contains, among other alkaloids, berberine, which is antibacterial. The Eclectics found it a powerful vulnerary, recommending "an alcoholic tincture of the root (3 ounces to 1 pint) will be found an unrivaled external application to prevent or subdue traumatic inflammations." Contact dermatitis has been reported. As stated above, the herb can be toxic and animals should be prevented from licking it, if used.

ARNICA, LEOPARDS BANE *(ARNICA MONTANA):* This herb is in popular use, both as the herb and as the homeopathic remedy. It was used to prevent and treat local inflammation and bruising, and also as a dressing for cuts, lacerations, and bruises. In vitro studies show that Arnica inhibits activation of NF-kappa B and NF-AT, which leads to release of cytokines and inflammatory mediators (Klaas, 2002). Arnica may have mild antibacterial activity (Iauk, 2003), although other studies show no effect. Arnica is a contact allergen that may cause dermatologic reactions in some patients with repeated use (Reider, 2001). It is toxic, and animals should be prevented from licking it.

CHAMOMILE *(MATRICARIA RECUTITA):* This herb has many traditional uses, including as treatment for ruptured abscesses. Few studies have been done, but one showed very mild anti-inflammatory activity in a trial of treatment for atopic eczema (Patzelt-Wenczler, 2000). Chamomile is a contact sensitizer in susceptible patients.

GOLDENSEAL *(HYDRASTIS CANADENSIS):* This treatment was particularly indicated in Eclectic medicine for "eczematous manifestations around the outlets of the body . . ."

SAINT JOHN'S WORT *(HYPERICUM PERFORATUM):* This is used in oil or ointment form for painful ulcers, tumors, and bruises. An extract reduced T-cell proliferation in healing wounds (and the authors concluded that this was possible support for traditional wound healing use) (Schempp, 2000). Another specis, *H. patulum,* may enhance wound contraction and epithelialization (Mukherjee, 2000). Oral and topical use may lead to skin photosensitization.

BAY LAUREL, SWEET BAY *(LAURUS NOBILIS):* This is the bay leaf used in cooking. The leaves have been used in powder or decoction form for "insect bites and stings, scalp eruptions." Contact hypersensitivity has been reported.

ROAST OR BOILED FIGS *(FICUS CARICA):* These have been used for infected ulcers, boils, and so forth. No medicinal principles from figs have been specifically investigated; however, the sugar may be active. Sugar and honey have been used as an antibacterial and vulnerary agent for burns and ulcers (Tanne, 1988; Okeniyi, 2005; Dunford, 2005). Figs were used as a poultice when the dried fruit was added to milk.

LOBELIA *(LOBELIA INFLATA):* This herb was considered useful for a wide variety of disorders, including "herpes, lichen, eczema, nettlerash, . . . sprains, bruises, rheumatic pains, erysipelas, and erysipelous inflammations, tetter, and other forms of cutaneous diseases."

FIGWORT *(SCROPHULARIA NODOSA):* Three compounds in this plant stimulate human fibroblast activity in vitro (Stevenson, 2002). It has been used for hemorrhoids, ringworm, vesicular eruptions, painful swellings, and so forth.

OTHER HERBS: Herbs used for indolent cutaneous ulcers, felons, or slow-healing abscesses or wounds include False sarsaparilla, small spikenard *(Aralia nudicaulis),* Copaiba *(Copaiba langsdorffii),* Daphne or Mezereum *(Daphne mezereum),* cataplasm of bruised Cyclamin *(Cyclamen hederifolium)* tubers, Wild carrot *(Daucus carota),* Epiphegus *(Epiphegus virginiana),* Galbanum *(Ferula galbaniflua),* Grindelia *(Grindelia robusta),* Ivy *(Hedera helix),* Bayberry *(Myrica cerifera),* Virginia stonecrop *(Penthorum sedoides),* Poke root *(Phytolacca americana),* Bearsfoot, Polymnia *(Polymnia uvedalia),* Potentilla, Tormentil *(Potentilla tormentilla),* Black alder bark and berries *(Prinus verticillatus),* Wild cherry bark *(Prunus serotina),* Yellow dock *(Rumex crispus),* Sorrel *(Rumex acetosa),* White willow *(Salix alba),* Pussy willow, Black willow *(Salix nigra),* Mossy stonecrop *(Sedum),* Chickweed *(Stellaria media),* Thuja *(Thuja occidentalis),* Red clover *(Trifolium pretense),* Blue whortleberry *(Vaccinium frondosum),* Mullein *(Verbascum thapsus),* Cramp bark, highbush cranberry *(Viburnum opulus),* and Black Haw *(Viburnum prunifolium).* A few of these plants are irritants to stimulate healing, and the reader is advised to understand them well before using them.

Useful Web Sites
King's American Dispensatory
www.ibiblio.org/herbmed/eclectic/kings/main.html
Botanical Dermatology Database
bodd.cf.ac.uk/
Paula Begoun's Cosmetic Dictionary
www.cosmeticscop.com/learn/dictionary.asp?TYPE=MAIN

Herbs cited in traditional literature for "various cutaneous affections" include Canada thistle root *(Cirsium arvense)*, Stoneroot *(Collinsonia canadensis)* as a poultice, Cynoglossum *(Cynoglossum officinale)*, Helenium, Frostwort *(Helianthemum canadense)*, Elecampane *(Inula helenium)*, Ox-eye daisy *(Chrysanthemum leucanthemum)*, Loosestrife, Lythrum *(Lythrum salicaria)*, Smartweed or Water pepper *(Polygonum hydropiper)*, Peru balsam tree *(Myroxylon pereirae)*, Jack-in-the-Pulpit *(Arisaema triphyllum)*, and Bellwort *(Uvularia perfoliata)*.

Herbs used for external inflammation, excoriations, and burns include Fringe tree bark *(Chionanthus virginicus)*, False bittersweet *(Celastrus scandens)*, American larch *(Larix americana)*, Meadow lily *(Lilium candidum)*, Bugleweed *(Lycopus virginicus)*, Catnip *(Nepeta cataria)*, and Passionflower *(Passiflora incarnata)*.

Herbs used for bruising and ecchymoses include the powdered flowers of Lily of the Valley *(Convallaria majalis)*, the bruised leaves of Navelwort, Cotyledon *(Cotyledon umbilicus)*, Hyssop *(Hyssopus officinalis)* leaves, and Pearly everlasting *(Antennaria margaritacea)*.

Herbs used for various chronic eruptions such as psoriasis, eczema, ringworm, leprosy, and ulcers include Cleavers *(Gallium aparine)*, Chaulmoogra, Gynocardia *(Hydnocarpus kurzii)*, Ivy *(Hedera helix)*, Jewelweed *(Impatiens pallida)* juice, Mountain laurel, Kalmia *(Kalmia latifolia)* leaves, Labrador tea *(Ledum latifolium)*, Sweet gum *(Liquidambar styraciflua)*, Kamala, Rottlera *(Mallotus phillipiensis, Echinus philippinensis, Rottlera tinctoria, Croton philippensis)*, Azedarach or Chinaberry tree *(Melia azedarach)*, Myrtle *(Myrtus communis)*, and Nettle *(Urtica dioica)*.

References

Abaineh D, Sintayehu A. Treatment trial of subclinical mastitis with the herb *Persicaria senegalense* (Polygonaceae). Trop Anim Health Prod 2001;33:511-519.

Abells Sutton G, Haik R. Efficacy of garlic as an anthelmintic in donkeys. Israel Journal Veterinary medicine Vol 54 (1), 1999.

Ackermann RT, Mulrow CD, Ramirez G, Gardner CD, Morbidoni L, Lawrence VA. Garlic shows promise for improving some cardiovascular risk factors. Arch Intern Med 2001;161:813-824.

ACP Australian College Phytotherapy. Course Notes, Module 4, Gastrointestinal System, 1999.

Ademola IO, Fagbemi BO, Idowu SO Anthelmintic activity of extracts of *Spondias mombin* against gastrointestinal nematodes of sheep: studies in vitro and in vivo. Trop Anim Health Prod 2005;37:223-235.

Adzet T, Camarasa J, Laguna JC. Action of an artichoke extract against CCl4-induced heptotoxicity in rats. Acta Pharm Jugosl 1987;37:183-187.

Ageel AM, Mossa JS, al-Yahya MA, al-Said MS, Tariq M. Experimental studies on antirheumatic crude drugs used in Saudi traditional medicine. Drugs Exp Clin Res 1989;15:369-372.

Ahmad N, Gupta S, Husain MM, Heiskanen KM, Mukhtar H. Differential antiproliferative and apoptotic response of sanguinarine for cancer cells versus normal cells. Clin Cancer Res 2000;6:1524-1528.

Ahsan SK, Tariq M, Ageel AM, al-Yahya MA, Shah AH. Effect of Trigonella foenum-graecum and Ammi majus on calcium oxalate urolithiasis in rats. J Ethnopharmacol 1989 Oct; 26(3):249-254.

Ajay M, Gilani AU, Mustafa MR. Effects of flavonoids on vascular smooth muscle of the isolated rat thoracic aorta. Life Sci 2003;74:603-612.

Akagi M, Fukuishi N, Kan T, Sagesaka YM, Akagi R. Anti-allergic effect of tea-leaf saponin (TLS) from tea leaves (*Camellia sinensis* var. sinensis). Biol Pharm Bull 1997;20:565-567.

Akhani SP, Vishwakarma SL, Goyal RK. Anti-diabetic activity of Zingiber officinale in streptozotocin-induced type I diabetic rats. J Pharm Pharmacol. 2004 Jan;56(1):101-105.

Akhondzadeh S, Naghavi HR, Vazirian M, Shayeganpour A, Rashidi H, Khani M. Passionflower in the treatment of generalized anxiety: a pilot double-blind randomized controlled trial with oxazepam. J Clin Pharm Ther 2001a;26:363-367.

Akhondzadeh S, Kashani L, Mobaseri M, Hosseini SH, Nikzad S, Khani M. Passionflower in the treatment of opiate withdrawal: a double-blind randomized controlled trial. J Clin Pharm Ther 2001b;26:369-373.

Akhondzadeh S, Kashani L, Fotouhi A, et al. Comparison of *Lavendula angustifolia* Mill. tincture and imipramine in the treatment of mild to moderate depression: a double-blind, randomized trial. Prog Neuropsychopharmacol Biol Psychiatry 2003a;27:123-127.

Akhondzadeh S, Noroozian M, Mohammadi M, Ohadinia S, Jamshidi AH, Khani M. *Melissa officinalis* extract in the treatment of patients with mild to moderate Alzheimer's disease: a double blind, randomised, placebo controlled trial. J Neurol Neurosurg Psychiatry 2003b;74:863-866.

Al-Ali M, Wahbi S, Twaij H, Al-Badr A. *Tribulus terrestris:* preliminary study of its diuretic and contractile effects and comparison with *Zea mays*. J Ethnopharmacol 2003;85:257-260.

Al-Qarawi AA, Abdel-Rahman HA, Ali BH, El Mougy SA. Liquorice (Glycyrrhiza glabra) and the adrenal-kidney-pituitary axis in rats. Food Chem Toxicol. 2002 Oct;40(10): 1525-1527

al-Zuhair H, el-Sayeh B, Ameen HA, al-Shoora H. Pharmacological studies of cardamom oil in animals. Pharmacol Res 1996; 34:79-82.

Alarcon-Aguilara FJ, Roman-Ramos R, Perez-Gutierrez S, Aguilar-Contreras A, Contreras-Weber CC, Flores-Saenz JL. Study of the anti-hyperglycemic effect of plants used as antidiabetics. J Ethnopharmacol 1998;61:101-110.

Alacrìn De La Lastra C, Martin MJ, Marhuenda E: Gastric Anti-Ulcer Activity Of Silymarin, A Lipoxygenase Inhibitor, In Rats. J Pharm Pharmacol 1992;44:929-931.

Alarcon de la Lastra AC, Martin MJ, Motilva V, Jimenez M, La Casa C, Lopez A. Gastroprotection induced by silymarin, the hepatoprotective principle of Silybum marianum in ischemia-reperfusion mucosal injury: role of neutrophils. Planta Med. 1995 Apr;61(2):116-119.

Albert-Puleo M. Fennel and anise as estrogenic agents. J Ethnopharmacol 1980;2:337-344.

Alexandrovich I, Rakovitskaya O, Kolmo E, Sidorova T, Shushunov S. The effect of fennel *(Foeniculum vulgare)* seed oil emulsion in infantile colic: a randomized, placebo-controlled study. Altern Ther Health Med 2003;9:58-61.

Ali M, Thomson M. Consumption of a garlic clove a day could be beneficial in preventing thrombosis. Prostaglandins Leukot Essent Fatty Acids 1995;53:211-212.

Allen FM. Blueberry leaf extract: physiologic and clinical properties in relation to carbohydrate metabolism. JAMA 1927;89: 1577-1581.

Amellal M, Bronner C, Briancon F, et al. Inhibition of mast cell histamine release by flavonoids and bioflavonoids. Planta Medica 1985;51:16-20.

Ammon HP, Safayhi H, Mack T, Sabieraj J. Mechanism of anti-inflammatory actions of curcumine and boswellic acids. J Ethnopharmacol 1993;38:113-119.

Amri H, Drieu K, Papadopoulos V. Transcriptional suppression of the adrenal cortical peripheral-type benzodiazepine receptor gene and inhibition of steroid synthesis by ginkgolide B. Biochem Pharmacol 2003;65:717-729.

Anand R, Patnaik G, Kulshreshtha D. Activity of certain fractions of *Tribulus terrestris* fruits against experimentally induced urolithiasis in rats. Indian J Exp Biol 1994;32:548-552.

Anderson J, Smith W. The antitussive activity of glycyrrhetinic acid and its derivatives. J Pharm Pharmacol 1961;13:396-404.

Anderson PM, Meyers DE, Hasz DE, et al. In vitro and in vivo cytotoxicity of an anti-osteosarcoma immunotoxin containing pokeweed antiviral protein. Cancer Res 1995;55:1321-1327.

Archana R, Namasivayan A. Antistressor effect of *Withania somnifera*. J Ethnopharmacol 1999;64:91-93.

Armanini D, Karbowiak I, Funder JW. Affinity of liquorice derivatives for mineralocorticoid and glucocorticoid receptors. Clin Endocrinol 1983;19:609-612.

Armanini D, Strasser T, Weber PC. Binding of agonists and antagonists to mineralocorticoid receptors in human peripheral mononuclear leucocytes. J Hypertens 1985;3(3):S157-159.

Arun N, Nalini N. Efficacy of turmeric on blood sugar and polyol pathway in diabetic albino rats. Plant Foods Hum Nutr. 2002 Winter;57(1):41-52.

Arzneimitteforschung 1996;46:389-394.

Atal CK, Sharma ML, Kaul A, Khajuria A. Immunomodulating agents of plant origin. I: Preliminary screening. J Ethnopharmacol 1986;18:133-141.

Auf'mkolk M, Kohrle J, Gumbinger H, et al. Antihormonal effects of plant extracts: iodothyronine deiodinase of rat liver is inhibited by extracts and secondary metabolites of plants. Horm Metab Res 1984a;16:188-192.

Auf'mkolk M, Ingbar JC, Amir SM, et al. Inhibition by certain plant extracts of the binding and adenylate cyclase stimulatory effect of bovine thyrotropin in human thyroid membranes. Endocrinology 1984b;115:527-534.

Austin S, Dale EB, DeKadt S. Long-term follow-up of cancer patients using Contreras, Hoxsey and Gerson therapies. Journal of Naturopathic Medicine 1994;5(1):74-76.

Awad R, Arnason JT, Trudeau V, et al. Phytochemical and biological analysis of skullcap *(Scutellaria lateriflora* L.*)*: a medicinal plant with anxiolytic properties. Phytomedicine 2003;10: 640-649.

Aydin S, Beis R, Ozturk Y, Baser KH. Nepetalactone: a new opioid analgesic from *Nepeta caesarea* Boiss. J Pharm Pharmacol 1998;50:813-817.

Baba K, Abe S, Mizuno D. Antitumor activity of hot water extract of dandelion, *Taraxacum officinale*—correlation between antitumor activity and timing of administration. Yagugaku Zasshi 1981;101:538-543.

Babu TD, Kuttan G, Padikkala J. Cytotoxic and anti-tumour properties of certain taxa of Umbelliferae with special reference to *Centella asiatica* (L.) Urban. J Ethnopharmacol 1995;48:53-57.

Backhauss C, Krieglstein J. Extract of kava *(Piper methysticum)* and its methysticin constituents protect brain tissue against ischemic damage in rodents. Eur J Pharmacol 1992;215:265-269.

Balasenthil S, Arivazhagan S, Ramachandran CR, Ramachandran V, Nagini S. Chemopreventive potential of neem *(Azadirachta indica)* on 7,12-dimethylbenz[a]anthracene (DMBA) induced hamster buccal pouch carcinogenesis. J Ethnopharmacol 1999;67:189-195.

Balasenthil S, Ramachandran CR, Nagini S. Prevention of 4-nitroquinoline 1-oxide-induced rat tongue carcinogenesis by garlic. Fitoterapia 2001;72:524-531.

Ballard CG, O'Brien JT, Reichelt K, Perry EK. Aromatherapy as a safe and effective treatment for the management of agitation in severe dementia: the results of a double-blind, placebo-controlled trial with Melissa. J Clin Psychiatry 2002;63:553-558.

Baltina LA. Chemical modification of glycyrrhizic acid as a route to new bioactive compounds for medicine [Review]. Curr Med Chem 2003;10:155-171.

Baluchnejadmojarad T, Roghani M. Endothelium-dependent and -independent effect of aqueous extract of garlic on vascular reactivity on diabetic rats. Fitoterapia 2003;74:630-637.

Banerjee SK, Maulik SK. Effect of garlic on cardiovascular disorders: a review. Nutr J 2002;1:4.

Barsanti JA, Finco DR, Mahaffey MM, et al. Effects of an extract of *Serenoa repens* on dogs with hyperplasia of the prostate gland. Am J Vet Res 2000;61:880-885.

Basch EM, Ulbricht CE. *Natural Standard Herb and Supplement Handbook: The Clinical Bottom Line*. St. Louis, Mo: Elsevier-Mosby; 2005.

Basit N, et al. In vitro effect of extracts of *Euphorbia hirta* Linn. on *Entamoeba histolytica*. Riv Parasitol 1977;38:259-262.

Baumann G, Felix S, Sattelberger U, Klein G. Cardiovascular effects of forskolin (HL 362) in patients with idiopathic congestive cardiomyopathy—a comparative study with dobutamine and sodium nitroprusside. J Cardiovasc Pharmacol 1990;16:93-100.

Beachey EH. Bacterial adherence: adhesin-receptor interactions mediating the attachment of bacteria to mucosal surface. J Infect Dis 1981;143:325-345.

Beaubrun G, Gray GE. A review of herbal medicines for psychiatric disorders. Psychiatr Serv. 2000 Sep;51(9):1130-1134.

Beaux D, Fleurentin J, Mortier F. Effect of extracts of *Orthosiphon stamineus* Benth., *Hieracium pilosella* L., *Sambucus nigra* L. and *Arctostaphylos uva-ursi* (L.) Spreng. in rats. Phytother Res 1999;13:222-225.

Beech J, Donaldson MT, Lindborg S. Comparison of *Vitex agnus castus* extract and pergolide in treatment of equine Cushing's syndrome. Proc AAEP 2002;48:177.

Beesley A, Hardcastle J, Hardcastle PT, Taylor CJ. Influence of peppermint oil on absorptive and secretory processes in rat small intestine. Gut 1996;39:214-219.

Beijamini V, Andreatini R. Effects of *Hypericum perforatum* and paroxetine in the mouse defense test battery. Pharmacol Biochem Behav 2003a;74:1015-1024.

Beijamini V, Andreatini R. Effects of *Hypericum perforatum* and paroxetine on rat performance in the elevated T-maze. Pharmacol Res 2003b;48:199-207.

Belford-Courtney R. Comparison of Chinese and Western uses of *Angelica sinensis*. Austral J Med Herbalism 1994;5:4,87-91.

Ben-Arye E, Goldin E, Wengrower D, Stamper A, Kohn R, Berry E. Wheat grass juice in the treatment of active distal ulcerative colitis: a randomized double-blind placebo-controlled trial. Scand J Gastroenterol 2002;37:444-449.

Bensoussan A; Talley NJ; Hing M; Menzies R; Guo A; Ngu M, 1998. Treatment of irritable bowel syndrome with Chinese herbal medicine: a randomized controlled trial. JAMA 11;280(18):1585-1589.

Bergner P. Immune treatment outcomes at Mexican cancer clinics: Hoxsey treatment may help some late stage cancer. Med Herbalism 1995;6:10.

Bergner P. Cardiotoxic effects of Blue Cohosh on a fetus. Available at: http://medherb.com/Materia_Medica/Caulophyllum_-_Cardiotoxic_effects_of_Blue_Cohosh_on_a_fetus.htm. Accessed June 13, 2005.

Bermejo Benito P, Abad Martinez MJ, Silvan Sen MJ. In vivo and in vitro antiinflammatory activity of saikosaponins. Life Sci 1998;63:1147-1156.

Bezakova L, Misik V, Malekova L, Svajdlenka E, Kostalova D. Lipoxygenase inhibition and antioxidant properties of bisbenzylisoqunoline alkaloids isolated from *Mahonia aquifolium*. Pharmazie 1996;51:758-761.

Bharani A, Ganguly A, Bhargava KD. Salutary effect of *Terminalia arjuna* in patients with severe refractory heart failure. Int J Cardiol 1995;49:191-199.

Bhatia N, Zhao J, Wolf DM, Agarwal R. Inhibition of human carcinoma cell growth and DNA synthesis by silibinin, an active constituent of milk thistle: comparison with silymarin. Cancer Lett 1999;147:77-84.

Bhattacharya SK, Mitra SK. Anxiolytic activity of *Panax ginseng* roots: an experimental study. J Ethnopharmacol 1991;34:87-92.

Bhattacharya SK, Satyan KS, Ghosal S. Antioxidant activity of glycowithanolides from *Withania somnifera*. Indian J Exp Biol 1997;35:236-239.

Bhattacharya SK, Ghosal S. Anxiolytic activity of a standardized extract of *Bacopa monniera:* an experimental study. Phytomedicine 1998;5:77-82.

Bhattacharya SK, Bhattacharya A, Sairam K, Ghosal S. Anxiolytic-antidepressant activity of *Withania somnifera* glycowithanolides: an experimental study. Phytomedicine 2000;7:463-469.

Bhattacharya SK, Muruganandam AV. Adaptogenic activity of *Withania somnifera:* an experimental study using a rat model of chronic stress. Pharmacol Biochem Behav 2003;75:547-555.

Bhuvaneswari V, Velmurugan B, Nagini S. Dose-response effect of tomato paste on 7,12-dimethylbenz[a]anthracene-induced hamster buccal pouch carcinogenesis. J Exp Clin Cancer Res 2004a;23:241-249.

Bhuvaneswari V, Rao KS, Nagini S. Altered expression of anti and proapoptotic proteins during chemoprevention of hamster buccal pouch carcinogenesis by tomato and garlic combination. Clin Chim Acta 2004b;350:65-72.

Bi ZQ, Bo YH, Duan JH. [Treatment of chronic renal failure with *Oenothera beinnis* L. in rats with subtotal nephrectomy.] Zhonghua Nei Ke Za Zhi 1992;31:7-10,59.

Bianchini F, Vainio H. Wine and resveratrol: mechanisms of cancer prevention? Eur J Cancer Prev 2003;12:417-425.

Birks J, Grimley EV, Van Dongen M. *Ginkgo biloba* for cognitive impairment and dementia. Cochrane Database Syst Rev 2002;4:CD003120.

Bisset NG, ed. *Herbal Drugs and Phytopharmaceuticals* (Wichtl M, ed. [German edition]). Stuttgart: Medpharm; 1994.

Bliddal H, Rosetzsky A, Schlichting P, et al. A randomized, placebo-controlled, cross-over study of ginger extracts and ibuprofen in osteoarthritis. Osteoarthritis Cartilage 2000;8: 9-12.

Block JR, Evans S. A review of recent results addressing the potential interactions of antioxidants with cancer drug therapy. JAMA 2001;4:11-19.

Blumenthal M, Busse WR, Goldberg A etal, eds. *The Complete German Commission E Monographs*. Austin, Tex: American Botanical Council; 1998.

Blumenthal M Busse WR, Goldberg A etal eds. *Herbal Medicine. Expanded Commission E Monographs*. Austin, Tex: American Botanical Council; 2000.

Bochorakova H, Paulova H, Slanina J, et al. Main flavonoids in the root of *Scutellaria baicalensis* cultivated in Europe and their comparative antiradical properties. Phytother Res 2003;17:640-644.

Boik J. *Cancer and Natural Medicine: A Textbook of Basic Science and Clinical Research*. Princeton, Minn: Oregon Medical Press; 1996.

Boik J. *Natural Compounds in Cancer Therapy*. Princeton, Minn: Oregon Medical Press; 2001.

Bomser J, Madhavi DL, Singletary K, Smith MA. In vitro anticancer activity of fruit extracts from *Vaccinium* species. Planta Med 1996;62:212-216.

Bond R, Lloyd DH. A double blind comparison of olive oil and a combination of evening primrose oil and fish oil in the management of canine atopy. Vet Rec. 1992;131(24):558-60.

Bond R, Lloyd DH. Combined treatment with concentrated essential fatty acids and prednisolone in the management of canine atopy. Vet Rec. 1994;134(2):30-32.

Bone K. *Clinical Applications of Ayurvedic and Chinese Herbs—Monographs for the Western Herbal Practitioner*. Warwick, Queensland, Australia: Phytotherapy Press; 1996:94.

Bone K. *Clinical Applications of Ayurvedic and Chinese Herbs—Monographs for the Western Herbal Practitioner*. Warwick, Queensland, Australia: Phytotherapy Press; 1997.

Bone K. Echinacea: when should it be used? Alt Med Rev 1997;2:451-458.

Bone K. Echinacea: useful for autoimmune disease? Eur J Herbal Med 1997-1998;3:13-17.

Bone K. Automimmune disease. Townsend Lett 1999;193:94-98.

Bone K. *A Clinical Guide to Blending Liquid Herbs*. St. Louis, Mo: Churchill Livingstone; 2003:197.

Bone K. Phytotherapy for autoimmune disease. Townsend Lett 2004;250.

Bonnett B, Poland C. Preliminary results of a randomized, double blind, multicenter, controlled clinical trial of two herbal therapies, acetylsalicylic acid and placebo for osteoarthritic dogs. Proceedings of the American Holistic Veterinary Medical Association. Burlington, Vt: AHVMA; 1996:143-147.

Borges LM, Ferri PH, Silva WJ, Silva WC, Silva JG. In vitro efficacy of extracts of *Melia azedarach* against the tick *Boophilus microplus*. Med Vet Entomol 2003;17:228-231.

Bradley PR, ed. *British Herbal Compendium*, vol 1. Bournemouth: British Herbal Medicine Association; 1992.

Bradley RR, Cunniff PJ, Pereira BJ, Jaber BL. Hematopoietic effect of *Radix angelicae sinensis* in a hemodialysis patient. Am J Kidney Dis 1999;34:349-354.

Braquet P. The ginkgolides: potent platelet-activating factor antagonists isolated from *Ginkgo biloba* L.: chemistry, pharmacology and clinical applications. Drugs Future 1987;12:643-699.

Braun JM, Ko HL, Schierholz JM, Beuth J. Standardized mistletoe extract augments immune response and down-regulates local and metastatic tumor growth in murine models. Anticancer Res 2002;22:4187-4190.

Braun L, Lester S, Kuzma AB, Hosie SC. Gastric dilatation-volvulus in the dog with histological evidence of preexisting inflammatory bowel disease: a retrospective study of 23 cases. J Am Anim Hosp Assoc 1996;32:287-290.

Brinker FJ. *Herb Contraindications and Drug Interactions*. Oregon: Eclectic Institute; 1997:104-106.

British Herbal Medicine Association. *A Guide to Traditional Herbal Medicines*. Bournemouth: British Herbal Medicine Association Publishing, 2003.

British Herbal Pharmacopoeia. Keighley: British Herbal Medicine Association; 1983.

Brousseau M, Miller SC. Enhancement of natural killer cells and increased survival of aging mice fed daily Echinacea root extract from youth. Biogerontology 2005;6:157-163.

Bruhwiler K, Frater-Sroder M, Kalbermatten R, et al. Golden Rod effective for urinary tract inflammation. International Congress on Phytotherapy; Munich, Germany; September 1992.

Bruneton J. *Pharmacognosy, Phytochemistry, Medicinal Plants.* Paris, France: Lavoisier Publishing; 1995:604.

Buck AC. Is there a scientific basis for the therapeutic effects of *Serenoa repens* in benign prostatic hyperplasia? Mechanisms of action. J Urol 2004;172:1792-1799.

Buffington CA, Blaisdell JL, Komatsu Y, Kawase K. Effects of choreito consumption on struvite crystal growth in urine of cats. Am J Vet Res 1994;55:972-975.

Buffington CA, Blaisdell JL, Komatsu Y, Kawase K. Effects of choreito and takushya consumption on in vitro and in vivo struvite solubility in cat urine. Am J Vet Res 1997a;58: 150-152.

Buffington CA, Blaisdell JL, Kawase K, Komatsu Y. Effects of choreito consumption on urine variables of healthy cats fed a magnesium-supplemented commercial diet. Am J Vet Res 1997b;58:146-149.

Burger AM, Mengs U, Schuler JB, Fiebig HH. Anticancer activity of an aqueous mistletoe extract (AME) in syngeneic murine tumor models. Anticancer Res 2001;21:1965-1968.

Busquets S, Carbo N, Almendro V, Quiles MT, Lopez-Soriano FJ, Argiles JM.Curcumin, a natural product present in turmeric, decreases tumor growth but does not behave as an anticachectic compound in a rat model. Cancer Lett. 2001 Jun 10;167(1):33-38.

Butterweck V. Mechanism of action of St John's wort in depression: what is known? CNS Drugs. 2003;17(8):539-562.

Calle J, Toscano M, Pinzon R, Baquero J, Bautista E. Antinociceptive and uterine relaxant activities of *Viburnum toronis* alive (Caprifoliaceae). J Ethnopharmacol 1999;66:71-73.

Cao J, Xu Y, Chen J, Klaunig JE. Chemopreventive effects of green and black tea on pulmonary and hepatic carcinogenesis. Fundam Appl Toxicol 1996;29:244-250.

Caron ME, White CM. Evaluation of the antihyperlipidemic properties of dietary supplements. Pharmacotherapy 2001;21: 481-487.

Carpinella MC, Defago MT, Valladares G, Palacios SM. Antifeedant and insecticide properties of a limonoid from *Melia azedarach* (Meliaceae) with potential use for pest management. J Agric Food Chem 2003;51:369-374.

Casto BC, Kresty LA, Kraly CL, et al. Chemoprevention of oral cancer by black raspberries. Anticancer Res 2002;22:4005-4015.

Cernakova M, Kost'alova D, Kettmann V, Plodova M, Toth J, Drimal J. Potential antimutagenic activity of berberine, a constituent of *Mahonia aquifolium*. BMC Complement Altern Med 2002;2:2.

Chainani-Wu N. Safety and anti-inflammatory activity of curcumin: a component of tumeric *(Curcuma longa)*. J Altern Complement Med 2003;9:161-168.

Chakurski I, Matev M, Stefanov G, Koichev A, Angelova I. Treanntment of duodenal ulcers and gastroduodenitis with a herbal combination of Symphitum officinalis and Calendula officinalis with and without antacids. Vutr Boles. 1981b; 20(6):44-47.

Chakurski I, Matev M, Koichev A, Angelova I, Stefanov G. [Treatment of chronic colitis with an herbal combination of *Taraxacum officinale, Hypericum perforatum, Melissa officinalis, Calendula officinalis,* and *Foeniculum vulgare.*] Vutr Boles 1981b;20:51-54.

Chan TY. Interaction between warfarin and danshen *(Salvia miltiorrhiza)*. Ann Pharmacother 2001;35:501-504.

Chandler RF. Licorice, more than just a flavour. Can Pharm J 1985;118:420-424.

Chang HM, But PPH, eds. *Pharmacology and Applications of Chinese Materia Medica,* vol 1. Singapore: World Scientific Publishing; 1986:366-369.

Chang HM, But PPH, eds:*Pharmacology and Applications of Chinese Materia Medica,* vol 2. Singapore: World Scientific Publishing; 1987.

Chang CK, Lin MT. DL-Tetrahydropalmatine may act through inhibition of amygdaloid release of dopamine to inhibit an epileptic attack in rats. Neurosci Lett 2001;307:163-166.

Chauhan DP. *Chemotherapeutic Potential of Curcumin for Colorectal Cancer. Current Pharmaceutical Design.* Hilversum, Netherlands: Bentham Science Publishers BV; 2002:1695-1706.

Chen CF, Chen SM, Lin MT, Chow SY. In vivo and in vitro studies on the mechanism of cardiovascular effects of Wu-Chu-Yu (Evodiae fructus). Am J Chin Med 1981;9:39-47.

Chen QM, Ye YC, Chai FL, Jin KP. [Protoscolicidal effect of some chemical agents and drugs against *Echinococcus granulosus.*] Zhongguo Ji Sheng Chong Xue Yu Ji Sheng Chong Bing Za Zhi 1991;9:137-139.

Chen J, Stavro PM, Thompson LU. Dietary flaxseed inhibits human breast cancer growth and metastasis and downregulates expression of insulin-like growth factor and epidermal growth factor receptor. Nutr Cancer. 2002;43(2):187-192.

Cheng XD, Hou CH, Zhang XJ, et al. Effects of huangqi (hex) on inducing cell differentiation and cell death in K562 and HEL cells. Acta Biochim Biophys Sin (Shanghai) 2004;36:211-217.

Cheshier JE, Ardestani-Kaboudanian S, Liang B, et al. Immunomodulation by pycnogenol in retrovirus-infected or ethanol-fed mice. Life Sci 1996;58:87-96.

Cheung ZH, So KF, Lu Q, et al. Enhanced survival and regeneration of axotomized retinal ganglion cells by a mixture of herbal extracts. J Neurotrauma 2002;19:369-378.

Chew BP, Wong MW, Wong TS. Effects of lutein from marigold extract on immunity and growth of mammary tumors in mice. Anticancer Res 1996;16:3689-3694.

Chew EC. Yunnan bai yao–induced platelet release in suspensions of washed platelets. Comp Med East West 1977;5:271-274.

Choi SW, Son BW, Son YS, Park YI, Lee SK, Chung MH. The wound-healing effect of a glycoprotein fraction isolated from aloe vera. Br J Dermatol 2001;145:535-545.

Christina AJ, Joseph DG, Packialakshmi M, et al. Anticarcinogenic activity of *Withania somnifera* Dunal against Dalton's ascitic lymphoma. J Ethnopharmacol 2004;93:359-361.

Cibere J, Deng Z, Lin Y, et al. A randomized double blind, placebo controlled trial of topical *Tripterygium wilfordii* in rheumatoid arthritis: reanalysis using logistic regression analysis. J Rheumatol 2003;30:465-467.

Cicero AF, Derosa G, Brillante R, Bernardi R, Nascetti S, Gaddi A. Effects of Siberian ginseng *(Eleutherococcus senticosis maxim.)* on elderly quality of life: a randomized clinical trial. Arch Gerontol Geriatr Suppl 2004;9:69-73.

Clavin ML, Gorzalczany S, Mino J, et al. Antinociceptive effect of some Argentine medicinal species of Eupatorium. Phytother Res 2000;14:275-277.

Clouatre DL. Kava kava: examining new reports of toxicity. Toxicol Lett 2004;150:85-96.

Coats BC, Holland RE, Ahola R. *Creatures in Our Care: The Veterinary Uses of Aloe Vera.* Published by the authors. 1985.

Coldren CD, Hashim P, Ali JM, Oh SK, Sinskey AJ, Rha C. Gene expression changes in the human fibroblast induced by *Centella asiatica* triterpenoids. Planta Med 2003;69:725-732.

Cometa MF, Mazzanti G, Tomassini L, 1998. Sedative and spasmolytic effects of *Viburnum tinus* L. and its major pure compounds. Phytotherapy research, 12 (suppl.1): S89-S91.

Conklin KA. Dietary antioxidants during cancerchemotherapy: impact on chemotherapeutic effectiveness and development of side effects. Nutr Cancer 2000;37:1-18.

Cook W. The Physiomedical Dispensatory. 1869. Available online at Henriette's Herbal Homepage: http://www.henriettesherbal.com/eclectic/cook/index.htm

Costello CH, Butler CL. An investigation of Piscidia erythrina (Jamaica Dogwood). J Am Pharm Assoc 1948;37:89-96.

Cropley M, Cave Z, Ellis J, Middleton RW. Effect of kava and valerian on human physiological and psychological responses to mental stress assessed under laboratory conditions. Phytother Res 2002;16:23-27.

Cruz T, Jimenez J, Zarzuelo A, Cabo MM. The spasmolytic activity of the essential oil of *Thymus baeticus* Boiss in rats. Phytother Res 1989;3:106-108.

Currier NL, Miller SC. *Echinacea purpurea* and melatonin augment natural-killer cells in leukemic mice and prolong life span. J Altern Complement Med 2001;7:241-251.

D'Angelo L, Grimaldi R, Caravaggi M, Marcoli M, Perucca E, Lecchini S, Frigo GM, Crema A Double-blind, placebo-controlled clinical study on the effect of a standardized ginseng extract on psychomotor performance in healthy volunteers. Journal of ethnopharmacology, 1986;16:15-22.

Dadkar VN, Ranadive NU, Dhar HL. Evaluation of antistress (adaptogen) activity of *Withania somnifera* (Ashwgandha). Ind J Clin Biochem 1987;2:101-108.

Danesch UC. *Petasites hybridus* (Butterbur root) extract in the treatment of asthma—an open trial. Altern Med Rev 2004;9: 54-62.

Darbinyan V, Kteyan A, Panossian A, Gabrielian E, Wikman G, Wagner H. *Rhodiola rosea* in stress induced fatigue—a double blind cross-over study of a standardized extract SHR-5 with a repeated low-dose regimen on the mental performance of healthy physicians during night duty. Phytomedicine 2000; 7:365-371.

Das P. Antiinflammatory and antiarthritc activity of varuna. Journal of Research Indian Medicine 1974;9:49.

Datta A, Sukul NC. Antifilarial effect of Zingiber officinale on Dirofilaria immitis. J Helminthol. 1987 Sep;61(3):268-270.

Daykin PW. *Veterinary and Applied Pharmacology and Therapeutics.* Bailliere: Tindall & Cox; 1960:78.

Deepak M, Handa SS. Antiinflammatory activity and chemical composition of extracts of Verbena officinalis. Phytother Res 2000;14:463-465.

DeFeudis FV. *Ginkgo biloba. From Chemistry to Clinic.* Wiesbaden, Germany: Ullstein Medical; 1998.

DeFeudis FV, Papadopoulos V, Drieu K. *Ginkgo biloba* extracts and cancer: a research area in its infancy. Fundam Clin Pharmacol 2003;17:405-417.

Dehpour AR, Zolfaghari ME, Samadian T, Kobarfard F, Faizi M, Assari M. Antiulcer activities of licorice and its derivatives in experimental gastric lesion induced by ibuprofen in rats. Int J Pharmaceut 1995;119:133-138.

de la Motte S, Bose-O'Reilly S, Heinisch M, Harrison F. Double-blind comparison of an apple pectin-chamomile extract preparation with placebo in children with diarrhea. Arzneimittelforschung 1997;47:1247-1249.

de Moura NF, Morel AF, Dessoy EC, et al. Alkaloids, amides and antispasmodic activity of *Zanthoxylum hyemale.* Planta Med 2002;68:534-538.

De Sanctis R, De Bellis R, Scesa C, Mancini U, Cucchiarini L, Dacha M. In vitro protective effect of *Rhodiola rosea* extract against hypochlorous acid–induced oxidative damage in human erythrocytes. Biofactors 2004;20:147-159.

De Smet PAGM, Keller K, Hänsel R, et al, eds. *Adverse Effects of Herbal Drugs.* Berlin, Germany: Springer Verlag; 1993.

Della Loggia R, Tubaro A, Redaelli C. Evaluation of the activity on the mouse CNS of several plant extracts and a combination of them. Riv Neurol 1981;51:297-310.

Della Loggia R, Traversa U, Scarcia V, Tubaro A. Depressive effects of *Chamomilla recutita* (L.) Rausch. tubular flowers, on central nervous system in mice. Pharmacological Research Communications 1982;14:153-162.

Della Loggia R, Zilli C, Del Negro P, Redaelli C, Tubaro A. Isoflavones as spasmolytic principles of *Piscidia erythrina.* Prog Clin Biol Res 1988;280:365-368.

Deng Y, Yang L. Effect of *Angelica sinensis* (Oliv.) on melanocytic proliferation, melanin synthesis and tyrosinase activity in vitro. Di Yi Junyi Daxue Xuebao 2003;23:239-241.

Deshpande P, Sahu M, Kumar P. *Crataeva nurvala* Hook and Forst (Varun): the Ayurvedic drug of choice in urinary disorders. Indian J Med Res 1982;76(suppl):46-53.

Desplaces A, Choppin J, Vogel G, Trost W. The effects of silymarin on experimental phalloidine poisoning. Arzneimittelforschung 1975;25:89-96.

Devasena T, Menon VP. Fenugreek affects the activity of beta-glucuronidase and mucinase in the colon. Phytother Res 2003;17:1088-1091.

Devi PU, Sharada AC, Solomon FE, Kamath MS. In vivo growth inhibitory effect of *Withania somnifera* (Ashwagandha) on a transplantable mouse tumor, sarcoma 180. Indian J Exp Biol 1992;30:169-172.

Devi PU, Sharada AC, Solomon FE. In vivo growth inhibitory and radiosensitizing effects of withaferin A on mouse *Ehrlich ascites* carcinoma. Cancer Lett 1995;95:189-193.

Dhananjay G, Jayadev R, Baquer NZ. Modulation of some gluconeogenic enzyme activities in diabetic rat liver and kidney: effect of antidiabetic compounds. Indian J Exp Biol 1999;37:2,196-199.

Dhawan K, Kumar S, Sharma A. Anxiolytic activity of aerial and underground parts of *Passiflora incarnata.* Fitoterapia 2001;72:922-926.

Dhawan K. Drug/substance reversal effects of a novel tri-substituted benzoflavone moiety (BZF) isolated from *Passiflora incarnata* Linn.—a brief perspective. Addict Biol 2003;8: 379-386.

Dhawan K, Dhawan S, Sharma A. Passiflora: a review update. J Ethnopharmacol 2004;94:1-23.

Didry N, Pinkas M. A propos du Buchu. Plantes Méd et Phyothér 1982;16:249-252.

Dimitrov M, Georgiev P, Vitanov S. [Use of tribestan on rams with sexual disorders.] Vet Med Nauki 1987;24:102-110.

Doan DD, Nguyen NH, Doan HK, et al. Studies on the individual and combined diuretic effects of four Vietnamese traditional herbal remedies (*Zea mays, Imperata cylindrica, Plantago major* and *Orthosiphon stamineus*). J Ethnopharmacol 1992; 36:225-231.

Dolara P, Corte B, Ghelardini C, et al. Local anaesthetic, antibacterial and antifungal properties of sesquiterpenes from myrrh. Planta Med 2000;66:356-358.

Dombradi CA, Foldeak S. Screening report on the antitumor activity of purified *Arctium lappa* extracts. Tumori 1966; 52:173.

Duan P, Wang ZM. [Clinical study on effect of Astragalus in efficacy enhancing and toxicity reducing of chemotherapy in patients of malignant tumor.] Zhongguo Zhong Xi Yi Jie He Za Zhi 2002;22:515-517.

Dunford C. The use of honey-derived dressings to promote effective wound management. Prof Nurse. 2005 Apr;20(8):35-8. Review.

Duwiejua M, Zeitlin IJ, Waterman PG, Gray AI. Anti-inflammatory activity of *Polygonum bistorta, Guaiacum officinale* and *Hamamelis virginiana* in rats. J Pharm Pharmacol 1994;46:286-290.

Eickstedt KWV, Rahmann R. Psychopharmakolgische Wirkungen von Valepotriaten. Arzneim-Forsch 1969;19:316-319.

Ek O, Waurzyniak B, Myers DE, Uckun FM. Antitumor activity of TP3(anti-p80)-pokeweed antiviral protein immunotoxin in hamster cheek pouch and severe combined immunodeficient mouse xenograft models of human osteosarcoma. Clin Cancer Res 1998;4:1641-1647.

Elhajili M, Baddouri K, Elkabbaj S, Meiouat F, Settaf A. Diuretic activity of the infusion of flowers from *Lavendula officinalis*. [French] Reprod Nutr Dev 2001;41:393-399.

Ellingwood F. The American Materia Medica, Therapeutics and Pharmacognosy, 1919. Available online at Henriette's Herbal Homepage: http://www.henriettesherbal.com/index.html

EMEA (European Medicines Evaluation Agency). Herbal Medicinal Products Working Party Draft Core Summary of Product Characteristics for Valerian and Ispaghula. http://www.emea.eu.int/ Accessed February 20, 2002.

Eng ET, Ye J, Williams D, et al. Suppression of estrogen biosynthesis by procyanidin dimers in red wine and grape seeds. Cancer Res 2003;63:8516-8522.

Erdelmeier CA, Cinatl J Jr, Rabenau H, Doerr HW, Biber A, Koch E. Antiviral and antiphlogistic activities of *Hamamelis virginiana* bark. Planta Med 1996;62:241-245.

Ernst E, Pittler MH. Efficacy of ginger for nausea and vomiting: a systematic review of randomized clinical trials. Br J Anaesth 2000a;84:367-371.

Ernst E, Chrubasik S. Phyto-anti-inflammatories: a systematic review of randomized placebo controlled double blind trials. Rheumatic Dis Clin North Am 2000b;26:13-27.

Ernst E, Schmidt K. Ukrain—a new cancer cure? A systematic review of randomised clinical trials. BMC Cancer. 2005 Jul 1;5(1):69.

ESCP (European Scientific Cooperative on Phytotherapy). *Monographs on the Medicinal Uses of Plant Drugs,* Fascicules 1 and 2 (1996), Fascicules 3, 4, and 5 (1997), Fascicule 6 (1999). Exeter: European Scientific Cooperative on Phytotherapy.

Farnsworth NR, Kinghorn AD, Soefarto DD, et al. Siberian ginseng *(Elutherococcus senticosis):* current status as an adaptogen. In: Farnsworth NR, et al, eds. *Economic and Medicinal Plant Research,* vol 1. London: Academic Press; 1985:157.

Felter HW, Lloyd JU. King's American Dispensatory, 1898. Available online at Henriette's Herbal Homepage at: http://www.henriettesherbal.com/eclectic/kings/index.html

Felter HW. The Eclectic Materia Medica, Pharmacology and Therapeutics, 1922. Reprint by Eclectic Medical Publications, Sandy OR.

Ferger B, Boonen G, Haberlein H, Kuschinsky K. In vivo microdialysis study of (+/−)-kavain on veratridine-induced glutamate release. Eur J Pharmacol 1998;347:211-214.

Fernandez-Banares F, Hinojosa J, Sanchez-Lombrana JL, et al. Randomized clinical trial of *Plantago ovata* seeds (dietary fiber) as compared with mesalamine in maintaining remission in ulcerative colitis. Spanish Group for the Study of Crohn's Disease and Ulcerative Colitis (GETECCU). Am J Gastroenterol 1999;94:427-433.

Ferreira PR, Fleck JF, Diehl A, Barletta D, Braga-Filho A, Barletta A, Ilha L. Protective effect of alpha-tocopherol in head and neck cancer radiation-induced mucositis: a double-blind randomized trial. Head Neck. 2004 Apr;26(4):313-321.

Fiebich BL, Grozdeva M, Hess S, et al. *Petasites hybridus* extracts in vitro inhibit COX-2 and PGE2 release by direct interaction with the enzyme and by preventing p42/44 MAP kinase activation in rat primary microglial cells. Planta Med 2005;71:12-19.

Fields AM, Richards TA, Felton JA, et al. Analysis of responses to valerian root extract in the feline pulmonary vascular bed. J Altern Complement Med 2003;9:909-918.

Fintelmann V, Menssen HG. Artichoke leaf extract. Current knowledge concerning its efficacy as a lipid-reducer and antidyspeptic agent. Dtsch Apoth Ztg 1996;136:1405-1414.

Fitzi J, Furst-Jucker J, Wegener T, Saller R, Reichling J, 2002. Phytotherapy of chronic dermatitis and pruritis of dogs with a topical preparation containing tea tree oil (Bogaskin®). Schweiz Arch Tierheilk 144(5):223-231.

Flausino OA Jr, Zangrossi H Jr, Salgado JV, Viana MB. Effects of acute and chronic treatment with *Hypericum perforatum* L. (LI 160) on different anxiety-related responses in rats. Pharmacol Biochem Behav 2002;71:251-257.

Floersheim GL, Eberhard M, Tschumi P, Duckert F. Effects of penicillin and silymarin on liver enzymes and blood clotting factors in dogs given a boiled preparation of Amanita phalloides. Toxicol Appl Pharmacol. 1978 Nov;46(2):455-62.

Forslund T, Fyhrquist F, Froseth B, Tikkanen I. Effects of licorice on plasma atrial natriuretic peptide in healthy volunteers. J Intern Med 1989;225:95-99.

Fratkin J. Leaky gut syndrome: treating intestinal candidiasis and dysbiosis. Proceedings of the American Holistic Medical Association Conference; May 1996; New York, NY.

Fronczek FR, Caballero P, Fischer NH, Fernandez S, Hernandez E, Hurtado LM. The molecular structure of 3'-demethoxynorisoguaiacin triacetate from creosote bush *(Larrea tridentata).* J Nat Prod 1987;50:497-499.

Fujikawa T, Soya H, Hibasami H, et al. Effect of *Acanthopanax senticosus* Harms on biogenic monoamine levels in the rat brain. Phytother Res 2002;16:474-478.

Fulder S. Garlic and the prevention of cardiovascular disease. Cardiol Pract 1989;7:30-35.

Gaffney BT, Hugel HM, Rich PA. The effects of *Eleutherococcus senticosus* and *Panax ginseng* on steroidal hormone indices of stress and lymphocyte subset numbers in endurance athletes. Life Sci 2001;70:431-442.

Gafner S, Bergeron C, Batcha LL, et al. Inhibition of [3H]-LSD binding to 5-HT7 receptors by flavonoids from *Scutellaria lateriflora.* J Nat Prod 2003;66:535-537.

Gauthaman K, Ganesan AP, Prasad RN. Sexual effects of puncturevine *(Tribulus terrestris)* extract (protodioscin): an evaluation using a rat model. J Altern Complement Med 2003;9: 257-265.

Gebhardt R. Inhibition of cholesterol biosynthesis in primary cultured rat hepatocytes by artichoke *(Cynara scolymus* L.) extracts. J Pharmacol Exp Ther 1998;286:1122-1128.

Georgiev P, Dimitrov M, Vitanov S. The effect of the preparation Tribestan on the plasma concentration of testosterone and spermatogenesis of lambs and rams. Vet Sb 1988;3: 20-22.

Ghannam N, Kingston M, Al-Mshaal IA, et al. The antidiabetic activity of aloes; preliminary clinical and experimental observations. Horm Res 1986;24:288-294.

Ghazanfar SA. Handbook of Arabian medicinal plants. Boca Raton, FL, CRC Press, 1994.

Ghelardini C, Galeotti N, Salvatore G, Mazzanti G. Local anaesthetic activity of the essential oil of *Lavandula angustifolia.* Planta Med 1999;65:8,700-703.

Gholap S, Kar A. Effects of *Inula racemosa* root and *Gymnema sylvestre* leaf extracts in the regulation of corticosteroid induced diabetes mellitus: involvement of thyroid hormones. Pharmazie 2003;58:413-415.

Glatzel von H, Hackenberg K. Röntgenologische untersuchungen der wirkungen von bittermitteln auf die verdauunogsorgane. Planta Med 1967;15:223-232.

Gleitz J, Friese J, Beile A, Ameri A, Peters T. Anticonvulsive action of (+/−)-kavain estimated from its properties on stimulated synaptosomes and Na+ channel receptor sites. Eur J Pharmacol 1996a;315:89-97.

Gleitz J, Beile A, Peters T. (+/–)-Kavain inhibits the veratridine- and KCl-induced increase in intracellular Ca2+ and glutamate-release of rat cerebrocortical synaptosomes. Neuropharmacology 1996b;35:179-186.

Gleitz J, Beile A, Peters T. Kavain inhibits non-stereospecifically veratridine-activated Na+ channels [letter]. Planta Med 1996c;62:580-581.

Gloor M, Reichling J, Wasik B, Holzgang HE. Antiseptic effect of a topical dermatological formulation that contains *Hamamelis* distillate and urea. Forsch Komplementarmed Klass Naturheilkd 2002;9:153-159.

Goel V, Lovlin R, Barton R, et al. Efficacy of a standardized echinacea preparation (Echinilin) for the treatment of the common cold: a randomized, double-blind, placebo-controlled trial. J Clin Pharm Ther 2004;29:75-83.

Gong QM, Wang SL, Gan C. [A clinical study on the treatment of acute upper digestive tract hemorrhage with wen-she decoction.] Zhong Xi Yi Jie He Za Zhi 1989;9:272-273,260.

Gong Z, Yuan Y, Lou K, Tu S, Zhai Z, Xu J. Mechanisms of Chinese herb emodin and somatostatin analogs on pancreatic regeneration in acute pancreatitis in rats. Pancreas 2002;25: 154-160.

Gorbacheva AV, et al. Anti-ulcerogenic characteristics of Filipendula ulmaria (L.) Maxim. [Russian] Rastitel'nye Resursy. Nauka, Sankt-Peterburg, St. Petersburg, Russia: 2002. 38:2,114-119.

Granados-Soto V. Pleiotropic effects of resveratrol. Drug News Perspect. 2003 Jun;16(5):299-307.

Grases F, Melero G, Costa-Bauza A, Prieto R, March JG. Urolithiasis and phytotherapy. Int Urol Nephrol 1994;26:507-511.

Grases F, Ramis M, Costa-Bauza A, March JG. Effect of *Herniaria hirsuta* and *Agropyron repens* on calcium oxalate urolithiasis risk in rats. J Ethnopharmacol 1995;45:211-214.

Gray RD, Haggart K, Lee DK, Cull S, Lipworth BJ. Effects of butterbur treatment in intermittent allergic rhinitis: a placebo-controlled evaluation. Ann Allergy Asthma Immunol 2004; 93:56-60.

Gresswell, George; Gresswell Charles, and Gresswell, Albert, 1887. The Veterinary Pharmacopeia, Materia Medical And Therapeutics. Bailliere, Tindall and Cox, London.

Grieve M. A Modern Herbal. Dover Publications NY 1931.

Griffiths P. The role of cranberry juice in the treatment of urinary tract infections. Br J Community Nurs 2003;8:557-561.

Grigoleit HG, Grigoleit P. Gastrointestinal clinical pharmacology of peppermint oil. Phytomedicine. 2005a Aug;12(8):607-611.

Grigoleit HG, Grigoleit P. Pharmacology and preclinical pharmacokinetics of peppermint oil. Phytomedicine. 2005b Aug;12(8):612-616.

Grochulski VA, Borkowski B. Influence of chamomile oil on experimental glomerulonephritis in rabbits. Planta Med 1972;21:289-292.

Grossarth-Maticek R, Kiene H, Baumgartner SM, Ziegler R. Use of Iscador, an extract of European mistletoe *(Viscum album),* in cancer treatment: prospective nonrandomized and randomized matched-pair studies nested within a cohort study. Altern Ther Health Med 2001;7:57-66,68-72,74-6.

Grover JK, Yadav SP. Pharmacological actions and potential uses of *Momordica charantia:* a review. J Ethnopharmacol 2004;93: 123-132.

Guan YJ, Hu Z, Hou-Chung-Kuo Chung Hsi i Chieh Ho Tsa Chih M, [Effect of *Cordyceps sinensis* on T-lymphocyte subsets in chronic renal failure.] Chinese J Integrated Med 1992;12:323, 338-339.

Guerrini VH, Kriticos CM. Effects of azadirachtin on *Ctenocephalides felis* in the dog and the cat. Vet Parasitol 1998;74: 289-297.

Gumbinger HG, Winterhoff H, Sourgens H, et al. Formation of compounds with antigonadotropic activity from inactive phenolic precursors. Contraception 1981;23:661-666.

Guodong L, Zhongqi L. Effects of ginseng saponins on insulin release from isolated pancreatic islets of rats. Chin J Integr Trad Western Med 1987;7:326.

Gupta I, Gupta V, Parihar A, et al. Effects of *Boswellia serrata* gum resin in patients with bronchial asthma: results of a double-blind, placebo-controlled, 6-week clinical study. Eur J Med Res 1998;3:511-514.

Gupta R, Singhal S, Goyle A, Sharma VN. Antioxidant and hypocholesterolaemic effects of Terminalia arjuna tree-bark powder: a randomised placebo-controlled trial. J Assoc Physicians India 2001;49:231-235.

Gupta S, George P, Gupta V, et al. *Tylophora indica* in bronchial asthma—a double blind study. Ind J Med Res 1979;69:981-989.

Gupta SS, Variyar MC. Experimental studies on pituitary diabetes IV. Effect of *Gymnema sylvestre* and Cocciniaindica against the hyperglycemia response of somatotropin and corticotrophin hormones. Indian J Med Res 1964;52:200-207.

Gupta SS. Inhibitory effect of *Gymnema sylvestre* (Gurmar) on adrenaline induced hyperglycemia in rats. Indian J Med Sci 1961;15:883-887.

Gupte S. Use of berberine in treatment of giardiasis. Am J Dis Child 1975;129:866.

Guslandi M. Ulcer-healing drugs and endogenous prostaglandins. Int J Clin Pharmacol Ther Toxicol 1985;23:398-402.

Habtemariam S. Antiinflammatory activity of the antirheumatic herbal drug, gravel root (Eupatorium purpureum): further biological activities and constituents. Phytother Res 2001;15:687-690.

Hacker B, Medon PJ. Cytotoxic effects of *Eleutherococcus senticosus* aqueous extracts in combination with N6-(delta 2-isopentenyl)-adenosine and 1-beta-D-arabinofuranosylcytosine against L1210 leukemia cells. J Pharm Sci 1984;73:270-272.

Hajhashemi V, Ghannadi A, Sharif B. Anti-inflammatory and analgesic properties of the leaf extracts and essential oil of *Lavandula angustifolia* Mill. J Ethnopharmacol 2003;89:67-71.

Halcon L, Milkus K. *Staphylococcus aureus* and wounds: a review of tea tree oil as a promising antimicrobial. Am J Infect Control. 2004 Nov;32(7):402-408.

Halder A, Raychowdhury R, Ghosh A, De M. Black tea *(Camellia sinensis)* as a chemopreventive agent in oral precancerous lesions. J Environ Pathol Toxicol Oncol 2005;24:141-144.

Halliwell RE. Dietary allergy and intolerance in the dog: new concepts. ASAVA Dermatology 1995 Australian Veterinary Association Annual Conference Proceedings.

Hamada H, Hiramatsu M, Edamatsu R, Mori A. Free radical scavenging action of baicalein. Arch Biochem Biophys 1993; 306:261-266.

Hammer KA, Carson CF, Riley TV. In vitro activities of ketoconazole, econazole, miconazole, and Melaleuca alternifolia (tea tree) oil against Malassezia species. Antimicrob Agents Chemother. 2000 Feb;44(2):467-469.

Hänsel R, Wohlfart R Coper H. Narcotic action of 2-methyl-3-butene-2-ol contained in hops. Zhurnal der Natuerforschungen 1980;35:1096-1097.

Hänsel R, Wagener HH. Versuche, sedativ-hypnotische Wirkstoffe im Hopfen nachzuweisen. Arzneim Forsch/Dru Res 1967;17:79-81.

Harney JW, Barofsky IM, Leary JD. Behavioral and toxicological studies of cyclopentanoid monoterpenes from *Nepeta cataria.* Lloydia 1978;41:367-374.

Harvey RG. A comparison of evening primrose oil and sunflower oil for the management of papulocrustous dermatitis in cats. Vet Rec. 1993a;133(23):571-573.

Harvey RG. Effect of varying propositions of evening primrose oil and fish oil on cats with crusting dermatosis (miliary dermatitis). Vet Rec. 1993b;133(9):208-211.

Harris C, Pierce K, King G, Yates KM, Hall J, Tizard I. Efficacy of acemannan in treatment of canine and feline spontaneous neoplasms. Mol Biother 1991;3:207-213.

Hart BL, Leedy MG. Analysis of the catnip reaction: mediation by olfactory system, not vomeronasal organ. Behav Neural Biol. 1985 Jul;44(1):38-46.

Hartz AJ, Bentler S, Noyes R, et al. Randomized controlled trial of Siberian ginseng for chronic fatigue. Psychol Med 2004; 34:51-61.

Hase K, Kasimu R, Basnet P, Kadota S, Namba T. Preventive effect of lithospermate B from *Salvia miltiorhiza* on experimental hepatitis induced by carbon tetrachloride or D-galactosamine/lipopolysaccharide. Planta Med. 1997 Feb;63(1):22-26.

Hasenohrl RU, Topic B, Frisch C, Hacker R, Mattern CM, Huston JP. Dissociation between anxiolytic and hypomnestic effects for combined extracts of *Zingiber officinale* and *Ginkgo biloba,* as opposed to diazepam. Pharmacol Biochem Behav 1998;59: 527-535.

Hawrelak J. Giardiasis pathophysiology and management. Alt Med Rev 2003;8:129-142.

Hayashi I, Ohotsuki M, Suzuki I, Watanabe T. Effects of oral administration of *Echinacea purpurea* (American herb) on incidence of spontaneous leukemia caused by recombinant leukemia viruses in AKR/J mice. Nihon Rinsho Meneki Gakkai Kaishi 2001;24:10-20.

Hazelhoff B, Malingre TM, Meijer DK. Antispasmodic effects of valeriana compounds: an in-vivo and in-vitro study on the guinea-pig ileum. Arch Int Pharmacodyn Ther 1982;257:274-287.

Heber D, Yip I, Ashley JM, Elashoff DA, Elashoff RM, Go VL. Cholesterol-lowering effects of a proprietary Chinese red-yeast-rice dietary supplement. Am J Clin Nutr 1999;69:231-236.

Helms S. Cancer prevention and therapeutics: Panax ginseng. Alt Med Rev 2004 9:259-274.

Hiai S, Yokoyama H, Oura H, Yano S. Stimulation of pituitary-adrenocortical system by ginseng saponin. Endocrinol Jpn. 1979 Dec;26(6):661-665.

Hirano T, Gotoh M, Oka T. Natural flavenoids and lignans are potent cytostatic agents against human leukemic HL-60 cells. Life Sci 1994;55:1061-1069.

Hobbs C. Sarsaparilla: a literature review. Herbalgram 1988;17: 10.

Hobbs C. Echinacea: a literature review. HerbalGram 1994; 30(suppl):33-47.

Hoffman D. The New Holistic Herbal Element, Brisbane, 1992.

Hoffman D (2004) Medical Herbalism, The Science Principles and Practices Of Herbal Medicine Healing Arts Press, Rochester, Vermont.

Hofmann D, Hecker M, Volp A. Efficacy of dry extract of ivy leaves in children with bronchial asthma—a review of randomized controlled trials. Phytomedicine 2003;10:213-220.

Holetz FB, et al. Screening of some plants used in the Brazilian folk medicine for the treatment of infectious diseases. Mem Inst Oswaldo Cruz 2002;97:1027-1031.

Hollander D. Intestinal permeability, leaky gut, and intestinal disorders. Curr Gastroenterol Rep 1999;1:410-416.

Homady MH. The influences of some medicinal plant extracts on the aggressivity and fertility of male mice. Philippine J Sci 2001;130:2,119-126.

Hook I, McGee A, Henman H. Evaluation of dandelion for diuretic activity and variation in potassium content. Int J Pharmacog 1993;31:29-34.

Hordegen P, Hertzberg H, Heilmann J, Langhans W, Maurer V. The anthelmintic efficacy of five plant products against gastrointestinal trichostrongylids in artificially infected lambs. Vet Parasitol 2003;117:51-60.

Horhammer L, Wagner H, Reinhardt H. New methods in pharmacognosy. XI. Chromatographic evaluation of commercial Viburnum drugs. Deutsche Apotheker Zeitung 1965;105:1371-1372.

Horhammer L, Wagner H, Reinhardt H. Chemistry, pharmacology, and pharmaceutics of the components from *Viburnum prunifolium* and *V. opulus*. Botanical Magazine (Tokyo) 1966; 79:510-525.

Hosford D, Mencia-Huerta JM, Page C, Braquet P. Natural antagonists of platelet-activating factor. Phytother Res 1988;2:1-17.

Howell AB, Vorsa N, Der Marderosian A, Foo LY. Inhibition of the adherence of P fimbriated *Escherichia coli* to uroepithelial-cell surfaces by proanthocyanidin extracts from cranberries. N Engl J Med 1998;339:1085-1086.

Hsiang CY, Lai IL, Chao DC, Ho TY. Differential regulation of activator protein 1 activity by glycyrrhizin. Life Sci 2002;70: 1643-1656.

Hsieh CL, Tang NY, Chiang SY, Hsieh CT, Lin JG. Anticonvulsive and free radical scavenging actions of two herbs, *Uncaria rhynchophylla* (MIQ) Jack and *Gastrodia elata* Bl., in kainic acid-treated rats. Life Sci 1999;65:2071-2082.

Hsieh CL, Chiang SY, Cheng KS, et al. Anticonvulsive and free radical scavenging activities of *Gastrodia elata* Bl. in kainic acid-treated rats. Am J Chin Med 2001;29:331-341.

Hu S, Cai W, Ye J, Qian Z, Sun Z. Influence of medicinal herbs on phagocytosis by bovine neutrophils. Zentralbl Veterinarmed A 1992;39:593-599.

Hu S, Concha C, Johannisson A, Meglia G, Waller KP. Effect of subcutaneous injection of ginseng on cows with subclinical Staphylococcus aureus mastitis. J Vet Med B Infect Dis Vet Public Health. 2001 Sep;48(7):519-528.

Huang KC. *The Pharmacology of Chinese Herbs*. Boca Raton: CRC Press; 2000.

Huang MT, Ho CT, Wang ZY, et al. Inhibition of skin tumorigenesis by rosemary and its constituents carnosol and ursolic acid. Cancer Res 1994;54:701-708.

Huang WM, Yan H, Jin JM, Yu C, Zhang H. Beneficial effects of berberine on hemodynamics during acute ischemic left ventricular failure in dogs. Chin Med J 1992;105:1014-1019.

Hughes-Formella BJ, Filbry A, Gassmueller J, Rippke F. Anti-inflammatory efficacy of topical preparations with 10% hamamelis distillate in a UV erythema test. Skin Pharmacol Appl Skin Physiol 2002;15:125-132.

Hui KM, Huen MS, Wang HY, et al. Anxiolytic effect of wogonin, a benzodiazepine receptor ligand isolated from Scutellaria baicalensis Georgi. Biochem Pharmacol 2002;64:1415-1424.

Hussain Z, Waheed A, Qureshi RA, et al. The effect of medicinal plants of Islamabad and Murree region of Pakistan on insulin secretion from INS-1 cells. Phytother Res 2004;18:73-77.

Hwang BY, Roberts SK, Chadwick LR, Wu CD, Kinghorn AD. Antimicrobial constituents from goldenseal (the Rhizomes of *Hydrastis canadensis*) against selected oral pathogens. Planta Med 2003;69:623-627.

Iauk L, Lo Bue AM, Milazzo I, Rapisarda A, Blandino G. Antibacterial activity of medicinal plant extracts against periodontopathic bacteria. Phytother Res 2003;17:599-604.

Idris UE, Adam SE, Tartour G. The anthelmintic efficacy of *Artemisia herba-alba* against *Haemonchus contortus* infection in goats. Natl Inst Anim Health Q (Tokyo) 1982;22:138-143.

Iizuka N, Hazama S, Yoshimura K, et al. Anticachectic effects of the natural herb Coptidis rhizoma and berberine on mice bearing colon 26/clone 20 adenocarcinoma. Int J Cancer 2002;99:286-291.

Ikram M. Medicinal plants as hypocholesterolemic agents. J Pak Med Assoc 1980;30:278-282.

Ilarionova M, et al. Cytotoxic effect on leukemic cells of the essential oils from rosemary, wild geranium and nettle and concret of royal bulgarian rose. Anticancer Res 1992;12:1915.

Innes JF, Fuller CJ, Grover ER, Kelly AL, Burn JF. Randomised, double-blind, placebo-controlled parallel group study of P54FP for the treatment of dogs with osteoarthritis. Vet Rec 2003;152:457-460.

Inouye H, Takeda Y, Uobe K, Yamauchi K, Yabuuchi N, Kuwano S. Purgative activities of iridoid glycosides. Planta Med 1974; 25:285-288.

Ishani A, MacDonald R, Nelson D, Rutks I, Wilt TJ.Pygeum africanum for the treatment of patients with benign prostatic hyperplasia: a systematic review and quantitative meta-analysis. Am J Med. 2000 Dec 1;109(8):654-664.

Islam MS, Rahman MT, Rouf AS, Rahman F. Evaluation of neuropharmacological effects of *Rumex maritimus* Linn. (Polygonaceae) root extracts. Pharmazie 2003;58:738-741.

Ito H. Effects of the antitumor agents from various natural sources on drug-metabolizing system, phagocytic activity and complement system in sarcoma 180-bearing mice Jpn J Pharmacol 1986;40:435-443.

Itokawa H, Mihashi S, Watanabe K, et al. Studies on the constituents of crude drugs having inhibitory activity against contraction of the ileum caused by histamine or barium chloride. I. Screening test for the activity of commercially available crude drugs and the related plant materials. Shoyakugaku Zasshi 1983;37:223-228.

Ivetic V, Popovic M, Mimica-Dukic N, Barak O, Pilija V. St. John's Wort (Hypericum perforatum L.) and Kindling Epilepsy in Rabbit Phytomedicine. 2002 Sep;9(6):496-499.

Jacker H-J, et al. Zum antiexsudativen Verhalten einiger Triterpensaponine. Pharmazie 1982;37:380-382.

Jackson B, Hicks LE. Effect of cranberry juice on urinary pH in older adults. Home Healthc Nurse 1997;15:198-202.

Jackson CM, Lee DK, Lipworth BJ. The effects of butterbur on the histamine and allergen cutaneous response. Ann Allergy Asthma Immunol 2004;92:250-254.

Jager AK, Hutchings A, van Staden J. Screening of Zulu medicinal plants for prostaglandin-synthesis inhibitors. J Ethnopharmacol 1996;52:95-100.

Jagtap AG, Shirke SS, Phadke AS. Effect of polyherbal formulation on experimental models of inflammatory bowel diseases. J Ethnopharmacol 2004;90:195-204.

Jamieson DD, Duffield PH. The antinociceptive actions of kava components in mice. Clin Exp Pharmacol Physiol 1990;17: 495-507.

Jana S, Esser MJ, Reid AR. Antidepressants as analgesics: an overview of central and peripheral mechanisms of action. J Psychiatry Neurosci 2001;26:21-29.

Janssen G, Bode U, Breu H, Dohrn B, Engelbrecht V, Gobel U. Boswellic acids in the palliative therapy of children with progressive or relapsed brain tumors. Klin Padiatr 2000;212:189-195.

Jarred RA, Keikha M, Dowling C, et al. Induction of apoptosis in low to moderate-grade human prostate carcinoma by red clover-derived dietary isoflavones. Cancer Epidemiol Biomarkers Prev 2002;11:1689-1696.

Jarrett RH, Norman EJ, Squires RA. Liquorice and canine Addison's disease. N Z Vet J 2005;53:214.

Jeffrey SL, Belcher HJ. Use of Arnica to relieve pain after carpal-tunnel release surgery. Altern Ther Health Med 2002;8:66-68.

Jellin JM, Batz F, Hitchens K. Pharmacists Letter/Prescribers Letter Natural Medicines Comprehensive Database. Stockton, Calif: Therapeutic Research Faculty; 1999.

Jensen et al. cited on http://www.froytang.no/html/cattle.htm accessed July 2005.

Jewell D, Young G. Interventions for nausea and vomiting in early pregnancy.The Cochrane Database of Systematic Reviews 2006,(1). available on for fee basis at: http://www.mrw.interscience.wiley.com/cochrane/clsysrev/articles/CD000145/frame.html

Jiang J, Xu Q. Immunomodulatory activity of the aqueous extract from rhizome of *Smilax glabra* in the later phase of adjuvant-induced arthritis in rats. J Ethnopharmacol 2003; 85:53-59.

Jones E. *Cancer: Its Causes, Symptoms and Treatment.* Wenatchee, Wash: Healing Mountain Publishing, Inc; 2001 (reprinted from 1911).

Jost M. Calendula as a healing plant for mastitis in dairy cows. Biodynamics 1984;152:7-19.

Kaemmerer K, Fink J. Untersuchungen von Eleutherococcus-Extrakt auf trophanabole Wirkungen bei Ratten. Der praktische Tierarzt 1980;61:748-753.

Kalin P. [The common butterbur (Petasites hybridus)—portrait of a medicinal herb.]Forsch Komplementarmed Klass Naturheilkd. 2003 Apr;10 (Suppl) 1:41-44.

Kamaldeep D, Suresh K, Anupam S. Evaluation of central nervous system effects of *Passiflora incarnata* in experimental animals. Pharmaceut Biol 2003;41:2,87-91.

Kamei J, Nakamura R, Ichiki H, Kubo M. Antitussive principles of *Glycyrrhizae radix,* a main component of the Kampo preparations Bakumondo-to (Mai-men-dong-tang). Eur J Pharmacol 2003;469:159-163.

Kamtchouing P, Mbongue Fandio GY, Dimo T, Jatsa HB. Evaluation of androgenic activity of *Zingiber officinale* and *Pentadiplandra brazzeana* in male rats. Asian J Androl 2002; 4:299-301.

Kang DG, Yun YG, Ryoo JH, Lee HS. Anti-hypertensive effect of water extract of danshen on renovascular hypertension through inhibition of the renin angiotensin system. Am J Chin Med 2002;30:87-93.

Kang H, Ahn KS, Cho C, Bae HS. Immunomodulatory effect of *Astragali radix* extract on murine TH1/TH2 cell lineage development. Biol Pharm Bull 2004;27:1946-1950.

Kaplan EI. The prophylactic effect of *Eleutherococcus senticosus* in craniocerebral trauma in animals. Lek Sredstva Dal'nego 1965;7:77-79.

Kar A, Panda S, Bharti S. Relative efficacy of three medicinal plant extracts in the alteration of thyroid hormone concentrations in male mice. J Ethnopharmacol 2002;81:281-285.

Kardosova A, Ebringerova A, Alfoldi J, Nosal'ova G, Franova S, Hribalova V. A biologically active fructan from the roots of *Arctium lappa* L., var. Herkules. Int J Biol Macromol 2003; 33:135-140.

Karthikeyan K, Bai BR, Gauthaman K, Sathish KS, Devaraj SN. Cardioprotective effect of the alcoholic extract of *Terminalia arjuna* bark in an in vivo model of myocardial ischemic reperfusion injury. Life Sci 2003;73:2727-2739.

Kassir ZA. Endoscopic controlled trial of four drug regimens in the treatment of chronic duodenal ulceration. Irish Med J 1985;78:153-156.

Kast A, Hauser SP. [Helixor—mistletoe preparation for cancer therapy. Documentation No. 19.] Schweiz Rundsch Med Prax 1990;79:291-295.

Katiyar SK, Mukhtar H. Tea antioxidants in cancer chemoprevention. J Cell Biochem Suppl 1997;27:59-67.

Kaur P, Sharma M, Mathur S, et al. Effect of 1-oxo-5beta, 6beta-epoxy-witha-2-ene-27-ethoxy-olide isolated from the roots of *Withania somnifera* on stress indices in Wistar rats. J Altern Complement Med 2003;9:897-907.

Kawai T, Kinoshita K, Koyama K, Takahashi K. Anti-emetic principles of *Magnolia obovata* bark and *Zingiber officinale* rhizome. Planta Med 1994;60:17-20.

Keene JL, Noakes, DLG; Moccia, RD; Soto, CG. The efficacy of clove oil as an anaesthetic for rainbow trout, *Oncorhynchus mykiss* (Walbaum). Aquaculture Res 1998;29:2,89-101.

Kempe C, Gruning H, Stasche N, Hormann K. [Icelandic moss lozenges in the prevention or treatment of oral mucosa irritation and dried out throat mucosa.] [In German] Laryngorhinootologie 1997;76:186-188.

Kempski HW. On the causal therapy of chronic helminthic bronchitis. Med Klin. 1967 Feb 17;62(7):259-260.

Kennedy DO, Scholey AB, Tildesley NT, Perry EK, Wesnes KA. Modulation of mood and cognitive performance following acute administration of *Melissa officinalis* (lemon balm). Pharmacol Biochem Behav 2002;72:953-964.

Kennedy DO, Scholey AB. Ginseng: potential for the enhancement of cognitive performance and mood. Pharmacol Biochem Behav 2003a;75:687-700.

Kennedy DO, Wake G, Savelev S, et al. Modulation of mood and cognitive performance following acute administration of single doses of *Melissa officinalis* (Lemon balm) with human CNS nicotinic and muscarinic receptor-binding properties. Neuropsychopharmacology 2003b;28:1871-1881.

Kennedy DO, Little W, Scholey AB. Attenuation of laboratory-induced stress in humans after acute administration of *Melissa officinalis* (Lemon balm). Psychosom Med 2004;66:607-613.

Khan N, Sultana S Inhibition of two stage renal carcinogenesis, oxidative damage and hyperproliferative response by *Nigella sativa*. Eur J Cancer Prev 2005;14:159-168.

Khayyal MT, el-Ghazaly MA, Kenawy SA, Seif-el-Nasr M, Mahran LG, Kafafi YA, Okpanyi SN. Antiulcerogenic effect of some gastrointestinally acting plant extracts and their combination. Arzneimittelforschung 2001;51(7):545-53.

Kiefer D, Pantuso T. *Panax ginseng*. Am Fam Physician 2003;68: 1539-1542.

Kim DH, Moon YS, Jung JS, et al. Effects of ginseng saponin administered intraperitoneally on the hypothalamo-pituitary-adrenal axis in mice. Neurosci Lett 2003;343:62-66.

Kim H, Lee E, Lee S, Shin T, Kim Y, Kim J. Effect of *Rehmannia glutinosa* on immediate type allergic reaction. Int J Immunopharmacol 1998;20:231-240.

Kim KS, Rhee KH, Yoon JH, Lee JG, Lee JH, Yoo JB. *Ginkgo biloba* extract (EGb 761) induces apoptosis by the activation of caspase-3 in oral cavity cancer cells. Oral Oncol 2005;41:383-389.

Kim MJ, Kim HN, Kang KS, et al. Methanol extract of *Dioscoreae rhizoma* inhibits pro-inflammatory cytokines and mediators in the synoviocytes of rheumatoid arthritis. Int Immunopharmacol 2004;4:1489-1497.

Kim DC, Kim SH, Choi BH, etal, Curcuma longa extract protects against gastric ulcers by blocking H2 histamine receptors. Biol Pharm Bull. 2005 Dec;28(12):2220-2224.

Kim MJ, Kim HN, Kang KS, Baek NI, Kim DK, Kim YS, Jeon BH, Kim SH.Methanol extract of Dioscoreae Rhizoma inhibits pro-inflammatory cytokines and mediators in the synoviocytes of rheumatoid arthritis. Int Immunopharmacol. 2005b Mar;5(3):629.

Kim-Park S, Ku DD. Garlic elicits a nitric oxide-dependent relaxation and inhibits hypoxic pulmonary vasoconstriction in rats. Clin Exp Pharmacol Physiol 2000;27:780-786.

Kimura Y, Sumiyoshi M. Effects of various *Eleutherococcus senticosus* cortex on swimming time, natural killer activity and corticosterone level in forced swimming stressed mice. J Ethnopharmacol 2004;95:447-453.

King GK, Yates KM, Greenlee PG, et al. The effect of acemannan immunostimulant in combination with surgery and radiation therapy on spontaneous canine and feline fibrosarcomas. J Am Anim Hosp Assoc 1995;31:439-447.

Kingwatanakul P, Alon US. Cranberries and urinary tract infection. Child Hosp Q 1996;8:69-72.

Kirk H. Index of Treatment in Small-Animal Practice. The Williams and Wilkins Company, Baltimore, 1948.

Kitts D, Hu C. Efficacy and safety of ginseng. Public Health Nutr 2000;3:473-485.

Klaas CA, Wagner G, Laufer S, et al. Studies on the anti-inflammatory activity of phytopharmaceuticals prepared from Arnica flowers. Planta Med 2002;68:385-391.

Kline RM, Kline JJ, DiPalma J, Barbero G. Enteric coated, pH dependent peppermint oil capsules for the treatment of irritable bowel syndrome in children. J Pediatr. 2001;138:125-128.

Klouchek-Popova E, Popov A, Pavlova N, Krusteva S. Influence of the physiological regeneration and epithelialization using fractions isolated from *Calendula officinalis*. Acta Physiol Pharmacol Bulg 1982;8:63-67.

Knuesel O, Weber M, Suter A. *Arnica montana* gel in osteoarthritis of the knee: an open, multicenter clinical trial. Adv Ther 2002;19:209-218.

Kobayashi Y, Nakano Y, Inayama K, Sakai A, Kamiya T. Dietary intake of the flower extracts of German chamomile (*Matricaria recutita* L.) inhibited compound 48/80-induced itch-scratch responses in mice. Phytomedicine 2003;10:657-664.

Kobayashi Y, Takahashi R, Ogino F. Antipruritic effect of the single oral administration of German chamomile flower extract and its combined effect with antiallergic agents in ddY mice. J Ethnopharmacol 2005;101:308-312.

Koc RK, Akdemir H, Kurtsoy A, et al. Lipid peroxidation in experimental spinal cord injury. Comparison of treatment with *Ginkgo biloba*, TRH and methylprednisolone. Res Exp Med (Berl) 1995;195:117-123.

Koch HP, Lawson LD, eds. *Garlic. The Science and Therapeutic Application of* Allium sativum *L. and Related Species*. 2nd ed. Baltimore, Md: Williams and Wilkins; 1996.

Koh JH, Kim KM, Kim JM, Song JC, Suh HJ. Antifatigue and antistress effect of the hot-water fraction from mycelia of *Cordyceps sinensis*. Biol Pharm Bull 2003;26:691-694.

Konopa J, Jereczek, E., Matuszkiewicz, A., et al. Screening of antitumor substances from plants. Arch Immunol Ther Exp 1957;15:129.

Kovar KA, Gropper B, Friess D, Ammon HP. Blood levels of 1,8-cineole and locomotor activity of mice after inhalation and oral administration of rosemary oil. Planta Med 1987;53:315-318.

Krack A, Sharma R, Figulla HR, Anker SD. The importance of the gastrointestinal system in the pathogenesis of heart failure. Eur Heart J 2005;26:2368-2374.

Kraft K. Therapeutisches Profil eines Spitzwegerichekraut-Fluidextraktes bei akuten repsiratorischen Erkrankungen im Kindes- und Erwachsenenalter. In: Loew D, Rietbrock N, Hrsg. *Phytopharmaka III: Forschung und klinische Anwendung*. Darmstadt: Steinkopff Verlag; 1997a:199-209.

Kraft K. Artichoke leaf extract—recent findings reflecting effects on lipid metabolism, liver and gastrointestinal tracts. Phytomedicine 1997b;4:369-378.

Krazhan IA, Garazha NN. Treatment of chronic catarrhal gingivitis with polysorb-immobilized calendula. Stomatologiia (Mosk). 2001;80(5):11-13.

Kreydiyyeh SI, Usta J. Diuretic effect and mechanism of action of parsley. J Ethnopharmacol 2002;79:353-357.

Krishnaswamy K, Goud VK, Sesikeran B, Mukundan MA, Krishna TP. Retardation of experimental tumorigenesis and reduction in DNA adducts by turmeric and curcumin. Nutr Cancer 1998;30:163-166.

Kudi AC, Myint SH, 1999. Antiviral activity of some Nigerian medicinal plant extracts. J Ethnopharmacol 1999 Dec 15;68(1-3):289-294.

Kumar V, Singh PN, Bhattacharya SK. Anti-inflammatory and analgesic activity of Indian *Hypericum perforatum* L. Indian J Exp Biol 2001;39:339-343.

Kuo CL, Chou CC, Yung BYM. Berberine complexes with DNA in the berberine-induced apoptosis in human leukemic HL-60 cells. Cancer Lett 1995;93:193-200.

Kupchan SM, Karim A. Tumor inhibitors. 114. *Aloe emodin:* antileukemic principle isolated from *Rhamnus frangula* L. Lloydia 1976;39:223-224.

Kurashige S, Akuzawa Y, Endo F. Effects of astragali radix extract on carcinogenesis, cytokine production, and cytotoxicity in mice treated with a carcinogen, N-butyl-N′-butanolnitrosoamine. Cancer Invest 1999;17:30-35.

Kwon YS, Jang KH, Jang IH. The effects of Korean red ginseng (ginseng radix rubra) on liver regeneration after partial hepatectomy in dogs. J Vet Sci. 2003 Apr;4(1):83-92.

Labriola D, Livingston R. Possible interactions between dietary antioxidants and chemotherapy. Oncology 1999;13:1003-1011.

Lahiri-Chatterjee M, Katiyar SK, Mohan RR, Agarwal R. A flavonoid antioxidant, silymarin, affords exceptionally high protection against tumour promotion in the SENCAR mouse skin tumorigenic model. Cancer Res 1999;59:622-632.

Lambert JD, Yang CS. Mechanisms of cancer prevention by tea constituents. J Nutr. 2003 Oct;133(10):3262S-3267S.

Lamson DW, Brignall MS. Antioxidants in cancer therapy: their actions and interactions with oncologic therapies. Altern Med Rev 1999;4:304-329.

Lamson DW, Brignall MS. Antioxidant and cancer therapy II: quick reference guide. Altern Med Rev 2000;5:152-163.

Langmead L, Dawson C, Hawkins C, Banna N, Loo S, Rampton DS. Antioxidant effects of herbal therapies used by patients with inflammatory bowel disease: an in vitro study. Aliment Pharmacol Ther 2002;16:197-205.

Langmead L, Feakins RM, Goldthorpe S, et al. Randomized, double-blind, placebo-controlled trial of oral aloe vera gel for active ulcerative colitis. Aliment Pharmacol Ther 2004a;19: 739-747.

Langmead L, Makins RJ, Rampton DS. Anti-inflammatory effects of aloe vera gel in human colorectal mucosa in vitro. Aliment Pharmacol Ther 2004b;19:521-527.

Larsson B, Jonasson A, Fianu S. Prophylactic effect of UVA-E in women with recurrent cystitis: a preliminary report. Curr Ther Res 1993;53:441-443.

Lau BHS Adetumbi MA, and Sanchez A *Allium sativum* (garlic) and atherosclerosis: a review. Nutr Res 1983;3:119-128.

Lau BH, Ruckle HC, Botolazzo T, Lui PD. Chinese medicinal herbs inhibit growth of murine renal cell carcinoma. Cancer Biother 1994;9:153-161.

Lau CB, Ho CY, Kim CF, et al. Cytotoxic activities of Coriolus versicolor (Yunzhi) extract on human leukemia and lymphoma cells by induction of apoptosis. Life Sci 2004;75:797-808.

Lee KM Jung JS, Song DK, et al. Effects of Humulus lupulus extract on the central nervous system in mice. Planta Med 1993; 59: A691.

Lee SM, Li ML, Tse YC, et al. *Paeoniae radix,* a Chinese herbal extract, inhibits hepatoma cell growth by inducing apoptosis in a p53 independent pathway. Life Sci 2002;71:2267-2277.

Lee DK, Carstairs IJ, Haggart K, Jackson CM, Currie GP, Lipworth BJ. Butterbur, an herbal remedy, attenuates adenosine monophosphate induced nasal responsiveness in seasonal allergic rhinitis. Clin Exp Allergy 2003;33:882-886.

Lee DK, Haggart K, Robb FM, Lipworth BJ. Butterbur, an herbal remedy, confers complementary anti-inflammatory activity in asthmatic patients receiving inhaled corticosteroids. Clin Exp Allergy 2004a;34:110-114.

Lee DK, Gray RD, Robb FM, Fujihara S, Lipworth BJ. A placebo-controlled evaluation of butterbur and fexofenadine on objective and subjective outcomes in perennial allergic rhinitis. Clin Exp Allergy 2004b;34:646-649.

Lee AN, Werth VP. Activation of autoimmunity following use of immunostimulatory herbal supplements. Arch Dermatol 2004c;140:723-727.

Leeney H. *Home Doctoring for Animals.* London: MacDonald & Martin; 1921.

Legnani C, Frascaro M, Guazzaloca G, Ludovici S, Cesarano G, Coccheri S. Effects of a dried garlic preparation on fibrinolysis and platelet aggregation in healthy subjects. Arzneimittelforschung 1993;43:119-122.

Lehrl S. Clinical efficacy of kava extract WS 1490 in sleep disturbances associated with anxiety disorders. Results of a multicenter, randomized, placebo-controlled, double-blind clinical trial. J Affect Disord 2004;78:101-110.

Lenartz D, Dott U, Menzel J, Schierholz JM, Beuth J. Survival of glioma patients after complementary treatment with galactoside-specific lectin from mistletoe. Anticancer Res 2000;20:2073-2076.

Lenau H, Muller A, Maier-Lewz H. Efficacy and Tolerance of a mixture of plant extracts and alpha tocopherol acetate in patients with irritable bladder and or urinary incontinence. Therapiewoche 1984;34:6054-6059.

Leng-Peschlow E. *Plantago ovata* seeds as dietary fibre supplement: physiological and metabolic effects in rats. Br J Nutr 1991;66:331349.

Leung AY. *Encyclopedia of Common Natural Ingredients Used in Food, Drugs and Cosmetics.* New York-Chichester: Wiley; 1980.

Lewis WH, Zenger VE, Lynch RG. No adaptogen response of mice to ginseng and *Eleutherococcus* infusions. J Ethnopharmacol 1983;8:209-214.

Li W, Zhou CH, Lu QL. [Effects of Chinese materia medica in activating blood and stimulating menstrual flow on the endocrine function of ovary-uterus and its mechanisms.] Zhongguo Zhong Xi Yi Jie He Za Zhi 1992;12:165-168,134.

Li MH, Zhang HL, Yang BY. [Effects of ginkgo leave concentrated oral liquor in treating asthma.] Zhongguo Zhong Xi Yi Jie He Za Zhi 1997;17:216-218.

Li N, Chen X, Han C, Chen J. [Chemopreventive effect of tea and curcumin on DMBA-induced oral carcinogenesis in hamsters.] Wei Sheng Yan Jiu 2002;31:354-357.

Li CZ, Cao ZG, Yang R, Shang ZH, Jin LJ, Cobert EF. [Effects of baicalin on the expression of pro-MMP-1 and MMP-3 in human gingival fibroblasts and periodontal ligament cells.] Zhonghua Kou Qiang Yi Xue Za Zhi 2004;39:197-200.

Li YP, Wang YM. Evaluation of tussilagone: a cardiovascular-respiratory stimulant isolated from Chinese herbal medicine. Gen Pharmacol. 1988;19(2):261-263.

Lin JH, Lo YY, Shu NS, et al. Control of preweaning diarrhea in piglets by acupuncture and Chinese medicine. Am J Chin Med 1988;16:75-80.

Lin RT. [An experimental study of dan sheng improving the mandibular bone fracture healing.] Zhonghua Kou Qiang Yi Xue Za Zhi 1992;27:215-216,256.

Lin CC, Lu JM, Yang JJ, Nabba T, Hatton M. Anti-inflammatory and radical scavenge effects of *Arctium lappa.* Am J Chin Med 1996a;24:127-137.

Lin CC, Shieh DE. The anti-inflammatory activity of *Scutellaria rivularis* extracts and its active components, baicalin, baicalein and wogonin. Am J Chin Med 1996b;24:31-36.

Lin MT, Wang JJ, Young MS. The protective effect of dl-tetrahydropalmatine against the development of amygdala kindling seizures in rats. Neurosci Lett 2002;320:113-116.

Lin J, Dong HF, Oppenheim JJ, Howard OM. Effects of astragali radix on the growth of different cancer cell lines. World J Gastroenterol. 2003 Apr;9(4):670-673.

Lis-Balchin M, Hart S, Simpson E. Buchu *(Agathosma betulina* and *A. crenulata,* Rutaceae*)* essential oils: their pharmacological action on guinea-pig ileum and antimicrobial activity on microorganisms. J Pharm Pharmacol 2001;53:579-582.

Lis-Balchin M, Hart S. Studies on the mode of action of the essential oil of lavender (*Lavandula angustifolia* P. Miller). Phytother Res 1999;13:540-542.

Lissoni P, Giani L, Zerbini S, Trabattoni P, Rovelli F. Biotherapy with the pineal immunomodulating hormone melatonin versus melatonin plus aloe vera in untreatable advanced solid neoplasms. Nat Immun 1998;16:27-33.

Liu J, Liang P, Yin C, et al. Effects of several Chinese herbal aqueous extracts on human sperm motility in vitro. Andrologia 2004;36:78-83.

Lloyd JU. History of the Vegetable Drugs of the Pharmacopoeia of the United States, 1911. Available online at Henriette's Herbal Homepage: http://www.henriettesherbal.com/eclectic/lloyd-hist/index.html

Lo HC, Tu ST, Lin KC, Lin SC. The anti-hyperglycemic activity of the fruiting body of *Cordyceps* in diabetic rats induced by nicotinamide and streptozotocin. Life Sci 2004;74:2897-2908.

Loeper ME. Mistletoe *(Viscum album)*. The Longwood Herbal Task Force, The Centre for Holistic Pediatric Education and Research, 1999. Available at: www.mcp.edu/hebal/default.htm. Accessed June 2005.

Long D, Ballentine NH, Marks JG, Jr. Treatment of poison ivy/oak allergic contact dermatitis with an extract of jewelweed. Am J Contact Dermatitis 1997;8:150-153.

Lorenz J, Ferlinz R. Expektoranzien: pathophysiologie und therapie der mukostase. Arzneimitteltherapie 1985;3:22-27.

Louis M, Kowalski SD. Use of aromatherapy with hospice patients to decrease pain, anxiety, and depression and to promote an increased sense of well-being. Am J Hosp Palliat Care 2002;19:381-386.

Lu H, Liu GT. Anti-oxidant activity of dibenzocyclooctene lignans isolated from Schisandraceae. Planta Med 1992;58:311-313.

Lu Y, Chen D, Deng J, Tian L. Effect of *Smilax china* on adjunctive arthritis mouse. Zhong Yao Cai. 2003;26:344-346.

Lupattelli G, Marchesi S, Lombardini R, Roscini AR, Trinca F, Gemelli F, Vaudo G, Mannarino E. Artichoke juice improves endothelial function in hyperlipemia. Life Sci. 2004 Dec 31;76(7):775-782.

Madabushi R, Frank B, Drewelow B, Derendorf H, Butterweck V. Hyperforin in St. John's wort drug interactions. Eur J Clin Pharmacol. 2006 Feb 14;:1-9

Madar Z, Stark AH. New legume sources as therapeutic agents. Br J Nutr 2002;88(suppl 3):S287-S292.

Magistretti MJ, Conti, Cristoni A. Antiulcer activity of an anthocyanidin from *Vaccinium myrtillus.* Arzneimittelforschung 1988;38:686-690.

Magliulo E, Scevola D, Carosi GP. Investigations on the actions of silybin on regenerating rat liver. Effects on Kupffer's cells. Arzneimittelforschung 1979;29:1024-1028.

Magura EI, Kopanitsa MV, Gleitz J, Peters T, Krishtal OA. Kava extract ingredients, (+)-methysticin and (+/–)-kavain inhibit voltage-operated Na+-channels in rat CA1 hippocampal neurons. Neuroscience 1997;81:345-351.

Mahady GB, Pendland SL, Yun GS, Lu ZZ, Stoia A. Ginger (*Zingiber officinale* Roscoe) and the gingerols inhibit the growth of Cag A+ strains of *Helicobacter pylori.* Anticancer Res 2003;23:3699-3702.

Makino T, Ito M, Kiuchiu F, Ono T, Muso E, Honda G. Inhibitory effect of decoction of *Perilla frutescens* on cultured murine mesangial cell proliferation and quantitative analysis of its active constituents. Planta Med 2001;67:24-28.

Malhotra CL, Mehta VL, Das PK, Dhalla NS. Studies on Withania-ashwagandha, Kaul. V. The effect of total alkaloids (ashwagandholine) on the central nervous system. Indian J Physiol Pharmacol 1965;9:127-136.

Malik ZA, Siddiqui S. Hypotensive effect of freeze dried garlic *(Allium sativum)* sap in dog. J Pak Med Assoc 1981;31:12-13.

Manez S, Recio MC, Gil I, et al. A glycosyl analogue of diacylglycerol and other antiinflammatory constituents from Inula viscosa. J Nat Prod 1999;62:601-604.

Mann C, Staba EJ. The chemistry, pharmacology, and commercial formulations of chamomile. In: Craker LE, Simon JE, eds. *Herbs, Spices, and Medicinal Plants: Recent Advances in Botany, Horticulture, and Pharmacology,* vol 1. Arizona: Oryx Press; 1986:235-280.

Manning R. *The Illustrated Stock Doctor.* Sydney: Pacific Publishing Company; 1883.

Mao SP, Cheng KL, Zhou YF [Modulatory effect of *Astragalus membranaceus* on Th1/Th2 cytokine in patients with herpes simplex keratitis.] Zhongguo Zhong Xi Yi Jie He Za Zhi 2004;24:121-123.

Maquart FX, Chastang F, Simeon A, Birembaut P, Gillery P, Wegrowski Y. Triterpenes from *Centella asiatica* stimulate extracellular matrix accumulation in rat experimental wounds. Eur J Dermatol 1999;9:289-296.

Marcilhac A, Dakine N, Bourhim N, et al. Effect of chronic administration of *Ginkgo biloba* extract or Ginkgolide on the hypothalamic-pituitary-adrenal axis in the rat. Life Sci 1998;62:2329-2340.

Maros T, Racz G, Katonai B, Kovacs VV. Wirkungen der *Cynara scolymus*—Extrakte auf die Regeneration der Rattenleber. Arzneimittelforschung 1966;16:127-129.

Marsella R, Nicklin CF, Melloy C. The effects of capsaicin topical therapy in dogs with atopic dermatitis: a randomized, double-blinded, placebo-controlled, cross-over clinical trial. Vet Dermatol 2002;13:131-139.

Martarelli D, Martarelli B, Pediconi D, Nabissi MI, Perfumi M, Pompei P. Hypericum perforatum methanolic extract inhibits growth of human prostatic carcinoma cell line orthotopically implanted in nude mice. Cancer Lett. 2004 Jul 8;210(1):27-33.

Martin N, Bardisa L, Pantoja C, Roman R, Vargas M. Experimental cardiovascular depressant effects of garlic *(Allium sativum)* dialysate. J Ethnopharmacol 1992;37:145-149.

Martin HB, McCallum M, Stofer WD, Eichinger MR. Kavain attenuates vascular contractility through inhibition of calcium channels. Planta Med 2002;68:784-789.

Martin KW, Ernst E. Herbal medicines for treatment of bacterial infections: a review of controlled clinical trials. J Antimicrob Chemother 2003;51:241-246.

Martinez Conesa C, Vicente Ortega V, Yanez Gascon MJ, Garcia Reverte JM, Canteras Jordana M, Alcaraz Banos M. [Experimental model for treating pulmonary metastatic melanoma using grape-seed extract, red wine and ethanol.] Clin Transl Oncol 2005;7:115-121.

Marzocco S, Piacente S, Pizza C, et al. Inhibition of inducible nitric oxide synthase expression by yuccaol C from Yucca schidigera roezl. Life Sci 2004;75:1491-1501.

Massoco CO, Silva MR, Gorniak SL, Spinosa MS, Bernardi MM. Behavioral effects of acute and long-term administration of catnip *(Nepeta cataria)* in mice. Vet Hum Toxicol 1995;37:530-533.

Matev M, Angelova I, Koichev A, Leseva M, Stefanov G. [Clinical trial of a *Plantago major* preparation in the treatment of chronic bronchitis.] Vutr Boles 1982;21:133-137.

Mathur R, Gupta SK, Singh N, Mathur S, Kochupillai V, Velpandian T. Evaluation of the effect of *Withania somnifera* root extracts on cell cycle and angiogenesis.: J Ethnopharmacol. 2006 Jan 9.

Matsuda H, Nakamura S, Shiomoto H, Tanaka T, Kubo M. [Pharmacological studies on leaf of *Arctostaphylos uva-ursi* (L.) Spreng. IV. Effect of 50% methanolic extract from *Arctostaphylos uva-ursi* (L.) Spreng. (bearberry leaf) on melanin synthesis.] Yakugaku Zasshi 1992a;112:276-282.

Matsuda H, Nakamura S, Tanaka T, Kubo M. [Pharmacological studies on leaf of *Arctostaphylos uva-ursi* (L.) Spreng. V. Effect of water extract from *Arctostaphylos uva-ursi* (L.) Spreng. (bearberry leaf) on the antiallergic and antiinflammatory activities of dexamethasone ointment.] Yakugaku Zasshi 1992b;112:673-677.

Matsuda H, Yamazaki M, Asanuma Y, Kubo M. Promotion of hair growth by *Ginseng radix* on cultured mouse vibrissal hair follicles. Phytother Res 2003;17:797-800.

Mazzanti MF, Cometa G, Tomassini L. Sedative and spasmolytic effects of *Viburnum tinus* L. and its major pure compounds. Phytother Res 1998;12:S89-S91.

McDaniel S, Goldman GD. Consequences of using escharotic agents as primary treatment for nonmelanoma skin cancer. Arch Dermatol 2002;138:1593-1596.

McHarg T, Rodgers A, Charlton K. Influence of cranberry juice on the urinary risk factors for calcium oxalate kidney stone formation. BJU Int 2003;92:765-768.

Mechirova E, Domorakova I.NADPH-diaphorase activity in the spinal cord after ischemic injury and the effects of pretreatment with *Ginkgo biloba* extract (EGb 761). Acta Histochem 2002;104:427-430.

Mehlhorn H, Schmahl G, Schmidt J. Extract of the seeds of the plant Vitex agnus castus proven to be highly efficacious as a repellent against ticks, fleas, mosquitoes and biting flies. Parasitol Res. 2005 Mar;95(5):363-5. Epub 2005 Jan 29.

Mehta AK, Binkley P, Gandhi SS, Ticku MK. Pharmacological effects of *Withania somnifera* root extract on GABAA receptor complex. Indian J Med Res 1991;94:312-315.

Merriam EA, Campbell BD, Flood LP, Welsh CJR, McDaniel HR, Busbee DL. Enhancement of immune function in rodents using a complex plant carbohydrate which stimulates macrophage secretion of immunoreactive cytokines. In: Klatz RM, ed. *Advances in Anti-Aging Medicine,* vol 1. Larchmont, NY: Mary Ann Liebert, Inc.; 1995:181-203.

Meybe R, ed. *The Complete New Herbal.* London: Elm Tree Books; 1988.

Milkowska-Leyck K, Filipek B, Strzelecka H. Pharmacological effects of lavandulifolioside from *Leonurus cardiaca.* J Ethnopharmacol 2002;80:85-90.

Milks, HJ. Practical Veterinary Pharmacology, Materia Medica and Therapeutics. Alex Eger, Inc., Chicago, 1949.

Miller DM, Brodell RT. Human papillomavirus infection: treatment options for warts. Am Fam Physician 1996;53:135-143,148-150.

Miller AL. Botanical influences on cardiovascular disease. Altern Med Rev 1998;3:422-431.

Mills S. *The Complete Guide to Modern Herbalism.* London: Thorsons; 1989:22.

Mills S. Acupharmacology: a fundamental approach to herbal therapeutics, part 2. Mod Phytother 1997;3.

Mills S, Bone K. *Principles and Practice of Phytomedicine.* Sydney: Churchill Livingston; 2000.

Min KT, Koo BN, Kang JW, Bai SJ, Ko SR, Cho ZH. Effect of ginseng saponins on the recombinant serotonin type 3A receptor expressed in xenopus oocytes: implication of possible application as an antiemetic. J Altern Complement Med. 2003 Aug;9(4):505-510.

Mitchell J, Rook A. *Botanical Dermatology—Plants and Plant Products Injurious to the Skin.* Vancouver: Greengrass; 1979.

Mittman P. Randomized,double-blind study of freeze-dried *Urtica dioica* in the treatment of allergic rhinitis. Planta Med 1990;56:44-47.

Mittra S, Datta A, Singh SK, Singh A. 5-Hydroxytryptamine-inhibiting property of Feverfew: role of parthenolide content. Acta Pharmacol Sin 2000;21:1106-1114.

Miyamoto K, Katsuragi T, Abdu P, Furukawa T. Effects of baicalein on prostanoid generation from the lung and contractile responses of the trachea in guinea pig. Am J Chin Med 1997;25:37-50.

Moalic S, Liagre B, Corbiere C, et al. A plant steroid, diosgenin, induces apoptosis, cell cycle arrest and COX activity in osteosarcoma cells. FEBS Lett 2001;506:225-230.

Momin RA, Nair MG. Antioxidant, cyclooxygenase and topoisomerase inhibitory compounds from *Apium graveolens* Linn. seeds. Phytomedicine 2002;9:312-318.

Moon EJ, Lee YM, Lee OH, et al. A novel angiogenic factor derived from *Aloe vera* gel: beta-sitosterol, a plant sterol. Angiogenesis 1999;3:117-123.

Mooreville M, Fritz RW, Mulholland SG. Enhancement of the bladder defense mechanism by an exogenous agent. J Urol 1983;130:607-609.

Moorhead LD. Contributions to the physiology of the stomach. XXVIII. Further studies on the action of the bitter tonic on the secretion of gastric juice. J Pharmacol Exp Ther 1915;7:577-589.

Morazzoni P, Bombardelli E. *Silybum marianum (Carduus marianus).* Fitoterapia 1995;66:3-42.

Morisset T, Cote NG, Panisset JC. Evaluation of the healing activity of hydrocotyle tincture in the treatment of wounds. Phytother Res 1987;1:117-121.

Morris J, Burke V, Mori TA, Vandongen R, Beilin LJ. Effects of garlic extract on platelet aggregation: a randomized placebo-controlled double-blind study. Clin Exp Pharmacol Physiol 1995;22:414-417.

Mors WB, do Nascimento MC, Pereira BMR, Pereira NA. Plant natural products active against snake bite—the molecular approach. Phytochemistry 2000;55:627-642.

Motomura N, Sakurai A, Yotsuya Y. Reduction of mental stress with lavender odorant. Percept Mot Skills 2001;93:713-718.

Moxley RA, Schneider NR. Apparent toxicosis associated with lily-of-the-valley *(Convallaria majalis)* ingestion in a dog. J Am Vet Med Assoc 1989;195:485-487.

Mukherjee PK, Verpoorte R, Suresh B. Evaluation of in-vivo wound healing activity of *Hypericum patulum* (Family: hypericaceae) leaf extract on different wound model in rats. J Ethnopharmacol 2000;70:315-321.

Mukhopadhyay A, Basu N, Ghatak N, Gujral PK. Antiinflammatory and irritant activities of curcumin analogues in rats. Agents Actions 1982;12:508-515.

Mulak A, Bonaz B. Irritable bowel syndrome: a model of the brain-gut interactions. Med Sci Monit. 2004 Apr;10(4):RA55-62.

Mulla MS, Su T. Activity and biological effects of neem products against arthropods of medical and veterinary importance. J Am Mosq Control Assoc 1999;15:133-152.

Muller-Limmroth W, Frohlich HH. [Effect of various phytotherapeutic expectorants on mucociliary transport.] Fortschr Med 1980;98:95-101.

Munday PL, Wilson SK. Comparative efficacy of clove oil and other chemicals in anaesthetization of *Pomacentrus amboinensis,* a coral reef fish. J Fish Biol 1997;51:931-938.

Murch SJ, Simmons CB, Saxena PK. Melatonin in feverfew and other medicinal plants. Lancet 1997;350:1598-1599.

Murphy LL, Lee TJ. Ginseng, sex behavior, and nitric oxide. Ann N Y Acad Sci 2002;962:372-377.

Murray MT. The Healing Power of Herbs. 2nd ed. Rocklin California: Prima Publishing; 1995:56.

Nadkarni AK, Dr KM. Nadkarni's Indian Materia Medica, vol 1. 3rd ed. Reprinted Bombay: Popular Prakashan; 1976.

Nagata M. Efficacy of commercial hypoallergenic diets in canine allergic dermatosis. Jpn J Vet Dermatol 1999;5:25-29.

Nagle TM, Torres SM, Horne KL, Grover R, Stevens MTA Randomized, Double-Blind, Placebo-Controlled Trial to Investigate the Efficacy and Safety of a Chinese Herbal Product (P07P) for the Treatment of Canine Atopic Dermatitis. Vet Dermatol 12[5]:265-274.

Nagourney RA. Garlic: medicinal food or nutritional medicine? J Medicinal Foods 1998;1:13-28.

Nammi S, Gudavalli R, Babu BS, Lodagala DS, Boini KM. Possible mechanisms of hypotension produced 70% alcoholic extract of Terminalia arjuna (L.) in anaesthetized dogs. BMC Complement Altern Med. 2003 Oct 16;3:5.

Nathan PJ, Clarke J, Lloyd J, et al. The acute effects of an extract of *Bacopa monnieri* (Brahmi) on cognitive function in healthy normal subjects. In: *Human Psychopharmacology, Clinical and Experimental*. Chichester, United Kingdom: John Wiley & Sons; 2001:345-351.

Newall CA, Anderson LA, Phillipson JD. *Herbal Medicines: A Guide for Health-Care Professionals*. London: Pharmaceutical Press; 1996:124-126.

Ng TB, Li WW. Effects of ginsenosides, lectins and *Momordica charantia* insulin–like peptide on corticosterone production by isolated rat adrenal cells. J Ethnopharmacol 1987;21: 21-29.

Ni JD, Ding RK, Lu GH. [Protective effect of dansheng injection on experimental rabbits' spinal cord injury.] Hunan Yi Ke Da Xue Xue Bao 2002;27:507-508.

Nicholson JA, Darby TD, Jarboe CH. Viopudial, a hypotensive and smooth muscle antispasmodic from *Viburnum opulus*. Proc Soc Exp Biol Med 1972;140:457-461.

Nocerino E, Amato M, Izzo AA. The aphrodisiac and adaptogenic properties of ginseng. Fitoterapia 2000;71(suppl 1):S1-S5.

Noorlander DO. US Patent 4670263 1987: Nontoxic, germicide and healing compositions. Cited in Australian College of Phytotherapy notes.

Nosal'ova G, Strapkova A, Kardosova A, Capek P, Zathurecky L, Bukovska E. Antitussive efficacy of the complex extract and the polysaccharide of marshmallow (*Althaea officinalis* L. var. Robusta). Pharmazie 1992;47:224-226.

Obertreis B, Ruttkowski T, Teucher T. Benke B, Schmitz H. Ex vivo, in vitro inhibition of lipopolysaccharide stimulated tumour necrosis factor alpha and interleukin 1 beta secretion in human whole blood by extractum urticae diocae folorum. Arzneimittelforschung 1996;46(4):389-394.

Obertreis B, Giller K, Teucher T. Benke B, Schmitz H. Anitinflammatory effect of *Urtica dioica* folia extract in comparison to caffeic malic acid. Arzneimitteforschung 1996;46:52-56.

Office of Technology Assessment (OTA). Essiac. Unconventional Cancer Treatments: A Report of the Office of Technology Assessment to the United States Congress. Washington, D.C.: US Government Printing Office, 1990. Report No.: Reprinted by the Commonweal Research Institute.

Ogle CW, Dai S, Ma JC. The haemostatic effects of the Chinese herbal drug Yunnan Bai Yao: a pilot study. Am J Chin Med 1976;4:147-152.

Ogle CW, Dai S, Cho CH. The hemostatic effects of orally administered Yunnan Bai Yao in rats and rabbits. Comp Med East West 1977;5:155-160.

Ohashi Y, Tsuchiya Y, Koizumi K, Sakurai H, Saiki I. Prevention of intrahepatic metastasis by curcumin in an orthotopic implantation model. Oncology. 2003;65(3):250-258.

Ohtaki Y, et al. Deoxycholic Acid as an Endogenous Risk Factor for Hepatocarcinogenesis and Effects of Gomisin A, a Lignan Component of Schizandra Fruits. Anticancer Res. Mar 1996; 16(2):751-755.

Ohyama K, Akaike T, Hirobe C, Yamakawa T.. (a) Cytotoxicity and apoptotic inducibility of *Vitex agnus-castus* fruit extract in cultured human normal and cancer cells and effect on growth. Biol Pharmaceut Bull. 2003;26:10-18.

Okeniyi JA, Olubanjo OO, Ogunlesi TA, Oyelami OA. Comparison of healing of incised abscess wounds with honey and EUSOL dressing. J Altern Complement Med. 2005 Jun;11(3):511-513.

Okimasu E, Moromizato Y, Watanabe S, et al. Inhibition of phospholipase A2 and platelet aggregation by glycyrrhizin, an anti-inflammation drug. Actu Med Okayama 1981;37:457-463.

Ooi VE, Liu F. Immunomodulation and anti-cancer activity of polysaccharide-protein complexes. Curr Med Chem 2000;7:715-729.

Osterhoudt KC, Lee SK, Callahan JM, Henretig FM. Catnip and the alteration of human consciousness. Vet Hum Toxicol 1997;39:373-375.

Ozaki Y. Vasodilative effects of indole alkaloids obtained from domestic plants, *Uncaria rhynchophylla* Miq. and *Amsonia elliptica* Roem. et Schult. Nippon Yakurigaku Zasshi 1990;95:47-54.

Paez X, Hernandez L. Topical hemostatic effect of a common ornamental plant, the geraniaceae *Pelargonium zonale*. J Clin Pharmacol 2003;43:291-295.

Paladini AC, Marder M, Viola H, Wolfman C, Wasowski C, Medina JH. Flavonoids and the central nervous system: from forgotten factors to potent anxiolytic compounds. J Pharm Pharmacol 1999;51:519-526.

Panda S, Kar A. Changes in thyroid hormone concentrations after administration of ashwagandha root extract to adult male mice. J Pharm Pharmacol 1998;50:1065-1068.

Panda S, Kar A. *Withania somnifera* and *Bauhinia purpurea* in the regulation of circulating thyroid hormone concentrations in female mice. J Ethnopharmacol 1999;67:233-239.

Pandian RS, Anuradha CV, Viswanathan P. Gastroprotective effect of fenugreek seeds (Trigonella foenum graecum) on experimental gastric ulcer in rats. J Ethnopharmacol. 2002 Aug;81(3):393-397.

Panossian A, Wikman G, Wagner H. Plant adaptogens III.* Earlier and more recent aspects and concepts on their mode of action. Phytomedicine 1999;6:287-300.

Panossian AG, Oganessian AS, Ambartsumian M, Gabrielian ES, Wagner H, Wikman G. Effects of heavy physical exercise and adaptogens on nitric oxide content in human saliva. Phytomedicine. 1999b;6:17-26.

Pantoja CV, Chiang LC, Norris BC, Concha JB. Diuretic, natriuretic and hypotensive effects produced by *Allium sativum* (garlic) in anaesthetized dogs. J Ethnopharmacol 1991;31:325-331.

Patočka J. Biologically active pentacyclic triterpenes and their current medicine: signification. J Appl Biomed 2003;1:7-12.

Patzelt-Wenczler R, Ponce-Poschl E. Proof of efficacy of Kamillosan® cream in atopic eczema. Eur J Med Res 2000;5:171-175.

Paulova J, Dvorak M, Kolouch F, Vanova L, Janeckova L. [Verification of the hepatoprotective and therapeutic effect of silymarin in experimental liver injury with tetrachloromethane in dogs]: overeni hepatoprotektivniho a terapeutickeho ucinku silymarinu pri experimentalnim poskozeni jater tetrachlormetanem u psu. Vet Med (Praha) 1990;35:629-635.

Pawlowski Z, Chwirot E. (1970). 5th Int Knogr Infektionskr: 277.

Peeters E, Driessen B, Steegmans R, Henot D, Geers R. Effect of supplemental tryptophan, vitamin E, and a herbal product on responses by pigs to vibration. J Anim Sci. 2004 Aug; 82(8):2410-2420.

Peigen X, Keji C. Recent advances in clinical studies of Chinese medicinal herbs. 1. Drugs affecting the cardiovascular system. Phytother Res 1987;1:53-57.

Peng A, Gu Y, Lin SY. Herbal treatment for kidney disease. Ann Acad Med Singapore 2005;34:44-51.

Peoa, N., Aurx, A. and Sumano, H.: A comparative trial of garlic, its extract and ammonium-potassium tartrate as anthelmintics in carp. J. Ethnopharmacol. 24: 199-203, 1988.

Percival SS. Use of echinacea in medicine. Biochem Pharmacol 2000;60:155-158.

Peredery O, Persinger MA. Herbal treatment following post-seizure induction in rat by lithium pilocarpine: *Scutellaria lateriflora* (Skullcap), *Gelsemium sempervirens* (Gelsemium) and *Datura stramonium* (Jimson Weed) may prevent development of spontaneous seizures. Phytother Res 2004;18:700-705.

Perfumi M, Santoni M, Ciccocioppo R, Massi M. Blockade of gamma-aminobutyric acid receptors does not modify the inhibiton of ethanol intake induced by *Hypericum perforatum* in rats. Alcohol Alcohol 2002;37:540-546.

Petersen FJ. Materia Medica and Clinical Therapeutics, 1905. Available online at Henriette's Herbal Homepage: http://www.henriettesherbal.com/eclectic/petersen/index.html

Petrowicz O, Gebhardt R, Donner M, et al. Effects of artichoke leaf extract (ALE) on lipoprotein metabolism in vitro and in vivo. Atherosclerosis 1997;129:147.

Piao BK, Wang YX, Xie GR, et al. Impact of complementary mistletoe extract treatment on quality of life in breast, ovarian and non-small cell lung cancer patients. A prospective randomized controlled clinical trial. Anticancer Res 2004;24:303-309.

PinDer D. Antioxidant activity of burdock (*Arctium lappa* linne): its scavenging effect on free radical and active oxygen. J Am Oil Chem Soc 1998;75:4,455-461.

Pittler MH, Ernst E. Kava extract for treating anxiety. The Cochrane Database of Systematic Reviews 2003.

Pizzorno JE, Murray MT. *Hydrastis canadensis, Berberis vulgaris, Berberis aquifolium* and other berberine containing plants. In: *Textbook of Natural Medicine*. Seattle: John Bastyr College Publications; 1985 (looseleaf).

Pocta J. Therapeutic use of lobeline Spofa. Cas Lek Cesk 1970;109:865 [in Czech].

Polesuk J, Ameodeo JM, Ma TS (1973) Microchemical Investigation of Medicinal Plants. X. Analysis of the Chinese Herbal Drug Yunnan Bai Yao. Mikrochim Acta 4, 507-517.

Poncemacotela M, Navarro-Alegria I, Martinez-Gordillo MN, Alvarez-Chacon R. In vitro effect against giardia of 14 plant extracts. Rev Invest Clin 1994;46:343-347. [In Spanish]

Prabhakar Y, Kumar S. *Crataeva nurvala:* an Ayurvedic remedy for urological disorders Br J Phytother 1997;4:103-109.

Prakash AO, Mather S, Mather R. Effect of feeding *Gymnema sylvestre* leaves on blood glucose in berylliumnitrate treated rats. J Ethnopharmacol 1986;18:143-146.

Preininger V. The pharmacology and toxicology of the Papaveraceae alkaloids. In: Manske RHF, Holmes HL, eds. *The Alkaloids,* vol 15. New York: Academic Press; 1975:239.

Pryme IF, Bardocz S, Pusztai A, Ewen SW, Pfuller U. A mistletoe lectin (ML-1)-containing diet reduces the viability of a murine non-Hodgkin lymphoma tumor. Cancer Detect Prev 2004;28:52-56.

Rackova L, Majekova M, Kost'alova D, Stefek M. Antiradical and antioxidant activities of alkaloids isolated from *Mahonia aquifolium.* Structural aspects. Bioorg Med Chem. 2004;12: 4709-4715.

Rácz-Kotilla, Racz G, Solomon A. The action of *Taraxacum officinale* extracts on the body weight and diuresis of laboratory animals. Planta Med 1974;26:212-217.

Rafatullah S, Tariq M, Al-Yahya MA, Mossa JS, Ageel AM. Evaluation of turmeric (Curcuma longa) for gastric and duodenal antiulcer activity in rats. J Ethnopharmacol. 1990 Apr;29(1): 25-34.

Rahman K, Billington D. Dietary supplementation with aged garlic extract inhibits ADP-induced platelet aggregation in humans. J Nutr 2000;130:2662-2665.

Rahman MT, Alimuzzaman M, Ahmad S, Chowdhury AA. Antinociceptive and antidiarrhoeal activity of *Zanthoxylum rhetsa.* Fitoterapia 2002;73:340-342.

Rai D, Bhatia G, Palit G, Pal R, Singh S, Singh HK. Adaptogenic effect of *Bacopa monniera* (Brahmi). Pharmacol Biochem Behav 2003a;75:823-830.

Rai D, Bhatia G, Sen T, Palit G. Anti-stress effects of *Ginkgo biloba* and *Panax ginseng:* a comparative study. J Pharmacol Sci 2003b;93:458-464.

Ramamoorthy L, Tizard IR. Induction of apoptosis in a macrophage cell line RAW 264.7 by acemannan, a β-(1,4)-acetylated mannan. Molecular Pharma 1998;53:415-421.

Ramaswamy AS, et al. Pharmacological studies on *Centella asiatica* Linn. *(Brahma manduki)* (N.O. Umbelliferae). J Res Indian Med 1970;4:160-175.

Randall C, Randall H, Dobbs F, Hutton C, Sanders H. Randomized controlled trial of nettle sting for treatment of base-of-thumb pain. J R Soc Med 2000;93:305-309.

Reichling J, Schmokel H, Fitzi J, Bucher S, Saller R. Dietary support with Boswellia resin in canine inflammatory joint and spinal disease. Schweiz Arch Tierheilkd 2004;146:71-79.

Reid G, Sobel JD. Bacterial adherence in the pathogenesis of urinary tract infection: a review. Rev Infect Dis 1987;9:470-487

Reider N, Komericki P, Hausen BM, Fritsch P, Aberer W. The seamy side of natural medicines: contact sensitization to arnica (*Arnica montana* L.) and marigold (*Calendula officinalis* L.). Contact Dermatitis 2001;45:269-272.

Remington JP, Wood HC. The Dispensatory of the United States of America 1918. Available at: www.henriettesherbal.com. Accessed June 2005.

Reynolds JEF, ed. Martindale: The Extra Pharmacopoeia. 28th ed. London: The Pharmaceutical Press; 1982.

Reynolds JEF, ed. Martindale: The Extra Pharmacopoeia. 29th ed. London: The Pharmaceutical Press; 1989.

Ribes G, Sauvaire Y, Da Costa C, et al. Effects of fenugreek seeds on endocrine pancreatic secretions in dogs. Ann Nutr Metab 1984;28:37-43.

Ribes G, Sauvaire Y, Da Costa C, Baccou JC, Loubatieres-Mariani MM. Anitidiabetic effects of subfractions from fenugreek seeds in diabetic dogs. Proc Soc Exp Biol Med 1986;182:159-166.

Riccioppo Neto F. Electropharmacological effects of berberine on canine cardiac Purkinje fibres and ventricular muscle and atrial muscle of the rabbit. Br J Pharmacol 1993;108:534-537.

Richardson MA, Russell NC, Sanders T, Barrett R, Salveson C. Assessment of outcomes at alternative medicine cancer clinics: a feasibility study. J of Alternative & Complementary Medicine. 2001;7(1):19-32.

Richardson MA, Ramirez T, Tamayo C, Perez C, Palmer JL. Flor-Essence Herbal tonic use in North America. Herbalgram 2000;50:40-6.

Riehemann K, Behnke B, Schulze-Osthoff K. Plant extracts from stinging nettle *(Urtica dioica),* an antirheumatic remedy, inhibit the proinflammatory transcription factor NF-kappaB. FEBS Lett 1999;442:89-94.

Rieli Mendes F, Mattei R, de Araujo Carlini EL. Activity of *Hypericum brasiliense* and *Hypericum cordatum* on the central nervous system in rodents. Fitoterapia 2002;73:462-471.

Rigelsky JM, Sweet BV. Hawthorn: pharmacology and therapeutic uses. Am J Health Syst Pharm. 2002 Mar 1;59(5):417-422.

Riggs DR, DeHaven JI, Lamm DL. *Allium sativum* (garlic) treatment for murine transitional cell carcinoma. Cancer 1997;79:1987-1994.

Roberts A, Williams JM. The effect of olfactory stimulation on fluency, vividness of imagery and associated mood: a preliminary study. Br J Med Psychol 1992;65:197-199.

Rogala E, Skopinska-Rozewska E, Sawicka T, Sommer E, Prosinska J, Drozd J. The influence of *Eleuterococcus senticosus* on cellular and humoral immunological response of mice. Pol J Vet Sci 2003;6(3 suppl):37-39.

Rolland A, Fleurentin J, Lanhers MC, et al. Behavioural effects of the American traditional plant *Eschscholzia californica:* sedative and anxiolytic properties. Planta Med. 19915:212-216.

Rolland A, Fleurentin J, Lanhers MC, Misslin R, Mortier F. Neurophysiological effects of an extract of *Eschscholzia californica* Cham (Papaveraceae). Phytother Res 2001;15:377-381.

Roodenrys S, Booth D, Bulzomi S, et al. Chronic effects of Brahmi *(Bacopa monnieri)* on human memory. Neuropsychopharmacology 2002;27:279-281.

Rudakewich M, Ba F, Benishin CG. Neurotrophic and neuroprotective actions of ginsenosides Rb(1) and Rg(1). Planta Med 2001;67:533-537.

Sairam K, Rao CV, Goel RK. Effect of *Centella asiatica* Linn on physical and chemical factors induced gastric ulceration and secretion in rats. Indian J Exp Biol 2001a;39:137-142.

Sairam K, Rao CV, Babu MD, Goel RK. Prophylactic and curative effects of *Bacopa monniera* in gastric ulcer models. Phytomedicine 2001b;8:423-430.

Sairam K, et al. Antidepressant activity of standardized extract of *Bacopa monniera* in experimental models of depression in rats. Phytomedicine 2002;9:207-211.

Samuelsen AB. The traditional uses, chemical constituents and biological activities of *Plantago major* L. A review. J Ethnopharmacol 2000;71:1-21.

Sancho R, Lucena C, Macho A, et al. Immunosuppressive activity of capsaicinoids: capsiate derived from sweet peppers inhibits NF-kappaB activation and is a potent antiinflammatory compound in vivo. Eur J Immunol 2002;32:1753-1763.

Sander O, Herborn G, Rau R. [Is H15 (resin extract of Boswellia serrata, "incense") a useful supplement to established drug therapy of chronic polyarthritis? Results of a double-blind pilot study.] Z Rheumatol 1998;57:11-16.

Sandler BI. The influence of Eleutherococcus extract on cerebral circulation in patients with acute cranio-cerebral trauma after rheoencephalography, 1972;11:109-113 Lek Sredstva Dal'nego, Vostoka, USSR.

Sandler BI, Sandler TV. Influence of Eleutherococcus on ceratin clinico-biochemical indexes in the blood of patients with acute craniocerebral trauma. 1972;11:114-19. Lek Sredstva Dal'nego, Vostoka, USSR.

Santini F, Vitti P, Ceccarini G, et al. In vitro assay of thyroid disruptors affecting TSH stimulated adenylate cyclase activity. J Endorcrinol Invest 2003;26:950-955.

Sastravaha G, Yotnuengnit P, Booncong P, Sangtherapitikul P. Adjunctive periodontal treatment with *Centella asiatica* and *Punica granatum* extracts. A preliminary study. J Int Acad Periodontol 2003;5:106-115.

Satoh K, Yasuda I, Nagai F, Ushiyama K, Akiyama K, Kano I. The effects of crude drugs using diuretic on horse kidney (Na+ + K+)-adenosine triphosphatase. Yakugaku Zasshi. 1991 Feb; 111(2):138-145.

Satoh H, Nishida S. Electropharmacological actions of *Ginkgo biloba* extract on vascular smooth and heart muscles. Clin Chim Acta 2004;342:13-22.

Satrija F, Nansen P, Bjorn H, Murtini S, He S. Effect of papaya latex against *Ascaris suum* in naturally infected pigs. J Helminthol 1994;68:343-346.

Satyanarayana S, et al. Evaluation of herbal preparations for hypoglycemic activity in normal and diabetic rabbits. Pharmaceut Biol. 2003;41:6,466-472.

Scarff DH, Lloyd DH. Double blind, placebo controlled, crossover study of evening primrose oil in the treatment of canine atopy. Vet Rec. 1992;131(5):97-99

Schapowal A. Petasites Study Group. Randomized controlled trial of butterbur and cetirizine for treating seasonal allergic rhinitis. BMJ 2002;324:144-146.

Schempp CM, Winghofer B, Ludtke R, Simon-Haarhaus B, Schopf E, Simon JC. Topical application of Saint John's Wort (*Hypericum perforatum* L.) and of its metabolite hyperforin inhibits the allostimulatory capacity of epidermal cells. Br J Dermatol 2000;142:979-984.

Schirrmacher K, et al. Effects of (+/–)-kavain on voltage-activated inward currents of dorsal root ganglion cells from neonatal rats. Eur Neuropsychopharmacol 1999;9:171-176.

Schliebs R, Liebmann A, Bhattacharya SK, Kumar A, Ghosal S, Bigl VLC, Singh BB, Dagenais S. Systemic administration of defined extracts from *Withania somnifera* (Indian Ginseng) and Shilajit differentially affects cholinergic but not glutamatergic and GABAergic markers in rat brain. Neurochem Int 1997;30: 181-190.

Schmidgall J, Schnetz E, Hensel A. Evidence for bioadhesive effects of polysaccharides and polysaccharide-containing herbs in an ex vivo bioadhesion assay on buccal membranes. Planta Med. 2000 Feb;66(1):48-53.

Schmidt CF, et al. Experiments with Chinese drugs. 1. Tang-kuei. Chin Med J 1924;38:362.

Schmidt D, Sobota A. An examination of the anti-adhernce activity of cranberry juice on urinary and nonurinary bacterial isolates. Microbios 1988;55:173-181.

Scholar EM, Wolterman K, Birt DF, Bresnick E. The effect of diets enriched in cabbage and collards on murine pulmonary metastasis. Nutr Cancer 1989;12:121-126.

Schramm HM. Iscador Clinical Documentation Summary and Expert Report, January 15, 2001.

Schulz V, Hänsel R, Tyler V. *Rational Phytotherapy.* 4th ed. Berlin: Springer; 2001.

Schulze-Tanzil G, de SP, Behnke B, Klingelhoefer S, Scheid A, Shakibaei M. Effects of the antirheumatic remedy hox alpha—a new stinging nettle leaf extract—on matrix metalloproteinases in human chondrocytes in vitro. Histol Histopathol 2002;17:477-485.

Scott DW, Miller WH, Decker GA, Wellington JR. Comparison of the clinical efficacy of two commercial fatty acid supplements (Efa Vet and DVM Derm caps), evening primrose oil, and cold water marine fish oil in the management of allergic pruritis in dogs: A double blinded study. Cornell Vet. 1992;82(3):319-329.

Seifen E, Adams RJ, Riemer RK. Sanguinarine: a positive inotropic alkaloid which inhibits cardiac Na+,K+-ATPase. Eur J Pharmacol 1979;60:373-377.

Seitz U, Ameri A, Pelzer H, Gleitz J, Peters T. Relaxation of evoked contractile activity of isolated guinea-pig ileum by (+/–)-kavain. Planta Med 1997;63:303-306.

Self H. Hilton Herbs—Latest News: Equine Cushing's disease results, 2003 Available online at: http://www.

hiltonherbs.com/news_details.cfm?itemid=171&cfid=562777 &cftoken=19285394 (accessed 7-6-05).

Seo K, Jung S, Park M, Song Y, Choung S. Effects of leucocyanidines on activities of metabolizing enzymes and antioxidant enzymes. Biol Pharm Bull 2001;24:592-593.

Seth SD, Jagdeesh G. Cardiac action of *T.terrestris* L. Indian J Med Res 1976;64:1821.

Shanmugasundaram KR, Panneerselvam C, Samudram P, Shanmugasundaram ER. Enzyme changes and glucose utilisation in diabetic rabbits: the effect of Gymnema sylvestre R. Br J Ethnopharmacol 1983;7:205-234.

Shanmugasundaram ER, Gopinath KL, Radha Shanmugasundaram K, Rajendran VM. Possible regeneration of the islets of Langerhans in streptozotocin-diabetic rats given *Gymnema sylvestre* leaf extracts. J Ethnopharmacol 1990;30:265-279.

Shao CR, Chen FM, Tang YX. [Clinical and experimental study on *Ligusticum wallichii* mixture in preventing and treating bronchial asthma.] Zhongguo Zhong Xi Yi Jie He Za Zhi 1994;14:465-468.

Sharada AC, Solomon FE, Devi PU, Udupa N, Srinivasan KK. Antitumor and radiosensitizing effects of withaferin A on mouse Ehrlich ascites carcinoma in vivo. Acta Oncol 1996;35:95-100.

Sharifi AM, Darabi R, Akbarloo N. Investigation of antihypertensive mechanism of garlic in 2K1C hypertensive rat. J Ethnopharmacol 2003a;86:219-224.

Sharifi AM, Darabi R, Akbarloo N. Study of antihypertensive mechanism of *Tribulus terrestris* in 2K1C hypertensive rats: role of tissue ACE activity. Life Sci 2003b;73:2963-2971.

Sharma RD. An evaluation of hypocholesterolemic factor of fenugreek seeds *(T. foenum graecum)* in rats. Nutr Rep Int 1986;33:669-677.

Sharma ML, Bani S, Singh GB. Anti-arthritic activity of boswellic acids in bovine serum albumin (BSA)-induced arthritis. Int J Immunopharmacol 1989;11:647-652.

Sharma SS, Kochupillai V, Gupta SK, Seth SD, Gupta YK. Antiemetic efficacy of ginger *(Zingiber officinale)* against cisplatin-induced emesis in dogs. J Ethnopharmacol 1997;57:93-96.

Sheets MA, Unger BA, Giggleman GF Jr, Tizard IR. Studies of the effect of acemannan on retrovirus infections: clinical stabilization of feline leukemia virus-infected cats. Mol Biother 1991;3:41-45.

Sheldon JP. *Dairy Farming: Being the Theory Practice, and Methods of Dairying.* London: Cassell and Company; 1880 (575 pages).

Sheng Y, Pero RW, Amiri A, Bryngelsson C. Induction of apoptosis and inhibition of proliferation in human tumor cells treated with extracts of Uncaria tomentosa. Anticancer Res 1998;18:3363-3368.

Sherry CJ, Hunter PS. The effect of an ethanol extract of catnip *(Nepeta cataria)* on the behavior of the young chick. Experientia 1979;35:237-238.

Shi M, Chang L, He G. Stimulating action of Carthamus tinctorius L., Angelica sinensis (Oliv.) Diels and Leonurus sibiricus L. on the uterus. Zhongguo Zhong Yao Za Zhi. 1995 Mar;20(3): 173-175, 192

Shi JF, Zhu HW, Zhang C, Bian F, Shan JP, Lu WI. Therapeutic effect of Astragalus on patients with chronic glomerulonephritis. Acta University Medicinalis Secondae Shanghai 2002;22:245-248.

Shi Jing-Shan1, Yu Jun-Xian, Chen Xiu-Ping, Xu Rui-Xia. Pharmacological actions of *Uncaria* alkaloids, rhynchophylline and isorhynchophylline. Acta Pharmacol Sin 2003;24:97-101.

Shi M, Chang L, He G. Stimulating action of Carthamus tinctorius L., Angelica sinensis (Oliv.) Diels and Leonurus sibiricus L. on the uterus. Chung Kuo Chung Yao Tsa Chih 1995;20:173-175.

Shidoji Y, Ogawa H. Natural occurrence of cancer-preventive geranylgeranoic acid in medicinal herbs. J Lipid Res 2004;45(6): 1092-1093. Epub April 1, 2004.

Shin WL. Sedative action of flavonoids and saponins from the seeds of *Zizyphus vulgaris* var. spinosa Bunge. Saengyak Hakhoechi 1981;12:23-27.

Shiota G, et al. Rapid Induction of Hepatocyte Growth Factor mRNA after Administration of Gomisin A, a Lignan Component of Shizandra Fruits. Res Commun Mol Pathol Pharmacol. Nov1996; 94(2):141-146.

Shipochliev T. [Uterotonic action of extracts from a group of medicinal plants.] Vet Med Nauki 1981;18:94-98.

Shivpuri DN, Menon MPS, Prakash D. A crossover double-blind study on *Tylophora indica* in the treatment of asthma and allergic rhinitis. J Allergy 1969;43:145-150.

Shivpuri DN, Singhal SC, Parkash D. Treatment of asthma with an alcoholic extract of *Tylophora indica:* a cross-over, double-blind study. Ann Allergy 1972;30:407-412.

Shukla B, Visen PK, Patnaik GK, Dhawan BN. Choleretic effect of andrographolide in rats and guinea pigs. Planta Med. 1992 Apr;58(2):146-149.

Sievenpiper JL, Arnson JT, Vidgen E, et al. A systematic quantitative analysis of the literature of the high variability in Ginseng (*Panax* spp). Diabetes Care 2004;27:839-840.

Sindrup SH, Madsen C, Bach FW, Gram LF, Jensen TS. St. John's wort has no effect on pain in polyneuropathy. Pain 2001;91: 361-365.

Singh A, Saxena E, Bhutani KK. Adrenocorticosterone alterations in male, albino mice treated with *Trichopus zeylanicus, Withania somnifera* and *Panax ginseng* preparations. Phytother Res. 2000;14:122-125.

Singh B, Chandan BK, Gupta DK. Adaptogenic activity of a novel withanolide-free aqueous fraction from the roots of *Withania somnifera* Dun. (Part II). Phytother Res 2003a;17:531-536.

Singh B, Saxena AK, Chandan BK, Gupta DK, Bhutani KK, Anand KK. Adaptogenic activity of a novel, withanolide-free aqueous fraction from the roots of *Withania somnifera* Dun. Phytother Res 2001;15:311-318.

Singh BB, Mishra LC, Vinjamury SP, Aquilina N, Singh VJ, Shepard N. The effectiveness of *Commiphora mukul* for osteoarthritis of the knee: an outcomes study. Altern Ther Health Med 2003b;9:74-79.

Singh N, Singh SP, Nath R etal. Prevention of induced lung adenomas by Withania somnifera (L) Dunal in albino mice. Int J Crude Drug Res 1986 24:90-100.

Singh NP, Lai HC. Artemisinin induces apoptosis in human cancer cells. Anticancer Res 2004;24:2277-2280.

Singh R. Evaluation of antilithic properties of varun *(Crataeva nurvala),* an indigenous drug. J Res Indian Med 1991;10: 35-39.

Singh RB, Niaz MA, Ghosh S. Hypolipidemic and antioxidant effects of *Commiphora mukul* as an adjunct to dietary therapy in patients with hypercholesterolemia. Cardiovasc Drugs Ther 1994;8:659-664.

Singh RP, Dhanalakshmi S, Agarwal C, Agarwal R. Silibinin strongly inhibits growth and survival of human endothelial cells via cell cycle arrest and downregulation of survivin, Akt and NF-kappaB: implications for angioprevention and antiangiogenic therapy. Oncogene. 2005 Feb 10;24(7):1188-1202.

Singh YN, Singh NN. Therapeutic potential of kava in the treatment of anxiety disorders. CNS Drugs. 2002;16:731-743.

Singletary K. Inhibition of DMBA-induced mammary tumorigenesis by rosemary extract. FASEB J 1991;5:5A927.

Skalisz LL, Beijamini V, Andreatini R. Effect of *Hypericum perforatum* on marble-burying by mice. Phytother Res 2004;18:399-402.

Soh C. The effects of natural food preservative substances on the development and survivial of intestinal Helminth eggs and larvaeII Action on Ancylostoma caninum larvae. American Jounral of tropical medicine and hygiene 1960 9:8-10

Song Z, Kharazmi A, Wu H, et al. Effects of ginseng treatment on neutrophil chemiluminescence and immunoglobulin G subclasses in a rat model of chronic *Pseudomonas aeruginosa* pneumonia. Clin Diagn Lab Immunol 1998;5:882-887.

Sotnikova R, Kettmann V, Kostalova D, Taborska E. Relaxant properties of some aporphine alkaloids from *Mahonia aquifolium*. Methods Find Exp Clin Pharmacol 1997;19:589-597.

Soto CG, Burhanuddin S. Clove oil as a fish anaesthetic for measuring length and weight of rabbitfish *(Siganus lineatus)*. Aquaculture 1995;136:149-152.

Spain Ward P. History of Hoxsey treatment. Contract report submitted to US Congress, Office of Technology Assessment, May 1988.

Spasov AA, Wikman GK, Mandrikov VB, Mironova IA, Neumoin VV. A double-blind, placebo-controlled pilot study of the stimulating and adaptogenic effects of *Rhodiola rosea* SHR-5 extract on the fatigue of students caused by stress during an examination period with a repeated low-dose regimen. Phytomedicine 2000;85-89.

Srimal RC. Dhawan BN pharmacology of diferuloyl methane (curcumin), a nonsteroid antiinflammatopry agent. J Pharm Pharmacol 1973;25:447-452.

Srivastava R, Srimal RC. Modification of certain inflammation induced biochemical changes by curcumin. Indian J Med Res 1985;81:215-223.

Staumont G, Fioramonti J, Frexinos J, Bueno L. Changes in colonic motility induced by sennosides in dogs: evidence of a prostaglandin mediation. Gut 1988;29:1180-1187.

Stephensen 1974 cited on http://www.froytang.no/html/cattle.htm accessed July 2005.

Stewart PM, Wallace AM, Valentino R, et al. Mineralocorticoid activity of liquorice: 11-beta-hydroxysteroid dehydrogenase deficiency comes of age. Lancet 1987;ii:821-824.

Stevenson PC, Simmonds MS, Sampson J, Houghton PJ, Grice P. Wound healing activity of acylated iridoid glycosides from *Scrophularia nodosa*. Phytother Res 2002;16:33-35.

Stocker HR. Sedative und hypnogene Wirkung des Hopfens. Schweizer Brauerei Rundschau 1967;78:80-80.

Stoss M, Michels C, Peter E, Beutke R, Gorter RW. Prospective cohort trial of Euphrasia single-dose eye drops in conjunctivitis. J Altern Complement Med 2000;6:499-508.

Streffer JR, Bitzer M, Schabet M, Dichgans J, Weller M. Response of radiochemotherapy-associated cerebral edema to a phytotherapeutic agent, H15. Neurology 2001;56:1219-1221.

Stull CL, Spier SJ, Aldridge BM, Blanchard M, Stott JL. Immunological response to long-term transport stress in mature horses and effects of adaptogenic dietary supplementation as an immunomodulator. Equine Vet J 2004;36:583-589.

Subbotina MD, Timchenko VN, Vorobyov MM, Konunova YS, Aleksandrovih YS, Shushunov S. Effect of oral administration of tormentil root extract (Potentilla tormentilla) on rotavirus diarrhea in children: a randomized, double blind, controlled trial. Pediatr Infect Dis J. 2003 Aug;22(8):706-711

Suguna L, Sivakumar P, Chandrakasan G. Effects of *Centella asiatica* extract on dermal wound healing in rats. Indian J Exp Biol 1996;34:1208-1211.

Suleyman H, Demirezer LO, Kuruuzum UA. Analgesic and antipyretic activities of *Rumex patientia* extract on mice and rabbits. Pharmazie 2001;56:815-817.

Sun Y, Hersh EM, Talpaz M, Lee SL, Wong W, Loo TL, Mavligit GM. Immune restoration and/or augmentation of local graft versus host reaction by traditional Chinese medicinal herbs. Cancer 1983:52(1):70-73.

Sundaram SG, Milner JA. Impact of organosulfur compounds in garlic on canine mammary tumor cells in culture. Cancer Lett 1993;74:85-90.

Sunila ES, Kuttan G. Immunomodulatory and antitumor activity of *Piper longum* Linn. and piperine. J Ethnopharmacol 2004;90:339-346.

Surh YJ, Lee E, Lee JM. Chemoprotective properties of some pungent ingredients present in red pepper and ginger. Mutat Res 1998;402:259-267.

Suzuki M, Yoshino K, Maeda-Yamamoto M, Miyase T, Sano M. Inhibitory effects of tea catechins and O-methylated derivatives of (-)-epigallocatechin-3-O-gallate on mouse type IV allergy. J Agric Food Chem 2000;48:5649-5653.

Swaim SF, Riddell KP, McGuire JA. Effects of topical medications on the healing of open pad wounds in dogs. J Am Anim Hosp Assoc 1992;28:499-502.

Swanston-Flatt SK, Day C, Bailey CJ, Flatt PR. Evaluation of traditional plant treatments for diabetes: studies in streptozotocin diabetic mice. Acta Diabetol Lat 1989;26:51-55.

Szelenyi I, Isaac O, Thiemer K. [Pharmacological experiments with compounds of chamomile. III. Experimental studies of the ulcerprotective effect of chamomile (author's transl)]. Planta Med. 1979;35:218-227.

Szentmihályi K, Kery A, Then M, et al. Potassium-sodium ratio for the characterization of medicinal plant extracts with diuretic activity. Phytother Res 1998;12:163-166.

Tachikawa E, Kudo K. Proof of the mysterious efficacy of ginseng: basic and clinical trials: suppression of adrenal medullary function in vitro by ginseng. J Pharmacol Sci 2004;95:140-144.

TajuddinA S, Latif A, Qasmi IA:. Aphrodisiac activity of 50% ethanolic extracts of *Myristica fragrans* (Houtt) (nutmeg) and *Syzygium aromaticum* (L.) (Merr and Perry) (clove) in male mice: a comparative study. BMC Complementary and Alternative Medicine 2003;3:6.

Tamaya MD, et al. Possible mechanism of steroid action of the plant herb extracts glycyrrhizin, glycyrrhetinic acid, and paeoniflorin: Inhibition by plant herb extracts of steroid protein binding in the rabbit. Am J Obstet Gynecol 1986;155:1134-1139.

Tanner AG, Owen ER, Seal DV. Successful treatment of chronically infected wounds with sugar paste. Eur J Clin Microbiol Infect Dis. 1988 Aug;7(4):524-525.

Tao X, Lipsky PE. The Chinese anti-inflammatory and immunosuppressive herbal remedy *Tripterygium wilfordii* Hook F. Rheum Dis Clin North Am 2000;26:29-50, viii.

Tao X, Younger J, Fan FZ, Wang B, Lipsky PE. Benefit of an extract of *Tripterygium wilfordii* Hook F in patients with rheumatoid arthritis: a double-blind, placebo-controlled study. Arthritis Rheum 20021;46:1735-1743.

Taylor LH, Kobak KA. An open-label trial of St. John's Wort *(Hypericum perforatum)* in obsessive-compulsive disorder. J Clin Psychiatry 2000;61:575-578.

Terris MK, Issa MM, Tacker JR. Dietary supplementation with cranberry concentrate tablets may increase the risk of nephrolithiasis. Urology 2001;57:26-29.

Thiruvengadam KV, Haranatii K, Sudarsan S, et al. *Tylophora indica* in bronchial asthma: a controlled comparison with a standard anti-asthmatic drug. J Indian Med Assoc 1978;71:172-176.

Thompson Coon JS, Ernst E. Herbs for serum cholesterol reduction: a systematic view. J Fam Pract 2003;52:468-478.

Tian J, Chen XM, Li LS. Effects of *Cordyceps sinensis* on renal cortical Na-K-ATPase activity and calcium content in gentamicin nephrotoxic rats. J Am Soc Nephrol 1991a;2:670.

Tian J, Chen XM, Li LS. Use of *Cordyceps sinensis* in gentamicin induced ARF: a preliminary animal experimentation and observation of cell culture. JAMA 1991b;2:670. Abstract 83P.

Tian J, Yang JY, Li LS. Observation of effects of *Cordyceps sinensis* in isolated perfused kidney of gentamicin nephrotoxic rats. J Am Soc Nephrol 1991c;2:671.

Tilak JC, Banerjee M, Mohan H, Devasagayam TP. Antioxidant availability of turmeric in relation to its medicinal and culinary uses. Phytother Res 2004;18:798-804.

Tisserand R, Balacs T. *Essential Oil Safety.* Edinburgh: Churchill Livingstone; 1995.

Tita B, Bello U, Faccendini P, Bartolini, R., Bolle, P. Taraxacum officinale W.: pharmacological effect of ethanol extract. Pharmacol Res 1993;27:23-24.

Titus Nelson N, 1862. The American Eclectic Practice Of Medicine, As Applied To The Diseases Of Domestic Animals. Baker and Godwin, New York. Also available online at the David Winston's Herbal Therapeutics Research homepage: http://www.herbaltherapeutics.net/DomesticAnimalDiseases.pdf

Toda N, Usui H, Nishino N, Fujiwara M. Cardiovascular effects of capsaicin in dogs and rabbits. J Pharm Exp Ther 1972;181:512-521.

Tohda C, Kuboyama T, Komatsu K. Dendrite extension by methanol extract of Ashwagandha (roots of *Withania somnifera*) in SK-N-SH cells. Neuroreport 2000;11:1981-1985.

Topic B, Hasenöhrl RU, Häcker R, Huston JP Enhanced conditioned inhibitory avoidance by a combined extract of *Zingiber officinale* and *Ginkgo biloba*. Phytother Res 2002;16:312-315.

Tort L, Puigcerver, M.; Crespo, S.; Padrós, F. Cortisol and haematological response in sea bream and trout subjected to the anaesthetics clove oil and 2-phenoxyethanol. Aquaculture Res 2002;33:11,907-910.

Touvay C, Etienne A, Braquet P. Inhibition of antigen-induced lung anaphylaxis in the guinea-pig by BN 52021 a new specific PAF-acether receptor antagonist isolated from Ginkgo biloba. Agents Actions 1986;17:371-372.

Treasure J. Urtica semen reduces serum creatinine levels. J Am Herbalists Guild 2003;4:22-25.

Tripathi RM, Sen PC, Das PK. Further studies on the mechanism of the anti-anaphylactic action of Albizzia lebbeck, an Indian indigenous drug. J Ethnopharmacol 1979a;1:397-400.

Tripathi RM, Sen PC, Das PK. Studies on the mechanism of action of *Albizzia lebbeck,* an Indian indigenous drug used in the treatment of atopic allergy. J Ethnopharmacol 1979b;1:385-396.

Trovato A, Raneri E, Kouladis M, Tzakou O, Taviano MF, Galati EM. Anti-inflammatory and analgesic activity of *Hypericum empetrifolium* Willd. (Guttiferae). Farmaco 2001;56:455-457.

Tsukada K, Tokunaga K, Iwama T, Mishima Y, Tazawa K, Fujimaki M. Cranberry juice and its impact on peristomal skin conditions for urostomy patients. Ostomy Wound Manage 1994;40: 60-62, 64, 66-68.

Tsung PK. *Allergy and Chinese Herbal Medicine,* Monograph. Long Beach, Calif: Oriental Healing Arts Institute; 1987.

Tyler VE. *The Honest Herbal.* 3rd ed. Philadelphia: Strickley; 1993.

Uddin S, Hussain AR, Manogaran PS, et al. Curcumin suppresses growth and induces apoptosis in primary effusion lymphoma. Oncogene 2005;24:7022-7030.

Udintsev SN, Shakhov VP, Borovskoi IG, Ibragimova SG. The effect of low concentrations of adaptogen solutions on the functional activity of murine bone marrow cells in vitro. Biofizika 1991;36:105-108.

Uehara M, Sugiura J, Sakurai K. A trial of oolong tea in the management of recalcitrant atopic dermatitis Arch Dermatol 2001;137:42-43.

Uglyanitsa KN, Nefyodov LI, Doroshenko YM, et al. Ukrain: a novel antitumor drug. Drugs Exp Clin Res 2000;26:341-356.

Umehara K, Nakamura M, Miyase T, Kuroyanagi M, Ueno A. Studies on differentiation inducers. VI. Lignan derivatives from *Arctium fructus*. Chem Pharm Bull (Tokyo) 1996;44:2300-2304.

Umezu T. Behavioral effects of plant-derived essential oils in the Geller type conflict test in mice. Jpn J Pharmacol. 2000;83: 2,150-153.

Upton R, Hawthorn Berry (Crataegus spp): Analytical, Quality Control and Therapeutic Monograph. American Herbal Pharmacopeia, Scotts Valley, CA. 1999.

Usow V. Farmakologiia i toxikologiia. 1958;21:31-34.

Vacca DD, Walsh RA. The antibacterial activity of an extract obtained from *Ascophyllum nodosum*. J Am Pharm Assoc 1954;43:24-26.

Van Den Broucke CO, Lemli JA. Spasmolytic activity of the flavonoids from *Thymus vulgaris*. Pharm World Sci 1983;5:9-14.

Van den Hoven R, Zappe H, Zitterl-Eglseer K, Jugl M, Franz C. Study of the effect of Bronchipret on the lung function of five Austrian saddle horses suffering recurrent airway obstruction (heaves). Vet Rec 2003;152:555-557.

Varalakshmi P, Shamila Y, Latha E. Effect of *Crataeva nurvala* in experimental urolithiasis. J Ethnopharmacol 1990;28:313-321.

Vazquez B, Avila G, Segura D, Escalante B. Antiinflammatory activity of extracts from Aloe vera gel. J Ethnopharmacol 1996;55:69-75.

Velasco G, Galve-Roperh I, Sanchez C, Blazquez C, Guzman M. Hypothesis: cannabinoid therapy for the treatment of gliomas? Neuropharmacology 2004;47:315-323.

Viana AF, Heckler AP, Fenner R, Rates SM. Antinociceptive activity of *Hypericum caprifoliatum* and *Hypericum polyanthemum* (Guttiferae). Braz J Med Biol Res 2003;36:631-634. Epub April 22, 2003.

Vikas Kumar, Singh PN, Muruganandam AV, Bhattacharya SK. Effect of Indian *Hypericum perforatum* Linn. on animal models of cognitive dysfunction. J Ethnopharmacol. 2000;72:1-2,119-128.

Vikas Kumar, Singh PN, Bhattacharya SK. Anti-stress activity of Indian *Hypericum perforatum* L. Indian J Exp Biol 2001;39: 4,344-349.

Viola H, Wasowski C, Levi M, Wolfman C, *Silveira R,* Dajas F, Medina J, Paladini A. Apigenin, a component of *Matricaria recutita* flowers, is a central benzodiazepine receptor-ligand with anxiolytic effects. Planta Med 1995;61:213-216.

Vogel G; Tuchweber B; Trost W; Mengs U. Protection by silibinin against *Amanita phalloides* intoxication in beagles. Toxicol Appl Pharmacol 1984;73:355-362.

Volate SR, Davenport DM, Muga SJ, Wargovich MJ. Modulation of aberrant crypt foci and apoptosis by dietary herbal supplements (quercetin, curcumin, silymarin, ginseng and rutin). Carcinogenesis 2005;26:1450-1456.

Vykusova B. New technologies and new species in aquaculture. Proceedings of a Special International Conference. Vurh Vodnany 2003;39:1-2,1-148.

Wagner H, Horhammer L, Frank U. Lithospermic acid, the antihormonally active principle of *Lycopus europaeus* L. and *Symphytum officinale* L. Arzneimittelforschung 1970;20:705-712.

Wagner H, Jurcic K. On the spasmolytic activity of valeriana extracts. Planta Med 1979;37:84-86.

Walker AF, Marakis G, Morris AP, Robinson PA. Promising hypotensive effect of hawthorn extract: a randomized double-blind pilot study of mild, essential hypertension. Phytother Res 2002;16:48-54.

Wang SM Lee LJ, Lin WW, Chang CM, Effects of a water-soluble extract of *Cordyceps sinensis* on steroidogenesis and capsular morphology of lipid droplets in cultured rat adrenocortical cells. J Cell Biochem 1998;69:483-489.

Wang X, Wei L, Ouyang JP, et al. Effects of an angelica extract on human erythrocyte aggregation, deformation and osmotic fragility. Clin Hemorrheol Microcirc 2001;24:201-205.

Wang H, Li J, Yu L, Zhao Y, Ding W. Antifibrotic effect of the Chinese herbs, *Astragalus mongholicus* and *Angelica sinensis,* in a rat model of chronic puromycin aminonucleoside nephrosis. Life Sci 2004;74:1645-1658.

Wang LS, Zhou G, Zhu B, Wu J, Wang JG, Abd El-Aty AM, Li T, Liu J, Yang TL, Wang D, Zhong XY, Zhou HH, St John's wort induces both cytochrome P450 3A4-catalyzed sulfoxidation and 2C19-dependent hydroxylation of omeprazole. Clin Pharmacol Ther 75:191, 2004

Ward P, Fasitsas S, Katz SE. Inhibition, resistance development, and increased antibiotic and antimicrobial resistance caused by nutraceuticals. J Food Prot 2002;65:528-533.

Wasser SP, Weis AL. Therapeutic effects of substances occurring in higher Basidiomycetes mushrooms: a modern perspective. Crit Rev Immunol 1999;19:65-96.

Wei F, Zou S, Young A, Dubner R, Ren K. Effects of four herbal extracts on adjuvant-induced inflammation and hyperalgesia in rats. J Altern Complement Med 1999;5:429-436.

Weijl NI, Elsendoorn TJ, Lentjes EG, Hopman GD, Wipkink-Bakker A, Zwinderman AH, Cleton FJ, Osanto S. Supplementation with antioxidant micronutrients and chemotherapy-induced toxicity in cancer patients treated with cisplatin-based chemotherapy: a randomised, double-blind, placebo-controlled study. Eur J Cancer. 2004 Jul;40(11):1713-1723.

Weiss RF, Volker F. *Herbal Medicine.* 2nd ed. Stuttgart, Germany: Thieme; 1988.

Weizman Z, Alkrinawi S, Goldfarb D, Bitran C. Efficacy of herbal tea preparation in infantile colic. J Pediatr. 1993 Apr;122(4):650-652.

Wende K, Krenn L, Unterrieder I, Lindequist U. Red clover extracts stimulate differentiation of human osteoblastic osteosarcoma HOS58 cells. Planta Med 2004;70:1003-1005.

Werk, W. 1994, "Wasser ausleiten: elektrolytneutral", Erfahrungsheilkunde, vol. 11, pp. 712-714

Weseler A, Geiss HK, Saller R, Reichling J. Antifungal effect of Australian tea tree oil on Malassezia pachydermatis isolated from canines suffering from cutaneous skin disease. Schweiz Arch Tierheilkd. 2002 May;144(5):215-221.

Westerhof W, Das PK, Middelkoop E, Verschoor J, Storey L, Regnier C. Mucopolysaccharides from psyllium involved in wound healing. Drugs Exp Clin Res 2001;27:165-175.

White DJ, Billingham C, Chapman S, et al. Podophyllin 0.5% or 2.0% v podophyllotoxin 0.5% for the self treatment of penile warts: a double blind randomised study. Genitourin Med 1997;73:184-187.

Widy-Tyszkiewicz E, Piechal A, Joniec I, Blecharz-Kin K. Long term administration of *Hypericum perforatum* improves spatial learning and memory in the water maze. Biol Pharm Bull 2002;25:1289-1294.

Wilburn AJ, King DS, Glisson J, Rockhold RW, Wofford MR. The natural treatment of hypertension. J Clin Hypertens (Greenwich) 2004;6:242-248.

Willard T. The Wild Rose Scientific Herbal Wild Rose College of Natural Healing Calgary 1991 p95.

Williamson EW, Evans FJ. Bradford, England: Health Science Press; 1975.

Willuhn G. Violae tricoloris herba. In: Bissett NG, ed. *Herbal Drugs and Phytopharmaceuticals.* Stuttgart: Medpharm; 1994: 527-529.

Wimer BM, Mann PL. Apparent pokeweed mitogen cure of metastatic gum melanoma in an older dog. Cancer Biother Radiopharm 2000;15:201-205.

Winking M, Sarikaya S, Rahmanian A, Jödicke A, Böker DK. Boswellic Acids Inhibit Glioma Growth: A New Treatment Option? J. Neuro-Onc 46(2):97-103, 2000.

Winslow K. Veterinary Materia Medica and Therapeutics, 1908. William R. Jenkins, New York.

Winston D. Herbal Therapeutics: Specific Indications for Herbs and Herb Formulas, ed 8, Herbal Therapeutics Research Library, Broadway, NJ, 2003.

Winterhoff H, Gumbinger HG, Vahlensieck U, et al. Endocrine effects of *Lycopus europaeus* L. following oral application. Arzneimittelforschung 1994;44:41-45.

Wohlfart R, Hänsel R, Schmidt H. An investigation of sedative-hypnotic principles in hops, Part 3. Planta Med 1982;45: 224.

Wohlfart R, Hänsel R, Schmidt H. The sedative-hypnotic principle of hops. Planta Med 1983;48:120-123.

Wolfson P, Hoffmann DL. An investigation into the efficacy of *Scutellaria lateriflora* in healthy volunteers. Altern Ther Health Med 2003;9:74-78.

Woo KC, Park YS, Jun DJ, et al. Phytoestrogen cimicifugoside-mediated inhibition of catecholamine secretion by blocking nicotinic acetylcholine receptor in bovine adrenal chromaffin cells. J Pharmacol Exp Ther 2004;309:641-649. Epub February 2, 2004.

Wood M. *Herbalism: Basic Doctrines, Energetics, and Classification.* Berkeley, Calif: North Atlantic Books; 2004.

Wren RC. Potter's New Cyclopedia of Botanical Drugs and Preparations, 1907 (revised, 1988) Potter & Clarke, 1985.

Wu G, Yamamoto K, Mori T, Inatomi H, Nagasawa H. Improvement by guan-mu-tong *(Caulis aristolochiae manshuriensis)* of lactation in mice. Am J Chin Med 1995;23:159-165.

Wuttke W, Jarry H, Christoffel V, Spengler B, Seidlova-Wuttke D. Chaste tree *(Vitex agnus-castus):* pharmacology and clinical indications. Phytomedicine 2003;10:348-357.

Wynn S, Marsden S. *Manual of Natural Veterinary Medicine.* Sydney: Mosby; 2003:158.

Xia Z, Gu J, Ansley DM, Xia F, Yu J. Antioxidant therapy with *Salvia miltiorrhiza* decreases plasma endothelin-1 and thromboxane B2 after cardiopulmonary bypass in patients with congenital heart disease. J Thorac Cardiovasc Surg 2003;126:1404-1410.

Xie SS. Immunoregulatory effect of polysaccharide of *Acanthopanax senticosus* (PAS). I. Immunological mechanism of PAS against cancer. [In Chinese] Zhonghua Zhong Liu Za Zhi 1989;11:338-340.

Yamaguchi N, Yoshida J, Ren LJ, et al. Augmentation of various immune reactivities of tumor-bearing hosts with an extract of Cordyceps sinensis. Biotherapy 1990;2:199-205.

Yamamoto H, Ogawa T. Antimicrobial activity of perilla seed polyphenols against oral pathogenic bacteria. Biosci Biotechnol Biochem 2002;66:921-924.

Yan ZY. Effect of radix Salviae miltiorrhizae on gastric mucosal barrier. Zhonghua Wai Ke Za Zhi. 1990 May;28(5):298-301, 319.

Yan L, Yee JA, Li D, McGuire MH, Thompson LU. Dietary flaxseed supplementation and experimental metastasis of melanoma cells in mice. Cancer Lett 1998;124:181-186.

Yang IW, Chou CC, Yung BYM. Dose-dependent effects of berberine on cell cycle pause and apoptosis in Balb/c 3T3 cells. Naunyn-Schmiedeberg's Arch Pharmacol 1996;354:102-106.

Yang CS, Liao J, Yang GY, Lu G. Inhibition of lung tumorigenesis by tea. Exp Lung Res 2005;31:135-144.

Yokozawa T, Liu ZW, Chen CP. Protective effects of *Glycyrrhizae radix* extract and its compounds in a renal hypoxia (ischemia)-reoxygenation (reperfusion) model. Phytomedicine 1999;6: 6,439-445.

Yongchaiyudha S, Rungpitarangsi V, Bunyapraphatsara N, Chokechaijaroenporn O. Antidiabetic activity of Aloe juice. I. Clinical trial in new cases of diabetes mellitus. Phytomedicine 1996:3:241-243.

Yoshida Y, Wang MQ, Liu JN, Shan BE, Yamashita U. Immunomodulating activity of Chinese medicinal herbs and *Oldenlandia diffusa* in particular. Int J Immunopharmacol 1997;19:359-370.

Yoysungnoen P, Wirachwong P, Bhattarakosol P, Niimi H, Patumraj S. Antiangiogenic activity of curcumin in hepatocellular carcinoma cells implanted nude mice. Clin Hemorheol Microcirc 2005;33(2):127-135.

Youn HJ, Noh JW. Screening of the anticoccidial effects of herb extracts against *Eimeria tenella*. Vet Parasitol 2001;96:257-263.

Yuan Y, Hou S, Lian T, Han Y. [Studies of *Rehmannia glutinosa* Libosch. f. hueichingensis as a blood tonic.] Zhongguo Zhong Yao Za Zhi 1992;17:366-368.

Yuan A, Liu C, Huang X. [Treatment of 34 cases of chronic aplastic anemia using prepared *Rehmannia* polysaccharide associated with stanozolol.] Zhongguo Zhong Xi Yi Jie He Za Zhi 1998;18:351-353.

Yuan SL, Wang XJ, Wei YQ. [Anticancer effect of tanshinone and its mechanisms.] Ai Zheng 2003;22:1363-1366.

Yuan CS, Mehendale SR, Wang CZ, et al. Effects of *Corydalis yanhusuo* and *Angelicae dahuricae* on cold pressor-induced pain in humans: a controlled trial. J Clin Pharmacol 2004;44:1323-1327.

Yun TK. Experimental and epidemiological evidence on non-organ specific cancer preventive effect of Korean ginseng and identification of active compounds. Mutat Res 2003;523:63-74.

Yun JH, Pang EK, Kim CS, et al. Inhibitory effects of green tea polyphenol (-)-epigallocatechin gallate on the expression of matrix metalloproteinase-9 and on the formation of osteoclasts. J Periodontal Res 2004;39:300-307.

Yushu H, Yuzhen C. The effect of *Panax ginseng* extract (GS) on insulin and corticosteroid receptors. J Trad Chin Med 1988;8:293-295.

Yang SH, Lin JK, Huang CJ, Chen WS, Li SY, Chiu JH. Silibinin inhibits angiogenesis via Flt-1, but not KDR, receptor up-regulation. J Surg Res. 2005 Sep;128(1):140-146.

Zafar Iqbal, A Jabbar, MS Akhtar, G Muhammad, M Lateef. In vitro anthelmintic activity of *Allium sativum, Zingiber officinale, Cucurbita mexicana* and *Ficus religiosa*. Int J Agric Biol 2001;3:454-457.

Zanoli P, Rivasi M, Baraldi C, Baraldi M. Pharmacological activity of hyperforin acetate in rats. Behav Pharmacol 2002;13: 645-651.

Zarkova S. Tribestan experimental and clinical investigations. Sofia, Bulgaria: Sopharma Chemical Pharmaceutical Research Institute 1981.

Zarkova S. Steroid saponins of *Tribulus terrestis* L having a stimulant effect on the sexual functions. Rev Port Ciencias Vet 1984;79:117-126.

Zeng XH, Zeng XJ, Li YY. Efficacy and safety of berberine for congestive heart failure secondary to ischemic or idiopathic dilated cardiomyopathy. Am J Cardiol 2003;92:173-176.

Zenner L, Callait MP, Granier C, Chauve C. In vitro effect of essential oils from Cinnamomum aromaticum, Citrus limon and Allium sativum on two intestinal flagellates of poultry, Tetratrichomonas gallinarum and Histomonas meleagridis. Parasite. 2003 Jun;10(2):153-157.

Zhang WR, et al. Protective effect of Ginkgo extract on rat brain with transient middle cerebral artery occlusion. Neurol Res 2000;22:517-521.

Zhang X. Influence of *Cordyceps sinensis* on pancreatic islet beta cells in rats with experimental liver fibrogenesis. [In Chinese] Chung Hua Kan Tsang Ping Tsa Chih 2003a;11:93-94.

Zhang M, Ning G, Shou C, Lu Y, Hong D, Zheng X. Inhibitory effect of jujuboside A on glutamate-mediated excitatory signal pathway in hippocampus. Planta Med 2003b;69:692-695.

Zhang R, Zhou J, Jia Z, Zhang Y, Gu G. Hypoglycemic effect of *Rehmannia glutinosa* oligosaccharide in hyperglycemic and alloxan-induced diabetic rats and its mechanism. J Ethnopharmacol 2004;90:39-43.

Zhang XP, Li ZF, Liu XG, et al. Effects of emodin and baicalein on rats with severe acute pancreatitis. World J Gastroenterol 2005;11:2095-2100.

Zhao KS, Mancini C, Doria G. Enhancement of the immune response in mice by *Astragalus membranaceus* extracts. Immunopharmacology 1990;20:225-233.

Zhao J, Sharma Y, Agarwal R. Significant inhibition by the flavonoid antioxidant silymarin against 12-O-tetradecanoylphorbol 13-acetate caused modulation of anti oxidant and inflammatory enzymes and cyclooxygenase 2 and interleukin-1 alpha expression in SENCAR mouse epidermis: implications in the prevention of stage I tumour promotion. Mol Carcinogen 1999;26:321-333.

Zhao YQ, Li GQ, Guo CX, Lian X. Evaluation of the effect of TNF alpha RBC immunological function and improvement on renal function by Astragalus root in patients with chronic renal failure. J Mudanjiang Coll 2000;21:5-6.

Zhou JG. Tianjin medical journal, 1960, 2:131.

Zhou DH, Lin LZ. [Effect of Jinshuibao capsule on the immunological function of 36 patients with advanced cancer.] Chungkuo Chung His I Chieh Ho Tsa Chih 1995;15:476-478.

Zhou Q. Journal of Chinese Materia Medica. 1999;30(5):386-388.

Zhou W, Chai H, Lin PH, Lumsden AB, Yao Q, Chen C. Clinical use and molecular mechanisms of action of extract of *Ginkgo biloba* leaves in cardiovascular diseases. Cardiovasc Drug Rev 2004a;22:309-319.

Zhou W, Chai H, Lin PH, Lumsden AB, Yao Q, Chen CJ. Molecular mechanisms and clinical applications of ginseng root for cardiovascular disease. Med Sci Monit 2004b;10:RA187-RA192. Epub July 23, 2004b.

Zhou YM, Huang ZQ, Hu MH, et al. Clinical study on the effect of Shengxueling on idiopathic thrombocytopenic purpura. Chin J Integr Med 2005;11:60-64.

Zhu DPQ. Dong guai. Am J Chin Med 1987;15:117-125.

Zhu YP. *Chinese Materia Media: Chemistry, Pharmacology, and Applications*. Australia: Harwood Academic Publishers; 1998a: 445-448.

Zhu JS, Halpern GM, Jones K. The scientific rediscovery of an ancient Chinese herbal medicine: *Cordyceps sinensis*. Part II. J Altern Complement Med 1998b;4:429-457.

Zi X, Simoneau AR. Flavokawain A, a novel chalcone from kava extract, induces apoptosis in bladder cancer cells by involvement of Bax protein-dependent and mitochondria-dependent apoptotic pathway and suppresses tumor growth in mice. Cancer Res 2005;65:3479-3486.

Ziauddin M, Phansalkar N, Patki P, et al. Studies on the immunemodulatory effects of ashwagandha. J Ethnopharmacol 1996;50:69-76.

Zou L, Harkey MR, Henderson GL. Effects of herbal components on cDNA-expressed cytochrome P450 enzyme catalytic activity, Life Sci 71:1579, 2002

Herbal Medicine in Equine Practice

CHAPTER

Joyce C. Harman

I have an earache . . .
2000 BC—Here, eat this root.
1000 AD—That root is heathen. Here, say this prayer.
1850 AD—That prayer is superstition. Here, drink this potion.
1940 AD—That potion is snake oil. Here, swallow this pill.
1985 AD—That pill is ineffective. Here, take this antibiotic.
2000 AD—That antibiotic is artificial. Here, eat this root.
From the Internet

The use of herbs in equine medicine is increasing, and clients are using them more often than veterinarians. Horse owners find herbs appealing and information readily available, even if the quality of this information is poor. Herbs are relatively easy to obtain. Veterinarians are learning more about herbs, but few courses are available to help them learn about medical application of herbs; this causes a lack of knowledge and confidence in prescribing. In addition, very little equine-specific herbal research is being conducted, so most available information on the use of herbal medicine in the treatment of horses is anecdotal.

Herbs are suited to equine practice because horses are natural herbivores. In addition, clients like to add herbs to the feed or use them topically. Most data and research from other species probably apply to the horse, but some known species-specific influences must be taken into account. A few recent studies have been performed; these are listed in the *Materia medica* for each herb, provided later in this chapter.

CURRENT USE OF HERBS IN EQUINE PRACTICE

Most herbs used today in the treatment of horses in the United States are selected by the client or recommended by another horse owner. Veterinarians are most often out of the picture. Consequently, the use of herbal therapy in the equine suffers from overuse and incorrect use. Owners may believe that if a little is good, a lot must be better. In addition, horses often have multiple problems, so a new formula is added to the feed for each new problem. The horse then may have 25 different herbs in the feed, and the client may wonder why treatment results are poor.

Most of those who call themselves equine herbalists are people with inadequate training, often not even professionally-qualified herbalists, who combine herbs but have no understanding of disease pathophysiology or equine medicine. This represents the biggest hurdle that must be overcome before herbs can be accepted into mainstream veterinary practice—many veterinarians recognize that herbal prescribing practices are of dubious quality and decide not to become involved with herbal medicine.

However, as more veterinarians become knowledgeable about herbs, the quality of herbal prescribing is improving. Ideal suppliers of herbal medicines use ethically harvested herbs and quality formulas prepared by educated herbalists. Many of these formulas can be safely and successfully used by veterinarians who have had basic herbal medicine training.

Client Considerations

Herbal medicine can be used successfully along with other forms of medicine, conventional or complementary. Clients must understand that herbs need to be fed in dry or fresh form for at least several weeks before clinical improvement may be seen, and months of use may be required before complete resolution has occurred. Herbal extracts usually work much faster, but are more costly. Some diseases and conditions cannot be cured with herbs, as is true of all medicine.

Horse compliance is as important as client compliance. Some horses will not eat herbs under any circumstances; others will eat them with inducement. In this author's opinion, a horse's refusal to eat herbs may mean that the formula is not correct. If a formula is not eaten, the case is revisited and a new formula selected. In most instances, the horse will eat the correct formula. An example of how this works was demonstrated by a mare that had been on a formula to help regulate her heat cycles. The formula contained valerian root *(Valeriana officinalis)*. The mare experienced mild colic, and after the colic passed, she completely refused to eat the original formula. The valerian was removed because it was the only herb in the formula known to possibly have an adverse effect on the intestinal tract; after that, the mare consumed the rest of the herbs. Valerian is considered to be a safe herb with relaxing and intestinal antispasmodic action. It is also known for producing paradoxical effects (Holmes, 1997; Tilford, 1999). This author has seen several clinical gastrointestinal cases in which valerian was fed over a long time. Removal of valerian cleared all cases. It is also a strong smelling herb which may deter some patients from eating it voluntarily.

EQUINE ZOOPHARMACOGNOSY

The field of zoopharmacognosy is expanding, as the interest in herbs is growing (Engel, 2002). This is the study of how animals self-select plants and other materials such as minerals, possibly in order to address disease or discomfort. Animal behaviorists, ecologists, pharmacologists, anthropologists, geochemists, and parasitologists have all contributed to this truly multifaceted discipline (Biser, 1998; Buchanan, 2002).

Most owners have noticed that horses rarely eat the rich grass next to feces. Research has shown that many domestic species avoid parasites as they graze. For example, sheep avoided eating patches of vegetation with higher fecal burdens than were found in uncontaminated patches. Further study has shown that sheep avoid the consumption of grass infected with larvae, even though it may offer them higher intake rates (Hutchings, 1999). This is particularly the case for animals that are naive to parasites. Also, hungry animals are more likely to eat at the expense of larval ingestion. These studies appear to demonstrate that domestic animals might assess the costs, as well as the benefits, of their foraging decisions.

One study of ponies showed that they apparently are able to learn a taste aversion—although incompletely (Houpt, 1990). Illness was created with the use of apomorphine when the pony ate one type of feed (corn, alfalfa pellets, sweet feed, or a complete pellet) when other feeds were offered simultaneously. Ponies learned to avoid all feeds except the complete feed when apomorphine injection immediately followed consumption of the feed. However, they did not learn to avoid a feed when apomorphine was delayed for 30 minutes after feed consumption. They could learn to avoid alfalfa pellets, but not corn, when these feeds were presented with the familiar "safe foods"—oats and soybean meal. This study demonstrated that ponies have some ability to distinguish between safe and unsafe foods.

Few scientific observations of equine species have been reported. Most observations of horses apparently self selecting herbs have been made by traditional herbalists and indigenous people who pass their knowledge along to interested individuals. Many herbal formulas and individual herbs have been selected on the basis of these observations.

Consideration of the environment where wild horses live, both presently and in the past, suggests that little "grass" or green pasture is available. In fact, this author's observations of wild horse environments have revealed that grass is scarce compared with the lush pastures of the civilized world. Even during the peak growing season, horses in native environments walk between every bite and are often surrounded by known toxic plants that they eat around. In winter, most natural environments offer little to eat at all; horses subsist on dried plant material of any sort that they can find.

Yet the modern horse owner assumes that horses require grass. When horses (that evolved to survive in relatively tough conditions) are placed in rich, lush, and fertilized fields without adequate exercise, they frequently become overweight and unfit. Other wild animals have been observed to become fat and unhealthy when they are given access to too much rich, unnatural food; it is easy to picture what would happen if the bears and monkeys in every national park were given access to junk food (Sapolsky, 1989).

Historically, it was recognized that "as regards to exercise, it is indispensable. No man or horse can ever enjoy good health unless habituated to daily exercise; it tends toward their health and strength, assists and promotes a free circulation of the blood, determines morbific matter to the various outlets, develops the muscular powers, creates a natural appetite, improves the wind, and finally invigorates the whole system" (Dadd, 1854). Medicine should not be given to prevent disease; "health is best preserved by the proper regulation of diet, exercise, and cleanliness" (Lawson, 1824). One of the fastest growing equine health problems is obesity and its associated illnesses.

Historical Perspective

Throughout this chapter, references will be made to several herbalists from the last 2 centuries. The two primary veterinarians were Robert McClure and George Dadd. Robert McClure, MD, VS, was a professor at the Veterinary College of Philadelphia who was well published in the early 1900s. He was the author of several books, an editor of *The Horse in the Stable and Field,* and a prize-winning essayist to the US Department of Agriculture, among his many accomplishments. He also appeared to practice primarily herbal medicine because that is what he wrote about.

George H. Dadd, MD, was a veterinary surgeon and author of at least two medical texts, including *The Anatomy and Physiology of the Horse* and *The Reformed Cattle Doctor.* He practiced eclectic medicine in the mid 1800s near Boston. His philosophy was to use whatever form of medicine worked. His writings were primarily based on herbs.

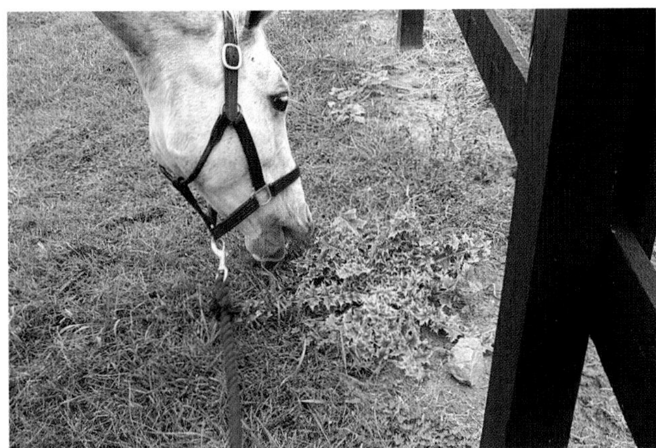

Figure 21-1 The Editor has observed horses in a training barn with access to rich pastures also eating chickweed, plantain, and privet bark. This thoroughbred was observed eating a bull thistle—note that the lip is elevated as if he is trying to avoid being stung by the spines. He ate thistle only for a limited time, then stopped.

Horses kept in fields will preferentially eat the grasses and legumes most of the time. However, horses grazing in a pasture in which a selection of plants is provided will eat a greater variety. At certain times of the year, for example, the tops of the yarrow in this author's field are eaten. Whether these are eaten by horses or by deer has yet to be determined. When horses are removed from the field and are allowed to graze along the fence rows, yarrow is sometimes eaten and sometimes not. Dandelions are always eaten in the spring—but only occasionally at other times of the year. Most horses crave spring dandelions, and some will eat the dirt while trying to get at the roots, especially if they have been ill through the winter (Figure 21-1).

Horses readily adapt to native and nonnative grasses, legumes, and plants in a given area. If horses are moved to a different part of the country, they generally can adapt to new forage. If the new forage is significantly richer in quantity or carbohydrate content than the forage on which they have been raised, the transition may be difficult or, at times, impossible. In many cases, horses must be removed from the rich pasture they were raised on and placed in dirt lots with very little forage to eat because they cannot handle the high carbohydrate content of rich grasses.

It would be interesting to study the behavior of horses in poor health when placed in a healthy, unfertilized pasture with a large selection of native grasses, herbs, and weeds. Detailed observations, including regular clinical examination, hematology and biochemistry should document any changes in health over time. It might then be possible to say whether horses actually self-medicate purposefully.

However, if domestic horses are raised in an artificial environment—exposed only to rich monoculture grass—it is possible that those horses will not instinctively know enough to self-medicate. Zoopharmacognosy researchers have tested the theory that animals learn which plants to eat by watching others of the same species (Huffman, 2001). Thus, a wild horse or a domesticated horse that has been raised with a natural, varied diet may be adept at determining which plants it should eat. These factors would need to be considered in research.

Author observation and information from toxicologists indicate that horses will not eat most toxic plants if they are well fed and do not graze in overcrowded pastures (Knight, 2001). Most poisonings occur when animals are exposed to unfamiliar plants, or when little safe plant material is available to graze. Certain plants such as red maple *(Acer rubrum)* and cherry *(Prunus* spp*)* become extremely toxic when the leaves are wilted. Domestic horses will often eat the wilted leaves; however, in most cases of poisoning, pasture overstocking has been found. Certain ornamental plants such as Yew may be unfamiliar enough to horses that they will eat them. Horses starved for green forage, as most confined horses are, will often eat indiscriminately anything green. Many "weeds" growing in barnyards are medicinal herbs or toxic plants; the vast majority of horses will never eat the toxic ones.

Ranching and grazing researchers have studied details about the grazing habits of livestock. Investigators examined which grasses were most palatable, and when they were most likely to be eaten (Fehmi, 2002). If given a choice of grasses to eat, cattle will select only what is at the peak of nutritive value and will leave the rest until it reaches peak. This indicates that cattle can make decisions about what is best to eat. Peak nutrition varies according to type of grass, season of the year, and climatic conditions. Research such as this does not show that animals are self-medicating, but rather that they recognize differences in the grasses they eat.

McClure wrote that horses should most often be fed hay if they are not being worked; corn and oats can be fed when they are working. Vetches and cut grass should be fed to horses that cannot graze in the spring. He believed that vetches and grass had cooling and refreshing qualities that were almost medicinal in effect (McClure, 1917).

Most modern horses have no idea what a day's work is; many are ridden less than an hour at a time and only a few days a week. They are fed large quantities of processed grain while they stand in a small stall or pen. In nature, horses walk about 20 hours a day and sleep less than 4 hours (Pascoe, 2000). Many modern stabled horses are almost never fed fresh greens—a fact that has increased the incidence of vitamin E deficiency diseases such as equine motor neuron disease, as well as fertility problems (Divers, 2003).

DRUG TESTING AND HERBS

Equine veterinarians working with competition horses may be asked whether a specific herb or formula will cause a positive drug test. Practitioners are responsible for any positive tests if they prescribe or approve an herb, and they should be cautious. No set answer exists regarding which herbs are legal because new tests are devised regularly. Any list published here or on any Web site should be considered partial. Positive test results are possible with herbs, so practitioners should consult with manufacturing companies and drug testing laboratories for advice. If there is any question, it is better to withdraw the herb rather than risk a positive drug test.

Herbs fed in extract or tincture form may contain higher levels of forbidden compounds because of the increased concentrations. However, other compounds may actually be present in lower quantities because some compounds are not soluble in alcohol or glycerin. Currently, no data are available on the concentrations of forbidden compounds in extracts versus raw herbs, so caution must be used if extracts are used regardless of whether the raw herb sources are forbidden.

Herbs that contain salicylates such as white willow bark *(Salix alba)* and others that can be sold under the name of white willow—crack willow *(Salix fragilis)*, purple willow *(Salix purpurea)*, and violet willow *(Salix daphnoides)*, along with meadowsweet *(Filipendula ulmaria)* *Betula* (birch) spp, *Populus* (poplar) spp, and bilberry *(Vaccinium myrtillus)*—have strong potential for producing a positive drug test. Salicylic acid is illegal in competition. Metabolism of plant-based salicylic acid precursors has not been studied in horses; however in humans these compounds undergo hepatic conversion into salicylic acid. It is unknown whether the concentration of salicylic acid precursors in these herbs are great enough to create a positive test. Willow bark and meadowsweet are the only herbs containing salicylates that are specifically listed as forbidden (United States Equine Federation, 2005).

The herb valerian is specifically singled out as an illegal compound in competition, with a 7-day recommended withdrawal time. Many horses do receive large quantities of valerian at shows, and a few positive tests have apparently been recorded. This herb should not be included in competition horses' formulas. Other herbs that have quieting effects have been used without reported positive tests; however, their use is not without risk as new tests are being developed regularly.

Essential oils and herbs with strong odors or mixed with ingredients such as peppermint *(Mentha piperita)*, camphor *(Cinnamomum camphora)*, menthol *(Mentha* spp*)*, rosemary *(Rosmarinus officinalis)*, and thymol *(Thymus vulgaris)*—typically used externally—may produce a positive test result if the horse ingests the compound through licking. These compounds are often considered masking agents for other illegal drugs, so they themselves are listed as illegal.

The guidelines that are available for compounds that may cause a positive drug test state, "Any product is forbidden if it contains an ingredient that is a forbidden substance, or is a drug which might affect the performance of a horse and/or pony as a stimulant, depressant, tranquilizer, local anesthetic, psychotropic (mood and/or behavior altering) substance, or might interfere with drug testing procedures (USEF, 2005)." These regulations also provide ". . . just some of the examples of the hundreds and perhaps thousands of examples of herbal/natural or plant ingredients that would cause a product to be classified as forbidden . . . ," indicating that in the future, possible testing may be available for any herb. Herbs specifically listed as prohibited in the United States are included in Table 21-1. In Australia, listed prohibited herbs include white willow, kola, kava, guarana, and valerian, but other herbs may be tested for. Chinese herbs with known compounds that can test positive are listed in Table 21-2 (Xie, 2003). Other Chinese herbs may consist of similar compounds but are not specifically listed as prohibited.

TABLE 21-1

Herbs Specifically Prohibited in Competition in the United States

Common Name	Scientific Name
Arnica, wolfsbane	*Arnica montana*
Cayenne (capsaicin, derivative)	*Capsicum annuum*
Chamomile (species is not specified in regulations)	*Matricaria* spp, *Ormenis mixta/multicola, Anthemis nobilis*
Comfrey	*Symphytum officinale*
Devil's claw	*Harpagophytum procumbens*
Hops	*Humulus lupulus*
Kava kava	*Piper methysticum*
Laurel	*Laurus nobiles*
Lavender	*Lavandula* spp
Lemon balm	*Melissa officinalis*
Leopard's bane (listed in regulations under this name), Arnica	*Arnica montana*
Night shade	*Solanum* spp
Passionflower	*Passiflora incarnata*
Rauwolfia	*Rauvolfia serpentina*
Red poppy	*Papaver rhoeas, P. somniferum*
Skullcap	*Scutelleria lateriflora*
Valerian	*Valeriana officinalis*
Vervain	*Verbena officinalis*

TABLE 21-2

Chinese Herbs That May Be Forbidden in the Racing Community in the United States

Herb	Chinese Name	Substances Forbidden by Rules
Ephedra	Ma huang	Ephedrine
Papaver	Yin su ke	Morphine
Strychnos	Ma qian zi	Strychnine
Datura	Yang jin hua	Atropine
Acacia	Er cha	Theophylline

From Xie, 2003.

QUALITY CONTROL ISSUES

Because of the large volume of herbs needed to treat even one horse, the temptation may be great for a company to use less-than-ethically harvested herbs. Herb quality and manufacture is as important today as it was in the past. Even in 1843, Youatt warned herbalists to stay away from powdered ginger because it was usually adulterated with bean meal or sawdust, then was made warm and pungent with capsicum; he recommended purchasing the whole root and grinding it (Youatt, 1843). To this day, the natural products industry is largely unregulated, and many poor-quality products are sold (Butters, 2003). A company without much knowledge of herbs can easily purchase poor-quality products without even being aware of it. The reader is referred to Chapter 17 on sustainable harvesting and endangered species, as this is another very important issue.

Well-informed clinicians should investigate the companies they intend to use by asking questions about purity, sources of ingredients, and independent testing practices. A formula is only as good as the formulator, so the clinician should learn the credentials behind product developers. Formulators, whether veterinarians or nonveterinarian herbalists, should have had extensive education in botanical medicine, as well as equine experience. Clients who choose to use herbal preparations on their own initiative should be counseled about the advisability of obtaining products from reputable companies with a strong dedication to research, quality control, and ethical harvesting.

In the United States, practitioners who must find out which companies are committed to quality control should contact the National Animal Supplement Council (National Animal Supplement Council, 2005). This is an alliance of companies dedicated to quality control and self-regulation and opposed to unnecessary government regulation. These companies work to raise the standards within an industry that often profits from the use of poor-quality raw materials. No such industry alliances have yet been formed in other parts of the world, to this author's knowledge.

ADVERSE REACTIONS

An adverse or toxic reaction to a substance occurs when an unfavorable, harmful, destructive, or deadly outcome occurs (Brown, 2001). An adverse or toxic reaction is one that is known to occur with the administration of a particular substance, for example, diarrhea after the administration of aloe. An idiosyncratic reaction is one that occurs when a compound that is routinely safely administered causes unique symptoms in one individual, for example, hives after the administration of meadowsweet.

Because no database is available widely to document adverse events related to herbal medicine in the equine, it may be impossible for a practitioner to know whether an herb is responsible or some unique reaction has occurred. VBMA (Veterinary Botanical Medicine Association) has the facility to record reported cases and is available at www.vbma.org. Consultation with an experienced equine herbalist may be helpful. In all cases, when any adverse event occurs, possible contributing factors such as concomitant drugs, diet and doses should be recorded. The product should be discontinued immediately. If the clinical sign subsides rapidly and was mild when it occurred, the product may be administered again at a lower dose after a week; if the sign then recurs, the product should be discontinued completely.

In the author's experience, most good-quality herbal preparations used judiciously have proved to be relatively safe. However, compromised health status (e.g., impaired liver or kidney function) may alter response to such products. It must be remembered that any animal can have an idiosyncratic reaction to any substance—even if the compound has a long history of safe use.

The veterinarian should also remember that many people do not view herbal preparations as substances that need to be mentioned to the veterinarian. Many do not appreciate that herbs have the potential to alter a horse's response to a drug, or that the potential for serious adverse events exists.

The reader should remember the proverb, "the dose makes the poison." Several reasons can be proposed for an adverse event associated with an herbal preparation:

- There may be an adverse event from concurrent drug administration, diet or new infection or disease process.
- A plant with a history of safe use when given to excess may provoke toxicity.
- A consumer may willfully disregard safety information.
- A plant of unknown or uncertain safety may be used or substituted.
- The plant in the preparation may not be the plant listed on the label.
- The plant or the product may be contaminated.
- Food or drug interactions may occur.
- The formulation itself, rather than the plant, may elicit an adverse response (Bruneton, 1999).
- The product may be deliberately adulterated with a pharmaceutical agent.

CAUTIONS WITH HERBS

False Information

Old wives' tales are abundant in equine practice and in the literature. In England and Australia particularly, flax *(Linum usitatissimum)* is considered toxic unless it is well cooked. Flax does contain cyanogenic glycosides; however, the quantity is small and no clinical symptoms have resulted when it is fed at high levels for long periods (personal experience, and Knight, 2001). Horses, because of their acid stomachs, are rarely affected by any type of cyanide poisoning (Knight, 2001). Even when cattle are fed the raw cake (by-product of linseed manufacturing), 10 minutes' boiling time is all that is needed, contrary to some claims that it must be boiled for an extended period in preparation for equine consumption.

Many claims have also been made about the toxicity of garlic *(Allium sativum)*. Garlic has the potential for toxicity in dogs and especially in cats. The toxic compound is N-propyl-disulfide, and some evidence in the literature supports the claim of toxicity (Knight, 2001). One equine case of urticaria associated with dry garlic feeding has been reported (Miyazawa, 1991). A few reports can be found in the literature regarding onion toxicity in the bovine. Acute hemolytic anemia caused by wild onion poisoning was reported in horses (Pierce, 1972). No significant toxicities have been reported for garlic specifically, although a few practitioners believe that they have seen horses that have become anemic through chronic ingestion of garlic.

In any pasture, garlic and onion leaves are eaten readily by horses, even when they have plenty of other food. In this author's practice, no horses have developed clinical anemia when garlic is fed in a sensible manner. It must be remembered that many clients will overfeed supplements, and garlic is more likely to be overfed than some other herbs because clients feed it to help control flies. The truth is that in most cases, flies are less of a problem for horses than they are for owners.

Internal

When black walnut *(Juglans nigra)* is given, a substance in the wood shavings or the heartwood can cause laminitis (Uhlinger, 1989; Minnick, 1987). Oral administration of the seed and bark appears safe clinically. The constituent juglone, which has been thought to be the cause of the laminitis, is present in the bark and nuts—but not in the heartwood, so juglone is probably not the poisonous principle (Knight, 2001). Although some practitioners believe it is safe to feed the seeds and bark, in this author's opinion, the risk is too great to make the chance worth taking. Other anthelmintic herbs are available as alternatives to black walnut.

Topical

Arnica has long been recognized as a skin irritant when used on open wounds or abrasions. Topical arnica is available in herbal form as an oil, ointment, or poultice. It is also commonly used as a homeopathic topical preparation with a low concentration of arnica. The same cautions apply in all forms. It is safe when used on intact skin.

PREGNANCY

A number of herbs are contraindicated in pregnancy because (1) they have the potential to cause uterine contractions, such as black cohosh *(Cimicifuga racemosa),* (2) they may alter hormones in a manner that can result in risk to the pregnancy, such as fenugreek *(Trigonella foenum-graecum)* (Gruenwald, 2000; Blumenthal, 2000; Brinker, 2000), or (3) they are teratogenic, such as comfrey *(Symphytum officinale)* (Gruenwald, 2000; Brinker, 2000) (Table 21-3). Because no specific research has been undertaken to investigate the equine, it is best for the practitioner to assume that an herb that is specifically contraindicated for use in pregnancy in humans or other species because of known biochemistry should not be used in the equine.

HERB/DRUG INTERACTIONS

At the present time, very little, if any, research has been conducted in the equine concerning herb/drug interactions and adverse reactions. However, it is possible and desirable for the practitioner to examine the data collected for other species and to at least consider that they may be applicable to the horse (Brinker, 2001; Harman, 2002). This is especially true for herb/drug interactions because the drugs used in horses have similar biochemical effects in other species. Some of the adverse reactions seen in other species may not occur in the equine because the digestive tract is designed to handle a large variety of plant material.

PRACTICAL USES OF HERBS

Horses are herbivores and as such are designed to eat unprocessed herbs (fresh or dried). The horse's cecum breaks down plant fiber very effectively. No studies show the digestibility of dried herbs in horses versus tinctures or extracts. In this author's experience, all forms work well. However, if an extract or tincture is very concentrated and was made from many more pounds of herbs than would normally be fed, the extract appears to act more rapidly.

Horses can be fed herbs in the whole, unprocessed state or as powders. For roots, powders are best because whole roots may be too hard to chew properly—even for the horse. Alcohol extracts are expensive but easy to give mixed in with food; however, some horses may not like the alcohol taste. If alcohol tincture is administered directly into the mouth, horses that dislike the taste will become very difficult to dose. It is better to dilute with some water, vinegar, or other liquid to offset the alcohol, or to use glycerin extracts.

Horses lend themselves well to topical applications of herbs—especially on their legs, which are highly prone to injury. Ointments, salves, liniments, gels, washes, paints, sweats, and poultices all can be applied under a bandage or with no bandage. Topical herbs are usually well tolerated by most horses, but some are sensitive to any medication. If irritation, scurf, or peeling of the skin is seen, one should remove the bandage, decrease the frequency of application (to every other day or once a week), or discontinue use.

Horses are more sensitive to, and require smaller quantities of, many food and drug items per pound of body weight than are small animals with a higher metabolic rate. This is true of many larger species of animals. Dosing in modern times has been based on experience and extrapolation from the old texts. However, doses derived according to McClure in 1917 were also empirical and approximate and were determined without a specific reason—they were just what had been found to work (McClure, 1917).

It is interesting to hear the experiences of Dr. Huisheng Xie (personal communication), the noted Chinese herbal-

TABLE 21-3

Some Common Herbs Contraindicated in Pregnancy

Plant	Clinical Result*
Chaste Berry *(Vitex agnus-castus)*	Uterotropic effects, emmenagogue (DerMarderosian, 2000; Blumenthal, 2000)
Black cohosh *(Actaea racemosa)*	Uterine stimulant, spontaneous abortions; except in 1st trimester—may decrease uterine spasms, antiabortive, hormonal effects (DerMarderosian, 2000; Gruenwald, 2000; Blumenthal, 2000; Brinker, 2000)
Burdock *(Arctium lappa)*	Uterine stimulant, especially first trimester, oxytocic effects (Blumenthal, 2000; Brinker, 2000)
Chamomile *(Matricaria chamomilla* or *recutita)*	Possible abortifacient in early pregnancy, emmenagogue (Blumenthal, 2000; Brinker, 2000; DerMarderosian, 2000); claims that there are no contraindications in pregnancy
Comfrey *(Symphytum officinale)*	Teratogenic, mutagenic, fetotoxin, chromosome damage to human lymphocytes (DerMarderosian, 2000; Blumenthal, 2000; Brinker, 2000)
Fenugreek *(Trigonella foenum-graecum)*	Oxytocic action, emmenagogue, abortifacient (DerMarderosian, 2000; Blumenthal, 2000; Brinker, 2000)
Garlic *(Allium sativum)*	Large doses can serve as uterine stimulant, emmenagogue effects (DerMarderosian, 2000; Gruenwald, 2000; Blumenthal, 2000; Brinker, 2000)
Goldenseal *(Hydrastis canadensis)*	Uterine stimulant, equivocal data for pregnancy complications, emmenagogue (Blumenthal, 2000)
Lavender *(Lavendula angustifolia)*	Emmenagogue (Blumenthal, 2000; Brinker, 2000; DerMarderosian, 2000; Gruenwald, 2000)
Parsley fruit *(Petroselinum crispum)* (roots and leaves are safe)	High doses increase contractility of smooth muscle—abortifacient. Low doses increase uterine tone; could be emmenagogue (DerMarderosian, 2000; Brinker, 2000; Gruenwald, 2000) no stated problem
Red clover *(Trifolium pretense)*	Estrogenic activity possible (Brinker, 2000)
Rosemary *(Rosmarinus officinalis)*	Can be used externally during pregnancy. Contains volatile oils; contraindicated in pregnancy because of uterine stimulation, emmenagogue, abortifacient (Gruenwald, 2000; Blumenthal, 2000; Brinker, 2000)
Sage *(Salvia officinalis)*	Emmenagogue (alcohol extract and essential oil) (Blumenthal, 2000); abortifacient, uterine stimulant (Gruenwald, 2000; Brinker, 2000)
Thyme *(Thymus vulgaris)*	Emmenagogue, early pregnancy (DerMarderosian, 2000; Gruenwald, 2000; Blumenthal, 2000; Brinker, 2000)
Turmeric *(Curcuma longa, aromatica)*	Emmenagogue, abortifacient, uterine stimulant (DerMarderosian, 2000; Gruenwald, 2000; Blumenthal, 2000; Brinker, 2000)
Wormwood tops, leaves *(Artemisia absinthum)*	Emmenagogue, abortifacient, uterine stimulant (possible) (Brinker, 2000)
Yarrow *(Achillea millefolium)*	Emmenagogue, abortifacient, uterine stimulant (possibly only some constituents) (DerMarderosian, 2000; Gruenwald, 2000; Brinker, 2000)

*This is not a complete listing of all herbs known to have effects on pregnancy, but it includes most of the ones commonly used in equine practice.

ist, after he came to the United States. In China, veterinarians received the lowest-grade herbs for use with animals, while the high-quality herbs were sent to export and to human hospitals. In the United States, only high-quality human-grade herbs are used (those that were exported), in his experience, and the doses required to get results dropped dramatically, to a level that is only a few times higher than the human dose.

Personal clinical experience has shown that a good rule of thumb for veterinarians to follow is to treat horses with two to four times the human dose of any given herb. Some modern herbal literature often uses a "handful" of leafy herbs as one dose (deBairacli-Levy, 1976; Ferguson, 2002; Self, 1996). Measured a bit more exactly, this dose is approximately 30 grams or 1 ounce (Self, 1996).

Doses are usually administered twice a day at feeding time. More frequent dosing might produce a faster response, especially in acute situations. In most cases, compliance will go down significantly if owners are asked to dose too frequently. Most formulas are designed to be fed for several months, although in acute cases or with the use of more toxic herbs, treatment times may be shorter. Horses should be introduced to herbs slowly if they are at all suspicious of the additions to the feed.

A number of older methods of dosing are not used much today but certainly have potential. Dadd usually made mixtures of herbs in a liquid drench with something to make it palatable, such as caraway seeds or honey. McClure used flax oil, spirits of turpentine, warm ale, or aloes in a solution. He would fill an old champagne bottle and tip it up, giving the solution slowly without any force, to allow time for the horse to swallow. Perhaps in modern times, a plastic bottle could more safely be used. Dadd definitely had a gentle approach to the horse compared with others of his time.

Another common way to administer herbs at the turn of the last century was with the use of a ball, sometimes called a "Physic ball". The ball was made with powdered herbs, linseed meal, treacle (pale cane syrup) or honey, and a bit of palm oil. These ingredients were mixed into a ball, with some being fairly hard, others slightly soft. Dadd believed this was bulky and difficult to give, that it required force to pull the tongue out and shove the bolus down the throat, and that it was slow to dissolve and deliver the active compound. Lawson and Clater used balls, frequently mixing in licorice powder to improve the consistency (Lawson, 1824; Clater, 1817).

FORMULA SELECTION

The selection of a formula should be based on a complete history and physical examination, as should any prescription. A complete health history covering the entire life of the horse is beneficial. However, it must be noted that many horses have been owned by the current caretaker for only 2 to 4 years, so information on past history may be difficult to obtain.

For instance, a horse with summer skin eruptions may have been purchased in winter and may have no history of previous skin disease. Horse trading has never been totally honest, so one does not know whether the previous owner is ignorant of, or lying about, skin problems. Other horses have passed through several owners, and they may genuinely not know the past history. For example, a history of pneumonia as a foal may signal weakness in the immune system, and lead to fibrosis in the lungs, or the residual effects of a large quantity of drugs such as antibiotics that may affect long-term health.

If the practitioner has been trained to observe tongue color and feel pulse, as is practiced in Chinese herbal medicine, that information can be added to the physical examination findings. McClure provided great detail about feeling the pulse on the angle of the jaw. He described pulse characteristics in various types of diseases. He accurately indicated how inflammatory diseases are associated with increases in pulse strength and rate, and how debility was associated with decreased pulse strength. He also recognized that sometimes the pulse was quicker in animals with debilitating disease. Although he offered no explanation for this variation of the pulse in debility, an understanding of Chinese medicine would suggest that he is describing a Yin deficiency.

Lawson, a practitioner who was active in the early 1800s, described in detail pulses felt at the jaw line (Lawson, 1824). The normal pulse felt perfectly elastic, neither hard nor soft, but in fever, it was increased. With fever, the pulse felt hard and rigid, and it resisted pressure from the fingers. He recommended bleeding until the pulse felt softer. The Chinese also used bleeding techniques when monitoring results by checking the pulse. Although this text does not discuss Chinese medicine, it is interesting to note that some early herbalists in this country used the same type of information (Table 21-4).

Once the diagnosis has been made, an individual herb or formula can be selected. Experienced herbalists can customize a single herb or a formula for individual cases. For many veterinarians, a prepared formula will be the preferred choice. The choice of which company's formulas to use should depend on the quality of the company's herbalist and the herbs themselves (see above, and Chapter 8 for more information). A formula can be selected on the basis of the clinical picture and fed for at least a month (about 2 weeks if the formula is in tincture form) before a reevaluation is undertaken to determine whether there has been a response.

Energetic or Traditional Chinese Veterinary Medicine (TCVM) Signs

The tongue and pulse are used by TCVM practitioners to detect internal imbalances. These characteristics can help the practitioner determine which type of herb or formula to select. Although they are not easy techniques to learn, tongue and pulse diagnosis can be very useful tools. Tongue color is examined in natural daylight. The pulse is felt at the base of the neck over the jugular vein. The reader is referred to Chinese medical texts and training for more detailed information (Xie, 2002). The basic presentations are listed here, along with examples of herbs that fit these patterns (Holmes, 1997). The first priority when examining a case is to decide whether the animal has an excess or deficient condition; then, the practitioner must decide which type of excess or deficiency is present.

PRESCRIBING CONSIDERATIONS

If a well-selected herb or formula is not working, it is important for the practitioner to reevaluate the case. Is the diagnosis correct? Is more information needed? Is the formula incorrect, or still appropriate after partial changes in the clinical condition have occurred? Is the horse consuming the full dose? Is the client paying attention to how much the horse is eating? Has the formula been given enough time to work? Is the horse under a heavy load of stress (showing, rough training, crowding in the pasture) which might be an obstacle to improvement? Is the horse's digestive system fully functional?

One of the most likely reasons for a well-selected formula or herb not to work is that the digestive tract is functioning poorly. Horses are often fed large quantities of antibiotics for every cut, scrape, nasal discharge, and bug bite. They are also commonly fed extremely large quantities of nonsteroidal anti-inflammatory agents, the most common of which—phenylbutazone—leads to sig-

TABLE 21-4

Traditional Chinese Veterinary Medicine Patterns

TCVM Pattern	Tongue	Pulse	Symptoms	Herbs That May Be Appropriate
1. Excess	May appear normal, red or purple	Strong	Animal is strong, often young, but does not have to be; signs appear quickly and are of short duration	
Heat	Deep red	Rapid, strong, often bounding	Signs of heat, inflammation, hemorrhage in any organ system	Gentian root, chicory root, goldenseal root, Oregon graperoot, echinacea root, willow bark
Cold	Normal or slightly pale or purple	May be tight, wiry, and often slow	Can have sudden onset, very painful, worse with cold, better with heat, ears are cold	Thyme, rosemary leaf, juniper berry, garlic, cinnamon essential oil
Wind	May have thin coating	Superficial, floating	Symptoms move, change location	Passionflower, hops flower, valerian root, black cohosh root, ginger, chamomile flower
Damp	May have a pale, lusterless color, with or without a greasy coating	Slow, soft	Slower onset than cold symptoms, not as severe, better with warmth, moves slow, stiff stiff	Burdock root, celery seed, red clover flower, cleavers herb, garlic, meadowsweet
Summer heat	Red, dry, with a yellow coating	Fast, strong	Fevers, thirst, sweating, dry mouth	Goldenseal root, chaparral leaf, wild indigo root
Dryness	Dry, pale or red	Variable pulse, can be wiry	Dry nose, manure, skin, dry cough	Licorice root, chickweed herb, slippery elm bark, marshmallow root, mullein leaf
2. Deficiency	Can be variable, depending on the type	Weak	Horse is usually older but does not have to be; signs usually appear over extended period or have been present for a long time	
Yin (deficiency heat)	Red, dry, with no coating	Weak but rapid and thready, often weaker on the left side	Inflammation, prone to sweating more easily, especially at night, worse in warm weather	Licorice root, borage leaf, mullein leaf, aloe gel, comfrey, marshmallow root, slippery elm bark, red clover flower
Yang	Pale, moist, may be quite large in the older animal	Pulse is weak, especially on the right side	Very common in older animals, stiff, worse in cold weather	Cinnamon bark, ginger, cayenne pepper, rosemary leaf, mint, meadowsweet, horseradish root
Chi	Very moist, pale	Usually soft, weak	Weak overall, often has lost weight or muscle mass	Elecampane root, sage leaf, thyme, American ginseng, hawthorn berry, licorice root, fennel seed
Blood	Pale and dry	Weak	Poor or dry coat, cracked hooves, may be anemic on blood test	Sage leaf, dandelion root, milk thistle seed, hawthorn berry, microalgea, nettle

Common Causes of Gastrointestinal Tract Dysfunction

- Use of antibiotics
  In a healthy gut, friendly bacteria inhabit specific areas. Antibiotics are nonselective, so they can damage required beneficial bacteria, as well as pathogenic bacteria. Once the bacterial populations have become unbalanced, normal digestive processes usually performed by the beneficials are altered (Sullivan, 2001)
- Nonsteroidal drug (NSAID) use, leading to inflammation, ulceration, or increased intestinal permeability (Jenkins, 1991; MacAllister, 1993; Sigthorsson, 1998)
- Antiulcer medication
  Increases the pH of the stomach and decreases ionization of calcium, magnesium, manganese, and iron, thereby preventing proper absorption of minerals (Kimbrough, 1995)
- Parasite damage that can leave scars on the intestinal wall
- Overuse of dewormers
  Dewormers themselves may not damage the intestinal flora; however, overuse of them can lead to poor gut immunity against parasites. Clinically, this author has seen many horses that are eating a daily deworming product have high levels of parasites and poor response to any other product. Strategic deworming is the latest approach; it takes into account the parasite load in the pasture, the weather conditions, and the parasite load in the individual horse, to come up with a schedule that best meets the needs of the individual farm and horse (Briggs 2005)
- Stress
- Confinement, performance, training, and excess drug use (Lizko, 1987)

nificantly increased permeability of the intestinal tract wall (McAllister, 1993). Antibiotics change the bacterial flora, so digestion may not be as complete as in a horse whose beneficial bacteria and protozoa are intact (Rolfe, 1984; Zinn, 1993). Because bacteria and protozoa are important for cellulose or plant wall digestion, an unhealthy digestive tract may not process herbs optimally.

How does one recognize a horse with an underfunctioning digestive tract? Signs can be subtle. A horse with a poorly functioning digestive tract often appears unthrifty, even though his teeth and deworming program may be adequate. The horse may or may not carry enough weight, but the coat does not have a deep, rich color to it. The manure may be abnormal—too soft, too hard, or not enough of it. An individual horse's manure may be perfectly normal, yet the gastrointestinal tract may still be functioning suboptimally.

Many patients and herb formulas require 2 to 3 weeks before results become evident; it may take even longer for the full effects of treatment to be seen. If no response is seen at the end of 1 month, the practitioner should reevaluate the case, consider reformulation of the herbal therapy, or investigate the need for another form of therapy. If some positive response occurs, treatment should be continued for another month, at the end of which good response should be seen. If by the end of the second month, results are mediocre, critical reevaluation of the case should be undertaken.

FORMULAS FOR COMMON EQUINE CONDITIONS

In this section, treatments for some of the most common equine-specific conditions are presented from historical and modern perspectives. Conditions present in all species such as liver disease are discussed elsewhere in this text. Formulas can apply to the equine if the doses are adjusted. The number of commercial formulas available to treat equine disease is large and formulas given here are examples to build from, rather than to copy without thought. It would appear that herbalists at the turn of the century were as discouraged with much of the conventional medicine practiced then as herbalists are in the present time. Dadd and McClure were the main references for this section, unless otherwise noted (Dadd, 1854; McClure, 1917).

Sulphur is used in many old formulas. This mineral is currently deficient in many soils, and consequently, in horses as well. Horses readily eat sulphur when it is offered to them as a separate mineral, especially in the spring and fall as the coat changes. Sulphur is a key mineral that is required by the proteins common in hair and hooves. The herbalists of old times may have known something about mineral nutrition that should be incorporated into modern nutrition. Methylsulfonylmethane (MSM) (usual dose is 5-10g/day) is a readily available source of sulphur. Elemental sulphur can also be obtained and salt blocks with sulphur can be offered, but the latter may be unpalatable for some horses if the salt level is too high.

Many of the herbs in common use today are different from those described in old veterinary texts and modern information on herbal medicine is more often available in the current human literature. Although this approach (applying similar principles) to equine herbal medicine is a valid one, much can be learned from hundreds of years of experience. Historical formulas can be adapted to modern times in many ways. One way is to substitute nontoxic herbs in formulas for those that are no longer available (e.g., opium *[Papaver somniferum]*, aconite [*Aconite* spp]). It is not necessary for the herbalist to mix herbs in ale or even in treacle (syrup), as was formerly recommended, because sugar should be avoided or limited. Other types of ingredients may be omitted (e.g., carbonate of iron—iron deficiency is uncommon in the modern horse because it is plentiful in the diet). If iron supplementation is desired, blue-green algae and parsley are both high in iron. Experimentation over time with historical uses of herbs will expand the current *Materia medica*.

General Health and Tonics

Prevention of disease by improving overall health is an important concept in herbal medicine. Formulas have been used for centuries as tonics to maintain health, as well as to aid in the recovery of good health after a serious illness has resolved. In modern times, this thought is often taken too far, and basically, healthy horses are fed large quantities of herbs for extended periods without good reason. In England, commercial horse feeds that do NOT have herbs added to them are scarce. However, in nature, plants change with the seasons, becoming scarce or nonexistent in the winter, so the body gets a break from them. Because herbs are medicine, it is best for the body to have this rest period. Formulas fed on a long-term basis can be given 6 days a week or 3 weeks each month, to give the body a break.

General tonics can be fed periodically and are especially beneficial in the spring. In a natural environment, spring brings fresh growth of herbs, and horses desire them at this time. Horses kept inside most of the time with little fresh grass and few natural herbs should be fed a general tonic for several months each year. Herbs often included in modern tonics include nettle leaf, milk thistle, meadowsweet, garlic, marigold or calendula, fenugreek, burdock, dandelion root, mint, chamomile, echinacea, cleavers, rosehip, and celery seed.

Personal favorites for inclusion in a tonic are nettles, gentian, dandelion, garlic, turmeric, and astragalus. A simple spring tonic is made by mixing dandelion root, nettles, and marshmallow in equal parts; 30 to 40g per day should be fed for 2 to 3 months. If the horse has been treated for any problems in the winter, 1 part milk thistle should be added for 3 to 4 weeks because this practice may support detoxification pathways. A tonic of broader spectrum can be made by mixing 2 parts each of nettle, gentian, and marshmallow with 1 part each of turmeric and licorice. About 30g should be fed per day for 2 months or so. Horses that have been ill and need more support for their immune system do well with a blend of garlic, gentian, eleuthero, turmeric, and flax or hemp. Mushrooms are excellent immune system tonics, although they are expensive to feed to horses. Shiitake and reishi mushroom powders can be fed at 3 to 5 tablespoons per day for 1 to 2 months.

No section on tonics is complete without the addition of essential fatty acids in the form of flax or hemp as an oil, meal, or whole seed. This author uses both of these herbs as a tonic on a regular basis, along with many other forms of therapy. Although horses appear to digest the whole seed, it is unknown what portion of the oils is absorbed. Therefore, this author uses doses of 4 to 6 ounces twice a day when the whole seed is used, 2 to 4 ounces when naturally stabilized ground flax is used, and 1 to 3 ounces of oil, which must be refrigerated in warm weather.

Historically, the following tonic was used for horses that were thin or needed to restore their health: 1.5 ounces each of powdered gentian, sassafras, sulphur, ginger, and fine salt, with 1 pound oatmeal, mixed and divided into 12 parts, fed twice a day until it was gone (Dadd, 1854). An alterative formula for restoring secretions and excretions after an illness consisted of equal parts of powdered sulphur, bloodroot, sassafras, cream of tartar (by-product of grape fermentation, the major component of baking powder), and skunk cabbage. One-half ounce was given twice a day mixed in food. Another variation recommended by Dadd to restore health in thin, "hide-bound" (dry coat, dehydrated) horses was made up of the following: 3 ounces each sassafras bark, sulphur, and salt, with 2 ounces bloodroot and balmony and 1 pound oatmeal, divided into 12 parts, given daily.

Another tonic, taken from McClure, that is used to revive horses after an illness included ginger or gentian combined with sulphate of copper (an ingredient then considered a powerful tonic for the whole body). Several other tonic formulas to be given after illnesses included (1) 1 ounce Peruvian bark, ½ ounce dry opium, 20 drops oil of caraway, and enough treacle to form a ball; (2) 1 drachm (1.8g) gentian, ½ drachm (0.9g) ginger, 1 drachm (1.8g) cascarilla, with treacle and linseed meal to form a ball; and (3) 2 drachms (3.5g) myrrh, 1 drachm (1.8g) mustard flour, 5 grams cantharides, and 4 drachms (7.1g) chamomile, mixed with Venice turpentine to make up the liquid part of the ball. Another tonic for lean, unhealthy, and hidebound horses is taken from Lawson (Lawson, 1824): caraway seeds 1 ounce, 0.5 ounces each of gentian root, zeodary root, fenugreek seeds, and mithridate, mixed as a powder, then given with 1.5 pints of ale in the morning every 2 to 3 days (formulas must not be boiled with seeds).

Even Youatt, who was not an herbalist but a conventional practitioner of the time, claimed to use some herbs in his treatments (Youatt, 1843). He most often practiced the regular medicine of the day with mercury and arsenic. However, one of his herbal tonics was a combination of ginger and gentian beaten together and made into a ball with treacle; another consisted of 4 drachms (7.1g) gentian, 2 drachms (3.5g) chamomile, 1 drachm (1.8g) carbonate of iron (nonirritating, tasteless preparation of iron), and 1 drachm (1.8g) ginger made into a ball.

Arthritis and Rheumatism

Chronic degenerative joint disease (DJD) is one of the most common conditions that limit a horse's performance. Many different herbal formulas are available for arthritis. Simple ones with several key herbs are usually superior to the "kitchen sink" variety, to which inexperienced herbalists add every herb known to have action on the joints. Clinically, this author finds that different horses respond to different formulas, and success or failure may not depend on the formula itself. Each horse's pathology is different, so herbal treatment results will vary. For example, one horse may respond very well to a formula that contains devil's claw or meadowsweet, and the next horse may have little response to the same formula. This holds true for most herbs; no one formula works every time.

It is also important that the owner keep the horse on a generally healthy diet without additives and other sources of potential toxins. Work in humans has shown that arthritis may be related to increased intestinal permeability resulting from the use of antibiotics or nonsteroidal anti-inflammatory drugs (NSAIDs) (Rolfe, 1984; Zinn, 1993; Darlington, 1991; Inman, 1991; O'Dwyer, 1988; Wells, 1991; Bjarnason, 1989). This author and other herbalists have noted that horses on poor diets respond less well to treatment (Harman, 2002). Workload, saddle fit, shoeing, and conformation also may contribute to outcomes in the treatment of horses with arthritis.

Modern formulas for arthritis may include white willow bark, meadowsweet, chamomile, devil's claw, cleavers, burdock, nettle, hawthorn, rosemary, lavender (as an essential oil), celery seed, juniper, horsetail, tansy, and comfrey. White French millet is used in Australia and New Zealand to provide silica for proper bone formation and to minimize exostosis.

A simple anti-inflammatory/antirheumatic formula consists of equal parts of meadowsweet, hawthorn, celery, turmeric, and milk thistle. For most arthritic conditions, this or any formula should be fed for an extended time, so a 6-day-a-week protocol is best after daily feeding is provided for the first 2 months. Faster action can be obtained by using extracts initially, although for maintenance, it is most common to use dried herbs. For all arthritic horses, the addition of 4 to 8 ounces flax or hemp seed is beneficial for its anti-inflammatory action.

Arthritis in aged horses is usually worse in cold, damp weather (Yang deficient, see Table 21-4), and horses may benefit from "warming" herbs. Warm herbs should not be used in animals with active inflammation because adding warm herbs to warm inflammation can worsen the condition. A formula for older animals is made with 2 parts each of meadowsweet, nettle, celery seed, burdock, dandelion, and hawthorn, and 1 part ginger. If the horse needs this formula through the summer months, when it is hot outside, it may be best to remove the ginger and add it back in late fall or as the weather cools, when the horse becomes stiffer again.

Externally, the following formula of oils can be carefully used: 45% comfrey infused oil, 45% linseed or flax oil, 5% arnica infused oil, and 1% wintergreen essential oil, with the final 4% unspecified; olive oil is usually used as a carrier (Beasley, 1861). Sometimes, the skin may be irritated by essential oils; resulting in flaking skin. Topically, plain lavender or other essential oils can be diluted by placing 10 to 12 drops of oil into 30 mL of a base oil such as flax or almond (deBairacli-Levy, 1976). For sore joints, this author uses *Arnica montana* topically, as an oil, tincture, or ointment; occasionally, it is used as a poultice with soaked herbs.

Historical advice (Dadd, 1854) included: (1) avoid cold water at all costs (which is the same advice given by Chinese herbalists), and (2) use warm baths and warm stalls. Bandages may be soaked in warm vinegar. From an herbal standpoint, a warming mixture was used to move circulation to all parts. One of Dadd's formulas consisted of 2 ounces each tincture of guaiacum, balm of gilead, and ginger combined with 6 ounces syrup of garlic and divided, with $^{1}/_{6}$th part given twice a day.

Colic

Veterinary herbalists rarely treat acute colic because herbs usually do not work as fast as drugs. Chronic colic is another matter and is often treated. Colics are more common in the spring and fall when the weather changes rapidly. According to Chinese medicine, the intestinal tract is extremely sensitive to environmental dampness and cold, so a sudden weather change toward cooler and damper weather can damage the spleen and stomach meridians, leading to digestive upset.

Chamomile and valerian are recommended by a number of herbalists for their antispasmodic action. One combination of herbs used to treat recurrent spasmodic colic comprises a mix of comfrey, marshmallow, slippery elm, licorice, and valerian (Beasley, 1861). An excellent formula for treating gassy colic is made up of two parts: chamomile and one part each fennel, peppermint, and marshmallow. This author uses high-quality probiotic supplements, along with any herbal treatment for digestive tract dysfunction. For chronic dry manure or mild constipation colic, the formula includes 4 to 6 ounces flax or hemp meal per day, 2 parts marshmallow root, and 1 part each dandelion root and fennel, combined with 2 ounces distilled aloe juice per day.

Historically, turpentine was frequently used in the treatment of acute colic (McClure, 1917; Youatt, 1843); although turpentine is a natural extract, it was considered too strong by some practitioners for use in the treatment of colic (Dadd, 1854). A simple peppermint tea was used instead.

One herbal formula for the treatment of acute colic comprised a combination of 1 tsp powdered grains of paradise *(Amomum melegueta),* $^{1}/_{2}$ tsp powdered caraway, 20 drops oil of peppermint, and 1 tbsp powdered slippery elm, mixed in a pint of hot water (Dadd, 1854). Another formula was used by Dadd when he suspected a twisted intestine, when the horse was colicky; but not dying (NB: this was probably a simple colic as we know now that a true torsion of the intestine will usually require surgery). The formula consisted of 2 ounces tincture of ginger, 20 drops oil of peppermint, and 2 drachms (7.4 mL) chloric ether (mix of chloride of sodium, manganese, sulphuric acid, and strong alcohol) combined with a half-pint (237 mL) thin gruel; this was provided along with rubbing of the belly and the administration of clysters (enemas) of salt and water.

Spasmodic colic caused by excessive cold (drinking cold water, washing in cold water, driving hot horses into a pond) was treated by warming the stomach and bowels with warm ale or porter with a bit of whiskey or 1 tablespoon ground ginger. If no relief was seen within a half-hour, a drench was given with 25 drops aconite root (*Aconite* spp) and 1 ounce spirit of turpentine mixed in a bottle of cold ale or porter (McClure, 1917).

Flatulent colic was, and still is, considered a swelling of the belly with passing of wind or gas; usually a result of indigestion or fermentation of food. One would start with oral administration or injection of warm water, soap, and table salt. If no response was observed, the practitioner mixed the following in cold water: 1 ounce aloe powder, 1 ounce sulphuric ether (ethyl sulphate), and 2 ounces tincture of opium. If pain was not relieved, chloroform was instilled into the nose on a rag, and if that did not work, the surgery of that time was trocarization performed to relieve gas; it worked on occasion but was probably unsuccessful most of the time given what we know about the inability of the horse to withstand abdominal contamination.

Flatulent colics were also treated simply with 2 to 6 drachms (3.5-10.6g or 0.125oz) ginger (Beasley, 1861). Ginger is readily available today and is easy for most clients to obtain. Because it has been used successfully historically (and is found in formulas today), ginger is an excellent herb for the client to use before the veterinarian arrives.

McClure believed that no case of colic could be cured without the use of "clysters or injections" (an enema), made with a quart of warm water, soap, and a handful of table salt. Another recipe for clysters consisted of a bucket of warm water at body temperature, 4 ounces common table salt, and enough soap to make a good lather. A total of 3 to 4 quarts was injected into the rectum every half-hour until the animal was better. Although enemas are seldom used today, their use may be considered in some cases of distal intestinal impaction because they stimulate the bowel. Herbal formulas given orally may take a while to reach the rectum or even the distal large bowel. Walking was also recommended to improve bowel motility; this is still considered important today.

Stercoral colic referred to impaction or constipation colic. McClure used 1 ounce powdered aloes, 25 drops tincture of aconite, and ½ ounce chloroform, mixed in a bottle of ale or porter and given in a drench through a stout horn or bottle. A note was made that some horses became wild with chloroform and others relaxed, so results were not always predictable.

Another formula used by McClure comprised 1 pint linseed/flaxseed oil with 2 ounces each turpentine and laudanum (an alcohol tincture of opium). In high doses, opium is constipating. However, in the homeopathic literature (Hering, 1993), homeopathically-prepared opium is an important treatment for impaction that has used successfully many times by this author, the opium tincture in this situation is most likely acting more as a homeopathic preparation.

This author rarely uses herbs to treat acute impaction because most true laxative herbs are somewhat toxic and provide a purgative action that clients do not appreciate. With some equine impactions, strong laxatives are also associated with the risk of bowel wall rupture. However, patients with chronic impaction need the support of herbs and generally respond well. Clinically, flax or hemp seed, 8 to 16 ounces divided two to three times daily, is excellent for impaction. Psyllium *(Plantago psyllium)* also works very well, although it should be obtained in its pure form. Many psyllium products manufactured for horses include undesirable additives. Oils added to small quantities of moist food such as bran mash or beet pulp are also very useful. Cold-pressed, ideally organic, olive oil is the best and most readily available; this author has used flax and hemp oil also, even though the seed is a better lubricant. A handful of herbs such as marshmallow and slippery elm are also easily added to wet food.

A simple formula that can be given over the phone to a client who is waiting for the arrival of the veterinarian is 100mL of cooled tea (use a good handful of herbs or tea bags, which people often have in the cupboard), to which 10 drops Rescue Remedy™ (Bach Flower Remedies Ltd, Oxfordshire, England) from the health food store is added; this is given to the horse every half-hour (Ferguson, 2002).

Enteritis

Herbs offer several excellent antibacterial and astringent choices for the treatment of patients with diarrhea. Probiotics should be included, even if antibiotics are also used. One part slippery elm and chamomile combined with two parts plantain may resolve mild cases. Dadd noted that in patients with enteritis, the pulse was full, firm, and quick, and it increased in volume and intensity as the disease progressed (Dadd, 1854). He was cautious about purging the bowels with very strong agents, as is commonly recommended in most of the old texts (Youatt, 1843), preferring the use of herbs or salt. His herbal mixtures included 4 drachms (14.8mL) pulverized aloe combined with 1 pint mucilage of slippery elm, or 8 ounces linseed oil (flax) mixed with 2 ounces lime water (a saturated aqueous solution of calcium hydroxide). For a cathartic, he used Epsom salts and a thin gruel, or plain salt and water. Although he wrote about not wanting to purge, his doses of aloe do have laxative effects. Another formula for the stomach in a "torpid condition" consisted of 2 ounces ginger, 1 ounce fine salt, and 1 ounce essence of peppermint, given as a drench. This was followed 4 hours later with drenches that had mucilaginous properties.

McClure (1917) used aconite tincture, 30 drops every 2 hours, to lessen the pain. (NB: Aconite given in these doses should be quite safe, and it is a potent pain reliever; however, it is not used currently because of its potential for toxicity.) Blankets soaked in boiling water were applied to the belly and renewed every 20 minutes. Warm water, soap, and a handful of table salt were given every 30 minutes as long as the horse was strong. This was considered a frequently fatal disease, yet no mention was made of using some of the herbs we now believe to be antibacterial.

Ulcers

Until recently, ulcers were not generally recognized as a problem in horses. However it has been known for many years that stabled horses under stress could develop ulcers and that racehorses suffer a high incidence of gastric ulceration. However, the reality today is that many types of horses are kept stabled and overfed on grain with inadequate green forage. The treatment of horses with ulcers must include changing the lifestyle of the horse, as has been discussed previously.

Formulas should contain only herbs; no antacids should be added. Antacids have been implicated as the cause of many digestive problems in humans (Russel, 1992; Gianella, 1979) and are being promoted, perhaps inappropriately, to clients in equine practice. Successful herbal formulas contain meadowsweet, licorice, milk thistle, slippery elm, marshmallow, comfrey, gotu kola, chamomile, marigold, marshmallow, Irish moss, oat powder, apple pectin *(Pirus malus)*, fenugreek, and aloe vera (as an extract or juice or distilled). Personal favorites are meadowsweet, licorice, marshmallow, calendula, slippery elm, chamomile, and aloe vera. In some cases, distilled aloe as a single herb is enough to treat patients with ulcers if the environment is also corrected. Flax or hemp seed (about 4-6 oz/day) is protective for the digestive tract; it provides an anti-inflammatory effect and supports the immune system.

A useful formula for ulcers consists of 2 parts meadowsweet, along with 1 part each chamomile, calendula, marshmallow root, raspberry leaf, and licorice.

Periodic Ophthalmia

Periodic ophthalmia, or "moon blindness," is a relatively common eye disease in horses that is difficult to treat, even with orthodox medicine, and it recurs easily. It can occur in horses kept in all sorts of environments, and leptospirosis infection may be at least one of the inciting factors. Periodic ophthalmia is the leading cause of blindness in the horse.

In this author's practice, bilberry *(Vaccinium myrtillus)* is clinically helpful in treating horses with this condition. Other beneficial herbs for the immune system include echinacea (aerial parts), astragalus, milk thistle, and dandelion. These latter two herbs support the liver, which, in Chinese medicine, is a primary influence for inflammation in the eye. A useful formula consists of 1 part each bilberry and echinacea flowers, combined with 2 parts each dandelion and milk thistle. Bilberry often works better as an extract with 25% anthocyanosides, given at 600 to 800 mg per day. Additionally 100 mg zinc picolinate supports the immune system in periocular tissues and contributes to a more successful therapeutic outcome.

A useful eyewash can be made with ¼ to ⅓ ounce saline and 10 drops calendula tincture. If the mixture is too strong, it will sting, and the horse will become difficult to treat. Several drops should be placed in the eye as many times a day as possible; four to six times daily is ideal.

Dadd believed that moon blindness was due to unclean conditions, so he recommended green fodder of any sort. He considered green feed to be an alterative that should be used as a primary part of the cure. The internal formula of the powdered herb consisted of 3 ounces each sassafras, skunk cabbage, and gentian, mixed with 2 ounces sulphur, 8 ounces elm bark, 2 ounces ginger, and 3 ounces salt, divided into 12 parts and administered once a day in the evening. A topical formula he considered antispasmodic included 1 ounce tincture of Indian hemp in 1 pint rain water. This was applied topically two to three times a day.

McClure (1917) considered this disease incurable but would treat it with 1 ounce cold water and 2 drachms (7.1 mL) tincture of opium to relieve pain. He preferred to puncture the bad eye to essentially remove it, claiming that the good eye would get brighter and healthier. Not all treatments were kind and gentle.

Laminitis

Laminitis is a complex disease with many causes and multiple treatments. In this author's practice, herbal therapy is critical to successful clinical outcome in most chronic cases (Self, 2003). However, herbs alone are often not enough to complete the treatment. It is beyond the scope of this chapter to detail the total approach to natural treatment of patients with laminitis; the reader is referred to other sources (Harman, 2001). Acute laminitis is not often treated by veterinary herbalists, other than with anti-inflammatory herbs that act to support other treatments.

Useful anti-inflammatory herbs include white willow bark, meadowsweet, devil's claw, hawthorn, cleavers, burdock, and nettle. Chronic cases often require the use of herbs to correct equine metabolic syndrome (EMS) or insulin resistance. The best way to approach a formula selection for laminitic horses is to be willing to change as the case progresses.

For simple acute cases or early-stage chronic cases that primarily need anti-inflammatory support, a formula of 2 parts each meadowsweet and dandelion, combined with 1 part each hawthorn, turmeric, licorice, and nettles, is useful. Later-stage cases with EMS may need a variety of different approaches to treatment. Older horses who are prone to have laminitis in the winter often can handle some warm herbs, although caution must be taken to monitor them for excessive signs of sweating, increased inflammation in the feet, or any other signs of excessive heat. One formula consists of 2 parts each dandelion and bilberry, along with 1 part each chaste berry *(Vitex agnus castus)*, meadowsweet, cinnamon, burdock, and hawthorn. To this formula, 6 to 10 ounces flax or hemp meal daily should be added, to enhance glucose metabolism and anti-inflammatory effects.

Hawthorn seems to be clinically very helpful, probably because it improves circulation. In several of the author's cases, hawthorn has increased healthy foot growth and reduced pain. Maca *(Lepidium meyenii)* is another herb that is clinically useful in the author's practice for chronically laminitic horses with insulin resistance.

Historically, aconite root was used as a painkiller—20 drops of tincture were given in a cupful of water every 4 to 6 hours for only 6 to 8 doses, because of its toxicity (McClure, 1917). Horses were encouraged to lie down and rest the feet in a big, clean stall. Because this was a "hot" disease with lots of inflammation, horses were cooled with ice water on the feet, shoes were removed, and they were given cold water to drink. Most veterinarians and horse owners use large doses of pain-relieving drugs to try to keep horses on their feet, which, in this author's clinical experience, is counterproductive because of extensive damage to the lamina.

Dadd used a different treatment. He packed the foot with a bandage that had been soaked in a weak arnica solution (8 oz tincture to 1 gal water). He supported the bottom of the foot with a flat sponge and 5 yards of bandage, to keep the foot moist for the next few days. For constitutional treatment, he fed thin gruel, scalded mashes, and boiled roots, with occasional doses of sulphur and cream of tartar. For horses in acute pain, he used drenches of hops or poppy heads. When inflammation was present, 20 drops of arnica tincture was given orally in water. Oral arnica is considered toxic, yet it was used in limited quantities for serious conditions. The drinking water was acidified with cream of tartar or a few drops of acetic acid.

Anxiety and Nervousness

Calming nervous horses is probably the number one reason why modern horse owners turn to herbal medicine. The biggest problem is that most horses stand in stalls, have greatly restricted exercise, and are fed too much, especially excessive amounts of high-sugar feeds. Pain is also another important factor that contributes to nervous behavior in that horses cannot focus on their riders when they are in pain. Discomfort from estrus cycles is another important cause of nervous behavior, and many formulas contain herbs that help regulate the hormonal cycle. The simplest answer to nervousness is to turn the horses out and treat them for pain. However, it is almost impossible to get owner compliance.

Many herbal formulas are sold to "calm" horses. No one formula is best because the reason for each horse being nervous is different. The best advice is to try one; if that does not work, try another with different ingredients. Most modern formulas contain several of these herbs: passionflower, valerian root, chamomile, hops, wood betony, goldenrod, marshmallow, meadowsweet, and hawthorn. Some formulas are designed primarily for mares with estrus behavior problems, but they often work with geldings and stallions. Herbs that may help regulate estrus-related behavior and hormones include chaste berry, skullcap, chamomile, vervain and raspberry leaves, black cohosh, wild lettuce, dandelion, and cramp bark.

Many of the more successful formulas contain valerian root, but use of this herb is known to produce a positive drug test. A nice combination of adaptogens, nervines and sedative herbs consists of 1 part each eleuthero, passionflower, hops, and kava kava. This formula can be made with or without valerian root. Kava and passionflower are on the list as herbs that could give a positive test; however, they have been used regularly (see section on drug testing).

McClure (1917) kept nervous horses in a quiet environment and would use 10 grains (65 mg) of opium and 1 drachm or 2 drachms (1.8-3.5 g) of powdered chalk about 30 minutes before riding. In Chinese medicine, calcium carbonate (chalk) is one of the most sedating medicines in the *Materia medica*. McClure also recommended stuffing the ears with cotton wool, which is routinely done today in the show ring but seldom by people who just want to trail ride.

Chronic Obstructive Pulmonary Disease, and Heaves

Chronic allergic lung disease currently goes by many different names, including heaves, broken wind, chronic obstructive pulmonary disease, and reactive airway disease. In this author's opinion, these are all variations on a similar theme. The airways have become reactive to something in the environment, possibly pollens, dusts, or molds. The seasonality of the disease varies and may help determine which formulas should be used and during which seasons they should be administered. In most horses that are treated with herbs, a maintenance dose will be needed during the horse's worst season, although treatment may not be required in the off-season.

The most important factor this author sees in determining which herbs should be used is what type of cough and expectoration is present. Different herbs are required for a wet cough versus a dry cough. The most common reason for treatment failure in Western herbal medicine occurs when moistening and drying herbs (as in the Chinese medicine system) are mixed together in a formula.

Herbs that moisten dry coughs include asparagus root, chickweed herb, comfrey leaf and root, licorice, coltsfoot, marshmallow, slippery elm, mullein leaf, borage leaf, aloe gel, and yarrow (Holmes, 1997; Ross, 2003). Herbs that dry dampness include angelica root, cowslip root, elder flower, eyebright, garlic, horseradish root, cayenne pepper, cardamom pod, elecampane root, sage leaf, and agrimony.

Some herbs, notably, thyme and plantain, simultaneously dry dampness and moisten a dry cough. Although ginger can dry damp conditions, it is very warming so would be contraindicated if the horse had any signs of excess or deficiency heat. A useful formula for a dry airway is made up of 2 parts mullein and 1 part each marshmallow, coltsfoot, plantain, and red clover. For treatment of a moist airway, equal parts plantain, garlic, yarrow, elecampane, and dandelion should be mixed together.

Historically, heaves and broken wind were similar, depending on who was describing the condition. Dadd called heaves difficult breathing without double respiration (second forced exhalation), and broken wind was a continual effort to breathe with double exhalation. He felt that the origin of this condition was related to the failure of digestion or respiration (a very similar concept to that of Traditional Chinese Medicine in which a spleen [digestive] deficiency can lead to a lung deficiency). Dadd (1854) believed that when heaves occurred, digestion was not supplying the lungs with nourishment and fuel (he called "innutrition"), or that the intestines failed first, and because of the "sympathy" between the lungs and digestion, the lungs failed.

Dadd's treatment was to give a tonic of aromatic sulphuric acid (an ether, formed by the reaction of alcohol with sulphuric acid), alcohol, ginger, and cinnamon dosed at 1 drachm (1.8 g) twice a day, which many horses would drink from a bucket. He added alteratives to strengthen the system and improve digestion. The alterative mixture consisted of equal parts of powdered ginger, gentian, sulphur, salt, cream of tartar, charcoal, licorice, elecampane, caraway seeds, and chopped balm of gilead buds. The dose was 1 ounce added to the food every night until improvement was seen. When the aromatic tonic was finished, a half-dose of the alterative was given, along with a bit of garlic and a few chopped cloves, every few days. The diet had to be changed, exercise improved, and environment corrected.

McClure (1917) believed that respiratory disease was caused by a "debility of the parvagum (NB: vagus) nerve," although visible changes could not be seen in the nerves. A treatment used by unscrupulous horse dealers was to give powdered sulphate of iron, gentian, and ginger root in large doses, which were repeated frequently. McClure believed that iron was injurious to the horse, but that it was good in that it enhanced the tone of the nerve. His preferred treatment was a 5-grain (325-mg) dose of arsenic, given once a day for 2 weeks, followed by a week's wait, then repetition of the treatment. Feed consisted only of a little hay.

Arsenic was used for a number of treatments in the past, although overdoses were not uncommon. From a homeopathic perspective, rather than an herbal one, *Arsenicum album* is a common and successful treatment for many horses with chronic obstructive pulmonary disease.

Sarcoids

Sarcoids are common tumors in horses. They are usually benign but may be invasive or may become malignant. Thuja *(Thuja occidentalis)* as part of an ointment has been applied topically with some degree of success, as has bloodroot in salve form. Bloodroot is discussed later in the *Materia medica*. General tonic herbs, such as burdock, meadowsweet, garlic, and cleavers, are also used to support the immune system. Burdock has demonstrated some action against tumors, and can even be fed as a single herb in these cases.

Scratches

Scratches are chronic lesions on the lower legs of horses that are most commonly seen in the winter. If the legs are white, the lesions may have resulted from photosensitization, so one must be careful not to use herbs such as Saint John's Wort, which may aggravate the problem. Topical ointments made up of many different herbs are used routinely, but the most effective treatment is an internal herbal formula that is used to support immune function, along with high levels of flax.

It is best not to wash the lesions with soap every day and pick the scabs off, as most clients are inclined to do. The skin must be allowed to heal, and scrubbing the skin does not allow that to happen. Water-based gels and creams or honey are better than lanolin or petroleum-based ointments, however ointments may help keep some of the moisture off of horses who are turned out on damp pastures.

Effective topical ingredients include chaparral, calendula, pau d'arco, aloe vera, vitamin E (natural source is best), comfrey, lavender, yarrow, tea tree oil, oregano oil, echinacea, and Saint John's Wort topical herbal salves may also be effective. (See the section on topical herbs in Chapter 20, A Systems-Based Approach)

Historically, Dadd used a poultice if the heels were hot and swollen; it consisted of ½ lb slippery elm powder combined with 2 ounces fine salt, mixed with hot water, then cooled and spread on a cotton cloth over the affected area. He also liked a mild cathartic with 4 drachms (7.1 g) powdered aloe, 2 drachms (3.5 g) powdered gentian, and 1 drachm ginger (1.75 g), mixed in a ball of honey or drenched with a pint of warm water.

McClure used glycerin on scratches and as a preventive when salt was dispersed to melt ice on the roads during winter.

Trauma, Bruises, and Sprains

Herbal treatment in cases of trauma generally centers around arnica. Because many injuries in horses occur on the legs, it is easy to apply liquids and poultices made from herbs and to keep a bandage on the injury to protect the horse from eating the formula or removing a poultice. Upper parts of the body may be more difficult to apply a poultice to, but liquids and ointments can be painted on and left unbandaged.

Lavender essential oil, witch hazel, comfrey, and rue are also used clinically as topical treatments for injuries.

McClure (1917) used 2 ounces of aconite root tincture in 4 ounces olive or sweet oil (usually made from almonds) combined with 1 ounce creosote, mixed together and applied topically to relieve inflammation, irritation, and pain. A diluted tincture of arnica was used for shoulder or other muscle strain. For extreme muscle pain, a fomentation of hops was used.

Wounds

Wounds are very common in horses, and many excellent commercial herbal treatments, topical and internal, are available. For deep, penetrating wounds, this author prefers to use a water-soluble gel or cream rather than an oil-based topical preparation. For all other wounds, almost any type of topical can be used (see the Chapter 20).

One study examined the effects of treatment with lavender and chamomile essential oils on chronic wounds. Five human patients used medical grade essential oil therapy, and three controls used only conventional therapy. Lavender (2 drops) and German chamomile (1 drop) were combined and diluted in one-half teaspoon of grapeseed oil to make a 6% solution. Twice daily, part of the mixture was applied directly to the wound and edges of the wound; the rest was placed on the gauze wound dressing. Wounds treated with essential oil healed faster than those that were treated only with conventional therapy. None of the patients acquired an infection during the course of the study, which the authors believed possibly demonstrated the antimicrobial effects of the oils. The authors concluded that essential oils have a promising role to play in chronic wound care, but randomized, controlled clinical trials are needed (Hartman, 2002).

McClure used 20 drops of aconite root tincture orally to suppress pain. Tincture of aloes was applied topically to wounds, or a mixture was made with aloes and myrrh. For unhealthy sores, a carrot poultice was made with washed carrots that were boiled until soft; the water was then strained and the carrots mashed into a fine pulp that was spread on a cloth over the wound.

For sores and wounds, another mixture consisted of a tincture of aloes and myrrh made from 1 ounce of powdered aloe, ½ ounce saffron, and ½ pint tincture of myrrh; this was macerated for 2 weeks and strained. Flaxseed cake or residue remaining after the oil was pressed was excellent for poultices on wounds. The flax was mixed with warm water.

Parasites

In evolutionary balance, parasites do not kill their hosts because this would deprive them of a place to live. When horses are confined and crowded with others of the same species, the intestinal immune system is stressed, and parasites can become a life-threatening problem. It is this author's belief that the reason many natural deworming protocols fail is the stress of modern horsekeeping. Dadd believed that infestation was the result of a perverted state of the organ that the parasite invaded. Healthy horses kept in low-stress environments can often successfully be dewormed for many years with natural products alone.

The horsekeeper should be advised to check fecal samples quarterly for the first 2 years of a natural program, then once or twice a year after that. If anything significant in the environment changes, such as the addition of a new horse, severe weather stress, or a move to another property, more frequent checks should be performed. Claims of herbal anthelmintic efficacy should be viewed with caution, and the ingredients should be known for any product used because many vermifugal herbs are relatively toxic.

This author has had the best success with natural deworming protocols that use a combination of diatomaceous earth, homeopathic combination remedies, and Chinese herbal vermifuges. Less success has occurred with Western herbal formulas. Most of the herbal formulas used in the past included a purgative of some sort to mechanically help remove the parasites. Lack of success with some horses in modern times may be related to the reluctance of herbalists and owners to purge the animals. Another possible reason may be the lack of herbal and immunologic support after the vermifuge is given. Dadd believed that worms could be expelled in a number of ways, but to prevent them from coming back, he used alteratives and vermifuges combined.

Herbs with vermifugal actions include agrimony, aloe resin (golden brown dried, powdered concentrate of the bitter-tasting juice), cinnamon, cloves, fennel, garlic, horseradish, hyssop, male fern, mugwort, parsley seed, peppermint, tansy, thyme, valerian, vervain, wormwood *(Artemisia absinthum)*, and wormseed *(Chenopodium ambrosioides)*. One study found that garlic (1 boiled bulb in 300 mL water per donkey) was unsuccessful as an anthelmintic in the treatment of 12 donkeys when compared with control and fenbendazole treatment groups. This failure may have been due to the method used to prepare the garlic, the dose used, or the method of evaluating the outcome; it may also suggest that garlic does not have anthelmintic activity in donkeys (Abells, 1999).

Dadd's formulas for expulsion of parasites included such herbs and products as wood ashes, poplar bark (balm of gilead, sulphur, salt, castor oil, turpentine, calomel (mercury chloride), tartar emetic (antimony tartrate), and aloes. One of the alterative/vermifuge combinations included 2 ounces of each of the following: white mustard seed (whole), powdered mandrake, sulphur, powdered wormseed, a salt, ginger, charcoal mix, and poplar bark, mixed together, and given 1 ounce morning and evening in the feed. A vermifuge used by Dadd that occasionally brought large amounts of parasites out was made up of 12 ounces castor oil, 1 ounce wormseed oil, and 3 drachms (11.1 mL) tansy tincture, given on an empty stomach and followed by mashes of fine feeds or "shorts," well seasoned with salt was repeated as needed until the parasites were expelled.

Juliet deBairacli-Levy fasted horses for 2 days, then used balls made from three or four grated whole bulbs of garlic combined with honey or treacle, followed by a pint of linseed oil an hour later (deBairacli-Levy, 1976). If linseed oil was not available, 4 pints cane molasses was mixed with 1 pint warm water and milk, to which 8 tablespoons castor oil was added. After this, the horse was fed a warm bran mash and was turned out on grass. Levy found male fern to be very effective for tapeworms, if it was given when the moon was approaching full. If that was not available, she used a combination of 4 teaspoons cayenne pepper and 2 teaspoons wormwood made into a ball with flour and honey.

Deworming formulas obviously did not work reliably; many were available and most contained some of the very toxic chemicals in common use around the turn of the last century. In 1861, a pharmacist named Beasley collected and published many recipes from a variety of practitioners. He used "worm balls," some of which were mostly herbal (Beasley, 1861). The first one consisted of 6 drachms (10.6 g) barbadoes aloes, 1½ drachm (0.9 g) ginger, 20 drops oil of wormwood, 2 drachms (3.5 g) subcarbonate of soda (sodium hydrogen carbonate—known as baking soda), and enough syrup to form a ball. This may be mixed with or without ½ to 1 drachm (0.9-1.8 g) calomel (mercurous chloride), added or given the previous night. This formula was given at intervals of 10 days, if needed.

Beasley also used a formula made from 2 drachms (3.5 g) asafoetida, 1 to 2 drachms (1.8-3.5 g) calomel, 1½ drachm (2.7 g) savin (also called juniper), and 20 drops oil of wormwood, combined with enough syrup to make a ball, given at night with a physic ball (purgative ball), then given in the morning. High doses of turpentine oil (2-4 oz or more) were used for vermifuge action. Wormwood is a bitter tonic and vermifuge; historically, a few drops of the essential oil was added to aloes for worms.

Clysters were made with 4 to 6 ounces salt and were used as a purgative to expel parasites. In small doses, salt was considered a tonic, a digestive aid, and an alterative, but in large doses, it was a purgative and a vermifuge. For bot control, injections of flaxseed oil were used but may not have been very effective because the bot fly larva resides in the stomach and "injections" refers to enemas.

MATERIA MEDICA OF HISTORIC AND CURRENT USES FOR HERBS

Herbs are listed here if they have a significant application in equine medicine today or in the past. Some herbs used extensively in the past have fallen by the wayside, because of their toxicity or because other herbs have been discovered that work as well or better. Perhaps herbalists should reexamine some of the nontoxic herbs that are no longer used. Herbs not listed here are probably usable in equine practice and have identical applications across animal species, so they are discussed elsewhere in this text. Equine research is included in the few instances where findings are available.

Aconitum napellus (Wolfsbane, Monkshood)

Historical use

The root was used; it is toxic and was known as one of the most powerful sedatives and pain relievers. It was used in treating almost all acute conditions. McClure (1917) highly recommended the herb, but he understood the toxicity and limited its use to a maximum of 6 to 8 doses at 25 or 20 drops each. Prostration and weakness would occur if too much was given. Afterward, it was important to follow up with iron and mineral salts to aid convalescence. Tincture of aconite root was made by combining 4 ounces dried and bruised root with $^1/_2$ pint alcohol; this mixture was macerated for 2 weeks, then strained.

Modern use

Use of this herb has been discontinued because of potential toxicity.

Atropa belladonna

Historical use

This was used to help dilate the eyes to prevent adhesions from forming (McClure, 1917); this practice is continued today with the use of atropine in the eye at any sign of injury or disease. This herb was also used for treating patients with colic, rheumatism, coughs, sore throats, bronchitis, influenza, and lockjaw (tetanus). Practitioners believed that it did not "bind up the gut" as opium did but was similar in action.

Modern use

This herb is considered too toxic for current use.

Vitex agnus-castus (Chaste Berry)

Historical use

Information was not found.

Modern use

Behavioral problems are related to hormonal cycles in mares; this herb is helpful with insulin resistance or EMS (previously called Cushing's syndrome) in horses.

Research

Hilary Self, in her dissertation, used a single dose, given in the morning, of a standard extract of *Vitus agnus castus* (10-mL dose of 1:5, 45%) compared with an untreated control group. Statistically significant improvement was noted in clinical signs (detailed notes were kept on each animal in the study) and in some blood parameters (e.g., cortisol, insulin, dexamethasone suppression test) (Self, 2003). Another study used a proprietary aqueous extract of *Vitus agnus castus* for the treatment of patients with equine Cushing's syndrome. Dosing was provided according to manufacturers' specifications (10 mL/200 lb). Study findings showed no improvement in clinical signs or blood parameters during the course of treatment, except in 1 of 14 horses (Beech, 2002). Blood insulin, adrenocorticotrophic hormone, and clinical signs were recorded. Horses were treated for 2 to 6 months, and some horses were removed from the trial because of worsening symptoms.

One possible reason for this discrepancy between results may be the different formulations; a great deal of variability has been reported in the quality and potency of herbal extracts.

Aloe spp (Aloe, Aloes)

Historical use

The juice was made from several species of the aloe plant (barbadoes, socotorine, cape, and hepatic). It was used as a purgative or cathartic for horses, and as topical treatment in tincture form alone or with myrrh (McClure, 1917). *A. barbadoes* is the safest form, with caution recommended against strong purging. A few loose stools were considered acceptable unless severe disease was present. Purges were administered in one dose only and were not to be repeated.

Modern use

The purgative actions of aloe occur when the whole plant is fed. Most commercial extracts now contain no anthroquinone glycosides and do not cause purging; thus, they are safe to use. This herb is used as a mild laxative, for fungal diseases, in wound healing for eyes and skin, for ulcerative colitis, and with stomach ulcers (particularly useful in distilled form for stomach ulcers, in this author's experience). Aloe is contraindicated in cases of intestinal obstruction—it can cause intestinal cramping. It has been used to help expel parasites. For topical use, the plants are easy to grow. The gel can be scraped out and applied directly to wounds.

Arnica montana

Historical use

Arnica was used primarily for bruises (e.g., 1 oz arnica tincture combined with 2 oz water; soak a cloth and apply topically) (McClure, 1917). Another formula recommended by Dadd (1854) consisted of 4 ounces arnica flowers in 1 pint new rum. This was macerated for 14 days; then, 1 ounce in a pint of water was used topically for all wounds, bruises, and saddle galls. A sedative drench was also made by Dadd for internal use, to decrease arterial "actation" (i.e., increased pulse rate): 4 drachms (14.8 mL) arnica mixed in 1 pint water; this was repeated as needed, but gradually, the dose was lessened.

Modern use

Arnica is used commonly in topical liniments or ointments for bruises, sprains, and contusions. Even more common than its topical use is its homeopathic use, in which the diluted preparation is taken internally to treat bruises. Internally, it is toxic in the herbal form (Brinker, 2001) but safe in the homeopathic preparation. In Europe, the internal form of arnica is banned (Brinker, 2000). The following is the topical formula for bruises: brew handful of flowers or whole plant as a tea in 2 cups water (not to be strained); then, massage onto injured parts (deBairacli-Levy, 1976).

Astragalus membranaceus (Huang Qi)

Historical use

This is a traditional Chinese herb that does not appear in historical Western *Materia medicas*. It is now in common use.

Modern use

This herb is used for immune modulation, viral and respiratory infections, and liver and kidney disease. It is useful clinically in horses, especially for respiratory disease.

Juglans nigra (Black Walnut)

Historical use

This herb has been used for parasitism, but details of its use in the equine are difficult to find.

Modern use

It is used for external and internal parasites and for constipation. The herb is rarely used because of the potential for laminitis caused by the heartwood (see earlier for discussion).

Actaea racemosa (Black Cohosh)

Historical use

This is not found in the veterinary historical literature.

Modern use

This herb is used to manage mare behavioral problems around cycles; it interacts with hormonal therapy. Prolonged use (>6 mo) should be avoided. It is also used for muscle spasm or injury as an antispasmodic.

Barosma betulina (Buchu)

Historical use

This herb has been used on the racetrack for urinary tract problems, whether real or perceived, often by horsemen who were not particularly interested in herbs and were just following what they thought was tradition. Much folklore has been passed along on the track about horses having kidney problems, when in fact, in modern times, urinary problems are known to be rare among horses, although lumbar back pain is common.

Modern use

This herb is used for any urinary infections, cystitis, and urethritis, as well as for diuretic purposes. Three to four fresh-dried leaves are given per day (Self, 1996).

Sanguinaria canadensis (Bloodroot)

Historical use

Apparently, this herb was not used much in the equine. Black salves were occasionally mentioned, but not salves made with bloodroot.

Modern use

Bloodroot cancer salves have become very popular in the treatment of patients with sarcoids, even among veterinarians who have little interest in herbs. Several are sold commercially, and clinically, they do remove many sarcoids. The salves include significant amounts (20%-50%) zinc chloride ($ZnCl_2$), which is caustic and probably accounts for a significant portion of the action. This caustic action can be very painful, and some horses will not tolerate application of the salve more than once or twice. It is recommended that the treated area be covered with a bandage. However, many parts of the horse are not amenable to bandaging, and it is possible to use the treatment without applying a bandage. Because these salves are caustic, they should not be used near the eyes or in an unbandaged area in which the eyes or other sensitive tissues are exposed.

Fagopyrum esculentum (Buckwheat)

Historical use

This herb is not found in the veterinary literature.

Modern use

This plant stimulates circulation in patients with arthritis and navicular disease. It strengthens blood vessel walls and is used in horses that have bleeding tendencies. Photosensitization is possible on white areas.

Calendula officinalis

Historical use

This herb was used as a blood tonic for stressed horses (Self, 1996).

Modern use

It is primarily known for its topical use as an antiseptic wound dressing; it can reduce scarring. In this author's practice, it is the primary topical agent used for wounds that produces excellent results. It can be used internally for stomach ulcers and other intestinal upsets.

Capsicum spp (Cayenne Pepper)

Historical use

This plant was used for loss of appetite, fever, and indigestion. Jamaica pepper or pimento/allspice was used for the same reason (McClure, 1917). Beasley used capsicum as a hot stimulant to treat patients with weakness of the stomach (10-20 g), flatulent colic, or a severe cold (20-60 g) (Beasley, 1861). It was also used topically for pain relief in patients with arthritis.

Modern use

It is used for gastrointestinal disorders, and topically, for arthritis and muscular pain.

Skin irritation or allergy is possible, especially among chestnut horses with sensitive skin. Potential adverse effects include gastrointestinal pain and diarrhea. However, the herb is very useful orally and is included in some joint formulas. It must be remembered that capsicum is a warming herb, so it will benefit older horses that tend to be cool or cold—similar to a Yang-deficient state in Chinese medicine (see Table 21-4). Capsicum may be contraindicated in horses that have been diagnosed with any hot conditions, that are Yin deficient in Chinese medicine, or that have a deficiency heat.

Matricaria chamomila, or *Recutita* (Chamomile)

Historical use

McClure (1917) considered this too mild a tonic to have much use in the horse; Beasley and even Youatt used it as an important mild tonic in any debilitated horse during late stages of fever or influenza: 1 to 4 drachms (1.8-7.1 g) dried flowers, or infusion of $\frac{1}{2}$ ounce dried flowers in 1 qt water. It was combined with ginger as the first herb given for convalescence.

Modern use

Chamomile appears in many formulas for calming nervous horses, and it excels there; however, its other uses are often forgotten. It is an excellent detoxification herb and was known historically as a blood cleanser and a mild tonic (as the historical use suggests); it is spasmolytic in the gastrointestinal tract and can be used in mild cases of colic. See the section on colic, earlier, for a chamomile tea recipe clients may use while waiting for the veterinarian to arrive on the farm.

Cinnamomum spp (Cinnamon)

Historical use

This herb was used as a carminative and a warm stimulant (Beasley, 1861).

Modern use

In recent times, this herb is gaining use in horses with metabolic syndrome and laminitis. Two studies published on cinnamon indicate that compounds are present that may potentiate insulin action and may be helpful in the treatment of people with diabetes and insulin resistance (Anderson, 2004; Khan, 2003). It must be noted that in Chinese medicine, cinnamon is a very warm herb. It may be contraindicated or less useful in horses that are showing hot signs (such as Yin deficiency or deficiency heat), but it may be very helpful in horses that are older and Yang deficient with overall cold signs (even though the laminitis that is often present is a hot condition). So far, the horses that have responded to this herb in the author's practice were older ones, although large numbers of cases are not yet available for evaluation.

Colchicum autumnale (Meadow Saffron)

Historical use

This herb was used for rheumatism in all joints and lumbago, as well as for eye disease (dose: 1-2 drachms [1.8-3.5 g] twice daily in feed for 1-2 wk) (McClure, 1917).

Modern use

Most modern uses are documented in the homeopathic *Materia medica,* rather than in equine herbal practice.

Galium aparine (Clivers, Cleavers)

Historical use

As popular as cleavers is today, no reference can be found to its use in veterinary equine medicine.

Modern use

This herb is used frequently as a tonic; it is high in silica—a mineral that is deficient in many soils and is required for bone health. It can be used as a circulatory tonic for the laminitis cases and is well known for its support of the lymphatic, so it has been used for horses with poor circulation and filled legs. It is also good for the skin and coat and to treat eczema, both topically and internally.

Symphytum officinale (Comfrey)

Historical use

A few mentions of its use for trauma can be found.

Modern use

This herb is used externally for sprains and fractures. Internally, it is used as an anti-inflammatory; it may support bone healing and is used as a demulcent for the intestinal and respiratory tracts, and for wounds. Horses voluntarily seek out and eat comfrey that is growing in pastures and demonstrate no ill effects, but it is considered to be potentially toxic when taken internally.

Taraxacum officinale (Dandelion)

Historical use

As popular as dandelion is today, no reference can be found to its use in historical texts on veterinary equine medicine.

Modern use

This laxative and diuretic is used for chronic colitis; it is an immune stimulant (Holmes, 1997), and it enhances the effects of insulin. The herb is known for its liver and kidney support. Horses crave these plants in the spring and will dig deep into the dirt at times to eat the roots at any time during the year, if they really want the plant. Dandelion is well known as a detoxifying herb.

Harpagophytum procumbens (Devil's Claw)

Historical use

This is an African herb that has recently become popular in Western herbal medicine, so it has no entrenched history in the Western *Materia Medica*.

Modern use

This herb has excellent anti-inflammatory properties for use in acute or chronic arthritis and joint pain. It is used in a number of preparations as a replacement for nonsteroidal anti-inflammatory drugs (NSAIDs), without the potential side effects of NSAIDS; however, it is contraindicated when gastric ulcers are present. It is poorly and unsustainably harvested, and unless it is grown and harvested properly, this herb should not be used. In many cases, response to treatment is poor, and this author suspects that the poor results are due to low quality products.

Research

A *Harpagophytum procumbens* preparation was tested with degeneration of the proximal intertarsal, distal intertarsal, and tarsometatarsal (hock) joints in 10 horses; treatment was compared with phenylbutazone given to a control group of 10 horses. Treatment was carried out for 90 days, and animals were regularly monitored for soundness for 120 days. Investigators concluded that the *H. procumbens* preparation is an effective alternative to phenylbutazone for the treatment of horses with bone spavin (Montavon, 1994).

Echinacea angustifolia/E. Purpurea

Historical use

This herb, which is very popular in modern times, has had little historical veterinary use.

Modern use

Clinical practice shows that echinacea is helpful in preventing and treating upper respiratory conditions and in supporting the immune system.

Research

In one of the few blinded, controlled studies performed on the equine, echinacea was shown to effectively stimulate immunocompetence (O'Neill, 2002b). A total of 8 horses were fed 30 mL of a standardized 1.4% echinacoside extract of echinacea, and, after 42 days of feeding on the herb, were compared with themselves in a placebo-controlled, crossover trial. Blood was drawn every 7 days for hematology, chemistry, and a phagocyte function test.

The echinacea extract improved the quality of blood by increasing hemoglobin levels and the number of erythrocytes. It also caused an increase in peripheral lymphocyte count and a decrease in circulating neutrophils that were presumed to have migrated to the tissues. In vitro tests showed that the neutrophils from treated horses consumed a greater quantity of yeast particles than were consumed by untreated controls (indicating greater phagocytic potential).

Inula helenium (Elecampane)

Historical use

The root of this plant was prized by horsemen of McClure's time for respiratory coughs and colds. Teas and decoctions were used.

Modern use

This herb is used by some practitioners as part of a respiratory formula because of its aromatic and mucilaginous content. It is not a popular herb, but perhaps, it should be used more often for patients with chronic, dry cough conditions.

Euphrasia officinalis (Eyebright)

Historical use

This herb was not found to have historical uses in veterinary medicine.

Modern use

It has excellent astringent, anticatarrhal, and anti-inflammatory properties, with a special affinity for the eye and for the digestive tract (Self, 1996). This herb is used topically and internally for eye ulceration and inflammation, and for blindness. It can be diluted in saline to make an eye wash, or a tea can be prepared and used as a compress. This herb is threatened, and others, such as tea, calendula, or chamomile, may be substituted for topical use.

Oenothera biennis (Evening Primrose Oil)

Historical use

This herb was not found to have historical uses in veterinary medicine.

Modern use

It is an excellent source of essential fatty acids (EFAs) and has anti-inflammatory properties. This herb is useful in mares with cycle-related behavioral problems, and in some horses with allergic itchy skin.

Research

Two studies investigated the use of evening primrose oil (EPO) in the horse. One explored the allergic dermatologic problem, "sweet itch" (Craig, 1997). EFA absorption and metabolism are species specific and have not been well researched in the horse. An interesting observation was made that no gamma-linoleic acid (GLA) was found in the plasma of any of the horses supplemented with EPO capsules, but rapid elevations in dihomogammalinoleic acid (DGLA) levels were observed after EPO was taken. The conclusion was that horses very rapidly and efficiently convert GLA to DGLA. Clinical signs were not significantly improved in the study; however, in practice, EPO and other EFA supplements are very effective in improving the condition of the skin in many of these cases.

The other controlled and blinded study documented the effects of EPO on the characteristics of the hoof wall. A total of 12 horses were fed 30 mL per day of an EPO solution for 12 weeks. A statistical difference was noted in perioplic lipid analysis, along with a significant reduction in free cholesterol in the periople of the horse's feet during weeks 4 to 8, but no changes were observed to occur in the stratum medium (Reilly, 1998).

Trigonella foenum-graecum (Fenugreek)

Historical use

This herb was recommended by Lawson (1824) as part of several tonics for debilitated horses.

Modern use

It is used to treat patients with constipation and gastritis; it is also used as a lymphatic stimulant to increase milk production, as an immune tonic, and as a topical agent for wound healing. DeBairacli-Levy claimed that all animals seek it out (deBairacli-Levy, 1976). Research in humans shows that it helps to control insulin resistance, and clinically, it appears to help some horses. Fenugreek is often recommended to be used with garlic to enhance its ability to fight infection.

Aspidium filix mas (Male Fern)

Historical use

This plant is used for deworming—1 pound of the root powder was given, followed by a purgative the next day (McClure, 1917).

Modern use

This herb is used occasionally for deworming, especially for tapeworms; a large root, sliced and boiled for 30 minutes, is given with $^{3}/_{4}$ pint of the boiling water, followed by a strong drench of castor oil (deBairacli-Levy, 1976). It is more commonly used for deworming in homeopathic form than in the herbal form.

Linum spp (Flaxseed)

Historical use

The herb was historically called linseed, and used for constipation, dermatitis, and gastritis. It has been considered a laxative and a tonic. All parts of the seed are used. Ground seed mixed in warm water was considered an excellent cooling food for horses—with aperient effects. Even though McClure added the seed to warm water, he considered the flax as a cooling food; it is a neutral food in Chinese medicine (Pitchford, 1993). Pressed juice or oil was a "certain and safe purgative" in quart quantities. For choking, $^{1}/_{2}$ pint was used to help lubricate the esophagus (McClure, 1917).

Modern use

Flax is used frequently for many of its excellent qualities. The omega-3 and omega-6 fatty acids clinically improve coat quality and immune function. Research in other species demonstrates its immune system support, anti-inflammatory actions, and anticancer properties. Clinically, in this author's practice, it is useful in insulin and glucose regulation in EMS (McCarty, 1998).

One study performed on horses demonstrated the efficacy of a milled flax *(Linum usitatissimum)* supplement in the skin-test response of atopic horses. Six horses that displayed a positive intradermal skin test for *Culicoides* spp participated in the 42-day, placebo-controlled, double-blind, crossover trial. They were fed 1 lb milled flax per 1000 lb. Blood was collected for routine chemistry; punch biopsies and hair samples were collected from the side opposite to the site of the skin test. A fatty acid profile was evaluated on the basis of biopsy findings. Results showed that supplementation with flaxseed for 42 days reduced the mean skin-test response and area of lesions. A significant decrease was observed in the long-chain saturated fatty acids in the hair, along with some other minor changes; the meaning of these effects is still open to speculation and further research (O'Neill, 2002a). The lack of hematologic change over the 42 study days suggests that feeding high levels of flax is safe.

Allium sativa (Garlic)

Historical use

Historically, garlic was used for coughs and asthma (Clater, 1817). It also has a reputation as a vermifuge but was not listed in the texts as such.

Modern use

Horses freely eat wild garlic leaves and stalks in fields. Garlic is administered for respiratory infection, flatulence, and gastrointestinal spasms, and to keep flies and other insects away. It seems to help many horses, but for others, it has no effect. Garlic has been used for deworming, to treat respiratory infection, and as a digestive tonic. In theory, it causes increased bleeding times or potentiates this effect in other drugs (see earlier section, "Cautions With Herbs).

Gentiana lutea (Gentian Root)

Historical use

This herb was extremely valuable as an appetite stimulant; as treatment for debility, weakness, and swelling of the legs; and in any illness associated with poor appetite (McClure, 1917). It was always used as a powder, not a tincture, and was put into all formulas used for conditioning horses. McClure combined it with iron to make a tonic. He would mix it with ammonia and pimenta berries to make a horse eat, even if it did not want to. The recommended dose was ½ to 1 ounce, given three times a day, mixed in a gruel or drenched.

Beasley used 2 to 4 drachms (3.1-7.1 g) powder, or ½ to 1 drachm (0.9-1.8 g) extract as a tonic for debilitated horses, usually combined with ginger.

Juliette deBairacli-Levy favored this herb.

Modern use

Although this herb was found in many of the old formulas, it is not seen in many of the modern ones. It is an excellent tonic, especially for the digestive tract and for poor eaters, so it deserves a much larger place in modern herbal medicine.

Zingiber officinale (Ginger Root)

Historical use

This herb was extremely useful as a digestive tonic. It was used by McClure for all colics and was put into all purgative formulas. It could be mixed with chalk for diarrhea. A dose of 2 ounces per day can be used as a tincture. Beasley used it as a stimulant and a carminative, as well as a general ingredient in tonics: 1 to 3 drachms (0.9-5.3 g) usually, but with flatulent colic, 2 to 6 drachms (3.1-10.6 g).

Modern use

This herb often helps practitioners treat horses that do not eat while trailering; this author believes that these horses have motion sickness, as the condition does occur in all other species. If the horse loads onto the trailer well (i.e., is not upset by trailering itself), but does not eat while moving, and may sweat or not, ginger generally helps to settle the nausea.

Panax ginseng (Korean Ginseng)

Historical use

This herb was historically used for lack of stamina, debility, recovery from illness, anxiety, and infertility.

Modern use

Currently, this herb is frequently used in formulas to increase racing speed, enhance fertility, and treat gastric ulcers, stress, and almost anything else one can think of. Many supportive studies of ginseng in other species show its usefulness across a broad spectrum of illnesses. Ginseng is an expensive herb, and it is often not sustainably produced. In many cases, the actual concentration may be too low for true clinical effects to be noted, or the quality may be so poor that again, little clinical benefit is derived from its use.

Different ginsengs have different properties; many Western formulators are not aware of this, so they use whatever type they can get, without regard for its action. Asian ginseng (ren shen) is a Qi tonic in Chinese herbal medicine, which is warming; American ginseng *(Panax quinquefolius)* is a Yin tonic, or a cooling herb.

Hydrastis canadensis (Goldenseal)

Historical use

This herb was not found in historical veterinary texts.

Modern use

Today, it is used to treat patients with gastric ulcer. This herb has excellent antibacterial properties and is used topically for wounds and infections, and as an eyewash. Internally, it has been used for respiratory infection. Extended use may cause digestive disorders, constipation, or diarrhea because of its very cold, energetic nature. Because goldenseal is an endangered species, most practitioners should use Oregon graperoot instead.

Crataegus oxyacantha (Hawthorn)

Historical use

This herb was not found to have historical uses in veterinary medicine.

Modern use

The herb does not appear in the older equine literature at all, yet it is gaining some use in modern times, both as a digestive tonic and as a circulatory herb for the hoof. Chinese literature supports the use of the berry for digestion and weight loss; Western herbalists use the leaf, twig, and berry for circulation. At present, its primary use is in EMS laminitis cases, and it shows promise in stimulating hoof growth and health.

Humulus lupulus (Hops)

Historical use

This herb was not found in historical veterinary texts.

Modern use

This herb is commonly used as a sedative or relaxing herb for tense or anxious horses, and occasionally for the relief of nerve pain and inflammation of the intestinal mucosa.

Piper methysticum (Kava Kava)

Historical use

Kava kava was not used in horses until recently.

Modern use

Kava kava is used in some equine anxiety formulas as a sedative, muscle relaxant, and analgesic. No liver problems in horses have been reported, although such reports can be found in the human literature; however, it must be mentioned that these herbs are generally administered to horses as whole or powdered raw herbs, so no other processing or ingredients are added. This herb is seen in some relaxing formulations; however, it is also on the list of herbs that could cause a positive drug test (see drug testing above).

Hypericum perforatum (Saint John's Wort)

Historical use

This herb was not found in historical veterinary texts.

Modern use

This herb is excellent for cleaning wounds, especially those with painful, damaged nerve endings. Hypericin, one of the active compounds in Saint John's Wort, may cause photosensitivity and may exacerbate photosensitivity caused by tetracyclines and sulfonamides. Lesions are usually seen on the white-skinned areas of the nose and legs. Saint John's Wort antagonizes the effects of reserpine (Brinker, 2001). It is most often used topically. If given internally, it is used as a nervine, to calm anxious horses.

Glycyrrhiza glabra (Licorice)

Historical use

Licorice was used as a tonic in many different applications (e.g., digestive, respiratory) and also as a binder to help make dosing balls (Lawson, 1824).

Modern use

This herb's primary use in the equine is to manage digestive tract and ulcer cases. It is also used in some respiratory formulas as a demulcent, antiviral, and immune stimulant, and it may be used to treat patients with liver disease.

Haematoxylon campechianum (Logwood)

Historical use

McClure mentioned this herb. It was considered one of the best for astringing diarrhea and dysentery cases: 2 ounces chips in 1 pint boiling water, strained, makes one dose that should be repeated, if needed. Perhaps one of the reasons this herb is rarely used now is that severe acute cases are seldom treated with herbs.

Modern use

Logwood is seldom found in the current literature.

Filipendula ulmaria (Meadowsweet)

Historical use

Historically, it was used for treatment of patients with fever and as a spring tonic.

Modern use

This herb is an antipyretic, analgesic, and antacid that is used in kidney and bladder disease and for gastric ulceration. It may potentiate the effects of NSAIDs. Because gastric ulcers are a significant problem in performance horses, meadowsweet is an important herb to consider for this condition.

Silybum marianum (Milk Thistle)

Historical use

This herb was not found in historical veterinary texts.

Modern use

This herb has an important place in modern horse keeping because of its hepatorestorative properties. Horses are often treated with multiple drugs, potentially stressing the liver's detoxification systems. Its use in the equine is very similar to that in other animals but deserves mention here because it is such an important herb. Horses can probably digest the whole seeds, but it is unknown how efficiently they digest them. In general, if no seeds are seen to pass in the manure, the horse is likely to get a significant percentage of the benefit offered by the herb. Clinically, in this author's practice, some horses do respond when they eat the seeds.

Mentha piperita (Peppermint)

Historical use

This herb was used for many purposes, primarily for digestive problems; it can be used in colics and was often given as a 1- to 2-pint carrier for other remedies. Oil of peppermint dose: 20 to 30 drops; 60 drops for oil of spearmint. A few drops of the oil can be given to help prevent griping from other medicines (Beasley, 1861).

Modern use

Horses will eat all mints readily, although it should be noted that because volatile oils are present, positive drug tests are possible. Some horses crave the mint/peppermint flavor, so it is used as treats, as well as to help disguise the flavor of other herbs that may not be so palatable. It is an excellent herb as part of digestive formulas and, particularly, in many ulcer formulas. Debate is ongoing as to whether it is a hot or a cooling herb; this can vary with the situation (Holmes, 1997). Clinically, for most common equine applications, the debate about the herb's energetics does not seem to be important.

If fed for a week or so, peppermint can also be used to help dry up a mare's milk at weaning time.

Commiphora molmol (Myrrh)

Historical use

Myrrh is a resin that was used on cuts made by the bit; it can be mixed with aloe. McClure and Beasley also used it for sores, especially in the mouth, and as a tonic, expectorant, and antiseptic.

Modern use

Myrrh is used occasionally as part of topical dressings, but it is an herb that probably deserves more frequent use. It is particularly useful for the mucous membranes of the mouth and gums, and for horses with sores from bit trauma, poor teeth, or gum disease (which is being recognized more frequently now). It improves the appetite, stimulates digestive processes, and acts as an astringent (Grieve, 1931).

Urtica dioica (Nettle Leaf)

Historical use

This herb was not found in historical veterinary texts.

Modern use

This herb is very useful in equine medicine; as a diuretic, antispasmodic, and expectorant, it is commonly used in modern formulas, but little is found in the old texts. It is an excellent tonic and alterative that is helpful in anemia, in part because of its high nutritive content. Horses readily eat it fresh in the fields. Horses can get a skin rash from brushing up against it in the pasture, or from eating it, although that occurs very infrequently.

Origanum vulgare (Oregano Oil)

Historical use

Oregano oil was used topically as a fomentation for the ulcers of Farcy, a disease with corrosive, watery tumors along the blood vessels that looked like round berries.

Modern use

This herb is very useful for thrush and white line disease or hoof wall separation; it has excellent antifungal and antibacterial properties, and it penetrates well up into the hoof wall to reach deep-seated infections. It can also be used topically on skin wounds, although it may need to be diluted for horses with sensitive skin.

Mahonia aquifolium (Oregon Graperoot)

Historical use

This herb was not found in historical veterinary texts.

Modern use

The use of this herb is similar to that of goldenseal; however, it is easily cultivated and much less expensive. Because of the larger amounts of herbs needed per dose for a horse, this is a much better choice for antibacterial action or most other properties for which one may select goldenseal.

Papaver somniferum (Opium Poppy)

Historical use

As the dried juices of the white poppy, opium was frequently used as a pain reliever. It worked best as a tincture or extract, rather than as the whole herb: 20 to 40 g per dose for horses in crude form, or 2 to 4 drachms (1.8-7.1 g) of the extract. This herb was replaced by aconite for popular use as a painkiller.

Modern use

This herb is not used currently because of controlled substance laws.

Passiflora incarnata (Passionflower)

Historical use

This herb was not found in historical veterinary texts.

Modern use

This herb is very commonly added to formulas that calm nervous horses. It can be effective alone, although it is usually combined with other herbs.

Prunus persica (Peach Leaf)

Historical use

The leaves made into a tea with 1 ounce leaves added to a pint of boiling water and applied topically helped relieve itchy skin (McClure, 1917).

Modern use

Horse owners need topical herbs that help relieve itchy skin. This formula is a simple one that can be effective in some cases. Some modern topical creams and ointments use peach leaves as an ingredient. The practitioner should make certain that the leaves have been harvested from trees that were handled organically because peach production is highly chemically intensive, with multiple sprayings each season.

Plantago major (Plantain)

Historical use

Plantain was used in the external treatment of Farcy. It was mixed with a handful each of oregano oil, wormwood, marshmallow roots, plantain leaves, and horseradish roots; then, 12 poppy heads were bruised and boiled in 3 gallons old urine or ale dregs (some liked the urine better). Lesions were fomented with a hot flannel wrung-out, twice daily, for an hour each time (Clater, 1817).

Modern use

Horses will readily eat this common plant, and they have been observed to eat it when they have digestive discomfort (deBairacli-Levy, 1976). It has been used to treat impactions and can be used topically as a drawing agent for wounds or on insect bites to relieve insect stings and swelling. Internally, it is used for cough, stomach ulcer, and dysentery.

Cucurbita spp (Pumpkin Seeds)

Historical use

This herb has been used for tapeworms (McClure, 1917).

Modern use

Its primary use in modern times is also for tapeworms, although it may need to be combined with other herbs to be effective.

Plantago ovata (Psyllium Seed)

Historical use

This herb was not found in historical veterinary texts.

Modern use

This herb is used to prevent and treat sand accumulation in the intestinal tract; however, one study has shown that sand removal does not occur (Hammock, 1998), which conflicts with the experience of those working in sandy areas of the country. This seed may decrease absorption of drugs.

Trifolium praetense (Red Clover)

Historical use

This herb was not found in historical veterinary texts.

Modern use

It is used for calming, general debility, and infertility. Photosensitization may be seen on white legs and faces. Clover is found in many pastures and may be one of the triggers for common lesions on the lower legs, usually referred to as scratches.

Rosmarinus officinalis (Rosemary)

Historical use

This herb was not found in historical veterinary texts.

Modern use

It contains volatile oils and may lead to a positive drug test. This anti-inflammatory, sedative, antibacterial, and antifungal is usually used externally or as an essential oil. Rosemary has been recommended in the performance horse to help the muscles recover from hard work and to promote circulation to the muscles and brain (McDowell 2003). The herb is useful as an anti-inflammatory in older, cold, damp, arthritic horses, but a positive blood test may occur.

Ruta graveolens (Rue)

Historical use

This herb is a stimulant, uterine antispasmodic, and vermifuge (Self, 1996). It can be used as decoction or infusion with 2 to 4 ounces fresh herb in water or beer for worms; it is also said to help prevent or antidote viper bites, farcy (given with diuretics), hydrophobia (given with box leaves) and lockjaw (given with camphor and opium). Bruised leaves were placed in a horse's ear for staggers.

Modern use

This herb is infrequently seen in modern formulas, but it could be used more often. It has some toxicity, as do many of the anthelmintics, so the doses used are lower than those of other herbs—one-half handful, or 1 ounce, with higher doses when used as a vermifuge (deBairacli-Levy, 1976). Rue is also used for external parasites such as lice. It contains rutin and strengthens blood vessels, bones, tendons, and ligaments, as well as nerves. It may have some use with bleeders (McDowell, 2003), and it can be used as an eyewash.

Laurus Sassafras (Sassafras)

Historical use

This is a favorite spring tonic for horses, and it is used as an appetite stimulant any time of the year. Powdered form, tea, or decoction may be used (McClure, 1917).

Modern use

This herb is not commercially available because of laboratory animal studies in which high doses of the single constituent, safrole, proved toxic.

Juniperus sabina (Savin)

Historical use

Oil of juniper was used for deworming (3-5 dr [11.1-18.5 mL]) (McClure, 1917). It was made into an ointment for blisters with 1 part fresh tops to 16 parts lard. It is an acrid stimulant (1-2 dr [3.7-7.4 mL]) with or without aloes to follow; it can be used for worms but with doubtful efficacy; it may be externally applied for warts in powder or ointment form; long-term use of it may cause hair loss.

Meleleuca alternifolia (Tea Tree Oil)

Historical use

This herb was not found in historical veterinary texts.

Modern use

Externally, it is very useful, especially for thrush and white line disease. This antimicrobial and antimycotic can be used for wound healing and insect bites; most horses tolerate it well.

Thymus vulgaris (Thyme)

Historical use

This herb was not found in historical veterinary texts.

Modern use

It is an expectorant, antimicrobial, and antispasmodic that contains volatile oils; drug tests may be positive.

Terebinthe (Turpentine)

Historical use

Many forms of turpentine have different uses and different plant origins (McClure, 1917). Turpentine is a semifluid or fluid oleoresin, primarily the exudation of the terebinth, or turpentine, tree *(Pistacia terebinthus)*, a native of the Mediterranean region. It is also obtained from many coniferous trees, especially species of pine, larch, and fir. Once collected as a naturally occurring mixture of resin and essential oil, it is distilled to make what we know as turpentine liquid. Doses are given mixed in relatively small quantities of pure liquids.

Common turpentine *(Pinus palustris* and *Pinus sylvestris)* is from North Carolina, Norway, and northern Europe. Venice turpentine *(Larix europa)* is from Europe. This is the most common form seen in barns today. Canadian balsam *(Abies balsamea)* is considered the purest form of turpentine.

Oil of turpentine is also known as spirit of turpentine. It is considered a powerful stimulant, diuretic, and antispasmodic that is used for colic and general debility. It can be used topically but should be carefully diluted with equal parts of sweet oil (usually made from almonds—*Prunus amygdalus*). The recommended dose is 1 to 2 ounces, always mixed with the same amount of plain or olive oil. Beasley used this in large doses (2-4 oz) as a vermifuge and in lower doses as a purgative.

Modern use

Turpentine is rarely used internally, although it may provide some benefits. It is applied topically to the hoof to dry and strengthen the hoof wall.

Nicotiana tabacum (Tobacco)

Historical use

This herb has been touted for its deworming qualities, but McClure found that it leaves the animal nauseous, weak, and sick, so he did not recommend it.

Modern use

It is occasionally seen in deworming formulas, but its efficacy is questionable. It is toxic.

Valeriana officinalis (Valerian)

Historical use

This herb was not found in historical veterinary texts.

Modern use

This sedative and muscle relaxant may have negative effects on the intestines, even though it is antispasmodic. Some horses can colic after receiving too much, or for too long a time. Diarrhea has also been seen in this author's practice; it may enhance the effects of tranquilizers and anesthetics. It may be prohibited for some competitive events.

Salix alba (White Willow Bark)

Historical use

This herb was used as an antipyretic, anti-inflammatory, and analgesic.

Modern use

This herb has the same uses in modern times. It is very effective as an anti-inflammatory herb in patients with arthritis and injury. It is contraindicated in gastric ulceration, may prolong bleeding times, and may interact with NSAIDs. Although these concerns have not been addressed experimentally in horses, it is important to consider the potential for herb-drug interaction if prescribing it.

Artemisia absinthum (Wormwood)

Historical use

This herb was used for parasite control.

Modern use

This herb is used for parasites, intestinal atony, and gastritis, and as an insect repellant; its use may lead to colic if is used with NSAIDs on a long-term basis. It may react with phenothiazines (Brinker, 2001).

Yucca Shidigera (Yucca)

Modern use

Yucca is a poorly investigated herb that is popular in equine joint formulas. The plant is included because of its popularity. The mechanisms of action are very poorly understood. Research in sheep, cattle, dogs, and cats shows an effect on digestive function. No research supports its use for arthritis. However, its positive effects on the intestinal tract may be helpful in arthritis. Research has shown a clear relationship between intestinal health and some forms of arthritis (Holden, 2003). However, the relationship between yucca, intestinal health, and arthritis improvement in the horse is only speculative at this point.

Yucca is commonly prescribed for patients with mild to moderate arthritis, with some clinical results, although in this author's experience, yucca is not one of the top choices. An accurate dose is unknown and will be established only by trial and error. Many products contain small amounts of yucca and may aid the digestive tract somewhat, but they are probably not that helpful for any significant case of arthritis. Products on the higher end of the dose range clinically help some horses to become more mobile (Table 21-4).

References

Abells S, Haik G. Efficacy of garlic as an anthelmintic in donkeys. Israel J Vet Med 1999;54:1.

Anderson RA, Broadhurst CL, Polansky MM, et al. Isolation and characterization of polyphenol type-A polymers from cinnamon with insulin-like biological activity. J Agric Food Chem 2004;52:65.

Beasley H. *The Druggist's General Receipt Book Comprising a Copious Veterinary Formulary.* 5th ed. London: John Churchill; 1861.

Beech J, Donaldson MT, Lindborg S. Comparison of *Vitex agnus castus* extract and pergolide in treatment of equine Cushing's syndrome. AAEP Proc 2002;48:175.

Biser JA. Really wild remedies—medicinal plant use by animals, 1998. Available at: http://nationalzoo.si.edu/Publications/ZooGoer/1998/1/reallywildremedies.cfm. Accessed March 2005.

Bjarnason I, Peters TJ. Intestinal permeability, non-steroidal anti-inflammatory drug enteropathy and inflammatory bowel disease: an overview. Gut 1989;30S:22.

Blumenthal M, Goldberg A, Brinkman J, eds. *Herbal Medicine, Expanded Commission E Monographs.* Newton: Integrative Medicine Communications; 2000.

Brinker F. *The Toxicology of Botanical Medicines.* Sandy: Eclectic Medical Publications; 2000.

Brinker F. Herb contraindications and drug interactions. Sandy: Eclectic Medical Publications; 2001.

Brown SD Jr, Landry FJ. Recognizing, reporting, and reducing adverse drug reactions. South Med J 2001;94:370.

Bruneton J (trans by Haton C). *Toxic Plants Dangerous to Humans and Animals.* Secaucus: Lavoisier Publishing Inc, c/o Sprenger Verlag; 1999.

Buchanan S. Zoopharmacognosy: animal self-medication, 2002. Available at: http://www.colostate.edu/Depts/Entomology/courses/en570/papers_2002/buchanan.htm. Accessed March 2005.

Butters DE, Whitehouse MW. Treating inflammation: some (needless) difficulties for gaining acceptance of effective natural products and traditional medicines. Inflammopharmacology 2003;11:97.

Clater F. *Every Man His Own Farrier; or the Whole of Farriery Laid Open.* 23rd ed.London: W. Lewis; 1817.

Craig JM, Lloyd DH, Jones RD. A double-blind, placebo-controlled trial of an evening primrose and fish oil combination vs. coconut oil in the management of recurrent seasonal pruritus in horses. Vet Derm 1997;8:177.

Dadd G. *The Modern Horse Doctor.* Cleveland, Ohio: Jewett, Proctor and Worthington; 1854.

Darlington LG. Dietary therapy for arthritis. Nut Rheum Dis/Rheum Dis Clin North Am 1991;17:273.

deBairacli-Levy J. *Herbal Handbook for Farm and Stable.* Emmaus, Pa: Rodale Press; 1976.

DerMarderosian A, ed. *The Review of Natural Products.* St Louis, Mo: Facts and Comparisons; 2000.

Divers TJ, Mohammed HO, Hintz HF, et al. Equine motor neuron disease: a review of clinical and experimental studies. Am Assoc Eq Pract Proc 2003;49:230.

Emerald Valley dosing protocol Available at: http://www.emeraldvalleybotanicals.com/dosing.htm. Accessed March 2005.

Engel C. *Wild Health: Lessons in Natural Wellness From the Animal Kingdom.* New York: Houghton Mifflin Company; 2002.

Fehmi JS, Karn JF, Ries RE, et al. Cattle grazing behavior with season-long free-choice access to four forage types. Appl Anim Behav Sci 2002;78:29.

Ferguson V. *The Practical Horse Herbal.* London: Carlton Books; 2002.

Gianella RA, Broitman SA, Zamcheck N. Influence of gastric acidity on bacterial and parasitic enteral infections. Ann Intern Med 1979;78:271.

Grieve M. *A Modern Herbal.* New York: Harcourt, Brace & Company; 1931.

Gruenwald J, Brendler T, Jaenicke C, eds. PDR for Herbal Medicines. 2nd ed. Montvale: Medical Economics; 2000.

Hammock PD, Freeman DE, Baker GJ. Failure of psyllium mucilloid to hasten evaluation of sand from the equine large intestine. Vet Surg 1998;27:547.

Harman JC. The toxicology of herbs in equine practice. Cl Tech Eq Pract 2002;1:74.

Harman JC, Ward M. The role of nutritional therapy in the treatment of equine Cushing's syndrome and laminitis. Alt Med Rev 2001;6S:S4.

Hartman D, Coetzee JC. Two US practitioners' experience of using essential oils for wound care. J Wound Care 2002;118:317.

Hering C. *The Guiding Symptoms of Our Materia Medica,* vol 8 (reprint of 1890 ed). New Delhi: B. Jain Pubishers Pvt, Ltd; 1993.

Holden W, Orchard T, Wordsworth P. Enteropathic arthritis. Rheum Dis Clin North Am 2003;29:513.

Holmes P. *The Energetics of Western Herbs,* vols 1 and 2. 3rd ed. Boulder: Snow Lotus Press; 1997.

Houpt KA, Zahorik DM, Swartzman-Andert JA. Taste aversion learning in horses. J Anim Sci 1990;68:2340.

Huffman MA, Caton JM. Self-induced gut motility and the control of parasite infections in wild chimpanzee. Int J Primatol 2001;22:329.

Hutchings MR, Kyriazakis I, Gordon IJ, et al. Trade-offs between nutrient intake and faecal avoidance in herbivore foraging decisions: the effect of animal parasitic status, level of feeding motivation and sward nitrogen content. J Anim Ecol 1999;68:310.

Inman RD. Antigens, the gastrointestinal tract and arthritis. Rheum Dis Clin North Am 1991;17:309.

Jenkins AP, Trew DR, Crump BJ, et al. Do non-steroidal anti-inflammatory drugs increase colonic permeability? Gut 1991;32:66.

Khan A, Safdar M, Ali Khan MM, et al. Cinnamon improves glucose and lipids of people with type 2 diabetes. Diabetes Care 2003;26:3215.

Kimbrough DR, Martinez N, Stolfus S. A laboratory experiment illustrating the properties and bioavailability of iron. J Chem Educ 1995;72:558.

Knight AP, Walter RG. *A Guide to Plant Poisoning of Animals in North America.* Jackson: Teton New Media; 2001.

Lawson A. *Modern Farrier, Curing the Disorders of Domestic Animals.* Newcastle Upon Tyne: Mackenzie and Dent; 1824.

Lizko NN. Stress and intestinal microflora. Nahrung 1987;31:443.

MacAllister CG, Morgan SJ, Borne AT, Pollet RA. Comparison of adverse effects of phenylbutazone, flunixen meglumine, and ketoprofen in horses. J Am Vet Med Assoc 1993;1202:71.

McCarty MF. Complementary measures for promoting insulin sensitivity in skeletal muscle. Med Hyp 1998;51:451.

McClure R. *McClure's American Horse, Cattle and Sheep Doctor.* Chicago: Frederick J. Drake and Co.; 1917.

McDowell R, Rowling D. *Herbal Horsekeeping.* North Pomfret: Trafalgar Square Publishing; 2003.

Minnick PD, Brown CM, Braselton WE, et al. The induction of equine laminitis with an aqueous extract of the heartwood of black walnut *(Juglans nigra).* Vet Hum Toxicol 1987;29:230.

Miyazawa K, Ito M, Ohsaki K. An equine case of urticaria associated with dry garlic feeding. J Vet Med Sci 1991;3:747.

Montavon S. Efficacy of a medicinal plant preparation based on *Harpagophytum procumbens* in cases of bone spavin of adult horses. Pratique-Veterinaire-Equine 1994;26:1994.

National Animal Supplement Council. Available at: http://www.nasc.cc/index.htm. Accessed March 2005.

O'Dwyer ST, Michie HR, Ziegler TR, Revhaug A, Smith RJ, Wilmore DW. A single dose of endotoxin increases intestinal permeability in healthy humans. Arch Surg 1988;123:1459.

O'Neill W, McKee S, Clarke AF. Flaxseed *(Linum usitatissimum)* supplementation associated with reduced skin test lesional area in horses with *Culicoides* hypersensitivity. Can J Vet Res 2002a;66:272.

O'Neill W, McKee S, Clarke AF. Immunological and haematinic consequences of feeding a standardized Echinacea *(Echinacea angustifolia)* extract to healthy horses. Equine Vet J 2002b;34:222.

Pascoe E. Equisearch: how horses sleep, 2002. Available at: http://www.equisearch.com/train/behavprobs/eqzzz629/index.html. Accessed March 2005.

Pierce KR, Joyce JR, England RB. Acute hemolytic anemia caused by wild onion poisoning in horses. J Am Vet Med Assoc 1972;160:323.

Pitchford P. *Healing With Whole Foods*. Berkeley: North Atlantic Books; 1993.

Reilly JD, Hopegood L, Gould L, Devismes L. Effect of a supplementary dietary evening primrose oil mixture on hoof growth, hoof growth rate and hoof lipid fractions in horses: a controlled and blinded trial. Equine Vet J Suppl 1998;9:58.

Rolfe RD. Interactions among microorganisms of the indigenous intestinal flora and their influence on the host. Rev Infect Dis 1984;67:S59.

Ross J. *Combining Western Herbs and Chinese Medicine*. Seattle: Greenfield's Press; 2003.

Russel RM. Changes in gastrointestinal function attributed to aging. Am J Clin Nutr 1992;55:1203S.

Sapolsky R. Junk food monkeys. Discover, September 1989.

Self HA. *Modern Horse Herbal*. Buckingham: Kenilworth Press; 1996.

Self HP. The application of the herb *Vitex agnus castus* for the symptomatic relief of hyperadrenocorticism in horses. Dissertation for BSC in Phytotherapy, College of Phytotherapy, Prifyscgol Cymru, University of Wales, 2003.

Sigthorsson G, Tibble J, Hayllar J, et al. Intestinal permeability and inflammation in patients on NSAIDs. Gut 1998;43:506.

Sullivan A, Edlund C, Nord CE. Effect of antimicrobial agents on the ecological balance of human microflora. Lancet Infect Dis 2001;1:101.

Tilford ML, Tilford GL. *All You Ever Wanted to Know About Herbs for Pets*. Irvine: Bowtie Press; 1999.

Uhlinger C. Black walnut toxicosis in ten horses. J Am Vet Med Assoc 1989;195:343.

United States Equine Federation. Summary of drug testing rules, 2005. Available at: http://www.usef.org/content/drugsMeds/. Accessed March 2005.

Wells CL, Jechorek RP, Gillingham KJ. Relative contributions of host and microbial factors in bacterial translocation. Arch Surg 1991;126:247.

Xie H. Drugs and performance in horses: overview. Adv Chinese Herb Med Notes 2003.

Xie H, Preast V. *Traditional Chinese Veterinary Medicine,* vol 1. Beijing: Jing Tang; 2002.

Youatt W. *The Horse*. New York: Levitt and Allen; 1843.

Zinn RA. Influence of oral antibiotics on digestive function in Holstein steers fed a 71% concentrate diet. J Anim Sci 1993;71:213.

Phytotherapy for Dairy Cows

Hubert J. Karreman

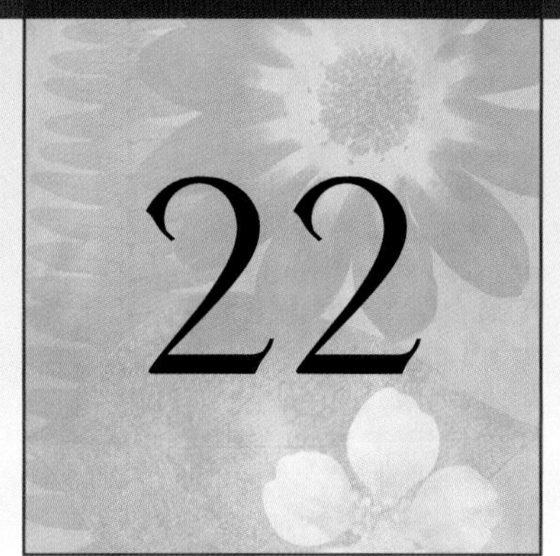

CHAPTER 22

Ruminant animals are classified in the family Bovidae and are obligate herbivores. The major species that are economically important to people globally, are milk- and meat-producing sheep, goats, and cows. Their development through the ages has hinged upon free access to plant materials for sustenance to promote basic maintenance, growth, and reproduction capabilities. When hunter-gatherer peoples began to settle down and grow crops, they also began to domesticate livestock, with ruminants most likely being among the first to be domesticated. Domestication probably coincided well with the growing of crops and the tending of grazing lands because these types of animals were accustomed to grass-based diets. Indeed, the bacteria and protozoa associated with the specialized forestomach digestive apparatus of the reticulum, rumen, and omasum—but especially, the rumen—require fibrous plant materials for their own growth and replication, which in turn, fuel the ruminant by producing volatile fatty acids, sugars, and other useful products. The intestinal enzymes of ruminants are well adapted to the breakdown products of plants, and they recognize plant primary metabolite compounds such as sugars and other carbohydrates, as well as vegetable proteins and fats.

Plants also make secondary metabolites, not so much because of their basic energy needs but more likely for protective purposes to fight off various pathogens. Some major classes of protective compounds include terpenoids, essential oils, saponins, alkaloids, phenolics, lectins, lactones, polypeptides, and polyacetylenes. Within the phenolics are found the more commonly known quinones, flavanoids, tannins, and coumarins. Undoubtedly, ruminants have encountered these types of substances in small amounts over time through their regular diet when grazing on fresh greens. It is not unreasonable to think that plant-based compounds, because they are easily recognized by an herbivorous system, may also be effective when applied to ruminants for reasons other than nourishment. For example, it was found that 1 gram of a combination of thymol, eugenol, vanillin, and limonene inhibited certain rumen microbial species and thus, the rate of deamination of amino acids in the rumen (McIntosh, 2003), which may affect the efficiency of protein use and nitrogen retention in ruminants. This could be beneficial for cattle in production. Alternatively, with the use of secondary metabolites such as essential oils, alkaloids, and tannins, some therapies may have beneficial effects for ruminants that are ill. However, it must always be kept in mind (as with all medicines, regardless of source) that the dose administered is what differentiates therapy from toxicity.

Modern ruminants, especially dairy cows, are not the same as they were when they lived free in the wild. Various traits (e.g., milk production) have been selected very carefully over the past few hundred years. The intense stresses placed on high-production dairy cows, especially those in modern confinement conditions, eclipse what these ruminant herbivores experienced centuries ago. Although it is beyond the scope of this chapter to discuss the many differences between confinement farming and intensive grazing management of cattle, it is reasonable to assume that dairy cows that are intensively grazed are more like their ancestors than are their cohorts that are kept inside, in total confinement. This is because the digestive systems of cows that take in fresh feeds while grazing—feeds containing chlorophyll, primary plant metabolites, and various secondary plant metabolites—keep their enzymatic systems actively responding to such substances. One study showed that dairy cows are healthier when they are actively grazing pasture swards than when they are confined and fed only fermented feeds (Karreman, 2000); thus, phytotherapy is, in a sense, unconsciously practiced by dairy farmers when cows are allowed to actively graze.

PARASITISM

Even so, intensively grazed cattle on a commercial dairy farm may have stresses due to parasitism simply because animals are kept on the same land base, whereas in the wild, they would freely roam and keep moving to fresh grasses and land. Parasites, when exposed to a captive population, can potentially explode in numbers and cause disease, especially among naïve young stock that have yet to establish lasting immunity while rotating through the pasture system. It is interesting to note that ruminants grazing birdsfoot trefoil *(Lotus corniculatus)* have been shown to have lower fecal egg counts (FECs), and ruminants grazing chicory *(Cichorium intybus)* had fewer adult abomasal helminths than those grazing a rye-grass/white clover mix (Marley, 2003). Similarly, feeding of sulla *(Hedysarum coronarium)* was associated with higher antibody titers against the secretory-excretory antigens of *Ostertagia circumcincta;* it also resulted in lower numbers of the adult parasite when compared with feeding alfalfa *(Medicago sativa)* (Niezen, 2002). Additionally, sainfoin *(Onobrychis viciifolia),* a legume forage with polyphenols and condensed tannins, had significant effects in vitro on third-stage larvae and abomasal adult worms of *Haemonchus contortus, Trichostrongylus colubriformis,* and lungworm *(Dictyocaulus viviparous)* (Paolini, 2004; Molan, 2000).

Prevention of parasitism should be a major goal for producers who lack access to or cannot afford to constantly use parasiticides, and for farmers who manage their herds under a certified organic program whereby conventional wormers are severely restricted. It is generally recognized that strong reliance on chemical wormers can lead to resistance. Even with the use of alternatives to chemotherapy, such as plant-based parasiticides, parasite resistance can still emerge because of reliance on a single product. Such plant-based products should still be used strategically.

Effective parasite control requires a holistic, multipronged approach that takes into account factors such as nutrition, pasture management, shelter, and water quality, even before a parasiticide is selected. If animals are kept in proper nutritional balance (i.e., not lacking major nutrients such as energy or minerals) and are rotated through well-managed pastures (with previously deposited manure in an advanced state of decomposition), with access to shelter from bad weather and fresh water of high quality, it is unlikely that strong parasite pressures will be present. At the least, the animals' immune systems will be able to cope with the parasite pressures in the best possible way. This situation contrasts with that of animals put onto ground with little to graze, drinking stagnant or slowly moving water in drainage ditches and having no shelter from the blazing sun or chilly rains. It is obvious that the latter conditions are poor and, even with chemical parasiticides, raising animals in this manner is unlikely to be productive or profitable. Efforts should be made to keep parasite infestation from occurring through good management of land and animals. Under such circumstances phytotherapies offer potential benefits in helping to protect animals from parasites.

Many studies conducted in the past decade have involved the use of plant extracts against various nematode infections. Some in vitro studies have used crude extracts or isolated compounds; in vivo studies have sometimes performed statistical comparisons between phytotherapy and conventional anthelmintics. Many studies are being conducted in tropical or developing countries by European, South American, African, or Indian researchers. In many cases, results are being published in well-known peer-reviewed journals; in other cases, lesser known scientific journals are documenting the findings. Few studies have been conducted in the United States, perhaps because of the lack of a tropical environment and because of the strong relationship between pharmaceutical firms and agribusiness.

The vast majority of investigations have studied phytotherapy-based parasiticides in sheep (or goats), probably because of their economic importance in developing parts of the world, and also because they are less expensive to maintain. Many, but certainly not all, of the parasite species that infect one type of ruminant also affect other ruminants. Thus, extrapolation, if needed, is justifiable. Results of studies must be considered with regard to whether the animals were naturally infected or were experimentally or artificially infected, and whether the researchers used crude extracts as made by traditional methods or isolated active ingredients. It is reasonable to consider that animals that are naturally infected may have adaptive capabilities that may somehow act synergistically with treatment; however, experimentally infecting an animal may jolt the system to a point at which adaptive mechanisms are absent (or not yet equilibrated), and thus certain treatments are hindered. Many studies have investigated phytotherapy targeted to *H. contortus* in sheep; the findings of these studies should be valuable for cattle as well, because these two animal species are both affected by *Haemonchus* species.

Summaries of in vivo research follow. It was shown that albendazole provided 100% fecal egg count reduction by day 4 posttreatment in an experimentally induced mixed infection (60% *Haemonchus* spp) in sheep; however, a botanical preparation of pyrethrum showed significant reductions by day 8 of treatment (Mbaria, 1998). Very favorable results were presented in two other studies that compared botanical products with albendazole in the treatment of patients with naturally occurring mixed nematode infection. With the use of 1600 mg/kg *Nauclea latifolia* stem bark extract orally for 5 consecutive days, Onyeyili and colleagues found significantly reduced fecal egg counts in sheep (93.8%). This reduction was equivalent to that attained with 5 mg/kg albendazole (94.1%). Gathuma and associates showed that *Myrsine afriacana, Albizia anthelmintica,* and *Hilderbrantia sepalosa* yielded 77%, 89.8%, and 90% efficacy, respectively, versus albendazole (100% efficacy) in sheep that were harboring mixed natural helminthosis. It is interesting to note that improved packed cell volume (Gathuma, 2004) and improved hemoglobin and leukocytosis (Onyeyili, 2001) were observed with phytotherapy. When examining *Moniezia* species, Gathuma found that herbal remedies were 100% efficacious versus 63% efficacy for albendazole. However, Githoria (2002, 2004) reported nine plants (including *M. africana*) that were not effective against sheep experimentally infected with *H. contortus.* In a study in which *Tinospora rumphii* was used to treat goats experimentally infected with *H. contortus,* the effective dose (ED_{50}) and lethal dose (LD_{50}) were identified, and 4.5

grams of a concentrated extract was found to be as effective as the commercial dewormer (mebendazole) (Fernandez, 2004).

In another study of five plant products tested against *Trichostrongylus* in artificially infected lambs, 183 mg/kg of an ethanol extract of *Fumaria parviflora* yielded a 100% reduction in fecal egg count, as well as 78% and 88% reductions in adult *H. contortus* and *T. colubriformis;* thus, according to the authors, it was as effective as pyrantel tartrate (Hordegen, 2003). Researchers in Egypt used a commercial compound (Mirazid®) that contained an oleoresin solution of *Commiphora molmol* as its active ingredient; they found that doses of 600 mg and 1200 mg cured 83% and 100%, respectively, of sheep with natural fascioliasis infection (Haridy, 2003); another group found that natural infection of sheep and goats with *Dicrocoeliasis dendriticum* was also cured by Mirazid containing *C. molmol* when the liquid equivalent of 2 capsules was given orally once daily for 4 consecutive days (Massaud, 2003).

After 6 weeks of experimental infection with *Schistosoma mansoni,* mice were given 200 mg/kg body weight of praziquantel daily or 200 mg/kg body weight of *Balantines aegyptiaca* fruits daily for 10 weeks; each treatment resulted in significant reduction of egg count per gram and egg burden in tissues, as well as recovery of adult worms from *S. mansoni* infection obtained from mice (Koko, 2004).

When the in vitro effects of plant materials against *H. contortus* were measured, it was shown that an essential oil and eugenol, both extracted from *Ocimum gratissimum,* caused maximal inhibition at 0.50% concentration in the egg hatch test from goat feces (Pessoa, 2002). The same laboratory found that ethyl acetate of *Spigelia anthelmia* used at 50 mg/mL inhibited 100% of egg hatching and 81% of larval development of *H. contortus,* and the methanolic extract inhibited 97% of egg hatching and 84% of larval development (Assis, 2003). As was mentioned previously, pasture plants such as birdsfoot trefoil and chicory contain tannins and possess anthelmintic attributes. Similarly, some woody plants known to contain tannins have been studied. Via the tannin inhibitor polyethylene glycol, it was shown that tannins, at least in part, are responsible for some anthelmintic effects observed within livestock (Paolini, 2004).

Protozoal parasites can cause disease, especially in neonatal young stock. Although garlic was shown to be helpful against cryptosporidiosis in a clinical trial of patients with acquired immunodeficiency syndrome (AIDS; Anonymous, 1996), a study of Holstein calves that were administered an allicin-based product (an active ingredient isolated from garlic) showed no effect on the duration of diarrhea, although with high doses, onset of diarrhea was delayed (Olson, 1998). However, other protozoal parasite infections do seem to be amenable to plant-based products, such as those derived from *Bertholletia excelsa* (Campos, 2004), *Ranunculus sceleratus, Coptis chinensis* (Schinella, 2002), and *Zanthoxylum liebmannianun* (Arrieta, 2001). An in vivo murine study demonstrated that 50% alcoholic extracts of *Xanthium strumarium* leaves, *Parthenium hysterophorus* flower, and *Nycanthes arbortristis* leaves at dosages of 100 and 300 mg/kg body weight were effectively trypanocidal (Dwivedi, 2004).

Overall, mixed results were obtained in studies that used phytotherapy for internal parasitism; however, these studies do not state how the animals were managed in terms of previous nutrition or pressure of exposure to nematodes. Sole reliance on therapeutic treatment (of whichever type) for parasitism is not good livestock management. It must be emphasized again that proper feed, water, and shelter contribute significantly to an animal's ability to emerge from an internal parasite problem. Given that phytotherapies thus far show more variable effects compared to known efficacy of anthelmintics, therapy that uses plant-based products will work best if management steps are also taken to improve pasture plant species, hasten manure decomposition, and provide proper nutrition, water, and shelter.

MASTITIS

A dairy cow's main role in life is to provide milk. Ideally, milk should have a low somatic cell count (SCC), the number of leukocytes per milliliter of milk). It is all too common for a cow or a number of cows to show increases in SCC. This is likely—but not always—due to pathogenic bacteria entering the teat canal. The usual ways in which bacteria gain entry into the mammary gland involve the environment (hot and humid weather), bad bedding, poor milking hygiene and milking technique, milking machine malfunction, and individual differences between immune systems in response to various other common stresses. When SCCs reach a particular point, visible abnormalities of the milk occur. This is called clinical mastitis; when abnormalities are confined solely to elevated SCC, these instances are considered subclinical mastitis. Bacteria associated with mastitis (or diagnosed as the etiologic agent) dictate which treatment measures should be taken. Environmental factors and milking machine problems *must* be corrected (if present) before medication is given because medications cannot effectively overcome major problems that are present in the environment.

Typically, mainstream dairy farmers infuse an antibiotic into a quarter that is exhibiting mastitis. This is often done empirically at the time of observed irregularities during milking. However, once the antibiotic does not seem to be effective, culture and sensitivity testing and selection of specific antibiotic treatment takes place. On organic farms that cannot use any antibiotics (otherwise the animal must be removed from the herd), alternative techniques are used to counter chronically elevated SCC or actual cases of mastitis. One rational technique is to stimulate the immune system of the animal, on the assumption that the immune system is integral to resolving infection in the mammary gland. Local irrigation of the gland via infusion of a medicinal substance makes sense as well. In addition, veterinarians working with organic cows can culture milk samples to identify the organism presumed to be the causative agent; this reveals proper management steps for stopping the spread or correcting other factors. Keeping a record of which bacteria are positively identified and recording the therapies used (any kind) helps to build data that do or do not support certain clinical therapies for a given animal or herd.

A common biologic (via extralabel usage) used to stimulate the immune system (and therefore lower SCC) is a US Department of Agriculture (USDA)-licensed product (Immunoboost®). It is derived from fractionation of the cell wall of a *Mycobacterium* species. When it is administered to an animal, the nonspecific branch of the immune system is enhanced by increased production of interferon-γ. It is often of clinical benefit in lowering the SCC of cows for a couple of months when they are subclinically infected by various *Streptococcus* species and coagulase-negative *Staphylococcus* species. One strain of *Staphylococcus, S. aureus,* produces a contagious type of mastitis that may cause large economic losses to the farmer because of poor milk quality and lost milk production by infected quarters. Cows are often culled, or they may be treated with relevant antibiotics at dry-off (when udder involution occurs), in the hope that the animal will clear the walled-off *S. aureus* microabscesses. Obviously, this is not an option for cows living on organic farms, where such antibiotic use (even in the dry period) necessitates that the animal be culled. It should be noted that in vitro sensitivity analysis of *S. aureus* usually indicates that any antibiotic will successfully kill that pathogen; invariably, however, the effectiveness of such antibiotics against *S. aureus* in vivo is universally disappointing.

In an in vivo experiment that used the extract from *Panax ginseng* (8 mg/kg body weight daily for 6 days) to treat cows infected with *S. aureus,* their innate immunity was activated, reducing *S. aureus* infection in quarters and lowering SCC (Hu, 2001). It is well known that the defense of the mammary gland against mastitis-causing pathogens is mediated primarily by cell-mediated immunity. One experiment (using *Echinacea purpura* and *Thuja occidentalis*) was carried out to see whether pharmacologic compounds from these phytopreparations have effects on bovine immune cells; it was found that flow cytometric characterization of neutrophil viability and shape changes constitute a reliable approach for quality testing of immunomodulating phytomedicines (Schuberth, 2002). In the ginseng experiment, it was demonstrated that neutrophil phagocytosis and oxidative burst, as well as the number of monocytes and lymphocytes, were significantly greater in the ginseng-treated cows than in saline controls (Hu, 2001). In another in vivo study in which 0.77 kg of dried Persicaria senegalense leaf powder was fed for 5 days, apparent cure of mastitis was better than with antibiotic treatment. The intramammary antibiotic was used for 3 consecutive days and consisted of 300,000 IU procaine penicillin G, 100 mg dihydrostreptomycin sulphate, 100 mg neomycin sulphate and 10,000 IU vitamin A propionate (Abaineh, 2001).

In a different in vivo study, an herbal gel containing *Cedrus deodara, Curcuma longa, Glycyrrhiza glabra,* and *Eucalyptus globulus* showed high levels of efficacy in the treatment of subclinical mastitis (Saxena, 1995). Promising results in a field study against mastitis were attained with a decoction of concentrated liquid *Herba taraxici* (dandelion leaf, *Taraxacum officinale), Flos lonicera* (honeysuckle flowers, species unspecified), *Radix isatidis* (Isatis root, species unspecified), *Radix scutellariae* (skullcap root, species unspecified), and *Radix angelica sinensis (Angelica sinensis,* or Chinese angelica root) (Hu, 1995). Another commercially available product (Masfrigao®, Vet Hon, China) contains *Herba violae* (violet leaf, species unspecified), *Flos lonicera* (honeysuckle flowers, species unspecified), *Radix angelica sinensis* (*Angelica sinensis,* or Chinese angelica root), *Radix angelicae dahuricae (Angelica dahurica* root), and *Flos fraxini* (flowers of the Korean ash tree) in *Oleum brassica campestris (Brassica campestris,* or field mustard oil). It is infused in the quarter every 12 hours for 4 doses. This product is convenient because it is dispensed in standard mastitis tubes, and farmers like the results they see, especially if it is used with a colostrum-whey product (Biocel CBT®, Agri-Dynamics, Pennsylvania, USA) that is injected subcutaneously.

Mastitis requires a two-prong approach if antibiotics are not used. Stimulation of the immune system in general and local infusion of affected quarters are both warranted. The in vivo studies cited earlier suggest that phytotherapy can be a useful tool in the treatment of subclinical and clinical mastitis. Phytotherapy for mastitis can be administered orally, subcutaneously, topically, or as intramammary infusion—route of administration selected hinges on product availability or farmer preference.

Because milk quality is of utmost importance, the use of phytotherapy, especially in relation to mastitis treatment, must be tempered by consideration of commercial end use. In other words, could residues be involved with the use of herbs? Because it is well recognized that phytotherapy most likely involves pharmacologically active substances, the answer needs to be, yes—but what types of residue are of concern, and what levels would be acceptable from a public health standpoint? Therefore, anytime that phytotherapy is used for mastitis, especially when it is infused directly into the mammary gland, milk from the treated quarter should not be co-mingled with other milk. In general, bad milk should never be put into the bulk tank; co-mingling of milk should not occur until the milk visually looks normal and is negative on a California Mastitis Test (CMT). Specifically, in relation to residues such as growth inhibitors (e.g., antibiotics) that affect cheese production, it is always wise to test the milk of cows treated by phytotherapy for antibiotic activity before milk is added to the bulk tank.

Various milk testing devices (Delvo®, Snap®, Charm II®) have been designed to detect the presence of antibiotics or growth inhibitors; each detects a specific panel of typical antibiotics that are commonly used. These devices should be used as needed. Information regarding potential toxic residues of public health concern is difficult to find. The US Food and Drug Administration (FDA) Food Animal Residue Avoidance Database (FARAD) is the best source of information concerning this in the United States. Yet only veterinarians and regulatory professionals can access FARAD. In Europe, the European Agency for the Evaluation of Medicinal Products (EMEA) would be a good starting point for such information because it delineates various plant concentrations and provides a strong section on the toxicology of each product. In the Summary Report of Substances, the EMEA includes sections on botanical name, parts used, known constituents, intended use, known toxicities, LD_{50} (especially genotoxicity or teratogenicity), margin of safety regarding concentration to be used as intended, and a formal conclusion and recommendation. The public Web site can be accessed at www.emea.eu.int/htms/vet/mrls/a-zmrl.htm. Substances that are generally recognized as safe (GRAS) by the FDA are of interest when questions arise regarding the safety of listed herbs. This list can be found in the US 21CFR182.1–21CFR182.50. It can be accessed on the Internet at www.cfsan.fda.gov/~lrd/FCF182.htm. Through the study of information regarding known potential toxicities, cross-referencing between FARAD and EMEA, and the use of cow side antibiotic/growth inhibitor assays, the use of phytotherapy for cows with elevated SCC or mastitis can be accomplished safely and with confidence.

REPRODUCTION

Issues of fertility and conception are major focus points in dairy herds because of the need for cows to become pregnant, give birth, and commence lactation. By ensuring proper nutrition and exercise during the dry period, many problems associated with reproduction can be minimized. Cows must calve, pass the placenta normally, and have the uterus completely involuted within about 3 weeks after calving so they can once again become fertile for another pregnancy. A cow is generally given about 2 months' time after calving before she is bred again to conceive for a subsequent lactation. A cow's normal gestation time is 9 months; it is possible therefore to have a cow calving again in about 11 months' time. Most farmers do not push for such a short calving interval because milk production tends to drop more precipitously once the cow is carrying a calf again (because of the metabolic demands of the new fetus). A common goal for farmers is to have a 12- to 13-month average calving interval for the entire herd, which indicates that most members of the herd are bred by 3 to 4 months into their current lactation (and are diagnosed as pregnant subsequent to that breeding). Of course, a few cows will always be very difficult to get bred; this often stems from uterine problems that occur early in lactation because of obstetric problems, but it may also be due to ovarian problems, such as cystic follicles or cystic corpora lutea, ovarian hypofunction due to negative energy balance from heavy milk production, and hormonal imbalance in the hypophoseal, anterior pituitary, and ovarian axis. By first diagnosing the problem, the practitioner can institute appropriate treatment to get the cow in estrus and ready to conceive.

The use of hormonal drugs in food animal agriculture seems to be continually expanding. With the discovery of the lysing action of prostaglandin $F_{2\alpha}$ ($PGF_{2\alpha}$) on the corpus luteum (CL), effective treatment for persistent pyometra was identified. Chronic pyometra had previously been a very difficult condition to effectively treat; however, with an injection of $PGF_{2\alpha}$, the cow cycles and pushes out the retained pus through an open cervix, thereby emptying the pathologic contents of the uterus that hindered conception. To take advantage of the presence of the CL at specific intervals, effective treatment may require repeated ($PGF_{2\alpha}$) injections given every 10 to 14 days. Use of ($PGF_{2\alpha}$) in this manner is a very effective therapy. However, ($PGF_{2\alpha}$) has not been confined to therapeutic use only. The fact that a CL can be lysed to bring a cow into estrus afforded theriogenologists the opportunity to shorten the estrus cycles of cows and to breed them sooner. Use of ($PGF_{2\alpha}$) in this manner is called "short cycling," that is, reducing the normal length of a cow's cycle from 21 days to 14 days. In the strongly driven economic world of dairy farming, this is of course an enticing opportunity to get cows back into lactation sooner. In short, all dairy economics is geared to having cows lactate as much as possible during their lifetimes so that as much milk as possible can be produced.

Gonadorelin (GnRH) is another hormonal drug that is used to treat cystic follicles. A cystic follicle is usually the result of a dominant follicle that has failed to release its oocyte during estrus. This upsets the normal cyclic activity of the cow, and a lack of estrus signs. Cystic follicles tend to respond to a single injection of GnRH, with the cow showing a heat in the next week or two. Intense research on the topic of modifying the use of these two hormonal drugs has given rise to a myriad of protocols that are available for dairy farmers and their veterinarians to employ. Details of these protocols are beyond the scope of this chapter. Research into and application of these hormonal drugs for reproduction are constantly being fine-tuned, with information rapidly disseminated and adopted by those in the mainstream dairy industry. Whether the use of these hormonal protocols purely for production purposes is valid when viewed under existing extralabel use laws (via the Animal Medicinal Drug Use Clarification Act [AMDUCA]) is open to debate because they were originally approved by the FDA only for therapy of pyometra ($PGF_{2\alpha}$) and cystic follicles (GnRH).

The use of synthetic hormones is not allowed on organic livestock farms; therefore, it is necessary to consider other ways to treat such chronic conditions as pyometra and cystic follicles. The reader should be made aware at this point that organic farmers must not withhold appropriate medication from an animal, merely to retain its organic status. Use of prohibited substances is required by the USDA National Organic Program to restore an animal to health—but that animal must then be culled from the herd. This is stated here now to distinguish the need for lifesaving measures that may employ a prohibited substance (like an antibiotic) for an organic cow versus the more chronic situation of an infertile organic cow that is otherwise eating and milking well.

Because uterine and ovarian conditions do not usually threaten the life of the cow, it is necessary here to discuss alternative therapies. However, one condition, metritis, can make a cow very ill, and although rare, death may result. Although antibiotics like penicillin are very effective, repeated intrauterine administration of iodine pills readily limits this condition to a localized problem, rather than a potentially overwhelming systemic problem, if not treated. Once the cervix closes to a diameter that does not allow the passage of iodine pills, infusions may become necessary. In the author's experience, infusion of 60 mL of a botanical combination of *Allium sativum, Echinacea angustifolia, Hydrastis canadensis, Berberis vulgaris,* and *Baptisia tinctoria* into the uterus every 24 to 48 hours is effective for normalizing the uterus, as evidenced by a more mucoid and clear discharge. This botanical combination is often extended (diluted) with a colostrum whey product. Before the era of synthetic antibiotics, common treatments included Lugol's iodine and a combination of activated charcoal and boric acid. Activated charcoal is a compound that contains ancient plant residues and undergoes some alterations during processing; its ability to adsorb toxins is nearly unmatched.

On organic farms in Lancaster County, Pennsylvania, in the United States, treatment of cows with metritis with the use of iodine pills from the fourth day to the eighth day postcalving, followed by infusion with the botanical combination from the eighth day to the fourteenth day postpartum, is in part responsible for statistically similar reproduction results between organic and conventional farms (Karreman, 2004). Another popular phytotherapy approach consists of infusion of the uterus with 60 to 120 mL of *Aloe barbadensis*. In reality, it is the experience of the author that *any* type of antiseptic or lavage eventually clears nearly all uterine infections. However, treatment must be started early, and the operator must be persistent. It is generally unrewarding to commence treatment to clear a pyometra when the cow is already 2 to 3 months postpartum. It cannot be emphasized enough that prompt treatment of metritis in early lactation is required if only phytotherapy and antiseptics are used. Through effective treatment of metritis, the usual sequelae of pyometra can be minimized. Chronic, low-grade pyometra should be avoided at all costs on all farms, but especially on organic farms, which must avoid unnecessary antibiotics and/or hormones.

Traditionally, farmers watch for behavioral signs of estrus (heat) twice daily. With the application of all the new hormonal protocols, this type of labor is no longer needed because the protocols rely strictly on timing, obviating the need to actually observe the animals for signs of heat. Farmers who do not wish to rely on hormone treatment to get cows bred are usually highly aware of which cows are not in estrus. This can become very frustrating, as economically they need to become pregnant for a future lactation. Rectal palpation or, better yet, ultrasound can be used to identify which structures are present or lacking in the ovary. Often, when a cow does not show signs of estrus, it is because of inactive ovaries (i.e., lacking any structures). This is most often found when a cow is milking really well (especially in still-growing first calf heifers) and is in a state of negative energy balance. The only real treatment for this condition is *time,* that is, allowing the animal to regain energy balance as milk production declines over a couple of months.

Another frustrating condition is when the veterinarian cannot find a reason why a cow does not show estrus yet is in good body condition (a reflection of energy balance). This can become chronic with certain cows, with a corpus luteum being palpated each time the cow is checked. Conventionally, $PGF_{2\alpha}$ would remedy this condition. However, in the author's experience, phytotherapy has shown very positive results. By using a combination botanical product (Spectra 305®, Integrative Therapeutics, Oregon, USA) that contains *Turnera diffusa, Dioscorea villosa, Mitchella repens, Actaea racemosa, Viburnum opulus, Angelica sinensis, Oenothera biennis,* and *Linum usitatissimum,* an overwhelming percentage of treated animals begin to show visible heat when they have not done so for months previously. This protocol consists of 10 tablets given every other day for 6 doses, beginning when a CL is detected on the ovary (midcycle). Sometimes, a cow that is started on this protocol shows heat before treatment has been completed. More often, a cow shows a good strong heat at the end of treatment, or shortly thereafter. Whenever a cow shows heat, she should be bred, regardless of the point in the protocol at which this occurs. Farmers sometimes describe how they saw the cow in heat right after treatment ended, bred the cow, and then the cow showed "a flaming heat" 3 weeks later, and they bred her again. Adherence to this treatment regimen almost always leads to the cow finally becoming pregnant, although the main point of this phytotherapy is to get the cow to show a heat when she has not done so for a long time. It is interesting to note that this particular therapy is not limited to cows with a CL. It has also shown positive effects in cows diagnosed with a cystic follicle on rectal palpation. However, in these cases, the protocol is extended to twice as long (12 doses over a total of 24 days). Results indicate that cows also show a heat and become pregnant if bred. Use of this botanical combination is a bit more expensive than the homeopathic methods that farmers tend to use first for cysts that cannot be gently ruptured. However, for those who wish to use neither homeopathy nor hormones, this phytotherapy protocol is beneficial, according to many farmers.

It would be interesting to study how this particular phytotherapy exerts its positive effects. It is already known that ingested phytoestrogens can affect the reproductive apparatus (Telefo, 2002), causing higher circulating levels of steroid hormones than endogenous estrogen alone (Mathieson, 1980; Zhu, 1996), thereby affecting target steroid receptors (Benie, 2003). It is likely that the treatment described to treat anestrus cows exerts its effects in a similar way. Study of the protocol described would probably require ultrasound verification of the presence of anatomic structures, as well as blood progesterone and estrogen assays performed both at the onset of treatment and throughout its course. A diagnosis followed by monitoring for a trend of regression of the CL, with changes in progesterone and estrogen during the course of administration of this botanical combination, would provide evidence for its continued use and for further research. At the time of this writing, one veterinary school had applied for a grant to study this particular phytotherapy in relation to ovarian and hormonal changes.

DIGESTIVE PROBLEMS

Unlike infectious problems (e.g., parasitism, mastitis), conditions associated with gut motility and normal passage of feed through the digestive tract do not require antibiotics, hormones, or parasiticides. If there is a fever further examination for a possible infection is needed. However, it is not uncommon to find rumen stasis or ileus with no obvious etiology. While conventional medicine is limited in treating rumen stasis or ileus (the primary agents are magnesium oxide, intravenous calcium, and mineral oil) phytotherapy may prove beneficial.

A look at what veterinarians used in an earlier era reveals that phytotherapy was employed for common digestive problems. Plant-derived "bitters" were widely used. Three classes of bitters were known—simple, aromatic, and astringent. Simple bitters are best represented by gentian *(Gentiana lutea)*, quassia *(Quassia amara)*, and Quaker button *(Nux vomica)*. The best known aromatic bitter is absinthum, with astringent bitters exemplified by cinchona (source of quinine) and cascarilla *(Clutia eluteria)*. A typical tonic prescription for simple indigestion in cows or horses follows:

Gentian	4 oz
Nux vomica	4 drachms
Ginger	4 oz
Sodium bicarbonate	4 oz

Powders are mixed and divided to make 8 doses; 1 dose should be given in feed 3 times daily (Milks, 1930).

Nux vomica provides use other than as an intense bitter; it is also known to be a stimulant to nerves and it increases intestinal peristalsis. Indigestion from exhaustion, perhaps best applicable to draft horses, carriage horses, oxen, and working dogs, was treated by the following mixture of quinine and *Nux vomica:*

Quinine sulphate	10 gr
Ferrous sulphate	20 gr
Nux vomica	2 gr

This can be mixed and formed into 20 pills, and 1 should be given after each meal (Milks, 1930).

Preferable to quinine sulphate was the compound tincture of cinchona, which consisted of 100 mL red cinchona, 80 mL bitter orange peel, 20 mL serpentaria (Virginia snakeroot), and 75 mL each glycerin, alcohol, and water to make 1000 mL. This preparation would contain 0.45% of alkaloids of cinchona. The recommended dose for a horse (or cow) was 60 to 120 mL, as needed (Winslow, 1919).

For excess gas retention (bloat) in ruminants, whether it affects many animals because of clover grazing or occurs as a solitary idiopathic incidence, vegetable oil (e.g., olive, canola, corn) works remarkably well. The farmer may elect to give 1 pint to an adult cow and repeat in 15 minutes. The gas can also be encouraged to move, through eructation or by peristalsis, by continuously walking the animal. A bloated animal should never be left tied in a stall. Use of *Nux vomica* tincture helps to induce needed peristalsis and carminatives can relieve pain by causing expulsion of gas from the stomach or intestines. Carminatives include capsicum, ginger, peppermint, sassafras, fennel, coriander, cloves, and asafetida, among others.

Diarrhea in ruminants can have many causes. On commercial dairy farms, simple diarrhea may be caused by a change in feedstuffs to which ruminal microorganisms must adapt. If this is the case and the cow is still eating, feeding of high-quality dry grass hay creates a good fiber mat and slows the rate of passage through the rumen. Feeding of fermented feeds, highly fermentable grains, and pasture, prolongs or exacerbates diarrhea. Infectious causes of diarrhea must be ruled out if the simple act of feeding hay does not resolve the situation. Differentials for acute diarrhea include Johne's disease, salmonellosis, clostridiosis, and rumen acidosis. If feeding of dry hay does not alleviate diarrhea in a cow that continues to eat, phytotherapy with astringent products may be warranted. Most astringents derive their action from tannins. Examples of plant-derived astringents include tannic acid, gallic acid, galls, kino, krameria, gambir, geranium, hematoxylon, *Rhus glabra*, and *Quercus rubor*.

FEVER AND INFLAMMATION

As mentioned before, cows that are off-feed are often feverish. The cause of fever certainly should be determined; however, reducing the fever itself with the use of antipyretics often causes the animal to feel better and resume eating. The simple act of eating, in turn, can lead to resumption of normal activity while homeostasis is regained (through further medical intervention or immune system adaption). Although many plants in the literature have antipyretic effects, not many were recorded in the veterinary literature before the synthetic drug era. The few vegetable or organic agents found in older veterinary textbooks were derived from cinchona, salix, and gaultheria. Active ingredients consisted of quinine, salicylic acid, and methyl salicylate, respectively, with methyl salicylate being nearly equivalent to salicylic acid. Methyl salicylate is also a constituent of betula (birch), which can be found in the old texts with gaultheria. One study showed that an alder birch *(Betula alnoides)* extract showed significant anti-inflammatory activity (Sur, 2002). Aspirin is the synthetic equivalent to salicylic acid derived from white willow (*Salix* spp). Another modern in vivo study showed that *Vernonia cinerea* had an equivalent antipyretic effect to paracetamol when the extract was taken at a dose of 500 mg/kg in rats (Gupta, 2003). *Vernonia cinerea* is used in combination with quinine in malarial fever.

Other botanical medicines act to reduce fever by affecting the heart rate or force and via vasodilation. These can be found in older veterinary and medical textbooks categorized as agents that affect circulation. They include aconite, gelsemium, veratrum, and bryonia. These medicines are administered with great caution orally or subcutaneously (if <5% alcohol), or they can be diluted and given intravenously. They were employed by all practitioners, that is, conventional doctors and veterinarians, as well as Eclectic practitioners, in the early part of the 20th century. Eclectic and Physiomedical physicians

TABLE 22-1

Phytotherapeutic Dosages Historically Used by Veterinarians

	Horse and Cow	Sheep and Swine
Aconite T.	2-6	2-1
Aloe	8-40	4-15
Areca nut	15-30	2-6
Arnica T.	15-30	4-8
Asafetida T.	60-120	8-15
Balsam Copaiba	15-60	2-8
Balsam Peru	15-60	4-8
Balsam Tolu	15-60	2-4
Belladonna leaves T.	15-30	4-8
Bryonia T.	15-30	2-4
Buchu leaves F.E.	30-60	2-4
Caffeine citrate	1-2	0.25-0.5
Calendula T.	15-30	4-8
Calumba T.	60-120	12-24
Cannabis indica T.	15-45	2-4
Cantharides	1-2	0.3-1
Capsicum	4-8	0.6-2
Cardamom T.	60-90	12-24
Cascara sagrada F.E	0.8-45	0.6-4
Cascarilla Bark F.E.	15-30	4-8
Castanea F.E.	30-60	8-15
Castor Oil	500	60-120
Catechu C/T.	30-60	8-15
Chamomile	30-60	4-8
Chaulmoogra Oil	2-12	0.3-2
Chenopodium Oil	6-12	0.6-1.3
Chimaphila F.E.	30-60	4-15
Cimicifuga T.	30-90	8-15
Cinchona C/T	0.60-120	15-30
Cinnamon Oil	2-6	0.3-0.6
Coca F.E.	30-120	15-30
Cocaine HCl	0.3-0.6 g	0.03-0.1 g
Cod Liver Oil	60-120	15-30
Codeine	0.4-2	0.3-2 g
Colchicum Root T.	15-45	4-6
Conium F.E.	4-8	0.6-1.3
Convallaria	4-8	0.6-1.3
Cotton Root Bark	15-60	4-8
Digitalis T.	12-24	3-10
Dioscorea F.E.	8-24	2-4
Echinacea F.E.	4-15	2-4
Ergot T.	15-60	4-15
Eriodictyon F.E.	15-60	2-8
Eucalyptus Oil	8-15	1.3-3.3
Fennel	30-60	8-12
Fenugreek	30-60	8-12
Gamboge	15-30	1.3-4
Gaultheria Oil	8-30	2-8
Gelsemium T.	15-60	4-12
Gentian F.E.	15-30	4-8
Geranium F.E.	8-30	2-4
Glycerin	30-60	8-15
Glycyrrhiza	15-60	4-15
Gossypium F.E.	8-30	2-8
Granatum F.E.	15-30	4-12
Guarana F.E.	8-30	2-4
Gum Tragacanth	60-90	15-30
Hamamelis F.E.	30-60	8-15
Helleborus F.E	4-15	0.6-2
Hematoxylin F.E.	15-45	6-12
Humulus T.	30-120	4-15
Hydrastis F.E.	8-30	4-8
Hydrastis Gly.	8-30	4-15
Hydrastis T.	30-60	4-15
Hyoscamus T.	30-90	8-15
Ignatia F.E.	2-4	1.3-2.6
Iodine T.	8-15	1.3-2.6
Ipecac F.E.	4-8	1-2
Jaborandi F.E.	8-15	2-4
Juniper Oil	4-8	0.6-2
Kamala F.E.	15-30	4-12
Kava kava F.E.	15-30	4-12
Kino F.E.	30-60	4-12
Kousso F.E.	15-60	4-12
Krameria F.E.	15-30	4-8
Lactucarium F.E.	8-30	1-4
Laudanum	15-60	4-15
Lobelia T.	30-60	4-12
Male Fern F.E.	12-24	4-8
Matico T.	30-60	8-15
Mentha piper. Oil	1-2	0.3-0.6
Morphine	0.2-0.6 g	<0.13 g
Myrrh T.	8-15	4-8
Nicotine	0.001-0.006	0.001-0.002
Nux vomica T.	4-24	1.3-2.6
Opium T. (paregoric))	60-120	15-30
Pepo (Pumpkin)	—	15-60
Physostigma F.E.	1-2	0.13-0.25
Phytolacca F.E.	4-8	1.3-3
Pichi F.E	8-24	2-4
Pilocarpus F.E.	8-15	2-4
Pipsissewa F.E.	30-60	4-15
Pomegranate	30-60	4-12
Polygonum F.E.	15-30	4-8
Prunus F.E.	15-60	4-8
Pulsatilla F.E.	2-8	0.3-0.6
Pyrethrum	15-30	2-6
Quassia F.E.	30-60	8-15
Quercus Alba F.E	15-30	4-8
Quinine (antipyretic)	8-15	1.3-2.6
Rhamnus F.E.	30-60	4-8
Rhubarb F.E.	30-60	4-8
Rhus glab. F.E.	15-30	4-8
Rumex F.E.	30-60	4-8
Ruta F.E.	15-30	15-30
Ruta Oil	2-4	0.13-0.6
Sabina F.E.	30-60	2-4
Sabina Oil	8-15	0.5-1
Sanguinaria F.E.	4-24	0.6-2

TABLE 22-1

Phytotherapeutic Dosages Historically Used by Veterinarians—cont'd

	Horse and Cow	Sheep and Swine		Horse and Cow	Sheep and Swine
Santal F.E.	15-60	8-12	Terebene	8-24	2-4
Santal Oil	4-12	0.6-3	Thiosimanin	2-4	0.5-1
Santonin	15-30	4-8	Thymol	2-8	0.3-2
Sarsaparilla F.E.	30-60	4-8	Tiglii Oil	1-2	0.3-0.6
Sassafras F.E.	30-60	4-8	Tonga F.E.	8-30	2-4
Sassafras Oil	2-8	0.3-0.6	Triticum F.E.	30-60	8-24
Scoparius F.E	15-30	4-8	Turpentine Oil		
Scutellaria F.E.	15-30	4-12	(carminative)	30-60	4-15
Senega F.E.	4-15	1-2	(anthelmintic)	60-120	15-30
Senna F.E.	120-150	30-60	Ustilago F.E.	15-60	2-4
Serpentaria F.E.	15-30	2-4	Uva ursi F.E.	60-120	8-15
Spigelia F.E.	4-30	2-4	Valerian F.E.	30-60	4-8
Squill F.E.	4-8	0.3-1.3	Valerian Oil	2-4	0.6-1.3
Squill T.	24-48	6-12	Veratrum vir F.E.	2-4	1.3-2
Stillingia F.E.	4-30	2-8	Veratrum vir T.	8-12	2.6-4
Stillingia T.	15-45	4-8	Viburnum Prun. F.E.	30-120	8-15
Stramonium F.E.	1.3-4	0.3-0.6	Vinegar	30-120	2-8
Stramonium T.	4-8	0.6-2	Whiskey	60-120	30-60
Strophanthus T.	4-15	0.3-1.3	Wintergreen Oil	8-30	2-8
Sumbul F.E.	8-24	1-4	Xanthoxylum F.E.	15-60	4-12
Sumbul T.	15-30	2-8	Zea F.E.	30-60	8-15
Tanacetum Oil	1.3-4	0.13-0.4	Zingiber F.E.	8-30	4-8
Taraxacum F.E.	30-60	8-15	Zingiber T.	30-60	8-15

From Fish, 1930.
C/T, compound tincture (mixture); F.E., fluidextract; T, tincture.
All doses are in cc's (ml's) to be given orally, unless otherwise noted ("g," grains), and may be administered up to 2-3 times daily.

based many of their therapies on botanical tinctures and fluid extracts of whole plant parts (not on isolated active compounds, similar to the conventional schools) and used them at lower concentrations. Therefore, although aconite, gelsemium, veratrum, and bryonia are avoided today because of their toxic potential, Eclectic practitioners used these compounds with careful consideration and in sufficiently small doses for them to be safe and effective. Indications were based on such physical findings as heart and pulse rates (strong, weak), skin temperature and moistness, mouth and tongue color and moistness, secretions (suppressed, deficient, free), pain experienced, age, and timing of presentation in the course of a disease (Ellingwood, 1919).

Much research has been conducted on phytotherapies that aim to alleviate inflammation, because use of conventional nonsteroidal anti-inflammatory drugs (NSAIDs) can lead to adverse events such as gastric ulceration. Most studies involved laboratory mice or rats as the model. Even though few studies have involved ruminants, these in vivo models of phytotherapies are worthy of consideration and extrapolation. It should be pointed out that local inflammation, especially in the udder of a cow with an acutely hot quarter during mastitis, can be easily cooled down with commercially available peppermint lotions. This cooling effect should not last longer than 24 to 48 hours, to allow lymphatic drainage to take place once the intense pain and heat are reduced, thus affording the animal relief.

Many pharmacognostic studies involve the analysis of plant parts via different extraction solvents. For instance, oral dosing of 200 mg/kg of a dried methanolic extract of fennel *(Foeniculum vulgare)* was evaluated by means of screening protocols that are widely used for testing NSAIDs; this treatment was found to cause significant inhibition of acute and subacute inflammatory disease, along with anti–type IV allergic and central analgesic activities, in mice and rats (Choi, 2004). In another study, a dried methanolic-petroleum ether extract (70/30, v/v) of lettuce seeds *(Lactuca sativa)* dissolved in sesame oil and administered at 4 g/kg intraperitoneally showed time- and dose-dependent analgesic effects (not mediated through the opioid system) in a standard formalin test, as well as a dose-dependent anti-inflammatory effect in a carrageenan model of inflammation (Sayyah, 2004). Black cumin seed *(Nigella sativa)* essential oil given intraperitoneally at 100, 200, and 400 μL/kg exerts significant analgesic effects, apparently through mechanisms other than opioid receptors because naloxone could not reverse the analgesic effects (Hajhashemi, 2004). Another study showed significant reduction in acute, subacute, and chronic inflammation with no adverse effects on gastric mucosa when an ethanolic extract of the bark of *Syzygium cumini* was used in mice, up to a dose of 10 g/kg

(Muruganandan, 2001). An interesting substance, crown gall (a tumor that affects *Eucalyptus globulus*), was screened for cytotoxic, antioxidant, anti-inflammatory, embryotoxic, and antimicrobial activities. It was found that all extracts (methanolic, acetone, and petroleum ether) were effective against inflammation and displayed predominantly antifungal activity against *Candida* species (Branter, 2003).

CONCLUSION

The information provided and studies cited in this chapter discuss many plant extracts used in aqueous, methanolic, ethanolic, volatile oil, or dry form that exert specified dose-dependent effects in vivo. It is noteworthy that because pharmacologically active substances are contained within plants, the clinical course of cure and attendant improvement in physical changes, whether biochemical or anatomic, are plausible and likely to be repeatable. Many of the plant-based drugs listed in the "Digestive Problems" section, for instance, were used by earlier generations of veterinarians and are now well studied regarding their constituents, activities, and uses. The time has come for veterinarians to begin to apply the findings of these studies to improve livestock health around the world.

References

Abaineh D, Sintayehu A. Treatment trial of subclinical mastitis with the herb *Persicaria senegalese* (Polygonaceae). Trop Anim Health Prod 2001;33:511-519.

Anonymous. Garlic for cryptosporidiosis? Treat Rev 1996;22:11.

Arrieta J, Reyes B, Calzada F, Cedilla-Rivera R, Navarrete A. Amoebicidal and giardicidal compounds from the leaves of *Zanthoxylum liebmannianun*. Fitoterapia 2001;72:295-297.

Assis LM, Bevilaqua CM, Morais SM, Vieira LS, Costa CT, Souza JA. Ovicidal and larvacidal activity in vitro of *Spigelia anthelmia* extracts on *Haemonchus contortus*. Vet Parasitol 2003;117:43-49.

Benie T, Thieulant M-L. Interaction of some traditional plant extracts with uterine estrogen or progestin receptors. Phytother Res 2003;17:756-760.

Brantner AH, Asres K, Chakraborty A, Tokuda H, Mou XY, Mukainaka T, Nishino H, Stoyanova S, Hamburger M. Crown gall—a plant tumor with biological activities. Phytother Res 2003;17:385-390.

Campos FR, Januario AH, Rosas LV, Nascimento SK, Pereira PS, Franca SC, Cordeiro MS, Toldo MP, Albuquerque S. Trypanocidal activity of extracts and fractions of Bertholletia excelsa (Fitoterapia). Available at: www.sciencedirect.com. Accessed November 17, 2004.

Choi EM, Hwang JK. Antiinflammatory, analgesic and antioxidant activities of the fruit of *Foeniculum vulgare*. Fitoterapia 2004;75:557-565.

Dwivedi SK. Evaluation of indigenous herbs as antitrypanosomal agents. Available at: www.vetwork.org.uk/pune13.htm. Accessed November 22, 2004.

Ellingwood F. *American Materia Medica, Therapeutics and Pharmacognosy*. Cincinnati, Ohio: Eclectic Medical Publications; 1919 (reprinted 1998).

Fernandez TJ. The potential of *Tinospora rumphii* as an anthelmintic against *H. contortus* in goats. Available at: www.vetwork.org.uk/pune13.htm. Accessed November 22, 2004.

Fish PA. Veterinary Doses and Prescription Writing. 6th ed. Ithaca: The Slingerland-Comstock Publishing Company; 1930.

Gathuma JM, Mbaria JM, Wanyama J, et al. Efficacy of Myrisine africana, Albizia anthelmintica and Hilderbrantia sepalosa herbal remedies against mixed natural sheep helminthosis in Samburu district, Kenya. J Ethnopharmacol 2004;91:7-12.

Githiori JB, Hoglund J, Waller PJ, Baker RL. Anthelmintic activity of preparations derived from *Myrsine africana* and *Rapanea melanophloeos* against nematode parasite, *Haemonchus contortus,* of sheep. J Ethnopharmacol 2002;80:187-191.

Githiori JM, Hoglund J, Waller PJ, Baker RL. Evaluation of anthelmintic properties of some plants used as live dewormers against *Haemonchus contortus* infections in sheep. Parasitology 2004;129(Pt 2):245-253.

Gupta M, Mazumder UK, Manikandan L, Bhattacharya S, Haldar PK, Roy S. Evaluation of antipyretic potential of *Veronia cinerea* extract in rats. Phytother Res 2003;17:804-806.

Hajhashemi V, Ghannadi A, Jafarabadi H. Black cumin seed essential oil, as a potent analgesic and antiinflammatory drug. Phytother Res 2004;18:195-199.

Haridy FM, El Garhy MF, Morsy TA. Efficacy of Mirazid *(Commiphora molmol)* against fascioliasis in Egyptian sheep. J Egypt Soc Parasitol 2003;33:917-924.

Hordegen P, Hertzberg H, Heilmann J, Langhans W, Maurer V. The anthelmintic efficacy of five plant products against gastrointestinal trichostrongylids in artificially infected lambs. Vet Parasitol 2003;117:51-60.

Hu S, Concha C, Johannisson A, Meglia G, Walker KP. Effect of subcutaneous injection of ginseng on cows with subclinical *Staphylococcus aureus* mastitis. J Vet Med B Infect Vet Dis Public Health 2001;48:519-527.

Hu SA, Liu HR. Medical herbs in treatment of bovine mastitis. In: *Proceedings of the 3rd International Mastitis Seminar.* Held May 28-June 1, 1995; Tel Aviv, Israel (V II, session 5, pages 128-129).

Karreman H-J. *Treating Dairy Cows Naturally: Thoughts and Strategies*. Berne, Ind: Paradise Publications; 2004.

Karreman H-J. Using serum amyloid A to screen dairy cows for sub-clinical inflammation. Vet Q 2000;22:175-178.

Koko WS, Abdalla HS, Gala M, Khalid, HS. Evaluation of oral therapy on mansonial schiostosomiasis using single dose of *Balantines aegyptiaca* fruits and praziquantel (Fitoterapia). Available at: www.sciencedirect.com. Accessed November 17, 2004.

Marley CL, Cook R, Keatinge R, Barrett J, Lampkin NH. The effect of birdsfoot trefoil and chicory on parasite intensities and performance of lambs naturally infected with helminth parasites. Vet Parasitol 2003;112:147-155.

Massaud A, Morsy TA, Haridy FM. Treatment of Egyptian dicrocoeliasis in man and animals with Mirazid. J Egypt Soc Parasitol 2003;33:437-442.

Mathieson RA, Kitts WD. Binding of phyto-estrogen and estradiol-17 beta by cytoplasmic receptors in pituitary gland and hypothalamus of the ewe. J Endocrinol 1980;85:317-325.

Mbaria JM, Maitho TE, Mitema ES, Muchiri DJ. Comparative efficacy of pyrethrum mare with albendazole against sheep gastrointestinal nematodes. Trop Anim Health Prod 1998;30:17-22.

McIntosh FM, Williams P, Losa R, Wallace RJ, Beever DA, Newbold CJ. Effects of essential oils on ruminal microorganisms and their protein metabolism. Appl Environ Microbiol 2003;69:5011-5014.

Milks HJ. *Practical Veterinary Pharmacology, Materia Medica and Therapeutics*. 4th ed. London, England: Bailliere, Tindall and Cox; 1930.

Molan AL, Hoskin SO, Barry TN, McNabb WC. Effect of condensed tannins extracted from four forages on the viability of the larva of deer lungworms and gastrointestinal nematodes. Vet Rec 2000;147:44-48.

Muruganandan S, Srinivasan K, Chandra S, Tandan SK, Lal J, Raviprakash V. Anti-inflammatory activity of *Syzygium cumini* bark. Fitoterapia 2001;72:369-375.

Niezen JH, Charleston WA, Robertson HA, Shelton D, Waghorn GC, Green R. The effect of feeding sulla *(Hedysarum coronarium)* or lucerne *(Medicago sativa)* on lamb parasite burdens and development of immunity to gastrointestinal nematodes. Vet Parasitol 2002;105:229-245.

Olson EJ, Epperson WB, Zeman DH, Fayer R, Hildreth MB. Effects of an allicin-based product on cryptosporidiosis in neonatal calves. J Am Vet Med Assoc 1998;212:987-990.

Onyeyili PA, Nwosu CO, Amin JD, Jibike JL. Anthelmintic activity of crude extract of *Nauclea latifolia* stem bark against ovine nematodes. Fitoterapia 2001;72:12-21.

Paolini V. In vitro effects of three woody plant and sanfoin extracts on 3rd stage larvae and adult worms of three gastrointestinal nematodes. Parasitology 2004;129(Pt 1):69-77.

Pessoa LM, Morais SM, Bevilaqua CM, Luciano JH. Anthelmintic activity of essential oil of *Ocimum gratissimum* and eugenol against *Haemonchus contortus*. Vet Parasitol 2002;109:59-63.

Saxena MJ, et al. Non-antibiotic herbal therapy for mastitis. In: *Proceedings of the 3rd International Mastitis Seminar.* Held May 28-June 1, 1995; Tel Aviv, Israel (V II, session 5, pages 79-80).

Sayyah M, Hadidi N, Kamalinejad M. Analgesic and anti-inflammatory activity of *Lactuca sativa* seed extract in rats. J Ethnopharmacol 2004;92:325-329.

Schinella GR, Tournier HA, Prieto JM, Rios JL, Buschiazzo H, Zaidenberg A. Inhibition of *Trypanosoma cruzi* growth by medical plant extracts. Fitoterapia 2002;73:569-575.

Schuberth HJ, Riedel-Caspari G, Leibold W. Flow cytometric testing of immunological effects of a phytomedicinal combination (equimun) and its compounds on bovine leucocytes. J Vet Med A Physiol Pathol Clin Med 2002;49:291-301.

Sur TK. Studies on the anti-inflammatory activity of *Betula alnoides* bark. Phytother Res 2002;16:669-671.

Telefo PB, Moundipa PF, Tchouanguep FM. Oestrogenicity and effect on hepatic metabolism of the aqueous extract of the leaf mixture of *Aloe buettneri, Dicliptera verticillata, Hibiscus macranthus* and *Justicia insularis*. Fitoterapia 2002;73:472-478.

Winslow K. *Veterinary Materia Medica and Therapeutics*. 8th ed. Chicago, Ill: American Veterinary Publishing Company; 1919.

Zhu M, Phillipson JD, Greengrass PM, Bowery NG. Chemical and biological investigation of the root bark of *Clerodendrum mandranorum*. Planta Med 1996;62:393-396.

Clinical Practice: Getting Started

CHAPTER

Susan G. Wynn and Barbara J. Fougère

Teachers frequently hear students complain that they are well educated but not confident to practice herbal medicine. It is a big subject, and in this chapter, the goal is to provide concrete starting points and resources.

WHY USE HERBAL MEDICINE?

This subject has already been covered earlier in this book; however, it is worth reviewing and perhaps looking at it from another angle. In terms of encouraging clients to try herbal medicine, it is worth knowing that in many cases, owners are interested in herbal medicine but will not divulge this to the practitioner—multiple studies have shown this to be the case in human medicine. Careful questioning during history taking may reveal that the owner is already using herbal medicine, giving the practitioner an opportunity to fine-tune that treatment when possible.

Clients are often willing to try herbal medicine for the following reasons:

- The perception is that it is natural
- Clients are likely to be using some form of natural medicine themselves
- Herbs can be used to treat subclinical conditions
- Herbs can be used in the absence of a medical diagnosis
- Herbs may be more effective than other agents for many chronic conditions intractable to conventional medication
- Herbs have actions that medications do not offer, such as adaptogenic activity, nutritional support, and immune stimulation
- Herbs can be used to treat particular organs like the liver, or systems such as the digestive system
- Herbal medicine is part of a holistic approach to animal health care.

The veterinarian can provide to clients a simple brochure that outlines what herbal medicine is about. A basic one can be found on the Veterinary Botanical Medicine Association Web site at www.vbma.org. When clients know that a particular veterinarian has an interest in herbal medicine, word spreads fast.

OBSTACLES TO PRACTICE

One of the greatest obstacles to the practice of veterinary herbal medicine is not lack of support from clients, but lack of support from other veterinarians. Colleagues might argue that the practice of herbal medicine is not evidence based, and that it is not known how it works, or whether it actually does. This is not true. The body of scientific validation is ever increasing, but clinical practice has validated the use of many herbs, in stark contrast to the lack of evidence for many novel drugs. When mechanisms of action are unknown, scientists cannot offer such an evidence base for conventional drugs. When a particular herb lacks scientific support, the traditional knowledge base provides some support.

Time and money are two other obstacles to the practice of veterinary herbal medicine. Herbal medicine does not generate the same revenue as is produced in regular practice, where a throughput of clients and a high average transaction fee caused by other services generate fees for the practice. Herbal medicine takes more time. Extended consultation may be needed for the practitioner to take a comprehensive history and perform a thorough examination of the patient. Clients must be taught to understand that an extended consultation is more expensive, and the veterinary herbalist must charge appropriate fees. The upside of this is the satisfaction that comes when health is restored in seemingly difficult cases, as well as the referrals that come from a job well done. Each practice must work out the best way that it can to deal with the financial restraints of this style of consulting.

Space for a dispensary can also be difficult to find. To begin with, the veterinary herbalist may meet with a local herbalist who can provide needed formulas or herbs.

SEEKING SUPPORT

Support consists of confidence building and reassurance when one is beginning work in veterinary herbal medicine. Where should the practitioner turn for quick, practical information on treating a case? What about ongoing mentorship to help him or her to develop the practice of veterinary herbal medicine? The following steps are suggested:

- Join a holistic veterinary group or veterinary herbal group. The Veterinary Botanical Medical Association (VBMA) is an organization of veterinary herbalists from around the world that provides an email listserv of professionals who can help on cases. An answer to a question is usually provided within 24 hours. This Association also provides a journal and regular continuing education meetings. For more information, the reader is referred to the VBMA Webpage at http://www.vbma.org.
- In each city, a network or organization of human herbalists can be located that is only too willing to assist with assessment of cases and with prescribing. A local herbalist can usually be identified who is very helpful in providing formulas and acting as the practice dispensary, at least in the beginning.
- Plenty of seminars and classes are available for the herbalist to join and participate in.
- Many herbal manufacturers and distributors are staffed by knowledgeable and helpful practitioners. These staff members can also help the herbalist to locate information or to find other practitioners who can assist.

DAY-TO-DAY LEARNING

Clearly, a basic herbal medicine library is essential; it may include both printed textbooks and bookmarked Internet sites (in the authors' opinion, the well-managed practice cannot function successfully without Internet access). It is useful to think of books as belonging to two general categories—those that provide detailed information on the herbs themselves (*Materia medica*–type books) and those that describe treatment strategies. Following are lists of useful texts and Internet sites:

Materia Medica Texts

Felter HW, Lloyd JU. *King's American Dispensatory* (1898). Available at: www.henriettesherbal.com/

Skenderi G. *Herbal Vade Mecum*. Rutherford, NJ: Herbacy Press; 2003.

Bone K, Mills S. *Principles and Practice of Phytotherapy*. St. Louis, Mo: Churchill Livingstone; 2000.

Bone K. *A Clinical Guide to Blending Liquid Herbs*. St. Louis, Mo: Churchill Livingstone; 2003.

Clinical Strategy Texts

Wynn S, Marsden S. *Manual of Natural Veterinary Medicine: Science and Tradition*. St. Louis, Mo: Mosby; 2003.

Weiss R. *Herbal Medicine*. 1st edition. Beaconsfield, England: Beaconsfield Publishers Ltd; 1988.

Hoffman D. *Medical Herbalism*. Rochester, VT: Healing Arts Press; 2003.

Although the practitioner can always expect to learn more with each major course in herbal medicine that is taken, it is useful to spend time with a colleague, watching diagnostic and prescription strategies used in his or her practice.

LENGTH OF CONSULTATIONS AND PRICING

The practice of herbal medicine is not simply about prescribing herbs; it requires a philosophy based on whole health, or holism. To begin with, the new herbalist should plan to allow 1 hour per patient to achieve this.

One of the very first considerations is what to charge for services and medicines. The first herbal consultation is usually a long one, ranging from 40 minutes to an hour; the practitioner may need to factor in time for dispensing unless he or she has hired trained staff. Follow-ups usually last from 20 to 30 minutes.

When the price of herbal medicines is considered in the fee, the practitioner must include the cost of the herbs, bottle, cap, and label, along with the time needed to dispense and order and maintain stock. A 100% markup is recommended to start. To start with, one should make up four or five formulas and calculate the time it takes to make them, as well as the costs of the herbs and materials. A consistent price for bottles of different sizes makes inventory easier, although for some herbs that are more expensive (e.g., *Panax ginseng*), or in cases in which formulas contain a larger number of herbs, a premium should be added to the price. In one author's practice (SW), every formula costs the same, but price is calculated in a way that ensures that the cost of the more expensive herbs is incorporated.

If pre-prepared formulas are used, a 50% to 100% mark-up is realistic.

Appointments should be scheduled according to the likely duration of the initial herbal prescription. When prescribing, one should work out the dose and decide how long the formula will last. A 2-week check-up and a follow-up visit usually provide enough time to indicate whether the formula is working; if it is not working, this plan allows the practitioner the opportunity to change the formula.

CASE SELECTION

Although herbal medicine can provide benefit in many types of cases, many prescribers will start by working with those patients that have not responded to conventional medication, or for which no conventional treatment is available. These generally involve chronic disease that is often immune mediated, along with cancer cases (Box 23-1). Owners are frequently willing to try something new for these animals.

The practitioner should warn the client that because of the chronicity of the problem, it may take some time for changes to be observed. In general, one should allow a month for each year the condition has been present.

BOX 23-1

Candidate Disorders for Herbal Medicine

Immune-mediated diseases
- Atopic dermatitis
- Inflammatory bowel disease
- Chronic allergic rhinitis
- Chronic bronchitis/asthma
- Autoimmune disease

Cancer
Digestive disturbances (especially diarrhea)
Chronic infection
Multiple problems of geriatric patients

Warning the owner of this and of the need to commit to the course of action can prevent early dissatisfaction while the herbal formulas are honed and change is implemented. With experience, a change is generally observed within 2 weeks, sometimes within days, although full health, if it can be restored, may take months.

If the patient is taking conventional medication, one should monitor the patient closely; often, readjustment of dose may be necessary. As health improves, the risks and benefits should be weighed, and, if appropriate (e.g., with dogs on long-term steroids, immune suppressives, or antibiotics), medications should be withdrawn. This step can be challenging for new herbalists but may be necessary for full vitality and health to be restored. One should warn the client that for some conditions, like autoimmune disease, recurrence is possible. It is hoped that the herbal prescription and process and generally improved health will prevent this.

HERBAL PHARMACY

A substantial investment is required for the development of a comprehensive herb pharmacy; however, new practitioners cannot efficiently take advantage of that breadth of choice anyway. The authors suggest a restricted number of remedies (Box 23-2) that can be used to treat a large percentage of chronic disorders among patients that are presented to general practices. Some herbal manufacturers help by providing a starter kit of smaller bottles at a lower cost. Manufacturer representatives serve as a good resource for information and help in many cases.

BOX 23-2

Herb Starter Kit

Tinctures
Ashwagandha
Astragalus
Burdock
Corydalis
Calendula
Dandelion
Devil's claw
Echinacea
Elecampane
Fennel
Fenugreek
Ginger root
Goldenseal
Kava
Licorice
Lobelia
Melissa
Milk thistle
Nettle seed
Panax ginseng
Peppermint
Prickly ash
Propolis
Siberian ginseng
Thyme
Turmeric
Valerian
Wild cherry bark

Other Forms
Tea tree essential oil
Slippery elm powder
Aloe plant for the clinic
Neem oil

Premade Formulas
Hoxsey formula
Choreito (zhu ling san)

STARTER EQUIPMENT

Tinctures represent an ideal form for use in the clinic because of the long shelf-life and ease of mixing. To make simple formulas, the dispenser should know the amount of formula to be dispensed. In general, 1-ounce, 2-ounce, 4-ounce, and 8-ounce bottles, or those that hold 25 mL, 50 mL, 100 mL, or 200 mL are needed.

The practitioner should consider the dose rate and total volume per week for each patient and should start by making up enough to last approximately 2 weeks. For example, a 20-pound dog (10 kg) with a formula that contains five herbs would need a dose of, say 2 mL daily; 2 × 14 = 28 mL, so a 1-ounce or 25-mL bottle should provide just enough formula, give or take a little, if the patient is scheduled to return in 12 days. Chapter 14 provides much greater detail on dispensing and should be studied carefully.

The piece of equipment that will be most needed is a graduated cylinder that can be used to measure amounts in milliliters. (A full dispensary equipment list is provided in Chapter 14.) The measure is held in the left hand, and the herbs are dispensed one at a time in a line. One should take care to line up the herbs or dispense them one at a time because it is easy for one to be interrupted and not remember what was last put in the cylinder. Herbs should be returned to the shelf in their correct

BOX 23-3

Minimum Dispensing Equipment

- Graduated cylinders—120-mL and 240-mL sizes
- Digital gram scale
- Funnels—two sizes
- Glass bottles—2-oz, 4-oz, and 8-oz sizes
- Funnel

places (alphabetical arrangement by Western name makes it easy to find them).

The practitioner may recall from laboratory days that a meniscus is read at eye level with the measure horizontal. To begin with, one herb at a time should be measured out and put into the dispensing bottle. As speed and confidence increase, the practitioner can measure all herbs in the graduated flask one after the other, then the total can be dispensed into the dispensing bottle. The risk that should be guarded against involves calculating incorrectly and adding too much or too little of an herb to a particular formula.

When the practitioner has decided that the patient needs more herbs than can be fit into a bottle or provided in therapeutic concentrations, he or she should consider providing some of those herbs in a tableted or fresh form. For example, high doses of bilberry can be given in a capsule form alongside a formula in a bottle.

A funnel is another useful piece of equipment for relaying herbs from the flask to the bottle. A steady hand can achieve this too. Herbs stain patient records and bench tops, so the practitioner should be prepared.

A formula is constructed in parts or percentages, up to the volume required by the patient. (A measuring cup is less precise but may work initially.) Funnels are helpful for pouring the tincture into dispensing bottles (Box 23-3).

DISPENSING AND LABELING

Registered and approved drugs are dispensed by professionals according to labeling guidelines that are strictly monitored. In the United States and Australia, a drug label must include the name and complete contact information of the dispensing practitioner; date dispensed; drug name, strength, and amount; and dosing instructions. It is suggested that labels for herbal medicines should contain the same information. When a custom formula is dispensed, the ingredients should be listed. Amounts of each herb in the formula may be listed on the label, although a list of included herbs will usually occupy much of the label. A complete list of ingredients with quantities must be written into the medical record.

CLIENT EDUCATION

Holistic practitioners spend a great deal of time on client education, which most medical consumers identify as a critical missing piece of their visits to doctors (lack of client interaction is another trigger that has fueled the Internet-supported self-help movement in medicine). Holistic practices typically schedule longer appointment times specifically for this purpose. This is not to say that the practitioner will be providing all client education—technicians should be part of the education process and can easily counsel clients in detail on such subjects as how to prepare homemade diets (working with the practitioner's prescription for diet type), how to administer herbs, and so forth. One must remember to warn clients that it may take a while for the herbs to work; the practitioner must ensure that clients can contact the practice in case they have difficulty administering the herbs. Client education handouts can also be provided.

At the time of this writing, most veterinary practices do not routinely send customized client instructions home. One excellent use of the longer appointment times used in holistic practice is to compose customized discharge instructions based on previously written templates. This is a value-added service that clients greatly appreciate; it can also serve as the basis for communication with colleagues.

COMMUNICATION WITH COLLEAGUES

Herbal medicine possesses the depth and breadth of a specialty; clients tend to find and use as a secondary or tertiary center of medicine those practitioners who choose to focus many of their interventions on the use of herbs. In cases like these, the veterinary herbalist is acting as a specialist and should communicate with the general practitioner. Whether this takes the form of a phone call or letter is dictated by the standard of practice in that locale. When computerized practice management programs allow, computerized templates that make use of the written medical record can facilitate composition of a referral letter.

In the authors' opinion, communication with colleagues is one of the best tools for educating the veterinary profession and the public on the potential benefits of herbal medicine; this approach should be considered by all herbalists who are acting as a member of the medical team in modern veterinary medicine.

RECORDKEEPING AND ACCURACY OF DIAGNOSIS

Accurate medical records should include the following for each case: (1) diagnosis (traditional and conventional), (2) herbs and proportions of herbs used, (3) dose of each herb or formula, (4) duration of treatment, (5) concurrent medications, diet, and treatments, and (6) patient response to treatment (when available). The veterinary herbalist should also document a conventional diagnosis when possible before initiating herbal therapies, or should note whether the client has not allowed diagnostics for this purpose. This information, along with knowledge of the natural history of the disease, will assist the herbalist in distinguishing adverse reactions, therapeutic effects, and the natural course of the disease. Other nonconventional diagnostic systems may be used as an adjunct to the conventional diagnosis.

The veterinary herbalist should also be knowledgeable about current case reports that discuss possible toxicologic effects or risks of a given herbal treatment; alternatively, he or she should possess personal experience with the dosing and individual contraindications of an herb before recommending its use. The client should give informed consent for the use of herbs in the treatment of a pet; this should be noted in the patient record.

ADVERSE EVENT REPORTING

Any suspected adverse events should be reported to www.vbma.org for the purpose of building a database of veterinary herbal experience, which can then be communicated to veterinary herbalists.

CODE OF ETHICS

A code of ethics for veterinary herbalists and for veterinary herbal medicine prescribing has been developed and is available at www.vbma.org.

FUN

Practicing veterinary herbal medicine is challenging, rewarding, and exciting and offers the most fun one can have in practice. Seeing a patient, gathering information, analyzing it, prescribing, and then making the medicine brings together all the veterinary skills one possesses, including some new ones. The plethora of medicines that are now available as herbs suggests that the pharmacy has expanded 100-fold. The herbs smell fantastic, even if they do not taste great. The greatest fun for the herbalist happens when the patient returns and demonstrates change, usually in a positive direction. For many of those cases in which the only available option was long term prednisolone, cyclosporine, azathioprine, chemotherapy, or nothing, the veterinary herbalist now has much more to offer.

Good luck!

Materia Medica

CHAPTER

INTRODUCTION

Thousands of medicinal plants are in use around the world. We have chosen the herbs in this section with a variety of purposes in mind. Those that are supported by a great deal of evidence and deserve additional veterinary research are discussed in the greatest detail, but we have also included herbs that are popular among pet owners, even if professional herbalists do not use or recommend them. We have included herbs that have almost no supporting evidence but that are commonly found in urban and suburban environments, so that herbalists may begin to explore their native (or introduced and invasive) plants. Animals may also accidentally ingest these plants, which is another good reason for one to become familiar with their purported effects.

The monographs in this chapter are organized in the following way:

Common Name:

This is the most common name, as indicated in *Herbs of Commerce* (McGuffin, 2000), the official authority recognized by the U.S. Food and Drug Administration and by the Therapeutic Goods Administration, the group that regulates medicine in Australia.

Botanical Name:

This is the taxonomic classification, with authority, that is generally agreed to indicate the correct species used in commerce, according to information from *Herbs of Commerce*.

Distribution:

This information is provided so that herbalists may know which plants are native to their areas and what plants may be grown locally. Please note that if a plant is invasive (which we try to note in the "Notes of Interest" section), it should *not* be planted, even if it can be grown locally. On the other hand, if the "Notes" section indicates that the plant is threatened or endangered, the authors encourage herbalists to plant it in their gardens and encourage local growers to produce it, so that populations will be increased and pressure on wild populations reduced.

Similar Species:

Occasionally (but less often than one might guess), a number of species in a single genus may be used for similar medical conditions. Whenever we could identify this similarity, the other species are listed in this section.

Other Common Names:

These are names that have been used historically or in languages other than English. They may or may not be in common use at this time.

Family:

This is the taxonomic classification that indicates related plants on the basis of morphologic structure. Knowledge of the plant family may assist the herbalist in identifying plants in the wild or as fresh or dried specimens.

Parts Used:

All parts of the plants used for medicine (and in most cases, those used for food) are listed.

Collection:

In general, herbalists recommend that when the roots of a plant are used, it is best to collect in spring before growth has started (so as to take advantage of a winter-long process of storing energy and manufacturing unique constituents that reside there). Late autumn is also considered acceptable. When the aerial parts are used, harvest should be accomplished during the growing season and when the plant is in bloom, where applicable. Barks and resins are sometimes harvested with special instructions in accordance with the experience of the grower. In cases where exceptions to these rules and special instructions are available, they have been included in this section. This information is included to educate herbalists on the complexities of harvest and preparation, and to guide them should they choose to prepare their own herbs for personal use. However, in this text, high-quality liquid extracts and tinctures are recommended for ease of formulating and for their concentration, which allows small doses to be used in animals.

Selected Constituents:

We have elected to include the more individually unique constituents here, as opposed to listing every possible constituent that may occur in a plant. Be aware that in plant medicine, no one constituent can be singled out as "the active constituent," and, even if all of the vitamins, minerals, proteins, fixed fats, and sugars in a plant are not listed, these are important active constituents as well.

Clinical Actions:

These are the actions for which the herb is best known through long traditional use and recent research findings.

History and Traditional Usage:

Here, we have tried to trace the use of the herb from its earliest recorded history but have concentrated on the more descriptive written records from the 1600s onward. We rely heavily on the literature of the Eclectic and Physiomedical doctors from the 1850s (approximately) through the 1930s. We have also scanned the veterinary literature from the late 1700s through the 1950s to determine how the herb was used in animals. These sources are listed in the reference section after each herb (although each claim in the text of the monographs has not been referenced).

Energetics:

Chapter 5 contains more detailed information to which this subheading refers. Briefly, energetics describes the taste of the herb and the end clinical effects that it has on patients, according to traditional understanding of the herb. Energetic characteristics may include reference to Heat, Damp, Cold, and Phlegm, and to Traditional Chinese Medicine (TCM) organs such as Spleen, Liver, Kidney, Heart, and Stomach; reference is not made to Western medicine organs of the same name.

Published Research:

In the interest of brevity, we have elected to review the information available on herbs in the following way.

With few exceptions, we have not described in detail studies on isolated constituents. Herbalists believe that the whole plant has broadly based benefits, and that studies of the whole plant are more likely to shed light on the traditional uses that humankind has come to know over the past few millennia. However, if experimental studies tended to confirm a traditional use, we may include a brief note on the subject.

In vitro studies are not emphasized, unless the herb is used topically and is not significantly metabolized. Examples include herbs used for cutaneous or gastrointestinal applications. Whole plants are metabolized in vivo to produce effects that are complex and unpredictable compared with those noted in in vitro trials.

We have placed little emphasis on laboratory animal studies, except when they might prove useful for the treatment of pocket pets. The studies frequently involve artificial models, whereas genetically identical groups of animals in controlled environments are subjected to chemical or surgical changes to create a model of a naturally occurring human or animal disease. Because the results of these studies translate inconsistently to real-life patients, we have not discussed them in detail and have not always referenced them.

Many herbs (especially traditional Chinese herbs) are commonly administered in formulas. Because the effect of a formula is different from the effect of a single constituent herb, we have not emphasized studies in which an herb was investigated as part of a formula, unless a particularly relevant clinical trial in a companion food or animal species was available.

When controlled clinical trials in humans or domestic animals, or even case series involving clinical patients, are available, we have highlighted these reports.

Indications:

These indications are based on solid traditional uses and evidence-based findings.

Suggested Veterinary Indications:

These indications are based on solid traditional uses and on evidence-based findings, as well as on the authors' experience. We did not always agree on the potential use of individual herbs for some indications, but this controversy reflects the current state of herbal practice until additional scientific studies have been completed.

We have used evidence from clinical trials in humans as fair support for use of herbs in companion and farm animals. Although the principles of evidence-based medicine relegate research in other species to a low priority, we consider this to be better evidence than that acquired through laboratory animal research.

Notes of Interest:

This section contains various points of interest, such as historical minutiae and conservation status. Maude Grieve's book, *A Modern Herbal,* contains many interesting historical and botanical notes and is available online at www.botanical.com. For more information on invasive species, see www.invasive.org. For information on threatened or endangered species, see the following Web sites:

- Convention on International Trade on Endangered Species of Wild Fauna and Flora
  http://www.cites.org
- United Plant Savers
  http://www.unitedplantsavers.org
- TRAFFIC
  http://www.traffic.org
- National Center for the Preservation of Medicinal Plants
  http://home.frognet.net/~rural8/frames2.html
- Australian Environment Protection and Biodiversity Conservation Act of 1999
  List of endangered species provided at: http://www.deh.gov.au/cgi-bin/sprat/public/publicthreatenedlist.pl?wanted=flora
- The Australian Network for Plant Conservation
  http://www.anbg.gov.au/anpc/
- National Park Service Medicinal Plant Working Group
  http://www.nps.gov/plants/medicinal/plants.htm

Contraindications; Toxicology and Adverse Effects; Drug Interactions:

Aside from information on commonly recognized effects found in the general literature on any specific herb, two primary references were used for this section. The Botanical Safety Handbook, published by the American Herbal Products Association, is an important collection of safety grades that was published in 1997. The grading system used was based on a critical review of world literature and is defined as follows:

- **Class 1:** Herbs that can be safely consumed when used appropriately
- **Class 2:** Herbs for which the following use restrictions apply, unless otherwise directed by an expert who is qualified in the use of the described substance:
  2a: For external use only
  2b: Not for use during pregnancy
  2c: Not to be used while nursing
  2d: Other specific use restrictions as noted
- **Class 3:** Herbs for which significant data exist for recommendation of the following labeling: "To be used only under the supervision of an expert qualified in the appropriate use of this substance." Labeling must include proper information about dosage, contraindications, potential adverse effects, drug interactions, and any other relevant information related to safe use of the substance.
- **Class 4:** Herbs for which insufficient data are available to allow classification.

The other reference used was Herr's *Herb–Drug Interaction Handbook*. This book is a comprehensive collection of the adverse events, contraindications, and drug interactions thought to be associated with individual herbs. It is one of the more up-to-date references available at this writing. Unfortunately, much of the information contained is purely theoretical and is based on an understanding of isolated constituents of herbs. In this section, we have attempted to present practical cautions but also to modulate the potential misinformation that may result from this last reference. It is critical for the reader to understand, however, that domestic animals may have unique problems with individual herbs, and that as these come into clinical use, we may discover new and unusual adverse effects, contraindications, and drug interactions.

Preparation Notes:

When herb pharmacists have determined that a particular preparation is endowed with the most potent activity, and others less, we note it here.

Dosage:

In addition to small animal doses, we have provided human doses. This is because they are better understood than animal doses, but also because they help the practitioner to derive animal doses for various available forms. Wherever possible, we have included doses from old veterinary texts, but most small animal doses are based on the authors' experience or on extrapolations from a number of the texts listed below, under Selected References, as well as manufacturers' recommendations for products that we use in our practices.

The reader will find that dose ranges are very wide, and that human and animal doses vary widely when the calculated total dry herb equivalents (explained below) for all forms are compared. This is because no optimal dose has been established in many cases; thus, we chose to present recommended doses from various authorities and manufacturers, and information on the forms that they recommend or use. Even the authors do not agree on optimal doses at this time! It will be up to future practitioners and researchers to determine optimal doses within these ranges.

Various forms of herbs can usually be converted to a dry herb equivalent. A 1:1 fluid extract, for instance, contains the soluble constituents of 1 g (1000 mg) of dried herb in 1 mL of solvent. A 1:5 extract, therefore, would contain ⅕ of that amount, or 0.2 g (200 mg) per mL. For the most part, with generally safe herbs, the most concentrated tinctures are recommended here (1:2-1:3). If the reader can obtain only more dilute tinctures (1:5), then the doses listed should be increased by approximately 25% to 50%. For extracts made from fresh herbs, although the water content may tend to produce a more dilute final product, the lack of processing and resultant retention of undamaged constituents may compensate, making them as potent as, if not more potent, than tinctures made from dried herbs. Therefore, in practice, there is little reason to modify doses when tinctures made from fresh versus dried herb are used.

The reader will also note that dried herb doses may be substantially higher than expected when dried herb equivalents in the extract forms are compared, particularly when the dose is tripled or quadrupled, as is suggested for dried unprocessed herbs. This is to be expected because dried herbs deteriorate more quickly than most extracts, so higher doses may be necessary to compensate for this effect.

We would like to especially thank Dr. Eric Yarnell for his assistance in making sense of the widely varying dose recommendations in the human literature. He tends to use the highest doses described here. As a general rule of thumb, safe herbs tinctured at 1:2 or 1:3 concentration are given to *humans* at a dose of 3 to 5 mL 3 times daily—up to 6 times daily for acute conditions. Dried herbs are given at a dose of 3 to 10 g 3 times daily—up to 6 times daily for acute conditions. For chronic conditions, smaller doses are usually used. Infusions and decoctions are made by using 5 to 30 g of herb per cup of water, with 1 cup of the tea given 3 times a day—up to 6 times daily acutely. Our dose recommendations span the lowest doses recommended by more conservative authors up to these higher doses.

Similarly, a general rule for small animals is 0.5 to 1.5 mL per 10 kg (20 lb) total daily dose, divided into two or three doses (assuming a 1:2 to 1:3 tincture). A total daily dose of a multiple herbs in a formula can be calculated by selecting a dose in the the given range for each herb and adding all doses together. Select the higher dose for herbs with the primary desired action or effect. Then, simply multiply the individual herb volume by the number of doses needed to arrive at the formula; round up or down to make dispensing easy. For example, if the daily dose for an herb is 0.5 to 1.5 mL daily for a 10-kg dog, the prescriber will, for instance, select 1 mL. For 14 doses (or 2 weeks of treatment), 14 mL is required, which can be rounded up to 15 mL. If the patient is 20 kg, you will need 30 mL in the formula. Infusions are made as for humans (5-30 g per cup of water) and administered at a rate of ½ cup to 1 cup per 10 kg (20 lb) per day, divided and added to meals or given by mouth. Dried herb extracts (assuming they have been extracted, then dried) are generally between 25 and 75 mg per kg per day, but this depends on the individual product. For simple dried herb, up to 4 times this dose may be indicated.

Note that the very highest doses and more frequent administrations are used over the short term in acute conditions; lower doses are used for weaker patients for longer periods. Also, note that human dosing frequencies are optimally every 4 to 8 hours. The pet caretaker should be advised as to how to divide the daily dosage into as many daily doses as is practical; twice daily is usually readily achievable by adding herbs to food at meal times.

For herbs with a high safety profile, the higher dose of the range can be used. When herbs are given in combination, the lower dose of the range can be used for each herb, and the key herb might be used at the higher end. Clearly, the exact dose depends not only on the weight of the patient and the concentration of the extract, but also on the patient's sensitivity to medication and relative strength (in terms of digestive and metabolic capacities).

If the practitioner lacks experience with a particular herb, it is wise to start with the lowest recommended dose and increase slowly (to the higher dose in the range). Experienced herbalists may use much higher doses for specific herbs than given here for various reasons. In general, a formula with mutiple herbs is dosed at the lower end of the range for individual herbs (so that the total volume is easy to administer and to take into account synergy). When in doubt, the prescriber should counsel owners that the initial dose is a low starting dose, and that if no results are seen within a few days to a week, the dose may be increased. Chapter 14 provides additional information on dose calculation and administration of herbs.

Combinations:

Occasionally, we include this section, wherein combinations with other herbs are uniquely effective or commonly used.

Selected References:

References most relevant to practical use of these medicinal herbs are included in this section. These may consist of scientific citations, as well as books, book chapters, Internet manuals, and Web sites. Much more information than is referenced in this section was gathered to generate each monograph. The sources used most heavily for the Materia Medica are as follows:

Bone K. *A Clinical Guide to Blending Liquid Herbs.* Sydney: Churchill Livingstone; 2003.

Brinker F. *Complex Herbs, Complete Medicines.* Sandy, Ore: Eclectic Medical Publications; 2004.

Evans WC. *Trease and Evans Pharmacognosy.* 15th edition. Philadelphia: WB Saunders; 2002.

Felter HW, Lloyd JU. *King's American Dispensatory* (1898). Available at: http://www.henriettesherbal.com (provided free on the Web on Henriette Kress's Herbal Homepage).

Grieg JR, Boddie GF. *Hoare's Veterinary Materia Medica and Therapeutics.* 6th edition. London: Bailliere, Tindall and Cox; 1942.

Grieve M. *A Modern Herbal* (1931). New York: Barnes and Noble Books; 1996. Also available online at www.botanical.com.

Herr SM. Herb-Drug Interaction Handbook, 2nd ed. Enst E, Young VSL, eds. Church Street Books, Nassau, NY, 2002.

Hoffmann D. *Medical Herbalism.* Rochester, Vt: Healing Arts Press; 2003.

Karreman H. *Treating Dairy Cows Naturally: Thoughts and Strategies.* Paradise, Pa: Paradise Publications; 2004.

Kirk H. *Index of Treatment in Small-Animal Practice.* Baltimore, Md: Williams and Wilkins; 1948.

Kuhn M, Winston D. *Herbal Therapy and Supplements: A Scientific and Traditional Approach.* Philadelphia, Pa: Lippincott, Williams and Wilkins; 2001.

Marsden S. *Foundations in Formula Design: Achieving Balance and Synergy with Western Herbs.* Thesis presented to the Faculty of the Department of Classical Chinese Medicine, National College of Naturopathic Medicine, Portland, Ore, 2000.

McGuffin M, Hobbs C, Upton R, et al. *Botanical Safety Handbook.* Boca Raton, Fla: CRC Press; 1997.

McGuffin M, Kartesz JT, Leung AY, et al. *Herbs of Commerce.* 2nd edition. Silver Spring, Md: American Herbal Products Association; 2000.

Milks HJ. *Practical Veterinary Pharmacology, Materia Medica and Therapeutics.* 6th edition. Chicago, Ill: Alex Eger, Inc; 1949.

Mills S, Bone K. *Principles and Practice of Phytotherapy: Modern Herbal Medicine.* New York: Churchill Livingstone; 2000.

Moerman DE. *Native American Ethnobotany.* Portland, Ore: Timber Press; 1998.

Skenderi G. *Herbal Vade Mecum: 800 Herbs, Spices, Essential Oils, Lipids, Etc. Constituents, Properties, Uses and Caution.* Rutherford, NJ: Herbacy Press; 2004.

Tierra M. *Planetary Herbology.* Twin Lakes, Wis: Lotus Press; 1988.

Van Wyk B-E, Wink M. *Medicinal Plants of the World: An Illustrated Scientific Guide to Important Medicinal Plants and Their Uses.* Pretoria, South Africa: Briza Publications; 2004.

Weiss RF. *Herbal Medicine.* Translated from the German 6th edition. Beaconsfield, England: Beaconsfield Publishers, Ltd; 1994.

Wichtl M. In: Bisset NG, ed. *Herbal Drugs and Phytopharmaceuticals: A Handbook for Practice on a Scientific Basis.* (English language edition, 1994.) Boca Raton, Fla: CRC Press; 1989.

Williamson EM, ed. *Major Herbs of Ayurveda.* United Kingdom: Churchill Livingstone; 2002.

Winslow K. *Veterinary Materia Medica and Therapeutics.* 6th edition. New York: William R. Jenkins Co; 1909.

Yarnell E. *Clinical Botanical Medicine.* Larchmont, NY: Mary Ann Liebert, Inc; 2003.

In addition, the following websites were indispensable and should be bookmarked on the reader's computer:

- Veterinary Botanical Medicine Association
  www.vbma.org
- Henriette's Herbal Homepage
  http://www.henriettesherbal.com
- Southwest School of Botanical Medicine
  www.swsbm.com
- Medline, of the National Library of Medicine
  www.pubmed.org
- David Winston's Herbal Therapeutics Research Library
  http://www.herbaltherapeutics.net/herbal_therapeutics_library.htm
- Veterinary Medicines Summary Reports from the European Medicines Agency
  http://www.emea.eu.int/index/indexv1.htm

Agrimony

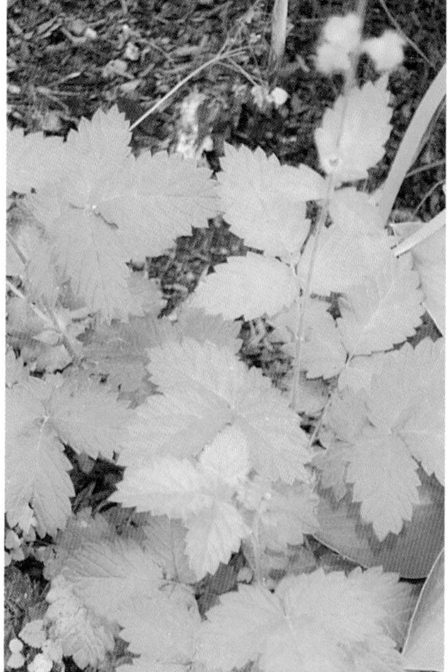

Agrimonia eupatoria • Agim-MOH-nee-uh yew-pat-TOH-ree-uh

Other Names: Church steeples, sticklewort, cockeburr, *Agrimoniae herba*. Should be distinguished from unrelated species known as hemp agrimony *(Eupatorium cannabinum)* and water agrimony *(Bidens tripartita)*. *Agrimonia pilosa* is a related plant used in Traditional Chinese Medicine.

Family: Rosaceae

Parts Used: Aerial parts

Selected Constituents: Tannins (up to 21%), flavonoids, triterpenes, coumarins, glycosidal bitters, polysaccharides

Clinical Actions: Astringent, antidiarrheal, antimicrobial, anti-inflammatory, hemostatic, mild choleretic, mild diuretic

Energetics: Slightly bitter, astringent, warm; affects primarily lung, liver, spleen (Tierra)

History and Traditional Usage: Grieve (1931) claims that sheep and goats eat the plant, but cattle, horses, and swine do not. Used since medieval times for wounds of all sorts and snakebites, this plant is an astringent antidiarrheal. Native American tribes used a native species *(Agrimonia gryposepala)* for similar purposes when astringents were called for—for diarrhea, for skin eruptions, as a styptic, and so forth. It has been used for a "relaxed throat" (in physiomedical philosophy) and has been used since the time of Dioscorides for liver problems. This astringent is also used for cystitis and urinary incontinence. Agrimony is considered when copious mucous secretions emerge from any mucous membrane.

Published Research: Older clinical trials using formulas containing agrimony in humans point to possible benefit in chronic gastroduodenitis and in cutaneous porphyria.

Potential Veterinary Indications: Acute diarrhea and gastritis. Hemorrhagic cystitis. May be useful for dogs with seasonal allergies that manifest as reverse sneezing and snoring. Stomatitis/gingivitis—as a mouthwash. Orally and topically (as a compress or dressing) for indolent ulcers, skin eruptions, and slowly healing wounds.

Contraindications: Pregnancy and lactation are usually listed as contraindications.

Toxicology and Adverse Effects: American Herbal Products Association (AHPA) class 1. *Potential but not reported*—photodermatitis and photosensitivity; acts as a hypoglycemic agent according to a single laboratory animal study and may complicate glycemic control in diabetics. Contains coumarins, so coagulation problems may surface during concurrent use with anticoagulant drugs.

Potential Drug Interactions: Theoretical interactions with hypoglycemic drugs and anticoagulants have been suggested.

Dosage:

Human:

Dried herb: 1-10 g TID, up to 6 times daily for acute conditions

Infusions and decoctions: 5-15 g per cup of water, with ¼-1 cup of the tea given TID, up to 6 times daily acutely

Tincture (commonly 35%-45% alcohol; some pharmacies use some glycerin to prevent precipitation by tannins): 1:2 or 1:3: 1-5 mL TID, up to 6 times daily for acute conditions

Small Animal:

Dried herb: 25-300 mg/kg divided daily (optimally TID)

Infusion: 5 g per cup of water, administered at a rate of ¼-½ cup per 10 kg (20 lb), divided daily (optimally TID)

Tincture (commonly 35%-45% alcohol; some pharmacies use some glycerin to prevent tannin precipitation): 1:2-1:3: 0.5-1.5 mL per 10 kg (20 lb), divided daily (optimally TID) and diluted or combined with other herbs for up to 1 week. Higher doses may be appropriate if the herb is used singly and is not combined in a formula.

Combinations: David Hoffmann suggests use with carminatives for gastrointestinal (GI) problems. It has also been used with yarrow for bladder inflammation and hematuria.

Selected Reference

Grieve M. *A Modern Herbal*. London: C.F. Leyel; 1931.

Albizia

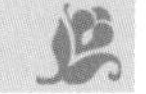

Albizia lebbeck [L.] Benth. • Al-BIZ-ee-uh LEB-ek

Other Names: Siris, siris tree, albizzia, pit shirish

Family: Fabaceae

Parts Used: Stem bark, leaves, and seeds (flowers also used)

Distribution: Albizia is a large deciduous tree common throughout India and used as an ornamental tree elsewhere.

Selected Constituents: Saponins, cardiac glycosides, tannins, flavonoids

Clinical Actions: Antiallergic, antimicrobial, anticholesterolemic

Energetics: Cooling, dry

History and Traditional Usage: It has been used for bronchitis, leprosy, paralysis, and helminth infections and by Ayurvedic physicians for bronchial asthma and eczema. Albizia seeds have been used in the treatment of patients with diarrhea and dysentery. The leaves are nutritious and palatable and can be used as fodder.

Published Research: Albizia has antidiarrheal activity, which supports the historical use of the seeds in the treatment of patients with diarrhea and dysentery. An extract potentiated the activity of loperamide (1 mg/kg intraperitoneally [ip]). Naloxone (0.5 mg/kg ip) significantly inhibited the antidiarrheal activity as well as the loperamide did, suggesting a role in the opioid system (Besra, 2002). Albizia has some nootropic activity involving monoamine neurotransmitters (Chintawar, 2002). The antiallergic activity of albizia was investigated, showing a significant action on mast cells and inhibiting early sensitization and synthesis of reaginic-type antibodies. The active ingredients of the bark appear to be heat stable and water soluble (Tripathi, 1979).

Indications: Albizia is reported to have antiseptic, antidysenteric, and antitubercular properties. It is indicated for use in asthma, allergic rhinitis, eczema, urticaria, and high cholesterol.

Potential Veterinary Indications: Allergic bronchitis, allergic skin disease, mast cell tumors

Toxicology and Adverse Effects: May depress T and B lymphocyte activity. Some data suggest an antifertility effect in animals.

Potential Drug Interactions: Caution with inotropic heart medications—may be synergistic

Dosage:

Human:

Dried herb: 3-10 g TID

Tincture: 1:2 or 1:3: 1-5 mL TID

Small Animal:

Dried herb: 25-200 mg/kg, divided daily (optimally TID)

Tincture: 1:2-1:3: 0.5-1.0 mL per 10 kg (20 lb), divided daily (optimally TID) and diluted or combined with other herbs

References

Besra SE, Gomes A, Chaudhury L, Vedasiromoni JR, Ganguly DK. Antidiarrhoeal activity of seed extract of *Albizzia lebbeck* Benth. Phytother Res 2002;16:529-533.

Chintawar SD, Somani RS, Kasture VS, Kasture SB. Nootropic activity of *Albizzia lebbeck* in mice. J Ethnopharmacol 2002; 81:299-305.

Tripathi RM, Sen PC, Das PK. Studies on the mechanism of action of *Albizzia lebbeck*, an Indian indigenous drug used in the treatment of atopic allergy. J Ethnopharmacol 1979;1:385-396.

Alfalfa

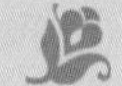

Medicago sativa L. • Med-DIK-ah-go sa-TEE-vuh

Other Names: Lucerne, luzerne, Spanish clover

Family: Fabaceae

Parts Used: Leaf used medicinally. Sprouted seeds used as food.

Selected Constituents: Proteins, cellulose, triterpenoid saponins, phytosterols, flavonoids, coumarins, amino acids, chlorophyll, carotenoids, vitamins, minerals, organic acids, porphyrins

Clinical Actions: Nutritive

Energetics: Sweet, pungent, cool; nourishes Yin, moistens dryness (Marsden)

History and Traditional Usage: Used mostly as food.

Published Research: No relevant clinical trials found.

Indications: Generally used as a nutritional supplement. Has been used as a source of phytoestrogens in the treatment of women with hot flashes in menopause. Is a recognized estrogenic agent in ruminants.

Potential Veterinary Indications: As a source of vitamins, minerals, flavonoids, and amino acids for chronically ill or geriatric animals.

Contraindications: In humans, pharmacognosists warn against using the herb in the presence of estrogen receptor–positive tumors because of the potential estrogen-like effects of coumarins and isoflavones (daidzein and formononetin). The amino acid canavanine (in sprouts) has been implicated in causing flare-ups of lupus.

Toxicology and Adverse Effects: None reported. AHPA class 1. Generally recognized as safe (GRAS) classification by U.S. Food and Drug Administration (FDA).

Potential Drug Interactions: Theoretical interactions have been suggested with estrogenic drugs, anticoagulants, lipid-lowering drugs, hypoglycemic drugs, and drugs or herbs that induce photosensitivity.

Preparation Notes: Dried herb usually has a very acceptable taste to dogs and cats.

Dosage:

Human:

Dried herb: 1-10 g TID

Infusions and decoctions: 5-30 g per cup of water, with 1 cup of the tea given TID, up to 6 times daily acutely

Tincture (usually prepared in 35% ethanol): 1:2 or 1:3: 1.5-5 mL TID, up to 6 times daily for acute conditions

Small Animal:

Dried herb: 50-500 mg/kg, divided daily (optimally TID)

Infusion: 5-30 g per cup of water, administered at a rate of ¼-½ cup per 10 kg (20 lb), divided daily (optimally TID)

Tincture: 1:2-1:3: 1.0-2.5 mL per 10 kg (20 lb), divided daily (optimally TID) and diluted or combined with other herbs. This is a very safe herb that can be used at higher doses as a single prescription.

Aloe

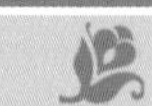

Aloe vera (L.) Burm. f., or its synonym, *Aloe barbadensis* Mill • AL-oh VER-uh *or* AL-oh bar-buh-DEN-sis

Also:

Aloe ferox Mill

Aloe perryi Baker (socotrine aloes)

Distribution: Native to Africa and introduced and naturalized in the Mediterranean region, the tropics, and warmer areas of the world, including America, Central America, Asia, China, and India.

Similar Species: *Aloe chinensis, Aloe elongata, Aloe indica, Aloe officinalis, Aloe perfoliata, Aloe rubescens*

Common Names: *Aloe capensis, aloe curacao,* Barbados aloe, cape aloe, Curaçao aloe, star cactus, aloès vrai, laloi, ecte aloe, sábila

Family: Aloaceae

Parts Used: Aloe vera gel is the viscous, colorless, transparent liquid from the inside of the leaf. Aloe vera juice arises from juice in the cells of the pericycle and adjacent leaf parenchyma and flows spontaneously from the cut leaf; it is usually dried. To obtain aloe gel, the leaf is processed and aloin is removed. The cape aloes preparation consists of dried latex from bundle sheath cells within the leaf, which is high in hydroxyanthrone derivatives of aloe emodin (such as aloin) and is the source of laxative preparations.
Constituents: Aloe vera gel consists primarily of water and polysaccharides (glucomannan, acemannan, mannose derivatives, pectin, hemicelluloses), as well as amino acids, lipids, sterols (campesterol, B-sitosterol, lupeol), and enzymes (Bruneton, 1995). Mannose-6-phosphate is a major sugar component (Davis, 1994). Cinnamoyl, p-coumaroyl, feruloyl, caffeoyl aloesin, and related compounds have been isolated from *Aloe* species. Aloe latex contains as its major and active principles hydroxyanthrone derivatives (Bruneton, 1995).

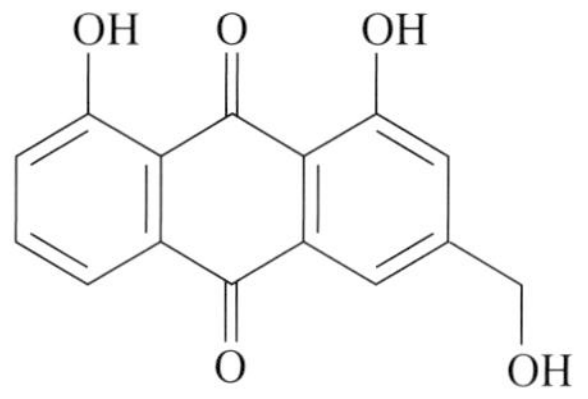

OH O OH

O OH

Emodin

Clinical Actions: Demulcent, vulnerary, stimulant laxative
Energetics: Gel slightly bitter; juice sour and very bitter
History and Traditional Usage: Aloe vera was used in the Middle East and Egypt as early as 1500 BC; it has been used for centuries as a topical treatment for various conditions and as a cathartic. Aloe vera gel is widely used for the external treatment of wounds, burns, and skin inflammation. Aloe vera has been described in folk medicine for a wide range of indications, including the treatment of patients with seborrheic dermatitis, peptic ulcer, tuberculosis, fungal infection, psoriasis, anemia, glaucoma, and blindness (WHO, 1999). American Eclectic doctors used aloe as a tonic, purgative, emmenagogue, and anthelmintic. The specific indication for its use was as follows: "Atony of large intestine and rectum, mucoid discharges, prolapsus ani, pruritis ani, ascaris vermicularis . . . difficulty in evacuating the lower bowel."

Modern clinical use of the gel began in the 1930s, with reports of successful treatment of x-ray and radium burns, which led to additional experimental studies that used laboratory animals in subsequent decades (Grindlay, 1986).

Modern veterinary usage was first reported in 1975 (Northway, 1975); however, in Europe, it was a popular ingredient of physic balls and was used in combination with ginger as a purgative for horses; it was used for horses that were coming off grass to undergo training. It was also a common ingredient in "condition" balls used to condition a horse for training, to aid assimilation of food, to improve skin, and to help condition the coat. Also used for the treatment of colic in horses (RCVS, 1920). In dogs, aloe was incorporated into "alterative balls" and condition pills (RCVS, 1920). Milks (1949) recommended aloe for whenever a "good brisk cathartic" is required, for instance, in "colic, hidebound, overloaded stomach or bowels, to expel worms after a vermicide, to promote excretion of waste products from the bowels and blood," or as a tonic. He also recommended it to stimulate wound healing and suggested that ruminants were less sensitive to it than horses, and that dogs and cats required as much as 5 to 10 times the dose a human should take!

It has been advocated for the treatment of farm animals with constipation, indigestion, worms, and urinary ailments and externally for the cure of corneal ulcers and keratitis (de Bairacli Levy, 1963). Aloe was used as a purgative for horses; it was also used in veterinary practice as a bitter tonic (in small doses) and "externally as a stimulant and desiccant" (Grieves, 1931). *Aloe nuttii* has been used to treat Newcastle's disease in poultry, worms, and dystocia; *Aloe perfoliata* has been used to treat pneumonia in livestock (Kambewa, 1997). *Aloe vera* is one of four major medical plants used to treat health problems in poultry in Trinidad and Tobago (Lans, 1998).

Published Research:

Laxative effect

Aloe's laxative mechanism of action is twofold. The juice (not the gel) stimulates colonic motility, augmenting propulsion and accelerating colonic transit, which reduces fluid absorption from the fecal mass and increases the water content in the large intestine (de Witte, 1993). The laxative effects are due to the glycosides aloin A and B (formerly known as barbaloin). These are hydrolyzed in the colon by intestinal bacteria and then reduced to active metabolites, which act as stimulants and irritants to the GI tract. The laxative effect of aloe is generally not observed before 6 hours after oral administration, and sometimes not until 24 hours or longer after administration (WHO, 1999).

Wound healing activity

Clinical studies indicate that aloe vera gel accelerates wound healing, and in vivo studies demonstrate that it promotes wound healing by directly stimulating macrophage and fibroblast activity (Davis, 1994). It is suggested that the polysaccharide mannose is responsible for the wound healing properties of the gel (Davis, 1994).

Other mechanisms of action include the hydrating, insulating, and protective properties of the gel (Bruneton, 1995). The gel inhibits thromboxane A2, a mediator of progressive tissue damage (Davis, 1994) produced in burned dermal tissue and pressure sores (Swaim, 1987, 1992). Angiogenesis is essential in wound healing, and the gel has been shown to be angiogenic (Moon, 1999). The constituent allantoin enhances epithelialization in suppurating wounds and resistant ulcers (Swaim, 1992). Another constituent, acemannan, stimulates macrophages to produce the cytokines interleukin-1 and tumor necrosis factor, which, in turn, stimulate angiogenesis, epithelialization, and wound healing (Cera, 1980). It also has anti-inflammatory and analgesic activities because of the presence of a salicylate-like substance (Swaim, 1987).

The effects of topical aloe gel have been compared with the therapeutic effects of systemic pentoxifylline in the treatment of frostbite on the ears of 10 New Zealand white rabbits. Pentoxifylline improved tissue survival (20%), as did aloe vera cream (24%), and the combination of both was best (30%) (Miller, 1995). Another study showed a 62.5% reduction in wound diameter in mice (with induced biopsy punch wounds) that received 100 mg/kg/day oral aloe, and a 50.8% reduction was recorded in animals that were given topical 25% aloe. These data suggest that aloe is effective through both oral and topical routes of administration (Davis, 1989).

Swaim (1992) compared the effects of aloe vera gel with those of triple antibiotic ointment on footpad wounds in dogs. Beagles were anesthetized, and a full-thickness 0.7-cm square defect was incised on one pad of each rear limb. In 12 dogs, one defect was treated with a dressing of aloe vera gel, and the other was treated with a dressing of triple antibiotic ointment. Three control dogs received no treatment. Monitoring of wound size occurred on days 7, 14, and 21. Although no differences were observed in wound size on days 14 and 21, the aloe-treated wounds were smaller on day 7. Compared with outcomes in controls, both treatments resulted in faster healing at day 14; however, control wounds were equivalent in size to treated wounds by day 21. Investigators concluded that aloe vera gel appears to stimulate early wound healing.

Inflammatory bowel disease

A double-blind, randomized, placebo-controlled trial of the efficacy and safety of aloe vera gel 100 mL twice daily was conducted for 4 weeks for the treatment of mildly to moderately active ulcerative colitis in humans. It produced a clinical response more often than placebo; it also reduced histologic disease activity and appeared to be safe (Langmead, 2004).

Ophthalmic activity

A study using pig cornea showed that biologically active aloe substances could not penetrate this biological barrier. Therefore, eyedrops that contain aloe and neomycin sulfate may be useful for the treatment of inflammation and infection of external parts of the eye, such as the conjuctiva, eyelid edges, lacrimal sac, and cornea (Kodym, 2002).

Burn treatment

Aloe vera inhibited the inflammatory process following burn injury in rats (Duansak, 2003) and promoted wound healing in second-degree burns in rats (Somboonwong, 2000). Aloe vera gel–treated guinea pigs with induced burns healed in 30 days compared with 50 days for controls and silver sulfadiazine and salicylic cream–treated animals (Rodriguez-Bigas, 1988). In a human placebo-controlled study, aloe vera gel–treated lesions healed faster (11.8 days) than burns treated with petroleum jelly gauze (18.2 days) (Visuthikosol, 1995). However, the aloe preparation may influence healing, as one preparation of aloe vera gel hindered the healing process of a burn wound model when compared with 1% silver sulfadiazine cream (Kaufman, 1988).

Antithyroid activity

Aloe vera (125 mg/kg) was investigated for the regulation of thyroid hormone concentrations in male mice. Serum levels of both triiodothyronine (T3) and thyroxine (T4) were inhibited by aloe; it was suggested that aloe may be used in the regulation of hyperthyroidism (Kar, 2002).

Grass sickness in horses

Brotizolam, acetylcysteine, and aloe vera gel were evaluated as ancillary treatments for 29 cases of equine grass sickness. None of the treatments had any significant beneficial effect on the survival of horses (Fintl, 2002).

Acemannan activity

Acemannan is the major carbohydrate fraction of the gel. Its therapeutic properties include acceleration of wound healing, inhibition of inflammation, and antiviral effects. It has also been shown to have antitumor activity; injection of acemannan has been shown to offer increased immune protection against implanted malignant tumor cells (Merriam, 1995). Acemannan in the presence of interferon-γ induces apoptosis in cancer cells (Ramamoorthy, 1998).

Acemannan and tumors in cats and dogs

Acemannan is believed to be an immunostimulant and is licensed by the U.S. Department of Agriculture (USDA) for the treatment of fibrosarcoma in dogs and cats. In an uncontrolled study, eight dogs and five cats with confirmed fibrosarcoma were treated with acemannan in combination with surgery and radiation therapy. These animals had recurring disease despite treatment, a poor prognosis for survival, or both. Of 13 animals, 7 remained alive and tumor free (range, 440+ to 603+ days) with a median survival time of 372 days. The authors suggested that an acemannan immunostimulant may be an effective adjunct to surgery and radiation therapy in the treatment of canine and feline fibrosarcoma (King, 1995).

In another uncontrolled study, 43 dogs and cats with spontaneous tumors were treated with acemannan administered through intraperitoneal and intralesional routes. Histopathology of tumors from 26 of these animals showed marked necrosis or lymphocytic infiltration. In all, 12 animals showed clinical improvement as assessed by tumor shrinkage, tumor necrosis, or prolonged survival; these included 5 of 7 animals with fibrosarcoma (Harris, 1991).

Acemannan and feline leukemia

Feline leukemia infection in persistently viremic cats can cause myeloproliferative disease, lymphoma, and ultimately, death. In a trial of symptomatic cats younger than 4 years of age, 2 mg of acemannan was administered intraperitoneally for 6 weeks. It significantly improved both quality of life and survival time for the 3 months of the trial (Sheets, 1991). This trial included historical controls because participating clients refused to allow placebo treatment in their sick cats. Treated cats showed nonsignificant rises in hematocrit and hemoglobin concentrations, and leukocyte and lymphocyte counts tended to normalize over the course of the trial.

Acemannan and feline immunodeficiency virus

Acemannan also has demonstrated antiviral activity in vitro against human immunodeficiency virus, Newcastle's disease virus, and influenza virus. A pilot study investigated the effects of acemannan in 49 feline immunodeficiency virus (FIV)-infected, symptomatic cats, 23 of which had severe lymphopenia. Acemannan was administered to cats by mouth daily, or intravenous or subcutaneous injection was provided once weekly for 12 weeks. The route of administration made no significant difference in efficacy among groups. A significant increase in lymphocyte count and a reduction in neutrophil count and in incidence of sepsis were observed over time. Cats that had lymphopenia on entering the trial were analyzed separately, and a much greater increase in lymphocyte counts was noted (235%) compared with nonlymphopenic cats (42%). The survival rate for all three groups was 75%. Of cats studied, 73% were alive 5 to 19 months post study entry. Acemannan therapy may be of benefit in FIV-infected cats that exhibit clinical signs of disease (Yates, 1992); however, FIV-infected cats are expected to live 8 or more years without treatment, so the clinical benefit of using acemannan to extend life expectancy is uncertain.

Acemannan and viral disease in chickens

Reovirus and infectious bursal disease virus are among the naturally occurring viruses that cause immunesuppression in chickens. They both cause necrotic lesions in the bursa of Fabricius and may destroy B cells, and both inhibit the mitogenic response of T cells. Early studies showed that pretreatment of chickens with acemannan reduced reovirus-induced inhibition of T cells (Sharma, 1994).

Acemannan has been shown to be an effective adjuvant in the vaccination of chickens against some avian viral diseases. It was able to produce a rapid and lasting increase in the activation capacity of macrophages (in particular, from the blood and spleen) after intramuscular inoculation in chickens (500 μg per 2-month-old bird). (Djeraba, 2000).

Acemannan and vaccination

An acemannan adjuvant formulation was compared with several others for the ability to potentiate primary and memory antibody responses in mice. Acemannan was not effective in increasing responses to feline leukemia virus (FeLV) and FIV, but it did increase primary response to the heartworm antigen more than 10-fold compared with control levels (Usinger, 1997).

Potential Veterinary Indications:

Aloe Vera Gel:

- Externally and internally, following surgery to aid wound healing. Allergies, eczema, abscesses, fungal infections, pyoderma, many types of dermatitis
- Conjunctivitis and keratitis (topically)
- Herpes conjunctivitis in cats (topically)
- Gingivitis, periodontal disease, extraction sites, acute mouth lesions, glossitis (topically)

Acemannan:

- FIV, feline leukemia
- Feline hyperthryroidism
- Fibrosarcoma and other tumors
- Adjuvant for vaccination
- Reoviruses in poultry

Aloe Juice:

- Uncomplicated constipation

Notes of Interest: Aloe is used as an ingredient in aquarium water conditioners.

Contraindications: Aloe-containing products for constipation should be used only when no effect can be attained through diet change or the use of bulk-forming products. Stimulant laxatives should not be used when abdominal pain, nausea, or vomiting is present, or in patients with intestinal obstruction or stenosis, atony, dehydration, or chronic constipation; nor should it be used for inflammatory intestinal disease (unlike the gel). It is also contraindicated in patients with cramps, colic, hemorrhoids, nephritis, or undiagnosed abdominal symptoms. Long-term use may cause dependence, electrolyte disturbances, and atonic colon.

NOTE: Laxatives that contain anthraquinone glycosides should not be used continuously or during pregnancy.

Toxicology and Adverse Effects:

Gel: AHPA class 1 for internal use, and AHPA class 2d for external use because of a reputation for delaying wound healing following laparotomy

Aloes (dried juice from pericyclic region of the leaves): AHPA classes 2b, 2c, and 2d

A few reports of contact dermatitis and burning skin sensations have been documented following topical application of aloe vera gel to dermabraded skin, probably associated with anthraquinone contaminants in the preparation (WHO, 1999). Dried aloe is a cathartic. Milks (1949) claimed that large doses "congest the pelvic viscera, irritate the rectum, and may cause abortion." *The Botanical Safety Handbook* lists that as little as 1 g given daily for several days has been reported to cause colon perforation, bleeding diarrhea, and kidney damage.

Acemannan was administered intravenously or intraperitoneally as a 1.0-mg/mL solution to mice, rats, and dogs. No significant signs of intoxication or deaths occurred in animals treated with a single injection of acemannan at dosages of 80 mg/kg IV or 200 mg/kg IP in mice, 15 mg/kg IV or 50 mg/kg IP in rats, and 10 mg/kg IV or 50 mg/kg IP in dogs (Fogelman, 1992a, 1992b). Acemannan was administered orally to rats for 14 days at 5% of the diet, for 6 months at up to 2000 mg/kg/day, and to beagle dogs for 90 days at up to 1500 mg/kg/day without significant effect on any parameter measured in either species (Fogleman, 1992).

Drug Interactions: Decreased intestinal transit time with aloe juice may reduce absorption of orally administered drugs. Hypokalemia from long-term use can potentiate cardiotonic glycosides and antiarrhythmic drugs. The induction of hypokalemia by diuretics, adrenocorticosteroids, and licorice root may be enhanced.

Preparation Notes: Fresh aloe vera gel is recommended for external use. Harvest leaves, and wash them with water. Remove the outer layers of the leaf, including the pericyclic cells, leaving a "fillet" of gel. Care should be taken not to tear the green rind, which can contaminate the gel with leaf exudates. Some herbalists simply cut a leaf and send it home with the owner to make fresh cuts daily. The yellow gel in the pericyclic tubules is dried into a red black mass and is used internally as a laxative.

Dosage:

External Use:

Fresh gel: may be applied topically as directed; when taken directly from a plant, the leaf should be cut lengthwise and the gel scraped out and applied

Juice: may be applied topically; because it degrades quickly, many herbalists simply keep an aloe plant in the office.

Internal use:

Human

Juice from leaf: 10-30 mL TID

Latex, dried: 500-1000 mg at bedtime (use for no longer than 10 days consecutively). (**Note:** The smallest amount needed for the desired effect is the correct dose!)

Acemannan: 500-1000 mg TID

Small Animals:

Juice from leaf: 0.5-1.5 mL per kg, divided daily

Acemannan: 15-30 mg/kg, divided daily

Tincture: 1:2-1:3: 0.5 mL per 10 kg (20 lb), divided daily (optimally TID) and diluted or combined with other herbs

References

Bruneton J. *Pharmacognosy, Phytochemistry, Medicinal Plants.* Paris: Lavoisier; 1995.

Cera LM, Heggers JP, Robson MC, et al. The therapeutic efficacy of *Aloe vera* cream (Dermaide aloe) in thermal injuries: two reports. J Am Anim Hosp Assoc 1980;16:768-772.

Davis RH, Leitner MG, Russo JM, Byrne ME.Wound healing. Oral and topical activity of Aloe vera. J Am Podiatr Med Assoc 1989;79:559-562.

de Bairacli Levy J. *Herbal Handbook for Farm and Stable.* London: Faber and Faber Limited; 1963.

de Witte P. Metabolism and pharmacokinetics of anthranoids. Pharmacology 1993;47(suppl 1):86-97.

Djeraba A, Quere P. In vivo macrophage activation in chickens with acemannan, a complex carbohydrate extracted from Aloe vera. Int J Immunopharmacol 2000;22:365-372.

Duansak D, Somboonwong J, Patumraj S. Effects of Aloe vera on leukocyte adhesion and TNF-alpha and IL-6 levels in burn wounded rats. Clin Hemorrheol Microcirc 2003;29:239-246.

Fintl C, McGorum BC. Evaluation of three ancillary treatments in the management of equine grass sickness. Vet Rec 2002;151: 381-383.

Fogleman RW, Shellenberger TE, Balmer MF, Carpenter RH, McAnalley BH. Subchronic oral administration of acemannan in the rat and dog. Vet Hum Toxicol 1992a;34:144-147.

Fogleman RW, Chapdelaine JM, Carpenter RH, McAnalley BH. Toxicologic evaluation of injectable acemannan in the mouse, rat and dog. Vet Hum Toxicol 1992b;34:201-205.

Grieve M. *A Modern Herbal.* London: Johnathan Cape; 1931 (Reprint 1975).

Grindlay D, Reynolds T. The Aloe vera phenomenon: a review of the properties and modern uses of the leaf parenchyma gel. J Ethnopharmacol 1986;16:117-151.

Harris C, Pierce K, King G, Yates KM, Hall J, Tizard I. Efficacy of acemannan in treatment of canine and feline spontaneous neoplasms. Mol Biother 1991;3:207-213.

Kambewa BM, Mfitilodze MW, Hüttner H, Wollny CB, Phoya RK. The use of indigenous veterinary remedies in Malawi in ethnoveterinary medicine: alternatives for livestock development. Proceedings of International Conference; November 4-6, 1997; Pune, India.

Kar A, Panda S, Bharti S. Relative efficacy of three medicinal plant extracts in the alteration of thyroid hormone concentrations in male mice. J Ethnopharmacol 2002;81:281-285.

Kaufman T, Kalderon N, Ullmann Y, Berger J. Aloe vera gel hindered wound healing of experimental second-degree burns: a quantitative controlled study. J Burn Care Rehabil 1988;9: 156-159.

King GK, Yates KM, Greenlee PG, et al. The effect of acemannan immunostimulant in combination with surgery and radiation therapy on spontaneous canine and feline fibrosarcomas. J Am Anim Hosp Assoc 1995;31:439-447.

Kodym A, Grzeskowiak E, Partyka D, Marcinkowski A, Kaczynska-Dyba E. Biopharmaceutical assessment of eye drops containing aloe (*Aloe arborescens* Mill.) and neomycin sulphate. Acta Pol Pharm 2002;59:181-186.

Langmead L, Feakins RM, Goldthorpe S, et al. Randomized, double-blind, placebo-controlled trial of oral aloe vera gel for active ulcerative colitis. Aliment Pharmacol Ther 2004;19: 739-747.

Lans C, Brown G. Observations on ethnoveterinary medicines in Trinidad and Tobago. Prev Vet Med 1998;35:125-142.

Merriam EA, Campbell BD, Flood LP, Welsh CJR, McDaniel HR, Busbee DL. Enhancement of immune function in rodents using a complex plant carbohydrate which stimulates macrophage secretion of immunoreactive cytokines. In: Klatz RM, ed. *Advances in Anti-Aging Medicine,* vol 1. Larchmont, New York: Mary Ann Liebert, Inc.; 1995:181-203.

Miller MB, Koltai PJ. Treatment of experimental frostbite with pentoxifylline and aloe vera cream. Arch Otolaryngol Head Neck Surg 1995;121:678-680.

Moon EJ, Lee YM, Lee OH, et al. A novel angiogenic factor derived from Aloe vera gel: beta-sitosterol, a plant sterol. Angiogenesis 1999;3:117-123.

Northway RB. Experimental use of aloe vera extract in clinical practice. Vet Med Small Anim Clin 1975;70:89.

Ramamoorthy L, Tizard IR. Induction of apoptosis in a macrophage cell line RAW 264.7 by acemannan, a β-(1,4)-acetylated mannan. 1998;53:415-421.

RCVS, Royal College of Veterinary Surgeons. *Veterinary Counter Practice: A Treatise on the Diseases of Animals and the Most Suitable Remedies for Them.* London: Ballantyne Press; 1920.

Rodriguez-Bigas M, Cruz NI, Suarez A. Comparative evaluation of aloe vera in the management of burn wounds in guinea pigs. Plast Reconstr Surg 1988;81:386-389.

Sharma JM, Karaca K, Pertile T. Virus-induced immunosuppression in chickens. Poult Sci 1994;73:1082-1086.

Sheets MA, Unger BA, Giggleman GF Jr, Tizard IR. Studies of the effect of acemannan on retrovirus infections: clinical stabilization of feline leukemia virus–infected cats. Mol Biother 1991;3:41-45.

Somboonwong J, Thanamittramanee S, Jariyapongskul A, Patumraj S. Therapeutic effects of Aloe vera on cutaneous microcirculation and wound healing in second degree burn model in rats. J Med Assoc Thai 2000;83:417-425.

Swaim SF, Lee AH. Topical wound medications: a review. J Am Vet Med Assoc 1987;190:1588-1593.

Swaim SF, Riddell KP, McGuire JA. Effects of topical medications on the healing of open pad wounds in dogs. J Am Anim Hosp Assoc 1992;28:499-502.

Usinger WR. A comparison of antibody responses to veterinary vaccine antigens potentiated by different adjuvants. Vaccine 1997;15:1902-1907.

Visuthikosol V, Chowchuen B, Sukwanarat Y, Sriurairatana S, Boonpucknavig V. Effect of aloe vera gel to healing of burn wound: a clinical and histologic study. J Med Assoc Thai 1995;78:403-409.

World Health Organization. *Monographs on Selected Medicinal Plants,* vol 1. Geneva, Switzerland: WHO; 1999.

Yates KM, Rosenberg LJ, Harris CK, et al. Pilot study of the effect of acemannan in cats infected with feline immunodeficiency virus. Vet Immunol Immunopathol 1992;35:177-189.

American Ginseng 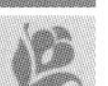

Panax quinquefolium L., *Panax quincefolius* L., (formerly *Aralia quinquefolium*) • PAN-ax kwin-kway-FOH-lee-um

Distribution: Eastern and Central North America; a woodland plant

Similar Species: *Panax ginseng*

Other Names: Sang, five fingers, tartar root, red berry, man's health

Family: Araliaceae

Parts Used: Root

Collection: The root of wild plants 3 to 6 years old is collected in the fall after the berries have ripened, and the berries are left to reseed the area. Most American ginseng is now cultivated.

Selected Constituents: Triterpenoid saponins known as ginsenosides are common to the *Panax* species. Quinquenosides I, II, III, IV, and V are ginsenosides unique to this species. *P. quinquefolium* also contains ginsenosides found in *P. ginseng*. Unique high-molecular-weight polysaccharides known as glycans (quinquefolans A, B, C), polyacetylenes, sesquiterpenes, sterols, flavonoids, and so forth.

Ginsenoside Rb1

Clinical Actions: Rejuvenative, adaptogen, mild stimulant, bitter tonic

Energetics: Sweet, slightly bitter, neutral or cooling. Yin tonic with an affinity for lung, stomach, and kidney channels. The Traditional Chinese Medicine view of *P. quinquefolium* activity includes generation of fluids, reduction of heat from deficiency, and tonifying of lung yin to address chronic lung deficiency coughs.

History and Traditional Usage: Cherokee Indians used this herb for headache, convulsions, and palsy; as a tonic and expectorant; and for colic, "weakness of the womb," nervous affections, and thrush. Other tribes had a wide variety of uses as well, including asthma, vomiting, rheumatism, earache, anorexia, and sore eyes; for strengthened mental powers; for worms; as a love charm, diaphoretic, or hemostatic for bleeding "cuts"; for "shortwindedness"; and for use when all other treatments have failed. One interesting use was "as a seasoner to render other remedies more powerful." Many Native American descriptions evoke the modern advertisement of ginseng as a panacea.

King's *American Dispensatory* has this to say: "A mild tonic and stimulant. Useful in loss of *appetite, slight nervous debility,* and *weak stomach.* Continued for some length of time, for its temporary administration gives but little benefit, it is a very important remedy in *nervous dyspepsia,* and in *mental exhaustion from overwork.*

This herb is similar to *P. ginseng* but is considered milder and safer for use in younger patients.

Published Research: *P. quinquefolium* has been subjected to less intense scrutiny than has *P. ginseng,* which was shown to enhance immune function and to improve cognitive dysfunction, chronic obstructive pulmonary disease, hepatic disease, and erectile dysfunction.

Immune function

Predy et al (2005) conducted a randomized, double-blind, placebo-controlled study to determine whether an extract of *P. quinquefolium* helped prevent colds in humans. The preparation was a poly-furanosyl-pyranosyl-saccharide–rich extract of the root. At the onset of influenza season, 323 subjects from 18 to 65 years of age were instructed to take 2 capsules daily of ginseng or a placebo. People who took ginseng had signficantly fewer colds, fewer days with cold symptoms, and and lower symptom scores.

Athletic performance

American ginseng has been investigated for its ability to improve exercise performance. Although performance of men on treadmills did not improve with supplementation, plasma creatine kinase was significantly reduced compared with that of subjects who were given placebo (Hsu, 2005).

The antioxidant properties of American ginseng were investigated in young and old rats fed a ginseng-supplemented diet for 4 months. Rats were randomly assigned to diet alone, or to a diet containing 0.5 g/kg or 2.5 g/kg dried powder for 4 months. Oxidant generation was significantly lower in heart, soleus, and vastus lateralis muscle tissues of young and old rats fed ginseng, with dose-dependent effects. In addition, antioxidant enzyme activity was increased in certain tissues of rats administered ginseng powder (Fu, 2003).

Effects on sex hormones

In male rats, administration of American ginseng significantly reduced plasma prolactin levels but did not affect luteinizing hormone or testosterone levels. At a dose of 100 mg/kg daily, male copulatory behavior was facilitated (Murphy, 1998). In vitro data suggest that *P. quinquefolium* extracts may regulate GABAergic neurotransmission (Yuan, 1998).

Diabetes

Multiple studies in diabetic mice have shown that American ginseng root has hypoglycemic activity (Oshima, 1987; Martinez, 1984). In vitro studies suggest a postabsorptive effect, with sulfonylurea-type activity (Rotsteyn,

2004). Recently, investigators have found that the berries of the plant also have hypoglycemic activity (at 150 mg/kg administered ip), and, in the obese mouse model used, they also had some weight-normalizing effects (Xie, 2004; Dey, 2003). Vuksan et al (2001, 2000a) found that when 1 to 9 g of American ginseng root was administered to normal humans 40 minutes before a glucose challenge, hyperglycemia was reduced. Lower doses were as effective as higher doses, and ginseng was effective only when given before the glucose challenge (Vuksan 2000b; Vuksan, 2001). According to studies conducted by the same group, a single preparation of *P. quinquefolius* suppresses postprandial hyperglycemia, but another does not. Possible explanations for this discrepancy include marked decrements in total ginsenosides and in the key ratios of protopanaxadiol ginsenosides to protopanaxatriol ginsenosides, ginsenoside Rb(1) to ginsenoside Rg(1), and ginsenoside Rb(2) to ginsenoside Rc.

Indications: Weakness and debility from chronic illness or stress, cough, "nervous stomach." Considered a relaxing tonic that also improves mental function. Diabetes.

Potential Veterinary Indications: Debility, immunesuppression, diabetes; for geriatric patients, to enhance vitality and cognitive function.

Notes of Interest: More of this plant is exported to China than is presently used in its native North America.

Contraindications: Safety in pregnancy and lactation has not been established. According to *The Botanical Safety Handbook* of the American Herbal Products Association, this is class 1, which means it is safe in pregnancy and lactation.

Toxicology and Adverse Effects: AHPA class 1. "Ginseng abuse syndrome" has been reported by some authors who cite a series of poorly described cases in which *P. ginseng* is used; it is found in the Chinese literature as well. Symptoms (e.g., diarrhea, edema, headache, hypertension, insomnia) have not been reported for *P. quinquefolius*.

Potential Drug Interactions: *P. quinquefolius* may have similar interactions to *P. ginseng*, but this has not been established. In vitro research indicated that *P. quinquefolius* may have synergistic effects with cyclophosphamide, methotrexate, paclitaxel, tamoxifen, and doxorubicin in inhibition of breast cancer cell growth. The hypoglycemic effect may add to the action of insulin in diabetic patients, but none of these interactions has been reported as a problem in clinical patients.

Preparation Notes: People can chew the root dried, or dried and candied.

Dosage:

Human:

Dried herb: 0.25-10 g TID, up to 6 times daily for acute conditions

Infusions and decoctions: 2.5-10 g per cup of water, with ¼-1 cup of the tea, given TID

Tincture (prepared with 30%-60% ethanol—doses are slightly lower with high-alcohol preparations): 1:2 or 1:3 in 30%: 3-5 mL TID, up to 6 times daily for acute conditions

Small Animal:

Dried herb: 25-300 mg/kg, divided daily (optimally TID)

Decoction and infusion: 2.5-10 g per cup of water, administered at a rate of ¼-½ cup per 10 kg (20 lb), divided daily (optimally, TID)

Tincture: 1:2-1:3 in 30%: 0.5-1.5 mL per 10 kg (20 lb), divided daily (optimally, TID) and diluted or combined with other herbs. Higher doses may be appropriate if the herb is used singly and is not combined in a formula

References

Dey L, Xie JT, Wang A, Wu J, Maleckar SA, Yuan CS. Anti-hyperglycemic effects of ginseng: comparison between root and berry. Phytomedicine 2003;10:600-605.

Fu Y, Ji LL. Chronic ginseng consumption attenuates age-associated oxidative stress in rats. J Nutr 2003;133:3603-3609.

Hsu CC, Ho MC, Lin LC, Su B, Hsu MC. American ginseng supplementation attenuates creatine kinase level induced by submaximal exercise in human beings. World J Gastroenterol 2005;11:5327-5331.

Martinez B, Staba EJ. The physiological effects of *Aralia, Panax* and *Eleutherococcus* on exercised rats. Jpn J Pharmacol 1984; 35:79-85.

Murphy LL, Cadena RS, Chavez D, Ferraro JS. Effect of American ginseng *(Panax quinquefolium)* on male copulatory behavior in the rat. Physiol Behav 1998;64:445-450.

Oshima Y, Sato K, Hikino H. Isolation and hypoglycemic activity of quinquefolans A, B, and C, glycans of *Panax quinquefolium* roots. J Nat Prod 1987;50:188-190.

Predy GN, Goel V, Lovlin R, Donner A, Stitt L, Basu TK. Efficacy of an extract of North American ginseng containing poly-furanosyl-pyranosyl-saccharides for preventing upper respiratory tract infections: a randomized controlled trial. CMAJ 2005;173:1043-1048.

Rotshteyn Y, Zito SW. Application of modified in vitro screening procedure for identifying herbals possessing sulfonylurea-like activity. J Ethnopharmacol 2004;93:337-344.

Sievenpiper JL, Arnason JT, Leiter LA, Vuksan V. Variable effects of American ginseng: a batch of American ginseng (*Panax quinquefolius* L.) with a depressed ginsenoside profile does not affect postprandial glycemia. Eur J Clin Nutr 2003;57:243-248.

Vuksan V, Sievenpiper JL, Wong J, Xu Z, Beljan-Zdravkovic U, Arnason JT, Assinewe V, Stavro MP, Jenkins AL, Leiter LA, Francis T. American ginseng (*Panax quinquefolius* L.) attenuates postprandial glycemia in a time-dependent but not dose-dependent manner in healthy individuals. Am J Clin Nutr 2001;73:753-758.

Vuksan V, Stavro MP, Sievenpiper JL, Beljan-Zdravkovic U, Leiter LA, Josse RG, Xu Z. Similar postprandial glycemic reductions with escalation of dose and administration time of American ginseng in type 2 diabetes. Diabetes Care 2000a;23:1221-1226.

Vuksan V, Sievenpiper JL, Koo VY, Francis T, Beljan-Zdravkovic U, Xu Z, Vidgen E. American ginseng (*Panax quinquefolius* L.) reduces postprandial glycemia in nondiabetic subjects and subjects with type 2 diabetes mellitus. Arch Intern Med 2000b;160:1009-1013.

Xie JT, Wu JA, Mehendale S, Aung HH, Yuan CS. Anti-hyperglycemic effect of the polysaccharides fraction from American ginseng berry extract in ob/ob mice. Phytomedicine 2004;11:182-187.

Yuan CS, Attele AS, Wu JA, Liu D. Modulation of American ginseng on brainstem GABAergic effects in rats. J Ethnopharmacol 1998;62:215-222.

Andrographis

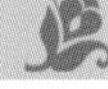

Andrographis paniculata Nees • An-dro-GRAF-us pan-ick-yoo-LAY-tuh *or* an-dro-GRAF-us pan-ick-yoo-LAH-tuh

Distribution: Widely found and cultivated in tropical and subtropical Asia, Southeast Asia, and India

Similar Species: *Justicia latebrosa, Justicia paniculata, Justicia stricta*
Common Names: Chuan xin lian, charita, chiretta, kalmegh
Family: Acanthaceae
Parts Used: Dried aerial parts
Selected Constituents: Diterpene lactones, including andrographolide, deoxyandrographolide, andrographiside, neoandrographiside, deoxyadnrographiside, and andropanoside

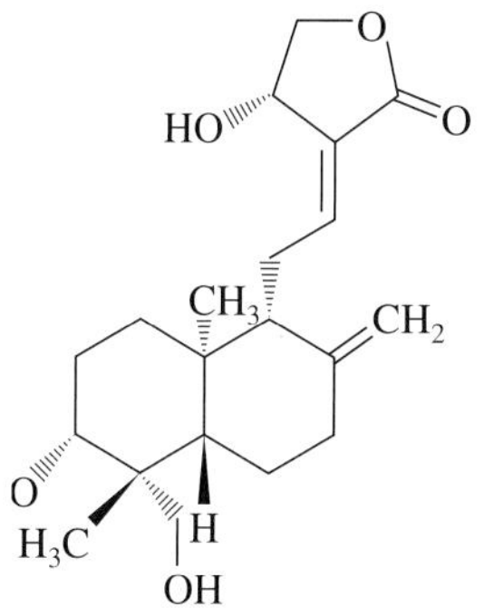

Andrographolide

Clinical Actions: Anti-inflammatory, antipyretic, antifertility, anthelmintic, immune stimulant, bitter tonic, cholagogue, antihepatotoxin, antimalarial
Energetics: Bitter and cold; clears Heat and relieves toxicity
History and Traditional Usage: *Andrographis paniculata* extract is traditionally used as a medicine to treat different diseases in India, China, and Southeast Asia (Ajaya, 2004). For treatment of dysentery, bronchitis, carbuncles, colitis, cough, dyspepsia, fever, hepatitis, malaria, mouth ulcer, sores, tuberculosis, venomous snakebites, otitis media, vaginitis, eczema, and burns (WHO, 1999).

The juice of the stem and whole plant is used to treat diarrhea, Newcastle's disease, and respiratory problems in poultry (IIRR, 2002). In India, plant leaves have been used to treat datura poisoning, maggots in wounds, worms in the eye and abdomen, liver fluke, glossitis, constipation, tuberculosis, pneumonia, contagious abortion of placenta, tetanus, and scabies in farm animals (Jha, 1992).

Published Research: Clinical data support the human use of andrographis for prophylaxis and the symptomatic treatment of upper respiratory tract infection such as the common cold and uncomplicated sinusitis, and for bronchitis and pharyngotonsillitis, lower urinary tract infection, and acute diarrhea (WHO, 1999).

Immunostimulatory activity

Oral administration of andrographis (as an ethanol extract at 25 mg/kg body weight) or purified andrographolides (1 mg/kg bw) in mice stimulated antibody production and delayed-type hypersensitivity response to sheep red blood cells. The ethanol extract also stimulated a nonspecific immune response in mice that was more effective than purified andrographolides, suggesting that other constituents may be responsible for the immunestimulant response (Puri, 1993).

Upper respiratory disease

Systematic reviews of the literature and meta-analyses of randomized controlled trials on the efficacy of *Andrographis paniculata* against upper respiratory tract infection have been published. Evidence from four studies (a total of 433 patients) suggests that *A. paniculata* extract alone or in combination with *Eleutherococcus senticosus* extract may be more effective than placebo and may provide appropriate treatment for uncomplicated acute upper respiratory tract infection (Poolsup, 2004). Evidence from 7 double-blind, controlled trials (a total of 896 patients) suggests that *A. paniculata* is better than placebo in alleviating symptoms of uncomplicated upper respiratory tract infection and may also have a preventive effect (Coon, 2004).

Hepatoprotective and choleretic activity

Andrographolide produces a significant, dose-dependent (1.5-12 mg/kg) choleretic effect (4.8%-73%), as noted by increases in bile flow, bile salt, and bile acids in conscious rats and anesthetized guinea pigs. Pretreatment with andrographolide significantly prevented paracetamol-induced decreases in volume and contents of bile and was found to be more potent than therapy with silymarin (Shukla, 1992). Several human studies have suggested that andrographis is effective against leptospirosis (Shanghai City Andrographis Research Group, 1976).

Acute hepatitis was induced in rats by means of a single dose of galactosamine (800 mg/kg, IP)/paracetamol (3 g/kg, orally [PO]) so that the hepatoprotective effects of andrographolide could be studied. Andrographolide treatment (400 mg/kg IP or 800 mg/kg PO) 48, 24, and 2 hours before galactosamine administration, or (200 mg/kg IP) 1, 4, and 7 hours after paracetamol, leads to complete normalization of toxin-induced increases in levels of hepatic enzymes and significantly reduced toxin-induced histopathologic liver changes in rats (Handa, 1990).

Effects on microfilaria in dogs

Andrographis paniculata (decoction of leaves) killed the microfilaria of *Dipetalonema reconditum* in 40 min in an in vitro study. Infected dogs were given three subcutaneous injections of the extract (0.06 mL per kg body weight), which reduced the number of microfilariae in blood by more than 85%. Additional injections did not eliminate the infection; however, a reduced microfilarial level persisted. Lethargy was observed for a week upon initiation of treatment, probably because of the mass killing of microfilariae. No toxicity was observed in rabbits given the extract (Dutta, 1982).

Cardioprotective effects

Studies on intravenous injection of *Andrographis* (water extract) in dogs have shown that it can limit myocardial ischemia and reperfusion injury and exert protective effects on reversible ischemia; it also has weak fibrinolytic action (Zhao, 1990). In another study, dogs were randomly divided into two groups; the treated group (n = 10) 45 min after ischemia received a slow iv bolus of 1 mg/kg of a refined extract, followed by an infusion of 80 µg/kg/min for 60 min; the control group (n = 10) was given only 5% glucose in saline. Previous findings were supported in that andrographis reduced the impact of ischemia on the myocardium, and in this study, prevented malignant arrhythmia. It was concluded that this extract may protect the myocardium from ischemic reperfusion injury (Guo, 1996).

Antifertility effects

Andrographis has an antifertility effect in rats and mice. Dried andrographis powder was mixed with animal food at a dose of 2 g/kg bw per day and was consumed daily by female mice for a period of 6 weeks. Compared with control female mice, which became pregnant (95.2%), none of the female mice that consumed andrographis became pregnant when they were mated with a male of proven fertility (Zoha, 1989).

Male rats fed a dry leaf powder of andrographis (20 mg per day for 60 days) demonstrated cessation of spermatogenesis, degenerative changes in the seminiferous tubules, regression of Leydig cells, and regressive or degenerative changes in the epididymis, seminal vesicle, ventral prostate, and coagulating gland. These changes suggest an antispermatogenic or an antiandrogenic effect of the plant (Akbarsha, 1990). Andrographis dried extract did not produce subchronic testicular toxicity effects in male rats (Burgos, 1997).

Potential Veterinary Indications: Fertility control in rats and mice, nonspecific immune stimulant, hepatoprotection: paracetamol-induced hepatotoxicity, uncomplicated upper respiratory tract infection

Contraindications: Because of potential anaphylactic reactions, crude extracts should not be injected.

Safety in pregnancy and lactation has not been established. Effects of the powdered extract of *Andrographis* leaves on blood progesterone content in rats were studied; it was found that high doses (30- to 300-fold higher than typical therapeutic doses) did not exhibit any effect on elevated levels of progesterone in blood plasma. Therefore, it is assumed that andrographis cannot induce progesterone-mediated termination of pregnancy (Panossian, 1999). Other theoretical contraindications have been proposed; these include bleeding disorders, hypotension, and male infertility.

Toxicology and Adverse Effects: AHPA class 2b. Large doses may cause gastric discomfort, vomiting, and loss of appetite (WHO, 1999).

Drug Interactions: Theoretical interactions have been proposed with anticoagulants, antihypertensives, immunesuppressants, and hypoglycemic drugs.

Dosage:

Human:

Dried herb: 0.5-10 g TID, up to 6 times daily for acute conditions (this is a bitter herb, and the higher doses are not usually required)

Standardized extract tablets (100 mg containing 5% andrographolide and deoxyandrographolide): 1-4 tablets TID

Infusions and decoctions: 2.5-10 g per cup of water, with ¼-1 cup of the tea given TID, up to 6 times daily acutely

Tincture (usually in 30% ethanol): 1:2 or 1:3: 2-5 mL TID, up to 6 times daily for acute conditions

Small Animal:

Dried herb: 25-300 mg/kg, divided daily (optimally, TID)

Standardized extract tablets (100 mg containing 5% andrographolide and deoxyandrographolide): ¼-9 tablets, divided daily (optimally, TID)

Infusion: 2.5-10 g per cup of water, administered at a rate of ¼-½ cup per 10 kg (20 lb), divided daily (optimally, TID)

Tincture: 1:2-1:3 in 30%: 0.5-1.5 mL per 10 kg (20 lb), divided daily (optimally, TID) and diluted or combined with other herbs

Selected References

Ajaya Kumar R, Sridevi K, Vijaya Kumar N, Nanduri S, Rajagopal S. Anticancer and immunostimulatory compounds from *Andrographis paniculata*. J Ethnopharmacol 2004;92:291-295.

Akbarsha MA, Manivannan B, Hamid KS, Vijayan B. Antifertility effect of *Andrographis paniculata* (Nees) in male albino rat. Indian J Exp Biol 1990;28:421-426.

Burgos RA, Caballero EE, Sanchez NS, Schroeder RA, Wikman GK, Hancke JL. Testicular toxicity assessment of *Andrographis paniculata* dried extract in rats. J Ethnopharmacol 1997;58:219-224.

Coon JT, Ernst E. *Andrographis paniculata* in the treatment of upper respiratory tract infections: a systematic review of safety and efficacy. Planta Med 2004;70:293-298.

Dutta A, Sukul NC. Filaricidal properties of a wild herb, *Andrographis paniculata*. J Helminthol 1982;56:81-84.

Guo Z, Zhao H, Fu L. Protective effects of API0134 on myocardial ischemia and reperfusion injury. J Tongji Med Univ 1996;16:193-197.

Handa SS, Sharma A.Hepatoprotective activity of andrographolide against galactosamine and paracetamol intoxication in rats. Indian J Med Res 1990;92:284-292.

IIRR, International Institute of Rural Reconstruction. 1994 Ethnoveterinary medicine in Asia. An information kit on traditional animal health care practices. Part 1 General information IIRR Silang Phillipines. In: Williamson E, ed. *Major Herbs of Ayurveda*. Sydney, Australia: Churchill Livingstone; 2002.

Jha M. 1992 folk veterinary medicine of Bihar—A research project. In: Williamson E, ed. *Major Herbs of Ayurveda*. Sydney, Australia: Churchill Livingstone; 2002.

Matsuda T, Kuroyanagi M, Sugiyama S, Umehara K, Ueno A, Nishi K. Cell differentiation-inducing diterpenes from *Andrographis paniculata* Nees. Chem Pharm Bull (Tokyo) 1994;42:1216-1225.

Panossian A, Kochikian A, Gabrielian E, et al. Effect of *Andrographis paniculata* extract on progesterone in blood plasma of pregnant rats. Phytomedicine 1999;6:157-161.

Poolsup N, Suthisisang C, Prathanturarug S, Asawamekin A, Chanchareon U. *Andrographis paniculata* in the symptomatic treatment of uncomplicated upper respiratory tract infection: systematic review of randomized controlled trials. J Clin Pharmacol Ther 2004;29:37-45.

Puri A, Saxena R, Saxena RP, Saxena KC, Srivastava V, Tandon JS. Immunostimulant agents from *Andrographis paniculata*. J Nat Prod 1993;56:995-999.

Shanghai City Andrographis Research Group. A study on water-soluble andrographolide. Newsletters of Chinese Herbal Medicine 1976;3:10-18.

Shukla B, Visen PK, Patnaik GK, Dhawan BN. Choleretic effect of andrographolide in rats and guinea pigs. Planta Med 1992;58:146-149.

World Health Organization. *Monographs on Selected Medicinal Plants,* vol 1. Geneva, Switzerland: WHO; 1999.
Zhao HY, Fang WY. Protective effects of *Andrographis paniculata* nees on post-infarction myocardium in experimental dogs. J Tongji Med Univ 1990;10:212-217.
Zoha MS, Hussain AH, Choudhury SA. Antifertility effect of *Andrographis paniculata* in mice. Bangladesh Med Res Counc Bull 1989;15:34-37.

Angelica

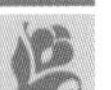

Angelica archangelica L. = *Angelica officinalis* Moench = *Angelica officinalis* (Moench) Hoffm • An-JELL-ik-uh ark-an-JELL-ik-uh

Other Names: Garden angelica, wild angelica, archangel, European angelica

Similar Species: *Angelica atropurpurea*

Family: Apiaceae

Parts Used: Root, rhizome

Selected Constituents: Volatile oil (containing alpha-angelica lactone, phellandrene, etc), coumarins (umbelliferone), furanocoumarins, phenolic acids, resins

Clinical Actions: Aromatic, diaphoretic, bitter tonic, antispasmodic, choleretic, cholagogue, carminative, emmenagogue, antimicrobial, diuretic, sedative

Energetics: Spicy, bitter, warm; action directed primarily toward the Lung, Stomach, Intestines

History and Traditional Usage: Popular for nonulcer dyspepsia, nausea, heartburn, anorexia, flatulence, borborygmus, menstrual cramps, colds, fever, headache, upper respiratory inflammation, or mouth inflammation. Used as a flavoring ingredient in some bitters, gin, and vermouth, and in the liqueurs Chartreuse and Benedictine.

Published Research: Angelica helped reduce gastric ulcer formation in rats given indomethacin in a dose-dependent manner; it reduced gastric acid output while increasing mucin secretion, thereby increasing prostaglandin E and decreasing leukotrienes (Khayyal, 2001).

Yeh et al (2003) investigated the antioxidant capacity of 10 mg/kg, 25 mg/kg, and 50 mg/kg of the extract. In mice given ethanol, the herb appeared to reduce transaminase elevation and oxidative damage.

A leaf extract from Angelica was administered to mice implanted with mouse breast cancer cells. A significant reduction in tumor growth was noted in those mice treated with the extract, in comparison with control mice (Sigurdsson, 2005).

Indications: Abdominal fullness, gas, mild cramps, nausea, cough, cystitis

Potential Veterinary Indications: Borborygmus, flatulence, mild abdominal pain, cough

Contraindications: Pregnancy and lactation, bleeding disorders

Toxicology and Adverse Effects: AHPA class 2b, 2d. Potential for photodermatitis; potential for interacting with anticoagulant drugs. Classified as GRAS by the FDA as a flavoring for beverages. The stalks can be served candied, and the leaf is used in salads. It is still probably best to avoid excessive exposure to sunlight if therapeutic amounts are used.

Potential Drug Interactions: Theoretical interactions with anticoagulants and photosensitizing drugs have been suggested.

Notes: Legend has it that angelica was revealed to humans by an angel as a cure for the plague, accounting for its name.

Dosage:

Human:

Dried herb: 0.5-10 g TID, up to 6 times daily for acute conditions

Infusions and decoctions: 5-30 g per cup of water, with 1 cup of the tea given TID, up to 6 times daily acutely

Tincture (from 45%-70% ethanol; lower doses are used for higher ethanol preparations): 1:2 or 1:3: 05-5 mL TID, up to 6 times daily for acute conditions

Small Animal:

Dried herb: 25-500 mg/kg, divided daily (optimally, TID)

Infusion: 5-30 g per cup of water, administered at a rate of 1/4-1/2 cup per 10 kg (20 lb) divided daily (optimally TID)

Tincture: 1:2-1:3: 0.5-2.5 mL per 10 kg (20 lb), divided daily (optimally, TID) and diluted or combined with other herbs.

References

Khayyal MT, el-Ghazaly MA, Kenawy SA, Seif-el-Nasr M, Mahran LG, Kafafi YA, Okpanyi SN. Antiulcerogenic effect of some gastrointestinally acting plant extracts and their combination. Arzneimittelforschung 2001;51:545-553.
Sigurdsson S, Ogmundsdottir HM, Hallgrimsson J, Gudbjarnason S. Antitumour activity of *Angelica archangelica* leaf extract. In Vivo. 2005;19:191-194.
Yeh ML, Liu CF, Huang CL, Huang TC. Hepatoprotective effect of *Angelica archangelica* in chronically ethanol-treated mice. Pharmacology 2003;68:70-73.

Arnica

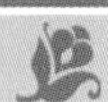

Arnica montana L. • ARN-ik-uh mon-TAN-uh

Other Names: Leopard's bane, wolf's bane, mountain tobacco, mountain snuff, mountain arnica

Similar Species: *Arnica latifolia*

Family: Asteraceae

Parts Used: Dried flower heads, rhizome

Selected Constituents: Flavonoid glycosides, terpenoids, sesquiterpene lactones, coumarins, carbohydrates, volatile oils, phytosterols, resins, tannins, carotenoids

Clinical Actions: Vulnerary, anti-inflammatory

Energetics: Unknown

History and Traditional Usage: Used almost exclusively externally for bruises, sprains, and traumatic injuries; as a mild pain reliever; and for insect bites, angina, and heart failure. Sheep and goats have been noted to eat the plant, but cattle did not.

Published Research: Arnica may have slight antibacterial activity against oral pathogens, and slight activity in preventing bacterial adherence and formation of glucans involved in periodontal disease. Studies examining the ability of arnica to reduce traumatic or joint swelling have had mixed results. Wagner (2004), using pig skin as a model, determined that the active sesquiterpene lactones were best absorbed from topically applied alcoholic tinctures of the whole plant. Isolated sesquiterpene lactones were not as well absorbed.

Indications: Externally as a mild pain reliever and anti-inflammatory, arnica is used for arthralgia, arthritis, and traumatic swelling, and to improve circulation. It is also used in hair tonics and as a dandruff remedy. The herb is too toxic to use internally, except in the low-dose homeopathic form.

Potential Veterinary Indications: Use should be limited to topical applications, and only if the animal can be prevented from licking the substance. Homeopathic forms (mother tincture, which is a 1:10 extract, or low potencies, under 12×) are more easily available in the United States. Low-potency homeopathic remedies should be safe for internal use. Primarily used for bruising and traumatic injury.

Contraindications: Not for use on damaged skin or open wounds; safety for topical use not established in pregnancy or lactation.

Toxicology and Adverse Effects: AHPA class 2d. Type IV allergic contact dermatitis has been reported frequently in sensitive persons or with prolonged use. Internal use may lead to stomach pain, vomiting, diarrhea, vomiting, kidney pain, dyspnea, tachycardia, cardiac arrest, and liver failure. One author (Kuhn, 2001) writes that a single gram dose can lead to heart damage and cardiac arrest in humans.

Potential Drug Interactions: Arnica contains some constituents that may change platelet function; theoretical interactions with anticoagulants have been suggested.

Notes: Plant may be threatened in the wild.

Dosage:

Topical Forms: Apply as directed by manufacturer. These generally contain 15% to 25% arnica oil.

Internal Use: **Not recommended.** Arnica should be used only by very experienced herbalists, who should also note that dose–response studies have never been conducted. The Eclectics used 1:10, 70% alcohol tinctures at 1 to 3 drops twice daily for an adult human. This dose is akin to that used internally by homeopaths. The **human** internal dose from one modern manufacturer is tincture, 1:2 fresh tops in 65% alcohol, 1-2 drops BID.

References

Kuhn M, Winston D. *Herbal Therapy and Supplements: A Scientific and Traditional Approach.* Philadelphia, Pa: Lippincott, Williams and Wilkins; 2001.

Wagner S, Suter A, Merfort I. Skin penetration studies of Arnica preparations and of their sesquiterpene lactones. Planta Med 2004;70:897-903.

Artichoke

Cynara scolymus L. • SIN-uh-ruh SKOL-ee-mus

Other Names: Globe artichoke, garden artichoke

Family: Asteraceae

Parts Used: Fresh or dried leaf

Selected Constituents: Sesquiterpene lactones (cynaropicrin), bitter principles (including cynaroside and cynarin, which are responsible for the hepatoprotection of artichoke). Flavonoids, volatile oils.

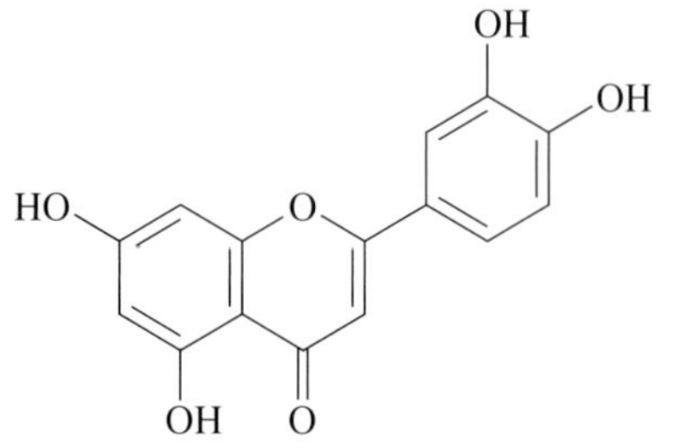

OH OH HO O OH O

Cynarin

Clinical Actions: Bitter tonic, antiemetic, diuretic, choleretic, hepatoprotective

Energetics: Cooling, slightly bitter, and salty, moist, and sweet.

History and Traditional Usage: Artichoke has long been cultivated as a vegetable; when introduced into England in the 16th century, it became popular as a food and as a mild diuretic and was used for appetite problems and dyspepsia. *Gerard's Herbal* (1597) says that the leaves of artichoke "containeth plenty of cholericke iuyce, and hath an hard substance, insomuch as of this is ingendred melancholy iuyce, and of that a thin and cholerick blood . . . they yield to the body a raw and melancholy iuice, and containe in them great store of winde."

Published Research: Artichoke leaf extract had choleretic activity (stimulation of bile production by hepatocytes) in rats equivalent to the bile salt, dehydrocholic acid (Saenz Rodriguez, 2002). Artichoke acts as an antioxidant, and its well-established hepatoprotective activity stems probably from phenolic derivatives. The leaf extract was studied in the treatment of patients with dyspepsia in a 6-week, double-blind, placebo-controlled multicenter trial; it was found to be significantly better than placebo in alleviating symptoms of indigestion (Holtmann, 2003). It significantly reduced serum cholesterol in humans (Thompson Coon, 2003).

Indications: Hyperlipidemia, steatorrhea due to choleretic action, nausea, flatulence, hepatoprotective, hepatic trophorestorative, bitter

Potential Veterinary Indications: Hyperlipidemia, cholestatic and other liver diseases, nausea, constipation

Contraindications: Biliary obstruction, gallstones, allergy to other plants in the daisy family

Toxicology and Adverse Effects: Used as food. Allergic reactions, contact dermatitis are possible in sensitive individuals.

Drug Interactions: May have additive effects with lipid-lowering drugs.

Dosage:

Human:

Dried herb: 0.5-10 g TID, up to 6 times daily for acute conditions

Dried extract: (12:1) 0.1-0.5 g QD

Infusions and decoctions: 5-30 g per cup of water, with 1 cup of the tea given TID

Fluid extract (1:1): 0.5-2 mL TID

Tincture (usually 30% ethanol): 1:2 or 1:3: 1-5 mL TID

Small Animal:

Dried herb: 25-250 mg/kg, divided daily (optimally, TID)

Dried extract (12:1): 10-50 mg/kg, divided daily (optimally, TID)

Infusion: 5-30 g per cup of water, administered at a rate of 1/4-1/2 cup per 10 kg (20 lb), divided daily (optimally, TID)
Fluid extract (1:1): 0.25-2.0 mL per 10 kg (20 lb), divided daily (optimally, TID)
Tincture: 1:2-1:3: 0.5-2.5 mL per 10 kg (20 lb), divided daily (optimally, TID) and diluted or combined with other herbs

References

Holtmann G, Adam B, Haag S, Collet W, Grunewald E, Windeck T. Efficacy of artichoke leaf extract in the treatment of patients with functional dyspepsia: a six-week placebo-controlled, double blind, multicentre trial. Aliment Pharmacol Ther 2003; 18:1099-1105.

Saenz Rodriguez T, Garcia Gimenez D, de la Puerta Vazquez R. Choleretic activity and biliary elimination of lipids and bile acid induced by an artichoke leaf extract in rats. Phytomedicine 2002;9:687-693.

Thompson Coon JS, Ernst E. Herbs for serum cholesterol reduction: a systematic view. J Fam Pract 2003;52:468-478.

Ashwagandha

Withania somnifera Dunal • Wi-THAY-nee-uh som-NIF-er-uh

Common Names: Winter cherry, sanskrit names: ashvagandha, hayahvaya, vajigandha. Hindi names: asgandh, Indian ginseng

Family: Solanaceae

Parts Used: Root, leaf, and whole plant

Distribution: Ashwagandha is a small woody shrub or herb that is indigenous to India, other Asian countries, and parts of Africa and is found widely on wasteland. Because of its wide range, considerable morphologic and chemotypical variations in terms of local species have been noted. Except for the bright red fruit, it is a fairly plain, nondescript plant.

Selected Constituents: The chemistry of withania has been well studied, and more than 35 phytochemicals have been identified, extracted, and isolated. Major constituents include steroidal lactones, alkaloids, and flavonoids, in addition to several amino acids and iron. Steroidal lactones (withanolides, withaferins), saponins (sitoindoside VII and VIII), and withanolides (sitoindoside IX and X) are found. Withanolides are found primarily in the leaves, and sitoindosides mainly in the root. Withania is also a rich source of iron (Mishra, 2000).

Withanolide

Clinical Actions: Tonic, adaptogen, nervine, sedative, antitumor in high doses, anti-inflammatory, anodyne

Energetics: Warm, pungent, and sweet

History and Traditional Usage: Withania is widely used in Ayurvedic medicine in India and in Unani and Middle Eastern traditional medicines, where it is highly regarded as a panacea, aphrodisiac, and rejuvenative. The use of ashwagandha in Ayurvedic medicine extends back more than 3000 to 4000 years (Upton, 2000). It has been widely extolled as a tonic, especially for emaciation in people of all ages, including babies, and enhances the reproductive function of both men and women. It has also been used for inflammation, especially in arthritic and rheumatic conditions, for asthma, and as a major tonic to counteract aging and promote youthful longevity. Some of its other traditional uses have been as a mild purgative for chronic constipation and for the treatment of swollen glands. It is prescribed for a wide range of musculoskeletal conditions and as a general tonic to increase energy, improve overall health and longevity, and prevent disease in athletes, the elderly, and pregnant women (Bone, 1996).

Ethnoveterinary Use: The plant is used in cough, dropsy, rheumatism, scabies, and sores. The roots are used to promote milk flow in ruminants (Williamson, 2002).

Published Research: Numerous studies on animals and humans have indicated that ashwagandha possesses anti-inflammatory, antitumor, antistress, antioxidant, immunomodulatory, hematopoietic, and rejuvenating properties. It also appears to exert a positive influence on the endocrine, cardiopulmonary, and central nervous systems. It is an ingredient in many formulations prescribed for a variety of musculoskeletal conditions and as a general tonic to increase energy, improve overall health and longevity, and prevent disease in athletes (Bone, 1996; Chatterjee, 1995). The combined alkaloids seem to exhibit calming, anticonvulsant, and antispasmodic properties against many spasmogenic agents in the intestinal, uterine, bronchial, tracheal, and blood vascular muscles. It is described as similar to but considerably weaker than papaverine and phenobarbitone (Bhatnagar, 1976).

Anti-inflammatory

Several studies support the anti-inflammatory use of Withania for a variety of musculoskeletal conditions (al-Hindawi, 1992; Sudhir, 1992). Although only few studies on the mechanism of anti-inflammatory action have been conducted, it appears that cyclooxygenase inhibition may be involved (Mishra, 2000; Somasundaram, 1983). As well, a direct musculotropic action of Withania accounts for the antispasmodic effects that produce relaxation (Malhotra, 1965a).

Antitumor

The antitumor and radiosensitizing effects of withania have been studied (Sharada, 1996; Devi, 1995). Withania root extract (greater than 400 mg/kg/day for 15 days) was associated with regression of induced sarcoma in mice. Cumulative doses of 7.5 to 10 g achieved by daily doses of 500 or 750 mg/kg seemed to produce a good response in this tumor. The 1000-mg/kg/day level produced some mortality (Devi, 1992).

Antistress

Withania root extracts have been evaluated for antistress activity (Singh, 2001; Singh, 2003). Withania induces a nonspecific increased resistance during stress; and several studies support the use of withania in nervous exhaustion due to stress and in cachexia to increase body weight (Mishra, 2000). Ashwagandha possesses adaptogenic, cardiotropic, cardioprotective, and anticoagulant properties, as evidenced by rats, which, when given the extract, showed increases in heart weight, glycogen content, and swimming time performance. No toxicity was seen at 100 mg/kg PO for 180 days (Dhuley, 2000); similarly, swimming time and muscle weight were increased in mice given ashwaganda (Grandhi, 1994). Withania also protects against stress-induced stomach ulcers in rats (Bhattacharya, 1987).

Central nervous system effects

In monkeys, cats, dogs, rats, and mice, withania alkaloids have exhibited a taming effect and a mild depressant (tranquilizer) effect on the central nervous system (Malhotra, 1965b; Bhattacharya, 1997). Withania extract contains an ingredient that has GABA-mimetic activity (Mehta, 1991). Cognition-enhancing and memory-improving effects of extracts from withania have been observed in animals and humans (Schliebs, 1997). Withania root extract (100 mg/kg) reduced morphine (10 mg/kg) tolerance and withdrawal (Kulkarni, 1997). Investigations support the use of withania as a mood stabilizer in clinical conditions of anxiety and depression in Ayurveda (Bhattacharya, 2000).

Antioxidant activity

Free radical damage may contribute to neuronal loss in cerebral ischemia and may be involved in normal aging and neurodegenerative disease (Mishra, 2000). Ashwagandha root powder (0.7 and 1.4 g/kg body weight/day) administered for 30 days produced a significant decrease in lipid peroxidation and an increase in superoxide dismutase and catalase activities in mice, thus demonstrating free radical scavenging activity (Panda, 1997). In another study, an aqueous extract of withania (100 mg/kg) reduced lipid peroxidation in mice and rabbits (Dhuley, 1998b).

Immunomodulatory

The use of withania as a general tonic to increase energy and prevent disease may be partially related to its effect on the immune system. Withania compounds produced significant mobilization and activation of peritoneal macrophages, phagocytosis, and increased activity of lysosomal enzymes, along with significant antistress activity in mice and rats. It also augmented learning acquisition and memory retention in old and young rats (Ghosal, 1989).

Myelosuppression in mice treated with cyclophosphamide, azathioprine, or prednisolone was prevented by ashwagandha. Significant increases in hemoglobin concentration, red blood cell count, white blood cell count, platelet count, and body weight were observed in treated mice as compared with untreated (control) mice (Ziauddin, 1996).

Ashwagandha (100 mg/kg/day for 7 days) enhanced survival of *Aspergillus fumigatus*–infected mice, apparently because of increased phagocytosis and intracellular killing of peritoneal macrophages (Dhuley, 1998a).

Hematopoietic

A total of 101 normal healthy male volunteers were given purified withania powder (3 g/day) for 1 year. Increased hemoglobin and red blood cell (RBC) count, along with improvement in hair melanin and seated stature, was observed in all subjects (Kuppurajan, 1980). A double-blind study of 60 healthy children on the growth-promoting effects of withania showed that the withania-treated group had a significant increase in hemoglobin at the end of 30 days (Venkataraghaven, 1980).

Chemoprotective activity

Mice treated orally with *Withania somnifera* extract (400 mg/kg body weight) for 15 weeks (1 week before injection of tumor-inducing agent) had significantly reduced tumor incidence and tumor volume and enhanced survival, compared with control mice. Tumor incidence was also delayed in the treatment group when compared with control mice. The mechanism of the chemopreventive activity of withania extract may be due to its antioxidant and detoxifying properties (Prakash, 2001).

Cyclophosphamide-induced urotoxicity and leukopenia, as well as gamma radiation–induced leukopenia, were reduced by withania in mice (Davis, 1998; Davis, 2000; Kuttan, 1996; Praveenkumar, 1994).

Thyroid-modulating activity

Withania increased serum T3 and T4 in mice dosed at 1.4 g/kg body weight (Panda, 1998; Panda, 1999).

Effects on the cardiopulmonary system

Withania may also be useful as a general tonic, in part because of its beneficial effects on the cardiopulmonary system. The effects of withania on the cardiovascular and respiratory systems of dogs and frogs have been studied. In dogs, the alkaloids had prolonged hypotensive, bradycardiac, and respiratory stimulant actions (Malhotra, 1981). An extract induced a significant decrease in arterial and diastolic blood pressure in normotensive pentobarbital-anesthetized dogs (Ahumada, 1991). Blood pressure fell in dogs with 5 mg/kg of a withania extract (blocked by atropine—not by mepiramine or propranolol). The compound is similar to the aglycones of cardiac glycosides (Budhiraja, 1983).

Indications: General debility, malnourishment, senile debility, arthritic conditions, nervous exhaustion, fatigue, senile dementia, muscular weakness, insomnia, general nerve tonic, skin disease.

Suggested Veterinary Indications: Aspergillosis, laboratory animal stress, osteoarthritis, cognitive dysfunction; adjunct to cyclophosphamide chemotherapy or long-term prednisolone therapy; anemia, convalescence, hypothyroid disease, and hypertension. Emaciation, chronic diseases, especially if inflammatory in nature. May have some preventive role in cancer.

Notes of Interest: The distinctive earthy odor and flavor of ashwagandha are due to the presence of certain steroidal lactones or withanolides (Bhatnagar, 1976). It is from this characteristic odor that its Sanskrit name, "like a horse," derives; "somnifera" comes from the use of the plant as a sedative.

Contraindications: Large doses of ashwagandha may possess abortifacient properties.

Toxicology and Adverse Effects: AHPA class 2b, 2d (for its potential for interacting with barbiturates). Ashwagandha is relatively safe when taken in the prescribed range of dosage. A daily dose of 100 mg/kg body weight for 30 days in rats resulted in no deaths and no changes to blood parameters (Sharada, 1993). Large doses, however, have been shown to cause gastrointestinal upset, diarrhea, and vomiting.

Drug Interactions: Caution is advised with use in conjunction with sedatives or anxiolytics. Ashwagandha has been found to potentiate the effects of barbiturates.

Preparation Notes: Ashwagandha is used in Ayurvedic medicine as a powder, decoction, medicated wine; it is mixed with clarified butter, combined with honey or sugar syrup, or used as medicated oil. For skin disease, a salve of ashwagandha can be made, or the powder may be mixed with sesame oil and applied topically.

Dosage:

Human:

Dried herb: 1-10 g TID, up to 6 times daily for acute conditions, can be mixed with ghee or honey

Infusions and decoctions: 5-30 g simmered in 1 cup cow's milk for 15-30 min, given TID

Tincture (generally prepared in 35%-45% ethanol): 1:2 or 1:3: 2-5 mL TID-QID, up to 6 times daily for acute conditions

Narayana taila oil: internally, 3-10 drops; or freely applied externally to painful, arthritic joints

Small Animal:

Dried herb: 50-125 mg/kg, divided daily (optimally, TID) if extracted and dried; triple or quadruple dose for unprocessed herb

Decoction: 5-30 g per cup of water, administered at a rate of ¼-½ cup per 10 kg (20 lb), divided daily (optimally, TID)

Tincture (generally prepared in 35%-45% alcohol): 1:2-1:3: 1.0-2.5 mL per 10 kg (20 lb), divided daily (optimally, TID) and diluted or combined with other herbs. Higher doses may be appropriate if the herb is used singly and not combined in a formula.

References

Ahumada F, Aspee F, Wikman G, Hancke J. *Withania somnifera* extract. Its effect on arterial blood pressure in anaesthetised dogs. Phytother Res 1991;5:111.

Al-Hindawi MK, al-Khafaji SH, Abdul-Nabi MH. Anti-granuloma activity of Iraqi *Withania somnifera*. J Ethnopharmacol 1992; 37:113-116.

Bhatnagar SS, ed. *The Wealth of India: A Dictionary of Indian Raw Materials and Industrial Products,* vol 10. New Delhi: Publicity and Information Directorate, Council of Social and Industrial Research; 1976:582-585.

Bhattacharya SK, Bhattacharya A, Sairam K, Ghosal S. Anxiolytic-antidepressant activity of *Withania somnifera* glycowithanolides: an experimental study. Phytomedicine 2000;7:463-469.

Bhattacharya SK, Goel RK, Kaur R, Ghosal S. Antistress activity of sitoindosides VII and VIII, new acylsterylglucosides from *Withania somnifera*. Phytother Res 1987;1:32-39.

Bhattacharya SK, Satyan KS, Ghosal S. Antioxidant activity of glycowithanolides from *Withania somnifera*. Indian J Exp Biol 1997;35:236-239.

Bone K. *Clinical Applications of Ayurvedic and Chinese Herbs. Monographs for the Western Herbal Practitioner.* Australia: Phytotherapy Press; 1996:137-141.

Budhiraja RD, Sudhir S, Garg KN. Cardiovascular effects of a withanolide from *Withania coagulans,* dunal fruits. Indian J Physiol Pharmacol 1983;27:129-134.

Chatterjee A, Pakrashi SC. *The Treatise on Indian Medicinal Plants.* 1995;4:208-212.

Davis L, Kuttan G. Suppressive effect of cyclophosphamide-induced toxicity by *Withania somnifera* extract in mice. J Ethnopharmacol 1998;62:209-214.

Davis L, Kuttan G. Effect of *Withania somnifera* on cyclophosphamide-induced urotoxicity. Cancer Lett 2000;148:9-17.

Devi PU, Sharada AC, Solomon FE. In vivo growth inhibitory and radiosensitizing effects of withaferin A on mouse Ehrlich ascites carcinoma. Cancer Lett 1995;95:189-193.

Devi PU, Sharada AC, Solomon FE, Kamath MS. In vivo growth inhibitory effect of *Withania somnifera* (Ashwagandha) on a transplantable mouse tumor, sarcoma 180. Indian J Exp Biol 1992;30:169-172.

Dhuley JN. Adaptogenic and cardioprotective action of ashwagandha in rats and frogs. J Ethnopharmacol 2000;70:57-63.

Dhuley JN. Therapeutic efficacy of Ashwagandha against experimental aspergillosis in mice. Immunopharmacol Immunotoxicol 1998a;20:191-198.

Dhuley JN.Ghosal S, Lal J, et al. Effect of ashwagandha on lipid peroxidation in stress-induced animals. J Ethnopharmacol 1998b;60:173-178.

Ghosal S, Jawahar L, Srivastva R, et al. Immunomodulatory and CNS effects of sitoindocides IX and X, two new glycowithanolides from *Withania somnifera*. Phytother Res 1989;3:201-206.

Grandhi A, Mujumdar AM, Patwardhan B. A comparative pharmacological investigation of Ashwagandha and Ginseng. J Ethnopharmacol 1994;44:131-135.

Kulkarni SK, Ninan I. Inhibition of morphine tolerance and dependence by *Withania somnifera* in mice. J Ethnopharmacol 1997;57:213-217.

Kuppurajan K, et al. J Res Ayu Sid 1980;1:247, as cited in Bone K. *Clinical Applications of Ayurvedic and Chinese Herbs. Monographs for the Western Herbal Practitioner.* Australia: Phytotherapy Press; 1996:137-141.

Kuttan G. Use of *Withania somnifera* Dunal as an adjuvant during radiation therapy. Indian J Exp Biol 1996;34:854-856.

Malhotra CL, Das PK, Dhalla NS, Prasad K. Studies on Withania ashwagandha, Kaul. III. The effect of total alkaloids on the cardiovascular system and respiration. Indian J Med Res 1981;49:448-460.

Malhotra CL, Mehta VL, Prasad K, Das PK. Studies on Withania ashwagandha, Kaul. IV. The effect of total alkaloids on the smooth muscles. Indian J Physiol Pharmacol 1965a;9:9-15.

Malhotra CL, Mehta VL, Das PK, Dhalla NS. Studies on Withania-ashwagandha, Kaul. V. The effect of total alkaloids (ashwagandholine) on the central nervous system. Indian J Physiol Pharmacol 1965b;9:127-136.

Mehta AK, Binkley P, Gandhi SS, Ticku MK. Pharmacological effects of *Withania somnifera* root extract on GABAA receptor complex. Indian J Med Res 1991;94:312-315.

Mishra LC, Singh BB, Dagenais S. Scientific basis for the therapeutic use of *Withania somnifera* (ashwagandha): a review. Altern Med Rev 2000;5:334-346.

Panda S, Kar A. Evidence for free radical scavenging activity of Ashwagandha root powder in mice. Indian J Physiol Pharmacol 1997,41:424-426.

Panda S, Kar A. Changes in thyroid hormone concentrations after administration of ashwagandha root extract to adult male mice. J Pharm Pharmacol 1998;50:1065-1068.

Panda S, Kar A. *Withania somnifera* and *Bauhinia purpurea* in the regulation of circulating thyroid hormone concentrations in female mice. J Ethnopharmacol 1999;67:233-239.

Prakash J, Gupta SK, Kochupillai V, Singh N, Gupta YK, Joshi S. Chemopreventive activity of *Withania somnifera* in experimentally induced fibrosarcoma tumours in Swiss albino mice. Phytother Res 2001;15:240-244.

Praveenkumar V, Kuttan R, Kuttan G. Chemoprotective action of Rasayanas against cyclophosphamide toxicity. Tumori 1994; 80:306-308.

Schliebs R, Liebmann A, Bhattacharya SK, et al. Systemic administration of defined extracts from *Withania somnifera* (Indian Ginseng) and Shilajit differentially affects cholinergic but not glutamatergic and GABAergic markers in rat brain. Neurochem Int 1997;30:181-190.

Sharada AC, Emerson SF, Uma DP. Toxocity of *Withania somnifera* root extract in rat and mice. Int J Pharmacognosy 1993;31:205.

Sharada AC, Solomon FE, Devi PU, Udupa N, Srinivasan KK. Antitumor and radiosensitizing effects of withaferin A on mouse Ehrlich ascites carcinoma in vivo. Acta Oncol 1996; 35:95-100.

Singh B, Chandan BK, Gupta DK. Adaptogenic activity of a novel withanolide-free aqueous fraction from the roots of *Withania somnifera* Dun. (Part II). Phytother Res 2003;17:531-536.

Singh B, Saxena AK, Chandan BK, Gupta DK, Bhutani KK, Anand KK. Adaptogenic activity of a novel, withanolide-free aqueous fraction from the roots of *Withania somnifera* Dun. Phytother Res 2001;15:311-318.

Somasundaram S, Sadique J, Subramoniam A. In vitro absorption of [14C]leucine during inflammation and the effect of antiinflammatory drugs in the jejunum of rats. Biochem Med 1983; 29:259-264.

Sudhir S, Budhiraja RD. Comparison of the protective effect of Withaferin-'A' and hydrocortisone against CCL4 induced hepatotoxicity in rats. Indian J Physiol Pharmacol 1992;36: 127-129.

Upton R, Booth SJ. Ashwagandha root, *Withania somnifera:* In: *American Herbal Pharmacopoeia and Therapeutic Compendium.* Santa Cruz, Calif: American Pharmacopoeia; 2000.

Venkataraghaven S, Seshadri C, Sundaresan TP, et al. The comparative effect of milk fortified with ashwaghanda and punarnava in children—a double blind study. J Res Ayur Sid 1980; 1:370-385.

Williamson EM, ed. *Major Herbs of Ayurveda.* Sydney, Australia: Churchill Livingstone; 2002:321.

Ziauddin M, Phansalkar N, Patki P, et al. Studies on the immunomodulatory effects of ashwagandha. J Ethnopharmacol 1996;50:69-76.

Astragalus

Astragalus membranaceus (Fisch. Ex Link) Bunge, *A. membranaceus* (Fische) Bge. var. mongholicus • Ass-TRA-gal-uss mem-bren-AY-shus

Other Names: Membranous milkvetch, astragalus root, huang-qi, milkvetch

Similar Species: *Astragalus floridus, Astragalus tonglensis,* and *Astragalus chrysopterus* are all used in trade, along with *A. membranaceus. Astragalus propinguus* is a similar species. These are considered adulterants.

Family: Fabaceae

Parts Used: Root

Distribution: Indigenous to China, Korea, Mongolia, and Siberia

Selected Constituents: Major constituents are triterpene saponins (astragalosides I-X and isoastragalosides I-IV) and polysaccharides (e.g., astragalan, astraglucan).

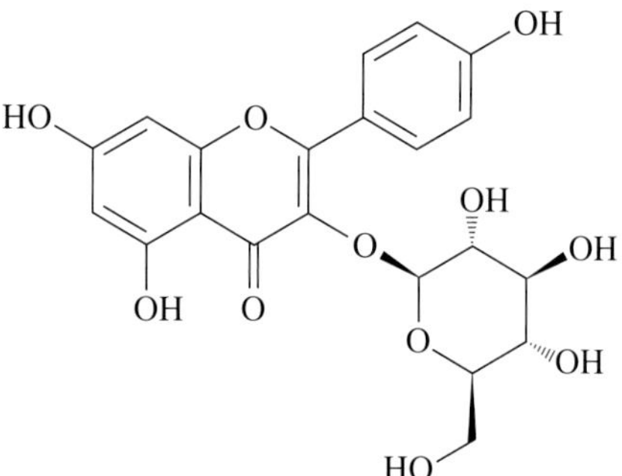

Astragalin

Clinical Actions: Immune enhancing, tonic, cardiotonic, diuretic, hypotensive

Energetics: Sweet and slightly warm

History and Traditional Usage: Astragalus has been used in Chinese medicine for thousands of years for increasing endurance. It has been used for gas and bloating and for reduction of night sweats, allergies, fatigue, anemia, ulcers, and uterine bleeding.

Published Research: Oral doses improve renal function in rats with experimental nephritis, and large doses are traditionally used in the treatment of chronic nephritis (Chang, 1987). Experimental diabetic nephropathy in rats is ameliorated by oral astragalus (Yin, 2004). It can increase albumin level in plasma, decrease the output of urinary protein, and increase muscle protein. This may improve dysfunctional protein metabolism in glomerulopathy and can effectively prevent glomerular sclerosis (Peng, 2005). The water decoction of astragalus (0.5 g/kg) administered to rats or to dogs under anesthesia, was found to have a significant diuretic effect. The water decoction (0.2 g/kg) also has a diuretic effect in humans (Modern TCM Pharmacology, 1997).

Astragalosides can delay senility in middle-aged mice and have an antiaging effect on induced senescent mice by improving brain function and having immunomodulatory effects (Lei, 2003). Immunologically astraglalan can enhance the phagocytic activity of mouse macrophages and increase the number of macrophagocytes. It can increase spleen size and promote antibody synthesis (Modern TCM Pharmacology, 1997).

Experiments show that astragalus can control a rise in blood pressure and lower the blood pressure of cats, dogs, and rats under anesthesia. Astragalus has positive cardiac effects and can increase coronary blood flow and decrease coronary circulation resistance and troponin-T release; it can also assist with postmyocardial infarction recovery (Modern TCM Pharmacology, 1997).

Astragalus has antiviral and anti-inflammatory effects (Modern TCM Pharmacology, 1997). It can significantly improve the immunity of mice with solid tumors and has antineoplastic effects (Kurashige, 1999).

Investigation into the effects of astragalus on the activity of dog small intestine indicated that it could strengthen movement and muscle tonus, especially in the jejunum (Yang, 1993).

Poultry: Antiparasitic effects

Compared with controls, an extract of *Astragalus membranaceus* significantly increased immunoglobulin (Ig)G and proliferation of antigen-specific splenocytes against *Eimeria tenella*–infected chickens. This study concluded that supplementation with the extract resulted in enhancement of both cellular and humoral immune responses in *E. tenella*–infected chickens (Guo, 2004a). Effects of astragalus extract on chicken growth and the cecal microbial ecosystem were also compared with those of the antibiotic apramycin. Chickens were naturally infected with avian *Mycoplasma gallisepticum*. In contrast to apramycin, the extract stimulated potentially beneficial bacteria (bifidobacteria and lactobacilli), while reducing potentially harmful bacteria (*Bacteroides* spp and *Escherichia coli*) (Guo, 2004b).

Indications: Chronic infection, immune deficiency, and cancer. Chronic wounds and lesions and chronic hepatitis. Hypertension, congestive heart disease, chronic debility, aging. Adjuvant to conventional cancer therapies.

Potential Veterinary Indications: Geriatric support, congestive heart failure, early heart failure, chronic infection, immune deficiency, renal disease, cancer

Contraindications: None known

Toxicology and Adverse Effects: AHPA class 1. Astragalus is a relative of locoweed (*Astragalus alpinus, Astragalus lentiginosus, Astragalus lambertii, Astragalus mollisimus, Astragalus emoryanus,* and *Astragalus miser*), aerial portions of which are toxic to livestock. The root of the Chinese species is nontoxic.

Preparation Notes: The traditional method of preparation is to decoct the dried root, or sometimes fry it with honey. Frying, however, negatively affects the triterpene content and decreases macrophage-stimulating activity. Some Western herb pharmacies supply tinctures that are a traditional decoction, preserved with alcohol. Simple hydroalcoholic extracts (as opposed to fluid extracts) are thought by some to be too weak to use.

Dosage:

Human:

Dried herb: 3-10 g TID

Infusions and decoctions: 5-30 g per cup of water, with 1 cup of the tea given TID, up to 6 times daily acutely

Tincture (usually in 25%-35% ethanol): 1 : 2 or 1 : 3: 1.5-5 mL TID

Small Animal:

Dried herb: 50-400 mg/kg divided daily (optimally, TID)

Decoction: 5-30 g per cup of water, administered at a rate of ¼-½ cup per 10 kg (20 lb), divided daily (optimally, TID)

Tincture: 1 : 2-1 : 3: 1.0-2.0 mL per 10 kg (20 lb), divided daily (optimally, TID) and diluted or combined with other herbs. Higher doses may be appropriate if the herb is used singly and is not combined in a formula.

References

Chang H, But P. *Pharmacology and Applications of Chinese Materia Medica,* vol 2. Singapore: World Scientific; 1987.

Guo FC, Kwakkel RP, Williams BA, et al. Effects of mushroom and herb polysaccharides on cellular and humoral immune responses of *Eimeria tenella*–infected chickens. Poult Sci 2004a; 83:1124-1132.

Guo FC, Kwakkel RP, Soede J, et al. Effects of mushroom and herb polysaccharides, as alternatives for an antibiotic, on the cecal microbial ecosystem in broiler chickens. Poult Sci 2004b;83: 175-182.

Kurashige S, Akuzawa Y, Endo F. Effects of astragali radix extract on carcinogenesis, cytokine production, and cytotoxicity in mice treated with a carcinogen, N-butyl-N′-butanolnitrosoamine. Cancer Invest 1999;17:30-35.

Lei H, Wang B, Li WP, Yang Y, Zhou AW, Chen MZ. Anti-aging effect of astragalosides and its mechanism of action. Acta Pharmacol Sin 2003;24:230-234.

Peng A, Gu Y, Lin SY. Herbal treatment for renal diseases. Ann Acad Med Singapore 2005;34:44-51.

Yang DZ. [Effect of *Astragalus membranaceus* on myoelectric activity of small intestine]. Chung Kuo Chung Hsi I Chieh Ho Tsa Chih 1993;13:582,616-617.

Yin X, Zhang Y, Wu H, et al. Protective effects of Astragalus saponin I on early stage of diabetic nephropathy in rats. J Pharmacol Sci 2004;95:256-266.

Atractylodes

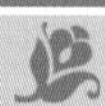

Atractylodes macrocephala Koidz • uh-TRAK-tuh-LO-deez mak-roh-SEF-uh-luh *or* uh-TRAK-tuh-LO-deez mak-roh-KEF-uh-luh

Other Names: Bai zhu

Family: Asteraceae

Distribution: China, Japan, and Korea

Parts Used: Root (dried rhizome)

Selected Constituents: Atractylol, atractylone (essential oil), phytochemicals: 2-furaldehyde, 3-beta-acetoxyatractylon, 3-beta-hydroxyatractrylon, acetylatractylodinol, atractylodin, atractylodinol, atractylon, beta-eudesmol, beta-selinene, calcium, copper, elemol, essential oil furfural, hinesol, iron, L-alpha-bisabolol, magnesium, manganese, potassium, scopoletin, sodium, zinc.

Atractylodes macrocephala has only 0.35% to 1.35% essential oil and even less after it is fried. Therefore, other active ingredients may explain its functions. Atractylenolide (sesquiterpene lactones) is found in atractylodes; this element increases with frying. Components may be antispasmodic agents.

Clinical Actions: Bitter tonic, digestive, adaptogen, diuretic, mild anticoagulant, diaphoretic

Energetics: Bitter, sweet, and warm. Tonifies Spleen *Qi,* dries dampness (fried form). For edema due to Spleen deficiency (raw form).

History and Traditional Usage: In China, atractylodes is traditionally used for dyspepsia, eczema, edema, and nyctalopia. In Japan, it is traditionally used for its balsamic, diaphoretic, diuretic, and stomachic actions. The main functions still recognized for atractylodes are its ability to overcome moisture accumulation and promote digestion. An indicator for the use of atractylodes in a diuretic formulation is limited urinary elimination with excessive sweating (Yang, 1998). When atractylodes turns deep brown after it is dry fried, it is called roasted bai zhu. This has the strongest effect in the stomach and is useful for treating those with a poor appetite, nausea, fullness in the stomach, and belching (Sionneau, 1995).

Published Research: In vitro studies show some hypoglycemic activity (Shan, 2003). The effect of *Atractylodes macrocephala* on the immune function of broiler chicks was investigated. Atractylodes was added to the basal diet at 1%, and the basal diet was supplemented with 50 mg/kg bacitracin zinc as the control. Birds were vaccinated against Newcastle's disease at 21 and 49 days of age. Serum antibody titers were significantly increased ($P < .05$) compared with those of controls, on days 28 and 49, which suggested that the plant could augment antibody formulation; as well, the plant demonstrated antiviral activity; no adverse effect on body weight was noted (Ma, 2003).

The plant also has antioxidant activity. Administered to mice for 4 consecutive weeks, atractylodes decoction enhanced the activity of blood; it was also observed to counteract red blood cell hemolysis through self-oxidation combined with clear active oxygen free radicals (Lu, 1996).

Indications: Anorexia, diarrhea, exhaustion, indigestion, intestinal bleeding, night blindness, edema, stress

Potential Veterinary Indications: Chronic debilitating disease, chronic gastroenteritis, diarrhea, stress

Contraindications: In Traditional Chinese Medicine terms, patients with endogenous heat due to yin deficiency and deficient body fluids should use with caution; therefore, avoid in patients for which dryness is a feature.

Toxicology and Adverse Effects: AHPA class 1. LD_{50} for mice is 13.3 g/kg of the decoction.

Drug Interactions: The herb has shown hypoglycemic activity in animal models; therefore, monitoring of diabetic patients who are administered this herb is advisable.

Dosage:

Human:

Dried herb: 2-10 g TID

Infusions and decoctions: 5-30 g per cup of water, with 1 cup of the tea given TID

Tincture: 1:2 or 1:3: 1-5 mL TID

Small Animal:

Dried herb: 25-200 mg/kg, divided daily (optimally, TID)

Decoction: 5-30 g per cup of water, administered at a rate of ¼-½ cup per 10 kg (20 lb), divided daily (optimally, TID)

Tincture: 1:2-1:3: 0.5-1.0 mL per 10 kg (20 lb), divided daily (optimally, TID) and diluted or combined with other herbs. Higher doses may be appropriate if the herb is used singly and is not combined in a formula.

References

Chen ZL. The acetylenes from *Atractylodes macrocephala*. Planta Med 1987;53:5,493-494.

Koo HN, Lee JK, Hong SH,et al. Herbkines increase physical stamina in mice. Biol Pharmaceut Bull 2004;27:1,117-119.

Lin YC, Jin T, Wu XY, et al. A novel bisesquiterpenoid, biatractylolide, from the Chinese herbal plant *Atractylodes macrocephala*. J Nat Prod 1997;60:1,27-28.

Ma DY, Shan Anshan, Li Q, et al. Effects of Chinese medicinal herb on growth and immunization of laying chicks. J Northeast Agric Univ (English Edition) 2003;10:2,121-125.

Shan JJ, Tian GY. Studies on physico-chemical properties and hypoglycemic activity of complex polysaccharide AMP-B from *Atractylodes macrocephala* Koidz [Chinese]. Acta Pharmaceut Sin 2003;38:6,438-441.

Sionneau P. *Pao Zhi: An Introduction to the Use of Processed Chinese Medicinals*. Boulder, CO: Blue Poppy Press; 1995.

Yang S. *The Divine Farmer's Materia Medica*. Boulder, Colo: Blue Poppy Press; 1998.

Bacopa

Bacopa monnieri (L) Pennell • Buh-KOH-puh mon-ee-ER-ee

Other Names: Brahmi (this is also the name used for *Centella asiatica* [gotu kola] in certain parts of India), Water Hyssop, Herb-of-Grace, Indian Pennywort

Family: Scrophulariceae

Parts Used: Dried whole plant, mainly leaves and stems

Selected Constituents: Alkaloids (brahmine and herpestine), saponins, d-mannitol, hersaponin acid A, and monnierin. Other constituents include betulic acid, stigmasterol, beta-sitosterol, and numerous bacosides and bacopasaponins. The constituents responsible for Bacopa's cognitive effects are bacosides A and B (Kapoor, 1990; Chakravarty, 2003; Hou, 2002).

Bacoside A.

Distribution: Native in tropical regions, including India and Australia
Clinical Action: Nervine tonic, spasmolytic, mild sedative, mental tonic, cardiotonic, digestive, antiasthmatic
Energetics: Cold, astringent in taste, slightly sweet
History and Traditional Usage: Bacopa has been used in the Ayurvedic system of medicine for centuries. Traditionally, it was used as a brain tonic to enhance memory development, learning, and concentration, and to provide relief to patients with anxiety or epileptic disorders (Chopra, 1958). The plant has also been used in India and Pakistan as a cardiac tonic and digestive aid and to improve respiratory function in cases of bronchoconstriction (Nadkarni, 1988).

Recent research has focused on the cognitive-enhancing effects of bacopa, specifically, memory, learning, and concentration; results support traditional Ayurvedic claims. Further research on anxiety, epilepsy, bronchitis and asthma, irritable bowel syndrome, and gastric ulcers supports the Ayurvedic uses of bacopa. Also, its antioxidant properties may offer protection from free radical damage in cardiovascular disease and certain types of cancer.

Ethnoveterinary practice involves use of the leaves and whole plants for the treatment of animals with seizures (Williamson, 2002).
Published Research: The antioxidant and free radical scavenging properties of bacopa may explain the reported antistress, immunomodulatory, cognition-facilitating, anti-inflammatory, and antiaging effects produced in experimental animals and in clinical situations (Russo, 2003). Potent adaptogenic activity has been demonstrated in stressed rats with a standardized extract of bacopa (Rai, 2003). It exerts cognition-enhancing effects in animals, especially rats, and reduced cognitive impairment when administered in conjunction with phenytoin (Vohora, 2000).

Bacopa has shown activity against depression, anxiety, and pain in laboratory animals. A study investigated the anxiolytic activity of a standardized extract (based on bacoside A) of bacopa (5, 10, and 20 mg/kg) given orally in rats; it elicited a response comparable with that of lorazepam at 0.5 mg/kg ip (Bhattacharya, 1998). Significant antidepressant activity in a rat model of depression was demonstrated with a standardized methanolic extract of Bacopa (bacoside A, 38.0+ or −0.9) at 20 and 40 mg/kg PO once daily for 5 days and was found to be comparable with that of imipramine (Sairam, 2002). Bacosine was found to have analgesic activity (opioidergic) but without barbiturate-type narcosis in rats and mice. Although analgesic activity was observed at 25 mg/kg IP, no mortality or untoward effects were observed at up to 300 mg/kg (Vohora, 1997).

Human clinical trials have shown benefits for cognitive function. In a double-blind, placebo-controlled clinical trial, people were tested for visual information processing, learning rate, anxiety, and memory consolidation after 5 and 12 weeks of administration of 300 mg of bacopa daily or placebo. Significant improvements were found following bacopa administration (Stough, 2001).

Bacopa may have a role in the treatment of those with hypothyroidism. Bacopa (200 mg/kg) increased T4 concentration in male mice, suggesting a thyroid-stimulating role. Bacopa increased T4 concentration by 41% without enhancing hepatic lipid peroxidation, thereby showing an antiperoxidative role (Kar, 2002).
Indications: Decreased mental acuity, depression, anxiety, stress
Potential Veterinary Indications: Epilepsy, for mild sedation, anxiolytic as a nervine, hypothyroidism, stressed laboratory rodents. Complementary therapy alongside anticonvulsant treatment. Stress-related bronchitis and diarrhea.
Contraindications: Bacopa has been noted in animal models to decrease the toxicity of morphine and phenytoin (Vohora, 2000). It has also been shown to have a slight sedative effect, so caution is advised in combination with sedatives. Because it may stimulate T4 activity at high doses, it can potentiate the activity of thyroid-stimulating drugs or inhibit the effects of thyroid-suppressant drugs.
Toxicology and Adverse Effects: Therapeutic doses of bacopa are not associated with any known adverse effects. A double-blind, placebo-controlled clinical trial of male volunteers investigated the safety of pharmacologic doses of isolated bacosides over a 4-week period. Concentrated bacosides in single (20-30 mg) and multiple (100-200 mg) daily doses were well tolerated and were associated with no adverse effects (Singh, 1997).

The LD_{50} values of bacopa extracts administered orally to rats were 5 g/kg for aqueous extracts and 17 g/kg for the alcohol extract. Neither resulted in gross behavioral changes (Martis, 1992).
Drug Interactions: Laboratory animal research suggests that bacopa may potentiate the effects of pentobarbitone and phenothiazines.
Dosage:
Human:
Dried herb: 2-10 g TID
Standardized extract (to 20% bacosides A and B): 100-400 mg daily in divided doses (for children, 100 to 200 mg daily in divided doses)
Syrup: 30 mL daily
Infusions and decoctions: 5-30 g per cup of water, with 1 cup of the tea given TID, up to 6 times daily acutely
Tincture (usually in 25%-40% ethanol): 1:2 or 1:3: 1-5 mL TID (2.5 to 6 mL per day for children aged 6 to 12)
Small Animal:
Dried herb: 50-300 mg/kg, divided daily (optimally, TID)
Standardized extract (to 20% bacosides A and B): 3-10 mg/kg daily in divided doses (optimally, TID)
Infusion and decoction: 5-30 g per cup of water, administered at a rate of ¼-½ cup per 10 kg (20 lb), divided daily (optimally, TID)
Tincture (usually in 25%-40% ethanol): 1:2-1:3: 1.0-3.0 mL per 10 kg (20 lb), divided daily (optimally, TID) and diluted or combined with other herbs. Higher doses may be appropriate if the herb is used singly and is not combined in a formula.

References

Bhattacharya SK, Ghosal S. Anxiolytic activity of a standardized extract of *Bacopa monniera:* an experimental study. Phytomedicine 1998;5:2,77-82.

Chakravarty AK, Garai S, Masuda K, Nakane T, Kawahara N. Bacopasides III-V: three new triterpenoid glycosides from *Bacopa monniera.* Chem Pharm Bull (Tokyo) 2003;51:215-217.

Chopra RN. *Indigenous Drugs of India.* 2nd ed. Calcutta, India: U.N. Dhur and Sons; 1958:341.

Hou CC, Lin SJ, Cheng JT, Hsu FL. Bacopaside III, bacopasaponin G, and bacopasides A, B, and C from *Bacopa monniera.* J Nat Products 2002;65:1759-1763.

Kapoor LD. *CRC Handbook of Ayurvedic Medicinal Plants.* Boca Raton, Fla: CRC Press Inc; 1990:61.

Kar A, Panda S, Bharti S. Relative efficacy of three medicinal plant extracts in the alteration of thyroid hormone concentrations in male mice. J Ethnopharmacol 2002;81:2,281-285.

Martis G, Rao A. Neuropharmacological activity of *Herpestis monniera.* Fitoterapia 1992;63:399-404.

Nadkarni KM. *The Indian Materia Medica.* Columbia, Mo: South Asia Books; 1988:624-625.

Rai D, Bhatia G, Palit G, Pal R, Singh S, Singh HK. Adaptogenic effect of *Bacopa monniera* (Brahmi). Pharmacol Biochem Behav 2003;75:823-830.

Russo A, Izzo AA, Borrelli F, Renis M, Vanella A. Free radical scavenging capacity and protective effect of *Bacopa monnieri* L. on DNA damage. Phytother Res 2003;17:870-875.

Sairam K, Dorababu M, Goel RK, Bhattacharya SK. Antidepressant activity of standardized extract of *Bacopa monniera* in experimental models of depression in rats. Phytomedicine 2002;9:3,207-211.

Singh HK, Dhawan BN. Neuropsychopharmacological effects of the Ayurvedic nootropic *Bacopa monniera* Linn. (Brahmi). Indian J Pharmacol 1997;29:S359-S365.

Stough C, Lloyd J, Clarke J, et al. The chronic effects of an extract of *Bacopa monniera* (Brahmi) on cognitive function in healthy human subjects. Psychopharmacology (Berl) 2001;156:481-484.

Vohora SB, Pal SN, Pillai KK. Analgesic activity of bacosine, a new triterpene isolated from *Bacopa monniera.* Fitoterapia 1997;68: 361-365.

Vohora D, Pal SN, Pillai KK. Protection from phenytoin-induced cognitive deficit by *Bacopa monniera,* a reputed Indian nootropic plant. J Ethnopharmacol 2000;71:383-390.

Baical Skullcap, Chinese Skullcap 

Scutellaria baicalensis Georgi • Skew-teh-LARE-ee-uh by-kol-EN-sis

Other Names: Huang quin. Although *Scutellaria baicalensis* is different from the related plant *Scutellaria laterifolia, S. laterifolia* was used for infectious diseases in the 1800s that were similar to those treated with Chinese scute.

Family: Lamiaceae

Parts Used: Root

Distribution: Native to China

Selected Constituents: Many flavonoids, including baicalein, baicalin, and wogonin

Baicalein

Wogonin

Clinical Actions: Anti-inflammatory, antiallergic, antibacterial, mild sedative, bitter, diuretic, hypotensive

Energetics: Bitter, cold

History and Traditional Usage: *Scutellaria baicalensis* is typically used in Traditional Chinese Medicine to "clear heat and dry dampness." It is used in herbal combinations to treat patients with inflammatory skin conditions, allergies, high cholesterol, and cancers, and as a sedative (Bone, 1996).

Published Research: The flavonoids baicalein, baicalin, and wogonin have been individually studied and shown to have anti-inflammatory activity (Chi, 2003), anxiolytic effects similar to diazepam without sedative and muscle relaxant adverse effects typical of benzodiazapenes (Hui, 2002), hepatoprotective effects against acetaminophen toxicity (Jang, 2003), and protective effects against amyloid beta proteins of nerve cells that may be useful in the prevention of Alzheimer's disease (Heo, 2004). *Scutellaria baicalensis* selectively and effectively inhibited cancer cell growth in vitro in human cell lines and in vivo in mice and could be an effective chemotherapeutic agent. Differences compared with baicalein suggest synergistic effects among components in *Scutellaria baicalensis* (Zhang, 2003).

Indications: Allergic conditions, chronic inflammatory conditions such as autoimmune disease, hypertension, atherosclerosis

Potential Veterinary Indications: *Anxiety, allergic conditions, inflammatory disorders, autoimmune disease*

Contraindications: None known

Toxicology and Adverse Effects: AHPA class 1

Dosage:

Human:

Dried herb: 3-10 g TID

Infusions and decoctions: 5-30 g per cup of water, with 1 cup of the tea given TID

Tincture (usually in 60% ethanol): 1:2 or 1:3: 2-5 mL TID

Small Animal:
Dried herb: 25-300 mg/kg, divided daily (optimally, TID)
Decoction: 5-30 g per cup of water, administered at a rate of ¼-½ cup per 10 kg (20 lb), divided daily (optimally, TID)
Tincture (usually in 60% ethanol): 1:2-1:3: 0.5-1.5 mL per 10 kg (20 lb), divided daily (optimally, TID) and diluted or combined with other herbs

References

Bone K, Morgan M. *Clinical Applications of Ayurvedic and Chinese Herbs: Monographs for the Western Herbal Practitioner.* Warick, Australia: Phytotherapy Press; 1996:75-79.

Chi YS, Lim H, Park H, Kim HP. Effects of wogonin, a plant flavone from *Scutellaria radix,* on skin inflammation: in vivo regulation of inflammation-associated gene expression. Biochem Pharmacol 2003;66:1271-1278.

Heo HJ, Kim DO, Choi SJ, Shin DH, Lee CY. Potent inhibitory effect of flavonoids in *Scutellaria baicalensis* on amyloid beta protein–induced neurotoxicity. J Agric Food Chem 2004;52: 4128-4132.

Hui KM, Huen MS, Wang HY, et al. Anxiolytic effect of wogonin, a benzodiazepine receptor ligand isolated from *Scutellaria baicalensis* Georgi. Biochem Pharmacol 2002;64:1415-1424.

Jang SI, Kim HJ, Hwang KM, et al. Hepatoprotective effect of baicalin, a major flavone from *Scutellaria radix,* on acetaminophen-induced liver injury in mice. Immunopharmacol Immunotoxicol 2003;25:585-594.

Zhang DY, Wu J, Ye F, et al. Inhibition of cancer cell proliferation and prostaglandin E2 synthesis by *Scutellaria baicalensis.* Cancer Res 2003;63:4037-4043.

Baptisia

Baptisia tinctoria L. Venten • Bap-TIZ-ee-uh tink-TOH-ree-uh
Other Names: Wild indigo
Family: Fabaceae
Distribution: Midwestern United States
Parts Used: Root, leaves
Selected Constituents: Alkaloids, isoflavones, coumarins, polysaccharides such as arabinogalactans
Clinical Actions: Immune modulator, antipyretic, chlolagogue
Energetics: Slightly bitter and pungent; clears toxic heat
History and Traditional Usage: Used by various North American tribes for cleaning cuts and ulcers, as a douche for gynecologic problems, for kidney and liver problems, for hemoptysis, and for rheumatism. The hallmark indication for its use by 19th century American herbalists was in stomatitis, typhoid, sepsis, and "putrid" inflammation and ulcerations in which tissue was dark or purple.
Published Research: No relevant clinical trials were found.
Indications: Common cold, stomatitis, gingivitis, pharyngitis, tonsillitis, pyorrhea; lymphadenitis; fever.
Potential Veterinary Indications: Stomatitis and periodontal disease, bacterial infections. Arabinogalactans may confer some immune stimulation properties.
Contraindications: Not for prolonged use, except under supervision
Toxicology and Adverse Effects: AHPA class 2b, 2d; none reported. Herbalists and the homeopathic *Materia Medica* note that some patients may have mental effects (hallucinations, mania, dementia). A rash was also reported.
Interesting Notes: The root of this plant was used to make blue (indigo) dye.
Dosage:
Human:
Dried herb is not used, as it has not been considered useful.
Tincture (25%-60% ethanol): 1:2 or 1:3: 0.25-2 mL TID, up to 6 times daily for acute conditions
Small Animal:
Tincture (usually in 25%-60% ethanol): 1:2-1:3: 0.5-1.5 mL per 10 kg (20 lb), divided daily (optimally, TID) and diluted or combined with other herbs
Combinations: For lymphadenopathy, may be combined with Pokeroot and Cleavers. For stomatitis, consider use with Myrrh and Agrimony.

Barberry

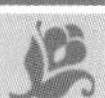

Berberis vulgaris L. • BEAR-ber-is vul-GAY-ris
Distribution: Native to Europe but naturalized over Asia and the United States
Similar Species: *Berberis canadensis* (American barberry), *Berberis aristata* (Indian barberry)
Other Common Names: European barberry
Family: Berberidaceae
Parts Used: Root, root or stem bark
Selected Constituents:
Bark: isoquinoline alkaloids such as berberine, chelidonic acid, resin
Berries: malic acid

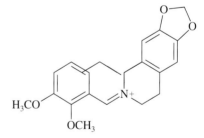

Berberine

Clinical Action: Bitter tonic, cholagogue, alterative, antidiarrheal, antibacterial, antifungal, antiprotozoal, diuretic
Energetics:
Bark: bitter and astringent
Berries: astringent
History and Traditional Usage: Native American Micmac, Mohegan, and Penobscot tribes found the bark and root useful for stomatitis and sore throat. The berries were used for fever. Barberry is considered a bitter tonic and is used for chronic diarrhea and "jaundice due to a congested state of the liver." Herbalists consider barberry a cholagogue that is useful for gallstones and cholecystitis. Specific indications include biliary disease and gastritis. The berries are astringent and are used for fever, diarrhea, and stomatitis.

Indian barberry is used in the treatment of patients with diarrhea and for repeat estrus in cows and buffalo, as well as for kidney stones. The leaf and stem are used for ocular conditions in ruminants and pigs (Williamson, 2002).

Published Research: Most of the clinical studies related to barberry actually use other species of *Berberis,* yet almost all concentrate on the common alkaloids and, in particular, berberine, as the most interesting component. Animal studies show that the ethanol extract of the root is anti-inflammatory, suppresses carrageenan- and zymosan-induced paw edema, and shows benefit in a rheumatoid arthritis model (Ivanovska, 1996).

The isolated alkaloid, berberine, is one of the best studied herbal extracts known. Berberine has been shown (among many things) to inhibit intestinal fluid accumulation, ion secretion, and smooth muscle contraction; reduce inflammation; suppress bacterial enterotoxin formation; inhibit malarial infection; inhibit platelet aggregation; stimulate bile and bilirubin secretion; and inhibit ventricular tachyarrhythmia. Recent clinical reports and clinical trials suggest that berberine administration may improve survival in human cardiac patients; it has cyclooxygenase (COX)-2 mediated anti-inflammatory activity that may be of use in the treatment of patients with certain cancers.

The alkaloid berberine showed strong nematocidal activity against *Toxocara canis* in vitro (Satou, 2002). It was found that 1% berberine sulphate inoculated intralesionally on four occasions at weekly intervals was highly effective against cutaneous leishmaniasis in domestic dogs (Ahuja, 1993). Bolus and infusion of berberine (1 mg/kg within 3 min, followed by 0.2 mg/kg/min at 30 min) in 18 dogs with ischemic left ventricular failure showed that berberine improved impaired left ventricular function through its positive inotropic effects and mild systemic vasodilatation (Huang, 1992).

Berberine hypochloride as an intrauterine preparation was given every second day over a 9-day period in cows with second-degree endometritis; a "cure" rate of 52% was compared with 81% for those treated with a combination of oxytetracycline, oleandomycin, neomycin, prednisolone, and chlorpheniramin maleate (Sinha, 1976).

Although the actions of one important constituent are of interest, whole plants are appreciated by herbalists for their spectra of effects, and Barberry provides one of the best studied examples of plant synergy. Stermitz (2000) discovered a multiple drug resistance pump inhibitor (5-methoxyhydnocarpin) that enhanced the plant's ability to kill *Staphylococcus aureus* by bypassing the bacterial strategy for drug resistance (Stermitz, 2000). The combination of the antibiotic berberine and the drug resistance pump inhibitor provides an example of additive action, and possibly synergy, within a plant.

Indications: Biliary catarrh with constipation and jaundice; gastritis, biliousness, debility during convalescence, ulcerative stomatitis, eczema of the hands

Potential Veterinary Indications: Gastritis, enteritis, dysbiosis, cholecystitis, hepatitis, stomatitis, giardia, endometritis, left ventricular heart failure, leishmaniasis

Contraindications: Not for use in pregnancy unless by a qualified practitioner. Some sources (Herr, 2002) list the traditional *indications* for barberry as *contraindications*, including "gallbladder disease, kidney disease, liver disease."

Toxicology and Adverse Effects: AHPA class 2b. Lethargy, skin and eye problems, cardiac effects, hypotension, dyspnea, GI distress, epistaxis, nephritis, nausea, vomiting, and stupor may theoretically result from consumption of large amounts of barberry. Berberine itself may lead to phototoxicity.

Drug Interactions: Berberine may inhibit some P450 enzymes. Some conservative sources suggest that berberine-containing herbs should be used cautiously with many drug types, including alpha-adrenergic agonists, antiarrhythmics, anticoagulants, antihypertensives, central nervous system depressants, cyclophosphamide, cardiac glycosides, general anesthetics, monoamine oxidase inhibitors, drugs that may cause photosensitivity, tetracyclines, and other antibiotics. The true risk of interaction with these drugs is unknown.

Dosage:

Human:

Dried herb: 0.25-5 g TID (this is a bitter herb, and the higher doses are not usually required)

Infusions and decoctions: 5-10 g per cup of water, with ½-1 cup of the tea given TID

Tincture (25%-60% ethanol have been used): 1:2 or 1:3: 0.25-4 mL TID

Small Animal:

Dried herb: 25-300 mg/kg, divided daily (optimally, TID)

Infusion and decoction: 5-10 g per cup of water, administered at a rate of ¼-½ cup per 10 kg (20 lb), divided daily (optimally, TID)

Tincture (usually in 25%-60% ethanol): 1:2-1:3: 0.5-1.5 mL per 10 kg (20 lb), divided daily (optimally, TID) and diluted or combined with other herbs

References

Ahuja A, Purohit SK, Yadav JS, Netra PR. Cutaneous leishmaniasis in domestic dogs. Indian J Public Health 1993;37: 29-31.

Ernst E, Young VSL, eds. *Herb-Drug Interaction Handbook.* 2nd edition. Nassau, NY: Church Street Books; 2002.

Huang WM, Yan H, Jin JM, Yu C, Zhang H. Beneficial effects of berberine on hemodynamics during acute ischemic left ventricular failure in dogs. Chin Med J (Engl) 1992;105: 1014-1019.

Ivanovska N, Philipov S. Study on the anti-inflammatory action of *Berberis vulgaris* root extract, alkaloid fraction and pure alkaloids. Int J Immunopharmacol 1996;18:553-556.

Sinha A, Singh B, Arneja D. Comparative studies on the efficacy of drugs against endometritis in cattle. Indian Vet J 1976; 53:430.

Stermitz FR, Lorenz P, Tawara JN, Zenewicz LA, Lewis K. Synergy in a medicinal plant: antimicrobial action of berberine potentiated by 5′-methoxyhydnocarpin, a multidrug pump inhibitor. Proc Natl Acad Sci U S A 2000;97:1433-1437.

Satou T, Akao N, Matsuhashi R, Koike K, Fujita K, Nikaido T. Inhibitory effect of isoquinoline alkaloids on movement of second-stage larvae of *Toxocara canis.* Biol Pharm Bull 2002;25: 1651-1654.

Williamson EM, ed. *Major Herbs of Ayurveda.* Sydney, Australia: Churchill Livingstone; 2002:321.

Bilberry

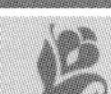

Vaccinium myrtillus L. • Vak-SIN-ee-um mir-TIL-us
Other Names: European blueberry, huckleberry, whortleberry
Family: Ericaceae
Parts Used: Ripe fruit and leaves
Distribution: Bilberry can be found in the mountains and forests of Britain, Europe, and northern United States.
Selected Constituents: Anthocyanoside flavonoids (anthocyanins), vitamins, sugars, and pectins are found in the berries; quercetin, catechins, tannins, iridoids, and acids are found in the leaves. The anthocyanosides are considered the most important active components. Anthocyanoside concentration in the fresh fruit is approximately 0.1% to 0.25%; concentrated bilberry extracts are usually standardized to 25% anthocyanosides (Baj, 1983). The berry's anthocyanoside content increases as the fruit ripens; the reverse is true of its leaf constituents (Morazzoni, 1996).

Anthocyanin

Clinical Actions: Vasoprotective, antioxidant, anti-inflammatory, astringent, antiedema
Energetics: Cool, dry
History and Traditional Usage: Bilberry has been used as food for centuries. Bilberry's history of medicinal use dates back to the Middle Ages, but it did not become widely known to herbalists until the 16th century, when its use was documented for treating patients with bladder stones, biliary disorders, scurvy, coughs, and lung tuberculosis (Grieve, 1971). Bilberry's modern reputation was sparked during World War II, when British Royal Air Force pilots noticed that their night vision was sharper than usual when they ate bilberry preserves before they started evening bombing raids. Subsequent research revealed that bilberries are powerful antioxidants, capable of protecting cells in the eye and other parts of the body against damage from free radicals. Currently, bilberry research is focused on the treatment of patients with ocular and vascular disorders, diarrhea, dysentery, and mouth and throat inflammation. Bilberry leaf decoctions have been used to lower blood sugar in diabetes (Grieve, 1971). It is recommended as a remedy in prolonged diarrhea or vomiting, as a mild vermifuge and remedy for throat ailments, and as a nerve tonic for animals (de Bairacli Levy, 1963).
Published Research: A review of placebo-controlled trials of bilberry anthocyanosides looked for evidence of positive effects on night vision. Of a total of 30 studies, 12 were placebo controlled. Four recent trials were randomized, controlled, and negative in outcome. Although the negative outcomes were associated with more rigorous methods, they also used lower dose levels and extracts from geographic sources that may differ in anthocyanoside composition. A fifth randomized, controlled trial, plus seven nonrandomized, controlled trials, reported positive effects on night vision. Evidence from methodologically weaker trials and animal studies and from trials of synthetic anthocyanosides and *Ribes nigrum* (black currant) anthocyanosides may warrant additional studies on *V. myrtillus* anthocyanosides in subjects with impaired night vision (Canter, 2004).

Recently, the effects of a supplemented control diet with 25% bilberry extract (BE, 20 mg/kg of body weight, including 4.5 mg of antocianidin) or vitamin E (40 mg/kg) on a rat model of early senile cataract and macular degeneration was investigated over 1.5 to 3 months. At 3 months, more than 70% of control rats had cataract and macular degeneration; the supplementation of BE completely prevented impairments in the lenses and retina. Vitamin E had no significant effects, but both antioxidants decreased lipid peroxides in the retina and serum of rats. This suggests that long-term supplementation with BE is effective in the prevention of macular degeneration and cataract (Fursova, 2005).

The results of one study indicated that anthocyanins in *V. myrtillus* exert multiple protective effects in endotoxic shock (Sautebin, 2004). An extract of bilberry possesses antiulcer activity, probably achieved by potentiating barriers of the gastrointestinal mucosa (Magistretti, 1988). Oral administration of an extract of *V. myrtillus* left significantly decreased plasma triglycerides and cholesterol levels and had no effect on the concentration of free fatty acids in the plasma of genetically hyperlipidemic rats. It was suggested that the leaves, reported to exhibit hypoglycemic activity, may also affect lipid metabolism (Cignarella, 1992).

V. myrtillus extract was found to be effective in inhibiting the growth of human leukemia cells and human colon carcinoma cells in vitro (Katsube, 2003).

A *V. myrtillus* preparation (25% anthocyanidins) demonstrated significant vasoprotective and antiedema properties in rabbits. Activity was more lasting than that of rutin or mepiramine (Lietti, 1976).
Indications: Retinal damage, night blindness, capillary fragility; evidence suggests that it is beneficial for diabetic retinopathy, macular degeneration, ulcers, and wound healing.
Potential Veterinary Indications: Progressive retinal atrophy, nuclear sclerosis, prevention of cataracts, capillary fragility, herbal antioxidant, geriatric patients. As a tea of the leaf for diarrhea.
Contraindications: None known
Toxicology and Adverse Effects: Leaves: AHPA class 4. Too little is known to rate the toxicity. Berries: AHPA class 1. Dosages as high as 400 mg/kg body weight have been administered to rats without toxicity. Long-term oral administration in humans of doses equivalent to 180 mg/kg anthocyanosides per day for 6 months produced no toxic effects. No mutagenic or carcinogenic effects were observed.

Bilberry extracts have antiplatelet aggregating properties; very high doses should be used cautiously in patients with hemorrhagic disorders and in those taking anticoagulant or antiplatelet drugs.

A review of studies comprising more than 2000 subjects who took bilberry extract reported only mild adverse effects that affected the gastrointestinal, cutaneous, or nervous system (Eandi, 1996).

Dosage:

Human:

Fresh berries: 10-100 g TID
Aqueous extract standardized to 25% anthocyanosides: 80-160 mg TID
Infusions: 5-30 g per cup of water, with 1 cup of the tea given TID
Fluid extract (1:1 in 25% ethanol): 3-5 mL daily
Tincture (20%-66% ethanol; higher doses used for lower ethanol products): 1:2 or 1:3: 3-5 mL TID

Small Animal:

Fresh berries: 5-100 g TID
Dried herb: 25-300 mg/kg, divided daily (optimally, TID)
Infusion: 5-30 g per cup of water, administered at a rate of ¼-½ cup per 10 kg (20 lb), divided daily (optimally, TID)
Dried aqueous extract standardized to 25% anthocyanosides: 2-4 mg/kg TID
Fluid extract (1:1 in 25% ethanol): 0.25-1.0 mL per 10 kg (20 lb), divided daily (optimally, TID)
Tincture (20%-66% ethanol; higher doses used for lower ethanol products): 1:2-1:3: 0.5-1.5 mL per 10 kg (20 lb), divided daily (optimally, TID) and diluted or combined with other herbs

References

Baj A, Bombardelli E, Gabetta B, et al. Qualitative and quantitative evaluation of *Vaccinium myrtillus* anthocyanins by high-resolution gas chromatography and high-performance liquid chromatography. J Chromatogr 1983;279:365-372.

Canter PH, Ernst E. Anthocyanosides of *Vaccinium myrtillus* (Bilberry) for night vision—a systematic review of placebo-controlled trials. Surv Ophthalmol 2004;49:38-50.

Cignarella A, Nastasi M, Cavalli E, et al. Hypolipidemic activity of *Vaccinium myrtillus* leaves in a new model of genetically hyperlipidemic rat. Planta Med 1992;58:A581-A582.

De Bairacli Levy J. *The Complete Herbal Handbook for Farm and Stable.* London: Faber and Faber; 1963.

De Bairacli Levy J. *The Complete Herbal Handbook for the Dog and Cat.* London: Faber and Faber; 1985.

Eandi M. Post-marketing investigation on Tegens' preparation with respect to side effects. Fitoterapia 1996;67:3-29.

Fursova AZh, Gesarevich OG, Gonchar AM, et al. [Dietary supplementation with bilberry extract prevents macular degeneration and cataracts in senesce-accelerated OXYS rats]. Adv Gerontol 2005;16:76-79.

Grieve M. *A Modern Herbal,* vol 1. New York, NY: Dover Publications; 1971:385-386.

Katsube N, Iwashita K, Tsushida T, Yamaki K, Kobori M. Induction of apoptosis in cancer cells by Bilberry *(Vaccinium myrtillus)* and the anthocyanins. J Agric Food Chem 2003; 51:68-75.

Lietti A, Cristoni A, Picci M. Studies on *Vaccinium myrtillus* anthocyanosides. I. Vasoprotective and antiinflammatory activity. Arzneimittelforschung 1976;26:829-832.

Magistretti MJ, Conti M, Cristoni A. Antiulcer activity of an anthocyanidin from *Vaccinium myrtillus.* Arzneimittelforschung 1988;38:686-690.

Morazzoni P, Bombardelli E. *Vaccinium myrtillus.* Fitoterapia 1996;67:3-29.

Sauebin L, Rossi A, Serraino I, Dugo P, Di Paola R, Mondello L, Genovese T, Britti D, Peli A, Dugo G, Caputi AP, Cuzzocrea S. Effect of anthocyanins contained in a blackberry extract on the circulatory failure and multiple organ dysfunction caused by endotoxin in the rat. Planta Med 2004;70:8,745-752.

Black Cohosh

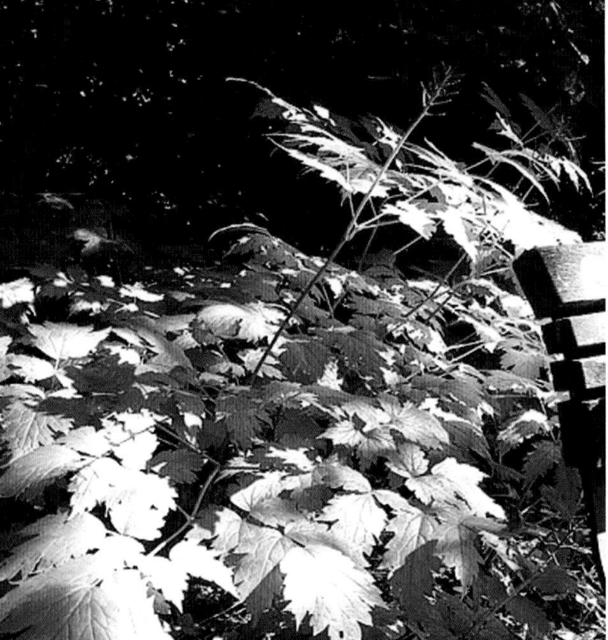

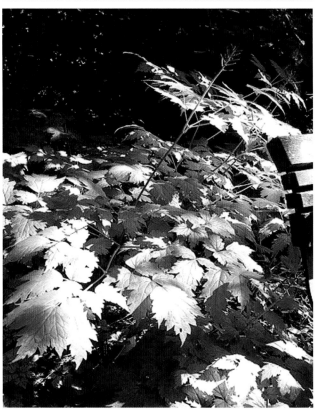

Actaea racemosa L. (formerly, *Cimicifuga racemosa* [L] Nutt.) • AK-tee-uh ray-see-MO-suh

Distribution: Indigenous to Canada and the United States

Common Names: Black cohosh, black bugbane, black snakeroot, squaw vine (considered extremely derogatory now), rattlesnake root, rheumatism weed

Family: Ranunculaceae

Parts Used: Rhizomes

Selected Constituents: Cimicifugin (a mixture of resins and bitters 15%-20%), triterpenoid glycosides (including cimifugoside, racemoside, and acteine). Isoflavones (including formononetin and kaemferol). Salicylic acid, tannins, alkaloids (including cytisine and methylecytisine)

Clinical Actions: Antispasmodic, anti-inflammatory, antirheumatic, emmenagogue, relaxing nervine, antitussive

Energetics: Bitter, pungent

History and Traditional Usage: Native Americans used black cohosh as a tonic, for rheumatism and coughs, and during and after childbirth, as well as for a range of gynecologic problems (such as amenorrhea and dysmenorrhea). Cherokee Indians used an infusion of the root to stimulate menstrual flow and to lessen menstrual pain; the Iroquois Indians used it for rheumatic pain and as a galactagogue. It was popularized by the Eclectics in the 19th century and as a pain-relieving remedy for muscular pain (including dysmenorrhea) and nerve pain. In Traditional Chinese Medicine and Traditional Japanese Medicine, black cohosh was considered a "female remedy" that was used to release the exterior, clear heat, relieve toxicity, and raise collapsed yang (associated with prolapses). Black cohosh has been used as therapy for pain and inflammation in Korean folk medicine.

Published Research: Black cohosh has been thought to contain constituents that, with long-term treatment, suppress luteinizing hormone (LH) release, constituents that bind estrogen receptors and suppress LH release, and compounds that are competitors for the estrogen receptor but have no effect on LH release (Duker, 1991). In whole plant studies, black cohosh caused a reduction in levels of LH and no changes in follicle-stimulating hormone (FSH). The triterpene glycosides affect the hypothalamic-pituitary axis, leading to a variety of secondary effects on the reproductive, nervous, and circulatory systems, as well as on bone density (Jarry, 1985a; Jarry, 1985b). Jarry suggests that these are estrogenic effects, i.e., binding to Erb receptors. The mechanism of action may involve estrogenic effects, but more recent studies dispute the estrogenic theory and indicates that extracts of black cohosh do not bind to the estrogen receptor, upregulate estrogen-dependent genes, or stimulate the growth of estrogen-dependent tumors in animal models (Lupu, 2003; Mahady, 2003). On the other hand, experiments have demonstrated that black cohosh does contain compounds with antiestrogenic properties (Zierau, 2002).

A wide range of clinical studies have used extracts of black cohosh, specifically, Remifemin, which is a 1:10 extract of *A. racemosa* that is marketed as an alternative to hormone replacement therapy (HRT) for women (Burdette, 2003). One critical review concluded that clinical benefit had not been convincingly demonstrated in quality trials, but that a central effect or an estrogenic effect could not be ruled out (Borelli, 2002). Another critical review of the effects of black cohosh on menopausal symptoms in women concludes, "Evidence for black cohosh is promising, albeit limited by the poor methodology of the trials" (Huntley, 2003).

Indications: Menopausal disorders, menopausal pain, migraine, and depression; osteoarthritis and rheumatoid arthritis, bronchitis, and coughs

Potential Veterinary Indications: Possibly osteoarthritis, rheumatism (muscular pain), bronchitis, tracheitis, and hormonally associated conditions in ovariectomized animals such as incontinence

Contraindications: Estrogen-sensitive cancers, pregnancy, lactation

Toxicology and Adverse Effects: AHPA class 2b, 2c. Published reports and herbalists are describing cases of hepatotoxicity with long-term use in women (Lynch, 2006). The main effects with long-term use have been mild to severe joint pain or headache, elevated liver enzymes, and adverse reactions in the liver caused by interaction with statins. This herb should not be used on a long-term basis (Lontos, 2003).

Potential Drug Interactions: In vitro potentiation of tamoxifen in cell lines (Freudenstein, 1999); in rats, enhanced effects of mestranol on induced ovulation

Dosage:

Human:

Dried herb: 100 mg-6 g TID

Standardized extract: 20-40 mg BID

Infusion: 5-10 g per cup of water, with ¼-1 cup of the tea given TID

Tincture (generally 60% ethanol): 1:2 or 1:3: 0.5-5 mL TID

Small Animal:

Dried herb: 25-300 mg/kg, divided daily (optimally, TID)

Infusion and decoction: 5-10 g per cup of water, administered at a rate of ¼-½ cup per 10 kg (20 lb), divided daily (optimally, TID)

Tincture (usually in 60% ethanol): 1:2-1:3: 0.5 mL per 10 kg (20 lb), divided daily (optimally, TID) and diluted or combined with other herbs. Higher doses may be appropriate if the herb is used singly and is not combined in a formula.

References

Borelli F, Ernst E. *Cimicifuga racemosa:* a systematic review of its clinical efficacy. Eur J Clin Pharmacol 2002;58:235-241.

Burdette JE, Liu J, Chen SN, et al. Black cohosh acts as a mixed competitive ligand and partial agonist of the serotonin receptor. J Agric Food Chem 2003;51:5661-5670.

Duker EM, Kopanski L, Jarry H, Wuttke W. Effects of extracts from *Cimicifuga racemosa* on gonadotropin release in menopausal women and ovariectomized rats. Planta Med 1991;57:420-424.

Huntley AL, Ernst E. A systematic review of herbal medicinal products for the treatment of menopausal symptoms. Menopause 2003;10:465-476.

Jarry H, Harnischfeger G, Duker E. [The endocrine effects of constituents of *Cimicifuga racemosa.* 2. In vitro binding of constituents to estrogen receptors]. Planta Med 1985a;4:316-319.

Jarry H, Harnischfeger G. [Endocrine effects of constituents of *Cimicifuga racemosa.* 1. The effect on serum levels of pituitary hormones in ovariectomized rats.] Planta Med 1985b;1:46-49.

Lontos S, Jones RM, Angus PW, Gow PJ. Acute liver failure associated with the use of herbal preparations containing black cohosh. Med J Aust 2003;179:390-391.

Lupu R, Mehmi I, Atlas E, et al. Black cohosh, a menopausal remedy, does not have estrogenic activity and does not promote breast cancer cell growth. Int J Oncol 2003;23: 1407-1412.

Lynch CR, Folkers ME, Hutson WR. Fulminant hepatic failure associated with the use of black cohosh: a case report. Liver Transpl 2006;12:989-992.

Mahady GB. Is black cohosh estrogenic? Nutr Rev 2003;61 (5 Pt 1):183-186.

Zierau O, Bodinet C, Kolba S, Wulf M, Vollmer G. Antiestrogenic activities of *Cimicifuga racemosa* extracts. J Steroid Biochem Mol Biol 2002;80:125-130.

Black Haw

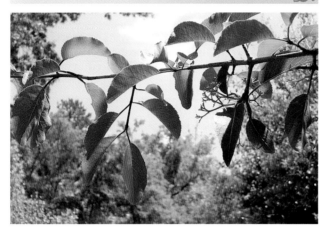

Viburnum prunifolium L. • Vy-BUR-num proo-ni-FOH-lee-um

Family: Caprifoliaceae

Other Common Names: Sloe, stag bush, sloe-leaved viburnum, nannybush

Distribution: Native to the United States, planted as an ornamental shrub in Europe

Part Used: Dried bark, root

Related Species: *Viburnum opulus* (Cramp bark) has similar properties.

Selected Constituents: Coumarins (including esculetin, scopoletin), flavones (such as amentoflavone), salicylic acid, triterpenes, phenolic acids, tannins, phytosterols (sitosterol)

Clinical Action: Anodyne, antispasmodic, astringent, bitter tonic, uterine sedative and tonic, nervine

Energetics: Bitter and cool

Traditional Uses: Delaware, Oklahoma, and Micmac American Indian tribes used the root as a gynecologic aid. The Cherokees used it to prevent recurrent spasms; as a diaphoretic; for fever, smallpox, and ague; and as a wash for sore tongue. The Eclectics viewed black haw as a nervine, antispasmodic, tonic, astringent, diuretic, and alterative, with affinity for the female reproductive system. Its most important uses were for painful uterine cramps, leg cramps, and threatened abortion. Black haw was also used for mouth ulcers, diarrhea, and heart palpitations. Modern herbalists generally use black haw for human menstrual disorders, to prevent miscarriage, and to take advantage of its antispasmodic activity in treating patients with asthma.

Published Research: Early in vitro and laboratory animal experiments confirm that black haw has spasmolytic activity on the uterine smooth muscle (Bissett, 1989).

Indications: Minor uterine cramps or painful dysmenorrhea, "spastic pregnancy"

Potential Veterinary Indications: Habitual or threatened abortion, skeletal muscle cramps

Contraindications: Those with a history of kidney stones should use this cautiously because of the high content of oxalates.

Toxicology and Adverse Effects: AHPA class 2d because of oxalate content. *King's* reported that large doses can cause nausea and vomiting in people. Contains coumarins, to which cats may have unique sensitivity.

Drug Interactions: None reported

Notes of Interest: A black haw cordial was described in *King's American Dispensatory*; it was used as an aid in treating women with menstrual disorders. It is prepared thus:

"Viburnum Cordial—Recent bark of root of black haw, 20 oz; recent bark of root of wild cherry, 40 oz; Ceylon cinnamon, 10 oz; cloves, 5 oz; sugar, 7½ lb; brandy, 2 gal; and water, 1½ gal. Mix the crushed drugs with the mixed brandy and water; add the sugar, and stir together for 14 days. Then, express and filter."

Dosage:

Human:

Dried herb: 1-10 g TID, up to 6 times daily for acute conditions

Infusions and decoctions: 5-30 g per cup of water, with 1 cup of the tea given TID, up to 6 times daily acutely

Tincture (30%-70% ethanol, sometimes with glycerin to prevent precipitation of tannins): 1:2 or 1:3: 4-5 mL TID, up to 6 times daily for acute conditions

Small Animal:

Dried herb: 25-200 mg/kg, divided daily (optimally, TID)

Infusion and decoction: 5-30 g per cup of water, administered at a rate of ¼-½ cup per 10 kg (20 lb), divided daily (optimally, TID)

Tincture (30%-70% ethanol, sometimes with glycerin to prevent precipitation of tannins): 1:2-1:3: 0.5-1.0 mL per 10 kg (20 lb), divided daily (optimally, TID) and diluted or combined with other herbs

Large Animals:

Fluid extract (1:1): 8-120 mL for farm animals (small ruminant to horse or cow)

Reference

Bissett NG. *Herbal Drugs and Phytopharmaceuticals: A Handbook for Practice on a Scientific Basis.* Boca Raton, Fla: CRC Press; 1989.

Black Walnut

Juglans nigra L. • JOO-glanz NY-gruh

Distribution: North America

Similar Species: *Juglans cinerea* (white walnut, or butternut) used as intestinal stimulant (found in North America); *Juglans regia* (European or English walnut) used as sweetmeat

Common Names: Black walnut, American walnut

Family: Juglandaceae

Parts Used: *Fruit rind or green hull:* for antimicrobial, anthelmintic actions

Nut: for food

Leaf and bark: as a gargle, or topically, for skin lesions; for GI disorders

Collection: The fruit is harvested when the rind is green. The leaves are dried.

Selected Constituents: *Nut/fruit:* alpha-hydrojuglone-4-glucoside, cobalt, ellagic acid, fat, iron, magnesium, manganese, myricetin, myricitrin, neosakurnin, niacin,

riboflavin, sakuranetin, sakuranin, selenium, silicon, sodium, tannin, thiamin, tin
Hull: aluminum, ascorbic acid, barium, calcium, chromium, phosphorus, potassium, zinc
Plant/root: juglone (5-hydroxy-alphanapthaquinone)

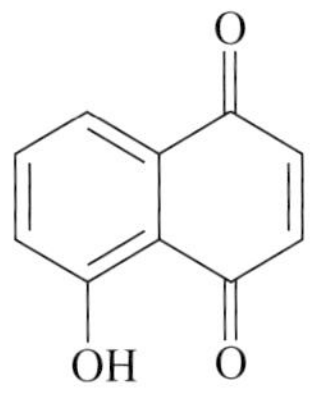

Juglone

Clinical Actions: *Bark:* laxative, alterative, astringent
Fruit: nutritive
Leaves: alterative
Energetics: Cool, sour, slightly bitter
History and Traditional Usage: Native North American tribes used the bark and leaves for all kinds of skin diseases, including ringworm; as an emetic and cathartic; for worms; and for dysentery. The leaves were scattered in dwellings to prevent fleas. The bark, leaves, and nuts were used to make green and black dyes, and the nuts were relished for many uses in cooking. The Eclectics used the juice of the fruit rind for ringworm, herpes, eczema, and other skin diseases; a decoction was used for worms. The hull and fruit were said to have mild sedative qualities. The bark and leaves are traditionally used for hemorrhoids, athlete's foot, gastroenteritis, and gastrointestinal helminths; topically for skin ailments; and as a gargle for toothache and ulcers. The bark was used as an astringent for GI inflammation and ulcers and for dyeing. It is said to be a mild purgative. The bark is used as a dentrifice in India and Pakistan, and it has been associated with dental staining. The fruit hull is also used externally for skin disease.

According to de Bairacli Levy (1963), Arabs use it as a supreme food for fertility in female animals. The residue after expression of the oil is a favored tonic for cattle and horses. Suggested uses in animals include treatment for worms, skin parasites, ringworm, skin ailments, abscesses, venereal disease, constipation, throat and mouth ulcers, and discharging ears; it is used externally as a douche in female ailments. The current use as a heartworm preventive and treatment is not based in tradition.
Published Research: One study on *Juglans regia* extract demonstrated some activity against *Microsporum canis* and *Tricophyton mentagrophytes.* A double-blind, randomized, case control study in people with hypertriglyceridemia indicated that 3 g daily of *J. regia* oil reduced plasma triglyceride concentrations by 19% to 33% from baseline in comparison with placebo treated patients ($P < .05$) (Zibaeenezhad, 2003).
Indications: Infusions or decoctions of leaves, hulls, and bark may be used topically for parasitic skin infections such as ringworm. The oil may be useful for the treatment of hypertriglyceridemia.
Potential Veterinary Indications: Topically for ringworm and focal inflammation, hot spots, and so forth. Possibly useful for diarrhea and gastrointestinal parasites. Black walnut hull has been advocated for the prevention and treatment of canine heartworm, but no traditional or scientific basis has been discovered for this use. Similar to fish oil, walnut oil, when substituted as a fat source in the diet, may be a useful adjunct in the treatment of patients with hyperlipidemia.
Notes of Interest: According to Maude Grieve *(A Modern Herbal),* in the "golden age, when men lived upon acorns, the gods lived upon walnuts, and hence the name of Juglans, Jovis glans, or Jupiter's nuts," pieces of walnut were apparently used to expedite fishing—adding hulls to the water was said to have a sedating effect.
Contraindications: None known. Safety of bark, leaves, and hull in pregnancy and lactation not established.
Toxicology and Adverse Effects: AHPA class 2d. Juglone (a constituent of roots and root bark) is a depressant and may cause severe pulmonary interstitial and alveolar edema in dogs (Boelkins, 1968). Black walnut wood shavings have been reported to cause laminitis in horses (Thomsen, 2000; Eaton, 1995; Galey, 1991; Galey, 1990; Galey, 1989; Minnick, 1987). Mouldy hulls and nuts may contain a neurotoxic mycotoxin, known as Penitrem A, which may have strychnine-like effects with tremors and hyperexcitability. If ingestion is recent, emesis can be induced and activated charcoal administered. If the patient is showing signs of toxicity, it should be anesthetized and gastric lavage performed—emesis is contraindicated because these patients may aspirate vomitus if neurologic effects have appeared. As well, inducing vomiting in patients who have ingested neurotoxins may lead to seizure activity.
Dosage:
Human:
Dried powdered hull: 125-250 mg TID
Infusion (5 g in 1 cup of water): 0.5-4 oz daily
Tincture (40% ethanol; some pharmacies include glycerin to prevent precipitation of tannins): 1:2 or 1:3 in 40% alcohol: 0.25-3 mL TID
Small Animal:
(**NOTE:** Veterinary herbalists do not use this herb often, so the doses are estimates. Long-term use is not recommended.)
Dried herb: 3-25 mg/kg, divided daily (optimally, TID)
Infusion: 5 g per cup of water, administered at a rate of ¼-½ cup per 10 kg (20 lb), divided daily (optimally, TID)
Tincture (40% ethanol; some pharmacies include glycerin to prevent precipitation of tannins): 2-1:3: 0.25-0.5 mL per 10 kg (20 lb), divided daily (optimally, TID) and diluted or combined with other herbs

References

De Bairacli Levy J. *The Complete Herbal Handbook for Farm and Stable.* London: Faber and Faber; 1963.

Eaton SA, Allen D, Eades SC, Schneider DA. Digital Starling forces and hemodynamics during early laminitis induced by an aqueous extract of black walnut *(Juglans nigra)* in horses. Am J Vet Res 1995;56:1338-1344.

Galey FD, Beasley VR, Schaeffer D, Davis LE. Effect of an aqueous extract of black walnut *(Juglans nigra)* on isolated equine digital vessels. Am J Vet Res 1990;51:83-88.

Galey FD, Beasley VR, Schaeffer DJ, Davis LE. Antagonism in isolated equine digital vessels of contraction induced by epinephrine in the presence of hydrocortisone and an aqueous extract of black walnut *(Juglans nigra)*. J Vet Pharmacol Ther 1989;12:411-420.

Galey FD, Whiteley HE, Goetz TE, Kuenstler AR, Davis CA, Beasley VR. Black walnut *(Juglans nigra)* toxicosis: a model for equine laminitis. J Comp Pathol 1991;104:313-326.

Grieve M. *A Modern Herbal,* vol 1. New York, NY: Dover Publications; 1971.

Minnick PD, Brown CM, Braselton WE, Meerdink GL, Slanker MR. The induction of equine laminitis with an aqueous extract of the heartwood of black walnut *(Juglans nigra)*. Vet Hum Toxicol 1987;29:230-233.

Thomsen ME, Davis EG, Rush BR. Black walnut induced laminitis. Vet Hum Toxicol 2000;42:8-11.

Zibaeenezhad MJ, Rezaiezadeh M, Mowla A, Ayatollahi SM, Panjehshahin MR. Antihypertriglyceridemic effect of walnut oil. Angiology 2003;54:411-414.

Web Sites:

Toxicology: http://vet.purdue.edu/depts/addl/toxic/plant45.htm

Botany, commerce, and tidbits: http://www.sfp.forprod.vt.edu/factsheets/walnut.pdf

Blackberry

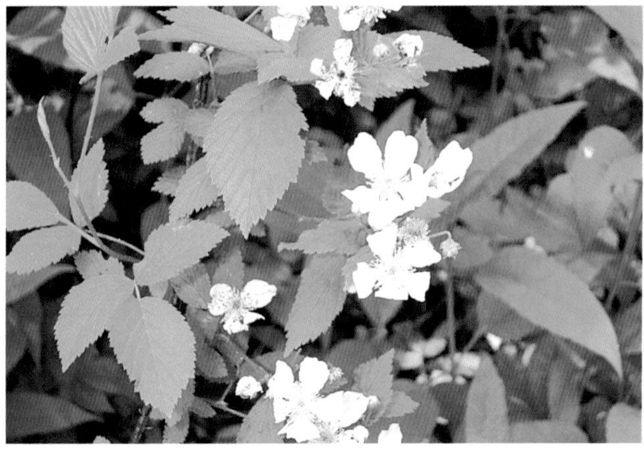

Botanical Name: *Rubus fruticosus* L., *R. villosus*, probably other *Rubus* spp

Other Names: Bramble, brambleberry, bramble-kite, brameberry, brummel, brymbyl, bumble-kite, bly, brombere, brombeere, cloudberry, dewberry, fingerberry, goutberry, scaldhead, thimbleberry

Family: Rosaceae

Parts Used: Leaf, root, bark, berry

Selected Constituents: Arbutin, hydroquinone, oxalic acid, tannins

Clinical Actions: Astringent, antidiarrheal

Energetic: Astringent, slightly bitter, cooling to GI and urinary tracts

History and Traditional Usage: Commission E recommends blackberry leaf for "Nonspecific, acute diarrhea, mild inflammation of the mucosa of the oral cavity and throat." Most species of blackberries were used by Native American tribes for a variety of indications, including diarrhea, hemorrhoids, skin eruptions, gynecologic uses, stomatitis, and rheumatism. The berries were used as food and contained enough vitamin C to prevent scurvy. A gypsy remedy for skin problems in horses was said to consist of blackberry leaf in red wine, applied topically. Some species of *Rubus* have been used to treat patients with diabetes in South America. The Eclectics and Physiomedicalists pronounced it indicated for watery diarrhea of gastrointestinal atony.

De Bairacli Levy (1985) recommended that blackberry leaf infusion be applied to the umbilical area of puppies, as well as to wounds and eczema; that an infusion be used for abrasions; and that it be taken internally for anemia and coughing.

Published Research: The berry is a powerful source of antioxidants. Blackberry and other *Rubus* species have been found to lower blood glucose in some (but not all) laboratory animal models (Jouad, 2002; Lemua, 2000).

Indications: Watery, voluminous diarrhea, stomatitis; as a sitz bath for gynecologic problems; cystitis; topically for skin eruptions

Potential Veterinary Indications: Root bark for watery diarrhea; berries as a nutritional tonic high in antioxidants; leaf for stomatitis and topically for skin eruptions

Contraindications: None described; may interact with hypoglycemic drugs. All astringents may coagulate proteins and interact with other drugs.

Toxicology and Adverse Effects: Leaf and fruit are AHPA class 1. No adverse effects described.

Preparation Notes: Decoction or tincture of root and leaves is most commonly used, as astringent components are best extracted through water techniques.

Dosage:

Human: Traditionally prepared as a syrup of the berries with a diluted ethanol extract of the root, and flavored with cinnamon, nutmeg, allspice, and cloves.

Dried herb: 3-10 g TID, up to 6 times daily for acute conditions

Infusions and decoctions: 10-30 g per cup of water, with ¼-1 cup of the tea given TID, up to 6 times daily acutely

Tincture (25%-40% ethanol; some pharmacies include glycerin to prevent precipitation of tannins): 1:2 or 1:3: 0.5-5 mL TID, up to 6 times daily for acute conditions

Small Animal:

Dried herb: 25-125 mg/kg, divided daily (optimally, TID) if extracted and dried; triple or quadruple dose for unprocessed herb

Infusion: 10-30 g per cup of water, administered at a rate of ¼-½ cup per 10 kg (20 lb), divided daily (optimally, TID)

Tincture (25%-40% ethanol; some pharmacies include glycerin to prevent precipitation of tannins): 1:2-1:3: 0.5-2.5 mL per 10 kg (20 lb), divided daily (optimally, TID) and diluted or combined with other herbs. Higher doses may be appropriate if the herb is used singly and is not combined in a formula.

Farm Animals:

Traditional sources suggest that 2 handfuls of leaves can be administered to farm animals daily for diarrhea. Large animals (small ruminants to horses and cows): 4-30 mL (10-20 minims) of the 1:1 fluid extract (Milks, 1949) and derived from (Karreman, 2004).

References

De Bairacli Levy J. *The Complete Herbal Handbook for the Dog and Cat.* London: Faber and Faber; 1985.

Jouad H, Maghrani M, Eddouks M. Hypoglycaemic effect of *Rubus fructicosis* L. and *Globularia alypum* L. in normal and streptozotocin-induced diabetic rats. J Ethnopharmacol 2002;81:351-356.

Karreman H. *Treating Dairy Cows Naturally: Thoughts and Strategies.* Paradise, Pa: Paradise Publications; 2004.

Lemus I, Garcia R, Delvillar E, Knop G. Hypoglycaemic activity of four plants used in Chilean popular medicine. Phytother Res 1999;13:91-94.

Milks HJ. *Practical Veterinary Pharmacology, Materia Medica and Therapeutics.* 6th edition. Chicago, Ill: Alex Eger, Inc; 1949.

Bladderwrack

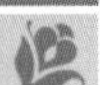

Fucus vesiculosis L. (synonomous to *F. quercus marina, Ascophyllum nodosum, F. scorphioides*) • FEW-kus ve-sik-yew-LOW-sus

Other Names: Kelp, fucus, sea-wrack, kelp-ware, Dyer's fucus, red fucus, rock-wrack, knotted wrack, black-tang, *Quercus marina,* cutweed, bladder fucus, *Fucus* (Varech) *vesiculeux,* blasentang, seetang, meeriche

Family: Fucaceae

Distribution: Bladderwrack grows on submerged rocks on the northern Atlantic and Pacific coasts of the United States and on the northern Atlantic coast and Baltic coast of Europe (north of the Mediterranean).

Parts Used: The main stem of bladderwrack, the thallus, is used medicinally. Dried mass of root and leaves can also be used. The thallus has tough, air-filled pods or bladders for flotation—thus, the name bladderwrack.

Selected Constituents: Major active constituents found in bladderwrack include polysaccharides (including algin, laminarin, fucoidan, fucose, mannitol), carotenoids (lutein, zeaxanthin, xanthophylls), and minerals, especially iodine. The amount of iodine is highly variable (Norman, 1987), resulting from different iodine concentrations in water according to location and season.

Alginic acid

Clinical Actions: Thyroid support; demulcent, emollient, diuretic

Energetics: Cool, salty; affecting most often the liver and stomach

History and Traditional Usage: Bladderwrack's mucilaginous thallus has been used to soothe irritated and inflamed tissues (Newall, 1996). It was also historically used as a bulk-forming laxative (Mills, 1991). People living near oceans or seas have a historically low rate of hypothyroidism, in part because of ingestion of iodine-rich food such as seafood and seaweeds like bladderwrack. It has also been used to counter obesity, possibly because of its reputation for stimulating the thyroid gland. Clinical research in this area has failed to confirm that seaweeds like bladderwrack help with weight loss (Björvell, 1986). According to Grieves (1971), bladderwrack is a valuable manure for potatoes and other crops and is used all along the British coast. In the Channel Islands, it is used to produce smoke for drying bacon and fish. Some cheeses, while drying, are covered with the salty ashes. Horses, cattle, and sheep have been fed with it. During the second World War, it was valued as a food for horses; it increased weight gain and improved the health of sick horses. It is interesting to note that fucus has a high digestibility and protein content (Applegate, 1995).

Kelp is prepared from several species of *Fucus* and from the deep-sea tangle, *Laminaria* species, especially *L. digitata.* The latter contain 10 times as much iodine as do the *Fuci* and are now practically the only kelps used in making iodine.

Published Research: Although studies have concentrated on the active fucoidin, to date, no human clinical trials have been conducted with whole bladderwrack.

Kelp, a variety of seaweed, has shown benefit against mastitis (Vacca, 1954), possibly being preventive rather than curative. In this 7-year study of twin cows, when the treatment group were supplemented with kelp, the incidence of mastitis was reduced in cows that received kelp compared with controls. Another early study conducted in Norway in 1968 by Jensen et al found the total milk yield to be around 6% higher than that of controls in dairy cows fed 3% *Ascophyllum nodosum* in a fortified seaweed meal over a 7-year period. The test concluded that the fortified seaweed meal was superior to standard mineral mixtures for milk production. In the seaweed group, the incidence of mastitis was markedly reduced (90% in the control group), a reduction in the number of services needed per conception and an increase in no returns were indicated, and a marked increase was observed in the iodine content of milk.

Because of its presumed iodine content, kelp is often used by dog owners for thyroid support. In some genetically predisposed people, increased iodine intake is associated with initiation of autoimmune thyroiditis (Lorini, 2003; Ruwhof, 2001). This is the most common form of hypothyroidism in dogs, so kelp supplementation may not be advisable in susceptible dogs.

Indications:

- For short-term use (a few days) to relieve constipation
- For gastritis or heartburn
- For people with insufficient iodine in their diet, bladderwrack may serve as a supplemental source of iodine. Some forms of hypothyroidism or goiter due to insufficient intake of iodine may improve with bladderwrack supplementation, although human studies have not confirmed this

Potential Veterinary Indications:

- Wound healing
- Nutritive in convalescence of large animals
- *Helicobacter pylori*
- Conditions responsive to mucilage administration

Contraindications: Bladderwrack is generally safe, although three potential problems have been associated with its consumption: acne, thyroid dysfunction, and heavy metal contamination. Iodine may cause or aggravate acne in some people (Harrell, 1976). Excessive iodine ingestion may cause hypothyroidism or hyperthyroidism and should be avoided (Okamura, 1978; Kim, 2000).

Bladderwrack and other seaweeds that grow in heavy metal–contaminated waters may contain high levels of these toxins (particularly, arsenic and lead). Use could lead to nerve damage (Walkiw, 1974), kidney damage (Conz, 1998), or other problems. Only bladderwrack known to have been harvested from clean water or labelled to indicate the absence of heavy metals or other contaminants should be consumed.

Toxicology and Adverse Effects: AHPA class 2b, 2c, 2d. Seaweed ingestion has been linked with chronic thyroiditis (Pye, 1992), and in these authors' opinion, should be avoided in dogs with immune-mediated thyroiditis. In humans, no more than 150 μg iodine should be consumed from all sources, including bladderwrack, per day (Blumenthal, 1998). Most bladderwrack products do not give iodine content. The safety of using bladderwrack during pregnancy and breastfeeding is unknown. People who are allergic to iodine may need to avoid bladderwrack. At the time of this writing, no well-known drug interactions with bladderwrack have been noted.

Preparation Notes: Bladderwrack is widely used in food and pharmaceuticals as a thickener and gelling agent (Lahaye, 1997).

The entire living plant is gathered from the rocks (not collected from the shore) about the end of June in the Northern hemisphere; it is rinsed and dried rapidly in the sun, when it becomes brittle and may be easily reduced to a coarse powder. If dried by artificial heat, it retains its hygroscopic qualities and does not become brittle (Grieves, 1931).

Dosage:

Human:

Dried herb: 3-10 g TID, up to 6 times daily for acute conditions

Infusions and decoctions: 10-30 g per cup of water, with ¼-1 cup of the tea given TID, up to 6 times daily acutely

Tincture (usually 25%-30% ethanol): 1:2 or 1:3: 3-6 mL TID, up to 6 times daily for acute conditions

Small Animal:

Dried herb: 50-500 mg/kg, divided daily (optimally, TID)

Infusion: 5-30 g per cup of water, administered at a rate of ¼-½ cup per 10 kg (20 lb), divided daily (optimally, TID)

Tincture (usually in 25%-30% ethanol): 1:2-1:3: 1.0-2.0 mL per 10 kg (20 lb), divided daily (optimally, TID) and diluted or combined with other herbs. Higher doses may be appropriate if the herb is used singly and is not combined in a formula.

References

Applegate RD, Gray PB. Nutritional value of seaweed to ruminants. Rangifer 1995;15:1,15-17.

Björvell H, Rössner S. Long-term effects of commonly available weight reducing programmes in Sweden. Int J Obes 1986;11: 67-71.

Blumenthal M, Busse WR, Goldberg A, et al, eds. *The Complete German Commission E Monographs: Therapeutic Guide to Herbal Medicines.* Austin: American Botanical Council; and Boston: Integrative Medicine Communications; 1998:315.

Conz PA, La Greca G, Benedetti P, et al. *Fucus vesiculosus:* a nephrotoxic alga? Nephrol Dial Transplant 1998;13:526-527 [letter].

Grieve M. *A Modern Herbal,* vol 1. New York, NY: Dover Publications; 1971.

Harrell BL, Rudolph AH. Kelp diet: a cause of acneiform eruption. Arch Dermatol 1976;112:560.

Jensen A, Nebb HS. *The Value of Norwegian Seaweed Meal as a Mineral Supplement for Dairy Cows.* Norsk Institutt for Tang-og Tareforskning, Rapport nr. 32, NTNU; 1968.

Kim JY, Kim KR. Dietary iodine intake and urinary iodine excretion in patients with thyroid diseases. Yonsei Med J 2000;41:22-28.

Lahaye M, Kaeffer B. Seaweed dietary fibres: structure, physico-chemical and biological properties relevant to intestinal physiology. Sci Aliment 1997;17:564-584 [review].

Lorini R, Gastaldi R, Traggiai C, Perucchin PP. Hashimoto's thyroiditis. Pediatr Endocrinol Rev 2003;1(suppl 2):205-211; discussion 211.

Mills SY. *Out of the Earth: The Essential Book of Herbal Medicine.* Middlesex, UK: Viking Arkana; 1991:514-516.

Newall CA, Anderson LA, Phillipson JD. *Herbal Medicines: A Guide for Health-Care Professionals.* London: Pharmaceutical Press; 1996:124-126.

Okamura K, Inoue K, Omae T. A case of Hashimoto's thyroiditis with thyroid immunological abnormality manifested after habitual ingestion of seaweed. Acta Endocrinol 1978;88:703.

Pye KG, Kelsey SM, House IM, et al. Severe dyserythropoiesis and autoimmune thrombocytopenia associated with ingestion of kelp supplements. The Lancet 1992;339:1540.

Ruwhof C, Drexhage HA. Iodine and thyroid autoimmune disease in animal models. Thyroid. 2001;11:427-436.

Vacca DD, Walsh RA. The antibacterial activity of an extract obtained from *Ascophyllum nodosum.* J Am Pharmaceut Assoc 1954;43:24-26.

Walkiw O, Douglas DE. Health food supplements prepared from kelp—a source of elevated urinary arsenic. Can Med Assoc J 1974;111:1301-1302 [letter].

Bloodroot

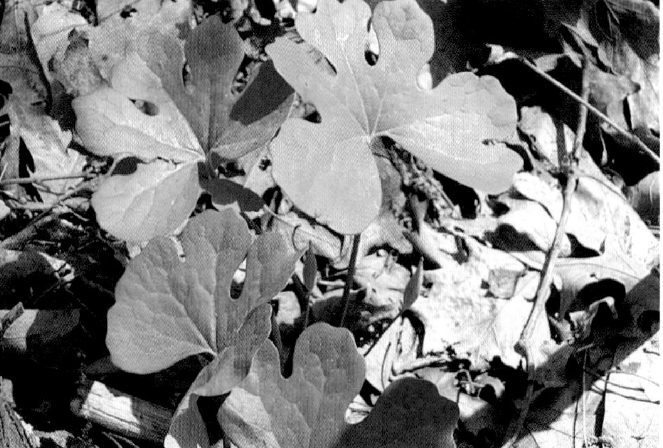

Sanguinaria canadensis L. • san-gwin-AR-ee-uh ka-na-DEN-sis

Other Names: Red puccoon, red turmeric, red root, kanadische blutwurzel, sanguinaire du Canada, *Sanguinaria canadensis rhizoma*
Family: Papaveraceae
Parts Used: Rhizome
Similar Species: *Macleaya cordata* (Plume poppy) and *Argemone mexicana* (Mexican poppy) also contain high levels of sanguinarine.
Selected Constituents: Benzophenanthridine (isoquinolone) alkaloids (sanguinarine, chelerythrine, allocryptopine, protopine, coptisine, etc.)
History and Traditional Usage: Expectorant, antispasmodic, emetic, cathartic, nervine, cardioactive, topical irritant. The alkaloids are believed to stimulate the vagus nerve, which may explain the emetic and expectorant qualities. Bloodroot was recommended for cough from many causes, for chronic nasal catarrh, and topically for conditions such as otitis media, anal fissure, "indolent ulcerative conditions," and epithelioma. The action was said to be specifically bronchorelaxant and expectorant.
Published Research: Sanguinarine intercalates DNA and binds to receptor proteins; it shows anti-inflammatory, antifungal, and antimicrobial actions. Controlled clinical trials indicate that sanguinarine suppresses the formation of dental plaque, and this alkaloid is included in some commercially available dentrifices.

Sanguinarine, at micromolar concentrations, imparts cell growth inhibitory response in human squamous carcinoma cells via induction of apoptosis (Ahmad, 2000). An important observation of this study was that sanguinarine treatment did not result in apoptosis of the normal human epidermal keratinocytes at similar concentrations. Sanguinarine also suppressed blood vessel formation in vivo and is thus an antiangiogenic product (Eun, 2004). Sanguinaria has also been investigated as an anticancer treatment in uterine cervical cancer (Ding, 2002). Sanguinarine induced growth inhibitory and antiproliferative effects in human prostate carcinoma cells (Adhami, 2004). The activation of human myeloid cells by tumor necrosis factor was completely suppressed by sanguinarine in a dose- and time-dependent manner (Chaturvedi, 1997).

Four cases in which patients had used bloodroot extracts (as "black salve") for the treatment of basal cell carcinomas were reported. One patient had a residual tumor, and another recurred deeply and required extensive surgery and subsequently metastasized; a third patient was cured but experienced severe scarring, and a fourth was lost to follow-up (McDaniel, 2002).
Indications: Chronic bronchitis, asthma, croup, laryngitis. As a mouthwash for gingivitis, stomatitis. Bloodroot is found in most escharotic salves.
Potential Veterinary Indications: Long-term oral use is not recommended. Possible uses include flare-ups of chronic bronchitis, COPD, asthma. Possibly for short-term use in cases of stomatitis. One author (BF) has used a combination blood root salve for effective removal of warts and small skin tumors; blood root salves have been used to remove equine sarcoids.
Contraindications: None reported.
Toxicology and Adverse Effects: May cause nausea, vomiting, mucosal irritation from contact, bradycardia, and hypotension at moderate doses. Laboratory animal studies have indicated that bloodroot is nontoxic for pregnant animals, but its use is best avoided because of the strength of the herb. Long-term use in dental preparations has led to leukoplakia, a precancerous lesion. When swine were fed the related species, *Macleaya cordata,* at an average daily oral dose of alkaloids up to 5 mg per 1 kg animal body weight, alkaloid accumulation in the gingivae and liver was noted, but no adverse effects were detected.
Notes: Bloodroot is an ingredient of compound white pine syrup, an Eclectic cough formula.
Dosage:
Human:
Dried herb: 30-300 mg TID. The lower dose was considered alterative, and the higher dose expectorant
Tincture (usually 60% ethanol; some pharmacies add vinegar to better extract alkaloids): 1:3-1:5: 0.25-0.5 mL TID (up to 1 mL TID for 1:10 extracts)
Small Animal:
Dried herb: 10-20 mg/kg, divided daily (optimally, TID)
Tincture (usually 60% ethanol; some pharmacies add vinegar to better extract alkaloids): 1:2-1:5: 0.25 mL per 10 kg (20 lb), divided daily (optimally, TID) and diluted or combined with other herbs

References

Adhami VM, Aziz MH, Reagan-Shaw SR, Nihal M, Mukhtar H, Ahmad N. Sanguinarine causes cell cycle blockade and apoptosis of human prostate carcinoma cells via modulation of cyclin kinase inhibitor-cyclin-cyclin-dependent kinase machinery. Mol Cancer Ther 2004;3:933-940.

Ahmad N, Gupta S, Husain MM, Heiskanen KM, Mukhtar H. Differential antiproliferative and apoptotic response of sanguinarine for cancer cells *versus* normal cells. Clin Cancer Res 2000;1524-1528, 2000.

Chaturvedi MM, Kumar A, Darnay BG, Chainy GBN, Agarwal S, Aggarwal BB. Sanguinarine (pseudochelerythrine) is a potent inhibitor of NF-κB activation, IκBκ phosphorylation, and degradation. J Biol Chem 1997;272:30129-30134.

Ding Z, Tang S, Weerasinghe P, Yang X, Pater A, Liepins A. The alkaloid sanguinarine is effective against multidrug resistance in human cervical cells via bimodal cell death. Biochem Pharmacol 2002;15;1415-1421.

Eun JP, Koh GY. Suppression of angiogenesis by the plant alkaloid, sanguinarine. Biochem Biophys Res Commun 2004; 317:618-624.

Kosina P, Walterova D, Ulrichova J, et al. Sanguinarine and chelerythrine: assessment of safety on pigs in ninety days feeding experiment. Food Chem Toxicol 2004;42:85-91.

McDaniel S, Goldman G. Consequences of using escharotic agents as primary treatment for nonmelanoma skin cancer. Arch Dermatol 2002;138;1593-1596.

Boneset

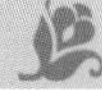

Eupatorium perfoliatum L. • Ew-puh-TOH-ree-um per-foh-lee-AY-tum
Distribution: Eastern North America
Similar Species: *Eupatorium purpureum* (Gravel root, Joe Pye weed) is also used medicinally, but for different indications

Other Names: Thoroughwort, agueweed, feverwort, Indian sage, herbe parfaite, durchwachsener, wasserhanf, eupatorio, tsé lan
Family: Asteraceae
Parts Used: Leaf and flowering parts
Selected Constituents: Sesquiterpene lactones (euperfolide, eupafolin, helenalin, etc.), polysaccharides, flavonoids (eupatorin, astragalin, quercetin, hyperoside, etc.), phytosterols, essential oils, and so forth; may contain pyrrolizidine alkaloids
Clinical Actions: Diaphoretic, aperient, immune stimulant, bitter tonic, expectorant, laxative
Energetics: Cold, dry, bitter; clears heat and resolves toxins, dries damp
History and Traditional Usage: Used by American Indian tribes for colds, flu, fever, and rheumatism, and to heal bones. The Iriquois used it to treat horses with fever. For mild fever, dyspepsia, upper respiratory infection, and especially for influenza. It has a reputation for relieving the pain in acute influenza infection, as well as the pain of periosteal inflammation and muscular rheumatism.
Published Research: In vitro evidence suggests that boneset may have immune-stimulating activity (Gassinger, 1981). A single trial that compared a homeopathic form of boneset (in D2 potency) with aspirin for people with common colds showed no difference in effect between the drugs (Wagner, 1985).
Indications: Fever, upper respiratory infection, flu, acute bronchitis, nasopharyngeal catarrh, possibly for bony or muscular pain
Potential Veterinary Indications: Fever, upper respiratory infection, possibly for bony or muscular pain. Fever in horses.
Contraindications: Pregnancy, lactation
Toxicology and Adverse Effects: AHPA class 4. At high doses, nausea, vomiting, diarrhea. May cause allergic reactions (contact dermatitis) in patients sensitive to other members of the Asteraceae family. Other members of this family contain pyrrolizidine alkaloids, although this species has not been reported to contain them, possibly because they have not yet been characterized.
Drug Interactions: None reported
Dosage:
Human:
Dried herb: 1-10gTID, up to 6 times daily for acute conditions
Infusions: 5-10g per cup of water, with ¼-1 cup of the tea given TID, up to 6 times daily acutely
Tincture (usually 35%-45% ethanol): 1:2 or 1:3: 3-5mL TID, up to 6 times daily for acute conditions
Small Animal:
Dried herb: 12.5-200mg/kg, divided daily (optimally, TID)
Infusion: 5-10g per cup of water, administered at a rate of ¼-½ cup per 10kg (20lb), divided daily (optimally, TID)
Tincture (usually in 35%-45% ethanol): 1:2-1:3: 0.25-0.5mL per 10kg (20lb), divided daily (optimally, TID) and diluted or combined with other herbs. Higher doses may be appropriate if the herb is used singly and is not combined in a formula.

References

Gassinger CA, Wunstel G, Netter P. A controlled clinical trial for testing the efficacy of the homeopathic drug eupatorium perfoliatum D2 inthe treatment of common cold. Arzneimittelforschung 1981;31:732-736. [German]

Wagner H, Proksch A, Riess-Maurer I, Vollmar A, Odenthal S, Stuppner H, Jurcic K, Le Turdu M, Fang JN. Immunostimulating action of polysaccharides (heteroglycans) from higher plants. Arzneimittelforschung 1985;35:1069-1075.

Boswellia

Boswellia serrata Roxb. *(formerly B. thurifera)* • Bos-WEL-ee-uh sair-AY-tuh
Similar Species: *Boswellia carteri* birdwood, *Boswellia sacra.* Considerable confusion is seen in the literature regarding which species is used most often (*B. serrata* or *B. carteri*), and whether the correct common name is boswellia, frankincense, or Indian frankincense.
Common Names: Indian frankincense (this is the standardized common name recommended by *Herbs of Commerce;* however, it is not in common use), frankincense (also used for the resin of *Boswellia carteri*), shallaki (Sanskrit), sallaki, salai, salai guggul, Indian olibanum, ru xiang *(B. carteri)*
Distribution: India
Family: Burseraceae
Parts Used: Resin, sometimes bark
Collection: A cut is made into the tree trunk, and resin is allowed to exude and harden before collection.
Selected Constituents: Gum, carbohydrates (4-O-methylglucuronoarabinogalactan, D-galactose, D-arabinose, D-xylose, and D-mannose), essential oils (alpha-pinene, alpha-phellandrene, p-cymene, alpha-thujene), diterpenes (incensole oxide, iso-incensole oxide, serratol, and others), triterpenes (α- and β-amyrins), pentacyclic triterpenic acids (α, β, and γ boswellic acids), tetracyclic triterpenic acids (tirucall-8,24-dien-21-oic acids), quercetin

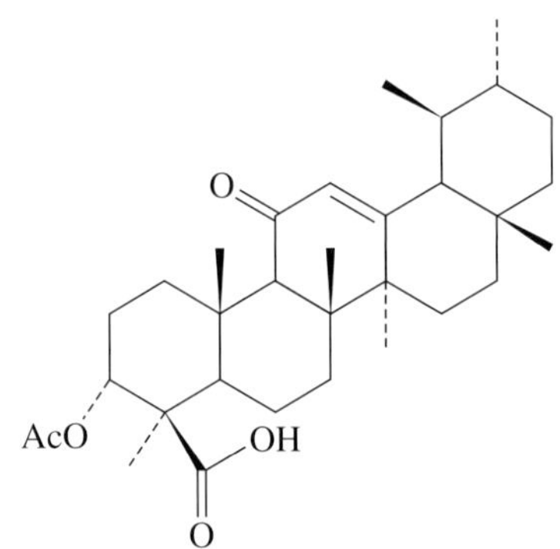

Boswellic acid

Clinical Actions: Anti-inflammatory, antirheumatic, diaphoretic, analgesic, antibacterial, immune suppressant, antidiarrheal, emmenagogue
Energetics: *Ayurvedic properties:* bitter, astringent, pungent, cooling; pacifies *Vata* and *Kapha doshas.*
History and Traditional Usage: Indian frankincense, or boswellia, is similar to both frankincense and myrrh,

which are resins that come from *B. sacra* and *Commiphora molmol*, respectively. Gums from any plant, known in general in India as guggul, were thought (as a group) to be useful in the treatment of patients with diarrhea, arthritis, and pulmonary and other disorders. Pliny is said to have claimed frankincense as an antidote to hemlock poisoning, and Dioscorides may have recommended vaginal pessaries made of the gum as a contraceptive. Avicenna recommended frankincense for treatment of tumors, stomatitis, vomiting, dysentery, and fever, and as part of a styptic formula. This gum was thought to render longevity, and when burned as incense, to drive away evil spirits. It has been used to enhance memory and for urinary disorders, obesity, diarrhea, skin conditions, colic, oral ulcers, ringworm, dysmenorrheal, and bone problems. In farm animals, it has been used for rinderpest, pox, and diarrhea.

Published Research: Boswellic and other organic acids control inflammation by mediating 5-lipoxygenase (Ammon, 1996; Ammon, 2002) and human leukocyte elastase production (Safayhi, 1997). Boswellia extracts may suppress or enhance 5-lipoxygenase activity, which may involve dose-dependent differences, or possibly, paradoxical actions of different constituents within the plant. Because of this recognized effect, consistent characterization of any single extract, formula, or herb source is important.

Ulcerative colitis

Krieglstein (2001) found that in experimental ileitis in rats, both boswellia extract and a single constituent, acetyl-11-keto-beta-boswellic acid, reduced tissue injury from indomethacin administration. However, boswellia extract was ineffective in controlling chemically induced colitis in two different murine models (Kiela, 2005). This study also documented hepatotoxicity when high doses were used. In a trial of 30 human patients with colitis, 20 were given boswellia gum extract, 300 mg TID for 6 weeks, and 10 served as controls and were given sulfasalazine, 1 g 3 times daily for 6 weeks. In this trial, boswellia extract was more effective than sulfasalazine, with a greater number of patients showing symptom improvement and more of the boswellia group achieving remission (Gupta, 2001). Another trial of 83 patients compared boswellia extract with mesalazine; boswellia showed efficacy and safety (Gerhardt, 2001).

Asthma

In a controlled study, 40 human patients with asthma were treated with boswellia gum resin (300 mg TID for 6 wk). In all, 70% of patients showed improvement in physical symptoms such as dyspnea, rhonchi, and frequency. Only 27% of control patients treated with lactose showed improvement (Gupta, 1998).

Arthritis

In a single study of 37 patients with rheumatoid arthritis, boswellia extract was indistinguishable from placebo treatment in terms of reduction in nonsteroidal anti-inflammatory drug (NSAID) use and in subjective, clinical, or laboratory measures (Sander, 1998).

Reichling (2004) studied 24 dogs seen by 10 different veterinarians for osteoarthritis of joints or spine in a prospective, open, multicenter clinical trial. Dogs that were given new herbal or nutraceutical treatment in the preceding 3 weeks, or diet changes or physical therapy within the preceding 2 weeks, were excluded. Dogs with neurologic disease, spinal tumors, septic conditions, and gastric ulcer, and those requiring surgical intervention (due to luxating patella and cruciate ligament rupture) were also excluded. The presence of chronic inflammatory joint or spinal disease was determined by clinical examination and confirmed by radiograph. Dogs were assessed according to nine common signs of arthritis: permanent and intermittent lameness, local pain, stiff gait, reduced range of motion, crepitation, increased filling of the joint, thickening of the capsule, muscle atrophy, and excess weight and effects of other external factors that aggravate lameness. A standardized boswellia resin extract (≥50% triterpenic acids) was given at a dose of 400 mg/10 kg body weight once daily in food for 6 weeks. No placebo control was included in this study. Final assessment of overall efficacy was graded simply as very good, good, moderate, or insufficient. Overall, 71% of the dogs that were assessed exhibited "good" or "very good" results at 2 and 6 weeks of treatment. Investigators claimed that after 6 weeks, anywhere from 40% to 70% of the dogs were symptom-free. Signs with statistically significant improvement (according to Bowker's test) included intermittent lameness ($P = .05$ at 2 weeks, not significant at 4 weeks; $P = .02$ at 6 weeks), local pain ($P = .02$ at 6 weeks), and stiff gait ($P = .05$ at 6 weeks). Significant improvements in external factor scores were noted; these included "lameness when moving" ($P = .001$) and "lameness after a long rest" ($P = .004$). Eleven of 29 dogs experienced adverse effects during the study; 5 had reversible diarrhea, but in only one dog was the study medication apparently suspected to be causative.

Brain tumor, cerebral edema

Two observational reports of patients undergoing treatment for brain tumor suggest that boswellia extract may assist in reducing cerebral edema (Janssen, 2000). Experimental and in vitro studies have shown that boswellia extract may slow growth and increase apoptosis of tumor cells implanted in the brains of experimental animals (Streffer, 2001).

Indications: Rheumatism, gout, gonorrhea, psoriasis, ulcers and cough, colitis, asthma, osteoarthritis, brain tumor

Potential Veterinary Indications: Rheumatism, osteoarthritis, bronchitis and asthma, ulcerative colitis, brain tumor

Contraindications: None reported

Toxicology and Adverse Effects: AHPA class 1. Most sources mention rash, diarrhea, and nausea as possible adverse effects, but adverse event reports are very rare in the medical literature.

Drug Interactions: None reported.

Preparation Notes: *Boswellia serrata* extract is prepared by alcoholic extraction of the oleogum resin. It does not combine well with other herbs and frequently precipitates upon mixing. Dried or tableted form may be preferable.

Dosage:
Small Animal:
Dried herb: 25-500 mg/kg divided daily (optimally TID)
Standardized extract to 20%-70% total organic acids or boswellic acids: 60 mg/kg divided daily (optimally TID)
Tincture: 1:2-1:3:1.5-2.5 mL per 10kg (20lb), divided daily (optimally TID) and diluted or combined with other herbs
Human:
Dried herb: 1-10 g TID
Standardized extract (to 20%-70% total organic acids or boswellic acids): 200-400 mg TID
Bark decoction (traditional): 15-100 mL, divided daily
Tincture: 1:2 or 1:3: 3-5 mL TID, up to 6 times daily for acute conditions
Combinations: With Curcuma (turmeric), boswellia is used for treatment of osteoarthritic pain.

References

Ammon HP. Salai guggal—*Boswellia serrata:* from an herbal medicine to a non-redox inhibitor of leukotriene biosynthesis. Eur J Med Res 1996;1:369-370.
Ammon HP. Boswellic acids (components of frankincense) as the active principle in treatment of chronic inflammatory diseases. Wien Med Wochenschr 2002;152:373-378.
Gerhardt H, Seifert F, Buvari P, Vogelsang H, Repges R. [Therapy of active Crohn disease with *Boswellia serrata* extract H 15] [article in German]. Z Gastroenterol 2001;39:11-17.
Gupta I, Gupta V, Parihar A, et al. Effects of *Boswellia serrata* gum resin in patients with bronchial asthma: results of a double-blind, placebo-controlled, 6-week clinical study. Eur J Med Res 1998;3:511-514.
Gupta I, Parihar A, Malhotra P, et al. Effects of gum resin of *Boswellia serrata* in patients with chronic colitis. Planta Med 2001;67:391-395.
Janssen G, Bode U, Breu H, et al. Boswellic acids in the palliative therapy of children with progressive or relapsed brain tumors. Klin Padiatr 2000;212:189-195.
Kiela PR, Midura AJ, Kuscuoglu N, Jolad SD, Solyom AM, Besselsen DG, Timmermann BN, Ghishan FK. Effects of Boswellia serrata in mouse models of chemically induced colitis. Am J Physiol Gastrointest Liver Physiol 2005;288:G798-G808.
Krieglstein CF, Anthoni C, Rijcken EJ, et al. Acetyl-11-keto-beta-boswellic acid, a constituent of a herbal medicine from Boswellia serrata resin, attenuates experimental ileitis. Int J Colorectal Dis 2001;16:88-95.
Monograph: *Boswellia serrata.* Altern Med Rev 1998;3:306-307.
Reichling J, Schmokel H, Fitzi J, et al. Dietary support with Boswellia resin in canine inflammatory joint and spinal disease. Schweiz Arch Tierheilkd 2004;146:71-79.
Safayhi H, Rall B, Sailer ER, Ammon HP. Inhibition by boswellic acids of human leukocyte elastase. J Pharmacol Exp Ther 1997;281:460-463.
Sander O, Herborn G, Rau R. [Is H15 (resin extract of *Boswellia serrata,* "incense") a useful supplement to established drug therapy of chronic polyarthritis? Results of a double-blind pilot study] [article in German]. Z Rheumatol 1998;57:11-16.
Streffer JR, Bitzer M, Schabet M, Dichgans J, Weller M. Response of radiochemotherapy-associated cerebral edema to a phytotherapeutic agent, H15. Neurology 2001;56:1219-1221.

Buchu

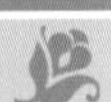

Agathosma betulina (Berg.) Pillans; formerly, *Barosma betulina* (Berg.) Bartl. and Wendl. • ag-ath-OHS-muh bet-yoo-LY-nuh
Other Names: *Barosma folium,* bucco, short buchu, round buchu
Related Species: *Agathosma crenulata* (long leaf buchu)
Family: Rutaceae
Distribution: Buchu is a small shrub native to South Africa.
Parts Used: Leaves, collected while plant is flowering and fruiting
Selected Constituents: Volatile oil 1.5% to 3.5%, including components diosphenol (main ingredient in oil), pulegone, menthone (carminative), and limonene. Sulphur-containing compounds (p-menthan-3-on-8-thiol) that give a black currant taste. Flavonoids (diosmin, rutin, quercetin, hesperidin); mucilage, resin
Clinical Actions: Stimulant diuretic, urinary disinfectant, diaphoretic
Energetics: Warm, mildly pungent
Traditional Use: Buchu has a long history of use for urinary tract infection, dysuria, cystitis, urethritis, prostatitis. Buchu leaves and oil of buchu were used by the indigenous peoples of South Africa for hundreds of years. Dutch settlers continued using buchu medicinally, and the herb was introduced into the pharmaceutical industry in the United Kingdom. Buchu preparations are used as diuretics, as well as for stomachache, rheumatism, bladder and kidney infection, colds, and cough (Simpson, 1998). It was introduced into Britain as an official medicine in 1821 for the treatment of patients with cystitis, urethitis, nephritis, and catarrh of the bladder.

Buchu appeared in veterinary pharmacopoeias until at least 1970 (Hungerford, 1970).
Published Research: No clinical studies, particularly on urinary antiseptic and diuretic effects, were found.
Indications: Urinary tract infection, prostatitis, rheumatism, minor digestive problems
Potential Veterinary Indications: Cystitis (best by infusion to increase fluid consumption), colic
Contraindications: Pregnancy, possibly a uterine stimulant because of the pulegone content. Should be used with caution in pregnancy and kidney disease.
Toxicology and Adverse Effects: AHPA class 2b, 2d (contraindicated when renal inflammation is present). Considered GRAS as a flavoring. No poisonings have been reported; however, it does contain pulegone (a hepatotoxin and oxytocic), volatile oil; also found in pennyroyal. May increase menstrual flow. Occasional gastrointestinal intolerance; avoid taking on empty stomach.
Drug Interactions: None identified
Notes of Interest: Buchu is considered a threatened species in South Africa.
Dosage:
Human:
Dried herb: 3-10 g TID, up to 6 times daily for acute conditions

Infusions (keep covered to retain essential oils): 5-15 g per cup of water, with ¼-1 cup of the tea given TID, up to 6 times daily acutely
Tincture (60%-90% ethanol; lower doses used for higher alcohol extracts): 1:2 or 1:3: 2-4 mL TID, up to 4 times daily for acute conditions
Small Animal:
Dried herb: 25-300 mg/kg, divided daily (optimally, TID)
Infusion (keep covered to retain essential oils): 5-15 g per cup of water, administered at a rate of ¼-½ cup per 10 kg (20 lb), divided daily (optimally, TID)
Tincture (60%-90% ethanol; lower doses used for higher alcohol extracts): 1:2-1:3: 0.5-1.0 mL per 10 kg (20 lb), divided daily (optimally, TID) and diluted or combined with other herbs. Higher doses may be appropriate if the herb is used singly and is not combined in a formula.
Historical Doses:
Dog (Hungerford, 1970)
Dried herb: 1-2 g per dose
Infusion: ½-20 oz per dose (RCVS, 1920)
Fluid extract (1:1): 5-30 minims (0.3-1.85 mL) per dose
Dog and cat (Kirk, 1949)
Tincture: 10-40 minims (0.6-2.5 mL) BID
Farm animal
Dried herb (Hungerford, 1970): Cattle, 30-60 g; horses, 30-60 g
Infusion: Horse, 2-4 oz; pig, ⅛-1 oz (RCVS, 1920)
Fluid extract (1:1) (Milks, 1949): Horse, 1-2 dr (3.7-7.4 mL)
Tincture: 2-60 mL daily
Combinations: May use with fennel if gastrointestinal tract intolerance occurs. Most herbalists consider it to be complementary to uva ursi.

References

Hungerford TG. *Veterinary Physicians Index.* Sydney: Angus & Robertson; 1970.

Kirk H. *Index of Treatment in Small-Animal Practice.* Baltimore, Md: Williams and Wilkins; 1948.

Milks HJ. *Practical Veterinary Pharmacology, Materia Medica and Therapeutics.* Chicago, Ill: Alex Eger, Inc; 1949.

Simpson D. Buchu—South Africa's amazing herbal remedy. Scott Med J 1998;43:189-191.

Bugleweed

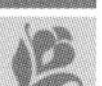

Lycopus europaeus L. • LIE-co-pus yoo-ROH-pay-us
Other Names: Virginia bugleweed, gypsy wort, *Lycopi herba,* water bugle, water horehound, sweet bugle
Similar Species: *Lycopus virginicus* often used interchangeably; also, *Lycopus americanus*
Family: Lamiaceae
Part Used: Leaf
Distribution: *L. virginicus* is a North American native. *L. europaeus* (also known as gypsy wort) refers to the perennial herbaceous plant native to Europe.
Selected Constituents: Lithospermic acid and other organic acids are believed to be responsible for bugleweed's activity (Wagner, 1970). Isopimarane diterpinoids (Hussein, 2000), phenolic compounds, rosmarinic acid (more than 3% of dry weight) (Lamaison, 1990), caffeic acid, cholorogenic acid, ellagic acid, flavone glycosides, including luteolin-7-glucaronide, bitter principle (Winterhoff, 1994), essential oil, manganese
Clinical Actions: Diuretic, astringent, nervine, antithyroid, antitussive
Energetics: Bitter
History and Traditional Usage: *Lycopus virginicus* (bugleweed) was recognized by the early Eclectics as an excellent sedative, subtonic, subnarcotic, and subastringent that had properties similar to digitalis without diuretic or adverse effects. It was also used as a remedy for diarrhea. It was thought to act chiefly on the blood vessels and was used in inflammatory states, particularly internal inflammation resulting from inebriety, and for cardiac disease. It was considered valuable for hemoptysis because of its action on the circulatory system as a sedative; it slowed the pulse and thereby allayed irritation and cough (Wren, 1988). *L. virginicus* and *L. europaeus* (European Bugleweed) have long had traditional use as sedatives and for cough and palpitations (Wren, 1988). Recently, bugleweed has been suggested as a treatment for patients with hyperthyroidism and mastodynia (breast pain). Bugleweed has been used in China for the treatment of gout.

Published Research

Effects on uric acid

Results of an in vitro study suggest that Lycopus extract exhibited almost 25% of the activity of allopurinol in the inhibition of xanthine oxidase (Kong, 2000).

Effects on thyroid function

Lycopus has been extensively studied in laboratory animals and its mode of action explored. It appears to inhibit thyroid-stimulating hormone and thyroid-stimulating IgG antibody, leading to a reduction in thyroid secretion; it also inhibits peripheral T3 production (Wagner, 1970; Winterhoff, 1994; Auf'mkolk, 1984; Auf'mkolk, 1985). However, a later study in rats found that administration of the extract did not affect thyroid hormone levels (Vonhoff, 2006).

Laboratory animal studies also suggest that Lycopus may reduce luteinizing hormone, testosterone, and prolactin levels. No controlled clinical trials in humans or companion animals were conducted.

Cardiovascular function

A hydroethanolic bugleweed extract was tested in rats (0.7 mg/kg BW i.p.) rendered hyperthyroid via administration of thyroxine during the previous week. Atenolol was used as positive control, and the test lasted 5½ weeks. The herb attenuated the increases in body temperature, heart rate, myocardial hypertrophy, and blood pressure. A reduction in beta-adrenergic receptor density was also observed, with activity equivalent to that of atenolol. No changes in weight loss, food intake, thyroid hormone, or TSH levels were noted (Vonhoff, 2006).

Indications: Mild thyroid hyperfunction, Graves' disease and associated symptoms, mild agitation or anxiety; tension and pain in the breast (mastodynia)

Potential Veterinary Indications:

- Feline hyperththyroid disease
- Urate urolithiasis in Dalmatians
- Equine pulmonary hemorrhage (although the [unproven] traditional use as a calming agent may complicate its use in athletes)

Contraindications and Cautions: Lycopus should not be taken by people with hypothyroidism, nor should it be used during pregnancy and breastfeeding (Brinker, 1990). It should not be combined with thyroid medications.

Toxicology and Adverse Effects: AHPA class 2b, 2c, 2d. Contraindicated in thyroid enlargement (presumably referring to hypothyroid goiter in people) or hypothyroidism, or during use of other thyroid treatments. Excessive intake of lycopus by people with thyroid disease or use by healthy people may cause a potentially harmful decrease in thyroid function. In rare cases, extended therapy and high doses have resulted in goiter; sudden discontinuation of bugleweed may cause increased symptoms of the disease (Blumenthal, 1998). Long-term use of lycopus is considered safe for people with hyperthyroidism (Weiss, 1988).

Preparation: Most research on the endocrine effects of lycopus extracts in experimental animals has explored parenteral application. However, oral administration of an ethanolic extract of *L. europaeus* produces longer-lasting effects on thyroid hormones. Differences in biological activity and dependence on the route of application may be explained by differences in absorption of plant constituents (Winterhoff, 1994). Extracts produced with ethanol show greater concentrations of phenolic compounds compared with pure aqueous extracts. The activity of lycopus is due to the oxidation and polymerization of phenolic compounds that occur during preparation of aqueous extracts (Harvey, 1996). It is therefore recommended that ethanol extracts or equivalents should be used in the treatment of patients with thyroid disease.

Dosage:

Human:

Dried herb: 1-2 g TID

Tincture (usually 25%-45% ethanol): 1:2 or 1:3: 2-3 mL TID

Small Animal:

Dried herb: 25-75 mg/kg, divided daily (optimally, TID)

Infusion: 5-30 g per cup of water, administered at a rate of ¼-½ cup per 10 kg (20 lb), divided daily (optimally, TID)

Tincture (usually in 25%-40% ethanol) 1:2-1:3: 0.5-1.5 mL per 10 kg (20 lb), divided daily (optimally, TID) and diluted or combined with other herbs

Notes of Interest: The name *Lycopus* originates from two Greek words—*lukus,* wolf; and *pous,* foot; hence, *wolf-foot,* so called because of a fancied resemblance of the cut leaves to a wolf's foot.

Combinations: Lycopus may be combined with other herbs used to treat mildly overactive thyroid function, including lemon balm *(Melissa officinalis)* and gromwell *(Lithospermum ruderale).*

References

Auf'mkolk M, Amir SM, Kubota K, et al. The active principles of plant extracts with antithyrotropic activity: oxidation products of derivatives of 3,4-dihydroxycinnamic acid. Endocrinology 1985;116:1677-1686.

Auf'mkolk M, Ingbar JC, Kubota K, et al. Extracts and auto-oxidized constituents of certain plants inhibit the receptor-binding and the biological activity of Graves' immunoglobulins. Endocrinology 1985;116:1687-1693.

Auf'mkolk M, Ingbar JC, Amir SM, et al. Inhibition by certain plant extracts of the binding and adenylate cyclase stimulatory effect of bovine thyrotropin in human thyroid membranes. Endocrinology 1984;115:527-534.

Auf'mkolk M, Kohrle J, Gumbinger H, et al. Antihormonal effects of plant extracts: iodothyronine deiodinase of rat liver is inhibited by extracts and secondary metabolites of plants. Horm Metab Res 1984;16:188-192.

Blumenthal M, Busse WR, Goldberg A, et al, eds. *The Complete Commission E Monographs: Therapeutic Guide to Herbal Medicines.* Boston, Mass: Integrative Medicine Communications; 1998:98-99.

Brinker F. Inhibition of endocrine function by botanical agents. I. Boraginaceae and Labiatae. J Naturopath Med 1990;1:10-18.

Gibbons S, Oluwatuyi M, Veitch NC, et al. Bacterial resistance modifying agents from *Lycopus europaeus.* Phytochemistry 2003;62:83-87.

Gumbinger HG, Winterhoff H, Sourgens H, et al. Formation of compounds with antigonadotropic activity from inactive phenolic precursors. Contraception 1981;23:661-666.

Gumbinger HG, Winterhoff H, Wylde R, et al. On the influence of the sugar moiety on the antigonadotropic activity of luteline glycosides. Planta Med 1992;58:49-50.

Harvey R. *Lycopus europaeus* L and *Lycopus virginicus* L: a review of scientific research. Br J Phytother 1996;4:55-65.

Hussein AA, Rodriguez B. Isopimarane diterpinoids from *Lycopus europaeus.* J Nat Prod 2000;63:419-421.

Kong LD, Cai Y, Huang WW, et al. Inhibition of xanthine oxidase by some Chinese medicinal plants used to treat gout. J Ethnopharmacol 2000;73:199-207.

Lamaison JL, Petitjean-Freytet C, Carnat A. Rosmarinic acid, total hydroxycinnamic derivatives and antioxidant activity of Apiaceae, Borraginaceae and Lamiceae medicinals. Ann Pharm Fr 1990;48:103-108.

Lamaison JL, Petitjean-Freytet C, Carnat A. Medicinal Lamiaceae with antioxidant properties, a potential source of rosmarinic acid. Pharm Acta Helv 1991;66:185-188.

Sourgens H, Winterhoff H, Gumbinger HG, et al. Antihormonal effects of plant extracts. TSH- and prolactin-suppressing properties of *Lithospermum officinale* and other plants. Planta Med 1982;45:78-86.

Vonhoff C, Baumgartner A, Hegger M, Korte B, Biller A, Winterhoff H. Extract of *Lycopus europaeus* L. reduces cardiac signs of hyperthyroidism in rats. Life Sci 2006;78:1063-1070.

Wagner H, Horhammer L, Frank U. Lithospermic acid, the antihormonally active principle of *Lycopus europaeus* L. and *Symphytum officinale.* Ingredients of medicinal plants with hormonal and antihormonal-like effects. Arzneimittelforschung 1970;20:705-713.

Weiss RF. *Herbal Medicine.* Beaconsfield, UK: Beaconsfield Publishers Ltd.; 1988:328-329.

Winterhoff H, Gumbinger HG, Vahlensieck U, et al. Endocrine effects of *Lycopus europaeus* L. following oral application. Arzneimittelforschung 1994;44:41-45.

Wren RC, Williamson EM, Evans FJ. *Potter's New Cyclopaedia of Botanical Drugs and Preparations.* Essex, UK: Saffron Walden, CW Daniel Co; 1988.

Bupleurum 

Bupleurum falcatum L. or *B. falcatum* L. var. *scorzonerifolium* (Willd.) Ledeb. • boo-PLUR-rum fal-KAY-tum

Other Names: *Radix bupleuri,* sickle-leaved hare's ear, beichaihu, bupleurum root, ch'ai hu, chaifu, chai hu, chaiku-saiko, juk-siho, kara-saiko, mishima-saiko, nan-chaihu, saiko, shi ho, shoku-saiko, wa-saiko, yamasaiko

Similar Species: *Bupleurum chinense* DC (Chinese thoroughwax)

Family: Apiaceae

Distribution: Indigenous to northern Asia, northern China, and Europe

Parts Used: Dried root

Selected Constituents: Triterpenoid saponins or saikosides (saikosaponins A-F, saikogenins A-G), fatty acids, polysaccharides, polyacetylenic compounds, lignans, sterols

Glc—Fuc—O ... CH_2OH ... OH ... H ... O

Saikosaponin

Clinical Actions: Anti-inflammatory, analgesic, antipyretic, diaphoretic, diuretic, carminative, hepatoprotective, mild sedative, alterative

Energetics: Bitter, cool, slightly acrid; releases the exterior, clears heat, stops shivers, harmonizes liver *Qi* stagnation; action primarily on the liver and gallbladder

History and Traditional Usage: Uses described in pharmacopoeias and in traditional systems of medicine include the treatment of patients with fever, pain, and inflammation associated with influenza and the common cold (Pharmacopoeia of the People's Republic of China, 1992; The Pharmacopoeia of Japan, 1991; Chang, 1987). The plant is also used as an analgesic for the treatment of distending pain in the chest and hypochondriac regions, and for amenorrhea (Pharmacopoeia of the People's Republic of China, 1992). Extracts have been used for the treatment of chronic hepatitis, nephrotic syndrome, and autoimmune diseases (Pharmacopoeia of the People's Republic of China, 1992; Chang 1987).

Uses described in folk medicine, not supported by experimental or clinical data, include the treatment of deafness, dizziness, diabetes, wounds, and vomiting (Chang, 1987).

Published Research: Laboratory animal studies support the traditional use for fever. Oral administration of a Bupleurum decoction (5 g/kg) to rabbits with a heat-induced fever decreased body temperature to normal levels within 1.5 hours (Chang, 1987). The anti-inflammatory and sedative activities of bupleurum have been demonstrated by in vivo studies (Chang, 1987). A number of studies in rats and mice have shown that bupleurum and its constituents may reduce hepatic damage caused by carbon tetrachloride (Arichi, 1978). *B. falcatum* also has antiallergy activity (Park Kwan Ha, 2002). Components of *B. falcatum* may decrease urine protein, lower blood lipids, and ameliorate pathologic glomerular changes in nephritis (Hattori, 1991). It has some antiulcer action caused by reinforcement of the protective mucosal barrier, as well as an antisecretory action on acid and pepsin (Shibata, 1974). *B. falcatum* is a potential immunomodulator and may be useful as an antitumor agent (Cho, 1994).

Indications: Chronic hepatitis, upper respiratory infection, colds, flu, dysmenorrhea, menopause, emotional swings, certain forms of depression, premenstrual syndrome, minor nervous tension

Potential Veterinary Indications: Liver disease, liver cancer, upper respiratory infection, fever

Contraindications: Traditional Chinese Medicine principles state that hyperactive liver yang and movement of endogenous liver wind is a contraindication. No data on teratogenic and nonteratogenic effects are available; therefore, Bupleurum should not be administered during pregnancy.

Toxicology and Adverse Effects: AHPA class 1. Reported adverse effects of bupleurum include mild lassitude, sedation, and drowsiness (Chang, 1987). Large doses have also been reported to decrease appetite and cause pronounced flatulence and abdominal distention. Herbalists call Bupleurum the "angry herb" because high doses have also been associated (anecdotally) with unexplained bouts of anger in people.

Potential Drug Interactions: The use of alcohol, sedatives, and other central nervous system depressants in conjunction with Bupleurum may cause synergistic sedative effects. No clinical studies have evaluated this possible interaction. Some concern exists about interactions between Bupleurum and interferon, although no supporting cases or data were found.

Dosage:

Human:

Dried herb: 3-10 g TID

Tincture (generally available as 40%-45% ethanol): 1:2 or 1:3: 2-3 mL TID, up to 6 times daily for acute conditions

Small Animal:

Dried herb: 50-400 mg/kg, divided daily (optimally, TID)

Tincture (usually in 40%-45% ethanol) 1:2-1:3: 1.0-2.0 mL per 10 kg (20 lb), divided daily (optimally, TID) and diluted or combined with other herbs

References

Arichi S, Konishi H, Abe H. Studies on the mechanism of action of saikosaponin. I. Effects of saikosaponin on hepatic injury induced by D-galactosamine. Kanzo 1978;19:430-435.

Chang HM, But PPH, eds. *Pharmacology and Applications of Chinese Materia Medica,* vol 2. Singapore: World Scientific Publishing; 1987.

Cho JG, Kim JM. Effect of *Bupleurum falcatum* on the immune system [Korean]. Korean J Vet Res 1994;34:4,769-779.

Hattori T, Ito M, Suzuki Y. [Studies on antinephritic effects of plant components in rats (1). Effects of saikosaponins original-type anti-GBM nephritis in rats and its mechanisms]. Nippon Yakurigaku Zasshi 1991;97:13-21.

Park KH, Park J, Koh D, Lim Y. Effect of saikosaponin-A, a triterpenoid glycoside, isolated from *Bupleurum falcatum* on experimental allergic asthma. Phytother Res 2002;16:359-363.

Pharmacopoeia of Japan XII. Tokyo: The Society of Japanese Pharmacopoeia; 1991.

Pharmacopoeia of the People's Republic of China [English ed]. Guangzhou: Guangdong Science and Technology Press; 1992.

Shibata M, et al. Pharmacological studies on the Chinese crude drug saiko, *Bupleurum falcatum.* Hoshi Yakka Daigaku Kiyo 1974;16:77.

Burdock

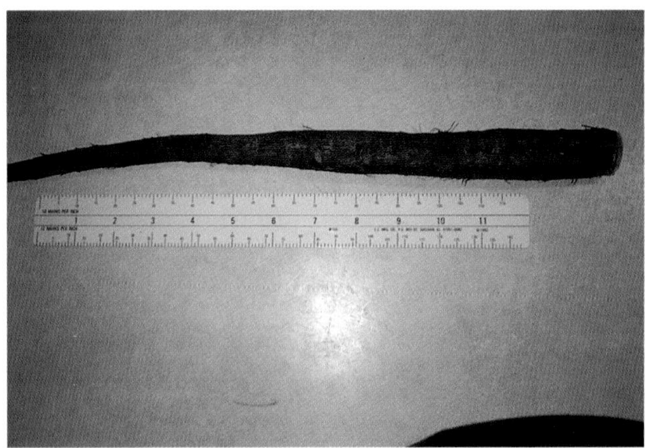

Arctium lappa L. • ARK-tee-um LAP-uh

Other Names: Great burdock, lappa, fox's clote, thorny burr, beggar's buttons, cockle buttons, love leaves, philanthropium, personata, happy major, clot-bur, dock, niu bang, niu bang zi, gobo, goboshi

Family: Asteraceae

Parts Used: Root, leaves, and fruits

Distribution: Burdock is common in Britain, Europe, and Asia Minor and was introduced to North America. It grows freely on roadsides, in wastelands, and in damp places. The plant varies considerably in appearance, and various subspecies or even separate species have been described.

Selected Constituents: Inulin, mucilage, sugar, flavonoids, bitter glycosides (including lappin, arctiopicrin), resin, fixed and volatile oils, tannic acid. The roots contain starch. Six compounds were isolated from the seeds of *Arctium lappa* L. The five compounds were identified as daucosterol (I), arctigenin (II), arctiin (III), matairesinol (IV), and lappaol F (V) combined with a lignan—neoarctin B (VI) (Wang, 1993).

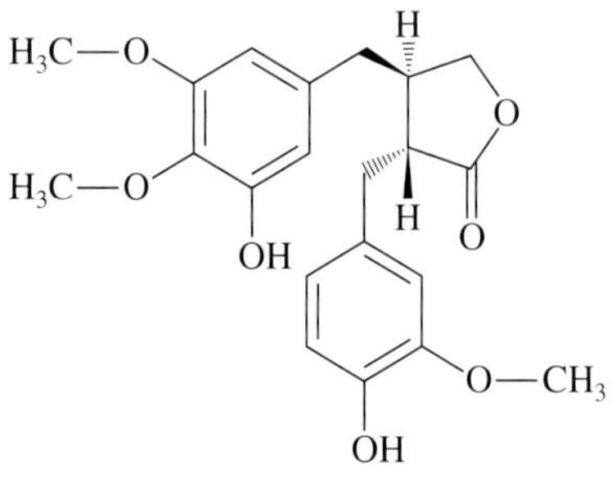

Arctigenin

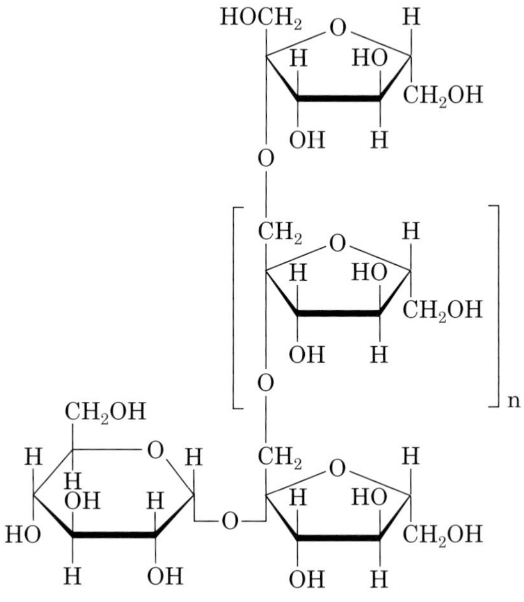

Inulin

Clinical Actions: Depurative, mild laxative, antioxidant, anticancer, mildly antiseptic; traditionally, an alterative

Energetics:

Root: bitter, slightly sweet, cool

Seed: bitter, sweet, cold

History and Traditional Usage: The root of *Arctium lappa* has been cultivated for a long time as a vegetable known as gobo. Burdock is traditionally used as a "tissue cleaner" (alterative, depurative) to eliminate accumulated toxins, for eczema and septic conditions, and for chronic inflammatory states. It is often used in combination with other alteratives such as nettles, cleavers, and yellow dock. Native Americans used the root as food, and the root, buds, and seeds as a blood purifier, for rheumatism, scurvy, gravel, venereal disease, and sores. The leaves were used as a poultice. Until 1916, burdock was officially identified in the US Pharmacopoeia as a diuretic and a diaphoretic. According to de Bairacli Levy (1963), animals, except for donkeys, will not graze burdock. The bruised leaves were suggested for the treatment of patients with ringworm and scabies, and the brewed fruits and roots for the treatment of those with burns.

Published Research: In vitro and experimental animal studies suggest that burdock has anti-inflammatory activity and activity against induced acute liver damage (Lin, 1996). One study suggested that *A. lappa* could protect liver cells against damage from CCl4 or acetaminophen and their toxic metabolites, perhaps through its antioxidative effects on hepatocytes (Lin, 2000). It may be useful in mammary carcinogenesis in female rats in that a protective effect against induced carcinogenesis has been documented (Hirose, 2000). Burdock is an excellent source of linoleic acid. In controlled studies, guinea pigs in which epidermal hyperproliferation was induced (as a model for psoriasis) were treated with *Arctium lappa* or safflower oil or water. Organic extracts of burdock were more effective than safflower oil in reversing epidermal hyperproliferation; this was attained through induction of high accumulations of LA in the epidermis of guinea pigs (Seong, 2003). One study investigated the effects of burdock on blood sugar, plasma lipids, and uric acid in rats. Rats were randomly assigned to one of four groups—control, hot water extract, water, and burdock tea. Blood was sampled after 4 weeks. Results showed that burdock did not affect fasting blood glucose, triglycerides, or uric acid. However, plasma cholesterol of rats in the burdock tea group was lower (Wang, 2000).

Antitussive activity in cats

An inulin isolate from the roots of *A. lappa* was tested for antitussive activity in cats. The fructan was found to be as active as some nonnarcotic, synthetic preparations used in clinical practice to treat cough (Kardosova, 2003).

Indications: Skin disease, including eczema and psoriasis, urticaria, and acne, as well as arthritis and gout

Veterinary Indications:

Chronic skin disorders

Disorders requiring improved elimination from the body

Potentially as a mild antitussive in cats

Contraindications: None known

Toxicology and Adverse Effects: AHPA class 1. A single case of toxicity in the literature was determined to be due to adulteration of the product. Contact dermatitis and anaphylaxis have been reported.

Potential Drug Interactions: None described.

Notes of Interest: "Burr tongue" in dogs can be caused by contact with the involucre of burdock. Granular stomatitis develops, characterized by the initial appearance of small papules, most often on the tip and edges of the tongue and the anterior part of the upper lip and gum. These lesions enlarge and develop necrotic centers, which later slough, leaving discrete ulcers. Treatment consists of deep and sometimes repeated currettage under general anesthesia (Thivierge, 1973).

Herb–Drug Interactions: None known.

Dosage:

Human:

Dried herb: 1-10 g TID

Infusions and decoctions: 5-30 g per cup of water, with 1 cup of the tea given TID

Tincture (usually as 25%-35% ethanol): 1:2 or 1:3: 1-5 mL TID, up to 6 times daily for acute conditions

Small Animal:

Dried herb: 25-500 mg/kg, divided daily (optimally, TID)

Infusion: 5-30 g per cup of water, administered at a rate of ¼-½ cup per 10 kg (20 lb), divided daily (optimally, TID)

Tincture (usually in 25%-35% ethanol) 1:2-1:3: 0.5-2.0 mL per 10 kg (20 lb), divided daily (optimally, TID) and diluted or combined with other herbs. Higher doses may be appropriate if the herb is used singly and is not combined in a formula.

References

De Bairacli Levy J. *The Complete Herbal Handbook for Farm and Stable*. London: Faber and Faber; 1963.

Hirose M, Yamaguchi T, Lin C, et al. Effects of arctiin on PhIP-induced mammary, colon and pancreatic carcinogenesis in female Sprague-Dawley rats and MeIQx-induced hepatocarcinogenesis in male F344 rats. Cancer Lett 2000;155:79-88.

Kardosova A, Ebringerova A, Alfoldi J, et al. A biologically active fructan from the roots of *Arctium lappa* L., var. 2003 Herkules. Int J Biol Macromol 2003;33:135-140.

Lin CC, Lu JM, Yang JJ, Chuang SC, Ujiiye T. Anti-inflammatory and radical scavenge effects of *Arctium lappa*. Am J Chin Med 1996;24:127-137.

Lin SC, Chung TC, Lin CC. Hepatoprotective effects of *Arctium lappa* on carbon tetrachloride-and acetaminophen-induced liver damage. Am J Chin Med 2000;28:163-173.

Pearson W, McKee S, Clarke AF. Effect of a proprietary herbal product on equine joint disease. Issues Studies 1999;35:31-46.

Seong K, et al. *Arctii fructus* is a prominent dietary source of linoleic acid for reversing epidermal hyperproliferation of guinea pigs [Korean]. Korean J Nutr 2003;36:819-827.

Thivierge G. Granular stomatitis in dogs due to burdock. Can Vet J 1973;14:96-97.

Wang BJ, et al. Effects of burdock on blood sugar, plasma lipid and uric acid of rats [Chinese]. Taiwan J Agric Chem Food Sci 2000;38:181-183.

Wang HY, Yang JS. Studies on the chemical constituents of *Arctium lappa* L [Chinese]. Yao Xue Xue Bao 1993;28:911-917.

Calendula

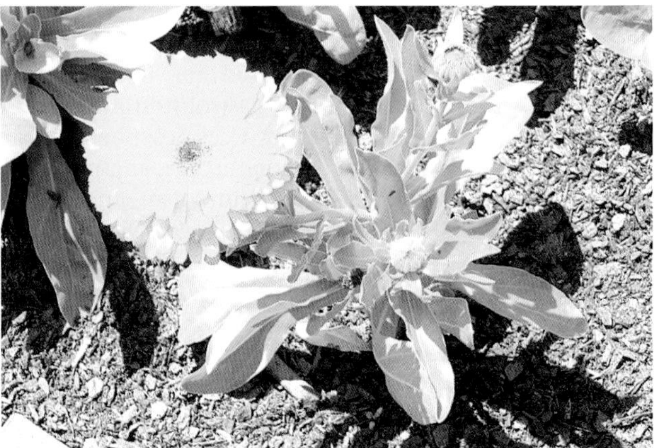

Calendula officinalis L. • Ca-LEN-dew-luh oh-fiss-ih-NAH-liss

Other Names: *Calendula officinalis,* Chinese safflower, fleur de calandule, gold-bloom, hen and chickens, holligold, körömvirag, marigold, mary-bud, souci, tousslat, xu xi, zubaydah (Boulos, 1983; Farnsworth, 1998; Bisset, 1994; Youngken, 1950).

Family: Asteraceae

Parts Used: Flowers

Distribution: Indigenous to Central, Eastern, and Southern Europe. Cultivated commercially in North America, the Balkans, Eastern Europe, and Germany (Bisset, 1994; Leung, 1996). Used extensively as a garden flower throughout the world.

Selected Constituents: Major constituents are triterpene saponins (2%-10%) based on oleanolic acid (calendulosides) and flavonoids (3-O-glycosides of isorhamnetin and quercetin), including astragalin, hyperoside, isoquercitrin, and rutin. Other constituents include essential oil, sesquiterpenes (e.g., caryophyllene), and triterpenes (eg, α- and β-amyrins, lupeol, and lupenone) (Farnsworth,

1998; Bisset, 1994; Bruneton, 1995). Immunostimulant polysaccharides have been reported (Varljen, 1989).

Clinical Actions: Antiseptic, lymphatic; reduces blood lipids; anti-inflammatory, astringent, spasmolytic, vulnery, cholagogue

Energetics: Neutral with cooling potential, dry

History and Traditional Usage: Although common in nearly every part of the world, calendula is believed to be native to Egypt. Ancient Egyptian records from 5000 years ago mention it, and hieroglyphics from the same period show stylized calendula flowers. Because calendula blooms almost continuously from early spring until the first frost, ancient Romans named it for their belief that new blooms appear on the first day, the "calend," of each month. Fresh calendula leaves or petals can be added to salads or dried for use in manufacturing or medicine. They produce a yellow dye that was used in the 1700s and 1800s to color cheese. Currently, calendula coloring may be used in beverage, cosmetic, food, and pharmaceutical products. Calendula petals may be substituted for saffron as a seasoning and coloring agent.

Uses described in traditional systems of medicine include external treatment of superficial cuts, minor inflammations of the skin and oral mucosa, wounds, varicosis, phlebitis, eczema, and acne; it is also included as part of treatment for dry skin, bee stings, and foot ulcers (British Herbal Pharmacopoeia, 1996; ESCOP, 1996; Blumenthal, 1998). Internally used for inflammatory conditions of internal organs, gastrointestinal ulcers, toothache, and eye inflammation. Uses described in folk medicine include treatment of amenorrhea, angina, fever, gastritis, hypotension, jaundice, rheumatism, and vomiting (British Herbal Pharmacopoeia, 1996; Farnsworth, 1998; Bisset, 1994).

According to de Bairacli Levy (1963), goats and sheep seek out calendula. It is a tonic and good heart medicine that provides restorative powers over the arteries and veins, which is why, she says, Arabs feed them to their racing horses. The leaves (raw) are useful for warts and tumors. She also suggests that as an infusion calendula can be used for alopecia in dogs (de Bairacli Levy, 1985).

Published Research: In vitro studies on antimicrobial activity show that the essential oil is more effective than ethanol, methanol, and water extracts (Rios, 1987; Dornberger, 1982; Acevedo, 1993; Gracza, 1987). Other in vitro studies suggest that a 70% ethanol extract has anti-inflammatory activity (Della-Loggia, 1994; Peyroux, 1981; Bezakova, 1996). The extract has significant antioxidant capacity. A crude extract of calendula exhibited significant antipyretic (74.95% inhibition at a dose of 300 mg/kg) and analgesic (27.42% inhibition at a dose of 40 mg/kg) activity in rat models. The extract at a dose of 20 mg/kg was as potent in its analgesic properties as acetylsalicylic acid is at 40 mg/kg (Shahnaz, 2000).

One study compared the effectiveness of calendula in a cream base with that of the commercial anti-inflammatory, trolamine, which is considered a reference topical agent. It was concluded that calendula is highly effective for the prevention of acute dermatitis with radiation treatment (Pommier, 2004). External application of an extract of Calendula accelerated the rates of contraction and epithelialization of excision wounds in rats (Rao, 1991). Duran (2005) investigated the effects of a calendula-containing ointment compared with a saline dressing on 21 people with lower leg venous ulcers. Total ulcer surface area was measured before and after 3 weeks of treatment. In the calendula group, ulcer surface area decreased by 41.71%, and surface area in the control group decreased by only 14.52%. More patients in the treatment group achieved complete epithelialization.

One Russian study investigated the treatment with topical calendula of patients with chronic catarrhal gingivitis and periodontal disease (Krazhan, 2001). The methanolic extract of Calendula flowers was found to show a hypoglycemic effect, inhibitory activity of gastric emptying, and gastroprotective effects (Yoshikawa, 2001). Extracts isolated from *Calendula officinalis* used perorally exerted an antiulcerous action on experimental ulcers (Iatsyno, 1978). Water-extracted calendula has demonstrated some uterine tone–enhancing activity (Shipochliev, 1981).

Indications: Mouthwash for gums, mucous membranes, and throat. Also for use in stomach infection and ulcers. Eyewash. Infections of the gastrointestinal tract, skin, and genitourinary tract. Inflamed skin, eczema, pruritus. Swollen glands. Elevated cholesterol and triglycerides. Wound dressing.

Potential Veterinary Indications: *Calendula officinalis* is used in bioorganic farming as a mastitis salve (Jost, 1984). For gingivitis, ulcers, erosions, eyewash, and dermatitis, and as a wound-cleansing agent (tea is appropriate)

Contraindications: When allergy to plants of the Asteraceae family (ESCOP, 1996) is known or suspected

Toxicology and Adverse Effects: AHPA class 1. No signs of toxicity have been exhibited with long-term use (18 months) of calendula extracts on mice, rats, and hamsters, nor have carcinogenic effects been observed (ESCOP, 1996; Yatsuno, 1978). Weak skin sensitization has been reported (Bruynzeel, 1992).

Potential Drug Interactions: None known.

Notes of Interest: One study showed that extracts of calendula (flowers and leaves) were effective against the snail *Lymnaea cailliaud,* with the flowers having greater molluskicidal activity than the leaf extract. The mortality rate of exposed snails was increased by longer exposure time, and the molluskicidal effect was the result of increased energy usage and nutrient consumption (Abd-El-Megeed, 1999).

Preparation Notes: The flowers require careful drying to avoid damp patches and overheating. Store in a well-closed container, protected from light (European Pharmacopoeia, 2000).

Dosage:

Externally:

Infusion: 1-2 g/150 mL of water (ESCOP, 1996)

Ointment: 2%-5% (Willuhn, 1992)

40% alcohol extract (1:1), or tincture (1:5) in 90% alcohol (British Herbal Pharmacopoeia, 1996): For the treatment of wounds, the tincture is applied undiluted; for compresses, the tincture is usually diluted at least 1:3 with sterile water (ESCOP, 1996; Willuhn, 1992; Van Hellemont, 1988).

Internally:

Human

Dried herb: 0.5-10 g TID

Infusions: 5-30 g per cup of water, with 1 cup of the tea given TID

Tincture (usually as 80%-90% ethanol) 1:2 or 1:3: 1-4 mL TID

Small Animal

Dried herb: 25-400 mg/kg, divided daily (optimally, TID)

Infusion: 5-30 g per cup of water, administered at a rate of ¼-½ cup per 10 kg (20 lb), divided daily (optimally, TID)

Tincture (usually in 80%-90% ethanol): 1:2-1:3: 0.5-2.0 mL per 10 kg (20 lb), divided daily (optimally, TID) and diluted or combined with other herbs

References

Abd-El-Megeed KN. Studies on the molluscicidal actvity of *Calendula micrantha officinalis* (Compositae) on fascioliasis transmitting snails. J Egypt Soc Parasitol 1999;29:183-192.

Acevedo JG, Lopez JL, Cortes GM. In vitro antimicrobial activity of various plant extracts used by purepecha against some Enterobacteriaceae. Int J Pharmacognosy 1993;31:61-64.

Bezakova L, Masterova I, Paulikova I, Psenak M. Inhibitory activity of isorhamnetin glycosides from *Calendula officinalis* L. on the activity of lipoxygenase. Die Pharmazie 1996;51:126-127.

Bisset NG. *Herbal Drugs and Phytopharmaceuticals.* Boca Raton, Fla: CRC Press; 1994.

Blumenthal M, Busse WR, Goldberg A, et al, eds. *The Complete German Commission E Monographs.* Austin, Tex: American Botanical Council; 1998.

Boulos L. *Medicinal Plants of North Africa.* Cairo: Reference Publications; 1983.

British Herbal Pharmacopoeia. London: British Herbal Medicine Association; 1996.

Bruneton J. *Pharmacognosy, Phytochemistry, Medicinal Plants.* Paris: Lavoisier; 1995.

Bruynzeel DP, van Ketel WG, Young E, van Joost T, Smeenk G. Contact sensitization by alternative topical medicaments containing plant extracts. Contact Dermatitis 1992;27:278-279.

Della-Loggia R, Tubaro A, Sosa S, et al. The role of triterpenoids in the topical anti-inflammatory activity of *Calendula officinalis* flowers. Planta Med 1994;60:516-520.

Dornberger K, Lich H. Screening for antimicrobial and presumed cancerostatic plant metabolites. Die Pharmazie 1982; 37:215-221.

Duran V, Matic M, Jovanovc M, Mimica N, Gajinov Z, Poljacki M, Boza P. Results of the clinical examination of an ointment with marigold *(Calendula officinalis)* extract in the treatment of venous leg ulcers. Int J Tissue React 2005;27:101-106.

ESCOP. *Monographs on the Medicinal Uses of Plant Drugs.* Fascicule 1. Elburg: European Scientific Cooperative on Phytotherapy; 1996.

European Pharmacopoeia. 3rd ed. Suppl 2000. Strasbourg: Council of Europe; 1999.

Farnsworth NR, ed. NAPRALERT Database. Chicago, Ill: University of Illinois at Chicago; 1998.

Gracza L. Oxygen-containing terpene derivatives from *Calendula officinalis.* Planta Med 1987;53:227.

Iatsyno AI, Belova LF, Lipkina GS, Sokolov SI, Trutneva EA. Pharmacology of calenduloside B, a new triterpene glycoside from the roots of *Calendula officinalis.* Farmakol Toksikol 1978;41:556-560.

Jost M. Calendula as a healing plant for mastitis in dairy cows. Biodynamics 1984;152:7-19.

Krazhan IA, Garazha NN. Treatment of chronic catarrhal gingivitis with polysorb-immobilized calendula [Russian]. Stomatologiia (Mosk) 2001;80:11-13.

Leung AY, Foster S. *Encyclopedia of Common Natural Ingredients Used in Food, Drugs, and Cosmetics.* 2nd ed. New York: John Wiley & Sons; 1996.

Mascolo N, Autore G, Capasso G, et al. Biological screening of Italian medicinal plants for antiinflammatory activity. Phytother Res 1987;1:20-31.

May G, Willuhn G. Antiviral activity of aqueous extracts from medicinal plants in tissue cultures. Arzneimittelforschung 1978;28:1-7.

Peyroux J, Rossignol P, Delareau P, et al. Anti-oedemic and anti-hyperhaemic properties of *Calendula officinalis* L. Plantes Médicinales et Phytotherapie 1981;15:210-216.

Pharmacopoeia Helvetica. 8th ed. Berne: Département Fédéral de l'Intérieur; 1997.

Pharmacopoeia Hungarica. 7th ed. Budapest: Hungarian Pharmacopoeia Commission, Medicina Konyvkiado; 1986.

Pommier P, Gomez F, Sunyach MP, D'Hombres A, Carrie C, Montbarbon X. Phase III randomized trial of *Calendula officinalis* compared with trolamine for the prevention of acute dermatitis during irradiation for breast cancer. J Clin Oncol 2004;22:1447-1453.

Rao SG, Laxminarayana AU, Saraswathi LU, et al. Calendula and Hypericum: two homeopathic drugs promoting wound healing in rats. Fitoterapia 1991;62:508.

Rios JL, Recio MC, Villar A. Antimicrobial activity of selected plants employed in the Spanish Mediterranean area. J Ethnopharmacol 1987;21:139-152.

Saify ZS, et al. Analgesic and antimicrobial activity of the leaves' extract of *Calendula officinalis.* Hamdard Med 2000;43:34-37.

Sarrell EM, Cohen HA, Kahan E. Naturopathic treatment for ear pain in children. Pediatrics 2003;111(5 Pt 1):e574-e579.

Schmidgall J, Schnetz E, Hensel A. Evidence for bioadhesive effects of polysaccharides and polysaccharide-containing herbs in an ex vivo bioadhesion assay on buccal membranes. Planta Med 2000;66:1,48-53.

Shahnaz A, et al. Antipyretic and analgesic activity in crude ethanolic extract of *Calendula officinalis* Linn. Pakistan J Sci Indust Res 2000;43:50-54.

Shipochliev T. Uterotonic action of extracts from a group of medicinal plants [Bulgarian]. Vet Med Nauki 1981;18:94-98.

Van Hellemont J. *Fytotherapeutisch Compendium.* 2nd ed. Utrecht, Bohn: Scheltema & Holkema; 1988:113-114.

Varljen J, Lipták A, Wagner H. Structural analysis of a rhamnoarabinogalactan and arabinogalactans with immunostimulating activity from *Calendula officinalis.* Phytochemistry 1989;28:2379-2383.

Willuhn G. Pflanzliche Dermatika, eine kritische Übersicht. Deutsche Apotheker Zeitung 1992;132:1873-1883.

Yatsuno AI, et al. Farmakol Toksikol (Moscow) 1978;41:556.

Yoshikawa M, Murakami T, Kishi A, et al. Medicinal flowers. III. Marigold. (1): Hypoglycemic, gastric emptying, inhibitory, and gastroprotective principles and new oleanane-type triterpene oligoglycosides, calendasaponins A, B, C, and D, from Egyptian *Calendula officinalis.* Chem Pharm Bull (Tokyo) 2001;49:863-870.

Youngken HW. *Textbook of Pharmacognosy.* 6th ed. Philadelphia, Pa: Blakiston; 1950.

California Poppy

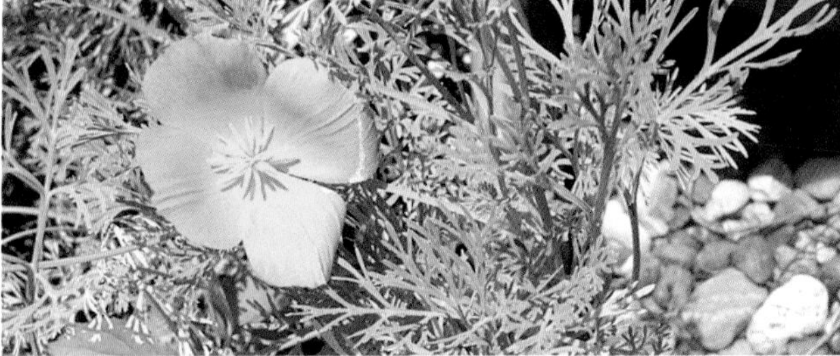

Eschscholzia californica Cham; possibly *E. mexicana* • es-SHOLT-zee-uh kal-ih-FOR-nik-uh

Distribution: Western North America

Similar Species: Unknown

Other Names: Globe du soleil, goldmohn, escolzia di California

Family: Papaveraceae

Parts Used: Aerial parts, when in flower

Selected Constituents: Alkaloids (californidine, escholzine, protopine, cryptopine, chelidonine), flavone glycosides, carotenoids

History and Traditional Usage: Various North American native tribes used the herb for the pain of toothache and headache. It was also used to help children sleep. The mashed seed pod and root juices were used to dry up mothers' milk. Used today for excitable children, and also for painful spasms, such as colic, gallbladder pain, irritable bowel.

Clinical Actions: Nervine, hypnotic, antispasmodic, anodyne

Energetics: Bitter, cool

Published Research: Alkaloids of California poppy bind certain 5HT receptors in vitro (Gafner, 2006). An aqueous extract was administered to mice and was found to confer anxiolytic and sedative properties, which were blocked with a benzodiazepine receptor antagonist. The extract also had peripheral analgesic effects (Rolland, 1991; Rolland, 2001).

Indications: Insomnia, abdominal pain due to spasm. Used most often in children for psychological problems.

Potential Veterinary Indications: Anxiety, insomnia, abdominal pain

Notes of Interest: This is the state flower of California, and picking the plant in that state is prohibited by law. Use of California poppy may result in a positive drug test.

Contraindications: Safety during lactation and pregnancy not established.

Toxicology and Adverse Effects: AHPA class 2b. No adverse effects reported, but Australian authorities warn not to exceed the recommended dose.

Drug Interactions: May have additive effects with drugs that have tranquilizer or sedative effects—binds benzodiazepine receptors and may have other anxiolytic mechanisms. May potentiate MAO inhibitors.

Dosage:

Human: (Last dose preferably given 30 minutes before bedtime if insomnia is being treated.)

Dried herb: 1-10 g TID

Infusions and decoctions: 5-30 g per cup of water, ¼-1 cup of the tea given TID

Tincture (available in 25%-60% ethanol preparations): 1:2 or 1:3: 0.25-5 mL TID, up to 6 times daily for acute conditions

Small Animal:

Dried herb: 25-400 mg/kg, divided daily (optimally, TID)

Infusion: 5-15 g per cup of water, administered at a rate of ¼-½ cup per 10 kg (20 lb), divided daily (optimally, TID)

Tincture (usually in 25%-60% ethanol): 1:2-1:3: 0.5-2.0 mL per 10 kg (20 lb), divided daily (optimally, TID) and diluted or combined with other herbs. Higher doses may be appropriate if the herb is used singly and is not combined in a formula.

References

Gafner S, Dietz BM, McPhail KL, et al. Alkaloids from *Eschscholzia californica* and their capacity to inhibit binding of [(3)H]8-hydroxy-2-(di-N-propylamino)tetralin to 5-HT(1A) receptors in vitro. J Nat Prod 2006;69:432-435.

Rolland A, Fleurentin J, Lanhers MC, et al. Neurophysiological effects of an extract of *Eschscholzia californica* Cham. (Papaveraceae). Phytother Res 2001;15:377-381.

Rolland A, Fleurentin J, Lanhers MC, et al. Behavioural effects of the American traditional plant *Eschscholzia californica:* sedative and anxiolytic properties. Planta Med 1991;57:212-216.

Cascara

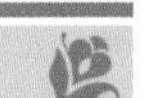

Frangula purshiana (DC) J.G. Cooper, *(Rhamnus purshiana* DC*);* also, *Rhamnus crocea, Rhamnus ilicifolia* • RAM-nus pur-shee-AH-nuh

Distribution: Native to the North American Pacific coast

Similar Species: *Rhamnus frangula* (Alder buckthorn)

Other Names: Cascara sagrada, *Rhamni purshianae* cortex, American buckthorn, cascara buckthorn, sacred bark, bitter bark, California buckthorn, chittem bark, purshiana bark, persiana bark, yellow bark, bearberry, amerikanisch faulbaum, sacrée

Family: Rhamnaceae

Parts Used: Bark; the berries were used by Native American tribes.

Collection: Bark is gathered in the spring and dried for 1 to 6 years.

Selected Constituents: Cascarosides A, B, C, D, E, F; aloe-emodin, barbaloin, frangulin, chrysalin, palmidin A, B, C; free aglycones

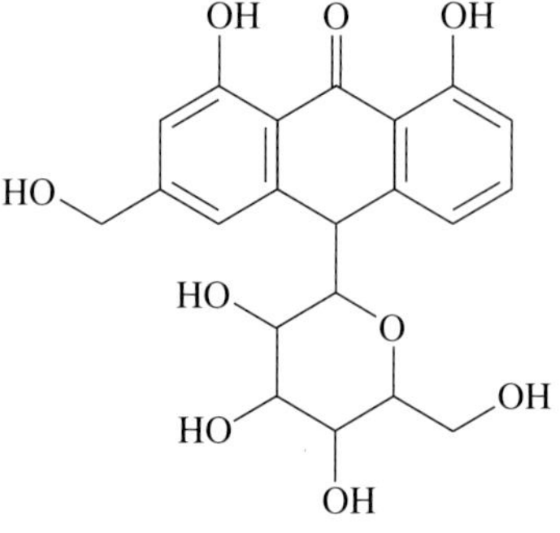

Barbaloin (syn. Aloin)

Clinical Actions: Laxative to purgative (dose dependent), alterative, hepatic, stomachic, febrifuge, nervine, antibilious, antidiabetic, peristaltic

Energetics: Bitter, cold, slightly acrid

History and Traditional Usage: Native American tribes used the bark as a laxative and emetic; it was also used topically for cuts and sores. *King's American Dispensatory* describes the specific indication as "constipation, . . . ; lesser ailments, depending solely upon constipation, with intestinal atony." In addition to use as a laxative, cascara was used in gallbladder disease, liver disease, dyspepsia, indigestion, gout, and "cardiac asthma" (Christopher, 1976).

Published Research: Cascara is one of the mildest of the class of laxatives that contain anthraquinone glycosides (senna is one of the strongest in this group). Anthraquinone glycosides stimulate water and electrolyte secretion into the large intestine and inhibit absorption of same, possibly through prostaglandin E_2-or nitric oxide–mediated mechanisms (Beubler, 1985; Izzo, 1997). The result is an increase in intestinal motility. Some anthrones are not converted to active forms until they have been metabolized by gut bacteria. Long-term use of anthranoid laxatives has been suggested to predispose to colorectal cancer (Siegers, 1993). Different anthraquinone precursors lead to various absorbed versus retained moieties. Cascara and buckthorn anthraquinones are not absorbed, which may suggest that they are preferred in cats, as some of the absorbed anthraquinones in other species require glucuronidation for elimination from the body (de Witte, 1990).

Indications: Constipation; painful conditions in which a softer stool is required to ease defecation (in people, anal fissures, hemorrhoids, rectal surgery, anal surgery). It is usually safer to try a bulk-forming laxative before a stimulant laxative like cascara is used.

Potential Veterinary Indications: For 1 to 2 weeks only in the treatment of constipation. Lactulose is a safer option for long-term use.

Contraindications: Ileus, GI obstruction, inflammatory GI disease, abdominal pain, pregnancy, lactation. Not recommended for use in the very young. (Literature from the late 1800s and as late as the 1970s, however, contains recommendations for doses to be given to pregnant mothers and small children.)

Toxicology and Adverse Effects: AHPA class 2b, 2c, 2d. With long-term use, loss of electrolytes (especially potassium) may occur. Anthraquinones are mutagenic and cause melanosis in the bowel with long-term use. Cascara has been shown to have milder adverse effects than other anthranoid-containing herbs such as senna and aloe. A case report associates use of cascara with cholestatic hepatitis (Nadir, 2000). Cardiac effects, chiefly caused by electrolyte abnormalities, have been noted. Albuminuria and hematuria have also been described with long-term use. Respiratory allergic signs have been reported in pharmacy workers who handle Cascara.

Drug Interactions: Laxatives may reduce intestinal absorption of other drugs. With regard to the long-term potential for electrolyte changes, concurrent use of antiarrhythmics, cardiac glycosides, corticosteroids, and diuretics should be considered carefully until cascara therapy is discontinued and the imbalance is corrected.

Preparation Notes: The anthrone and dianthrone glycosides present in fresh bark are emetic and can lead to severe colic. These compounds must be converted to safer anthraquinones through oxidation. This is accomplished by aging the bark for 1 year, or by heating it for several hours to 60° C to 100° C.

Dosage: (NOTE: Laxative herbs are usually given at bedtime, allowing the herb to progress through the GI tract, producing catharsis in the morning. The smallest amount needed for the desired effect is the correct dose!)

Human:

Dried herb: 1-3 g at bedtime

Infusions and decoctions: ½ tsp of the dried herb in 1 cup boiling water; dose is ⅛-½ cup BID

Tincture (generally as 25%-40% ethanol preparations): 1:2 or 1:3: 3-10 mL at bedtime

Small Animal:

Dried herb: 25-300 mg/kg, divided daily (optimally, TID)

Decoction: 2-5 g per cup of water, administered at a rate of ¼ cup per 10 kg (20 lb), divided daily (optimally, TID)

Tincture (usually in 25%-40% ethanol): 1:2-1:3: 0.5-1.5 mL per 10 kg (20 lb), divided daily (optimally, TID) and diluted or combined with other herbs

Farm Animal:

Fluid extract (1:1): 0.6-45 mL for farm animals from small ruminants to horses and cows

References

Beubler E, Kollar G. Stimulation of PGE2 synthesis and water and electrolyte secretion by senna anthraquinones is inhibited by indomethacin. J Pharm Pharmacol 1985;37:248-251.

Christopher JR. *School of Natural Healing.* Provo, Utah: BiWorld Publishers; 1976.

de Witte P, Lemli L. The metabolism of anthranoid laxatives. Hepatogastroenterology 1990;137:601-605.

Izzo AA, Sautebin L, Rombola L, Capasso F. The role of constitutive and inducible nitric oxide synthase in senna- and cascara-induced diarrhoea in the rat. Eur J Pharmacol 1997;323:93-97.

Nadir A, Reddy D, Van Thiel DH. Cascara sagrada–induced intrahepatic cholestasis causing portal hypertension: case report and review of herbal hepatotoxicity. Am J Gastroenterol 2000;95:3634-3637.

Siegers CP, von Hertzberg-Lottin E, Otte M, Schneider B. Anthranoid laxative abuse—a risk for colorectal cancer? Gut 1993;34:1099-1101.

Cat's Claw

Uncaria tomentosa (Willd.) *DC* • Un-KEH-ree-uh toh-men-TOH-suh

Distribution: Tropical South and Central America

Similar Species: *Uncaria rhynchophylla* is *Gou Teng* in Chinese medicine; it is used to extinguish wind and stop tremors. *Uncaria guiaensis* is another South American species that contains fewer of the constituents that are considered important for the therapeutic indications of *U. tomentosa.*

Other Names: Una de gato, katzenkralle, griffe du cat, samento, saventero, garabato Colorado (Loreto, Peru), uña de gato de altura (Ucayali, Peru), garabato amarillo (Inca), tsachik, paotati-mösha, misho-mentis, jjipotatsa, unganangui. The name "una de gato" is a common name for 12 or more different species of plants in Peru. *Acacia greggi* is a Southwestern American plant also called cat's claw; this plant is often sold in commercial trade instead of *Uncaria tomentosa,* but it is not related and is more toxic.

Family: Rubiaceae

Parts Used: Inner bark of the stem or root; best to purchase stem bark so that the plant's root is left to regenerate

Selected Constituents: Indole alkaloids (isopteropodine, pteropodine, rhynchophylline), triterpene saponins, flavonoids. The plant exists as two chemotypes—one that is high in pentacyclic alkaloids, and the other is high in tetracyclic alkaloids. These two groups of chemicals have opposing effects according to in vitro studies, with the pentacyclic oxindole alkaloids having immune-enhancing and anti-inflammatory activities, and the tetracyclic oxindole alkaloids having central nervous system activity and counteracting the immune stimulant activity of the pentacyclic alkaloids. Positive studies have used both chemotypes of the plant and their respective compounds. Commercial products are usually standardized to contain less than 0.02% tetracylic alkaloids.

Clinical Actions: Anti-inflammatory, astringent, antirheumatic, immune modulatory

Energetics: Slightly bitter

History and Traditional Usage: A South American tonic taken regularly to prevent illness, cat's claw was also traditionally used for cancer, rheumatism, and urinary tract problems; as an anti-inflammatory agent and contraceptive; and for stomach ulcers. The Ashaninka tribe of Peru is the source of most ethnobotanical data; in that tribe, cat's claw is understood and prescribed only by healer priests.

Published Research: Research on this herb has centered on its alkaloids, which appear to have anti-inflammatory and immune stimulant activities. The plant exhibited antimutagenic activity in early National Institutes of Health (NIH) cancer screening tests. One small 4-week trial found that 30 humans with knee osteoarthritis experienced significant relief from pain during daily activities when given *Uncaria guianensis,* but not at night or during rest; the control group, by comparison, had no pain relief (Piscoya, 2001). In a 52-week randomized, double-blind, placebo-controlled trial, an extract of *Uncaria tomentosa* reduced the number of painful joints in humans with rheumatoid arthritis (Mur, 2002). A water extract of *U. tomentosa* enhanced the immune response to pneumococcal vaccine in human subjects (Lamm, 2001).

Jones (1995) describes clinical observations by Peruvian veterinarians Victor Humberto Ruiz and Victor Fernandez, at the University of San Marcos. The preparation used most often was injectable (50% alcohol and 50% water extract) and was processed to remove tannins; the usual dose was 3 mL once daily. Teas, decoctions, dried bark powder, dried and fluid extracts, and a 1:5 tincture were used. The case descriptions are certainly anecdotal, but records are available for 53 cats and 135 dogs treated with the herb; many conditions treated are considered chronic or incurable. Many patients had mammary cancer, and Jones reports that more than 20 treated cats lived 3 to 4 years longer than untreated cats (presumably with the use of historical controls, but this is not explicitly stated). A similar increase in life expectancy was seen in more than 40 dogs with mammary cancer.

Ruiz also treated 15 dogs with parvovirus, using a distilled preparation at 1 mL/kg body weight BID. Ten of 15 dogs recovered from the disease. Cases described as osteoarthritis, hip dysplasia, and disk disease were said to have been provided significant pain relief (but no objective measurements of outcome were provided); improvements in haircoat were noted frequently in his diary. The dose used in most of these cases was 25 to 30 mg/kg of the powdered bark divided BID.

Jones also describes work by Keplinger that was presented at an AIDS conference in Vienna in 1991. Her group used injections of Krallendorn (a proprietary root extract) given at 0.3 mg IM on days 1, 3, and 5. Results of her studies are not well described; 85% of cats with symptomatic FIV were reported as improved, and 44% of "cats with leukemia" became aviremic by the end of the 20th week. Unfortunately, the original paper could not be located.

Indications: Cat's claw has been recommended for a very wide variety of problems, including asthma, gonorrhea, diverticulitis, Crohn's disease, peptic ulcer, colitis, gastritis, parasites, leaky gut, parasites, hemorrhoids, HIV, cancer, herpes, chronic fatigue, asthma, diabetes, arthritis, alzheimer's and cognitive disorders, circulatory problems, and as an immune stimulant and adaptogen.

Potential Veterinary Indications: Osteoarthritis, certain viral infections, chronic debility, and immune suppression. Interest in the potential for this herb to be used in the treatment of demodectic mange is apparent (Vega, 2003).

Contraindications: Pregnancy or use in the very young may be contraindicated.

Toxicology and Adverse Effects: AHPA class 4. Diarrhea and signs of bleeding may result if large doses are administered. Theoretically, cat's claw may cause hypotension. A case report describes acute renal failure in a patient with lupus who was taking cat's claw, but the role of the herb was not proved.

Drug Interactions: Although no clinical reports of interactions were found, cat's claw may alter the metabolism of drugs that are substrates of CYP3A4 enzymes (Budzinski, 2000). Cat's claw may theoretically add to the effects of antihypertensive drugs. For patients on immune suppressive drugs, the theoretical immune stimulant effect of cat's claw may be a problem.

Dosage:

Human:

Dried herb: 2-10 g TID

Decoction: 1 tsp pulverized root in 1 qt of water for 45 min: ¼-1 tsp on an empty stomach

Tincture (usually 50%-60% ethanol): 1:2 or 1:3: 1-3 mL TID

Small Animal:

Dried herb: 50-500 mg/kg, divided daily (optimally, TID)

Decoction: As above, ¼ cup per 10 kg (20 lb), divided daily (optimally, TID)

Tincture (usually in 50%-60% ethanol): 1:2-1:3: 1.0-2.5 mL per 10 kg (20 lb), divided daily (optimally, TID) and diluted or combined with other herbs

References

Budzinski JW, Foster BC, Vandenhoek S, Arnason JT. An in vitro evaluation of human cytochrome P450 3A4 inhibition by selected commercial herbal extracts and tinctures. Phytomedicine 2000;7:273-282.

Jones K. *Cat's Claw: Healing Vine of Peru.* Seattle, Wash: Sylvan Press; 1995:90-97.

Lamm S, Sheng Y, Pero RW. Persistent response to pneumococcal vaccine in individuals supplemented with a novel water soluble extract of *Uncaria tomentosa,* C-Med-100. Phytomedicine 2001;8:267-274.

Mur E, Hartig F, Eibl G, Schirmer M. Randomized double blind trial of an extract from the pentacyclic alkaloid–chemotype of *Uncaria tomentosa* for the treatment of rheumatoid arthritis. J Rheumatol 2002;29:678-681.

Piscoya J, Rodriguez Z, Bustamante SA, Okuhama NN, Miller MJ, Sandoval M. Efficacy and safety of freeze-dried cat's claw in osteoarthritis of the knee: mechanisms of action of the species *Uncaria guianensis.* Inflamm Res 2001;50:442-448.

Vega M. Tratamiento de la demodeccia con Uncaria tomentosa. Available at: http://www.portalveterinaria.com/sections.php?op=viewarticle&artid=160. Accessed June 27, 2003.

Chamomile

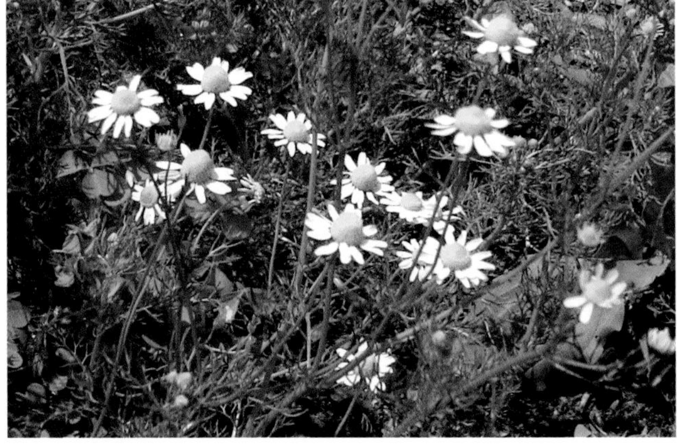

Matricaria recutita L., synonymous with *Chamomilla recutita* L. • mat-ri-KAR-ee-uh re-KOO-tee-ta

Related to *Anthemis nobilis* (Roman chamomile), which is also a widely used and accepted form of chamomile.

Other Names: Camomile, flos chamomillae, German chamomile, matricaire, matricaria flowers, pin heads, sweet false chamomille, sweet feverfew, wild chamomile

Family: Asteraceae

Parts Used: Dried flowering heads

Distribution: Chamomile is indigenous to northern Europe; it grows wild in central European countries and is abundant in eastern Europe. Also found in western Asia, the Mediterranean region of northern Africa, and the United States. It is cultivated in many countries.

Selected Constituents: Chamomile contains an essential oil (0.4%-1.5%) that has an intense blue color owing to its chamazulene content (1%-15%). Other major constituents include α-bisabolol and related sesquiterpenes (up to 50% of the oil). Apigenin and related flavonoid glycosides constitute up to 8% (dry weight) of the herb (Bruneton, 1995; Dölle, 1985).

(−)-α-Bisabolol

Clinical Actions: Carminative, spasmolytic, mild sedative, cholagogue, antiallergic, anti-inflammatory, healing, bitter tonic

Energetics: Slightly bitter and pungent, neutral

History and Traditional Usage: Uses described in pharmacopoeias and in traditional systems of medicine include the following: adjuvant in the treatment of minor inflammatory conditions of the gastrointestinal tract (Weiss, 1987); also as an antibacterial and antiviral agent, an emetic, and an emmenagogue. It is used to relieve eye strain, as an eyewash, and to treat patients with urinary infection and diarrhea (Tyler, 1988). The dried flower heads of *Matricaria recutita* L. (Asteraceae) are used to prepare a spasmolytic and a sedative tea (Viola, 1995).

According to de Bairacli Levy (1985), chamomile is a female remedy and a pregnancy herb; she suggests the use of chamomile tea to soak oat flakes for handrearing of puppies, for bathing discharging eyes (a mix of chamomile tea and milk), and for treating patients with diarrhea (2 tbsp of tea 3 times daily) and gastroenteritis (as much as the animal will drink). She suggests that it is good for inflamed gums, female ailments, wounds, and bruises; in the treatment of tumors (as a poultice) for blood and skin disorders; and for constipation (de Bairacli Levy, 1963).

Published Research: Chamomile extracts inhibited both cyclooxygenase and lipoxygenase (Wagner, 1986) and thus the production of prostaglandins and leukotrienes. Numerous in vivo studies have demonstrated the anti-inflammatory effects of chamomile extract, the essential oil, and isolated constituents (Kakovlev, 1979; Ammon, 1992; Albring, 1983; Della Loggia, 1985; Hempel, 1999; Safayhi, 1994). The principal anti-inflammatory and antispasmodic constituents of chamomile appear to be the terpene compounds matricin, chamazulene, α-bisabololoxides A and B, and α-bisabolol (Jakovlev, 1983). Chamazulene is actually an artifact formed during the heating of flowers when an infusion or the essential oil is prepared (Bruneton, 1995). Chamomile tea has significant antioxidant capacity, according to animal studies (Jung, 2003). In vitro studies show possible antibacterial and mild immune stimulating effects (Aggag, 1972; Chao, 2000; Laskova, 1992; Uteshev, 1999).

Mouth and throat lesions

Chamomile preparations have been found to be beneficial in the treatment of radiation mucositis following head and neck radiation and systemic chemotherapy (Carl, 1991). However, additional studies found conflicting results. A chamomile mouthwash was investigated for its putative ability to relieve stomatitis in people secondary to 5-flourouracil treatment. No difference was noted between people treated with chamomile and those treated with placebo mouthwash (Fidler, 1996). Two separate studies examined the effects of a chamomile spray or a gel used as a lubricant for endotracheal tubes. The authors hypothesized that chamomile could prevent postoperative sore throat and hoarseness. In both trials, no difference was observed between chamomile and placebo lubricants (Charulauxananan, 2004; Kyokong, 2002).

Skin inflammation

The therapeutic efficacy of chamomile extract was tested in a double-blind trial of 14 patients after dermabrasion from tattoos. Reduction of the weeping wound area, as well as improved drying tendency, was statistically significant (Glowania, 1987).

The efficacy of chamomile cream versus 0.25% hydrocortisone, 0.75% fluocortin butyl ester, and 5% bufexamac was tested in 161 patients with inflammatory dermatoses in a bilateral comparative study. Chamomile cream was as effective as hydrocortisone. It was superior to bufexamac and to fluocortin butyl ester. With neurodermitis, chamomile cream showed the same therapeutic effects as hydrocortisone and was superior to the other reference products (Aertgeerts, 1985).

The antipruritic effects of German chamomile on induced scratching in mice were examined. In mice fed a diet that contained (1.2 w/w% of ethyl acetate extract) dried flower of German chamomile for 11 days, scratching behavior was significantly suppressed with no effect on body weight. The inhibitory effects of the dietary intake of the German chamomile extracts were comparable with those of an antiallergic agent (Kobayashi, 2003).

Anxiety

Apigenin showed anxiolytic activity in mice, without sedation, muscle relaxant effects, or anticonvulsant action. A 10-fold increase in dosage produced a mild sedative effect (Viola, 1995). Chamomile depresses the central nervous system (Della Loggia, 1982), and the oil had significant sedative effects in mice (Wakame, 2003). One study found that inhaling chamomile oil vapor decreased stress-induced increases in plasma adrenocorticotropic hormone (ACTH) levels in ovariectomized rats. The plasma ACTH level decreased further when diazepam was administered along with inhalation of chamomile oil vapor (Yamada, 1996). Additional results suggest that chamomile oil may enhance GABAergic (gamma aminobutyric acid) activity in the central nervous system (Yamada, 2000). The spasmolytic activity of chamomile has been attributed to apigenin, apigenin-7-O-glucoside, and α-bisabolol, all of which have activity similar to that of papaverine (Bruneton, 1995; Della Loggia, 1990).

Chamomile and goats' milk

Six groups of goats were fed different rations that cotained variously black cumin, chamomile, garlic, fenugreek, or no supplementation. Gouda cheese was made from the milk of each treatment. The cheese was analyzed monthly for parameters such as moisture, fat, total protein, salt, acidity, and soluble nitrogen, as well as other properties. Sensory evaluation was also carried out. The attributes of the experimental cheeses were better than those of control cheese, and experimental cheeses were characterized by the absence of goaty flavor. The best treatments were derived from the milk of goats fed black cumin seeds and its straw or chamomile flowers (Mostafa, 1999).

A study determined whether the essential oils from these products could be detected in goat milk after goats were fed chamomile and caraway seed. Although relatively large quantities of chamomile were fed to goats over time, the characteristic essential oils of chamomile could not be detected in milk (Molnar, 1997).

Indications: ***Internal use:*** Dyspepsia, epigastric bloating, impaired digestion, flatulence, restlessness, and mild cases of insomnia due to nervous disorders. Well known as a remedy for the irritation and pain of teething. Also, for allergic reactions, including asthma, food intolerance, hayfever, anorexia, colic, irritable bowel syndrome, and diarrhea. ***Externally:*** Inflammation and irritation of the skin and mucosa (skin cracks, bruises, frostbite, and insect bites), irritations and infections of the mouth and gums, and hemorrhoids. Also inhaled for relief of irritation of the respiratory tract due to the common cold.

Potential Veterinary Indications: Eyewash, mild sedative, anxiolytic; for flatulence and mild colic, source of antioxidants, topical wound therapy, for pruritic mice and rats, odor reducer in goats' milk.

Contraindications: Chamomile is contraindicated in patients with a known sensitivity or allergy to plants of the Asteraceae (Compositae), such as ragweed, asters, and chrysanthemums (Carle, 1992). Chamomile may be contraindicated in cats because of the coumarin content.

Toxicology and Adverse Effects: AHPA class 1. The presence of lactones in chamomile preparations may cause allergic reactions in sensitive individuals; reports of contact dermatitis have also been documented (Dstychova, 1992; Subiza, 1990; Paulsen, 1993, 2001). Very few cases of allergy were specifically attributed to German chamomile (Hausen, 1984). A few cases of anaphylactic reaction to the ingestion of chamomile have been reported (Benner, 1973; Casterline, 1980; Reider, 2000; Subiza, 1989).

Means (2002) described a series of cases in which cats administered chamomile developed epistaxis and subcutaneous hemorrhage. Anticoagulant activity due to coumarin content was postulated. Details of the herb form were not provided.

Potential Drug Interactions: The concomitant use of opioid analgesics with the sedative herbal supplement chamomile may lead to increased central nervous system depression. It is suggested that further research is needed to confirm and assess the clinical significance of these potential adverse interactions (Abebe, 2002).

Dosage:

External Use:

Compresses, baths, vapor inhalations, rinses: 15-50 g flower/500 mL water, steep 15-30 min, or mix 10 mL fluid extract or 1:2 tincture into 500 mL water

Cream: apply to cover affected area BID-TID

Vapor inhalation: 1-5 drops of volatile oil per liter of water

Internal Use:

Human

Dried herb: 2-10 g TID, up to 6 times daily for acute conditions
Infusions and decoctions: 5-30 g per cup of water, with 1 cup of the tea given TID, up to 6 times daily acutely
Tincture (usually as 50%-60% ethanol): 1:2 or 1:3: 1-5 mL TID, up to 6 times daily for acute conditions
Child dose of flowers: 2 g TID, or a single dose of the fluid extract, 0.6-2 mL (British Herbal Pharmacopoeia, 1990). Should not be used by children younger than 3 years old

Dogs

Dried herb: 25-300 mg/kg, divided daily (optimally, TID)
Infusion: 5-30 g per cup of water, administered at a rate of ¼-½ cup per 10 kg (20 lb), divided daily (optimally, TID)
Tincture (usually in 50%-60% ethanol): 1:2-1:3: 0.5-1.5 mL per 10 kg (20 lb), divided daily (optimally, TID) and diluted or combined with other herbs. Higher doses may be appropriate if the herb is used singly and is not combined in a formula.

References

Abebe W. Herbal medication: potential for adverse interactions with analgesic drugs. J Clin Pharm Ther 2002;27:391-402.

Aertgeerts P, Albring M, Klaschka F et al. Comparative testing of Kamillosan cream and steroidal (0.25% hydrocortisone, 0.75% fluocortin butyl ester) and non-steroidal (5% bufexamac) dermatologic agents in maintenance therapy of eczematous diseases [German]. Z Hautkr 1985;60:270-277.

African Pharmacopoeia. 1st ed. Lagos: Organization of African Unity, Scientific, Technical & Research Commission; 1985.

Aggag ME, Yousef RT. Study of antimicrobial activity of chamomile oil. Planta Med 1972;22:140-144.

Albring M, Albrecht H, Alcorn G, et al. The measuring of the anti-inflammatory effect of a compound on the skin of volunteers. *Methods and findings in experimental and clinical pharmacology.* 1983;5:75-77.

Ammon HPT, Kaul R. Pharmakologie der Kamille und ihrer Inhaltsstoffe. Deutsche Apotheker Zeitung 1992;132(suppl 27):3-26.

Benner MH, Lee HJ. Anaphylactic reaction to chamomile tea. J Allergy Clin Immunol 1973;52:307-308.

British Herbal Pharmacopoeia. London: British Herbal Medicine Association; 1990.

Bruneton J. *Pharmacognosy, Phytochemistry, Medicinal Plants.* Paris: Lavoisier; 1995.

Carl W, Emrich LS. Management of oral mucositis during local radiation and systemic chemotherapy: a study of 98 patients. J Prosthet Dent 1991;66:361-369.

Carle R, Gomaa K. Chamomile: a pharmacological and clinical profile. Drugs Today 1992;28:559-565.

Casterline CL. Allergy to chamomile tea. JAMA 1980;244:330-331.

Chao SC, Young DG, Oberg CJ. Screening for inhibitory activity of essential oils on selected bacteria, fungi and viruses. J Essential Oil Res 2000;12:639-649.

Charuluxananan S, Sumethawattana P, Kosawiboonpol R et al. Effectiveness of lubrication of endotracheal tube cuff with chamomile-extract for prevention of postoperative sore throat and hoarseness. J Med Assoc Thai 2004;87(suppl 2):S185-S189.

Della Loggia R, Traversa U, Scarcia V, et al. Depressive effects of *Chamomilla recutita* (L.) Rausch. tubular flowers, on central nervous system in mice. Pharmacol Res Commun 1982; 14:153-162.

Della Loggia R Evaluation of the anti-inflammatory activity of chamomile preparations. Planta Med 1990;56:657-658.

Della Loggia R. Lokale antiphlogistische Wirkung der Kamillen-Flavone. Deutsche Apotheker Zeitung 1985;125(suppl 1):9-11.

Dölle B, Carle R, Müller W. Flavonoidbestimmung in Kamillenextraktpräparaten. Deutsche Apotheker Zeitung 1985; 125(suppl I):14-19.

Dstychova E, Zahejsky J. Contact hypersensitivity to camomile. Ceskoslovenska Dermatologie 1992;67:14-18.

Fidler P, Loprinzi CL, O'Fallon JR, et al. Prospective evaluation of a chamomile mouthwash for prevention of 5-FU-induced oral mucositis. Cancer 1996;77:522-525.

Glowania HJ, Raulin C, Swoboda M. Effect of chamomile on wound healing—a clinical double-blind study [German]. Z Hautkr 1987;62:1262,1267-1271.

Hausen BM, Busker E, Carle R. Über das Sensibilisierungsvermögen von Compositenarten. VII. Experimentelle Untersuchungen mit Auszügen und Inhaltsstoffen von *Chamomilla recutita* (L.) Rauschert und *Anthemis cotula* L. Planta Med 1984; 50:229-234.

Hempel B. CO2-extract from German chamomile—proposed medicinal use. Acta Horticulturae 1999;503:15-19.

Jung SeWon, Kim MiKyung. Effect of dried powders of chamomile, sage, and green tea on antioxidative capacity in 15-month-old rats [Korean]. Korean J Nutr 2003;36:699-710.

Kobayashi Y, Nakano Y, Inyama K, Sakai A, Kamiya T. Dietary intake of the flower extracts of German chamomile (*Matricaria recutita* L.) inhibited compound 48/80-induced itch-scratch responses in mice. Phytomedicine 2003;10:657-664.

Kyokong O, Charuluxananan S, Muangmingsuk V, et al. Efficacy of chamomile-extract spray for prevention of post-operative sore throat. J Med Assoc Thai 2002;85(suppl 1):S180-S185.

Laskova IL, Uteshev BS. Immunomodulating action of heteropolysaccharides isolated from camomile flower [Russian]. Antibiot Khimioter 1992;37:15-18.

Means C. Selected herbal hazards. Vet Clin North Am Small Anim Pract 2002;32:367-382.

Molnar A, Lemberkovics E, Spiller S. Detection of caraway and camomile components in goat milk [Hungarian]. Tejgazdasag 1997;57:22-27.

Mostafa MBM. Quality and ripening of Gouda cheese made from goat milk as affected by certain ovariectomized-rat under restriction stress. Biol Pharm Bull 1996;19:1244-1246.

Paulsen E, Andersen KE, Hausen BM. Compositae dermatitis in a Danish dermatology department in one year. Contact Dermatitis 1993;29:6-10.

Paulsen E, Andersen KE, Hausen BM. Sensitization and cross-reaction patterns in Danish Compositae–allergic patients. Contact Dermatitis 2001;45:197-204.

Reider N, Sepp N, Fritsch P, Weinlich G, Jensen-Jarolim E. Anaphylaxis to camomile: clinical features and allergen cross-reactivity. Clin Exp Allergy 2000;30:1436-1443.

Safayhi H, Sabieraj J, Sailer ER, Ammon HP. Chamazulene: an antioxidant-type inhibitor of leukotriene B4 formation. Planta Med 1994;60:410-413.

Subiza J, Subiza JL, Alonso M, et al. Allergic conjunctivitis to chamomile tea. Ann Allergy 1990;65:127-132.

Subiza J, Subiza JL, Hinojosa M, et al. Anaphylactic reaction after the ingestion of chamomile tea: a study of cross-reactivity with other composite pollens. J Allergy Clin Immunol 1989;84: 353-358.

Tyler VE, Brady LR, Robbers JE, eds. *Pharmacognosy.* 9th ed. Philadelphia: Lea & Febiger; 1988.

Uteshev BS, Laskova IL, Afanas'ev VA. The immunomodulating activity of the heteropolysaccharides from German chamomile *(Matricaria chamomilla)* during air and immersion cooling [Russian]. Eksp Klin Farmakol 1999;62:52-55.

Viola H, Wasowski C, Levi de Stein M, et al. Apigenin, a component of *Matricaria recutita* flowers, is a central benzodiazepine receptor ligand with anxiolytic effects. Planta Med 1995;61:213-216.

Wagner H, Wierer M, Bauer R. In vitro inhibition of prostaglandin biosynthesis by essential oils and phenolic compounds. Planta Med 1986;3:184-187.

Wakame K, Wagatsuma C, Miura T. Sedative, analgesic, and sleep-prolonging effects to the mouse of commercial essential oils [Japanese]. Aroma Res 2003;4:249-252.

Wolter H. Possibilities for homeopathic therapy of colic in the horse including helminth infections [German]. Praktische Tierarzt 1985;66:135-138.

Yamada K, Miura T, Mimaki Y, Sashida Y. Effect of inhalation of chamomile oil vapour on plasma ACTH level in ovariectomized rat under restriction stress. Biol Pharm Bull 1996; 19(9):1244-1246.

Yamada K, Ina H, Mimaki Y, Sashida Y. Effects of plant derived essential oils on plasma ACTH level in experimental menopausal rats. International Congress and 49th Annual Meeting for the Society for Medicinal Plant Research, Sept 2-6, 2001, Erlangen, Germany. Available at www.biologie.uni-erlangen.de/pharmbiol/abstract/Effects.htm/.

Chaste Tree

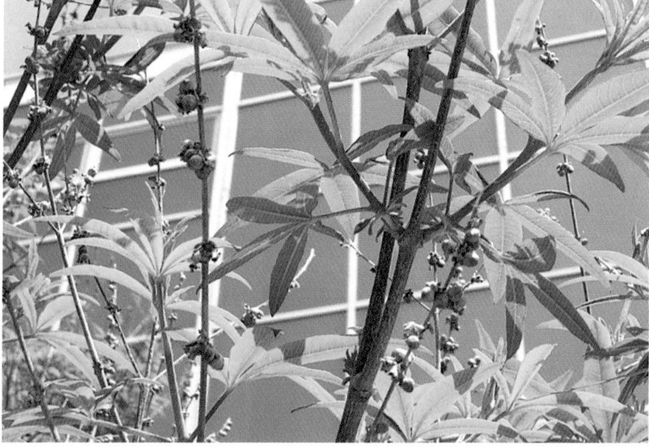

Vitex agnus castus L. • VY-teks AG-nus KAS-tus

Other Names: Chasteberry, vitex, monk's pepper

Family: Verbenaceae

Parts Used: Peppercorn-sized dried ripe fruit

Distribution: Native to Western Asia and Southwestern Europe. Now established throughout Asia, Europe (especially Mediterranean regions), and North America, often as a garden shrub

Selected Constituents: *Iridoid glycosides* (leaves), *flavonoids (leaves, flowers, and fruit):* including vitexin, isovitexin, isovitexin (Hirobe, 1997); *alkaloids:* viticin, volatile oil (berries), pinenes; *essential fatty acids:* palmitic acid, oleic acid, linoleic acid, stearic acid (Anonymous, 1998; Fleming, 1998; Du Mee, 1993). Monoterpenoids, diterpenes, sesquiterpenoids, iridoids (aucubin and agnuside), and the flavonoid casticin, which is an important marker; diterpenes are in the active, lipophilic fraction.

Clinical Actions: Regulates female hormonal activity, regulates latent hyperprolactinemia, dopaminergic

Energetics: *Neutral:* both cooling and warming potential, pungent, drying

History and Traditional Usage: Chaste tree derives its name from the belief that the plant inspires chastity. One of the first records of its medical use is by Hippocrates in the 4th century BC. It was used in ancient Greece and Rome to diminish sexual desire and by monks in the Middle Ages for the same purpose, giving it the name "Monk's pepper." In Persia, it was used to treat insanity, madness, and epilepsy. Chaste tree has been traditionally used to treat menstrual disorders and related hormonal problems, to promote breast milk flow, and as a digestive aid, sedative, and anti-infective (Christie, 1997).

Modern interest in chaste tree began in Germany in 1930, when Dr. Gerhard Madaus researched the plant's effects on the female hormonal system and developed a patent medicine. A standardized preparation has been available in Germany since the1950s and is used to treat ovarian insufficiency and uterine bleeding (Newall, 1996). In Iceland, hormonal imbalance and infertility in both sexes are often treated with herbal mixtures, including Chaste Tree (Veal, 1998).

Published Research

The cytotoxicity of chaste tree extract against human uterine cervical canal fibroblast, human embryo fibroblast, ovarian cancer, cervical carcinoma, breast carcinoma, gastric signet ring carcinoma, colon carcinoma, and small cell lung carcinoma cells was examined. The cytotoxic activity of chaste tree extract may be attributed to increased intracellular oxidation by chaste tree extract treatment, resulting in apoptosis (Ohyama, 2003a; Ohyama, 2003b).

Menstrual Disorders: A methanol extract of chaste tree berry was tested for its ability to displace radiolabeled estradiol from the binding site of estrogen receptors alpha and beta. The research suggested that linoleic acid from the fruits of chaste tree can bind to estrogen receptors and induce certain estrogen-inducible genes (Liu, 2004). The flavonoid apigenin was identified as an estrogenic flavonoid contained in chaste tree (Jarry, 2003).

In a prospective, multicenter trial, the efficacy of a chaste tree extract was investigated in 50 women with premenstrual syndrome. A single tablet (20 mg of extract) was taken daily during three menstrual cycles. At the end of the study, symptoms were reduced and gradually returned after treatment cessation. However, a difference from baseline remained (20%; $P < .001$) for up to 3 cycles. The study concluded that the main response to treatment is related to symptomatic relief, rather than to the duration of the syndrome (Berger, 2000). The treatment was also found to be well tolerated (Loch, 2000).

The clinical effects of chaste tree preparations are probably due to prolactin-inhibiting activity. Confirmation of efficacy in the treatment of patients with premenstrual syndrome, individual symptoms, and mastalgia has been supported by published double-blind studies plus several open and surveillance studies (Gorkow, 2002; Roemheld-Hamm, 2005).

The activity of unidentified constituents of the ethanol extract of chaste tree seed was localized within the pituitary-gonadal axis. Research in pituitary cell assays further elucidated the dopaminergic inhibition of prolactin synthesis or release (Odenthal, 1998). Clinical trials have demonstrated that serotonin reuptake inhibitors and extract of chaste tree are effective in the treatment of patients with premenstrual dysphoric disorder (PMDD). One study compared the efficacy of fluoxetine, a selective serotonin reuptake inhibitor, with that of Chaste Tree extract. A total of 41 patients with PMDD were randomized to fluoxetine or chaste tree for 2 months of single-blind, rater-blinded, prospective treatment. No statistically significant differences in response between groups were observed, suggesting that patients with PMDD respond well to treatment with both fluoxetine and chaste tree. However, fluoxetine was more effective for psychological symptoms, and chaste tree extract diminished physical symptoms (Atmaca, 2003).

Hyperadrenocorticism (Cushing's disease) in horses

Two commercial preparations of vitex have been tested for the treatment of horses with Cushing's disease. A clinical trial involving 25 horses and ponies diagnosed with Cushing's disease considered the action of chaste tree over a 3-month period when any animal still carrying a full winter coat could reasonably be said to have "failed to shed." Hirsutism is one of the most obvious clinical signs of Cushing's. The owners of the horses and ponies in the trial completed a detailed questionnaire before and at the end of the trial. Before and after photographs were taken to illustrate coat changes and changes in mood, behavior, energy, water intake, laminitic episodes, and so forth. Each of the trial animals was given a daily dose of *Vitex agnus-castus* for the duration of the trial. The study demonstrated the following: reduction of hirsutism with a subsequent reduction in hyperhidrosis; improved energy levels and mood; an apparent reduction in the incidence of laminitis; reduction in polyuria and polydipsia; and reduction in abnormal fat deposits (Self, 2003).

In another trial, Beech (2002) studied the effects of a commercially available vitex supplement (Evitex) on 14 horses with typical signs of Cushing's disease. ACTH and insulin levels were monitored, along with changes in hirsutism, fat distribution, weight, laminitis, lethargy, and abnormal estrus cycles. Horses were treated for 2 to 6 months (the shorter terms were due to worsening clinical signs) with the manufacturer's recommended dose (no information was provided to investigators about the concentration or ingredients of the product). Plasma ACTH levels decreased in only 1 of the 14 horses; in contrast, most horses subsequently given pergolide did improve.

Indications: Menstrual disturbances (with corpus luteum insufficiency), premenstrual syndrome, breast tenderness, menopausal complaints; to stimulate milk production. Relative progesterone deficiency

Potential Veterinary Indications: Infertility and hormonal problems caused by anovulatory cycles, low progesterone levels, and latent hyperprolactinemia. Moody mares. Equine Cushing's disease

Contraindications: None known.

Toxicology and Adverse Effects: AHPA class 2b, 2d (may counteract birth control pills in women). Adverse effects are rare and may include rash, gastrointestinal disorders, headache, and increased menstrual flow. No interactions with other drugs are known. Dioscorides reported its ability to bring on an early menstrual period in women. Effects on lactation are mixed: rat studies show inhibitory effects caused by prolactin suppression, and one human report shows increased milk, although these studies were poorly done.

Potential Drug Interactions: May interact with dopaminergic modulators; binds to opioid receptors and may potentiate medications that affect these receptors.

Dosage:

Human: It is usually recommended that chaste tree should be taken as a single daily dose first thing in the morning. Note that chaste tree is not fast acting and must be taken consistently for some time (6 months in humans), although Dr. Yarnell reports more rapid responses at higher doses.

Dried herb: 3-10 g TID (Yarnell); 20 mg BID (German Commission E)

Infusions and decoctions: 5-30 g per cup of water, 2-3 cups daily

Tincture (usually as 45%-60% ethanol): 1:2 or 1:3: 1-12 mL daily

Small Animal:

Dried herb: 12.5-200 mg/kg, divided daily (optimally, TID)

Infusion and decoction: 5-30 g per cup of water, administered at a rate of ¼-½ cup per 10 kg (20 lb), divided daily (optimally, TID)

Tincture (usually in 45%-60% ethanol): 1:2-1:3: 0.25-1.0 mL per 10 kg (20 lb), divided daily (optimally, TID) and diluted or combined with other herbs. Higher doses may be appropriate if the herb is used singly and is not combined in a formula.

Equine:

1:5 in 45% alcohol: 10-30 mL given once daily in the morning

References

Anonymous. Chaste tree. In: Dombek C, ed. *Lawrence Review of Natural Products*. St. Louis: Facts and Comparisons; 1998.

Atmaca M, Kumru S, Tezcan E. Fluoxetine versus *Vitex agnus castus* extract in the treatment of premenstrual dysphoric disorder. Human Psychopharmacol 2003;18:191-195.

Beech J, Donaldson MT, Lindborg S. Comparison of *Vitex agnus castus* extract and pergolide in treatment of equine Cushing's syndrome. AAEP Proceedings 2002;48:175-177.

Berger D, Schaffner W, Schrader E, Meier B, Brattstrom A. Efficacy of *Vitex agnus castus* L. extract Ze 440 in patients with pre-menstrual syndrome (PMS). Arch Gynecol Obstet 2000;264:150-153.

Christie S, Walker A. *Vitex agnus castus:* a review of its traditional and modern therapeutic use, current use from a survey of practitioners. Eur J Herb Med 1997;3:29-45.

Du Mee C. *Vitex agnus castus.* Aust J Med Herbalism 1993;5: 63-65.

Fleming T. *PDR for Herbal Medicines*. Montvale, NJ: Medical Economics Company, Inc.; 1998.

Gorkow C, Wuttke W, Marz RW. Effectiveness of *Vitex agnus-castus* preparations [German]. Wiener Medizinische Wochenschrift 2002;152:364-372.

Hirobe C, Qiao ZS, Takeya K, Itokawa H. Cytotoxic flavonoids from *Vitex agnus-castus*. Phytochemistry 1997;46:521-524.

Jarry H, Spengler B, Porzel A, Schmidt J, Wuttke W, Christoffel V. Evidence for estrogen receptor beta-selective activity of *Vitex agnus-castus* and isolated flavones. Planta Med 2003;69: 945-947.

Liu J, Burdette JE, Sun Y, et al. Isolation of linoleic acid as an estrogenic compound from the fruits of *Vitex agnus-castus* L. (chaste-berry). Phytomedicine 2004;11:18-23.

Loch EG, Selle H, Boblitz N. Treatment of premenstrual syndrome with a phytopharmaceutical formulation containing *Vitex agnus castus*. J Womens Health Gend Based Med 2000;9:315-320.

Newall CA, Anderson LA, Phillipson JD. *Herbal Medicines: A Guide for Health-Care Professionals*. London: Pharmaceutical Press; 1996: 296.

Odenthal KP. *Vitex agnus castus* L.—traditional drug and actual indications. Phytother Res 1998;12(suppl 1):S160-S161.

Ohyama K, Akaike T, Hirobe C, et al. Cytotoxicity and apoptotic inducibility of *Vitex agnus-castus* fruit extract in cultured human normal and cancer cells and effect on growth. Biol Pharmaceut Bull 2003a;26:10-18.

Ohyama K, Akaike T, Hirobe C, et al. Cytotoxic effects of *Vitex agnus-castus* fruit extract against human cultured uterine cervical fibroblast, breast cancer and ovarian cancer cells, and its biochemical mechanism. Acta Horticulturae 2003b;597: 167-176.

Roemheld-Hamm B. Chasteberry. Am Fam Physician 2005; 72:821-824.

Self H. Hilton herbs—Latest news: Equine Cushing's disease results. Available at: http://www.hiltonherbs.com/news_details.cfm?itemid=171&cfid=562777&cftoken=19285394 Accessed November 2003.

Veal L. Complementary therapy and infertility: an Icelandic perspective [Review]. Complementary Therapies in Nursing and Midwifery 1998;4:3-6.

Chickweed

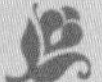

Stellaria media (L.) Vill. • stell-AR-ee-uh MEED-ee-uh

Other Names: Star chickweed, stichwort, scarwort

Family: Caryophyllaceae

Parts Used: Above-ground parts

Distribution: Native to Britain, cultivated in parts of Europe (the young, growing tips are edible). Introduced worldwide from Europe and Asia; declared noxious in some areas. Generally considered a common and invasive weed (Defelice, 2004).

Selected Constituents: Saponins, mucilage, organic acids, glycosides, flavonoids, vitamins (including vitamin C)

Clinical Actions: Antirheumatic, topically antipruritic, vulnerary, emollient

Energetics: Cool and moist

History and Traditional Usage: In traditional medicine, *Stellaria media* is used as a diuretic, cardioactive, and anti-inflammatory agent and is applied externally to treat patients with wounds, rheumatism, arthritis, dermatitis, and some other skin diseases (Kitanov, 1992).

According to de Bairacli Levy (1963), all animals should be encouraged to feed on it, but sheep and lambs that engorge on it can develop digestive upset. She suggests that it contains the same properties as slippery elm. She suggests it as a remedy for all stomach ailments and externally as an eye lotion and ointment for stiff joints. It can also be used to treat patients with gastric ulcers, skin disorders, and cramps. Dose is several handfuls of fresh herb per animal per day (eye lotion, 1 handful brewed in ¾ of a pint of water). de Bairacli Levy (1985) suggests 1 heaped dessertspoonful daily for adult dogs as part of the diet and as a rinse for discharging eyes.

Published Research: A *Stellaria media* extract demonstrated in vitro inhibition of xanthine oxidase and may be useful for antioxidant activity in the prevention of diseases related to aging and CNS disorders, and as a potential source of phytomedicines for treating patients with hyperuricemia and gout (Pieroni, 2002). *Stellaria media* inhibits tyrosinase (catechol oxidase) activity (Ren, 2003).

Indications:

External: As a poultice or cream for boils, eczema, psoriasis, indolent ulcers, sores, swellings, ulcers, pruritus

Internal: For gastrointestinal inflammation and ulceration

Potential Veterinary Indications: Poultice for abscesses, pruritus, eyewash, nutritive herb

Contraindications: None known.

Toxicology and Adverse Effects: AHPA class 1. The fruit is eaten by small birds, and the plant is eaten by pigs and rabbits. Although this is generally considered a "salad herb," young lambs have been poisoned after eating too many plants (ILPIN).

Photoaggravation has been seen with common chickweed on patch testing. In the essential oil obtained from common chickweed, the well-known contact allergens borneol, menthol, linalool, 1,8-cineole, and terpene are present.

Dosage:

Human:

Dried herb: 1-10 g TID

Succus (stabilized fresh juice): 2.5-6 mL daily, divided

Infusions and decoctions: 5-30 g per cup of water, with 1 cup of the tea given TID

Tincture (available as 35%-50% ethanol): 1:2 or 1:3: 3-5 mL TID, up to 6 times daily for acute conditions

Small Animal:

Dried herb: 25-400 mg/kg, divided daily (optimally, TID)

Succus (stabilized fresh juice): 0.5-1.0 per 10 kg (20 lb) daily, divided

Infusion: 5-30 g per cup of water, administered at a rate of ¼-½ cup per 10 kg (20 lb), divided daily (optimally, TID)

Tincture (35%-50% ethanol): 1:2-1:3: 0.5-2.0 mL per 10 kg (20 lb), divided daily (optimally, TID) and diluted or combined with other herbs. Higher doses may be appropriate if the herb is used singly and is not combined in a formula.

References

De Bairacli Levy J. *The Complete Herbal Handbook for Farm and Stable*. London: Faber and Faber; 1963.

De Bairacli Levy J. *The Complete Herbal Handbook for the Dog and Cat*. London: Faber and Faber; 1985.

Defelice MS. Common chickweed, *Stellaria media* (L.) Vill.—"mere chicken feed?" Weed Technol 2004;18:193-200.

Guil JL, Rodriguez-Garcia I, Torija E. Nutritional and toxic factors in selected wild edible plants. Plant Foods for Human Nutrition 1997;51:99-107.

Illinois Plant Information Network. ILPIN information on *Stellaria media*. Available at: http://www.fs.fed.us/ne/delaware/ilpin/2905.co. Accessed June 2005.

Kitanov GM. Phenolic acids and flavonoids from *Stellaria media* (L.) Vill. (Caryophyllaceae). Pharmazie 1992;47:470-471.

Pieroni A, Janiak V, Durr CM, Ludeke S, Trachsel E, Heinrich M. In vitro antioxidant activity of non-cultivated vegetables of ethnic Albanians in Southern Italy. Phytother Res 2002;16:467-473.

Ren BR, Wu Jl, Guo RI, et al. The effects of extracts from six plants on tyrosinase activities [Chinese]. J Plant Resources Environ 2003;12:58-59.

Cinnamon 

Cinnamomum verum J. Presl., synonym = *Cinnamon zeylanicum* Blume • sin-uh-MOH-mum VER-um

Other Names: *Cinnamomum cassia, Laurus cinnamomum,* L. *Cinnamomum aromaticum,* nees, abdalasini, blood-giving drops, kannel, wild cinnamon, zimtrinde, annan cinnamon, cassia, cassia bark, Chinese cassia, Chinese cinnamon, ching hua yu-kuei, gui zhi, keishi, rou gui, róugì, saleekha, canela, cannelle, zimt darchini

Family: Lauraceae

Parts Used: Dried inner bark

Distribution: Native to India and Sri Lanka; cultivated in parts of Africa, southeastern India, Indonesia, the Seychelles, South America, Sri Lanka, and the West Indies. Also found in China and Vietnam.

Selected Constituents: 1% to 2% v/w of volatile oil derived, containing 60% to 80% mainly cinnamaldehyde, the major constituent. Also contains cinnamic acid, coumarin, tannins, and methyl-eugenol diterpenes known as cinncassiols. Melatonin occurs naturally in the bark (Watanabe, 2002).

Clinical Actions: Spasmolytic, carminative, antidiarrheal, antimicrobial

Energetics: Warming and drying

History and Traditional Usage: Cinnamon and cassia, along with myrrh, were used by Egyptians for embalming, successfully perhaps because cinnamic acid (and also myrrh) has antibacterial effects. As a spice, cinnamon has had an illustrious history. The Venetians controlled the trade of cinnamon (or cassia) in the 13th and 14th centuries, which created great wealth for the city. Ceylonese trade in the 16th century was controlled by the Portuguese, and an increasing demand for cinnamon led to war between the Dutch and Portuguese in the mid-17th century. Sri Lanka's (Ceylon's) cinnamon trade was subsequently taken over by Holland. The cinnamon market was dominated and monopolized by the Dutch, and to prop up prices, they burned warehouses in Amsterdam in 1760 to create a shortage. Cinnamon is best known today for its culinary use and aroma; few would appreciate its huge economic significance and the struggles that surrounded its trade in history.

Traditional uses included treatment of patients with dyspepsia such as mild spastic conditions of the gastrointestinal tract, fullness and flatulence, and loss of appetite. Also used in China to treat those with abdominal pain with diarrhea and pain associated with amenorrhea and dysmenorrhea, and elsewhere in the treatment of patients with impotence, frigidity, dyspnea, inflammation of the eye, leukorrhea, vaginitis, rheumatism, neuralgia, wounds, and toothache (Farnsworth, 1995).

It has been used medicinally, usually in combination with other herbs, as a carminative, astringent, and local stimulant and antiseptic and for vomiting; it has been used for flatulence and, in combination with chalk and astringents, for diarrhea and hemorrhage of the womb (Grieve, 1975).

Milks (1949) provides two contemporary uses for cinnamon in volatile oil form—as a carminative, and in dentistry, as an antibacterial and analgesic.

Published Research: Antibacterial and antifungal activities of the essential oil have been demonstrated against *Escherichia coli, Staphylococcus aureus* (Janssen, 1986; George, 1949), *Salmonella typhimurium* (Sivaswamy, 1991), and *Pseudomonas aeruginosa* (Janssen, 1986). The essential oil of the bark has carminative activity (Harries, 1978) and decreases smooth muscle contractions in guinea pig trachea and ileum (Reiter, 1985), and in dog ileum, colon, and stomach (Plant, 1926). The active antispasmodic constituent of the drug is cinnamaldehyde. Reduced stomach motility in rats and dogs and intestinal motility in mice and decreased occurrence of stress- and serotonin-induced ulcers in mice have been described (Harada, 1975; Plant, 1921; Akira, 1986). The essential oil of *Cinnamomum cassia* (cassia) can regulate the activity of hepatic drug-metabolizing enzymes through the formation of a glutathione conjugate (Choi, 2001).

Cinnamon has hypoglycemic and lipid-lowering properties. In a placebo-controlled, randomized clinical study, 60 people with type 2 diabetes were divided into groups. Groups 1, 2, and 3 consumed 1, 3, or 6 g of cinnamon daily, respectively, and groups 4, 5, and 6 were given placebo capsules corresponding to the number of capsules consumed for the three levels of cinnamon. The cinnamon was consumed for 40 days, followed by a 20-day washout period. The results showed that intake of 1, 3, or 6 g of cinnamon per day reduced serum glucose (18%-29%), triglyceride (23%-30%), LDL cholesterol (7%-27%), and total cholesterol (12%-26%) levels in people with type 2 diabetes; no changes were observed in the placebo groups. This suggests that inclusion of cinnamon in the diet of people with type 2 diabetes may reduce risk factors associated with diabetes and cardiovascular disease (Khan, 2003).

In vitro studies confirm that bioactive compound(s) extracted from cinnamon potentiate insulin activity and, similar to insulin, affect protein phosphorylation–dephosphorylation reactions in the intact adipocyte. Thus, cinnamon compounds may find further use in studies of insulin resistance in adult-onset diabetes (Imparl-Radosevich, 1998).

Indications: Medicinally, it is used to "warm the organs" to treat patients with chronic diarrhea, indigestion, cramps or colic, gas, heart and abdominal pain, diabetes, coughing, wheezing, and lower back pain. In Chinese Medicine, the spicy, warming nature of cinnamon is specific for patients with type 2 diabetes who are overweight and tend to be cold and sluggish, whereas it may be contraindicated in many of those with type 1 diabetes who are not overweight and are yin deficient.

Potential Veterinary Indications: Warming for chilly patients; flavoring agent. Mild colic, diarrhea, and flatulence, diabetes, back pain.

Contraindications: The herb is contraindicated in cases of fever of unknown origin, pregnancy, and stomach or duodenal ulcer (German Commission E, 1990) and in patients with an allergy to cinnamon.

Toxicology and Adverse Effects: AHPA class 2b, 2d. Not for long-term use; do not exceed recommended dose because large doses have been reported to cause vasomotor center stimulation, methemoglobinemia, hematinemia, and possibly nephritis. Allergic reactions of the skin and mucosa have been reported (German Commission E, 1990; Nixon, 1995; Drake, 1976).

Herb–Drug Interactions: *Cinnamomum cassia* blume bark extract (2g in 100mL) (Chinese cinnamon or rou gui) markedly decreased the in vitro dissolution of tetracycline hydrochloride (Miyazaki, 1977). In the presence of *Cinnamomum cassia* blume bark, only 20% of tetracycline remained in solution after 30 minutes, in contrast to 97% when only water was used (Miyazaki, 1977). However, the clinical significance of this interaction has not been established.

Dosage:

Human:

Dried herb: 0.5-2 g TID

Volatile oil: 1-3 drops TID

Infusions and decoctions: 5 g per cup of water, with 1 cup of the tea given TID

Tincture (usually 60%-80% ethanol; some pharmacies include glycerin to prevent precipitation by tannins): 1:2 or 1:3: 3-5 mL TID if 30% alcohol tincture is used; 1-3 mL TID if 60% alcohol tincture is used

Small Animal:

Dried herb: 25-300 mg/kg, divided daily (optimally, TID)

Infusion and decoction: 5 g per cup of water, administered at a rate of ¼-½ cup per 10 kg (20 lb), divided daily (optimally, TID)

Tincture (60%-80% ethanol), some pharmacies include glycerin to prevent precipitation of tannins): 1:2-1:3: 0.5-1.5 mL per 10 kg (20 lb), divided daily (optimally, TID) and diluted or combined with other herbs. Use higher dose for low-alcohol preparations.

References

Akira T, Tanaka S, Tabata M. Pharmacological studies on the antiulcerogenic activity of Chinese cinnamon. Planta Med 1986;52:440-443.

Choi J, Lee KT, Ka H, Jung WT, Jung HJ, Park HJ. Constituents of the essential oil of the *Cinnamomum cassia* stem bark and the biological properties. Arch Pharmacol Res 2001;24:418-423.

Drake TE, Maibach HI. Allergic contact dermatitis and stomatitis caused by cinnamic aldehyde-flavored toothpaste. Arch Dermatol 1976;112:202-203.

Farnsworth NR, ed. NAPRALERT Database. Chicago: University of Illinois at Chicago; August 8, 1995 production.

George M, Pandalai KM. Investigations on plant antibiotics. Part IV. Further search for antibiotic substances in Indian medicinal plants. Indian J Med Res 1949;37:169-181.

German Commission E. Monograph, *Cinnamomi cassiae* cortex. Bundesanzeiger 1990;22:1.

Grieve M. *A Modern Herbal.* London: Jonathan Cape (1931); reprint 1975.

Harada M, Yano S. Pharmacological studies on Chinese cinnamon. II. Effects of cinnamaldehyde on the cardiovascular and digestive systems. Chem Pharmaceut Bull 1975;23:941-947.

Harries N, James KC, Pugh WK. Antifoaming and carminative actions of volatile oils. J Clin Pharmacol 1978;2:171-177.

I-Radosevich J, Deas S, Polansky MM, Baedke DA, Ingebritsen TS, Anderson RA, Graves DJ. Regulation of PTP-1 and insulin receptor kinase by fractions from cinnamon: implications for cinnamon regulation of insulin signalling. Horm Res 1998;50:177-182.

Janssen AM, Chin NLJ, Scheffer JJC, et al. Screening for antimicrobial activity of some essential oils by the agar overlay technique. Pharmaceut Weekbl (Sci ed) 1986;8:289-292.

Khan A, Safdar M, Ali Khan MM, Khattak KN, Anderson RA. Cinnamon improves glucose and lipids of people with type 2 diabetes. Diabetes Care 2003;26:3215-3218.

Milks HJ. *Practical Veterinary Pharmacology, Materia Medica and Therapeutics.* Chicago, Ill: Alex Eger, Inc.; 1949.

Miyazaki S, Inoue H, Nadai T. Effect of antacids on the dissolution behavior of tetracycline and methacycline. Chem Pharmaceut Bull 1977;27:2523-2527.

Nixon R. Vignette in contact dermatology. Cinnamon allergy in bakers. Austral J Dermatol 1995;36:41.

Plant OH. Effects of carminative volatile oils on the muscular movements of the intestine. J Pharmacol Exp Ther 1921;22:311-324.

Plant OH, Miller GH. Effects of carminative volatile oils on the muscular activity of the stomach and colon. J Pharmacol Exp Ther 1926;27:149.

Reiter M, Brandt W. Relaxant effects on tracheal and ileal smooth muscles of the guinea pig. Arzneimittel-Forschung 1985;35:408-414.

Sivaswamy SN, Balachandran B, Balanehru S, et al. Mutagenic activity of South Indian food items. Indian J Exp Biol 1991;29:730-737.

Watanabe H, Kobayashi T, Tomii M, et al. Effects of Kampo herbal medicine on plasma melatonin concentration in patients. Am J Chin Med 2002;30:65-71.

Cleavers

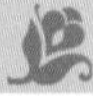

Galium aparine L. and other *Galium* spp • GAY-lee-um ap-air-EEN

Other Names: Clivers, bedstraw, goose grass, galium, burweed, barweed, catch weed, clike, click, clitheren, clithers, cleaverwort, coachweed, sticky-willie, gosling weed, love-man, stick-a-back, sweethearts, hayruff, hayriffe, hedge burs, erriffe, goosebill, hedgeheriffe, grip grass, catchweed, catchgrass, scratweed, mutton chops, robin-run-in-the-grass, everlasting friendship

Family: Rubiaceae (madder family)

Distribution: Europe, North Asia; introduced into temperate zones worldwide

Parts Used: Aerial parts—plant juice most commonly used form

Selected Constituents: Coumarin, asperuloside, monotropein, tannins, nicotinic acid, anthraquinone, flavonoids, and a red dye
Clinical Actions: Lymphatic, mildly diuretic, mildly astringent, anti-inflammatory, aperient
Energetics: Cool, neutral, slightly salty
History and Traditional Usage: Considered an important lymphatic alterative; used for lymphadenitis, tonsillitis, or any condition in which swollen lymph tissue is a problem. Cleavers has also been used for dry skin eruptions and as a remedy for ulcers and tumors. The plant is good when steamed as a vegetable. The roots produce a red dye, similar to that produced by its relative, madder.
Published Research: None found for cleavers. However, asperuloside and monotropein have been shown to cause a mild laxative effect in mice. The effect was reported to be approximately 15 times less potent than that of senna, and of shorter duration (Inouye, 1974).
Indications: Lymphadenitis, edema, psoriasis, cystitis, urinary calculi. Used as a vegetable.
Potential Veterinary Indications: Lymphadenopathy, dermatitis; topically for ulcerated lesions; has been used as a feed for poultry.
Contraindications: No contraindications reported.
Toxicology and Adverse Effects: AHPA class 1. No adverse effects reported.
Notes of Interest: This is considered an invasive species, so it should not be planted.
Dosage:
Human:
Dried herb: 3-10 g TID
Expressed juice: 1.25-15 mL daily
Infusions and decoctions: 5-30 g per cup of water, with 1 cup of the tea given TID
Fluid extract (1:1): 2-4 mL TID
Tincture (25%-35% ethanol): 1:2 or 1:3: 3-7 mL TID
Small Animal:
Dried herb: 50-400 mg/kg, divided daily (optimally, TID)
Infusion: 5-30 g per cup of water, administered at a rate of ¼-½ cup per 10 kg (20 lb), divided daily (optimally, TID)
Tincture (usually in 25%-35% ethanol): 1:2-1:3: 1.0-2.0 mL per 10 kg (20 lb), divided daily (optimally, TID) and diluted or combined with other herbs. Higher doses may be appropriate if the herb is used singly and is not combined in a formula.
Combinations:
Lymphatic swelling/congestion: Phytolacca, Echinacea, and Calendula
Dermatitis: Yellow dock and Burdock

Reference

Inouye H, Takeda Y, Uobe K, et al. Purgative activities of iridoid glucosides. Planta Med 1974;25:285-288.

Clove

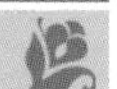

Syzygium aromaticum (L.) Merr. et L.M. Perry = *Eugenia caryophyllata* Thunb. • Siz-ZY-gee-um ar-oh-MAT-ih-kum
Other Names: *Caryophyllus aromaticus* L., *Flos caryophylli, Eugenia aromatica* (L.) Baill., *Eugenia caryophylla* Thunb., Caryophyllus *(C. spreng.)* Bull. et Harr., *Jambosa caryophyllus* (Spreng.) Nied., *Myrtus caryophyllus* Spreng. (African Pharmacopoeia, 1985; European Pharmacopoeia, 1996; Blaschek, 1998; Iwu, 1993; Bisset, 1994).
Family: Myrtaceae
Parts Used: Dried flower buds
Distribution: Indigenous to the Moluccas and Southern Philippines. Cultivated in many tropical areas, including Africa, South America, Indonesia, Malaysia, and Sri Lanka (Bisset, 1994; Farnsworth, 1998).
Selected Constituents: The major constituent (up to 20%) is an essential oil, which is characterized by the presence of eugenol (60%-95%), eugenol acetate (2%-27%) and α-and β-caryophyllene (5%-10%) (Bisset, 1994; Farnsworth, 1998; Bruneton, 1995; Leung, 1996).

CH_3
H_3C CH_3
H_2C

Caryophyllene

Clinical Actions: Aromatic, local anesthetic, antibacterial, antiviral, antifungal, antispasmodic, anti-inflammatory, astringent, antiulcer
Energetics: Warm, pungent; in TCM, used to warm the exterior and expel cold.
History and Traditional Usage: Traditional use includes external or local applications for the treatment of patients with toothache and minor infections of the mouth and skin. Also used as an antiseptic for dressing of minor wounds and as lozenges for sore throats and coughs associated with the common cold. The essential oil is used in mouthwashes (Iwu, 1993; Bruneton, 1996; Blumenthal, 1998). Other uses include the treatment of those with asthma, bleeding gums, dyspepsia, fever, and morning sickness (Farnsworth, 1998). It is used to treat children with measles in India (Singh, 1994).

de Bairacli Levy (1985) suggests the use of clove-infused oil for foreign bodies in ears and sore teeth. For vomiting, she advises a tea of peppermint, powdered clove, and ginger. Gresswell (1886) stated that the most common form (oil of clove) was used as a stomachic, carminative, stimulant, antispasmodic, and corrective, and that it was useful for colic in horses. Kirk (1948) recommended that the oil be applied directly to "carious teeth" for pain relief in animals.
Published Research: Ethanol extracts (95%), aqueous extracts, monoterpenes, the terpene eugenol, and juice have antimicrobial effects against a number of bacteria,

as well as some viruses and fungi (Khadija, 2003; Dorman, 2000; Juliani, 2004; Thirach, 2003; Nakatani, 2003). Anti-inflammatory action has been demonstrated, and eugenal inhibits cylooxygenase and lipoxynase activity in vitro, as well as the formation of prostaglandin and thromboxane (Naidu, 1995; Chen, 1996; Srivastava, 1993).

The essential oil had spasmolytic activity in vitro on isolated guinea pig trachea and intestine (Wagner, 1973; Reiter, 1985). Eugenol and caryophyllene had a narcotic effect after intravenous administration of high doses (200-400 mg/kg body weight) (Laekeman, 1990; Sell, 1976) and a sedative effect after intragastric administration of low doses (1-100 mg/kg body weight) to mice (Wagner, 1973). In a comparative study, ethanol extracts of nutmeg and clove were found to stimulate the mounting behavior of normal male mice and to significantly enhance their mating performance (Tajuddin, 2003).

Anesthesia of fish

Clove oil was tested for anesthesia induction, recovery time, hematology, and stress indicators in the gilthead sea bream and rainbow trout and was compared with 2-phenoxyethanol. Results showed only slight differences in anesthetic efficiency and physiologic effects, and that clove oil does not block cortisol response to stress as do other anesthetics (Tort, 2002; Vykusova, 2003). In a similar study, clove oil (85%-95% eugenol) was only slightly less effective than quinaldine and more effective than benzocaine, MS-222, and 2-phenoxyethanol. Clove oil had a much calmer induction to anesthesia than did quinaldine, but it had a recovery time that was 2 to 3 times longer (Munday, 1997).

The anesthetic effects of clove oil–derived eugenol were studied in juvenile rainbow trout. Times to induction and recovery from anesthesia were measured and compared with those for MS-222. Eugenol induced anesthesia, faster and at lower concentrations than did MS-222, and recovery times for eugenol were 6 to 10 times longer. Clove oil eugenol was determined to be an acceptable anesthetic for use in aquaculture and aquatic research. A dose of 40 to 60 ppm eugenol was found to induce rapid anesthesia with a relatively short time for recovery in juvenile trout (Keene, 1998). Juvenile rabbitfish were anesthetized, and their length and weight recorded on three separate occasions. Fish were fed shortly afterward, and no mortality was observed. Clove oil appeared to be highly effective as a fish anesthetic, with potentially few or no adverse effects (Soto, 1995).

Honeybees

Bactericidal and fungicidal effects of clove oil on the growth of two honeybee *(Apis mellifera)* pathogens—*Bacillus larvae* (American foulbrood) and *Ascosphaera apis* (chalkbrood)—and *Bacillus alvei* (a secondary invader in European foulbrood) were evaluated. Clove oil inhibited or reduced bacterial growth in a dose- and time-dependent manner. Results suggest that clove oil and other plant extracts may play a significant role in the management of honeybee disease (Calderone, 1994).

Indications: Local analgesia of mucous membranes

Potential Veterinary Indications: For abdominal pain or intestinal spasm as a carminative, following dental extractions for local pain relief, anesthesia of fish, preventive antimicrobial in apiary industry

Contraindications: Concentrated clove oil causes tissue irritation.

Toxicology and Adverse Effects: Allergic contact dermatitis has been reported in patients who were regularly exposed to clove products or who already had dermatitis of the fingertips (Seetharam, 1987).

Dosage:

Human: If using topically, dilute well.

Dried herb: 0.5-2 g TID

Volatile oil: 1-3 drops TID

Infusions and decoctions: 5 g per cup of water, with 1 cup of the tea given TID

Tincture (available from 25%-70% ethanol; doses are significantly lower for the high-alcohol preparations): 1:2 or 1:3: 3-5 mL TID if 30% alcohol tincture is used; 0.5-3 mL TID if 60% alcohol tincture is used

Small Animal:

Dried herb: 25-300 mg/kg, divided daily (optimally, TID)

Infusion: 5 g per cup of water, administered at a rate of ¼-½ cup per 10 kg (20 lb), divided daily (optimally, TID)

Tincture (usually in 25%-70% ethanol; doses are significantly lower for the high-alcohol preparations): 1:2-1:3: 0.5-1.5 mL per 10 kg (20 lb), divided daily (optimally, TID) and diluted or combined with other herbs

Historical Veterinary Doses: Gresswell recommended oil of cloves, 0.5 dr (1.8 mg) to 40 minims (2.5 mL) for horses, and 1-3 minims (0.06-0.18 mL) for dogs.

References

Bisset NG. *Herbal Drugs and Phytopharmaceuticals.* Boca Raton, Fla: CRC Press; 1994.

British Herbal Pharmacopoeia. London: British Herbal Medicine Association; 1996.

Bruneton J. *Pharmacognosy, Phytochemistry, Medicinal Plants.* Paris: Lavoisier; 1995.

Calderone NW, Shimanuki H, Allen-Wardell G. An in vitro evaluation of botanical compounds for the control of the honeybee pathogens *Bacillus larvae* and *Ascosphaera apis,* and the secondary invader *B. alvei.* J Essential Oil Res 1994;6: 279-287.

Chen SJ, Wang MH, Chen IJ. Antiplatelet and calcium inhibitory properties of eugenol and sodium eugenol acetate. Gen Pharmacol 1996;27:629-633.

De Bairacli Levy J. *The Complete Herbal Handbook for the Dog and Cat.* London: Faber and Faber; 1985.

Dorman HJ, Deans SG. Antimicrobial agents from plants: antibacterial activity of plant volatile oils. J Appl Microbiol 2000;88:308-316.

Iwu MM. *Handbook of African Medicinal Plants.* Boca Raton, Fla: CRC Press; 1993.

Juliani HR, Simon JE, Ramboatiana MMR, et al. Malagasy aromatic plants: essential oils, antioxidant and antimicrobial activities. Acta Horticulturae 2004;629:77-81.

Keene JL, Noakes DLG, Moccia RD, et al. The efficacy of clove oil as an anaesthetic for rainbow trout, *Oncorhynchus mykiss* (Walbaum). Aquaculture Res 1998;29:89-101.

Khadija R, et al. The mechanism of bactericidal action of oregano and clove essential oils and of their phenolic major components on *Escherichia coli* and *Bacillus subtilis*. J Essential Oil Res 2003;15:356-362.

Kramer RE. Antioxidants in clove. J Am Oil Chem Soc 1985; 62:111-113.

Laekeman GM, et al. Eugenol, a valuable compound for in vitro experimental research and worthwhile for further in vivo investigation. Phytother Res 1990;4:90-96.

Leung AY, Foster S. *Encyclopedia of Common Natural Ingredients Used in Food, Drugs, and Cosmetics*. 2nd ed. New York: John Wiley & Sons; 1996:174-177.

Munday PL, Wilson SK. Comparative efficacy of clove oil and other chemicals in anaesthetization of *Pomacentrus amboinensis*, a coral reef fish. J Fish Biol 1997;51:931-938.

Naidu KA. Eugenol—an inhibitor of lipoxygenase-dependent lipid peroxidation. Prostaglandins Leukot Essent Fatty Acids 1995;53:381-383.

Reiter M, Brandt W. Erschlaffende Wirkung auf die glatte Muskulatur von Trachea und Ileum des Meerschweinchens. Arzneimittelforschung 1985;35:408-414.

Seetharam KA, Pasricha JS. Condiments and contact dermatitis of the fingertips. Indian J Dermatol Venereol Leprol 1987;53:325-328.

Sell AB, Carlini EA. Anesthetic action of methyleugenol and other eugenol derivatives. Pharmacology 1976;14:367-377.

Singh MB. Maternal beliefs and practices regarding the diet and use of herbal medicines during measles and diarrhea in rural areas. Indian Pediatr 1994;31:340-343.

Soto CG, Burhanuddin S. Clove oil as a fish anaesthetic for measuring length and weight of rabbitfish *(Siganus lineatus)*. Aquaculture 1995;136:149-152.

Srivastava KC. Antiplatelet principles from a food spice clove (*Syzygium aromaticum* L.). Prostaglandins Leukot Essent Fatty Acids 1993;48:363-372.

Tajuddin AS, Latif A, Qasmi IA. Aphrodisiac activity of 50% ethanolic extracts of *Myristica fragrans* Houtt. (nutmeg) and *Syzygium aromaticum* (L) Merr. and Perry. (clove) in male mice: a comparative study. BMC Complement Altern Med 2003;3:6.

Thirach S, Tragoolpua K, Punjaisee S, et al. Antifungal activity of some medicinal plant extracts against *Candida albicans* and *Cryptococcus neoformans*. Acta Horticulturae 2003;597:217-221.

Tort L, Puigcerver M, Crespo S, et al. Cortisol and haematological response in sea bream and trout subjected to the anaesthetics clove oil and 2-phenoxyethanol. Aquaculture Res 2002;33:907-910.

Vykusova B. New technologies and new species in aquaculture. Bull Vurh Vodnany 2003;39:1-148.

Wagner H, Sprinkmeyer L. Über die pharmakologische Wirkung von Melissengeist. Deutsche Apotheker Zeitung 1973;113:1159-1166.

Wie MB, Won MH, Lee KH, et al. Eugenol protects neuronal cells from excitotoxic and oxidative injury in primary cortical cultures. Neurosci Lett 1997;225:93-96.

Zheng GQ, Kenney PM, Lam LK. Sesquiterpenes from clove *(Eugenia caryophyllata)* as potential anticarcinogenic agents. J Nat Prod 1992;55:999-1003.

Comfrey

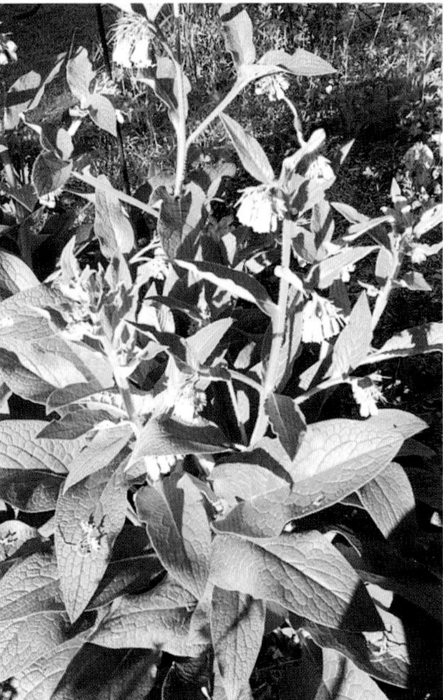

Symphytum officinale L. • sim-FY-tum oh-fiss-ih-NAH-lee

Botanical Names: *Symphytum officinale, Symphytum asperum, Symphytum caucasicum, Symphytum tuberosum, Symphytum* × uplandicum

Other Names: Comfrey, common comfrey, prickly comfrey, Russian comfrey, boneset, knitbone, consolida, blackwort, bruisewort, gum plant, healing herb, knitback, salsify, slippery root, wallwort, yalluc (Saxon), ass ear, nipbone

Family: Boraginaceae

Parts Used: Leaf, roots, rhizomes

Distribution: Grows in most damp areas of the United Kingdom, Europe, Western Asia, and the United States.

Selected Constituents: *Leaf:* Mucilage, tannin, allantoin, symphytine, echinidine, vitamin B_{12}. *Root:* Allantoin (0.6%-4.7%), about 29% mucilage, phytosterols, triterpenoid (isobauerenol), phenolic compounds (including caffeic, chlorogenic, and lithospermic acids), tannin, asparagine, pyrrolizidine alkaloids (including symphytine, cynoglossine, consolidine), inulin, resin, gum, starch. *Other:* Vitamins, including riboflavin, niacin, pantothenic acid, vitamin B_{12} (very rare in vegetable matter); vitamin A, vitamin C, and vitamin E.

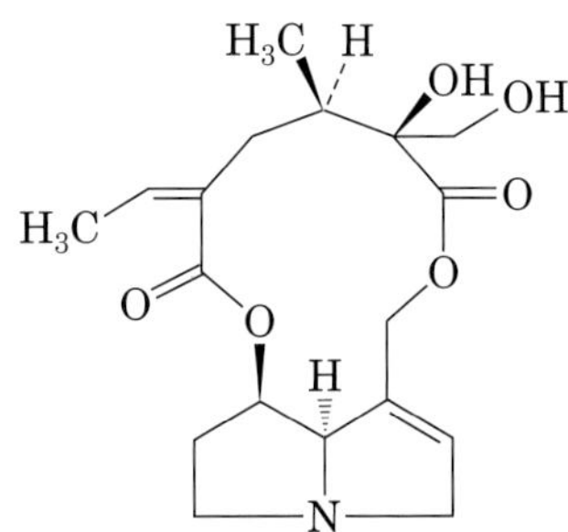

Pyrrolizidine alkaloid

Clinical Actions: *Leaf:* Vulnerary, demulcent, antihemorrhagic, antirheumatic, anti-inflammatory. *Root:* Vulnerary, demulcent, cell proliferant, astringent, antihemorrhagic, expectorant, antiulcer, hemostaic. *Symphytum* is an effective stimulant to fibroblast, chondroblast, and osteoblast activity.
Energetics: Sweet, bland, cool, moist
History and Traditional Usage: Gerard wrote in 1597 that Comfrey should be "... given to drinke against the paine of the backe, gotten by violent motion as wrestling." The name knitbone derives from its useful property of healing broken bones and wounds. Widespread use followed a faith in its ability to promote the healing of bruised and broken parts. Used for wounds, the pain of inflammation, tenderness, broken bones, fractures, and sprains, this property has been known at least since Roman times, when it was named *conferva,* meaning "to join together." Other traditional uses include raw indolent ulcers; wounds of the nerves, tendons, and arteries; cracked nipples; and bleeding from the lungs or bladder. Has been recommended as a preventive of foot and mouth disease in cattle.

The wound-healing properties of comfrey are partially due to the presence of allantoin, which stimulates cell proliferation, thereby accelerating defect healing both internally and externally. Allantoin is able to diffuse through the skin and tissues, hence its traditional use as an external application for the treatment of bone fractures. On the surface of the skin, its action is aided by the contracting "plaster" effect of the mucilage, tannins, and resins as they dry. In addition, comfrey is rich in demulcent mucilage, which augments the action of allantoin in gastric and duodenal ulcers and ulcerative colitis. The mild astringency of comfrey, due to its tannin content, helps arrest bleeding. The mucilage also explains the use of comfrey as a bulk laxative and as a soothing remedy for the lower gut; this may in turn operate by reflex to account for its usefulness in excessive menstrual bleeding, hematuria, and urinary spasm. Comfrey has been used with success in cases of bronchitis and irritable cough, in which it soothes and reduces irritation while enhancing expectoration. Spring harvested parts are higher in PAs than fall harvested parts; young leaves are higher than older leaves.

In Europe, comfrey has been applied for inflammatory disorders such as arthritis, thrombophlebitis, and gout, and as a treatment for diarrhea (Stickel, 2000).

According to de Bairacli Levy (1963), comfrey was widely cultivated as fodder. Sheep and cows sought it to eat. English gypsies would give a handful of comfrey leaves to their horses and cows in spring to "rid them of winter tupor and put them in fine bloom in one week." She recommended a drench of 1 pound of comfrey boiled in 1.5 pints of water for 1 hour, then adding a handful of ground ivy plant *(Glechoma hedera)* and 2 ounces of Spanish licorice. A half-pint is given 3 times daily. For bone healing, she suggested 2 handfuls of well-bruised roots daily. She also wrote that once hip dysplasia has developed, feeding of raw, finely minced leaves or comfrey tablets has achieved "cure" (1 tbsp at midday and evening); this was to be given 5 days a week until "cure" is achieved. She also recommended it as a cure for rickets, sprains, and arthritis, and for broken legs as an infusion (2 tbsp morning and night) with infused cloth wrapped around the fracture site; it was also recommended for the internal treatment of teeth (de Bairacli Levy, 1985).
Published Research: The anti-inflammatory and analgesic properties of topical comfrey preparations were investigated in a prospective, open, multicenter observational study in Germany. A topical preparation was applied to bruises, sprains, and distortions and painful conditions of the muscles and joints. Results of this study confirmed the effectiveness and tolerability of the topical comfrey preparation investigated in the treatment of bruises, sprains, and distortions, as well as for painful conditions affecting muscles and joints (Koll, 2002). In an open, uncontrolled study, 105 patients with locomotor system symptoms were treated twice daily with an ointment that contained comfrey. A clear therapeutic effect was noted and was most effective against muscle pain, swelling and overstrain, arthralgia/distortions, enthesopathy, and vertebral syndrome (Kucera, 2000).

Mastitis in cows

In a different study (Noorlander, 1987), topical applications of comfrey extract (in propylene glycol base with allantoin, ascorbic acid, and chlorophyll or carotene) applied to the teats of dairy cows and infusion of the extract into the udder resolved acute mastitis after two applications. Chronically infected cows did not respond as well. Seven cows with teat ends that were ruptured and cracked received topical application of this extract, which healed the tissue. Similar success rates were observed in another herd; cows with chapped teats and skin lesions healed in less than 3 days, and the tissue became softer. A deep cut on the surface of one teat of one cow healed within 5 days after treatment was provided. The same extract has also been used in the treatment of dairy cows with metritis. Treatment consisted of 90 mL of extract infused into the uterus every day for 3 days. No visible irritation to the mucous membrane or epithelial tissue was noted; a beneficial effect on the endometrium was observed (Noolander, 1987).
Indications: *Internal:* It is currently considered unsafe for internal use because of potential pyrrolizidine toxicity. Traditionally used for cough, irritable bowel syndrome, peptic ulcer disease, rheumatic pain, and arthritis. The root had been used internally for hematemesis, ulcers, and colitis.

External: Blepharitis, conjunctivitis; as a poultice, ointment, or fomentation for bruises, chronic skin ulcer, fracture, rashes, strains, sprains, thrombophlebitis, wounds, and mastitis.
Caution: Traditional texts warn that care should be taken with very deep wounds because the external application of comfrey can lead to the formation of tissue over the wound before it has healed deeper down, leading to the possibility of an abscess.
Contraindications: Pregnancy and lactation. Evidence for teratogenicity or transfer across placental membranes is lacking, and this contraindication is described by Brinker as speculative (Brinker, 1998).
Internal Use: Comfrey is potentially hepatotoxic when administered orally because of the pyrrolizidine alkaloid content. Comfrey is not recommended for internal use by

the AHPA (American Herbal Products Association). This caution is regarded as excessively stringent by some herbalists, especially for short-term use of comfrey leaf preparations. Assessment of hepatic detoxification status should be performed.

External use: Percutaneous absorption has been investigated; dermally absorbed alkaloids are not, or are to only a small extent, converted to free alkaloids in the animal at a rate approximately 20 times less than that observed in gastrointestinal absorption (Brauchli, 1982). In Australia, comfrey is restricted to dermal use on intact skin. It should not be used longer than 4 to 6 weeks over 1 year in humans; the daily dose applied should not exceed 100 µg.

Toxicity: AHPA class 2a, 2b, 2c. External application should be limited to 4 to 6 weeks. Contains hepatotoxic pyrrolizidine alkaloids (PAs) that are associated with hepatic veno-occlusive disease (Bach, 1989). Comfrey root contains a greater quantity of PAs than are found in the leaf. Evaluation of risks from ingestion of PA that contains herbs is a complex, controversial, and unresolved subject. PAs vary in toxicity, not only by distribution in different species of the same genera, but in their distribution in different plant parts (e.g., leaf, root) of the same species.

The carcinogenicity of *Symphytum officinale* L. was studied in inbred rats. Three groups of 19 to 28 rats each were fed comfrey leaves for 480 to 600 days; four additional groups of 15 to 24 rats were fed comfrey roots for varying lengths of time. A control group was given a normal diet. Hepatocellular adenomas were induced in all experimental groups that received the diets containing comfrey roots and leaves. Hemangioendothelial sarcoma of the liver was infrequently induced (Hirono, 1978).

Preparation: The roots should be unearthed in the spring or autumn, when allantoin levels are highest, then washed, chopped, and dried at a moderate temperature. The leaves are harvested after flowering in early summer.

Dosage:

External:

Ointment root: 10%-15% extractive in ointment base

Human

Note that internal use is not recommended, but published doses are provided here because some herbalists still use the herb orally. Even so, they limit use to no longer than 1 month. Australian GSL schedule 2: restricted to external use

Dried herb: 2-4 g TID

Infusions and decoctions: 5 g per cup of water, with 1 cup of the tea given TID

Tincture (leaf): 1 : 2 or 1 : 3: 1-5 mL TID

Fluid extract (root): 1 : 1: 2-4 mL TID

Small Animal: Caution is advised. Should be restricted to external use

References

Bach N, Thung SN, Schaffner F. Comfrey herb tea–induced hepatic veno-occlusive disease. Am J Med 1989;87:97-99.

Brinker F. *Herb Contraindications and Drug Interactions.* 2nd ed. Sandy, Ore: Eclectic Institute Inc; 1998.

De Bairacli Levy J. *The Complete Herbal Handbook for Farm and Stable.* London: Faber and Faber; 1963.

De Bairacli Levy J. *The Complete Herbal Handbook for the Dog and Cat.* London: Faber and Faber; 1985.

Grieve M. *A Modern Herbal.* London: C.F. Leyel; 1931.

Hirono I, Mori H, Haga M. Carcinogenic activity of *Symphytum officinale.* J Natl Cancer Inst 1978;61:865-869.

Koll R, Klingenburg S. [Therapeutic characteristance and tolerance of topical comfrey preparations. Results of an observational study of patients]. Fortschr Med Orig 2002;120:1-9.

Kucera M, Kalal J, Polesna Z. Effects of *Symphytum* ointment on muscular symptoms and functional locomotor disturbances. Adv Ther 2000;17:204-210.

Noorlander DO. US Patent 4670263. Nontoxic, germicide and healing compositions, cited in Australian College of Phytotherapy notes, 1987.

Stickel F, Seitz HK. The efficacy and safety of comfrey. Public Health Nutr 2000;3:501-508.

Coptis

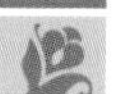

Coptis chinensis Franch. • kop-tiss chi-NEN-sis

Other Names: Coptis rhizome, chinese gold thread, huang lian

Family: Ranunculaceae

Parts Used: Dried rhizome

Distribution: China

Selected Constituents: The major constituents are berberine and related protoberberine alkaloids. Berberine occurs in the range of 4% to 8%, followed by palmatine, coptisine, and berberastine, among others (Ikuta, 1984).

Clinical Actions: Antimicrobial, antidiarrheal, hypoglycemic, hypocholesterolemic, anticancer

Energetics: Cold, bitter

History and Traditional Usage: Uses described in pharmacopoeias and in traditional systems of medicine: management of bacterial diarrheas, acute conjunctivitis (as an eyewash), gastroenteritis, boils, and cutaneous and visceral leishmaniasis. Other uses include treatment of patients with arthritis, burns, diabetes, dysmenorrhea, toothache, malaria, gout, and renal disease (Bruneton, 1995).

Published Research: Numerous in vitro studies support the antimicrobial activity of coptis mainly caused by berberine (Chang, 1987; Kaneda, 1991; Nakamoto, 1990); the antidiarrheal effects of berberine may be due to its antisecretory and antimicrobial actions (Shin, 1993; Swabb, 1981; Tai, 1981).

A study investigated the antibacterial effect of coptis on oral bacteria; it was concluded that it had an inhibitory effect on periodontal pathogens; the possibility of clinical application for the treatment of periodontal disease was suggested (Hu, 2000).

Coptis has been evaluated for its anti-inflammatory properties and was active only in the chronic phase (Cuellar, 2001). Serum cholesterol levels were reduced significantly in a dose-dependent manner in rats given coptis extract orally (50 and 100 mg/kg body weight/day) for 30 days. Results indicated that it lowered serum cholesterol levels and was effective in reducing the pathologic damage caused by hypercholesterolemia. The cholesterol level–lowering effect resulted from the reduction of cholesterol synthesis—not the enhancement of its excretion (Yokozawa, 2003).

The antiproliferative activities of coptis and its major component berberine were investigated in eight human pancreatic cancer cell lines (Iizuka, 2003). In transplanted nasopharyngeal carcinoma, tumor growth was inhibited by 29.5% after coptis was used for 30 days. It was concluded that coptis can affect gene expression in implanted tumors, and that inhibition of the growth of implanted tumors might be associated with control of gene expression (Wang, 2003). In mice with induced colon carcinoma, the anticachectic effect of coptis was investigated. Coptis significantly attenuated weight loss in tumor-bearing mice without changing food intake or tumor growth. It was therefore shown to exert an anticachectic effect, and it was suggested that this effect might be due to berberine (Iizuka, 2002). The effect of berberine in coptis was tested on lymph node metastasis of murine lung cancer. Oral administration of berberine for 14 days significantly inhibited mediastinal lymph node metastasis, but it did not affect tumor growth. Combined treatment with berberine and an anticancer drug resulted in marked inhibition of tumor growth and of lymphatic metastasis, as compared with either treatment alone (Mitani, 2001).

Indications: Gastroenteritis, infection

Potential Veterinary Indications: Infectious enteritis, adjunctive cancer care, hypercholesterolemia

Contraindications: Pregnancy

Toxicology and Adverse Effects: AHPA 2b (see Contraindication above). Berberine is reported to be well tolerated in therapeutic doses of 500 mg, with no intoxication in humans (Roth, 1998). One report noted nausea, vomiting, abdominal distortion, diarrhea, polyuria, and erythropenia after oral administration of coptis to human adults (Bao, 1983).

Dosage:

Human:

Dried herb: 1.5-6 g, divided daily (Pharmacopoeia of the People's Republic of China, 1992). American herbalists may use higher doses.

Small Animal:

Dried herb: 25-150 mg/kg, divided daily

References

Bao Y. Side effects of *Coptis chinensis* and berberine. Chin J Integrated Traditional Western Med 1983;3:12-13.

Bruneton J. *Pharmacognosy, Phytochemistry, Medicinal Plants.* Paris: Lavoisier; 1995.

Chang HM, But PPH, eds. *Pharmacology and Applications of Chinese Materia Medica,* vol 2. Singapore: World Scientific Publishing; 1987.

Cuellar MJ, Giner RM, Recio MC, Manez S, Rios JL. Topical anti-inflammatory activity of some Asian medicinal plants used in dermatological disorders. Fitoterapia 2001;72:221-229.

Hu JP, Takahashi N, Yamada T. *Coptidis rhizoma* inhibits growth and proteases of oral bacteria. Oral Dis 2000;6:297-302.

Iizuka N, Oka M, Yamamoto K, et al. Identification of common or distinct genes related to antitumor activities of a medicinal herb and its major component by oligonucleotide microarray. Int J Cancer 2003;107:666-672.

Iizuka N, Hazama S, Yoshimura K, et al. Anticachectic effects of the natural herb *Coptidis rhizoma* and berberine on mice bearing colon 26/clone 20 adenocarcinoma. Int J Cancer 2002;99:286-291.

Ikuta A, Kobayashi A, Itokawa H. Studies on the quantitative analysis of protoberberine alkaloids in Japanese, Chinese and other countries: Coptis rhizomes by thin-layer chromatography-densitometry. Shoyakugakuzasshi 1984;38:279-282.

Kaneda Y, Torii M, Tanaka T, Aikawa M. In vitro effects of berberine sulfate on the growth and structure of *Entamoeba histolytica, Giardia lamblia,* and *Trichomonas vaginalis.* Ann Trop Med Parasitol 1991;85:417-425.

Mitani N, Murakami K, Yamura T, Ikeda T, Saiki I. Inhibitory effect of berberine on the mediastinal lymph node metastasis produced by orthotopic implantation of Lewis lung carcinoma. Cancer Lett 2001;165:35-42.

Nakamoto K, Sadamori S, Hamada T. Effects of crude drugs and berberine hydrochloride on the activities of fungi. J Prosthet Dent 1990;64:691-694.

Pharmacopoeia of the People's Republic of China (English ed). Guangzhou: Guangdong Science and Technology Press; 1992.

Roth L, Daunderer M, Kormann K. *Giftpflanzen. Pflanzengifte.* 3rd ed. Landsberg: Ecomed; 1988:145-146,810.

Shen ZF, Xie MZ. Determination of berberine in biological specimens by high performance TLC and fluoro-densitometric method. Yao Hsueh Hsueh Pao 1993;28:532-536.

Shin DH, Yu H, Hsu WH. A paradoxical stimulatory effect of berberine on guinea-pig ileum contractility: possible involvement of acetylcholine release from the postganglionic parasympathetic nerve and cholinesterase inhibition. Life Sci 1993;53:1495-1500.

Swabb EA, Tai YH, Jordan L. Reversal of cholera toxin-induced secretion in rat ileum by luminal berberine. Am J Physiol 1981;241:G248-G252.

Tai YH, Feser JF, Marnane WG, Desjeux DF. Antisecretory effects of berberine in rat ileum. Am J Physiol 1981;241:G253-G258.

Wang GP, Tang FQ, Zhou JP. Effect of *Coptis chinensis* compound on the gene expression in transplanted tumor tissue in nasopharyngeal carcinoma cell line of CNE1 by cDNA microarray [Chinese]. Bull Hunan Med Univ 2003;28:347-352.

Yokozawa T, Ishida A, Cho EJ, Nakagawa T. The effects of *Coptidis rhizoma* extract on a hypercholesterolemic animal model. Phytomedicine 2003;10:17-22.

Cordyceps

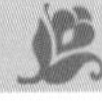

Cordyceps sinensis (Berk.) Sacc. • KOR-di-seps sye-NEN-sis

Other Names: Caterpillar fungus, dong zhong chang cao, dong chong xia cao (China), semitake (Japan)

Family: Claviceptaceae

Parts Used: Cordyceps consists of the dried fungus *Cordyceps sinensis* growing on caterpillar larvae.

Distribution: *C. sinensis* grows at altitudes of 3000 m or more in the cold, grassy Alpine marshlands of the mountainous regions of Tibet and China. Elsewhere, it occurs in Japan, Australia, New Zealand, Canada, the United States, Mexico, Russia, Norway, the Netherlands, Italy, Kenya, Tanzania, and Ghana. Advances in the cultivation of cordyceps in China have resulted in a number of aseptic mycelial products grown in culture from strains of the wild fungus as imperfect forms. These have been given different Latin binomials, such as *Cephalosporium sinensis* and *Paecilomyces sinensis,* to distinguish them from the natural wild form, *Cordyceps sinensis.*

Selected Constituents: Carbohydrates, including polysaccharides and galactomannans; various cyclic dipeptides, minerals, and vitamins B_1, B_2, B_{12}, E, and K; amino acids, including glutamic acid, l-tryptophan, l-arginine, and lysine; d-mannitol; sterols, including ergosterol and ergosterol derivatives, alkaloids, and fatty acids (mainly oleic, linoleic, palmitic, and stearic acids)
Clinical Actions: Hypocholesterolemic, lipid-lowering, hepatoprotective, nephroprotective, anticancer, antioxidant, antiasthma, hypoglycemic
Energetics: Sweet, warm
History and Traditional Usage: Cordyceps has been used in food and medicine in Asia for millennia. In China, it is eaten in soups (Pegler, 1994; Chamberlain, 1996) and cooked with meats (Zhu, 1998a). Traditionally, the powdered fungus is taken with other herbs, such as ginseng, or as a tea, or is soaked in alcohol as a tincture. Its main use is as a strengthening tonic following convalescence. Other traditional uses include the treatment of patients with cough, anemia, tuberculosis, lower back pain (Pegler, 1994), impotence, infertility, irregular menstruation, night sweats, and senile weakness. In Traditional Chinese Medicine, it is used as a mild tranquilizer or sedative (Liu, 1980; Guo, 1986). Cordyceps is also taken to keep lungs fit, strengthen kidneys, build up bone marrow, reduce phlegm, and stop hemorrhage (Liu, 1980). A Jesuit priest in France during the 18th century described its use for the treatment of patients with debility and fatigue, noting that it was used only by those who could afford the rare and costly medicine (Pereira, 1843). Wild cordyceps is still rare and costly and is endangered by overharvesting (Jones, 1997).
Published Research: Animal and human studies have repeatedly found that plasma triglyceride, low-density lipoprotein cholesterol, very low density lipoprotein cholesterol, and total cholesterol levels are lowered, and high-density lipoprotein cholesterol levels are increased, by the cultured mycelium extract (strain Cs-4) (Zhu, 1998b; Kiho, 1999; Koh, 2003a; Shao, 1990); cordyceps may reduce formation of atherosclerotic lesions induced by oxidative stress (Yamaguchi, 2000).

In clinical studies of cultured mycelium products of cordyceps, researchers have reported benefits in the treatment of patients with posthepatic cirrhosis and chronic hepatitis B (Gong, 2000). A hepatoprotective effect was observed in CCl4-induced liver cirrhosis in rats (Zhang, 2004b), and a study found that *Cordyceps sinensis* could inhibit hepatic fibrogenesis derived from chronic liver injury, retard the development of cirrhosis, and notably ameliorate liver function (Liu, 2003).

In vitro, cordyceps increases corticosteroid production, and the induction of corticosteroid production might explain the antirejection activity of cordyceps in organ transplant experiments (Wang, 1998). Researchers have reported the successful use of cordyceps (3 g/day) in a placebo-controlled study in 69 kidney transplant patients. The cordyceps + cyclosporine group showed a significant decrease in nephrotoxicity compared with the cyclosporine + placebo group, which indicated that cordyceps had a protective effect against cyclosporine (Xu, 1995). Cordyceps was used to replace the maintenance immunosuppressant azathioprine in seven kidney transplant patients who developed leukopenia as an adverse effect of the drug. Although they continued to receive prednisone and cyclosporine, leukocyte counts improved (Yu, 1994).

Cordyceps is regarded as an important "kidney tonic" in TCM; it may be of use in the treatment of patients with IgA nephropathy (Lin, 1996) or chronic renal failure, and as a nephroprotective agent. A randomized, placebo-controlled trial of cordyceps in 21 elderly patients receiving amikacin sulfate found less nephrotoxicity compared with the placebo group (Bao, 1994). It has been shown that cordyceps can prevent gentamicin-induced nephrotoxicity in animals and humans (Tian, 1991a, 1991b; Li, 1992). A comparative clinical study of cordyceps (3-5 g/day) was conducted in 51 patients with chronic renal failure. In all, 28 were given cordyceps and showed a significant increase in renal function and T-lymphocyte subsets, including the T helper cell ratio, compared with the control group (Guan, 1992).

In vivo studies demonstrate antimetastasis and antitumor activity of cordyceps (Nakamura, 1999a). *Cordyceps sinensis* (water extracts) might be beneficial in the prevention of tumor metastasis as an adjuvant agent in cancer chemotherapy (Nakamura, 2003). Controlled, open-label clinical studies found that cordyceps appeared to restore immune cell function in patients with advanced cancer given conventional cancer therapies (Zhou, 1995; Zhu, 1998a); more than 85% of cordyceps-treated patients undergoing chemotherapy and radiation showed more normal blood cell counts versus 59% of controls (Zhu, 1998a).

Animal and in vitro studies have shown that cordyceps fruit body and mycelial extracts are potent immune-stimulants (Nakamura, 1999b; Li, 1993; Yamaguchi, 1990). In a study on mice, the immunopotentiating effect was associated with increased interleukin-2 production, and stimulation of myocardial adenosine triphosphate (ATP) generation was paralleled by an enhancement in mitochondrial electron transport (Siu, 2004). However, immunosuppressive fractions of fruit bodies were shown to inhibit tumor necrosis factor, interleukin-2, and natural killer cell activity (Kuo, 1996). In an animal model of lupus, cordyceps (100 mg/kg po/day) significantly prolonged the survival time of mice and significantly inhibited production of antibodies. In preliminary studies in patients with systemic lupus erythematosus, cordyceps fruit body extract ameliorated the defective production of interleukin-2 (Chen, 1993).

Cordyceps is used for its antioxidation activity derived from cordyceps polysaccharides (Li, 2001; Li, 2003). In aged mice, cordyceps extract could significantly enhance learning and memory and improve the activity of red blood cells, brain, and liver, probably because of the effects of mitigating oxidative stress and removing free radicals (Wang, 2004).

Cordyceps has hypoglycemic effects in diabetic but not normal mice and rats (Kiho, 1999). One experiment showed that compared with placebo, rats fed the fruiting body of cordyceps exhibited reduced weight loss, polydipsia, and hyperglycemia, and it is suggested that the fruiting body of cordyceps has potential as a functional food for diabetes (Lo, 2004). Cordyceps increases the basal insulin level of pancreatic B cells in rats with induced liver fibrosis (Zhang, 2003).

Cordyceps is used in China for the treatment of those with general debility after sickness and for persons of advanced age (Chiou, 2000). Adaptogenic activity has been demonstrated in rats and mice. Cordyceps enhances endurance and performance (Koh, 2003b). Cordyceps alleviates fatigue and improves physical endurance, especially in elderly subjects (Dai, 2001). A double-blind, placebo-controlled clinical trial in 59 elderly patients (aged 60-84) with various symptoms of senescence found that an extract of cordyceps alleviated fatigue, along with other symptoms, in 92% of subjects (cited in Zhu, 1998a).

Clinical studies with the cultured mycelium extract have reported increased levels of estradiol, testosterone, and cortisol following a 40-day treatment (Guo, 1986). Cordyceps stimulated both in vitro and in vivo testosterone secretions in mice and may be useful for the treatment of those with reproductive problems caused by insufficient testosterone levels in human males (Hsu, 2003).

Cordyceps powder may have a role in the treatment of patients with asthma. A single study found that cordyceps at 5 g/kg significantly inhibited bronchial response to challenge with ovalbumin and inhibited antigen-induced increase of eosinophils in rats. Results suggested that cordyceps could be used in the prevention and management of asthma (Lin, 2001). A randomized, controlled study in 45 patients with respiratory disease, including chronic bronchitis, pulmonary heart disease, and pneumocystis, found that 86.7% of participants improved after taking a cultured cordyceps mycelium extract (Qu, 1995). Cordyceps improved symptoms of chronic bronchitis, despite the fact that 75% of patients had complications of pulmonary heart disease and emphysema, and all were elderly patients (Han, 1995). The therapeutic activity of cordyceps may be related to modulation of the function of TH1 and TH2 cells in the bronchial airway (Kuo, 2001).

Poultry growth promotion

One study indicated that cordyceps enhances physiologic activity in chicks and can be used as a substitute for antibiotic growth promoters. Broiler chicks were orally dosed with a hot water extract of mycelia from *Cordyceps sinensis* to assess possible substitution of avilamycin as an antibiotic growth promoter. The growth performance (body weight gain and survivability) and health index (microflora in the small intestines and antibody titer to Newcastle's disease virus) of chicks were significantly improved in the cordyceps group (600-mg/kg diet) and in the avilamycin (20-mg/kg diet)-fed group in comparison with the control group ($P < .05$). The avilamycin-fed group and the cordyceps-fed group had similar growth performances, but the latter had better microbial flora in the small intestine (Koh, 2003c).

Indications: Hyperlipidemia, chronic kidney disease, liver disease, cancer (as an adjuvant with conventional therapy), bronchitis, arteriosclerosis, male erectile dysfunction, decreased libido, and immune potentiation (Zhu, 1998a, 1998b; Jones, 1997)

Potential Veterinary Indications: Nephropathy, chronic renal failure, diabetes mellitus, lupus, adjunct to chemotherapy. Adjunct to gentamicin therapy to reduce adverse effects. To support chemotherapy patients with leukopenia, hypoadrenocorticoism. To increase feed efficiency

Contraindications: None found.

Toxicology and Adverse Effects: AHPA class 1. Possible adverse effects from cordyceps were reported in some hyperlipidemic patients who experienced dry mouth, skin rash, drowsiness, nausea, and diarrhea, in association with ingestion of an extract of the cultured mycelium (Shao, 1990).

Drug Interactions: Cordyceps may affect patients on blood thinning and antithrombotic medications. Because of corticosterol production–increasing activity in vitro (Wang, 1998) and use of cordyceps as a substitute for immunesuppressant medication in organ-transplanted patients (Lin, 1996), care should be taken with other corticosteroid use. Cultured cordyceps mycelium extracts have been reported to exhibit significant inhibition of monoamine oxidase type B in vitro (Zhu, 1998b); however, in vivo effects in patients taking MAO inhibitors are absent from the literature.

Dosage:

Human: Wild cordyceps is traditionally taken in a dosage of 5-10 g/day (Yen, 1992).

Another source states that 3 to 9 g is taken for sedative and invigorating effects, sexual impotence, debility following illness, anemia, night sweats, cough, and excessive tiredness, and that 15 g steamed with chicken is taken as a tonic (Liu, 1980).

Dried herb: 3-10 g TID

Infusions and decoctions: 5-30 g per cup of water, with 1 cup of the tea given TID

Tincture (27.5% ethanol): 1:2 or 1:3: 1-5 mL TID

Small Animal:

Dried herb: 25-500 mg/kg, divided daily (optimally, TID) if extracted and dried; triple or quadruple dose for unprocessed herb

Infusion: 5-30 g per cup of water, administered at a rate of ¼-½ cup per 10 kg (20 lb), divided daily (optimally, TID)

Tincture (usually in 27.5% ethanol; doses are significantly lower for the high-alcohol preparations): 1:2-1:3: 0.5-2.0 mL per 10 kg (20 lb), divided daily (optimally, TID) and diluted or combined with other herbs. Higher doses may be appropriate.

References

Bao ZD, Wu ZG, Zheng F. [Amelioration of aminoglycoside nephrotoxicity by *Cordyceps sinensis* in old patients]. Chin J Integrated Med 1994;14:259,271-273.

Chamberlain M. Ethnomycological experiences in South West China. Mycologist 1996;10:173-176.

Chen JR, Yen JH, Lin CC, et al. The effects of Chinese herbs on improving survival and inhibiting anti-ds DNA antibody production in lupus mice. Am J Chin Med 1993;21:257-262.

Chiou WF, Chang PC, Chou CJ, Chen CF. Protein constituent contributes to the hypotensive and vasorelaxant activities of *Cordyceps sinensis*. Life Sci 2000;66:1369-1376.

Dai G, Bao T, Xu C, Cooper R, Zhu JA. CordyMax Cs-4 improves steady-state bioenergy status in mouse liver. J Altern Complement Med 2001;7:231-240.

Gong HY, Wang KQ, Tang SG. [Effects of *Cordyceps sinensis* on T lymphocyte subsets and hepatofibrosis in patients with chronic hepatitis B] [Chinese]. Bull Hunan Med Univ 2000;25:248-250.

Guan YJ, Hu G, Hou M, et al. [Effect of *Cordyceps sinensis* on T-lymphocyte subsets in chronic renal failure]. Chin J Integrat Med 1992;12:323,338-339.

Guo YZ. [Medicinal chemistry, pharmacology, and clinical applications of fermented mycelia of *Cordyceps sinensis* and JinShuiBao capsule]. J Modern Diagn Ther 1986;1:60-65.

Han SR. [Experiences in treating patients with chronic bronchitis and pulmonary diseases with Cs-4 capsules]. J Admin Tradit Chin Med 1995;5(suppl):29-30.

Hsu CC, Huang JL, Tsai SJ, Sheu CC, Huang BM. In vivo and in vitro stimulatory effects of *Cordyceps sinensis* on testosterone production in mouse Leydig cells. Life Sci 2003;73:2127-2136.

Jones K. *Cordyceps: Tonic Food of Ancient China.* Seattle, Wash: Sylvan Press, Inc; 1997.

Kiho T, Ookubo K, Usui S, et al. Structural features and hypoglycemic activity of a polysaccharide (CS-F10) from the cultured mycelium of *Cordyceps sinensis.* Biol Pharm Bull 1999;22:966-970.

Koh JH, Kim KM, Chang UJ, Suh HJ. Hypocholesterolemic effect of hot-water extract from mycelia of *Cordyceps sinensis.* Biol Pharm Bull 2003a;26:84-87.

Koh JH, Kim KM, Kim JM, Song JC, Suh HJ. Antifatigue and antistress effect of the hot-water fraction from mycelia of *Cordyceps sinensis.* Biol Pharm Bull 2003b;26:691-694.

Koh JH, Suh HJ, Ahn TS. Hot-water extract from mycelia of *Cordyceps sinensis* as a substitute for antibiotic growth promoters. Biotechnol Lett 2003c;25:585-590.

Kuo YC, Tsai WJ, Shiao MS, Chen CF, Lin CY. *Cordyceps sinensis* as an immunomodulatory agent. Am J Chin Med 1996; 24:111-125.

Kuo YC, Tsai WJ, Wang JY, Chang SC, Lin CY, Shiao MS. Regulation of bronchoalveolar lavage fluid cell function by the immunomodulatory agents from *Cordyceps sinensis.* Life Sci 2001;68:1067-1082.

Li LS, Zheng F. Clinical protection of aminoglycoside nephrotoxicity by *Cordyceps sinensis* (CS). J Am Soc Nephrol 1992;3:726. Abstract 24P.

Li SP, Li P, Dong TT, Tsim KW. Anti-oxidation activity of different types of natural *Cordyceps sinensis* and cultured *Cordyceps mycelia.* Phytomedicine 2001;8:207-212.

Li SP, Zhao KJ, Ji SN, et al. A polysaccharide isolated from *Cordyceps sinensis,* a traditional Chinese medicine, protects PC12 cells against hydrogen peroxide-induced injury. Life Sci 2003;73:2503-2513.

Li Y, Chen GZ, Jiang DZ. Combined traditional Chinese and Western medicine: effect of *Cordyceps sinensis* on erythropoiesis in mouse bone marrow. Chin Med J 1993;106:313-316.

Lin CY, Shiao MS, Wang ZN. Active fractions of *Cordyceps sinensis* and method of isolation thereof. US Patent 5,582,828, December 10, 1996.

Lin XX, Xie QM, Shen WH, et al. [Effects of fermented Cordyceps powder on pulmonary function in sensitized guinea pigs and airway inflammation in sensitized rats] [Chinese]. Zhongguo Zhong Yao Za Zhi/Zhongguo Zhongyao Zazhi/China Journal of Chinese Materia Medica 2001;26:622-625.

Liu B, Bau YS. *Fungi Pharmacopoeia (Sinica).* Oakland, Calif: The Kinoko Co.; 1980:14-21.

Liu YK, Shen W. Inhibitive effect of *Cordyceps sinensis* on experimental hepatic fibrosis and its possible mechanism. World J Gastroenterol 2003;9:529-533.

Lo HC, Tu ST, Lin KC, Lin SC. The anti-hyperglycemic activity of the fruiting body of Cordyceps in diabetic rats induced by nicotinamide and streptozotocin. Life Sci 2004;74:2897-2908.

Nakamura K, Yamaguchi Y, Kagota S, Kwon YM, Shinozuka K, Kunitomo M. Inhibitory effect of *Cordyceps sinensis* on spontaneous liver metastasis of Lewis lung carcinoma and B16 melanoma cells in syngeneic mice. Jpn J Pharmacol 1999a;79:335-341.

Nakamura K, Yamaguchi Y, Kagota S, Shimozuka K, Kunitomo M. Activation of in vivo Kupffer cell function by oral administration of *Cordyceps sinensis* in rats. Jpn J Pharmacol 1999b;79:505-508.

Nakamura K, Konoha K, Yamaguchi Y, et al. Combined effects of *Cordyceps sinensis* and methotrexate on hematogenic lung metastasis in mice. Receptors Channels 2003;9:329-334.

Pegler DN, Yao YJ, Li Y. The Chinese 'Caterpillar Fungus.' Mycologist 1994;8(part 1):3-5.

Pereira J. Summer-plant-winter-worm. NY J Med 1843;1:128-132.

Qu ZY [Evaluation of therapeutic effect of JinShuiBao capsule for treatment of respiratory disease]. J Admin Tradit Chin Med 1995;29-30.

Shao G. Treatment of hyperlipidemia with *Cordyceps sinensis.* A double blind placebo control trial. Int J Orient Med 1990;15:77-80.

Siu KM, Mak DH, Chiu PY, Poon MK, Du Y, Ko KM. Pharmacological basis of 'Yin-nourishing' and 'Yang-invigorating' actions of Cordyceps, a Chinese tonifying herb. Life Sci 2004;76:385-395.

Tian J, Chen XM, Li LS. Effects of *Cordyceps sinensis* on renal cortical Na-K-ATPase activity and calcium content in gentamicin nephrotoxic rats. J Am Soc Nephrol 1991a;2:670.

Tian J, Chen XM, Li LS. Use of *Cordyceps sinensis* in gentamicin induced ARF: a preliminary animal experimentation and observation of cell culture. J Am Soc Nephrol 1991b;2:670. Abstract 83P.

Wang SM, Lee LJ, Lin WW, et al. Effects of a water-soluble extract of *Cordyceps sinensis* on steroidogenesis and capsular morphology of lipid droplets in cultured rat adrenocortical cells. J Cell Biochem 1998;69:483-489.

Wang YH, Ye J, Li CL, Cai SQ, Ishizaki M, Katada M. [An experimental study on anti-aging action of Cordyceps extract]. Zhongguo Zhong Yao Za Zhi 2004;29:773-776.

Xu F, Huang JB, Jiang L, et al. Amelioration of cyclosporin nephrotoxicity by *Cordyceps sinensis* in kidney-transplanted recipients. Nephrol Dial Transplant 1995;10:142-143.

Yamaguchi Y, et al. Inhibitory effects of water extracts from fruiting bodies of cultured *Cordyceps sinensis* on raised serum lipid peroxide levels and aortic cholesterol deposition in atherosclerotic mice. Phytother Res 2000;14:650-652.

Yen KY. *The Illustrated Chinese Materia Medica Crude and Prepared.* Taipei, Taiwan: SMC Publishing, Inc.; 1992:223.

Yu J. The application of cultivated *Cordyceps sinensis* in renal transplantation. J Am Soc Nephrol 1994;5:1016.

Zhang WY, Wang Y, Hou Y. Effects of Chinese medicinal fungus water extract on tumor metastasis and some parameters of immune function. Int Immunopharmacol 2004a;4:461-468.

Zhang X, Liu YK, Zheng Q, et al. Influence of *Cordyceps sinensis* on pancreatic islet beta cells in rats with experimental liver fibrogenesis [Chinese]. Chung Hua Kan Tsang Ping Tsa Chih 2003;11:93-94.

Zhang X, Liu YK, Shen W, et al. Dynamical influence of *Cordyceps sinensis* on the activity of hepatic insulinase of experimental liver cirrhosis. Hepatobil Pancreat Dis Int 2004b;3:99-101.

Zhou DH, Lin LZ. [Effect of Jinshuibao capsule on the immunological function of 36 patients with advanced cancer]. Chung-kuo Chung His I Chieh Ho Tsa Chih 1995;15:476-478.

Zhu JS, Halpern GM, Jones K. The scientific rediscovery of an ancient Chinese herbal medicine: *Cordyceps sinensis*. J Altern Complement Med 1998a;4:289-303.

Zhu JS, Halpern GM, Jones K. The scientific rediscovery of an ancient Chinese herbal medicine: *Cordyceps sinensis*. J Altern Complement Med 1998b;4:429-457.

Corn Silk

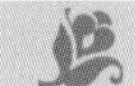

Zea mays L. • ZEE-uh maze

Other Names: Stigmata maydis, maidis stigmata, yu mi xu

Family: Poaceae

Parts Used: Stigmas and styles. Corn silk refers to stigmata from the female flowers of maize, fine soft threads 10 to 20 cm long. When fresh, they are like silk threads of a light green or yellow-brown color; when dry, they resemble fine, dark, crinkled hairs.

Distribution: Indigenous to Central America; now cultivated all over the world.

Selected Constituents: Maizenic acid (claimed to be an active ingredient), flavonoids (maysin, a glycoside of luteolin), rutin, anthocyanidins, flavon-4-ols, chlorogenic acid, saponins, volatile oil (alpha terpinol, menthol, carvacrol, thymol), fixed oil, resin, sugars, saponins, phytosterols, allantoin, mucilage, tannin, minerals (especially potassium).

Maysin

Clinical Actions: Mild diuretic, urinary demulcent, tonic, antilithic

Energetics: Sweet, cool, draining

History and Traditional Usage: Corn silk has a long history of use by Incas and Native Americans and was also recorded in early Chinese Medicine. Its first recorded use in Europe occurred in 1712. Traditionally, corn stigmata are used to treat patients with urinary tract disorders—dysuria, cystitis, urethritis, nocturnal enuresis, prostatitis and gonorrhea. Considered to have a soothing, diuretic action, corn silk was used for any irritation of the urinary system. The diuretic action is thought to be due in part to the high concentration of potassium.

French herbalists use it to thin the bile and promote bile flow, and Chinese research confirms this action. It is also believed to lower blood pressure. Corn silk, known as yu mi xu in China, is used as a treatment for edema. Pollen extract was used for prostate hyperplasia, and powdered pollen was taken for weakness and appetite loss. Hay flowers were used externally as hot compresses for arthritis. The Eclectics used it as a diuretic and for any inflammatory condition in the bladder. In 1949, Milks wrote that it had been abandoned in veterinary practice but was a "feeble diuretic" that was formerly used for inflammation of the genitourinary tract.

Published Research: The diuretic action confirmed in animals may be due to the high concentration of potassium (2.7%) (British Herbal Medicine Association, 1992). Maizenic acid is also claimed to act as a cardiotonic, stimulating diuretic action (Willard, 1991). Allantoin has vulnerary properties. Chlorogenic acid is antibacterial, antimutagenic, antiviral, antioxidant, and clastogenic (Harborne, 1995).

In rats, corn silk was investigated regarding risk factors for kidney stones; however, an extract did not influence citraturia, calciuria, or urinary pH (Grases, 1993). No influence was recorded for 12- and 24-hour urine output or for the sodium excretion of corn silk when tested under standardized conditions in a placebo-controlled double-blind crossover model (Doan, 1992).

Glycoproteins inhibit immunoglobulin (Ig)E formation in mice, perhaps supporting the traditional Chinese use of corn silk as an antiallergy remedy (Namba, 1993). Corn silk may possess antitumor potential as it was found to influence tumor necrosis factor-and lipopolysacchardise-mediated leukocyte adhesion and trafficking in vitro (Habtemariam, 1998).

Indications: Acute or chronic inflammation of the urinary tract, cystitis, prostatitis

Potential Veterinary Uses: IgE-mediated allergies in mice, cystitis, prostatitis

Contraindications: No contraindications are known.

Toxicology and Adverse Effects: AHPA class 1. None known.

Preparation Notes: Stigmata should be collected just before pollination occurs.

Dosage:

Human:

Dried herb: 2-10 g TID, up to 6 times daily for acute conditions

Infusions and decoctions: 10-30 g per cup of water, with 1 cup of the tea given TID, up to 6 times daily acutely

Syrup (British Herbal Compendium, 1923): 8-15 mL TID

Fluid extract (1:1): 2-8 mL TID

Tincture (usually 25%-35% ethanol): 1:2 or 1:3: 3-15 mL TID, up to 6 times daily for acute conditions

Small Animal:

Dried herb: 50-600 mg/kg, divided daily (optimally, TID)

Infusion: 5-30 g per cup of water, administered at a rate of ¼-½ cup per 10 kg (20 lb), divided daily (optimally, TID)

Fluid extract (1:1): 0.5-2.0 mL per 10 kg (20 lb)

Tincture (usually in 25%-35% ethanol): 1:2-1:3: 1.0-3.0 mL per 10 kg (20 lb), divided daily (optimally, TID) and diluted or combined with other herbs. Higher doses may be appropriate if the herb is used singly and is not combined in a formula.

Historical Veterinary Doses:

Dog (Milks, 1949)

Fluid extract (1:1): 0.5-2 dr (1.8-7.4 mL) per dose

References

British Herbal Medicine Association. Bradley P, ed. *British Herbal Compendium,* vol 1. Bournemouth: BHMA; 1992:69.

Doan DD, Nguyen NH, Doan HK, et al. Studies on the individual and combined diuretic effects of four Vietnamese traditional herbal remedies (*Zea mays, Imperata cylindrica, Plantago major* and *Orthosiphon stamineus*). J Ethnopharmacol 1992;36:225-231.

Grases F, Melero G, Costa-Brauza A, et al. The influence of *Zea mays* on urinary risk factors for kidney stones in rats. Phytother Res 1993;7:146-149.

Habtemariam S. Extract of cornsilk inhibits the tumour necrosis factor alpha and bacterial lipopolysaccharide induced cell adhesion and ICAM-1 expression. Planta Med 1998;64:314-318.

Harborne J, Baxter H, eds. *Phytochemical Dictionary. A Handbook of Bioactive Compounds from Plants.* London: Taylor & Francis; 1995.

Milks HJ. *Practical Veterinary Pharmacology, Materia Medica and Therapeutics.* Chicago, Ill: Alex Eger, Inc.; 1949.

Namba T, Xu H, Kadota S, et al. Inhibition of IgE formation in mice by glycoproteins from corn silk. Phytother Res 1993;7:227-230.

Willard T. *The Wild Rose Scientific Herbal.* Calgary: Wild Rose College of Natural Healing; 1991-1995.

Corydalis

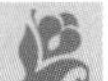

Corydalis ambigua., Corydalis yanhusuo. Corydalis turtschaninovii • kor-ee-DAH-liss am-big-yoo-uh *or* kor-ee-DAH-liss yan-hu-swo

Other Names: Yan huo suo, Chinese fumewort, fitweed

Family: Papaveraceae

Parts Used: Root

Distribution: Corydalis grows throughout the world, but the species *Corydalis yanhusuo* is native to the northern Chinese province of Zhejiang.

Selected Constituents: Alkaloids, including corydaline, tetrahydropalmatine (THP), dl-tetrahydropalmatine (dl-THP), protopine, tetrahydrocoptisine, tetrahydrocolumbamine, and corybulbine (Hsu, 1986). Corydalis also contains starch, mucilage, resins, volatile oil, and inorganic microelements.

Clinical Actions: Analgesic, cardioprotective, sedative, antiarrythmic

Energetics: Warm, bitter, pungent

History and Traditional Usage: Corydalis is one of the chief analgesics in Traditional Chinese Medicine; it is used to invigorate the blood, move energy through the body, and alleviate pain, including back, menstrual, abdominal, chest, traumatic, postpartum, arthritic, and hernial pain (Bensky, 1993). Corydalis has a mildly sedative and tranquilizing effect and is sometimes used for mood disorders and emotional disturbances. In folk medicine, because of its tendency to reduce spasms, corydalis was also used in the treatment of patients with Parkinson's disease.

Published Research: THP (tetrahydropalmatine) is the most intensively studied constituent and has been shown to exhibit a wide number of pharmacologic actions on the central nervous system, including analgesic and sedative effects (Zhu, 1998) and hypnotic actions (Zhu, 1991). THP is an effective antiepileptogenic and anticonvulsant agent (Lin, 2002). THP may act through inhibition of amygdaloid dopamine release to inhibit seizures (Chang, 2001). Corydalis strengthened the analgesia produced by electroacupuncture (Hu, 1994). It was noted that 75 mg THP daily was effective in reducing nerve pain in 78% of patients tested (Lin, 1990). Painful menstruation (dysmenorrhea), abdominal pain after childbirth, and headache have also been reported to be successfully treated with THP (Zhu, 1998).

THP has been found to exhibit a tranquilizing action in mice. It is suggested that THP blocks certain receptor sites (eg, dopamine) in the brain to cause sedation (Zhu, 1998). Human clinical trials with THP showed that insomnia was reduced by 100 to 200 mg THP taken on retiring, without adverse symptoms such as morning grogginess, dizziness, or vertigo (Chang, 1986).

In a large sample of patients with stomach and intestinal ulcers or chronic inflammation of the stomach lining, a 90- to 120-mg extract of corydalis per day (equal to 5-10 g crude herb) was found to improve healing and symptoms in 76% of patients (Chang, 1986).

A variety of plant constituents were tested in vitro for inhibitory action against human immunodeficiency virus type 1 (HIV-1). Alkaloids inhibited HIV-1 reverse transcriptase (Wang, 2001).

THP has been shown to decrease platelet adhesion, to protect against stroke (Xing, 1997), and to lower blood pressure and heart rate in animal studies (Lin, 1996). THP appears to exert antiarrhythmic action on the heart (eg, supraventricular premature beat; Xiaolin, 1998). Antiplatelet effects have been demonstrated (Ko, 1989). THP acts through dopamine receptor antagonism to induce hypotension and bradycardia in rats (Chueh, 1995).

Corydalis was effective in both acute and chronic phases of inflammation and can be considered to exert anti-inflammatory activity (Kubo, 1994b). A crude extract of corydalis inhibited aldose reductase, which may help in the prevention of cataracts associated with diabetes (Kubo, 1994a).

Indications: Pain, epilepsy, gastrointestinal ulceration, insomnia, cardiac arrythmia

Potential Veterinary Indications: Pain, mild anxiety, epilepsy, palliative pain relief in cancer care

Contraindications: Pregnancy. THP has been found to have antihypertensive effects. Corydalis may worsen weakened heart function in cardiac patients through calcium influx inhibition (Chan, 1999).

Toxicology and Adverse Effects: Corydalis is considered to be a safe herb. The LD_{50} of whole corydalis extract given intragastrically to mice was determined to be equivalent to 100 g/kg, indicating extremely low toxicity (Chang, 1986). AHPA class 2b, due to emmenagogue and uterine stimulant effects. THP toxicity, including acute hepatitis (Horowitz, 1996; Kaptchuk, 1995), has been reported, but these effects have not been reported with the whole herb. In addition, people who take Corydalis may experience vertigo, fatigue, and nausea.

Dosage:

Human:

Dried herb: 2-3 g TID

Tincture (60% ethanol): 1:2 or 1:3: 0.5-6 mL TID
Small Animal:
Dried herb: 50-250 mg/kg, divided daily (optimally, TID)
Infusion: 5-15 g per cup of water, administered at a rate of ¼-½ cup per 10 kg (20 lb), divided daily (optimally, TID)
Tincture (usually 60% ethanol): 1:2-1:3: 1.0-2.5 mL per 10 kg (20 lb), divided daily (optimally, TID) and diluted or combined with other herbs. Note that in palliative care, this dose may be tripled and divided into 4 doses, but sedation may occur.

References

Bensky D, Gamble A, Kaptchuk T. *Chinese Herbal Medicine Materia Medica.* Vista, Calif: Eastland Press; 1993:270.

Bone K. *Clinical Applications of Ayurvedic and Chinese Herbs.* Warwick, Queensland, Australia: Phytotherapy Press; 1996: 25-28.

Chan P, Chiu WT, Chen YJ, Wu PJ, Cheng JT. Calcium influx inhibition: possible mechanism of the negative effect of tetrahydropalmatine on left ventricular pressure in isolated rat heart. Planta Med 1999;65:340-342.

Chang CK, Lin MT. DL-Tetrahydropalmatine may act through inhibition of amygdaloid release of dopamine to inhibit an epileptic attack in rats. Neurosci Lett 2001;307:163-166.

Chang HM, But PPH. *Pharmacology and Applications of Chinese Materia Medica,* vol 1. Singapore: World Scientific, Inc.; 1986:521.

Chueh FY, Hsieh MT, Chen CF, Lin MT. DL-tetrahydropalmatine-produced hypotension and bradycardia in rats through the inhibition of central nervous dopaminergic mechanisms. Pharmacology 1995;51:237-244.

Horowitz RS, Feldhaus K, Dart RC, et al. The clinical spectrum of Jin Bu Huan toxicity. Arch Intern Med 1996;156:899-903.

Hsu HY. *Oriental Materia Medica: A Concise Guide.* Long Beach, Calif: Oriental Healing Arts Institute; 1986:448-450.

Hu J, Xie J, Hu J, Zhang Y, Wang J, Chen R. Effect of some drugs on electroacupuncture analgesia and cytosolic free Ca2+ concentration of mice brain [Chinese]. Zhen Ci Yan Jiu 1994;19:55-58.

Kaptchuk TJ, Woolf GM, Vierling JM. Acute hepatitis associated with Jin Bu Huan. Ann Intern Med 1995;122:636.

Ko FN, Wu TS, Lu ST, Wu YC, Huang TF, Teng CM. Antiplatelet effects of protopine isolated from Corydalis tubers. Thromb Res 1989;56:289-298.

Kubo M, Matsuda H, Tokuoka K, Kobayashi Y, Ma S, Tanaka T. Studies of anti-cataract drugs from natural sources. I. Effects of a methanolic extract and the alkaloidal components from Corydalis tuber on in vitro aldose reductase activity. Biol Pharm Bull 1994a;17:458-459.

Kubo M, Matsuda H, Tokuoka K, Ma S, Shiomoto H. Anti-inflammatory activities of methanolic extract and alkaloidal components from Corydalis tuber. Biol Pharm Bull 1994b;17: 262-265.

Lin DZ, Fang YS. *Modern Study and Application of Materia Medica.* Hong Kong: China Ocean Press; 1990:323-325.

Lin MT, Chueh FY, Hsieh MT, et al. Antihypertensive effects of dl-tetrahydropalmatine: an active principle isolated from corydalis. Clin Exper Pharm Physiol 1996;23:738-742.

Lin MT, Wang JJ, Young MS. The protective effect of dl-tetrahydropalmatine against the development of amygdala kindling seizures in rats. Neurosci Lett 2002;320:113-116.

Wang HX, Ng TB. Examination of lectins, polysaccharopeptide, polysaccharide, alkaloid, coumarin and trypsin inhibitors for inhibitory activity against human immunodeficiency virus reverse transcriptase and glycohydrolases. Planta Med 2001;67:669-672.

Xiaolin N, Zhenhua H, Xin M, et al. Clinical and experimental study of dl-tetrahydropalmatine effect in the treatment of supraventricular arrhythmia. J Xi'An Med Univ 1998;10: 150-153.

Xing JF, Wang MN, Ma XY, et al. Effects of dl-tetrahydropalmatine on rabbit platelet aggregation and experimental thrombosis in rats. Chin Pharm Bull 1997;13:258-260.

Zhu XZ. Development of natural products as drugs acting on central nervous system. Mem Inst Oswaldo Cruz 1991; 86(suppl 2):173-175.

Zhu YP. *Chinese Materia Media: Chemistry, Pharmacology, and Applications.* Australia: Harwood Academic Publishers; 1998:445-448.

Couch Grass

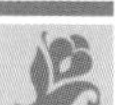

Elymus repens (L.) Gould • EL-ih-mus REE-penz
Common Names: Dog grass, couch grass, quack grass, triticum, *Graminis rhizome,* twitch grass, quick grass, scrutch, English couch
Family: Poaceae
Distribution: Temperate countries everywhere; found particularly on wasteland and abandoned gardens, roadsides, and field margins
Parts Used: Rhizome
Selected Constituents: Triticum 3% to 8%; a polysaccharide related to inulin mannitol; mucilage 8% to 10%; agropyrene, saponins, silica, silicic acid, and silicates, essential oil, lectin, inositol, vanilloside, vanillin, phenolcarboxylic acids. High in iron and many other minerals
Clinical Actions: Anti-inflammatory, diuretic, urinary antiseptic, urinary demulcent
Energetics: Cold, moist
History and Traditional Usage: Diuretic, irritability of the bladder; lessens frequency and pain of urination. Cystitis, dysuria, incipient nephritis. Valued in pyelitis and catarrhal and purulent urinary infections. Chronic prostatitis, hematuria, and stranguria. Also for gout, rheumatism, and jaundice. For preventing gravel, skin disorders, and coughs. *King's* lists the specific indications as "Irritation of the urinary apparatus; pain in the back; frequent and difficult or painful urination; gravelly deposits in the urine; catarrhal and purulent discharges from urethra." De Bairacli Levy recommends an infusion of root of couch grass for bladder troubles (stone and gravel, irritability, and inflammation) and notes that dogs will seek out couch grass and soon after ingesting it, will vomit as a "cleansing" method (de Bairacli Levy, 1985). Greig noted that the herb was recommended for cystitis and urethritis in dogs as late as 1942. He also noted that dogs seek out and eat couch grass (Greig, 1942).
Published Research: Couch grass does not appear to have any effect on the main urolithiasis risk factors in calcium oxalate urolithiais in rats (Grases, 1995). In sheep, couch grass is a source of crude protein fed as hay (Christen, 1990).
Indications: Urinary tract infection, arthritis, and rheumatism

Potential Veterinary Uses: Urinary tract infection, inflammation
Contraindications: None found
Toxicology and Adverse Effects: HPA class 1. Couch grass is a common cause of atopy in dogs (Mueller, 2000); use medicinally with caution if atopy is suspected.
Drug Interactions: None found
Dosage:
Human:
Dried herb: 3-10 g TID, up to 6 times daily for acute conditions
Infusions: 5-30 g per cup of water, with 1 cup of the tea given TID, up to 6 times daily acutely
Decoction: simmer 30 g of rhizome in 500 mL for 15 to 20 min
Fluid extract (1:1) in 25% ethanol: 3-8 mL TID
Tincture 1:2 or 1:3: 1-5 mL TID, up to 6 times daily for acute conditions
Small Animal:
Dried herb: 50-400 mg/kg, divided daily (optimally, TID)
Decoction: 30 g per cup of water, administered at a rate of ¼-½ cup per 10 kg (20 lb), divided daily (optimally, TID)
Tincture: 1:2-1:3: 1.0-2.0 mL per 10 kg (20 lb), divided daily (optimally, TID) and diluted or combined with other herbs. Higher doses may be appropriate if the herb is used singly and is not combined in a formula.
Historical Veterinary Doses:
Dog
Liquid extract (1:2): 1-2 dr (3.7-7.4 mL) (Greig, 1942)

References

Christen AM, Seoane JR, Leroux GD. The nutritive value for sheep of quackgrass and timothy hays harvested at two stages of growth. J Anim Sci 1990;68:3350-3359.

De Bairacli Levy J. *The Complete Herbal Handbook for the Dog and Cat.* London: Faber and Faber; 1985.

Grases F, Ramis M, Costa-Bauza A, March JG. Effect of *Herniaria hirsuta* and *Agropyron repens* on calcium oxalate urolithiasis risk in rats. J Ethnopharmacol 1995;45:211-214.

Grieg JR, Boddie GF. *Hoare's Veterinary Materia Medica and Therapeutics.* 6th edition. London: Bailliere, Tindall and Cox; 1942.

Mueller RS, Bettenay SV, Tideman L. Aero-allergens in canine atopic dermatitis in southeastern Australia based on 1000 intradermal skin tests. Aust Vet J 2000;78:392-399.

Cramp Bark

Viburnum opulus L. • vy-BUR-num OP-yoo-lus
Other Names: Guelder rose, European cranberry, snowball, high-bush cranberry
Family: Caprifoliaceae
Parts Used: Stem bark
Distribution: Indigenous to Canada and North America. Cramp bark grows wild in Europe, Britain, Russia, and Asia. The name Guelder Rose comes from Gueldersland, a Dutch province, where the tree was first cultivated.
Selected Constituents: Virburnin, a bitter glucoside, valerianic acid, salicosides, tannins, coumarins, resin, arbutin (Petricic, 1980)
Clinical Actions: Antispasmodic, sedative, astringent
Energetics: Cool, dry
History and Traditional Usage: A decoction made from the bark was traditionally used to provide relief from cramps and spasms of involuntary muscular contractions. It is used for menstrual cramps, to relax the uterus and alleviate cramping during miscarriage, and to relax intestinal cramping. Also taken for spasms of all kinds, such as convulsions, seizures, and lockjaw. It is used to calm hysteria and nervous debility and also for heart disease, palpitations, and rheumatism. *King's* lists the specific Eclectic indications as "Cramps; uterine pain, with spasmodic action; pain in thighs and back; bearing down, expulsive pains; neuralgic or spasmodic dysmenorrhea. As an antiabortive."
Published Research: The effects of a complex of oligomeric anthocyanidins from cramp bark were investigated in induced hepatic damage in rats. The hepatoprotectants legalon and pycnogenol were used as standards. The complex of oligomeric anthocyanidins showed pronounced antitoxic and antioxidant actions; it inhibited lipid peroxidation processes, normalized the level of antiradical hepatic activity, and had a gluthathione-sparing effect. It was concluded that the preparation can be used for the prevention and treatment of toxic hepatic lesions (Sprygin, 2003).

Immunestimulating properties were found in the polysaccharides from *V. opulus:* They enhanced phagocytosis, the phagocytic index, and secretion of lysosomal enzymes in peritoneal macrophages. Calcium ions were found to be necessary for the immunestimulating effect (Ovodova, 2000).

A digitalis-type cardiotonic action of aqueous extracts of bark, leaves, fruit, and flowers of *Viburnum lantana, V. opulus,* and *V. opulus* var. *sterilis* was demonstrated. The bark extract was found to be the most active (Vlad, 1977).
Indications: Muscle tension relaxant, especially active on smooth muscle; for threatened miscarriage, uterine dysfunction, ovarian and uterine pain, and partus preparatory
Potential Veterinary Indications: Muscle cramps, trigger points, due to smooth muscle spasm pain
Contraindications: None known.
Toxicology and Adverse Effects: AHPA class 1. None known.
Dosage:
Human:
Dried herb: 1-10 g TID, up to 6 times daily for acute conditions
Infusions and decoctions: 5-30 g per cup of water, with 1 cup of the tea given TID, up to 6 times daily acutely
Tincture (available as 30%-70% alcohol; some pharmacies include glycerin to prevent precipitation of tannins): 1:2 or 1:3: 1-5 mL TID, up to 6 times daily for acute conditions
Small Animal:
Dried herb: 25-200 mg/kg, divided daily (optimally, TID)
Infusion: 5-30 g per cup of water, administered at a rate of ¼-½ cup per 10 kg (20 lb), divided daily (optimally, TID)
Tincture (available as 30%-70% alcohol; some pharmacies include glycerin to prevent precipitation of tannins): 1:2-1:3:

0.5-1.0 mL per 10 kg (20 lb), divided daily (optimally, TID) and diluted or combined with other herbs. Higher doses may be appropriate if the herb is used singly and is not combined in a formula.

References

Ovodova RG, Golovchenko VV, Popov SV. [The isolation, preliminary study of structure and physiological activity of water-soluble polysaccharides from squeezed berries of Snowball tree *Viburnum opulus*] [Russian]. Bioorganicheskaia Khimiia 2000;26:61-67.

Petricic J, Stanic G. Flavonoids. saponins, tannins, and arbutin as constituents of leaves of *Viburnum tinus, V. opulus* and *V. lantana*. Acta Pharmaceut Jugoslav 1980;30:97-101.

Sprygin VG, Kushnerova NF, Rakhmanin IA, et al. Antioxidant action of oligomeric anthocyanidins isolated from *Viburnum opuli* on liver lesions caused by carbon tetrachloride and prevention of its toxic effects [Russian]. Gigiena i Sanitariya 2003;3:57-60.

Vlad L, Munta A, Crisan IG. Digitalis-type cardiotonic action of *Viburnum* species extracts [German]. Planta Med 1977;31: 228-231.

Zholobova ZP. Honeysuckle and viburnum as valuable food and medicinal plants [Russian]. Agrotekhnika i Selektsiya Sadovykh Kul'tur 1983;11:39-46.

Cranberry

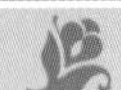

Vaccinium macrocarpon Aiton • vak-SIN-ee-um mak-roh-KAR-pon

Family: Ericaceae

Distribution: Native to North America and northern Asia, favoring acidic wet areas such as bogs and marshes

Parts Used: Fruit

Selected Constituents: Constituents of cranberry fruit or juice (not commercial cranberry juice or extracts) include proanthocyanidins (procyanidins and polyphenols), catechins, epicatechin, and cyadin. Also included are polyphenols, procyanidins, anthocyanins (fruit), and flavonoids such as quercetin and myricetin. Organic acids include quinic, malic, glucaronic, ascorbic, citric, and benzoic acids. Hippuric acid (derived from benzoic and quinic acids), amino acids, and peptides are included, as are the sugars fructose and D-mannose.

Clinical Actions: Antimicrobial

Energetics: Astringent

History and Traditional Usage: Used during the 17th century for blood disorders, stomach ailments, liver and gallbladder disorders, appetite loss and vomiting, cancer, and scurvy. Cranberry juice has been widely used for the treatment and prevention of urinary tract infection and is reputed to give symptomatic relief from these infections. Traditionally, the juice was thought to cause acidification of the urine, resulting in a bacteriostatic effect. However, recent research has demonstrated that a bacterial antiadhesion mechanism is responsible (Howell, 2002).

Published Research: Cranberry juice may have the ability to lower urinary pH (Jackson, 1997); however, urinary pH of an experimental group was 6.0 compared with the control value of 5.5, suggesting that urinary acidification is not the mechanism of action (Barry, 1997).

Cranberry concentrate at pH 7.0 irreversibly inhibited *Escherichia coli* adherence in vitro, probably by preventing proper attachment of fimbrial subunits or by preventing expression of normal fimbriae (Ahuja, 1998). Mice given cranberry juice in place of their normal water supply for a period of 14 days exhibited suppressed adherence of *E. coli* to uroepithelial cells by approximately 80% (Sabota, 1984). Cranberry juice cocktail provided anti-adherence activity toward gram-negative rods, including *Klebsiella, Enterobacter, Pseudomonas,* and *Proteus* (Schmidt, 1988).

In a randomized, double-blind, placebo-controlled trial, the use of a cranberry beverage (300 mL/day) reduced the frequency of bacteriuria with pyuria in older women (Avorn, 1994). Cranberry juice was a potent inhibitor of bacterial adherence in 15 of 22 subjects for up to 3 hours after drinking 15 oz cranberry juice (Sabota, 1984). Cranberry juice increased hippuric acid, but this is thought to be insufficient for bacteriostasis (Barry, 1997).

As a preventative, cranberry (as juice or capsule) significantly reduces the recurrence rate of urinary tract infection in women (based on a review of two randomly controlled trials). Evidence supports the use of cranberry to prevent urinary tract infection in some populations but none to support its use as a treatment (Griffiths, 2003).

Cranberry juice decreased catheter blockage (from excess mucus production), reduced pyuria, and improved urine odor in children (Rogers, 1991). Conversely, liquid cranberry products taken on a daily basis at the dosage employed (15 mL/kg/day) did not have any effect greater than that of water in preventing urinary tract infection in a pediatric neuropathic bladder population (Foda, 1995).

In a study undertaken to investigate the potential influence of cranberry juice on urinary risk factors associated with the formation of calcium oxalate kidney stones, the ingestion of cranberry juice significantly and uniquely altered three key urinary risk factors. Oxalate and phosphate excretion decreased, and citrate excretion increased. In addition, a decrease was noted in the relative supersaturation of calcium oxalate, which tended to be significantly lower than that induced by water alone. The study concluded that cranberry juice has antilithogenic properties and, as such, deserves consideration as a conservative therapeutic protocol in managing calcium oxalate urolithiasis (McHarg, 2003). However, paradoxically, cranberry juice has a moderately high concentration of oxalate, a common component of kidney stones, and should be limited in patients with a history of nephrolithiasis. In five healthy volunteers, urinary oxalate levels significantly increased by an average of 43.4% when cranberry tablets were taken. Excretion of the potentially lithogenic ions calcium, phosphate, and sodium also increased. On the other hand, quantities of inhibitors of stone formation, magnesium, and potassium increased as well (Terris, 2001).

Urostomy patients frequently suffer peristomal skin problems that may stem from alkaline urine. In a study on human urostomy, drinking of cranberry juice did not appear to acidify the urine as expected; however, improvements in skin condition were still seen among study participants, suggesting that drinking of cranberry juice positively affects the incidence of skin complications in these patients (Tsukada, 1994).

Indications: Prevention of urinary tract infection and treatment of urinary tract infection, bacteriuria, pyuria, and cystitis. Improvements in urinary odor, urinary tract mucous production, and peristomal skin conditions in patients that have undergone urinary tract surgery or those that are catheterized. Prevention of struvite and calcium carbonate, linked to alkaline urine (Leaver, 1996).

Potential Veterinary Uses: Prevention of urinary tract infection; possibly for prevention of struvite and calcium carbonate urolithiasis; as adjunct in acute and chronic cystitis, post urethrostomy surgery

Contraindications: Caution should be used in patients with renal insufficiency. In a study of normal and uremic men, cranberry increased renal excretion of hippuric acid and increased acid secretion in the nephron (Cathcart-Rake, 1975). Should also be avoided in patients with urate or calcium oxalate stones because of the high oxalate content of cranberry (Terris, 2001).

Toxicology and Adverse Effects: This food was not rated by the AHPA. None known.

Drug Interactions: None known.

Dosage

Human:

Fresh berries: 10-20 per day (the berry is quite tart and is usually prepared in some way with sugar)

Juice: 300-600 mL/day, 4-8 wk

Dried extract: 400 mg BID

Tincture: 1:2 or 1:3: 3-5 mL TID, up to 6 times daily for acute conditions

Small Animal:

Dried extract: 20 mg/kg, divided daily

Juice: 1 mL/kg per day, divided daily (may be diluted and added to food); use low-sugar products and aim for highest juice concentrate possible

Tincture: 1:2-1:3: 1.0-3.0 mL per 10 kg (20 lb), divided daily (optimally, TID) and diluted or combined with other herbs

Combinations: Bearberry, crataeva, buchu, urinary alkinizers

References

Ahuja S, Kaack B, Roberts J. Loss of fimbrial adhesion with the addition of *Vaccinium macrocarpon* to the growth medium of P fimbriated *Escherichia coli*. J Urol 1998;159:559-562.

Avorn J, Monane M, Gurwitz JH, Glynn RJ, Choodnovskiy I, Lipsitz LA. Reduction of bacteriuria and pyuria after ingestion of cranberry juice. JAMA 1994;271:751-754.

Barry P. Does cranberry juice play a therapeutic role in urinary tract infections? A literature review. J N Z Diet Assoc 1997; 51:17-18.

Cathcart-Rake W, Porter R, Whittier F, Stein P, Carey M, Grantham J. Effect of diet on serum accumulation and renal excretion of aryl acids and secretory activity in normal and uremic man. Am J Clin Nutr 1975;28:1110-1115.

Foda MM, Middlebrook PF, Gatfield CT, Potvin G, Wells G, Schillinger JF. Efficacy of cranberry in prevention of urinary tract infection in a susceptible pediatric population. Can J Urol 1995;2:98-102.

Griffiths P. The role of cranberry juice in the treatment of urinary tract infections. Br J Commun Nurs 2003;8:557-561.

Hamilton-Miller JM. Reduction of bacteriuria and pyuria using cranberry juice. JAMA 1994;272:588; author reply 589-590.

Howell AB. Cranberry proanthocyanidins and the maintenance of urinary tract health. Crit Rev Food Sci Nutr 2002;42 (3 suppl):273-278.

Jackson B, Hicks LE. Effect of cranberry juice on urinary pH in older adults. Home Health Nurse 1997;15:198-202.

Leaver RB. Cranberry juice. Prof Nurse 1996;11:525-526.

McHarg T, Rodgers A, Charlton K. Influence of cranberry juice on the urinary risk factors for calcium oxalate kidney stone formation. BJU Int 2003;92:765-768.

Rogers J. Pass the cranberry juice. Nurs Times 1991;87:36-37.

Sabota AE. Inhibition of bacterial adherence by cranberry juice: potential use for the treatment of urinary tract infections. J Urol 1984;131:1013-1016.

Schmidt D, Sobota A. An examination of the anti-adherence activity of cranberry juice on urinary and nonurinary bacterial isolates. Microbios 1988;55:173-181.

Terris MK, Issa MM, Tacker JR. Dietary supplementation with cranberry concentrate tablets may increase the risk of nephrolithiasis. Urology 2001;57:26-29.

Tsukada K, Tokunaga K, Iwama T, Mishima Y, Tazawa K, Fujimaki M. Cranberry juice and its impact on peristomal skin conditions for urostomy patients. Ostomy Wound Manage 1994; 40:60-62,64,66-68.

Damiana

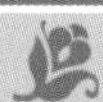

Turnera diffusa Willd ex. Schult. var. diffusa or *Turnera diffusa* Willd ex. Schult. var. aphrodisiaca (Ward) Urb. Syn. *Turnera aphrodisiaca* Ward • TER-ner-uh dy-FEW-suh

Other Names: Old woman's broom

Family: Turneraceae

Parts Used: Leaf

Distribution: Damiana prefers hot, humid climates and is native to Texas, Mexico, and Central America.

Selected Constituents: 0.5%-1% volatile oil, arbutin, tannin, damianin, gonzalitosin (cyanogenic glycoside), and beta-sitosterol

Clinical Actions: Antidepressant, mild purgative, stomachic

Energetics: Dry, neutral

History and Traditional Usage: Damiana, also called the "lover's herb" because of its ancient reputation as an aphrodisiac, is used in Europe to support both male and female sexuality; however, because it has a testosterone-like effect, it has been considered "the male herb."

Damiana has been used for orchitis, impotence, exhaustion, cystitis, nephritis, and enuresis. Damiana has further use as a mild purgative and a diuretic, and to treat patients with constipation and nervous afflictions, such as depression, lethargy, and nervous dyspepsia; it is specifically indicated in anxiety associated with sexuality. Milks (1949) lists damiana as an aphrodisiac for animals, theorizing that it acts as a general stimulant of the nervous system.

Published Research: *Turnera diffusa* was shown to have antibacterial activity against 14 bacterial strains that cause the most common gastrointestinal diseases in the Mexican population (Hernandez, 2003).

One study appeared to support the folk reputation of *Turnera diffusa* (Arletti, 1999). Male rats that were sexually potent or sexually sluggish/impotent were treated (PO) with different amounts of *Turnera diffusa;* it improved the copulatory performance of sexually sluggish or impotent rats but had no effect on sexually potent rats. The highest dose (1 mL/kg of fluid extract) increased the percentage of rats that achieved ejaculation and significantly reduced times for mounting, intromission, and ejaculation, as well as the postejaculatory and intercopulatory intervals.

Turnera diffusa (damiana) significantly decreased the glycemic peak and/or the area under the glucose tolerance curve in temporarily hyperglycemic rabbits, suggesting the validity of study toward clinical use in the control of diabetes mellitus (Alarcon-Aguilara, 1998).

Indications: Anxiety, depression, nervous dyspepsia, atonic constipation, decreased libido

Potential Veterinary Indications: Male reproductive disorders, mild aphrodisiac

Contraindications: None known.

Toxicology and Adverse Effects: AHPA class 1. No adverse effects known.

Dosage:

Human:

Dried herb: 3-10 g TID

Infusions and decoctions: 5-30 g per cup of water, with 1 cup of the tea given TID

Fluid extract (1:1): 3-15 mL TID (Felter, 1898; Bartram, 1995)

Tincture (usually in 60%-65% ethanol): 1:2 or 1:3: 1-5 mL TID

Small Animal:

Dried herb: 25-300 mg/kg, divided daily (optimally, TID)

Infusion: 5-30 g per cup of water, administered at a rate of ¼-½ cup per 10 kg (20 lb), divided daily (optimally, TID)

Tincture (usually in 60%-65% ethanol): 1:2-1:3: 0.5-1.5 mL per 10 kg (20 lb), divided daily (optimally, TID) and diluted or combined with other herbs

References

Alarcon-Aguilara FJ, Roman-Romas R, Perez-Gutierrez S, et al. Study of the anti-hyperglycemic effect of plants used as antidiabetics. J Ethnopharmacol 1998;61:101-110.

Arletti R, Benelli A, Cavazzuti E, et al. Stimulating property of *Turnera diffusa* and *Pfaffia paniculata* extracts on the sexual behavior of male rats. Psychopharmacology (Berl) 1999;143:15-19.

Bartram T. *Bartram's Encyclopedia of Herbal Medicine: The Definitive Guide to the Herbal Treatment of Diseases.* New York: Marlowe and Company, 1995.

Felter HW, Lloyd JU. *King's American Dispensatory* (1898). Available online at Henriette's Herbal Homepage at: http://www.henriettesherbal.com/eclectic/kings/index.html.

Hernandez T, Canales M, Avila JG, et al. Ethnobotany and antibacterial activity of some plants used in traditional medicine of Zapotitlan de las Salinas, Puebla (Mexico). J Ethnopharmacol 2003;88:181-188.

Milks HJ. *Practical Veterinary Pharmacology, Materia Medica and Therapeutics.* Chicago, Ill: Alex Eger, Inc.; 1949.

Dan Shen

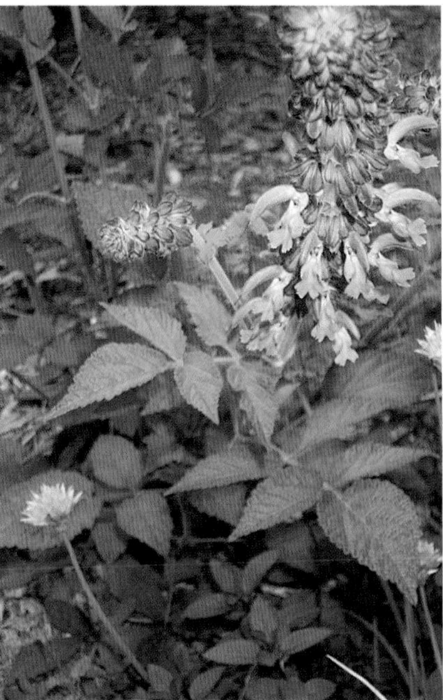

Salvia miltiorrhiza Bunge • SAL-vee-uh mil-tee-OOR-riza

Common Names: Red root sage

Family: Lamiaceae

Parts Used: Root

Distribution: China

Selected Constituents: Tanshinones (diterpine diketones) are the major lipid-soluble "active" constituents from dried roots.

O, O, CH_3, O, H_3C CH_3

Tanshinone IIA

Clinical Actions: Cardioprotective, hypotensive, antiplatelet, anticoagulant, hepatoprotective, fibrinolytic, antimicrobial, vulnery, antifibrotic

Energetics: Bitter, slightly cold; in TCM, a blood mover, blood stasis remover with sedative action

History and Traditional Usage: In China, Dan shen has a traditional use for cardiovascular and cerebrovascular disease and is currently used in Chinese hospitals (usually under the tongue or via injection) to treat patients with angina, acute heart attacks, hypertension, and recovery from stroke (Chang, 1986). Dan shen also has a traditional use in chronic hepatitis and hepatic fibrosis (Hase, 1997).

Published Research: Dan shen potentiates other cardiotonic herbs such as Astragalus but is not in itself cardiotonic, nor does it increase cardiac output (Zhu, 1987). It improves coronary blood flow, however, in dogs with experimental acute myocardial infarction. It has been suggested that it might do this by improving the formation of coronary collateral circulation and protecting the myocardium from ischemia (Liu, 1999). Dan shen has a mild vasodilatory action and causes a drop in blood pressure in rats. Angiotensin-converting enzyme (ACE) activity was inhibited in a dose-dependent manner by the addition of dan shen extract (Kang, 2002). Dan shen is a potent inhibitor of platelet activity; it improves blood flow and deaggregated red blood cells in rabbits with peripheral circulatory disturbances. This is thought to be due to the activity of tanshinone constituents (Chang, 1986). Dan shen yielded good results in disseminated intravascular coagulation, demonstrating anticoagulant and fibrinolytic activity and prolonging thrombosis time; the thrombus size is also reduced (Chang, 1986).

Dan shen is a potent antioxidant with free radical scavenging activity (Kang, 2003). It has been used in heart and lung bypass surgery to reduce myocardial damage (Xia, 2003). It protects rat hepatocytes against carbon tetrachloride (CCl4)-induced necrosis (Hase, 1997).

The effects of dan shen on canine gastric mucosa were investigated. Dan shen increases gastric mucosal blood flow and potential differences (reducing hydrogen ion back-diffusion) in normal tissue, thereby maintaining the integrity of the mucosal barrier and defense functions. However, in aspirin-induced gastric irritation, dan shen could only delay the advance of mucosal lesions. According to this observation, dan shen combined with cimetidine may be used as a prophylactic medicine (Yan, 1990).

Dan shen–injected rabbits with induced impacted vertebrae and spinal cord injury showed histologically less serious damage compared with controls. It was concluded that dan shen has a protective effect on spinal cord injury in the early stages (Ni, 2002). Dan shen caused early formation of dense callus in rabbits with experimental fracture. It increased osteoblast activity in an experimental group of rabbits with induced bone defects, compared with controls. Protein synthesis was also vigorous in fibroblasts. The study suggested that dan shen could enhance mandibular bone fracture healing (Lin, 2002).

Dan shen is used in China for the treatment of patients with cerebrovascular disease, including stroke. Tanshinone I showed in vivo anti-inflammatory activity (Kim, 2002). Tanshinones (16 mg/kg) readily penetrated the blood–brain barrier and reduced brain infarct volume by 30% and 37% 24 hours following treatment with tanshinones. This reduction in brain infarct volume was accompanied by a significant decrease in observed neurologic deficit (Lam, 2003).

In Chinese Medicine, dan shen is used to "nourish the heart and calm the spirit." It has been shown to be active orally as a tranquilizer in animals with some constituents of dan shen binding to the same sites as benzodiazepines do on the γ-aminobutyric acid (GABA) receptor complex. No acute muscle relaxant effect, induction of drug dependence, or withdrawal reactions after long-term administration were observed (Lee, 1991).

Administration of dan shen led to increased plasma estradiol, uterine weight, and ovarian prostaglandin$_{2\alpha}$ content in rats; it also stimulated ovulation in immature mice pretreated with gonadotropin. In pseudopregnant rats, dan shen inhibited the function of the corpus luteum and decreased the level of plasma progesterone (Lee, 1991).

Indications: *Cardiovascular, cerebrovascular, and hepatic disease:* ischemic heart disease, high blood pressure, impaired peripheral and cerebrovascular circulation, acute and chronic liver disease, promotion of healing of fractures and other injuries, nerve compression, autoimmune disease

Potential Veterinary Indications: Feline thrombosis, disseminated intravascular coagulation, ischemic injury, stroke, recovery from cerebrovascular accidents, in combination with H2 blockers or prophylaxis against nonsteroidal anti-inflammatory drug (NSAID)-induced gastritis, chronic active hepatitis in dogs, spinal injury, fracture healing, mild sedation.

Contraindications: Use with caution in patients on anticoagulant and antiplatelet medications or in animals with bleeding tendencies or pregnancy. May potentiate cardiovascular drugs and herbs.

Toxicology and Adverse Effects: AHPA class 1. Has been reported to cause pruritus, stomachache, and reduced appetite. Activated charcoal is effective in preventing absorption of dan shen from the gastrointestinal tract (Dasgupta, 2002).

Drug Interactions: *Salvia miltiorrhiza* can theoretically slow or speed up the metabolism of other drugs in vivo and in vitro because constituents of dan shen can inhibit and induce cytochrome P450, UDP-glucuronosyltransferase, and glutathione S-transferase (Yang, 2002). Three case reports in people—including one that was well documented—suggested that dan shen increased bleeding time through an additive effect with warfarin (Chavez, 2006).

Dosage:

Human:

Dried herb: 1-10 g TID, up to 6 times daily for acute conditions

Infusions and decoctions: 5-30 g per cup of water, with 1 cup of the tea given TID, up to 6 times daily acutely

Tincture: 1:2 or 1:3: 1.5-5 mL TID, up to 6 times daily for acute conditions

Small Animal:

Dried herb: 50-400 mg/kg, divided daily (optimally, TID)

Infusion and decoctions: 5-30 g per cup of water, administered at a rate of ¼-½ cup per 10 kg (20 lb), divided daily (optimally, TID)

Tincture: 1:2-1:3: 1.0-2.0 mL per 10 kg (20 lb), divided daily (optimally, TID) and diluted or combined with other herbs

References

Chang H, But P. *Pharmacology and Applications of Chinese Materia Medica,* vol 1. Singapore: World Scientific Publishing; 1986.

Chavez ML, Jordan MA, Chavez PI. Evidence-based drug-herbal interactions. Life Sci 2006;78:2146-2157.

Dasgupta A, Wahed A, Culton L, Olsen M, Wells A, Actor JK. Activated charcoal is more effective than equilibrium dialysis in removing Chinese medicines Chan Su and Dan Shen from serum, and activated charcoal also prevents further absorption of these agents from G.I. tract in mice: monitoring the effect in clinical laboratory by measuring digoxin activity in serum. Clin Chim Acta 2002;324:51-59.

Hase K, Kasimu R, Basnet P, Kadota S, Namba T. Preventive effect of lithospermate B from *Salvia miltiorrhiza* on experimental hepatitis induced by carbon tetrachloride or D-galactosamine/lipopolysaccharide. Planta Med 1997;63:22-26.

Kang DG, Yun YG, Ryoo JH, Lee HS. Anti-hypertensive effect of water extract of danshen on renovascular hypertension through inhibition of the renin angiotensin system. Am J Chin Med 2002;30:87-93.

Kang HS, Chung HY, Byun DS, Choi JS. Further isolation of antioxidative (+)-1-hydroxypinoresinol-1-O-beta-D-glucoside from the rhizome of *Salvia miltiorrhiza* that acts on peroxynitrite, total ROS and 1,1-diphenyl-2-picrylhydrazyl radical. Arch Pharm Res 2003;26:24-27.

Kim SY, Moon TC, Chang HW, Son KH, Kang SS, Kim HP. Effects of tanshinone I isolated from *Salvia miltiorrhiza* bunge on arachidonic acid metabolism and in vivo inflammatory responses. Phytother Res 2002;16:616-620.

Lam BY, Lo AC, Sun X, Luo HW, Chung SK, Sucher NJ. Neuroprotective effects of tanshinones in transient focal cerebral ischemia in mice. Phytomedicine 2003;10:286-291.

Lee CM, Wong HN, Chui KY, Choang TF, Hon PM, Chang HM. Miltirone, a central benzodiazepine receptor partial agonist from a Chinese medicinal herb *Salvia miltiorrhiza*. Neurosci Lett 1991;127:237-241.

Lin RT. [An experimental study of dan sheng improving the mandibular bone fracture healing]. Zhonghua Kou Qiang Yi Xue Za Zhi 1992;27:215-216,256.

Liu Q, Lu Z. Effect of *Salvia miltiorrhiza* on coronary collateral circulation in dogs with experimental acute myocardial infarction. J Tongji Med Univ 1999;19:40-41,69.

Liu T, Qin CL, Zhang Y, Kang LY, Sun YF, Zhang BL. [Effect of dan-shen, san-qi of different proportion on platelet aggregation and adhesion in normal rabbits]. Zhongguo Zhong Yao Za Zhi 2002;27:609-611.

Ni JD, Ding RK, Lu GH. [Protective effect of dansheng injection on experimental rabbits' spinal cord injury]. Hunan Yi Ke Da Xue Xue Bao 2002;27:507-508.

Xia Z, Gu J, Ansley DM, Xia F, Yu J. Antioxidant therapy with *Salvia miltiorrhiza* decreases plasma endothelin-1 and thromboxane B2 after cardiopulmonary bypass in patients with congenital heart disease. J Thorac Cardiovasc Surg 2003;126:1404-1410.

Yan ZY. [Effect of radix *Salviae miltiorrhizae* on gastric mucosal barrier]. Zhonghua Wai Ke Za Zhi 1990;28:298-301,319.

Yang XF, Wang NP, Zeng FD. [Effects of the active components of some Chinese herbs on drug metabolizing-enzymes]. Zhongguo Zhong Yao Za Zhi 2002;27:325-328.

Zhu BQ, Dai RH [Use of qi-replenishing and stasis-removing herbs in treating patients with heart failure of qi deficiency and blood stasis type]. Zhong Xi Yi Jie He Za Zhi 1987;7:580,591-593.

Dandelion

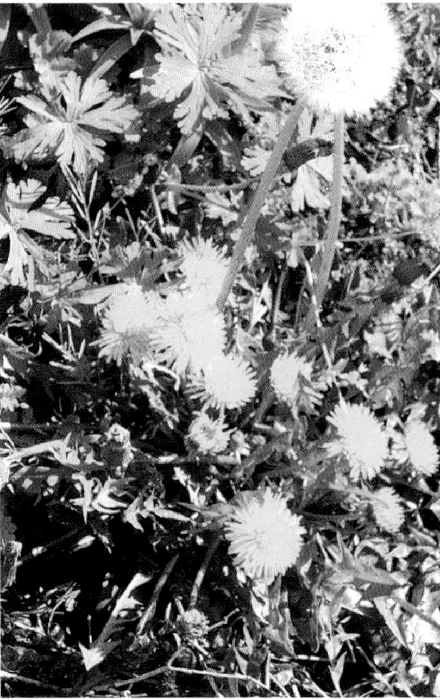

Taraxacum officinale Webster ex. F.H. Wigg. syn. *Taraxacum dens-leonis* Desf. and *Taraxacum vulgare* (Lam.) Schrank • ta-RAKS-uh-kum oh-fiss-ih-NAH-lee

Other Names: Lion's tooth, dent de lion, gemeiner lowenzahn, taraxaco

Family: Asteraceae

Parts Used: Root and leaves

Distribution: Native of western Europe; dandelion originated in Central Asia but now grows almost everywhere.

Selected Constituents: Sesquiterpene lactones such as taraxinic acids, triterpenes—beta-amyrin, taraxol, and taraxerol; carotenoids, including lutein; inulin; saponins; fatty acids such as myristic acid; flavonoids, including apigenin, luteolins, and chrysoeriol; minerals (up to 4.5% potassium); phenolic acids (chicoric and monocaffeyltartaric acids); coumarins (cichoriin and aesculin); sitosterol, stigmasterol, and taraxasterol; sugars; vitamin A; quercetin glycosides

Taraxasterol

Clinical Actions: *Leaf:* diuretic, cholagogue (although not as strong as the root). *Root:* laxative, cholagogue

Energetics: Bitter, cold, dry

History and Traditional Usage: As early as the 7th century, dandelion was recorded as a Chinese herbal medicine. By the 10th and 11th centuries, Arabian physicians referred to it as Taraxacon. The first recording of its use in Europe was around 1485, and its common name was invented by a 15th century surgeon, who compared the shape of the leaves to a lion's tooth—"dent-de-lion." Nicholas Culpeper wrote that a common name for the plant was "piss-a-beds," indicating that the diuretic effect had been noted. Native Americans used dandelions for food, for dermatologic and gastrointestinal problems, as a cure for sore throat, and as an analgesic, sedative, laxative, love potion, and general tonic. In Italy, dandelion sap was used for the treatment of patients with warts. *Taraxacum officinale* has been used as a remedy for women's diseases (e.g., breast and uterine cancer) and disorders of the liver and gallbladder (Koo, 2004). The Eclectics used dandelion root as a digestive bitter and aperient (mild laxative). De Bairacli Levy wrote that goats graze the plant and horses take quantities of the leaves when mixed with bran. She suggested using dandelion for skin eruptions, sluggish blood flow, weak arteries, all liver complaints, jaundice, and constipation (de Bairacli Levy, 1963). Winslow (1909) described dandelion root as a simple stomachic and bitter, and as a useful substitute in these uses for gentian or calumba.

Published Research: Dandelion may be a source of natural antidiabetic compounds. In vitro testing demonstrated that *Taraxacum officinale* showed insulin secretagogue activity (Hussain, 2004). *Taraxacum officinale* showed potent α-glucosidase inhibitory activity (Onal, 2005). However, dandelion did not significantly affect basal glucose and insulin, insulin-induced hypoglycemia, glycated hemoglobin, or pancreatic insulin concentration when given to streptozocin-diabetic mice (Swanston-Flatt, 1989).

Dandelion may be useful in the treatment of patients with acute pancreatitis. In rats with cholecystokinin-induced acute pancreatitis, *Taraxacum officinale* (10 mg/kg po) reduced interleukin-6, a principal mediator of acute phase response, and decreased TNF-α production, thus ameliorating the severity of induced pancreatitis (Seo, 2005).

Infusion of dandelion root in vitro stimulated the growth of 14 strains of bifidobacteria. Dandelion oligofructans were an important source of carbon and energy for bifidobacteria tested (Trojanova, 2004).

Dandelion leaf extract (given orally) had a strong diuretic effect (compared with furosemide) in an experimental model. With the use of high doses, long-term weight loss resulting from diuresis was observed. Dandelion leaf exhibited stronger activity than occurred with dandelion root (Racz-Kotilla, 1974). Diuretic activity was, however, not observed in another study after oral or intraperitoneal administration (Tita, 1993). Herbalists frequently claim that the potassium content in dandelion leaf prevents potassium depletion that occurs with other types of diuretics. However, assuming that a 1:2 tincture of the leaf (containing 4% potassium) supplies 20 mg of potassium per milliliter, at normal doses, the potassium content would not be enough to prevent depletion.

Indications: Leaf: oliguria, edema, cholecystitis
Root: cholecystitis, jaundice, constipation

Potential Veterinary Indications: Digestive tonic (root), liver tonic (root), pancreatitis, triaditis, edema (leaf); as a diuretic for adjunct management of urinary calculi (leaf)

Contraindications: Contraindicated in bile duct obstruction, acute gallbladder inflammation, and intestinal obstruction. The high mineral content of a single species of dandelion (*Taraxacum mongolium*) presents a potential problem for the absorption of quinolone antibiotics. A study was undertaken to discern the interaction between dandelion and ciprofloxacin in rats. Compared with control, maximum plasma concentration of ciprofloxacin was lowered by 73% in treated rats (Zhu, 1999).

Toxicology and Adverse Effects: AHPA class 2d—see contraindication described previously. Allergies to Asteraceae have been reported (Lovell, 1991).

Preparation: Felter and Lloyd note in *King's American Dispensatory* that dried root has very little medicinal activity. *Cook's Physiomedical Dispensatory* recommended preparing it by washing and slicing the fresh root, then mashing it with a mortar and pestle and tincturing it fresh.

Dosage:

Human:

Dried herb: 3-10 g TID, up to 6 times daily for acute conditions

Infusions and decoctions: 5-30 g per cup of water, with 1 cup of the tea given TID, up to 6 times daily acutely

Root tincture (available from 25%-70% ethanol): 1:2 or 1:3: 1-5 mL TID, up to 6 times daily for acute conditions

Leaf tincture (available from 25%-35% alcohol): 1:2 or 1:3: 2-5 mL TID up to 6 times daily for acute conditions

Whole plant tincture: 1:2 or 1:3: 1-5 mL TID up to 6 times daily for acute conditions

Small Animal:

Dried herb: Leaf, root or whole plant: 50-400 mg/kg, divided daily (optimally, TID)

Infusion: 5-30 g per cup of water, administered at a rate of ¼-½ cup per 10 kg (20 lb), divided daily (optimally, TID)

Tincture, root, or whole plant (usually in 25%-70% ethanol): 1:2-1:3: 0.5-1.5 mL per 10 kg (20 lb), divided daily (optimally, TID) and diluted or combined with other herbs. Higher doses may be appropriate if the herb is used singly and is not combined in a formula

Leaf (usually in 25%-35% ethanol): 1:2-1:3: 1.0-2.5 mL per 10 kg (20 lb), divided daily (optimally, TID) and diluted or combined with other herbs. Higher doses may be appropriate if the herb is used singly and is not combined in a formula

Historical Veterinary Doses:

Small Animal

Dried root: Dog, 1-2 dr (4-8 g)

Root juice and fluid extract: Dog, 5-20 grain (0.3-1.3 g) (Winslow, 1908)

Large Animal

Dried root: Horse and cow, 1-2 oz (30-60 g); sheep and swine, 2-4 dr (8-15 g)

Root juice and fluid extract: Horse and cow, 1-4 dr (4-15 g) (Winslow, 1908)

References

de Bairacli Levy J. *Herbal Handbook for Farm and Stable.* London: Faber and Faber; 1963.

Hussain Z, Waheed A, Qureshi RA, et al. The effect of medicinal plants of Islamabad and Murree region of Pakistan on insulin secretion from INS-1 cells. Phytother Res 2004;18:73-77.

Koo HN, Hong SH, Song BK, Kim CH, Yoo YH, Kim HM. *Taraxacum officinale* induces cytotoxicity through TNF-alpha and IL-1 alpha secretion in Hep G2 cells. Life Sci 2004;74:1149-1157.

Lovell CR, Rowan M. Dandelion dermatitis. Contact Dermatitis 1991;25:185-188.

Onal S, Timur S, Okutucu B, Zihnioglu F. Inhibition of alpha-glucosidase by aqueous extracts of some potent antidiabetic medicinal herbs. Prep Biochem Biotechnol 2005;35:29-36.

Racz-Kotilla E, Racz G, Solomon A. The action of *Taraxacum officinale* extracts on the body weight and diuresis of laboratory animals. Planta Med 1974;26:212-217.

Seo SW, Koo HN, An HJ, et al. *Taraxacum officinale* protects against cholecystokinin-induced acute pancreatitis in rats. World J Gastroenterol 2005;11:597-599.

Swanston-Flatt SK, Day C, Flatt PR, Gould BJ, Bailey CJ. Glycaemic effects of traditional European plant treatments for diabetes: studies in normal and streptozotocin diabetic mice. Diabetes Res 1989;10:69-73.

Tita B, Bello U, Faccendini P, et al. Evaluation of dandelion for diuretic activity and variation in potassium content. Int J Pharmacog 1993;31:29-34; Pharmacol Res 1993;27(suppl):23-24.

Trojanova I, Rada V, Kokoska L, Vlkova E. The bifidogenic effect of *Taraxacum officinale* root. Fitoterapia 2004;75:760-763.

Winslow K. *Veterinary Materia Medica and Therapeutics*. New York: William R. Jenkins; 1908.

Zhu M, Wong PY, Li RC. Effects of *Taraxacum mongolicum* on the bioavailability and disposition of ciprofloxacin in rats. J Pharm Sci 1999;88:632-634.

Dang Gui, Dong Quai

Angelica sinensis (Oliv.) Diels syn. *Angelica polymorpha* Maxim var. sinensis Oliv. • an-JEL-ee-kuh sye-NEN-sis

Other Names: Tang kuei, Chinese angelica, radix angelicae sinensis

Family: Apiaceae

Parts Used: Root: In Chinese medicine, the root is divided into three parts: dang gui shen (root body), dang gui tou (root head), and dang gui wei (root tail).

Distribution: Indigenous to China

Selected Constituents: *Essential oils:* ligustilide, butylidenephthalides, terpenes (also phenylpropanoids), coumarins, and umbelliferone (Hsu, 1986; Lin, 1998). Polysaccharides (Ma, 1988)

Clinical Actions: Uterine tonic, anti-inflammatory, regulator of heart rhythm, circulatory stimulant, antiallergic, antiseptic, vasodilator

Energetics: Sweet, acrid, bitter, warm

History and Traditional Usage: In Traditional Chinese Medicine, dang gui is considered a "blood tonic" and "blood mover" that was used in the treatment of menstrual disorders such as irregular menstruation, amenorrhea, and dysmenorrhea. It has been used in China as an analgesic for rheumatic arthralgia and abdominal pain, in the management of postoperative pain, and for the treatment of patients with constipation, anemia, chronic hepatitis, and liver cirrhosis (Pharmacopoeia of the People's Republic of China, 1997; Chang, 1986; Hsu, 1986; Mei, 1991). Other uses described in folk medicine include treatment for dehydration, lumbago, menopausal symptoms (including hot flushes), hypertonia, and nervous disorders (Buck, 1899; Duke, 1985).

Published Research: The polysaccharides of *Angelica sinensis* possess several pharmacologic effects. These include immunoregulation, antioxidation, antitumor activity, prevention of irradiation injury, promotion of hematopoiesis, and promotion of gastrointestinal wound healing in rats in vitro and in vivo (Liu, 2003). *Angelica sinensis* has a protective effect on immunologic colon injury in rats, which is probably due to the mechanisms of antioxidation, immunomodulation, and promotion of wound repair and may be useful in the treatment of patients with inflammatory bowel disease (Liu, 2003).

In vitro and in vivo studies have shown that extracts of dang gui inhibit platelet aggregation and have antithrombotic activity (Mei, 1991; Yang, 2002; Yin, 1980). In ulcerative colitis, platelets can be significantly activated, possibly because of vascular endothelial cell injury. In a study of three groups—39 patients with active ulcerative colitis (UC), 25 with remissive UC, and 30 healthy people—64 UC patients were divided into a routine treatment group and a group given dang gui injection + routine treatment for 3 weeks. Dang gui injection significantly inhibited platelet activation, relieved vascular endothelial cell injury, and improved microcirculation in ulcerative colitis (Dong, 2004).

A decoction of dang gui (11 mL/kg body weight) ameliorated galactosamine-induced hepatotoxicity in rats (Xiong, 1982). Ferulic acid, a constituent of dang gui, protected rat liver mitochondria against damage induced by oxygen free radicals (Lin, 1994).

Dang gui has nonspecific immunostimulatory effects on lymphocyte proliferation. The immunostimulatory effects of dang gui were consistently seen in cell-mediated immune response and in nonspecific lymphoproliferation in vitro (Wilasrusmee, 2002).

In vivo, a polysaccharide of dang gui possessed antitumor effects on experimental tumor models and inhibitory effects on invasion and metastasis of hepatocellular carcinoma cells in vitro (Shang, 2003).

The effects of dang gui injection on acute cerebral infarction were studied. In all, 1404 patients were treated. Group A patients were treated with Angelica injection (n = 692 patients), group B with compound salvia (n = 390 patients), and group C with low-molecular-weight dextran injection (n = 322 patients). Results (measurements on CT scan, infarct volume, and neurologic deficits) were as follows: group A = 78.7% improved, group B = 63.6% improved, and group C = 59.3% improved. Group A rates were significantly higher ($P < .05$). The authors concluded that Angelica injection has therapeutic effects in acute cerebral infarction (Liu, 2004).

Indications: Injury with pain and bruising, poor digestion, and liver disease

Potential Veterinary Indications: Ulcerative colitis, anemia, constipation, abdominal pain, and bruising

Contraindications: In Traditional Chinese Medicine, dang gui is contraindicated in patients with diarrhea, hemorrhagic disease, or hypermenorrhea and should not be used during pregnancy or lactation (Zhu, 1987). Decreased prothrombin times were reported in rabbits that received both a single subcutaneous dose of warfarin

(2 mg/kg) and a repeated oral dose of dang gui (2 g/kg BID for 3 days) (Lo, 1995).

Toxicology and Adverse Effects: AHPA class 2b. Not to be used during pregnancy unless specifically indicated according to the principles of Traditional Chinese Medicine. However, dang gui is specifically used in some cases of threatened miscarriage. Oral administration of dang gui is regarded generally as safe; however, headache may occur in sensitive individuals (Hirata, 1997; Chang, 1986). No adverse reactions were reported in 40 people who received an aqueous root extract by intravenous administration (240 mL/person) for 30 days (Chang, 1986)

Dosage:

Human:

Dried herb: 3-10 g TID (Yarnell); 4.5-9 g total daily dose (Pharmacopoeia of the People's Republic of China, 1997)

Infusions and decoctions: 5-30 g per cup of water, with 1 cup of the tea given TID

Tincture (usually as 50%-80% ethanol): 1:2 or 1:3: 1.5-5 mL TID, up to 6 times daily for acute conditions

Small Animal:

Dried herb: 50-400 mg/kg, divided daily (optimally, TID)

Infusion and decoctions: 5-30 g per cup of water, administered at a rate of ¼-½ cup per 10 kg (20 lb), divided daily (optimally, TID)

Tincture (usually in 50%-80% ethanol): 1:2-1:3: 1.0-2.0 mL per 10 kg (20 lb), divided daily (optimally, TID) and diluted or combined with other herbs

References

Buck P. Un nouveau remède spécifique contre la dysmenorrhée: l'eumenol. Belgique Méd 1899;2:363-365.

Chang HM, But PPH, eds. *Pharmacology and Applications of Chinese Materia Medica,* vol 1. Philadelphia, Pa: World Scientific Publishing; 1986.

Dong WG, Liu SP, Zhu HH, Luo HS, Yu JP. Abnormal function of platelets and role of *Angelica sinensis* in patients with ulcerative colitis. World J Gastroenterol 2004;10:606-609.

Duke JA, Ayensu ES. *Medicinal Plants of China,* vol 1. Algonac, Mich: Reference Publications; 1985.

Hirata JD, et al. Does dong guai have estrogenic effects in postmenopausal women? A double-blind, placebo-controlled trial. Fertil Steril 1997;68:981-986.

Hsu HY. *Oriental Materia Medica, A Concise Guide.* Long Beach, Calif: Oriental Healing Arts Institute; 1986.

Lin LZ, He XG, Lian LZ, King W, Ellrolt J. Liquid chromatographic-electrospray mass spectrometric study of the phthalides of *Angelica sinensis* and chemical changes of Z-ligustilide. J. Chromatography A, 1998;810:71-79.

Lin YH, Zhang JJ, Chen WW. [Protective effect of sodium ferulate on damage of the rat liver mitochondria induced by oxygen free radicals.] Yao Xue Xue Bao 1994;29(3):171-175.

Liu SP, Dong WG, Wu DF, Luo HS, Yu JP. Protective effect of *Angelica sinensis* polysaccharide on experimental immunological colon injury in rats. World J Gastroenterol 2003;9:2786-2790.

Liu YM, Zhang JJ, Jiang J. Observation on clinical effect of Angelica injection in treating acute cerebral infarction [Chinese]. Chin J Integrative Tradit West Med/Zhongguo Zhong Xi Yi Jie He Xue Hui, Zhongguo Zhong Yi Yan Jiu Yuan Zhu Ban 2004;24:205-208.

Lo A, Chan K, Yeung JH, Woo KS. Danggui *(Angelica sinensis)* affects the pharmacodynamics but not the pharmacokinetics of warfarin in rabbits. Eur J Drug Metab Pharmacokinet 1995;20:55-60.

Ma LF. The effect of *Angelica sinensis* polysaccharides on mouse bone marrow hemaopoiesis. Zhonghua Xinxuguanbing Zazhi 1988;9:148-149.

Mei QB, Tao JY, Cui B. Advances in the pharmacological studies of *Radix Angelica sinensis* (Oliv.) Diels (Chinese danggui). Chin Med J 1991;104:776-781.

Pharmacopoeia of the People's Republic of China, vol I (English edition). Beijing: Chemical Industry Press; 1997.

Shang P, Qian AR, Yang TH, Jia M, Mei QB, Cho CH, Zhao WM, Chen ZN. Experimental study of anti-tumor effects of polysaccharides from *Angelica sinensis.* World J. Gastroenterol 2003;9(9):1963-1967.

Wilasrusmee C, Sidaiqui J, Bruch D, Wilasrusmee S, Kittur S, Kittur DS. In vitro immunomodulatory effects of herbal products. Am Surg 2002;68(10):860-864.

Xiong X. The protective effect of radix *Angelicae sinensis* against acute liver damage by D-galactosamine in rats: a histochemical study. Wu-han I Hsyet Yuan Hsueh Pao 1982;11:68-72.

Yang T, Jia M, Mei Q, et al. Effects of Angelica polysaccharide on blood coagulation and platelet aggregation [Chinese]. Zhong Yao Cai 2002;25:344-345.

Yin ZZ. The effect of danggui *(Angelica sinensis)* and its ingredient ferulic acid on rat platelet aggregation and release of 5-HT. Acta Pharmaceut Sin 1980;15:321.

Zhu DPQ. Dong guai. Am J Chin Med 1987;15:117-125.

Devil's Claw

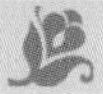

Harpagophytum procumbens (Burch.) DC ex Meisn. • har-pag-o-FY-tum pro-KUM-benz

Distribution: Namibia, Botswana, South Africa, Angola, Zimbabwe, Mozambique

Similar Species: Only two species have been identified in the *Harpagophytum* genus, along with five subspecies. The other species, *Harpagophytum zeyheri,* is commonly harvested and sold as *H. procumbens;* authorities suggest that it is similar in effect.

Other Names: *Radix harpagophyti, Harpagophyti tuberi,* beesdubbetje, duiwelsklou, grapple plant, grapple thorn, kanako, kamangu, kloudoring, ouklip, rankdoring, sengaparile, skerpioendubbeltje, teufelskralle, toutje, tou, tswana, tubercule de griffe du diable, woodspider

Family: Pedaliaceae

Parts Used: Secondary tubers

Selected Constituents: Iridoid glycosides (including harpagoside, harpagide, procumbide, and procumboside and their cinnamic and coumaric acid esters), phenolic glycosides (acteoside, isoacteoside, verbascoside), flavonoids, triterpenes (including oleaic and ursolic acids), polysaccharides (stachyose, raffinose), sterols

Harpagoside

Clinical Action: Bitter tonic, anti-inflammatory, antirheumatic, analgesic
Energetics: Bitter, cool
History and Traditional Usage: Rheumatism, arthritis, digestive complaints, anorexia, labor pains, fever, kidney and bladder ailments
Published Research: Devil's claw has been investigated extensively in humans for the treatment of nonspecific low back pain, arthritis, and rheumatism. Good evidence indicates that dried powders and aqueous extracts that provide more than 50 mg of harpagoside daily are effective for pain relief (Gagnier, 2006; Chrubasik, 2004; Wegener, 2003). In a single randomized, double-dummy, double-blind pilot study of acutely exacerbated low back pain, Doloteffin, a proprietary extract of Harpagophytum, was compared with rofecoxib, a selective cyclooxygenase (COX)-2 inhibitor. No differences were noted between groups for measures such as pain scores and adverse effects (Chrubasik, 2003).

Most authors recognize that the activity of devil's claw is attributable to more constituents than simply harpagoside. The activity of devil's claw is still not well characterized, but one in vitro study showed that it suppressed prostaglandin (PG)E_2 synthesis and nitric oxide production by inhibiting lipopolysaccharide-stimulated enhancement of COX-2 and inducible nitric oxide synthase mRNA expression (Jang, 2003).

A trial that compared a devil's claw formula with phenylbutazone was conducted in 20 horses with bone spavin. The other herbs in the granular formula included *Ribes nigrum* (black currant), *Equisetum arvense* (horsetail), and *Salix alba* (white willow). Ten horses were given phenylbutazone, and ten were given the herbal formula. Horses were evaluated clinically by means of observation for gait asymmetry and irregularity on movement in a 6-meter circle, a flexion test, and radiographic confirmation within the previous 6 months. Each test was rated 0 (undetectable lameness) to 4 (maximum lameness), and a composite score (with a maximum score of 12 for serious lameness) was given at each examination. Horses were given a composite score on days 0, 15, 30, 60, 90, and 120. By day 120, the horses given phenylbutazone had a group score of 8.6, and those given the herbal formula had a score of 6; this was a statistically significant difference (Montavon, 1994).
Indications: Arthritis, rheumatism, gout, low back pain, tendonitis, bursitis, digestive complaints, lack of appetite, liver congestion and gallbladder complaints, menstrual pain, hypertension, headache, antipyretic
Potential Veterinary Indications: Osteoarthritis, back pain, muscle pain (rheumatism); possibly as a tonic for older animals with flagging appetite; many types of pain
Notes of Interest: *H. procumbens* is probably a threatened species in Africa, in part because it was considered a pest by African farmers and stockmen before the medicinal value was recognized by the rest of the world. Attempts to have it placed on the CITES II Appendix met with resistance because of threats to the livelihood of local wildcrafters. Attempts at large-scale cultivation were reportedly under way in 2000 (Schippman, 2000).
Contraindications: *Gastric ulcers:* Devil's claw is believed to have the traditional activity of a digestive bitter (increasing secretion of gastric acid), which may worsen ulcers.
Toxicology and Adverse Effects: AHPA class 2d. The LD_{50} in mice is more than 13.5 g/kg body weight. Although one of the traditional indications for devil's claw is dyspepsia and loss of appetite, use in the presence of gastric or duodenal ulcer is contraindicated. Diarrhea and gastrointestinal distress are possible, but no serious adverse effects have been reported.
Drug Interactions: Devil's claw inhibits the activity of some CYP enzymes (Unger, 2004). Theoretical interactions include the following classes of drugs: antiarrhythmics (none reported), anticoagulants (concurrent use with warfarin-induced purpura), antihypertensives (because the plant has induced hypotension in laboratory animals), and cardiac drugs (herb can increase heart rate and contractility). No reports of clinical drug interactions have been published at the time of this writing.
Dosage:
Human:
Dried herb: 0.5-10 g TID, up to 6 times daily for acute situations
Standardized extract (to 1.5%-3% harpagosides): 1200-2400 mg daily in divided doses
Decoction: 5-30 g per cup of water, with 1 cup of the tea given TID, up to 6 times daily acutely
Decoction: Boil ½-1 tsp in 1 cup water; simmer 10-15 min and administer ¼-1 cup TID
Tincture (usually as 25%-50% ethanol): 1:2 or 1:3: 3-5 mL TID, up to 6 times daily for acute conditions
Small Animal:
Dried herb: 50-500 mg/kg, divided daily (optimally, TID)
Decoction: 5-30 g per cup of water, administered at a rate of ¼-½ cup per 10 kg (20 lb), divided daily (optimally, TID)
Tincture (usually in 25%-50% ethanol): 1:2-1:3: 1.0-2.5 mL per 10 kg (20 lb), divided daily (optimally, TID) and diluted or combined with other herbs

References

Chrubasik S, Conradt C, Roufogalis BD. Effectiveness of Harpagophytum extracts and clinical efficacy. Phytother Res 2004;18:187-189.
Chrubasik S, Model1 A, Black A, Pollak S. A randomized double-blind pilot study comparing Doloteffin® and Vioxx® in the treatment of low back pain. Rheumatology 2003;42:141-148.
Gagnier JJ, Chrubasik S, Manheimer E. *Harpagophytum procumbens* for osteoarthritis and low back pain: a systematic review. BMC Complement Altern Med 2004;4:13.
Jang MH, Lim S, Han SM, et al. *Harpagophytum procumbens* suppresses lipopolysaccharide-stimulated expressions of cyclooxygenase-2 and inducible nitric oxide synthase in fibroblast cell line L929. J Pharmacol Sci 2003;93:367-371.
Montavon S. Efficacy of a phytotherapeutic preparation based on *Harpagophytum procumbens* in case of bone spavin of adult horses [in French]. Prat Vet Equine 1994;26:49-53.
Schippman U. *Focus on Harpagophytum, Newsletter of the Medicinal Plant Specialist Group of the IUCN Species Survival Commission. Medicinal Plant Conservation,* vol 6. Gland, Switzerland: IUCN, The World Conservation Union; 2000.

Unger M, Frank A. Simultaneous determination of the inhibitory potency of herbal extracts on the activity of six major cytochrome P450 enzymes using liquid chromatography/mass spectrometry and automated online extraction. Rapid Commun Mass Spectrom 2004;18:2273.

Wegener T, Lupke NP. Treatment of patients with arthrosis of hip or knee with an aqueous extract of devil's claw (*Harpagophytum procumbens* DC). Phytother Res 2003;17:1165-1172.

Echinacea 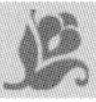

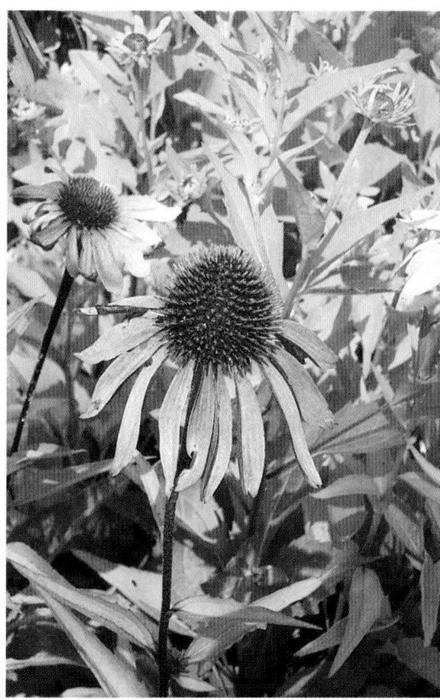

Echinacea purpurea (L.) *Moench and Echinacea angustifolia* DC (two different species but will be reviewed together here). *Echinacea pallida* is also found in trade. • ek-in-NAY-shuh poor-POOR-ee-uh; ek-in-NAY-shuh an-gust-if-FOH-lee-uh

Note Regarding the Historical and Scientific Information in this Monograph: The two species of echinacea in trade deserve separate monographs, which is beyond the scope of this survey. Much of the unreferenced information below is derived from Brinker (2004), where more recent and complete findings on the various echinacea species and preparations are reviewed. This reference is highly recommended for its authoritative comparison of the different species and their various extracts.

Distribution: Native to North America. Grows from Zone 3 southward in North America. Cultivated in other parts of the world.

Similar Species: *E. purpurea* is used interchangeably in trade with *E. angustifolia* and *Echinacea pallida. Echinacea atrorubens* may also be found in echinacea products. *Echinacea laevigata* and *Echinacea tennesseensis* are endangered species. *E. angustifolia* was originally used by the Eclectics, but when American use began to decline, Germans grew their own, which turned out to be *E. purpurea,* on which most current clinical research has been conducted.

Common Names: Purple coneflower, black root, Kansas snakeroot, black sampson, sampson root, Indian comb, Indian head, Kansas coneflower, *Echinacea herba* (pharmaceutical name for the aerial parts), *Echinacea radix* (pharmaceutical name for the root), sonnenhutkraut, igelkopf (German), solhat (Danish). Missouri snakeroot has been sold as echinacea, but it is a contaminant because it is of a different genus *(Parthenium integrifolium).* Western echinacea is *E. angustifolia.*

Family: Asteraceae

Parts Used: *E. angustifolia:* The root was used by early herbalists and is most commonly used today.

E. purpurea: Aerial parts (modern preparations) or 2- to 3-year-old roots (only the roots were used by early American herbalists).

E. angustifolia and *E. pallida* have deep tap roots (adapted to drier climates), and *E. purpurea* has a mass of smaller roots that adapt to wetter climates. This may explain why we more often use aerial parts of *E. purpurea* today.

Collection: Roots are dug in the fall or very early spring. Shoots and flowers are harvested just at the beginning of flowering.

Selected Constituents: *E. purpurea* and *E. angustifolia* are very similar but not identical. The most important constituents are the alkamides (a mixture of dodeca-2E,4E,8Z,10E/Z-tetraenoic acid, isobutylamides 8 and 9, and others), caffeic acid derivatives or phenylpropanoids (cichoric acid and others), echinacoside, cynarin (not in *E. purpurea*), polysaccharides (arabinogalactan, rhamnoarabinogalactan, inulin), and glycoproteins. Flavonoids such as quercetin and kaempferol are also present, as are volatile oils. Contrary to earlier literature, both echinacoside (0%-0.01%) and chlorogenic acid (<0.01%-0.08%) have been reported in aerial parts of *E. purpurea* by other investigators (Binns, 2002; Letchamo, 1999; Perry, 2001).

Cichoric acid

Clinical Action: Alterative, immunestimulant, antimicrobial, anti-inflammatory, local anesthetic, vulnerary, carminative

Energetics: Pungent, cooling, slightly bitter, and slightly sweet

Traditional and Historical Usage: Native Americans used echinacea species topically as an analgesic for toothache, sore throat (gargle), cough, gastrointestinal distress, and venereal disease, topically for wound and burn dressings, as a snakebite remedy, and for the treatment of patients with other skin lesions. Echinacea attracted attention in the 1880s, when the formulator for "Meyer's Blood Purifier" promoted *E. angustifolia* for more widespread study. It became popular for every type of infection, diphtheria, typhoid, measles, puerperal fever, and scarlet fever. One of the earliest clinical studies on echinacea was reported from the Eclectic Medical College in 1933. Students were administered the equivalent of less than 1 g of dried root, and increases in neutrophil and lymphocyte numbers were noted. Numerous case reports published in the early 1900s suggested that *E. angustifolia* was quite effective in the treatment of bacterial and viral infections in people. When European interest increased, a German supplier (Madaus) imported what he thought to be *E. angustifolia* seeds, but instead, they were *E. purpurea*. *E. angustifolia* boasts the most traditional use in the United States; however, *E. purpurea* is supported by most of the scientific research. The Eclectics used *E. pallida* interchangeably with *E. angustifolia*.

King's American Dispensatory states that *E. angustifolia* is useful for abscesses, furuncles, cellulite, swelling from snake or insect bites, septicemia from many sources, fever, ulcerative stomatitis, and a "tendency to malignancy in acute and subacute disorders." The text recommends it for topical pain relief for cancerous growths, as well as for internal use for mammary cancer and cancer cachexia. Case reports from the early 1900s indicated that when low-alcohol or fluid extracts were used as a nasal douche or swab, upper respiratory colds resolved within 24 hours.

The specific indication for echinacea was "to correct fluid deprivation, 'bad blood,' tendency to sepsis and malignancy, as in gangrene, sloughing and phagedenic ulcerations, carbuncles, boils, and various forms of septicaemia; foul discharges, with weakness and emaciation; deepened, bluish or purplish coloration of skin or mucous membranes, with a low form of inflammation; dirty-brownish tongue; jet-black tongue; [and] tendency to the formation of multiple cellular abscesses of semi-active character, with marked asthenia. Of especial importance in typhoid, septicaemic, and other adynamic fevers, and in malignant carbuncle, pulmonary gangrene, cerebrospinal meningitis, and pyosalpinx." Although modern research on echinacea focuses on the systemic treatment of patients with upper respiratory infection, it is interesting to note that traditional indications mention this not at all. Case reports from the early days of echinacea use suggest, on the other hand, that local treatment of nasal mucous membranes with the tincture resolved a simple cold within 24 hours. The Eclectics used mainly high-alcohol extracts, which would have been high in alkamides and phenolics and low in polysaccharides.

The "Specific Echinacea" (of *E. angustifolia*) determined by the Eclectics to be the most efficacious was a 1:1 fluid extract in 65% alcohol. *E. angustifolia* root disappeared from the National Formulary permanently in 1946 because antibiotics overtook it as preferred treatment for patients with bacterial infection.

Echinacea was first mentioned by early 18th century Virginia botanist John Clayton as "beneficial for saddle sores." It was apparently popular as a treatment for "horses with distemper" (strangles). Officially introduced into Eclectic medicine in the 1850s, it does not yet appear in Nelson N. Titus' 1865 classic, *The American Eclectic Practice of Medicine, As Applied to the Diseases of Domestic Animals*. A letter that appeared in a 1928 issue of *Veterinary Medicine* (p 712, no volume or issue available) contains information about echinacea from one Dr. E. L. Quitman. He stated that it was used for "canine distemper, septicemia, pyemia, furunculous and septic febrile conditions in general in all animals. Omphalophlebitis, etc."

Published Research: *Biochemical activity and laboratory animal studies*

A number of echinacea constituents appear to have immune modulating activity, many of them polysaccharides. One of the most well known is arabinogalactan, which has been shown to stimulate macrophage cytokine production and neutrophil and B-lymphocyte activity in vitro. Caffeic acid derivatives and alkylamides have also shown immune modulating activity. Isobutylamides are responsible for enhanced phagocytosis, anti-inflammatory activity, and the mild local anesthetic activity of echinacea. Polyphenolic caffeic acid derivatives inhibit hyaluronidase activity, which influences bacterial and tumor cell migration. Echinacoside appears to provide antibacterial and antiviral activity.

Animal models suggest that echinacea extracts may reduce inflammation and edema, possibly by inhibiting cyclooxygenase and lipoxygenase (Muller-Jakic, 1994). Mouse studies have also demonstrated increased phagocytosis by macrophages and neutrophils when animals were given *E. purpurea*, as well as slightly less activity with *E. pallida* and *E. angustifolia*. *E. angustifolia*, given to mice before they undergo challenge with an antigen, enhanced production of specific IgG. Melchart (1995) administered hydroethanolic extracts of *E. purpurea* root for 5 days to volunteers. Thirty drops TID of a root extract (equivalent to 1 g of root daily) stimulated phagocytosis more effectively than did a 70% ethanol extract from 95% aerial parts and 5% root. A root extract made with 50% alcohol and then dried was less effective than the same extract supplied as a liquid (Melchart, 1995).

Fungal infection

Pretreatment with echinacea extracts reduced infective loads of *Candida albicans* in mice. One human clinical trial (in women with vaginal candidiasis) suggests that concurrent use of topical econazole cream and oral use of *E. purpurea* may suppress *C. albicans* reinfection significantly better than the cream alone. The dose given to women in this trial was 30 drops of plant juice TID (Coeugniet, 1986).

Upper respiratory infection

E. purpurea: Various forms of this plant have been investigated in the treatment and prevention of colds and flu. In one trial, a proprietary combination of *E. purpurea* dried root extract (6:1) along with *E. purpurea* and *E. angustifolia* leaves, flowers, and stems, was given to people in the form of a tea. People drank 8 oz of the infusion from 1 teabag 5 to 6 times on the first day and reduced the dosage to 1 cup of tea by the fifth day. Compared with those who drank a control tea of other herbs (peppermint, fennel, ginger, rose hips, papaya leaf, alfalfa, and cinnamon), people taking echinacea had significantly greater symptom relief and shorter duration of symptoms (Lindenmuth, 2000). Another group compared the efficacy of fresh whole plant hydroethanolic extract in tablet form with that of a root extract and a placebo in patients with colds. The whole plant extract was more effective in the 2 doses tested—6.78 mg and 48.27 mg (Brinkeborn, 1999). The expressed juice of the plant, preserved in alcohol, has been shown effective in reducing the severity and duration of colds in double-blind studies of people (Hoheisel, 1997; Schoneberger, 1992). Dose frequency in these last two studies ranged from 20 drops every 2 hours on day 1 and then 3 times daily, to 4 mL twice daily. *E. purpurea* root, 1:5 in 55% alcohol, has been shown to improve flu symptoms dose dependently (compared with placebo) when given to people (Braunig, 1992).

E. purpurea juice may have a role in preventing upper respiratory infection. Two placebo-controlled trials in people given 8 mL daily suggested that treatment may reduce the incidence of infection (Berg, 1998; Grimm, 1999). A modest benefit was seen in Melchart's trial (1998), in which a 1:11 30% alcohol extract was given, 1 mL twice daily 5 days weekly, to prevent colds. The most recent Cochrane Review (Linde, 2006) suggests that evidence is available that preparations of aerial parts may be effective in the early treatment of patients with colds, but that differences in preparations studied may account for inconsistencies in clinical trial results to date.

E. Angustifolia: Dried root of Western echinacea (492 mg) was given, in combination with dried *E. purpurea* roots and aerial parts (496 mg), to people with colds 6 times daily on the first day of symptoms, then 3 times daily for up to 10 days. Despite this seemingly adequate dose and frequency, no difference was observed between people taking echinacea and those taking placebo. The dried root was not a traditional preparation for these herbs (early American herbalists used only the hydroethanolic extracts). Considering that the study of *E. purpurea* given in tea form (above) was more successful, one wonders whether encapsulating the herb does not mitigate some of its effects. It is possible that direct exposure to oropharyngeal tissue is necessary for the herb to better influence immune function.

Oral preparations of Western echinacea that included a low dose (50 drops BID) of low alcohol (1:11 in 30%) extracts have shown little efficacy in preventing upper respiratory infection (Melchart, 1998).

Cancer

Human case series in which terminal patients were given echinacea or combinations did not report improvements in survival times. Echinacea may provide protective effects against the development of cancer. Mice who received dietary echinacea daily throughout life—from youth until late middle age—demonstrated significant longevity/survival differences, as well as differences in various populations of immune/hematopoietic cells. Regular intake of echinacea maintains elevated levels of natural killer cells (Brousseau, 2005).

Wound healing

Animal trials suggest that echinacin (fresh, stabilized, expressed juice of *E. purpurea* aerial parts and root) accelerated wound healing (Meissner, 1987; Kinkel, 1984). Large case series in humans have been reported, but no controlled trials have been undertaken.

Horses: Changes in hematologic measurements

The standardized *Echinacea angustifolia* product Echi-Fend™ (Equine Formulated Echinacea; Bioniche Animal Health, Canada) was administered to eight horses in this double-blind, placebo-controlled, crossover trial. This product is a 1:3 powdered root extract of *E. angustifolia.* Each horse received 1000 mg of the extract in sucrose syrup BID or a placebo of sucrose syrup. At the end of 42 days, horses were not treated for an additional 14 days; then, they were crossed over to receive the other treatment. Results of this study indicated that administration of 1000 mg Echi-Fend BID to horses increased circulating lymphocyte and neutrophil numbers and enhanced neutrophil activity.

Feed efficiency in pigs

In a study of growing pigs, echinacea appeared to increase feed efficiency and growth when supplied at up to 3% of the diet. One hundred pigs were divided into 5 pens and were fed a positive control diet that contained the antibiotic Mecadox® (Carbadox; Pfizer Inc, New York, NY) or one of four different concentrations of echinacea (0%, 0.1%, 0.5%, 2%). The species of echinacea was not reported. In weeks 0 to 2, echinacea at higher levels gave better results. In 3 to 4 weeks, 0.5% and 2% echinacea diets resulted in greater feed efficiency, but by the end of the trial, no difference in growth was noted between the Mecadox and echinacea groups (Holden, 2002).

Immune function in pigs

Echinacea purpurea powder (determined to contain 1.35% cichoric acid) was administered to 120 weaned pigs; its effects on performance, viremia, and the development of the humoral antibody response against porcine reproductive and respiratory syndrome virus (PRRSV) infection were assessed. PRRSV-naive pigs were randomly alloted to one of eight pens in two separate rooms; each pen contained five pigs. Pigs in each of the four pens in each room were administered a different diet. These diets were isocaloric and isolysinic, and they were formulated in the following way: (1) basal diet composed of corn, soybean meal, whey, and essential vitamins and minerals; (2) basal diet plus carbadox (0.055 g/kg of diet; as-fed basis); (3) basal diet plus echinacea 2% (2% of the total diet); and (4) basal diet plus echinacea 4% (4% of the total diet). After 7 days on their diets, pigs were inoculated with PRRSV, and body weight and blood samples were obtained at 7-day intervals. All challenged pigs were infected with PRRSV; unchallenged pigs did not show infection with PRRSV. Blood samples were analyzed for PRRSV and PRRSV-specific antibodies. No difference was observed in average daily gain (ADG), average daily food intake (ADFI), or gain:feed ratio between unchallenged, challenged, and challenged treated with echinacea groups. Echinacea had no effect on the rate or level of antibody response detected by enzyme-linked immunosorbent assay (ELISA). Investigators concluded that *E. purpurea* powder did not enhance growth, exhibit antiviral activity against PRRSV, or increase antibody resistance to the virus (Hermann, 2003).

Upper respiratory infection in dogs

Reichling and associates investigated a powdered *E. purpurea* root extract (1:3) in an open, multicentered clinical trial that compared signs of respiratory disease in dogs before and after treatment. A total of 41 dogs were enrolled and were noted to have at least one of the following chronic or seasonal conditions as listed by the authors: "kennel cough, bronchitis, pharyngitis/tonsillitis, and nonthriving young animals"; these signs were expected to persist for at least 8 weeks if untreated. Dogs were not enrolled if they had received antibiotics, steroids, nonsteroidal anti-inflammatory drugs, anabolic steroids, or other herbal products over the preceding 2 weeks. Signs were noted at time zero and at 4 and 8 weeks post treatment initiation; dogs were given one of four possible scores for improvement: very good, good, moderate, or insufficient. In all, 38 dogs stayed in the trial to its end, and analysis suggested that 92% of them had "good" or "very good" improvement at 4 weeks, which increased to 95% at 8 weeks. With the rather subjective clinical parameters and no proof of actual infection, along with the lack of a control group in this study, it was impossible to assess the efficacy of echinacea.

Indications: Most human clinical trials support the use of *E. purpurea* aerial parts and root for oral use, and the juice of fresh aerial parts to enhance wound healing. *E. angustifolia* has been less well investigated. Popular and traditional uses of all three common echinacea species include the following: topically and internally for snakebites and insect bites, infected injury, focal or generalized infection, septicemia, fever, upper respiratory catarrh, respiratory infection, and digestive disorders such as dyspepsia and ulcerative stomatitis, and orally, for vaginal candidiasis. As a local pain reliever for ulcers, dental pain, and tumors.

Potential Veterinary Indications: Acute and chronic bacterial and viral infections, septicemia; perhaps as a synergistic combination with antibiotics as necessary; stomatitis; topically and perhaps orally for painful skin, ear and wound infections, snakebites, and ulcerated tumors

Notes of Interest: *E. purpurea* and *E. angustifolia* may be adulterated with *Parthenium integrifolium* (American feverfew). Overharvesting of wild echinacea has led to concern about the plant's survival in the wild. North Dakota and Montana have enacted laws that prohibit the harvesting of echinacea on private land.

Contraindications: Allergy to members of the daisy family. Possibly contraindicated in patients with autoimmune disease, although this oft-stated contraindication has not been proved. Most texts recommend the use of echinacea for no longer than 8 weeks, but this warning appears to be unsubstantiated. The Eclectics reported no problems with longer-term use. On the basis of theoretical concerns about stimulating abnormal immune function, the German Commission E stated that echinacea is contraindicated when autoimmune disorders are present, and that it should not be used longer than 2 weeks at a time. Although the occasional case report confirms that echinacea should be used with caution in individuals who have autoimmune disease (Bergner, 1997; George, 2006), concern about the duration of use is less important. In human trials in which *E. purpurea* was taken for 10 to 12 weeks, no adverse effects were reported. A prospective trial was published that compared 206 women who had taken echinacea during pregnancy with 206 women who had not taken echinacea. No difference in live birth rate or malformations was noted between groups (Gallo, 2000).

Toxicology and Adverse Effects: AHPA class 1. Echinacea is very safe. Rare allergic hypersensitivity reactions have been reported. Worsening of immune-mediated signs (such as in asthma) may reflect allergies to this relative of the daisy. A single case report of a 51-year-old woman who was taking buproprion and a combination of vitamins and herbs, including echinacea, suggests that her supplements may have been associated with mild leukopenia. The report notes that buproprion is associated with leukopenia in company literature, so this patient appears to have experienced an unusual drug interaction instead of a clear adverse event related to echinacea.

Drug Interactions: Echinacea may alter the metabolism of drugs that are substrates of CYP3A4 enzymes (e.g., clomipramine, corticosteroids, cyclosporine, diltiazem, fentanyl, imipramine, doxorubicin, ketoconazole, ondansetron, tacrolimus, vinblastine, vincristine), but results of in vitro trials and clinical studies may conflict (Brinker, 2004). It is possible (but has not been proved) that echinacea may counteract immune suppressant drugs.

Preparation Notes: (See important information on echinacea preparations in Chapter 7.) Low-alcohol preparations concentrate the polysaccharides, which have immune modulating and anti-inflammatory properties. Higher alcohol tinctures contain more of the alkamides, which are probably responsible for immune modulating, anti-inflammatory, prophagocytic, and analgesic properties. For oral use, high-alcohol tinctures are probably best.

Quality control of echinacea products has been reported to be variable, but the American Herbal Pharmacopeia is working to standardize analysis procedures. The example below from ConsumerLab.com illustrates the problem that may occur when validated analysis procedures are not recognized and widely adopted:

> "In summary, out of the 25 products originally purchased, only 14 products (56%) passed this review. It is possible that the products that did not contain the expected levels of markers were made from other types or parts of Echinacea, or, perhaps, contained other ingredients altogether. This analysis was determined internally and did not conform with recommended validation procedures. It was based on the constituent profile of *E. purpurea* aerial parts and then applied to *E. purpurea, E. angustifolia,* and *E. pallida* root and aerial products. In this analysis, very high quality *E. angustifolia* and

E. pallida would fail, and poor-quality *E. purpurea* would pass. Most of these findings are questionable without clear caveats regarding their pass-fail criteria and testing parameters."

Dosage:

Human: For infection (especially upper respiratory infection), most herbalists prefer to give this plant at high doses, frequently, at least TID, and up to every 2 to 4 hours in the acute stages

Dried herb: 3-10g TID, up to 6 times daily for acute conditions

Fresh plant juice of E. purpurea: 6-10mL daily po, in divided doses

Infusions and decoctions: 5-30g per cup of water, with 1 cup of the tea given TID, every 2-4 hours acutely

Tincture (usually as 40%-70% ethanol): 1:2 or 1:3: 3-5mL TID, up to 6 times daily for acute conditions

Small Animal: On the basis of human studies and traditional preparations, hydroethanolic liquid extracts may be preferred.

Dried herb: 25-300mg/kg, divided daily (optimally, TID); can be given at higher doses and more frequently in acute stages of infection

Infusion and decoctions: 5-30g per cup of water, administered at a rate of ¼-½ cup per 10kg (20lb), divided daily (optimally, TID)

Tincture (usually in 40%-70% ethanol): 1:2-1:3: 0.5-1.5mL per 10kg (20lb), divided daily (optimally, TID) and diluted or combined with other herbs (acute infections may require more frequent high doses that exceed this range)

Large Animals:

Fluid extract (1:1) (Karreman, 2004): 2-15mL

Historic Veterinary Doses: Fluid extract (1:1) or tincture as noted by Quitman (quoted previously) states that the dose for dogs is 2 to 30 minims and usually no more than 15 minims (0.1-1.8mL), and for horses, 0.5 to 4oz, and for cattle, 1 to 4oz. Quitman notes that the best results in acute septic conditions were obtained when small or moderate doses were given every 2 hours.

Combinations: Echinacea is frequently combined with herbs that are specific for different body systems to treat patients with infections in those systems. Marsden recommends echinacea with baptisia and commiphora for severe upper respiratory infection; with hydrastis and commiphora for milder infection; and with althaea, glycyrrhiza, geranium, agrimonia, baptisia, and hydrastis for bleeding gastric ulcer.

Meyer's Blood Purifier (circa 1886) was a combination of echinacea, hops, and wormwood. Meyer believed this remedy to be useful for various stings and bites, and for serious local and systemic infection.

References

Berg A, Northoff H, König D, Weinstock C, Grathwohl D, Parnham MJ, Stuhlfauth I, Keul J. Influence of Echinacin (EC31) treatment on the exercise-induced immune response in athletes. J Clin Res 1998;1:367-380.

Bergner P. Echinacea: cautions in autoimmune disease? Med Herb 1997;9:17,20.

Binns SE, Purgina B, Bergeron C, Smith ML, Ball L, Baum BR, Arnason JT. Light-mediated antifungal activity of Echinacea extracts. Planta Med 2000;66:241-244.

Braunig B. *Echinacea purureae* radix for strengthening the immune response in flu-like infections. Z Phytother 1992;13:7-13.

Brinkeborn RM, Shah DV, Degenring FH. Echinaforce and other Echinacea fresh plant preparations in the treatment of the common cold. Phytomedicine 1999;6:1-5.

Brinker F. *Complex Herbs, Complete Medicines.* Sandy, Ore: Eclectic Medical Publications; 2004.

Brousseau M, Miller SC. Enhancement of natural killer cells and increased survival of aging mice fed daily Echinacea root extract from youth. Biogerontology 2005;6:157-163.

Coeugniet E, Kuhnast R. Recurrent candidiasis: adjuvant immunotherapy with different formulations of Echinacin®. Therapiewoche 1986;36:3352-3358.

Gallo M, Sarkar M, Au W, et al. Pregnancy outcome following gestational exposure to echinacea: a prospective controlled study. Arch Intern Med 2000;160:3141-3143.

George L, Ioannis E, Radostina T, Antonios M. Severe thrombotic thrombocytopenic purpura (TTP) induced or exacerbated by the immunostimulatory herb Echinacea. Am J Hematol 2006;81:224.

Grimm W, Muller HH. A randomized controlled trial of the effect of fluid extract of *Echinacea purpurea* on the incidence and severity of colds and respiratory infections. Am J Med 1999;106:138-143.

Hermann JR, Honeyman MS, Zimmerman JJ, Thacker BJ, Holden PJ, Chang CC. Effect of dietary *Echinacea purpurea* on viremia and performance in porcine reproductive and respiratory syndrome virus–infected nursery pigs. J Anim Sci 2003;81:2139-2144.

Hoheisel O. Echinagard treatment shortens the course of the common cold: a double blind, placebo controlled clinical trial. Eur J Clin Res 1997;9:261-268.

Holden P. Botanicals as feed additive substitutes in nursery swine diets. Presented at: Third Annual Nutraceutical Alliance Symposium; 2002; Guelph, Ontario.

Karreman HJ. *Treating Dairy Cows Naturally: Thoughts and Strategies.* Paradise, Pa: Paradise Publications; 2004.

Kinkel HJ. Verifiable effect of echinacin ointment on wound healing. Med Klin 1984;79:580-583.

Letchamo W. Cichoric acid and isobutylamide content in *Echinacea purpurea* as influenced by floer developmental stages. In: Janick J, ed. *Perspectives on New Crops and New Uses.* Alexandria, Va: ASHA Press; 1999.

Linde K, Barrett B, Wolkart K, Bauer R, Melchart D. Echinacea for preventing and treating the common cold. Cochrane Database Syst Rev 2006;1:CD000530.

Lindenmuth G, Lindenmuth EB. The efficacy of Echinacea compound herbal tea preparation on the severity and duration of upper respiratory and flu symptoms: a randomized double-blind placebo-controlled study. J Alt Compl Med 2000;6:327-334.

Meissner FK. Experimental studies of the mode of action of herba recens *Echinacea purpurea* on skin flap. Arzneimittelforschung 1987;37:17-20.

Melchart D, Linde K, Fischer P, Kaesmayr J. Echinacea for preventing and treating the common cold. Cochrane Database Syst Rev 2000;2:CD000530.

Melchart D, Linde K, Worku F, Sarkady L, Holzmann M, Jurcic K, Wagner H. Results of five randomized studies on the immunomodulatory activity of preparations of Echinacea. J Alt Compl Med 1995;1:145-160.

Melchart D, Walther E, Linde K, Brandmaier R, Lersch C. Echinacea root extracts for the prevention of upper respiratory tract infections. Arch Fam Med 1998;7:541-545.

Muller-Jakic B, Breu W, Probstle A, Redl K, Greger H, Bauer R. In vitro inhibition of cyclooxygenase and 5-lipoxygenase by alkamides from Echinacea and Achillea species. Planta Med 1994;60:37-40.
O'Neill W, McKee S, Clarke AF. Immunological and haematinic consequences of feeding a standardised Echinacea *(Echinacea angustifolia)* extract to healthy horses. Equine Vet J 2002;34: 222-227.
Percival SS. Use of echinacea in medicine. Biochem Pharmacol 2000;60:155-158.
Perry NB, Burgess EJ, Glennie VL. Echinacea standardization: analytical methods for phenolic compounds and typical levels in medicinal species. J Agric Food Chem 2001;49:1702-1706.
Reichling J, Fitzi J, Furst-Jucker J, Bucher S, Saller R. Echinacea powder: treatment for canine chronic and seasonal upper respiratory tract infections. Schweiz Arch Tierheilk 2003;145:223-231.
Schoneberger D. The influence of immune-stimulating effects of pressed juice from *Echinacea purpurea* on the course and severity of colds. Forum Immunol 1992;8:2-12.
Upton R. *Echinacea purpurea Root. American Herbal Pharmacopeia and Therapeutic Compendium.* Scotts Valley, Calif: American Herbal Pharmacopeia; 2004.
Wichtl M; Norman Granger Bisset, ed. *Herbal Drugs and Phytopharmaceuticals: A Handbook for Practice on a Scientific Basis.* Boca Raton, Fla: CRC Press; 1989.

Websites

Echi-Fend. Available at: http://www.nutraceuticalalliance.com/research_echinachea2.htm. Accessed March 2, 2005.
Herb Research Foundation's Green Paper on Echinacea. Available at: http://www.herbs.org/greenpapers/echinacea.html. Accessed March 6, 2005.
Longwood Herbal Task Force Monograph on Echinacea. Available at: http://www.mcp.edu/herbal/echinacea/echinacea.htm. Accessed March 6, 2005.

Elder

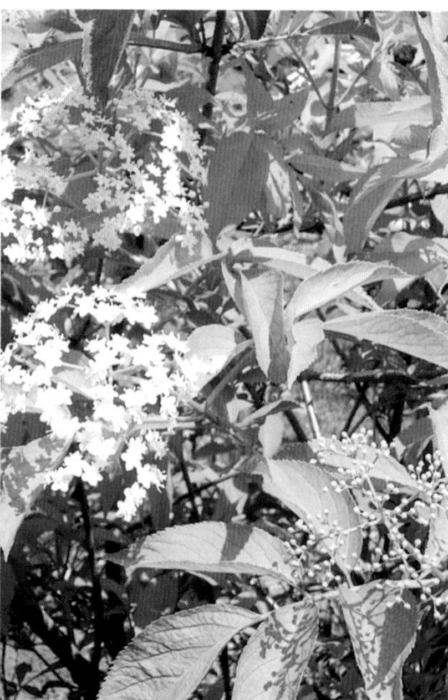

Sambucus nigra L. • sam-BYOO-kus NY-gruh

Other Names: European elder, holunder, black elder, sureau, sauco, sambreco

Flowers: Sambuci flos, bourtree flowers, holunderblüten, aalhornblüten, fliedertee, schwitztee

Berries: Sambuci fructus, baccae, holunderbeeren, baies de Sureau

Family: Caprifoliaceae

Similar Species: *Sambucus canadensis*

Parts Used: Usually the flowers for their diaphoretic effects, but historically also, the leaves and bark; the fruit has been used most often for food but also for medicinal effects, as an antiviral agent.

Selected Constituents: High in rutin. Other flavonoids (e.g., isoquercitrin, hyperoside, astragalin), tannins, mucilage, essential oil, fixed oils, triterpenes, organic acids. Bark and leaf contain the cyanogenic glycoside sambunigrin.

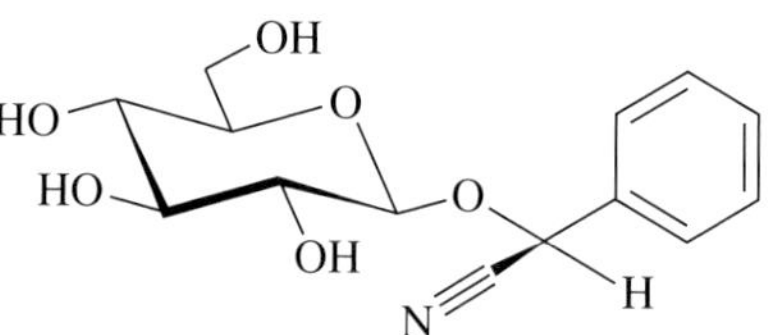

Sambunigrin

Energetics: *Flowers:* pungent, bitter, cool; expel wind. *Berries:* cooling, slightly sweet and acidic

History and Traditional Usage: The leaf is considered purgative, diuretic, expectorant, vulnerary, emollient, and diaphoretic. The flower is diaphoretic, anticatarrhal, and antispasmodic. The berry is diaphoretic, diuretic, laxative, and antirheumatic.

S. canadensis was used internally and topically by various Native American tribes and by the Eclectics. According to *King's,* the fresh inner bark was preferred, although the US Pharmacopoeia (USP) recognized only the flowers at that time. Natives used the bark and roots as an emetic and laxative and topically for skin lesions; flowers were used for fever, as a laxative, and for colic in babies. Berries were used in food and beverages, including wine, as a laxative, and for rheumatism. *S. nigra* is a traditional European herb used by the Cherokee Native Americans for flu, the common cold, and sinusitis; as a gargle for tonsillitis and sore throat; and for coughs and mild constipation. Externally, the leaf is used for focal skin inflammation. It has also been used for sciatica and neuralgia.

Dr. John Clarke, in the *Dictionary of the Materia Medica* (1900), opined: "If sheep or farm animals with footrot have access to the bark and young leaves, they soon cure themselves."

Published Research: A standardized extract has shown significant activity in vitro (via reduced hemagglutination [HI] and suppressed replication) against numerous strains of human influenza virus, as well as Northern European turkey and porcine strains (Zakay-Rones, 1995). In a placebo-controlled, double-blind trial in humans, the same extract resulted in higher titers (via HI), and symptom improvement was reported in those taking the extract (Zakay-Rones, 2004)

Indications: Influenza, colds, sinusitis, and rhinitis. Also used as demulcent tea for tonsillitis and pharyngitis.
Potential Veterinary Indications: Main indications are acute and chronic sinusitis and rhinitis, along with upper respiratory infection.
Contraindications: None reported.
Toxicology and Adverse Effects: AHPA class 1. Leaf and flower are GRAS (generally recognized as safe)-classified flavorings or seasonings. Ingestion of raw or inadequately cooked berries may result in vomiting and diarrhea.
Drug Interactions: May interact with other drugs that are metabolized via CYP3A4 enzymes.
Preparation Notes: Stem pedicles are considered toxic and should be cut out if the bark is used.

The diaphoretic effect is disputed because it is very hot tea that is administered to people with fever, which alone would cause sweating.
Notes of Interest:
Basic Elderberry Wine Recipe: (From Paul Teclaff's Web Page, http://www.patch-work.demon.co.uk/elder.htm#A. Accessed October 11, 2004)
Ingredients
- 4 lb elderberries
- 5 L (1 gal) boiling water
- 3 lb granulated sugar
- A "claret" yeast sachet
- 8 oz chopped raisins
- Juice of 1 lemon
- Juice of 1 orange
- 1 vitamin B tablet
- 1 tsp yeast nutrient

Procedure:
1. Strip the berries from the umbels into a large primary fermentation vessel with a fork.
2. Add 8 oz chopped raisins, juice of the lemon, juice of the orange, a vitamin B tablet, and a teaspoon of yeast nutrient.
3. Add the boiling water and stir well.
4. When cool enough to handle, squeeze fruit with hands to extract juice.
5. Leave for 1 day to infuse.
6. Add 2½ lb sugar and activated yeast, and leave covered for 3 days.
7. Strain off liquid into demijohns; top up with another ¼ lb of sugar in each and, if necessary, with cooled boiled water.
8. Leave to ferment in a warm (65°-75°), dark place.
9. Rack into a clean vessel when bubbling has subsided.
10. Rack again 6 weeks later.
11. Bottle in dark green bottles when wine is clear (use a lamp to shine from the other side) and there has been no activity for some time.
12. Mature for at least 6 months before drinking.

Dosage:
External Use:
Ointment of fresh elder leaf: heat 3 parts leaf with 6 parts melted ointment (homemade, or Vaseline) until the leaves are crisp, then strain.
Internal Use:
Human
Dried herb: 3-10 g TID, up to 6 times daily for acute conditions
Infusion, hot: 5-30 g per cup of water, with 1 cup of the tea given TID, up to 6 times daily acutely
Tincture (available as 25%-60% ethanol; lower doses are used with higher ethanol preparations): 1:2 or 1:3: 3-5 mL TID, up to 6 times daily for acute conditions
Small Animal:
Dried herb: 25-300 mg/kg, divided daily (optimally, TID)
Infusion: 5-30 g per cup of water, administered at a rate of ¼-½ cup per 10 kg (20 lb), divided daily (optimally, TID)
Tincture (usually in 25%-60% ethanol) (lower doses are associated with higher ethanol preparations): 1:2-1:3: 0.5-1.5 mL per 10 kg (20 lb), divided daily (optimally, TID) and diluted or combined with other herbs. Higher doses may be appropriate if the herb is used singly and is not combined in a formula.

References

Zakay-Rones Z, Thom E, Wollan T, Wadstein J. Randomized study of the efficacy and safety of oral elderberry extract in the treatment of influenza A and B virus infections. J Int Med Res 2004;32:132-140.

Zakay-Rones Z, Varsano N, Zlotnik M, et al. Inhibition of several strains of influenza virus in vitro and reduction of symptoms by an elderberry extract (*Sambucus nigra* L.) during an outbreak of influenza B Panama. J Altern Complement Med 1995;1:361-369.

Elecampane 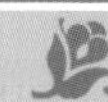

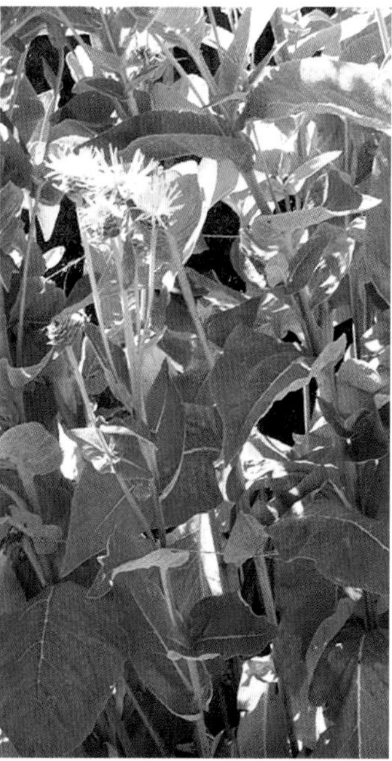

Inula helenium L. • IN-yoo-luh hel-EE-nee-um
Distribution: Native to Southeastern Europe and Asia; naturalized to Europe and the United States
Similar Species: None found.
Other Names: Scabwort, alantwurzelstock, rhizome d'aunee, radix enulae, radix inulae, rhizoma helenii, *Inula campana,* alant, elf dock, elfwort, horse-elder, horseheal, velvet dock, yellow starwort
Family: Asteraceae
Parts Used: Root/rhizome

Collection: The root should be collected in fall, early winter, or early spring.
Selected Constituents: Inulin, mucilage, sterols, and aromatic oils, including the sesquiterpene lactone alantolactone (also known as helenalin)

Helenalin

Inulin

History and Traditional Usage: Expectorant, emmenagogue, diuretic, hepatic, carminative, cholagogue, diaphoretic. Used for "... chronic pulmonary affections, weakness of the digestive organs, hepatic torpor, atonic dyspepsia, with flatus, and internally and externally in tetter, itch, and other cutaneous diseases ... cough of a teasing, persistent character ... catarrhal discharges" *(King's Dispensatory)*. Has also been used against intestinal parasites and as both topical and systemic treatment for skin problems.
Energetics: Aromatic stimulant and tonic, warming, moves *Qi*
Published Research: Studies from the 1940s and 1950s suggest that elecampane root is diuretic, secretolytic, and choleretic (Wichtl, 1994). Most citations in the National Library of Medicine refer to the skin-sensitizing activity of the sesquiterpenes. A dearth of clinical research has been conducted on this herb.
Indications: Productive cough, chronic bronchitis, digestive disturbances due to inactivity/ileus
Potential Veterinary Indications: Chronic bronchitis, asthma, chronic diarrhea or flatus
Notes of Interest: Has been suggested by some herbalists as a substitute for the highly endangered Asian herb, *Saussurea costus,* or for *Saussurea lappa.*
Contraindications: None reported.
Toxicology and Adverse Effects: AHPA class 2b, 2c. Large doses may cause vomiting, diarrhea, spasms, and paralysis. Allergy possible in susceptible individuals.

Drug Interactions: None reported. The possibility that inulin may inhibit glucose absorption from the gut has led some pharmacists to caution patients with diabetes to be aware of interactions with their hypoglycemic drugs.
Dosage:
Human:
Dried herb: 0.25-10 g TID
Infusion, cold: 5-30 g per cup of water, with 1 cup of the tea given TID
Tincture (available as 25%-60% ethanol preparations, lower doses are used for higher ethanol extracts): 1:2 or 1:3: 0.25-5 mL TID, up to 6 times daily for acute conditions
Small Animal:
Dried herb: 25-300 mg/kg, divided daily (optimally, TID)
Infusion: 5-30 g per cup of water, administered at a rate of ¼-½ cup per 10 kg (20 lb), divided daily (optimally, TID)
Tincture (usually in 25%-60% ethanol): 1:2-1:3: 0.5-1.5 mL per 10 kg (20 lb), divided daily (optimally, TID) and diluted or combined with other herbs. Higher doses may be appropriate if the herb is used singly and is not combined in a formula.

Selected Reference

Wichtl M, NG Bisset, eds. Helenii radix. In: *Herbal Drugs and Phytopharmaceuticals.* (English translation by Norman Grainger Bisset.) Stuttgart: CRC Press; 1994:254-256.

Eleuthero, Siberian Ginseng, Eleutherococcus

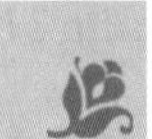

Eleutherococcus senticosus (Rupt and Maxim) Maxim. Formerly, *Acanthopanax senticosus, Hedera senticosus* • el-ew-ther-oh-KOK-us sen-tih-KOH-sus
Other Names: Devil's bush, many prickle, thorny ginseng, touch-me-not, devil's shrub, wild pepper
Family: Araliaceae
Parts Used: Dried bark from the roots and rhizomes
Distribution: Indigenous to North China, Southeast Asia, Japan, Korea, and Southeast Russia
Selected Constituents: *Phenyl propanoids:* syringin (eleutheroside B), caffeic and chlorogenic acids, and esters; *Lignans:* eleutherosides D, E, B4; coumarins: eleutheroside B1; *sterols:* beta-sitosterol, eleutheroside A, polysaccharides, heteroglycans (eleutherans A-G), simple sugars (Bradley, 1992)

An eleutheroside

Clinical Actions: Immune modulating, adaptogenic
Energetics: Acrid, sweet, bitter, warm
History and Traditional Usage: Uses described in pharmacopoeias and in traditional systems of medicine: treatment of patients with rheumatoid arthritis, insomnia, and dream-disturbed sleep (Pharmacopoeia of the People's Republic of China, 1997). Folk medicine uses included treatment for acute and chronic gastritis (as a carminative), as a diuretic, to treat impotence, and to regulate blood pressure (Farnsworth, 1998). Clinical data support use as a tonic (both prophylactic and restorative) for improving mental and physical capacities in weak, exhausted, and tired patients and during convalescence (Farnsworth, 1998; Asano, 1986; Bohn, 1987; Blumenthal, 1998).
Published Research: The mechanism of the antistress or adaptogenic activities of eleuthero is thought to be threefold. Extracts of the roots have an adaptogenic effect that produces a nonspecific increase in the body's defense against exogenous stress factors and noxious chemicals (Farnsworth, 1985; Brekhman, 1969). The roots also stimulate the immune system and promote overall improvement in physical and mental performance (Farnsworth, 1985). A clinical trial investigated the effects of eleuthero on endurance athletes in training. Results suggested that eleuthero increased rather than decreased hormonal indices of stress. This may be consistent with animal research that suggests a threshold of stress below which eleuthero increases the stress response and above which it decreases the stress response, overall, damping or normalizing excessive stress responses (Gaffney, 2001).

A study that used rabbits found that eleuthero increased glycogen storage of the liver by 82% and of the muscles by 32% more than was noted in control animals (Bykhovtzeva, 1966). A later study found that eleuthero extract enhanced the muscle restoration of normal glycogen, adenosine triphosphate (ATP), creatine phosphate, and lactic and pyruvic acid levels after a 2-hour stress/swim test (Brekhman, 1971).

Administration of eleuthero was found to reduce the pathologic effects of cerebral lesions in mice (Kaplan, 1965). A several-year study examined eleuthero in 124 people, half with severe brain injuries. The test group received eleuthero extract ½ hour before meals, and the control group received a placebo. Eleuthero caused a normalizing effect on brain activity and resulted in a higher functional level of recovery. Alleviation of neurodynamic disturbances in the vestibular apparatus and normalizing effects on cerebral hemodynamics, cortical neurodynamics, unconditioned reflex vasculomotor reactions, and leukocyte counts were found (Sandler, 1972a).

The effects of eleuthero polysaccharide against cancer and its immunoregulatory function were studied. Results indicated that its ability to inhibit tumor growth and prolong survival time of tumor-bearing mice was significantly related to the enhanced immune response (Xie, 1989).

A total of 75 people with cancers of the lip and mouth who were to receive radiation therapy were studied. In all, 38 received eleuthero for 2 weeks and 37 controls received a placebo. Eleuthero was taken 1 hour before radiation was administered. The test group reported better sleep, improved appetite, and a renewed interest in life. Better normalization of pulse, blood pressure, and respiration was observed. Tumors receded for both groups; however, wounds in the treatment group healed up to 1 month sooner. Complete lip restoration occurred in 24 test members but in only 14 controls. All patients were observed for 2 years; in the control group, four recurrences and two metastases occurred, and in the test group, no recurrence was observed (Katnashvili, 1964).

Eleuthero given to rats daily for 30 days protected against thrombogenesis induced by intravenous administration of tissue thromboplastin. The effect of the adaptogen was more obvious after a 60-day treatment period (Bazaz'ian, 1987).

A double-blind, placebo-controlled study of 36 diabetic non–insulin-dependent patients was conducted. Patients were treated for 8 weeks with eleuthero (100 or 200 mg) or placebo, and efficacy was evaluated. It was found that use of eleuthero was associated with elevated mood, improved psychophysical performance, and reduced fasting blood glucose and body weight. Patients given the 200-mg dose also experienced improved glycated hemoglobin levels, serum profiles, and levels of physical activity (Sotaniemi, 1995).

Veterinary studies

Eleuthero extracts were found to increase sperm count and volume of ejaculate in bulls (Collison, 1991; Farnsworth, 1985). They were noted to enhance the reproductive capacity of bulls and to increase their semen production by 28% (Maxsimov, 1967). Studies on mink found that eleuthero reduced the number of sterile females and the number of stillborn cubs (Brekhman, 1970).

Research has been undertaken on the efficacy and safety of various eleuthero supplements on the productivity of farm animals of different species and age groups. Supplements were given at the following critical periods only: within the first 10 days of lactation for cows and pigs; from 4.5 to 5.5 months for calves; and 8 days before weaning for suckling pigs. Hens received eleuthero 20 days before expected egg laying. It was found that the milk yield of cows increased by 20%, and this effect continued for a year. Calves grew faster than in the control group and at 18 months surpassed controls by 14 to 16 kg. The milk yield of pigs increased, and suckling pigs were heavier and healthier and weaned more easily. Hens began laying eggs 6 to 11 days earlier; their productivity increased and they became healthier (Protasov, 2000).
Indications: Stress, chemotherapy protection, fatigue, hypertension, ischemic heart disease, immune compromise, infertility, menopause, recuperation from disease or surgery, radiation protection. Tonic for geriatric patients. Possibly useful in cancer, diabetes, depression, alcoholism, and mental disorders. Considered to be less stimulating than *Panax ginseng*.
Potential Veterinary Indications: To aid recovery from acute and chronic disease, for shelter animals under undue stress, to improve performance of athletic animals, as prophylaxis against stress, for improving productivity in food animals, for allergic skin disease, for head and

brain injuries, as an adjunct to radiation therapy, as an adjunct therapy for cancer to reduce adverse effects of conventional therapy, for thrombosis in cats, for disseminated intravascular coagulation (DIC) or pulmonary thromboembolism, for increasing fertility in bulls, for non–insulin dependent diabetes

Contraindications: Some sources claim that eleuthero should not be used during pregnancy or by patients with blood pressure in excess of 180/90 mmHg (24/12 kPa) (Farnsworth, 1998). Long-term use is not recommended (Blumenthal, 1998; Bradley, 1992).

Toxicology and Adverse Effects: AHPA class 1. Negligible toxicity. LD_{50} (po) in dogs >33 mL/kg for ethanolic extract. The incidence of adverse effects is low. Reports include insomnia, irritability, anxiety, tachycardia, palpitations, and headaches (Newall, 1996). Anecdotally, has caused breakthrough menstrual bleeding in some women. A case of elevated serum digoxin level in a patient taking Siberian ginseng and digoxin has been reported. The mechanism remains unclear, and because the electrocardiogram (ECG) was unchanged, it is possible that the herb interfered with the digoxin assay only (McRae, 1996).

Dosage:

Human: If insomnia or agitation occurs, do not administer any doses after 5 PM; if insomnia persists, reduce dose by half

Dried herb: 3-10 g TID

Infusions and decoctions: 5-30 g per cup of water, with 1 cup of the tea given TID

Fluid extract (1:1): 1-2 mL TID

Tincture (usually as 25%-35% ethanol) 1:2 or 1:3: 1-5 mL TID

Small Animal:

Dried herb: 25-400 mg/kg, divided daily (optimally, TID)

Infusion and decoctions: 5-30 g per cup of water, administered at a rate of ¼-½ cup per 10 kg (20 lb), divided daily (optimally, TID)

Tincture (usually in 25%-35% ethanol): 1:2-1:3: 0.5-2.0 mL per 10 kg (20 lb), divided daily (optimally, TID) and diluted or combined with other herbs. Higher doses may be appropriate if the herb is used singly and is not combined in a formula.

References

Asano K, Takahashi T, Miyashita M, et al. Effect of *Eleutherococcus senticosus* extracts on human physical working capacity. Planta Med 1986;4:175-177.

Bazaz'ian GG, Liapina LA, Pastorova VE, et al. Effect of Eleutherococcus on the functional status of the anticoagulation system in older animals [Russian]. Fiziol Zh SSSR Im I M Sechenova 1987;73:1390-1395.

Blumenthal M, Busse WR, Goldberg A, eds. *The Complete Commission E Monographs: Therapeutic Guide to Herbal Medicines.* Boston, Mass: Integrative Medicine Communications; 1998.

Bohn B, Nebe CT, Birr C. Flow-cytometric studies with *Eleutherococcus senticosus* extract as an immunomodulatory agent. Arzneimittelforschung 1987;37:1193-1196.

Bradley PR, ed. *Eleutherococcus* in British Herbal Compendium, vol 1. Bournemouth, Dorset, UK: British Herbal Medicine Association; 1992.

Brekhman II. Eleutherococcus experimental and clinical data. Moscow, USSR: Foreign Trade Publication No. 28017/2; 1970:26.

Brekhman II, Dardymov IV. Mechanism of increasing organism resistance under the effect of ginseng and Eleutherococcus preparations. Sb Rab Inst Tsitol 1971;14:82-85.

Brekhman II, Dardymov IV. Pharmacological investigation of glycosides from ginseng and Eleutherococcus. Lloydia 1969;31:46-51.

Bykhovtzeva TL, Polozhentzeva MI. On the question of the effect of Eleutherococcus on certain metabolic processes. In: *A Summarized Review of the Study of Eleutherococcus in the Soviet Union.* Vladivostok, USSR: The Academy of Sciences; 1966.

Collison RJ. Siberian ginseng (*Eleutherococcus senticosus* Maxim). Br J Phytother 1991;2:61-71.

Farnsworth NR, Kinghorn AD, Soejarto DD, et al. Siberian ginseng *(Eleutherococcus senticosus):* current status as an adaptogen. In: Wagner H, Hikino H, Farnsworth NR, eds. *Economic and Medicinal Plant Research,* vol 1. London: Academic Press; 1985b:217-284.

Gaffney BT, Hugel HM, Rich PA. The effects of *Eleutherococcus senticosus* and *Panax ginseng* on steroidal hormone indices of stress and lymphocyte subset numbers in endurance athletes. Life Sci 2001;70:431-442.

Kaplan EI. The prophylactic effect of *Eleutherococcus senticosus* in craniocerebral trauma in animals. Vostoka, USSR: Lek Sredstva Dal'nego; 1965:77-79.

Katnashvili TM. Trial of the use of the fluid extract of Eleutherococcus in the treatment of patients with lip and mouth cancer. In: *Materials for the Conference on Problems of Medicinal Therapy at the Oncology Clinic.* Leningrad, USSR: 1964.

Maxsimov YL. Eleutherococcus as a vegetable stimulator of the reproductive functions of horned cattle. In: *Eleutherococcus in the Animal Breeding Industry.* Vladivostok, USSR: The Academy of Sciences; 1967:96-102.

McRae S. Elevated serum digoxin levels in a patient taking digoxin and Siberian ginseng. CMAJ 1996;155:293-295.

Newall C, Anderson L, Phillipson JD. *Herbal Medicines: A Guide for Health-Care Professionals.* London: The Pharmaceutical Press; 1996.

Pharmacopoeia of the People's Republic of China, vol I (English edition). Beijing: Chemical Industry Press; 1997.

Protasov BI. *Stress Reduces Animal Productivity.* St. Petersburg: All-Russian Research Institute of Genetics and Breeding of Farming Animals; 2000.

Sandler BI. The influence of Eleutherococcus extract on cerebral circulation in patients with acute cranio-cerebral trauma after rheoencephalography. Lek Sredstva Dal'nego 1972a;11:109-113.

Sotaniemi EA, Haapakoski E, Rautio A. Ginseng therapy in non–insulin-dependent diabetic patients. Diabetes Care 1995;18:1373-1375.

Xie SS. Immunoregulatory effect of polysaccharide of *Acanthopanax senticosus* (PAS). I. Immunological mechanism of PAS against cancer [Chinese]. Zhonghua Zhong Liu Za Zhi 1989;11:338-340.

Eyebright

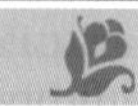

Euphrasia rostkoviana F. Hayne and *Euphrasia stricta* J.P. Wolff ex J.E. Lehm (formerly, *Euphrasia officinalis* L.) • Yew-FRAY-jhuh oh-fiss-ih-NAH-liss

Distribution: Europe

Similar Species: This herb's name is ambiguous and does not denote a single species. *Herbs of Commerce* lists only

E. rostkoviana, F. Hayne and *E. stricta* J.P. Wolff ex J.E. Lehm as the species used in trade. *E. rostkoviana, Euphrasia montana, E. stricta, Euphrasia minima,* and *Euphrasia nemorosa* have all been used, but considerable confusion is revealed in the literature as to which of these species is the "official" one, as well as some question as to whether *E. rostkoviana* and *E. montana* are the same.

Other Names: Euphrasia, bright-eye, birds-eye, meadow eyebright, red eyebright, augentrost, casse-lunettes, oogentroost, eufrasia, adhil, herbal degli occhi

Family: Scrophulariaceae

Parts Used: Above-ground parts

Selected Constituents: Iridoids (e.g., aucubin, euphroside), flavonoids, tannins, phenolic acids, phenylethanoid glycosides (e.g., eukovoside), phytosterols, lignans

Aucubin

History and Traditional Usage: Anti-inflammatory, anticatarrhal, astringent, mild antimicrobial, and bitter tonic. For mucous membranes of eyes, nose, mouth—conjunctivitis, keratitis, rhinitis, sneezing, sore throat, cough—primarily when lacrimation or nasal discharge is watery. Also, for minor skin inflammation and upper gastrointestinal inflammation.

Energetics: Bitter, cold, slightly sour; dries damp and clears heat

Published Research: A recent uncontrolled trial that investigated the efficacy and tolerability of euphrasia eyedrops in humans with conjunctivitis yielded positive results, with only one case of worsening symptoms reported in 65 patients. The authors recommend 1 drop TID in affected eyes (Stoss, 2000).

Indications: Primarily as a tea for eye inflammation; to a lesser extent, for hayfever or allergic rhinitis

Potential Veterinary Indications: Allergic rhinitis (orally), allergic conjunctivitis, keratitis (topically)

Notes of Interest: This herb is harvested from the wild because it is very difficult to cultivate and is sensitive in its environment. Reasonable substitutes should be explored in practice. These might include *Ambrosia* spp (ragweed), *Lythrum salicaria* L. (purple loosestrife), tea *(Camellia sinensis),* chamomile *(Matricaria recutita),* galbanum *(Ferula galbaniflua),* calendula *(Calendula officinalis),* sage, Chinese coptis, and yarrow.

Contraindications: None reported.

Toxicology and Adverse Effects: AHPA class 1. None reported.

Drug Interactions: None reported.

Preparation Notes: The potential for tea to harbor bacteria or other possible pathogens that can colonize the eye should be considered. It should be made fresh daily and kept ***refrigerated*** when not in use. Sterile saline can be used to infuse the herb.

Dosage:

Human:

Dried herb: 3-10 g TID, up to 6 times daily for acute conditions

Infusions and decoctions: 5-10 g per cup of water, with 1 cup of the tea given TID, up to 6 times daily acutely

Tincture (usually 35%-45% ethanol): 1 : 2 or 1 : 3: 0.25-5 mL TID, up to 6 times daily for acute conditions

Small Animal:

Dried herb: 25-200 mg/kg, divided daily (optimally, TID)

Infusion: 5-30 g per cup of water, administered at a rate of $\frac{1}{4}$-$\frac{1}{2}$ cup per 10 kg (20 lb), divided daily (optimally, TID)

Tincture (usually in 35%-45% ethanol): 1 : 2-1 : 3: 0.5-1.0 mL per 10 kg (20 lb), divided daily (optimally, TID) and diluted or combined with other herbs. Higher doses may be appropriate if the herb is used singly and is not combined in a formula.

Selected Reference

Stoss M, Michels C, Peter E, Beutke R, Gorter RW. Prospective cohort trial of Euphrasia single-dose eye drops in conjunctivitis. J Altern Complement Med 2000;6:499-508.

Fennel

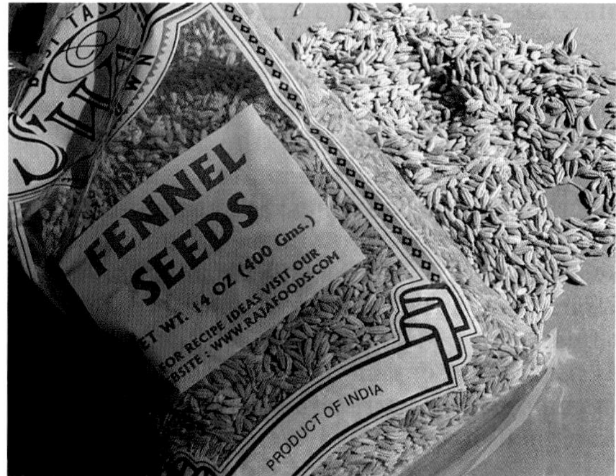

Foeniculum vulgare Mill • fen-IK-yoo-lum vul-GAY-ree

Distribution: Indigenous to the Mediterranean, now growing wild or cultivated worldwide

Similar Species: Two species that are difficult to separate because they hybridize, commonly known as sweet fennel and bitter fennel, are cultivated under the name *Foeniculum vulgare. Foeniculum dulce* is Finnochio, which is cultivated as a vegetable.

Common Names: Fennel, sweet fennel, fenchel, fenkel, bitterfenchel (German), fenouil (French), finnochio (Italian), xiao hui xiang

Family: Apiaceae

Parts Used: Fruits (which are mistakenly called seeds); juice of the fresh plant. The root and dried plant are used for food.
Collection: Fennel can be confused with poison hemlock, so if found in the wild, care should be taken in proper plant identification.
Selected Constituents: Volatile oil, phenylpropanoids (including anethole and estragole), phenolic acids (including caffeic acid), flavonoids, furanocoumarins, fixed oil

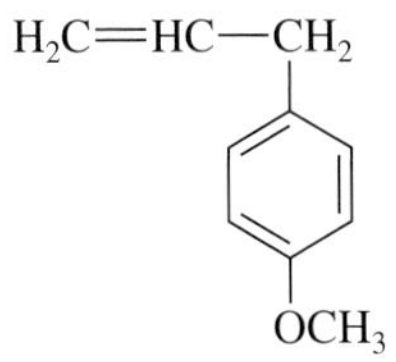

$H_2C{=}HC{-}CH_2$

OCH_3

Estragole

Clinical Actions: Aromatic, stomachic, antispasmodic, carminative, expectorant, galactagogue, antimicrobial
Energetics: Pungent, warm; regulates Qi
History and Traditional Usage: Herbalists as early as Pliny through early English history believed that fennel was good for the eyesight. English herbalists praised fennel for its ability to help people lose weight, and the ancient Greek name for the herb, marathron (from "maraino"—to grow thin), reflects this old belief. It is most commonly used as a remedy for intestinal gas and colic, cough, and conjunctivitis or blepharitis. Fennel was also highly regarded throughout history for stimulating milk production in women.
Published Research: Some fennel constituents (e.g., anethole) are structurally similar to catecholamines, and they possess similar activities, such as bronchodilation and weight loss. Rat studies have shown that various fennel extracts have hypotensive activity (El Bardai, 2001). Fennel relieves inflammation and has inhibitory effects against acute and subacute inflammatory diseases and type IV allergic reactions; it has exhibited a central analgesic effect (Choi, 2004). Tanira et al (1996) showed that fennel extract had diuretic, analgesic, antipyretic, and cholagogue activity in experimental rat studies. Doses up to 3 g/kg were given; at this dose, depression and piloerection were noted. Fennel essentially prevented liver damage in a rat model when CCl4 was used (Ozbek, 2003).

Gastrointestinal effects

Mahadi (2005) investigated the in vitro efficacy of a variety of herbal extracts against *Helicobacter pylori* and found that fennel had a moderate effect, with a mean inhibitory concentration (MIC) of 50 µg/mL. Fennel has long been used to relieve the pain of intestinal spasm. Although the mechanism of action is unknown, fennel and other carminatives are thought to relax smooth muscle spasms that occur in response to filling of the bowels with gas, leading to relief of intestinal cramping. In animals given a fennel infusion, peristalsis tone and amplitude decreased from 2 to 30 minutes after administration. In vitro studies and animal models have indicated that fennel extracts modulate calcium availability and metabolism. Alexandrovich (2003) studied the effects of a fennel oil emulsion for colic in babies. In this multicenter, randomized, placebo-controlled trial, fennel significantly relieved symptoms of colic (defined as a decrease in the number of hours weekly spent crying) compared with placebo.

Respiratory effects

The German Commission E approved fennel for use in upper respiratory catarrh. Fennel tea increased mucociliary transport activity in frog respiratory epithelium in vitro (Muller-Limmroth, 1980). Aerosolized fennel oil suppressed cough initiated mechanically in guinea pigs (Misawa, 1990). In rabbits given anethole and fenchone, respiratory tract fluid was increased in volume and decreased in thickness (Boyd, 1971). The ethanolic extract and essential oil of fennel were shown to relax guinea pig tracheal muscle, but the aqueous extract had no such effect. The authors suggest that the effect is mediated through potassium channels (Boskabady, 2004).

Estrogenic effects

Because fennel was reputed to increase milk production, enhance libido, and promote menstruation, it has been investigated for estrogenic effects. The fennel constituents dianethole and photoanethole resemble stilbene and diethylstilbestrol; anethole is structurally similar to catecholamines—a characteristic that may influence secretion of prolactin. In a study on goats, fennel oil benefited milk production and fat content. Fennel extracts appear to induce estrus in rats (Mills, 2000). A case report describes the effects of ingestion of large amounts of fennel and anise tea on human infants. Mothers drank more than 2 L daily of combination tea to stimulate lactation; their infants were presented for vomiting; weakness in suckling, muscle tone, and crying; and a reduced pain response. Blood test results were normal, and all signs resolved when mothers discontinued the tea (Rosti, 1994). One group investigated the effect of fennel on male pattern hair growth in women with normal menstrual cycles. A 2% alcohol extract applied as a cream resulted in a significant reduction in hair diameter compared with placebo in this double-blind, placebo-controlled trial (Javidnia, 2003). In another study, 60 women with dysmenorrhea were treated with a fennel extract, mefenamic acid, or placebo. In this study, fennel was effective (although less so than mefenamic acid) in relieving pain. A greater number of women in the fennel group withdrew from the study, primarily because of odor, although one woman reported a mild increase in flow (Namavar, 2003).
Indications: Chronic digestive problems, bloating, flatulence, infantile colic, dyspepsia, irritable bowel syndrome, suppressed lacation
Potential Veterinary Indications: Flavoring agent for formulas for colic, flatulence, abdominal pain, chronic cough, inflammatory bowel disease, reduced lactation

Contraindications: Essential oil and concentrated extracts should be used with caution in pregnant animals, but infusions appear to be safe. Very high doses should be avoided in those with liver disease.

Toxicology and Adverse Effects: AHPA class 1. GRAS (generally regarded as safe) as a spice or flavoring. Photodermatitis and contact dermatitis have been reported. A cross-reactivity known in humans as celery-carrot-mugwort-condiment syndrome suggests that an allergic individual may react to other members of the Apiaceae. Seizures resulted when sustained high doses were used, according to a single report.

Drug Interactions: None reported, although theoretical cautions regarding the use of diuretics, blood pressure medication, and ciprofloxacin (Zhu, 1999) have been raised.

Notes of Interest: Fennel given to laying hens gave an aromatic flavor to the eggs (Richter, 2002).

Dosage:

Human:

Dried herb: 2-10 g TID, up to 6 times daily for acute conditions

Infusions and decoctions: 5-30 g per cup of water, with 1 cup of the tea given TID, up to 6 times daily acutely

Tincture (usually 60% ethanol): 1:2 or 1:3: 1-5 mL TID, up to 6 times daily for acute conditions

Small Animal:

Dried herb: 25-300 mg/kg, divided daily (optimally, TID) if extracted and dried; triple or quadruple dose for unprocessed herb

Infusion: 5-30 g per cup of water, administered at a rate of ¼-½ cup per 10 kg (20 lb), divided daily (optimally, TID)

Tincture (usually in 60% ethanol): 1:2-1:3: 0.5-1.5 mL per 10 kg (20 lb), divided daily (optimally, TID) and diluted or combined with other herbs. Higher doses may be appropriate if the herb is used singly and is not combined in a formula.

Historic Veterinary Doses:

Farm animals (Karreman): 30-60 mL for horses and cows; 8-12 mL for sheep and goats

Selected References

Alexandrovich I, Rakovitskaya O, Kolmo E, et al. The effect of fennel *(Foeniculum vulgare)* seed oil emulsion in infantile colic: a randomized, placebo-controlled study. Altern Ther Health Med 2003;9:58-61.

Boskabady MH, Khatami A, Nazari A. Possible mechanism(s) for relaxant effects of *Foeniculum vulgare* on guinea pig tracheal chains. Pharmazie 2004;59:561-564.

Boyd EM, Sheppard EP. An autumn-enhanced mucotropic action of inhaled terpenes and related volatile agents. Pharmacology 1971;6:65-80.

Choi EM, Hwang JK. Antiinflammatory, analgesic and antioxidant activities of the fruit of *Foeniculum vulgare*. Fitoterapia 2004;75:557-565.

El Bardai S, Lyoussi B, Wibo M, Morel N. Pharmacological evidence of hypotensive activity of *Marrubium vulgare* and *Foeniculum vulgare* in spontaneously hypertensive rat. Clin Exp Hypertens 2001;23:329-343.

Javidnia K, Dastgheib L, Mohammadi Samani S, Nasiri A. Antihirsutism activity of Fennel (fruits of *Foeniculum vulgare*) extract: a double-blind placebo controlled study. Phytomedicine 2003;10:455-458.

Karreman H. *Treating Dairy Cows Naturally: Thoughts and Strategies*. Paradise, Pa: Paradise Publications; 2004.

Mahady GB, Pendland SL, Stoia A, Hamill FA, Fabricant D, Dietz BM, Chadwick LR. In vitro susceptibility of *Helicobacter pylori* to botanical extracts used traditionally for the treatment of gastrointestinal disorders. Phytother Res 2005;19:988-991.

Mills S, Bone K. *Principles and Practice of Phytotherapy: Modern Herbal Medicine*. New York, NY: Churchill Livingstone; 2000.

Misawa M, Kizawa M. Antitussive effects of several volatile oils especially of cedar leaf oil in guinea pigs. Pharmacometrics 1990;39:81-93.

Muller-Limmroth W, Frohlich HH. Effect of various phytotherapeutic expectorants on mucociliary transport. Fortschr Med 1980;98:95-101.

Namavar Jahromi B, Tartifizadeh A, Khabnadideh S. Comparison of fennel and mefenamic acid for the treatment of primary dysmenorrhea. Int J Gynaecol Obstet 2003;80:153-157.

Ozbek H, Ugras S, Dulger H, Bayram I, Tuncer I, Ozturk G, Ozturk A. Hepatoprotective effect of *Foeniculum vulgare* essential oil. Fitoterapia 2003;74:317-319.

Richter T, Braun P, Fehlhaber K. [Influence of spiced feed additives on taste of hen's eggs.] Berl Munch Tierarztl Wochenschr 2002;115:200-202.

Rosti LA, Nardini M, Rosti D. Toxic effects of a herbal tea mixture in two newborns. Acta Paediatr 1994;83:683.

Tanira MOM, Shah AH, Mohsin A, Ageel AM, Qureshi S. Pharmacological and toxicological investigations on *Foeniculum vulgare* dried fruit extract in experimental animals. Phytother Res 1996;10:33-36.

Zhu M, Wong PY, Li RC. Effect of oral administration of fennel *(Foeniculum vulgare)* on ciprofloxacin absorption and disposition in the rat. J Pharm Pharmacol 1999;51:1391-1396.

Fenugreek

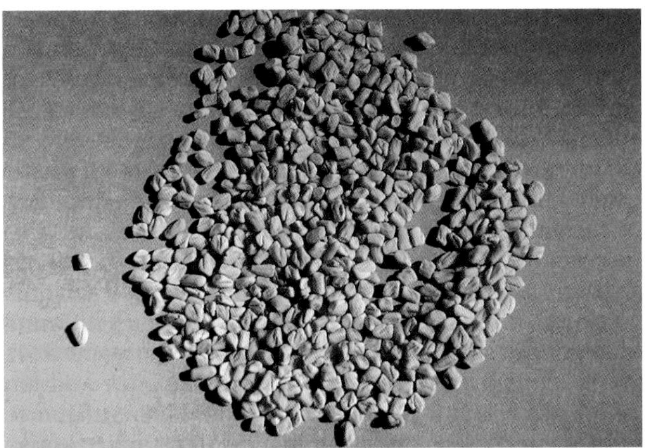

Trigonella foenum-graecum L. • try-go-NEL-uh FEN-um GRAY-kum

Family: Fabaceae

Parts Used: Seed and leaf used most often as food and flavoring in India, the Middle East, and Central Europe

Distribution: Originally from Southeastern Europe and Western Asia, fenugreek now grows and is cultivated commercially in many parts of the world, including India, Northern Africa, Australia, and America.

Other Names: Many, including bird's foot, hulba, fenegriek, fenugreko, trigonelle, trigonella, kasoori methi (leaves), klabat, greco, shambala, triplat, meeti, ho lo ba

Selected Constituents: Fenugreek seeds contain a strong-smelling bitter oil (~5%); other constituents include the alkaloids trigonelline and choline; the steroidal saponins diosgenin, yamogenin, tigogenin, and neotigogenin; mucilaginous fiber (~28%); protein (~22%), which is high in lysine; L-tryptophan; and phosphates, lecithin, and nucleoalbumin (which contains iron in a readily absorbed organic form).

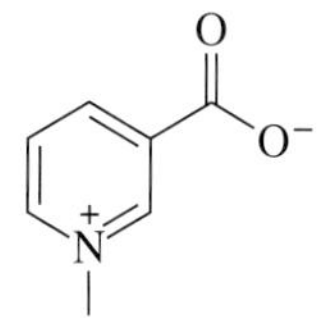

Trigonelline

Clinical Actions: Alterative, carminative, demulcent, hypoglycemic, laxative, nutritive, expectorant, galactagogue. Topically, vulnerary.

Energetics: Warm, pungent, bitter

History and Traditional Usage: Fenugreek seeds have been used medicinally by persons of many cultures, including the Egyptians, Greeks, and Romans. Fenugreek is traditionally used for bronchitis, arthritis, and diabetes, as well as for gastritis and enteritis. Externally, the seeds are used as a poultice for wounds, abscesses, boils, and carbuncles. Traditional Chinese herbalists used fenugreek for kidney problems and problems of the male reproductive tract. It has been used to treat scrofula, rickets, anemia, and debility following infectious disease. Fenugreek was commonly used in condition powders for horses and cattle by early veterinarians, and it was used to flavor cattle forage and to make hay palatable. De Bairacli Levy (1985) recommends fenugreek seeds as a treatment for patients with anal gland problems and for fattening horses; she also recommends it for all gastric weaknesses and ailments, nerves and neuralgia, female ailments such as failing milk supply, and externally as a poultice for relief of abscesses, boils, and running sores (1963). Winslow (1909) stated that the main use of fenugreek was as a condition powder—a claim that was repeated verbatim by Greig in 1942. Fenugreek plants have also been used as livestock feed; they provide 16% to 18% protein.

Despite this, American herbalists apparently did not have so high an opinion of it. From *King's American Dispensatory* (1898): "The only property worth mentioning is its emolliency. A poultice (or plaster or ointment) of the powdered seeds, or a decoction, has been used on inflamed parts, and the latter has been used as a rectal and vaginal wash to soothe *irritation* or *inflammation;* it has likewise been used to allay irritation of the throat and breathing passages . . ."

In ethnoveterinary medicine, the seeds are mixed with cottonseed and given to cattle to enhance milk production, and they are used in the manufacture of nutritional supplements. In rural India, the seeds are applied over swellings and wounds in cattle. Seeds are also given to ruminants and poultry with diarrhea and are considered useful in ruminants after calving (Williamson, 2002).

Published Research: Fenugreek and isolated fenugreek fractions have been shown to act as hypoglycemic and hypocholesterolemic agents in dog, rat, and human studies. In dogs rendered diabetic with alloxin, fenugreek lowered blood and urine glucose, improved responses to glucose tolerance testing, and suppressed blood glucogen and somatostatin levels (Ribes, 1986). In human clinical trials, fenugreek seeds reduced blood glucose levels as well as blood lipid levels (Gupta, 2001; Sharma, 1990; Madar, 1998; Thompson Coon, 2003). The dietary fiber composition and high saponin content in Fenugreek may be responsible for these therapeutic properties (Ribes, 1984; Valette, 1984).

The immunomodulatory activity of fenugreek (aqueous extract) has been studied in mice. A significant increase in relative organ weight of thymus and liver was observed, but levels of liver function test enzymes were unchanged. A significant increase was noted in the delayed-type hypersensitivity response with Fenugreek doses of 50 and 100 mg/kg. An elevated humoral immunity response was seen, and the phagocytic capacity of macrophages was significantly increased (Bin-Hafeez, 2003).

Fenugreek seeds were compared with omeprazole for their effects on induced gastric ulcer in rats. An aqueous extract and a gel fraction from fenugreek seeds showed significant ulcer protective effects because of antisecretory action and its effects on mucosal glycoproteins. The soluble gel fraction was more effective than omeprazole in preventing lesion formation (Pandian, 2002).

Powdered fenugreek seed was incorporated into the diet of rats at a dose of 2 g/kg body weight and was fed for 30 weeks. Compared with controls, the study showed that fenugreek inhibited colon carcinogenesis by modulating the activities of β-glucuronidase and mucinase. The beneficial effects may be attributed to the presence of fiber, flavonoids, and/or saponins (Devasena, 2003).

The anti-inflammatory and antipyretic effects of fenugreek leaf extract were examined. Although it has nonsteroidal anti-inflammatory drug (NSAID)-like effects with anti-inflammatory, analgesic, and antipyretic properties, a different mechanism for the extract is suspected because of the presence of alkaloids, the absence of other effective compounds, and the analgesic effect not usually produced by NSAIDs (Ahmadiani, 2001).

In rats, an aqueous extract of seeds and a suspension of powdered seeds of fenugreek were investigated for wound healing. Results indicated that both extracts promoted significant wound healing activity in excision, incision, and dead space wound models, and the seed suspension was more potent than the aqueous seed extract (Taranalli, 1996).

Meloidogyne javanica is a root knot nematode that parasitizes many staple crops and is of major economic importance in developing countries. Nematocidal activity against this parasite has been demonstrated with the methanol-soluble fraction eluted from pure distilled water (>92% nematicidal activity) (Zia, 2001).

Indications: Diabetes, high cholesterol, hyperlipidemia, anorexia, gastritis, diarrhea, convalescence, atherosclerosis, constipation, suppressed milk production, bronchitis, topically for wounds

Potential Veterinary Indications: Diabetes, galactagogue, immune modulation, diabetes, hyperlipidemia, poultice for wounds, bronchitis, gastric ulceration, especially in horses, convalescence, adjunct in colonic cancer, anorexia (as a digestive bitter)

Contraindications: High doses are not recommended in patients with low thyroid activity. No adverse effects are expected. Fenugreek is traditionally used to promote lactation but should not be used during pregnancy.

Toxicology and Adverse Effects: AHPA class 2b. Not to be used during pregnancy. US Food and Drug Administration (FDA) GRAS (generally regarded as safe) when used as spice or flavoring.

Fenugreek caused myopathy in ruminants (Shlosberg, 1983). Excessive consumption of seeds has been linked to anemia because of the iron binding effect. In a survey of patients with food allergy, two cases of severe allergy to fenugreek were found (Patil, 1997). When fenugreek seeds are used in animal nutrition, a good protein supply and sufficient vitamin E should be considered to compensate for the potential hemolytic effects of fenugreek sapogenins (Elmadfa, 1980).

Preparation Notes: If mucilage is desired, it is extracted with water as a decoction or cold infusion. The aromatic and bitter principles extract well in alcohol. For a poultice, the seed can be boiled and made into a thick paste. Fenugreek seeds can be soaked in warm water, 2 tablespoons to 1 cup or more for 24 hours; then the liquid can be given as a drink and the seeds mixed with food.

Notes of Interest: The Ebers papyrus mentions fenugreek for inducing childbirth. *Foenum graecum* means "Greek hay," which indicates how long the plant has been used as livestock feed. Fenugreek contains coumarins, which give it the ability to "rehabilitate" the aroma and flavor of bad hay. Cattle do not immediately take to the flavor of pure fenugreek hay; however, they have been reported to habituate to it after about 7 days.

Dosage:

External Use: Powdered seeds are stirred with hot water to produce a paste that is used for poultices, boils, and carbuncles at 50 g powdered seeds/250 mL water (Blumenthal, 1998; Bisset, 2001)

Internal Use:

Human

Dried herb: 3-10 g TID, up to 90 g daily

Infusions and decoctions: 5-30 g per cup of water, with 1 cup of the tea given TID, up to 6 times daily acutely

Tincture (45% alcohol): 1:2 or 1:3: 1-5 mL TID, up to 6 times daily for acute conditions

Small Animal

Dried herb: 25-500 mg/kg, divided daily (optimally, TID)

Infusion: 5-30 g per cup of water, administered at a rate of ¼-½ cup per 10 kg (20 lb), divided daily (optimally, TID)

Tincture (45% ethanol): 1:2-1:3: 0.5-2.0 mL per 10 kg (20 lb), divided daily (optimally, TID) and diluted or combined with other herbs. Higher doses may be appropriate if the herb is used singly and is not combined in a formula.

Historic Veterinary Doses

Seeds: dogs, 1 tbsp (de Bairacli Levy, 1975); dogs, 1-2 g (RCVS, 1920); horses, 15-45 g; pigs, 2-7.5 g (RCVS, 1920)

References

Ahmadiani A, Javan M, Semnanian S, Barat E, Kamalinejad M. Anti-inflammatory and antipyretic effects of *Trigonella foenum-graecum* leaves extract in the rat. J Ethnopharmacol 2001;75:283-286.

Bin-Hafeez B, Haque R, Parvez S, et al. Immunomodulatory effects of fenugreek (*Trigonella foenum graecum* L.) extract in mice. Int Immunopharmacol 2003;3:257-265.

Bisset NG, Wichtl M. *Herbal Drugs and Phytopharmaceuticals.* 2nd ed. Stuttgart (Germany): Medpharm GmbH Scientific Publishers; 2001.

Blumenthal M, Busse WR, Goldberg A, et al, eds. *The Complete German Commission E Monographs: Therapeutic Guide to Herbal Medicines.* Austin, Tex: American Botanical Council; 1998.

De Bairacli Levy J. *The Complete Herbal Handbook for Farm and Stable.* London: Faber and Faber; 1963.

De Bairacli Levy J. *The Complete Herbal Handbook for the Dog and Cat.* London: Faber and Faber; 1985.

Devasena T, Menon VP. Fenugreek affects the activity of beta-glucuronidase and mucinase in the colon. Phytother Res 2003;17:1088-1091.

Elmadfa I, Koken M. Effect of vitamin E and protein quality on the haemolytic action of Trigonella sapogenins in rats [German]. Zeitschrift fur Ernahrungswissenschaft 1980;19:280-289.

Pandian RS, Anuradha CV, Viswanathan P. Gastroprotective effect of fenugreek seeds *(Trigonella foenum-graecum)* on experimental gastric ulcer in rats. J Ethnopharmacol 2002;81:393-397.

Patil SP, Niphadkar PV, Bapat MM. Allergy to fenugreek *(Trigonella foenum graecum).* Ann Allergy Asthma Immunol 1997;78:297-300.

RCVS (Royal College of Veterinary Surgeons). *Veterinary Counter Practice.* Sydney: Ballantyne Press; 1920.

Ribes G, Sauvaire Y, Baccou JC, et al. Effects of fenugreek seeds on endocrine pancreatic secretions in dogs. Ann Nutr Metab 1984;28:37-43.

Ribes G, Sauvaire Y, Da Costa C, Baccou JC, Loubatieres-Mariani MM. Antidiabetic effects of subfractions from fenugreek seeds in diabetic dogs. Proc Soc Exp Biol Med 1986;182:159-166.

Shlosberg A, Egyed MN. Examples of poisonous plants in Israel of importance to animals and man. Arch Toxicol Suppl 1983;6:194-196.

Taranalli AD, Kuppast IJ. Study of wound healing activity of seeds of *Trigonella foenum graecum* in rats. Indian J Pharmaceut Sci 1996;58:117-119.

Thompson Coon JS, Ernst E. Herbs for serum cholesterol reduction: a systematic view [Review]. J Fam Pract 2003;52: 468-478.

Williamson A, ed. *Major Herbs of Ayurveda.* London: Churchill Livingstone; 2002.
Winslow K. *Veterinary Materia Medica and Therapeutics.* New York: William R. Jenkins; 1908.
Valette G, Sauvaire Y, Baccou JC, Ribes G. Hypocholesterolaemic effect of fenugreek seeds in dogs. Atherosclerosis 1984;50:105-111.
Zia T, Siddiqui IA, Nazrul H. Nematicidal activity of *Trigonella foenum-graecum* L. Phytother Res 2001;15:538-540.

Feverfew

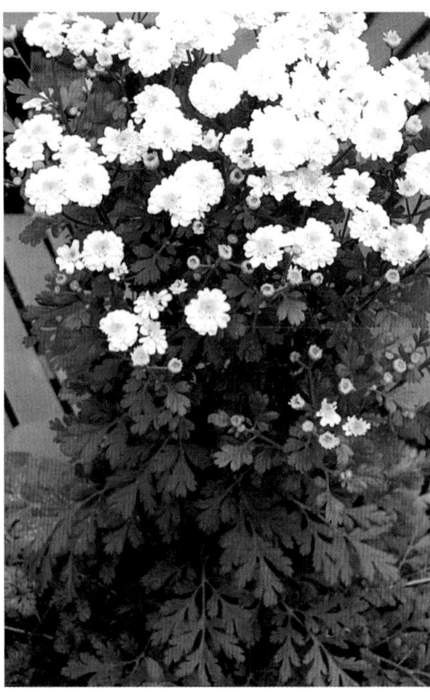

Tanacetum parthenium (L.) Schultz-Bip.
Syn: Chrysanthemum parthenium (L.) Berhn., formerly, *Leucanthemum parthenium, Matricaria eximia, M. parthenium* L., *Pyrethrum parthenium.* • TAN-uh-SEE-tum par-THEN-ee-um

Other Names: Camomilla, featherfew, featherfoil, febrifuge plant, flirtwort, midsummer daisy, santa maria

Family: Asteraceae

Parts Used: Leaf

Distribution: Indigenous to Southeast Europe and commonly found throughout Europe and the United States of America

Selected Constituents: The major constituent is sesquiterpene lactones, including parthenolide (up to 0.9%) (Awang, 1998; Heptinstall, 1992). Monoterpenes, flavonoids, and polyacetylenes (US Pharmacopoeia, 1998; Bruneton, 1995)

Clinical Actions: Tonic, carminative, emmenagogue, vermifuge, stimulant

Energetics: Bitter, cool

History and Traditional Usage: Uses described in folk medicine include treatment of patients with anemia, arthritis, asthma, common cold, constipation, diarrhea, dysmenorrhea, dyspepsia, edema, fever, indigestion, insect bites, rheumatism, sciatica, tinnitus, toothache, and vertigo (Farnsworth, 1998; Berry, 1984; Heptinstall, 1998; Pugh, 1988). Scudder summarizes the Eclectic uses of the herb: "It influences the entire intestinal tract, improves the appetite and digestion, and stimulates secretion." De Bairacli Levy (1963) describes feverfew as one of the most important herbal aids for female ailments; "It exerts remarkable powers over the uterus." Her suggested uses include "female irregularities, inflamed or weak uterus, abortion, difficult labor, and retained afterbirth (2 handfuls of the herb fed to farm animals twice daily, or made into a brew and used as a douche in addition to internal medicine)."

Published Research: The efficacy of feverfew for migraine prevention and its safety profile were investigated in a systematic review. Only randomized, placebo-controlled, double-blind trials of feverfew preparations for the prevention of migraine in human subjects were included. Six trials met the inclusion/exclusion criteria. Most favored feverfew over placebo, and the data suggested that feverfew is likely to be effective in the prevention of migraine and is associated with only mild and transient adverse effects and no major safety issues (Ernst, 2000).

Oral administration of feverfew *(Tanacetum parthenium)* extract led to significant antinociceptive and anti-inflammatory effects in mice and rats (Jain, 1999). An extract of feverfew produced a dose-dependent inhibition of histamine release from rat peritoneal mast cells and contained a mast cell inhibitor (Hayes, 1987). Anti-inflammatory effects in human synovial fibroblasts have been observed (Piela-Smith, 2001).

The capacity for parthenolide to prevent papilloma formation was studied in vivo. When compared with the placebo group, mice fed parthenolide (1 mg/day) showed delayed onset of papilloma incidence and significant reductions in papilloma multiplicity and sizes (Won, 2004).

Indications: Prevention of migraine headaches, arthritis, allergies, mild gastrointestinal problems

Potential Veterinary Indications: Allergies in rats, papillomas, headache (although veterinarians do not often recognize headache in animals, it probably occurs)

Contraindications: Feverfew may be contraindicated in cases of known allergy to plants of the *Asteraceae* family. The use of feverfew during pregnancy is contraindicated because of its uterotonic activity in vivo (Newall, 1996).

Toxicology and Adverse Effects: AHPA class 2b. Not for use in pregnancy. Intragastric administration of 100 times the normal daily dose for humans of powdered feverfew leaf to rats did not result in loss of appetite or weight (Hausen, 1994).

Dizziness, heartburn, indigestion, and weight gain have been reported. Contact hypersensitivity may manifest as inflammation of the mouth and tongue with swelling of the lips, loss of taste, and mouth ulceration (Hausen, 1994). Abdominal bloating, heart palpitations, constipation, diarrhea, flatulence, increased menstrual flow, nausea, and skin rash have been reported to a lesser degree (Murphy, 1988; De Weerdt, 1996). Allergic reactions such as contact dermatitis have been reported (Hausen, 1994; Paulsen, 2002). Cross-sensitivity between pollen allergens of other members of the Asteraceae family such as American feverfew and ragweed has been reported (Sriramarao, 1993).

Dosage:

Human:

Dried herb: 3-10 g TID, up to 6 times daily for acute conditions; 50-200 mg daily (British Herbal Compendium, 1992)

Standardized extract (to at least 0.6 mg parthenolide): 150 mg BID (Mills, 2000)

Infusions and decoctions: 5-30 g per cup of water, with 1 cup of the tea given TID, up to 6 times daily acutely

Tincture (usually 60% ethanol): 1:2 or 1:3: 0.5-5 mL TID, up to 6 times daily for acute conditions

Small Animal:

Dried herb: 12.5-200 mg/kg, divided daily (optimally, TID)

Infusion: 5-30 g per cup of water, administered at a rate of ¼-½ cup per 10 kg (20 lb), divided daily (optimally, TID)

Tincture (60% ethanol) 1:2-1:3: 0.5-1.0 mL per 10 kg (20 lb), divided daily (optimally, TID) and diluted or combined with other herbs

References

Berry MI. Feverfew faces the future. Pharmacy J 1984;232:611-614.

Bradley PR, ed. *British Herbal Compendium,* vol 1. Bournemouth, UK: British Herbal Medicine Association; 1992.

Bruneton J. *Pharmacognosy, Phytochemistry, Medicinal Plants.* Paris: Lavoisier; 1995.

De Bairacli Levy J. *The Complete Herbal Handbook for Farm and Stable.* London: Faber and Faber; 1963.

De Weerdt CJ, Bootsma HPR, Hendriks H. Herbal medicines in migraine prevention: randomized double-blind placebo-controlled crossover trial of a feverfew preparation. Phytomedicine 1996;3:225-230.

Ernst E, Pittler MH. The efficacy and safety of feverfew (*Tanacetum parthenium* L.): an update of a systematic review. Public Health Nutr 2000;3:509-514.

Farnsworth NR, ed. NAPRALERT database. Chicago, Ill: University of Illinois at Chicago; February 9, 1998 production.

Hausen BM. Sesquiterpene lactones—*Tanacetum parthenium.* In: De Smet PAGM, et al, eds. *Adverse Effects of Herbal Drugs.* Berlin: Springer-Verlag; 1994.

Hayes NA, Foreman JC. The activity of compounds extracted from feverfew on histamine release from rat mast cells. J Pharm Pharmacol 1987;39:466-470.

Heptinstall S, Awang DVC. Feverfew: a review of its history, its biology and medicinal properties, and the status of commercial preparations of the herb. In: Lawson L, Bauer R, eds. *Phytomedicines of Europe: Chemistry and Biological Activity.* Washington, DC: American Chemical Society; 1998:158-175 (ACS Symposium Series).

Heptinstall S, Awang DV, Dawson BA, Kindack D, Knight DW, May J. Parthenolide content and bioactivity of feverfew (*Tanacetum parthenium* [L.] Schultz Bip.): estimation of commercial and authenticated feverfew products. J Pharm Pharmacol 1992;44:391-395.

Jain NK, Kulkarni SK. Antinociceptive and anti-inflammatory effects of *Tanacetum parthenium* L. extract in mice and rats. J Ethnopharmacol 1999;68:251-259.

Mills S, Bone K. *Principles and Practice of Phytotherapy: Modern Herbal Medicine.* New York: Churchill Livingstone; 2000.

Murphy JJ, Heptinstall S, Mitchell JRA. Randomized double-blind placebo controlled trial of feverfew in migraine prevention. Lancet 1988;8604:189-192.

Newall CA, Anderson LA, Phillipson JD. *Herbal Medicines: A Guide for Healthcare Professionals.* London: Pharmaceutical Press; 1996.

Paulsen E, Christensen LP, Andersen KE. Do monoterpenes released from feverfew *(Tanacetum parthenium)* plants cause airborne Compositae dermatitis? Contact Dermatitis 2002;47:14-18.

Piela-Smith TH, Liu X. Feverfew extracts and the sesquiterpene lactone parthenolide inhibit intercellular adhesion molecule-1 expression in human synovial fibroblasts. Cell Immunol 2001;209:89-96.

Pugh WJ, Sambo K. Prostaglandin synthetase inhibitors in feverfew. J Pharm Pharmacol 1988;40:743-745.

Sriramarao P, Rao PV. Allergenic cross-reactivity between Parthenium and ragweed pollen allergens. Int Arch Allergy Immunol 1993;100:79-85.

US Pharmacopeia. *National Formulary.* Rockville, Md: US Pharmacopeial Convention; 1998.

Won YK, Ong CN, Shi X, Shen HM. Chemopreventive activity of parthenolide against UVB-induced skin cancer and its mechanisms. Carcinogenesis 2004;25:1449-1458. Epub 2004 Mar.

Forskohlii

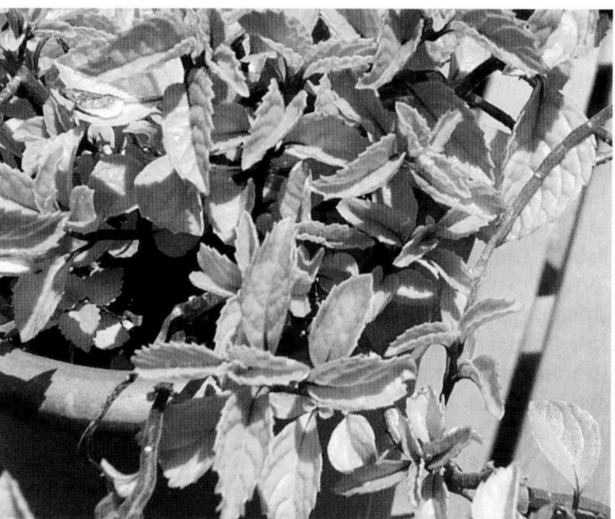

Plectranthus barbatus Andrews. Formerly, *Coleus barbatus* (Andrews) Benth. *Coleus forskohlii* (auct) • plek-TRAN-thus bar-BAY-tus

Other Names: Makandi

Family: Lamiaceae

Parts Used: Root

Selected Constituents: Diterpenes (forskolin, colforsin), plectrin, plectrinone.

Forskolin

Clinical Actions: Carminative
Energetics: Neutral, bitter
History and Traditional Usage: Forskohlii is a pleasantly pungent member of the mint family that is cultivated in India for food. The leaves are eaten and the roots made into pickles. It was used as a folk medicine for digestive upset such as gas and abdominal bloating, as a diuretic, and for respiratory problems such as asthma and cough.
Published Research: The single constituent forskolin has been used in physiology research for its ability to activate adenyl cyclase. It is a positive inotrope, peripheral vasodilator, antihypertensive, and antispasmodic; it inhibits platelet aggregation and lowers intraocular pressure. Recent clinical trials suggest that it is useful in controlling high blood pressure, supporting cardiovascular function in heart failure, and encouraging weight loss. However, no studies were found that used the whole herb, so whether these effects apply to the whole herb is unknown.
Indications: Asthma, cough, abdominal pain, and gas. Unknown whether the whole herb is useful for the same indications as forskolin (i.e., heart disease, hypertension, and weight loss).
Potential Veterinary Indications: Asthma and bronchitis, abdominal pain, bloating and gas
Contraindications: None found.
Toxicology and Adverse Effects: None reported.
Drug Interactions: May have effects that are additive to those of anticoagulants and hypotensives
Dosage:
External Use:
Topically for glaucoma: 4-8 drops 1:1 extract in an eye bath (Bone, 1996) (eye baths should be sterile and well filtered)
Internal Use:
Human:
Dried herb: 1-10 g TID
Infusions and decoctions: 5-30 g per cup of water, with 1 cup of the tea given TID
Tincture (generally 50% ethanol): 1:2 or 1:3: 1-5 mL TID
Small Animal:
Dried herb: 50-500 mg/kg, divided daily (optimally, TID)
Infusion: 5-30 g per cup of water, administered at a rate of ¼-½ cup per 10 kg (20 lb), divided daily (optimally, TID)
Tincture (50% ethanol): 1:2-1:3: 1.0-2.5 mL per 10 kg (20 lb), divided daily (optimally, TID) and diluted or combined with other herbs

References

Bone K. *Clinical Applications of Ayurvedic and Chinese Herbs.* Warwick, Queensland, Australia: Phytotherapy Press; 1996.
Chakraberty C. *A Comparative Hindu Materia Medica.* Delhi: Low Price Publications; first published 1923, reprinted 1998.

Fringe Tree

Chionanthus virginicus, L. • kye-oh-NAN-thus vir-JIN-ih-kus
Other Names: White fringetree, old man's beard, snowdrop tree, white ash, poison ash, arbre de neige, virginischer schneeflockenstrauch, albero della neve
Family: Oleaceae
Parts Used: Bark of the root
Selected Constituents: Saponins, lignan glucoside (phillyrin), a phenol glycoside (syringin)

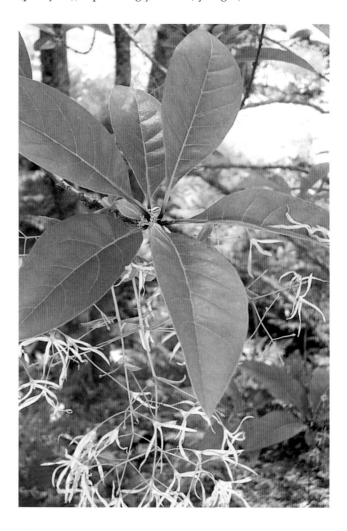

Clinical Actions: Alterative, diuretic, tonic, cholagogue
Energetics: Bitter and cool
History and Traditional Usage: Native Americans used decoctions and poultices of the bark to treat patients with infected wounds and ulcers. The Eclectics used this herb primarily for jaundice, hepatitis, hepatic congestion, duodenitis, and "hepatic pain." It was also found useful in pancreatitis and nephritis. It was considered a tonic and was used for "convalescence from exhaustive diseases," for local application in ulcers and wounds, and as a digestive tonic to aid digestion and improve the appetite.
Published Research: None found.
Indications: Icterus (especially with sensitivity in the abdomen), nausea, and light-colored loose or dry stools. Gallbladder symptoms. Pancreatitis. Externally as a wash or compress for wounds, abrasions, or lacerations. Some sources suggest that a hypoglycemic effect makes this herb useful in diabetes.
Potential Veterinary Indications: Hepatitis, pancreatitis, triaditis, inflammatory bowel disease, and possibly topically for ulcers, abrasions, etc.

Contraindications: No contraindications have been reported.
Toxicology and Adverse Effects: AHPA class 1. No adverse effects have been reported, but *King's* states that ptyalism was sometimes seen with its use.
Dosage:
Human:
Dried herb: 2-10 g TID
Infusions and decoctions: 5-30 g per cup of water, with 1 cup of the tea given TID (*King's* warned that the water extract may not be effective)
Tincture (generally as 40%-60% ethanol): 1:2 or 1:3: 0.25-5 mL TID
Small Animal:
Dried herb: 25-300 mg/kg, divided daily (optimally, TID)
Infusion: 5-30 g per cup of water, administered at a rate of ¼-½ cup per 10 kg (20 lb), divided daily (optimally, TID)
Tincture (usually in 40%-60% ethanol): 1:2-1:3: 0.5-1.5 mL per 10 kg (20 lb), divided daily (optimally, TID) and diluted or combined with other herbs. Higher doses may be appropriate if the herb is used singly and is not combined in a formula.

Reference

Bartram T. Bartram's Encyclopedia of Herbal Medicine. New York: Marlowe Company; 1995.

Garlic 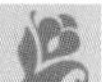

Allium sativum L. • AL-ee-um sa-TEE-vum
Common Names: Ail, allium, dasuan, dawang, lasun, pa-se-waa, rasum, stinking rose, velluli
Family: Liliaceae
Parts Used: Bulb
Distribution: Indigenous to Asia but commercially cultivated in most countries
Selected Constituents: Alliin (10 mg/g fresh weight or 30 mg/g dry weight); the enzyme alliinase (10 mg/g fresh—converts alliin to allicin); allicin (the main thiosulfinate in crushed garlic—typically 75%); other thiosulfinates, diallyl sulfide, and other allyl sulfides; ajoene, vinylthiins, S-allylcysteine, S-allyl-mercaptocysteine, and many other sulfur-containing compounds; amino acids; glycosides; vitamins; minerals; and trace elements, including calcium, selenium, and germanium. High levels of fructans (approximately 65% of dry weight), fructose polymers of 10 to 60 U (fructans increase mineral absorption, support beneficial bacteria within the digestive tract, and help to eliminate pathogenic gut bacteria and yeast). Fresh garlic has a sulfur content of approximately 3 mg/g.

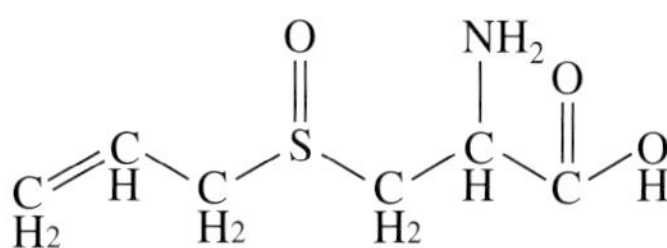

Alliin

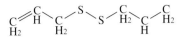

Diallyl disulphide

Clinical Actions: Antiplatelet, anticholesterolemic, antiseptic, mucolytic, vasodilator
Energetics: Pungent, acrid, warm
History and Traditional Usage: Traditionally, garlic has been used in humans for abnormal growths, bronchitis, pneumonia, digestive problems, intestinal infection, tuberculosis, dysentery, earache and ear infection, vascular disorders of many kinds, and poor circulation. French priests used it to treat and prevent the Bubonic Plague, and during World War I, European soldiers applied it to their wounds. It was also known as Russian penicillin because of its ability to treat infection. In China, garlic is used to prevent influenza, relieve toxicities, and kill parasites such as roundworms and tapeworms (Bensky, 1993).

In Ireland, one of the most consistent uses of garlic was in the treatment of a cow that was unable to rise after calving. Tradition required that the "worm in the tail" should be removed. Typically, an incision was made over the base of the cow's tail, and cloves of garlic were inserted under the skin, or a garlic poultice was applied to the site; "if it was a milking beast, you could taste the garlic in her milk that night" (Doherty, 1999). Garlic "is often employed by farriers as a remedy for coughs and thickness of wind" (*A Treatise on Veterinary Medicine,* by James White, 1826). It was rumored for many years that garlic could be used to acidify urine, but when it was tested in cat food, the pH of patient urine increased from 6.7 to 7.1—the opposite effect (Lewis, 1987).

de Bairacli Levy (1985) suggested that garlic can be used for coccidiosis in poultry, for coughing and bronchitis in dogs, for insect bites (applied topically and removed after 1 hour), for breast tumors on dogs (topically), for distemper, for jaundice, for rheumatism, and for thyroid complaints and worms. In large animals, she recommended 2 bulbs or 2 handfuls of leaves given twice daily in bran mash with molasses. For fever and pulmonary complaints, one should make a brew and add honey. Garlic-infused oil should be massaged into arthritic joints, and de Bairacli Levy (1963) recommended that milking animals should be dosed at milking time to avoid flavoring at the next milking.

In Indian ethnoveterinary use, the bulb is used for fungal infection and swelling of the tongue, oral blisters and wounds, rheumatism, contagious abortion, tetanus, milky diarrhea, abdominal pain, asthma, polyuria, sores, compound fracture, epilepsy, and swelling of the kidney (Williamson, 2002). Kirk noted that garlic was reported useful for gangrene of the lungs because the aromatic oil is excreted via the lungs. He recommended garlic oil, 0.5 to 2 minims (0.03-0.12 mL), given in a capsule twice daily for this purpose (Kirk, 1948).
Published Research: Garlic's long reputation as an important herb for treatment or prevention of disease, includ-

ing cancer and cardiovascular disease, has been supported by medical science. Recent studies have revealed a variety of pharmacologic activities of garlic, such as lowering of cholesterol, inhibition of platelet aggregation, immune enhancement, reduction of systolic and diastolic blood pressure, and antithrombotic and antioxidant activities (Agarwal, 1996; Augusti, 1996; Kiesewetter, 1993).

The hypolipidemic effects of garlic powder were screened in dogs and Presbytis monkeys. Following intravenous administration of garlic powder, progressive decreases in cholesterol, triglycerides, and phospholipids were evident for 48 hours. Garlic powder (25 mg/kg body weight) was more effective in lowering serum cholesterol and triglycerides than was guggul in this study (Dixit, 1980).

Garlic extract (garlic dialysate) was investigated for its effects on arrhythmias induced in anesthetized dogs and in rat left atria in vitro. Results suggested that garlic dialysate has an antiarrhythmic effect on ventricular and supraventricular arrhythmias (Martin, 1994).

In one experiment, pulmonary vascular responses to allicin (0.1-1.0 mg) were studied in the intact chest of an anesthetized cat and in the isolated lung of the rat under constant flow conditions. Results showed that allicin has significant vasodilator activity in the pulmonary vascular bed of the cat and the rat (Kaye, 1995). In vivo, allicin dilates the mesenteric circulation of the cat independent of prostaglandin release or a β-adrenergic mechanism (Mayeux, 1988).

Garlic plays a significant role in the reduction of deaths caused by malignant disease, according to epidemiologic and case control studies. Many investigators have examined garlic and garlic constituents for their antitumor and cytotoxic actions in vitro and in laboratory animals. Evidence points to the ability of allyl sulfides from garlic to suppress tumor proliferation in vitro and in vivo (Knowles, 2000). Results from investigations suggest that garlic contains several potentially important agents with antitumor and anticarcinogenic properties (Agarwal, 1996). Oil-soluble organosulfur compounds (diallyl sulfide, diallyl disulfide, and diallyl trisulfide) markedly inhibited growth of canine mammary tumor cells in vitro (Sundaram, 1993). Garlic was also investigated in induced transitional cell carcinoma in mice. Garlic was given orally at doses of 5 mg, 50 mg, and 500 mg per 100 mL in drinking water. Mice that received 50 mg oral garlic had significant reductions in tumor volume when compared with controls, and mice that received 500 mg oral garlic had significant reductions in tumor volume and mortality (Riggs, 1997).

The pharmacokinetics of S-allylcysteine (SAC) was investigated after oral administration to rats, mice, and dogs. It was rapidly and easily absorbed from the gastrointestinal tract and distributed mainly in plasma, liver, and kidney. Bioavailability was 98.2%, 103.0%, and 87.2% in rats, mice, and dogs, respectively. SAC was excreted mainly into urine in the N-acetyl form in rats; however, mice excreted SAC and the N-acetyl form. The half-life of SAC was longer in dogs than in rats and mice (Nagae, 1994).

Encapsulated garlic powder was administered intragastrically to anesthetized dogs. It induced dose-dependent (2.5-15 mg/kg) natriuresis and diuresis that peaked 30 to 40 minutes after administration and fell to basal levels after 100 to 150 minutes. It also reduced arterial blood pressure, which continued past the 250-minute mark. High garlic doses (15 and 20 mg/kg) provoked bradycardia and T-wave inversion during the first 10 to 15 minutes of the experiment; these returned to normal for the remainder of the experiment (Pantoja, 1991).

In vitro, various compounds isolated from the aqueous ethanol extract of garlic induced methemoglobin formation and subsequent oxidation of canine erythrocytes (Yang, 2003). Four healthy adult mixed-breed dogs were given 1.25 mL garlic extract/kg of body weight (5 g of whole garlic/kg) intragastrically once a day for 7 days, to determine whether dogs given garlic extract developed hemolytic anemia. (Note: This is an extremely high dose.) The remaining four control dogs received water instead of garlic extract. Erythrocyte count, hematocrit, and hemoglobin concentration decreased to a minimum value on days 9 to 11 in dogs given garlic extract. At the same time, Heinz body formation, an increase in erythrocyte-reduced glutathione concentration, and eccentrocytes were also detected in these dogs. However, no dog developed hemolytic anemia per se. Study investigators concluded that the constituents of garlic have the potential to oxidize erythrocyte membranes and hemoglobin and to induce hemolysis associated with the appearance of eccentrocytes in dogs. Eccentrocytosis appears to be a major diagnostic feature of garlic-induced hemolysis in dogs (Lee, 2000). It has been suggested that foods that contain garlic should not be fed to dogs (Hu, 2002; Lee, 2000); however, it is difficult to relate the doses used in this study to those given as a flavor enhancer or medicinal remedy to dogs.

The effects of three garlic preparations—raw garlic powder (RGP), boiled garlic powder (BGP), and aged garlic powder (AGE)—on the gastric mucosa of dogs were investigated with the use of an endoscopic air powder delivery system (40 mg powder was sprayed on the mucosal site). Of the three preparations, RGP caused severe mucosal damage, including erosion. BGP also caused reddening of the mucosa, whereas AGE caused no undesirable effects on the mucosa (Hoshino, 2001). Direct administration of pulverized enteric-coated garlic products also caused reddening of the mucosa, and, when an enteric-coated tablet was administered orally (40 mg of pulverized commercial tablet), it caused a loss of epithelial cells at the top of the crypts in the ileum. These results indicate that the safety of enteric-coated products is a matter of concern (Hoshino, 2001). It is important to note that the various garlic products tested vary significantly in their chemistry and activity

Garlic has been used in the treatment of patients with roundworm *(Ascaris strongyloides)* and hookworm *(Ancylostoma caninum* and *Necator americanus)*. Allicin appears to be an anthelmintic constituent, and diallyl disulphide was not effective (Kempski, 1967; Soh, 1960). Minced garlic has been reported successful in reducing parasitism by *Capillaria* species in carp (Peoa, 1988) and as a mosquito larvicide (Amonkar, 1970). Garlic (1 boiled bulb in 300 mL water per donkey) was unsuccessful in reducing fecal strongyle ova counts in 12 donkeys when compared with control and fenbendazole treatment groups. This failure may have been due to the method used to prepare the garlic, the dose used, the method of evaluating the outcome, or the fact that it does not have anthelmintic activity in donkeys (Abells, 1999).

A brief abstract from ethnoveterinary conference proceedings suggested that Sarcoptic mange in dogs was susceptible to local application of crude extracts of garlic, neem, and sitaphalas 1:10 (v/w). Recovery rates for the three plants were 54%, 67%, and 44%, respectively, and the average numbers of days required for complete cure were 22 ± 0.6, 27 ± 1.7, and 28 ± 1.9 days. All treatments were ineffective in treating *Demodex* species infection (Dakshinkar, 1997).

Garlic essential oil may be an effective preventive or curative treatment against several flagellated poultry parasites. *Allium sativum* bulbs were investigated in vitro on *Tetratrichomonas gallinarum* and *Histomonas meleagridis;* the major active ingredients were diallyl trisulfide and disulfide (79%). It appears that these oils may be useful as therapeutic agents against several poultry parasites (Zenner, 2003). Three battery tests were conducted to study the anticryptosporidial efficacy of diclazuril and toltrazuril, along with a garlic extract. The efficacy of garlic extract was 24.4%. It was concluded that garlic oil cannot be recommended for prophylaxis or for therapy of cryptosporidiosis in chickens (Sreter, 1999).

Northern fowl mites (NFMs) are external parasites that can lower egg production and cause anemia and even death in laying hens. An experiment was conducted with New Hampshire red and single comb white leghorn laying hens. Hens were individually caged and were given a complete laying diet and water ad libitum. Hens were assigned to groups in a way that assured that treatments, within each breed, would be applied to comparable numbers of birds with light and heavy mite infestations. Each hen was sprayed around the vent with water or 10% garlic juice in water. Spraying continued each week for 3 weeks. During the fourth week, each bird was scored for the presence of NFM on its skin and feathers. Significantly fewer NFMs were found on birds treated with garlic juice compared with controls. Topical application of garlic juice may be an effective way to decrease NFM in laying hens (Birrenkott, 2000).

Studies were conducted to evaluate the effects of dietary garlic on egg yolk cholesterol concentrations and overall performance in different layer hen strains. Performance was unchanged and no different among strains over a 6-week period; however, yolk weight responded to increasing levels of dietary garlic and differed among strains. Both serum and egg yolk cholesterol concentrations decreased linearly with increasing levels of dietary garlic and serum, and egg yolk cholesterol concentrations differed among different strains. The research concluded that garlic paste in the diets of laying hens reduced serum and yolk cholesterol concentrations. It was also concluded that dietary garlic paste had no adverse effects on layer performance (Chowdhury, 2002).

Garlic has a broad range of antibacterial and antifungal activities. Essential oil, water and ethanol extracts, and juice inhibit in vitro growth of *Bacillus* species, *Staphylococcus aureus, Escherichia coli, Pasteurella multocida, Proteus* species, *Pseudomonas aeruginosa, Candida* species, and *Cryptocococcus* species. Antimicrobial activity has been attributed to allicin; however, allicin is relatively unstable and highly reactive and may not have activity in vivo. Ajoene and diallyl trisulphide also have antibacterial and antifungal activities (WHO, 1999).

Garlic has been proposed as a substitute for antimicrobials in swine diets because of potential natural antibiotic activity. In 1997, a trial was conducted with the use of inclusion levels of garlic at 0.0%, 0.5%, 2.5%, and 5% in the diet. Garlic generally reduced feed intake and average daily gain in nursery pigs and depressed feed performance compared with the control diet. In addition, muscle samples from garlic-fed pigs had very or extremely "objectionable" flavors (Holden, 1998). A more recent trial with inclusion levels of 0.0%, 0.1%, 0.25%, and 0.5% demonstrated significantly poorer performance than a standard feed additive, and the addition of garlic did not enhance performance (Holden, 2000). However, dietary inclusion of garlic and cinnamon resulted in decreased mortality in nursery pigs (Peet-Schwering, 2000).

Indications: Hyperlipidemia, atherosclerosis, hypertension, cough and respiratory infection, poor circulation

Potential Veterinary Indications: Adjunct treatment for cancer, poultry husbandry, carp husbandry, respiratory infection in large animals, cough, hyperlipidemia, thrombosis

Contraindications: Evidence suggests that caution must be used when animals are treated with garlic; monitoring of blood parameters (RBC and morphology) is recommended. Use should be avoided in conditions in which the gastric mucosa is inflamed.

Dog breeds such as Akitas and Shibas, with high erythrocyte levels of reduced glutathione and potassium, are especially susceptible to the hemolytic effects of oxidants such as N-propyl disulphide (Yamoto, 1992) and so may be at greater risk of allium toxicity. Cats are more susceptible to the effects of garlic because their hemoglobin contains a greater number of sites for oxidation than are found in humans or dogs.

Toxicology and Adverse Effects: AHPA class 2c. Should not be used in nursing animals, although a single study of nursing children showed that they nursed for longer periods than children whose mothers were not eating garlic. Several species may be susceptible to the adverse effects of garlic. Suspected wild garlic poisoning has been reported in sheep (Stevens, 1984). An equine case of urticaria associated with dry garlic feeding was reported (Miyazawa, 1991). Acute hemolytic anemia caused by wild onion poisoning was reported in horses (Pierce, 1972), but little primary documentation is available for garlic as a cause of hemolytic anemia at normal doses. Caution should be used with regard to safety and effectiveness when a garlic preparation is selected, because some preparations may have undesirable effects, including gastrointestinal problems and potentially hemolysis (Hoshino, 2001; Hu, 2002; Lee, 2000).

Drug Interactions: Garlic may interact with antiplatelet and anticoagulant drugs. It can reduce blood glucose, so patients on insulin may require insulin dose adjustments (Brinker, 1988).

Preparation Notes: The chemistry of garlic is complex. Processing triggers the formation of other compounds, and various types of processing techniques produce different constituents in their preparations (Yan, 1993; Yu, 1993); thus, various preparations may exhibit different health benefits and safety profiles. Preparations are divided into the following five main groups: (1) dried garlic powder, which is the preparation that has been used most often in clinical research. Drying preserves the compound alliin and the enzyme allinase. On distintegration of the tablet or capsule, alliin contacts allinase and is converted to allicin. This is the same process that occurs when fresh garlic is crushed. Allicin is unstable and further degrades into compounds such as diallyl sulphides, ajoene, and others; (2) steam distillations of garlic (garlic oil) that are rich in diallyl sulphides; (3) aged garlic extracts, which are "odorless" and are produced by fermentation. They contain modified sulphur compounds, for example, S-allylcysteine, but no allicin or its derivatives; (4) fresh or raw garlic; and (5) ethanol-extracted garlic liquid extracts or tinctures..

Dosage:

Human:

Dried herb: 3-10 g TID

Garlic oil: 10 mg per day, equivalent to 3-4 g or 1 moderately sized fresh clove

Standardized extract (to 6 mg allicin potential): 1-6 times daily

Tincture: 1 : 2 or 1 : 3: 2-5 mL TID

Small Animal:

Fresh garlic: 1 clove (approximately 3-4 g) per 20-25 kg as a guide has not resulted in anemia in the authors' experience.

Dried herb: 15-20 mg/kg, divided daily (optimally, TID). (Cats and small dogs, 50-100 mg garlic; small dogs, 50-100 mg; medium dogs, 100-300 mg; large dogs, 300-600 mg; and giant dogs 600-900 mg)

Tincture (usually in 25%-40% ethanol): 1 : 2-1 : 3: 0.5 mL per 10 kg (20 lb), divided daily (optimally, TID) and diluted or combined with other herbs

References

Abells SG, Haik R. Efficacy of garlic as an anthelmintic in donkeys. Israel J Vet Med 1999;54:1. Available online at: http://www.isrvma.org/article/54_1_5.htm.

Agarwal KC. Therapeutic actions of garlic constituents. Med Res Rev 1996;16:111-124.

Amonkar SV, Reeves EL. Mosquito control with active principle of garlic, *Allium sativum.* J Econ Entomol 1970;63:1172-1175.

Augusti KT. Therapeutic values of onion (*Allium cepa* L.) and garlic (*Allium sativum* L.). Indian J Exp Biol 1996;34:634-640.

Bensky D, Gamble A. Herbs that expel parasites. In: *Chinese Herbal Medicine: Materia Medica.* Seattle, Wash: Eastland Press Inc.; 1993:441-444.

Birrenkott GP, Brockenfelt GE, Greer JA, Owens MD. Topical application of garlic reduces northern fowl mite infestation in laying hens. Poult Sci 2000;79:1575-1577.

Brinker F, ed. *Herb Contraindications and Drug Interactions.* 2nd ed. Sandy, Ore: Eclectic Medical Publications; 1998:74-75.

Chowdhury SR, Chowdhury SD, Smith TK. Effects of dietary garlic on cholesterol metabolism in laying hens. Poult Sci 2002;81:1856-1862.

Dakshinkar N, Sarode D. Therapeutic evaluation of crude extracts of indigenous plants against mange of dogs: ethnoveterinary medicine: alternatives for livestock development. In: Ethnoveterinary Medicine: Alternatives for livestock development *Proceedings of an International Conference;* November 4-6, 1997; Pune, India. Available at: http://www.vetwork.org.uk/pune20.htm.

De Bairacli Levy J. *The Complete Herbal Handbook for Farm and Stable.* London: Faber and Faber; 1963.

De Bairacli Levy J. *The Complete Herbal Handbook for the Dog and Cat.* London: Faber and Faber; 1985.

Dixit VP, Joshi S, Sinha R, Bharvava SK, Varma M. Hypolipidemic activity of guggal resin *(Commiphora mukul)* and garlic (*Allium sativum* linn.) in dogs *(Canis familiaris)* and monkeys (*Presbytis entellus entellus* Dufresne). Biochem Exp Biol 1980;16:421-424.

Doherty M. Folklore: a veterinary perspective. Available at: www.clonmany.com/mcglinchey/magazines/1999/mdohertyref.shtml. Accessed July 7, 2005.

Holden P, McKean JD. *Botanicals for Pigs—Garlic ASL R1559, ISU Swine Research Report AS 640.* Ames, Iowa: Iowa State University; 1998:23-26.

Holden P, McKean JD. *Botanicals for Pigs—Garlic II (ASL-R648) ISU Swine Research Report.* Ames, Iowa: Iowa State University; 2000:19.

Hoshino T, Kashimoto N, Kasuga S. Recent advances on the nutritional effects associated with the use of garlic as a supplement: effects of garlic preparations on the gastrointestinal mucosa. *J Nutr* 2001;131:1109S-1113S.

Hu Q, Yang Q, Yamato O, Yamasaki M, Maede Y, Yoshihara T. Isolation and identification of organosulfur compounds oxidizing canine erythrocytes from garlic *(Allium sativum).* J Agric Food Chem 2002;50:1059-1062.

Kaye AD, Nossaman BD, Ibrahim IN, et al. Analysis of responses of allicin, a compound from garlic, in the pulmonary vascular bed of the cat and in the rat. Eur J Pharmacol 1995;276:21-26.

Kempski H. Zur kausalen Therapie chronischer. Helminthien-Bronchitis Medizinische Klinik 1967;62:259-260.

Kiesewetter H, Jung F, Jung EM, Mroweitz C, Koscielny J, Wenzel E. Effect of garlic on platelet aggregation in patients with increased risk of juvenile ischaemic attack. Eur J Clin Pharmacol 1993;45:333-336.

Kirk H. *Index of Treatment in Small-Animal Practice.* Baltimore, Md: Williams and Wilkins; 1948.

Knowles LM, Milner JA. Allyl sulfides modify cell growth. Drug Metab Drug Interact 2000;17:81-107.

Lee KW, Yamato O, Tajima M, Kuraoka M, Omae S, Maede Y. Hematologic changes associated with the appearance of eccentrocytes after intragastric administration of garlic extract to dogs. Am J Vet Res 2000;61:1446-1450.

Lewis LD, Morris ML, Hand MS. *Small Animal Clinical Nutrition IIL.* Topeka, Ks: Mark Morris Associates; 1987:9-27.

Martin N, Bardisa L, Pantoja C, Vargas M, Quezada P, Valenzuela J. Anti-arrhythmic profile of a garlic dialysate assayed in dogs and isolated atrial preparations. J Ethnopharmacol 1994;43:1-8.

Mayeux PR, Agrawal KC, Tou JS, et al. The pharmacological effects of allicin, a constituent of garlic oil. Agents Actions 1988;25:182-190.

Miyazawa K, Ito M, Ohsaki K. An equine case of urticaria associated with dry garlic feeding. J Vet Med Sci 1991;53:747-748.

Nagae S, Ushijima M, Hatono S, et al. Pharmacokinetics of the garlic compound S-allylcysteine. Planta Med 1994;60:214-217.

Pantoja CV, Chiang LC, Norris BC, Concha JB. Diuretic, natriuretic and hypotensive effects produced by *Allium sativum* (garlic) in anaesthetized dogs. J Ethnopharmacol 1991;31:325-331.

Peet-Schwering C, Swinkles J. Enteroguard as an alternative feed additive to antibiotics in weanling piglet diets (abstract). J Anim Sci 2000;78(suppl 1):184.

Peoa N, Aur A, Sumano H. A comparative trial of garlic, its extract and ammonium-potassium tartrate as anthelmintics in carp. J Ethnopharmacol 1988;24:199-203.

Pierce KR, Joyce JR, England RB, Jones LP. Acute hemolytic anemia caused by wild onion poisoning in horses. J Am Vet Med Assoc 1972;160:323-327.

Riggs DR, DeHaven JI, Lamm DL. *Allium sativum* (garlic) treatment for murine transitional cell carcinoma. Cancer 1997;79:1987-1994.

Soh C. The effects of natural food preservative substances on the development and survivial of intestinal Helminth eggs and larvae. II. Action on *Ancylostoma caninum* larvae. Am J Trop Med Hyg 1960;9:8-10.

Sreter T, Szell Z, Varga I. Attempted chemoprophylaxis of cryptosporidiosis in chickens, using diclazuril, toltrazuril, or garlic extract. J Parasitol 1999;85:989-991.

Stevens H. Suspected wild garlic poisoning in sheep. Vet Rec 1984;115:363.

Sundaram SG, Milner JA. Impact of organosulfur compounds in garlic on canine mammary tumor cells in culture. Cancer Lett 1993;74:85-90.

Williamson E. *Major Herbs of Ayurveda.* London: Churchill Livingstone; 2002.

World Health Organization. *Monographs on Selected Medicinal Plants,* vol 1. Geneva, Switzerland: WHO; 1999.

Yamoto O, Maaede Y. Susceptibility to onion induced haemolysis in dogs with hereditary high erythrocyte reduced glutathione and potassium concentrations. Am J Vet Res 1992;53:134-137.

Yan X, Wang Z, Barlow P. Quantitative determination and profiling of total sulphur compounds in garlic health products using a simple GC procedure. Food Chem 1993;47:289-294.

Yang Q, Hu Q, Yamato O, Lee KW, Maede Y, Yoshihara T. Organosulfur compounds from garlic *(Allium sativum)* oxidizing canine erythrocytes. Z Naturforsch [C] 2003;58:408-412.

Yu TH, Wu CM, Ho CT. Volatile compounds of deep-oil fried, microwave-heated, and oven-baked garlic slices. J Agric Food Chem 1993;41:800-805.

Zenner L, Callait MP, Granier C, Chauve C. In vitro effect of essential oils from *Cinnamomum aromaticum, Citrus limon* and *Allium sativum* on two intestinal flagellates of poultry, *Tetratrichomonas gallinarum* and *Histomonas meleagridis.* Parasite 2003;10:153-157.

Ginger

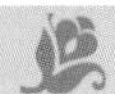

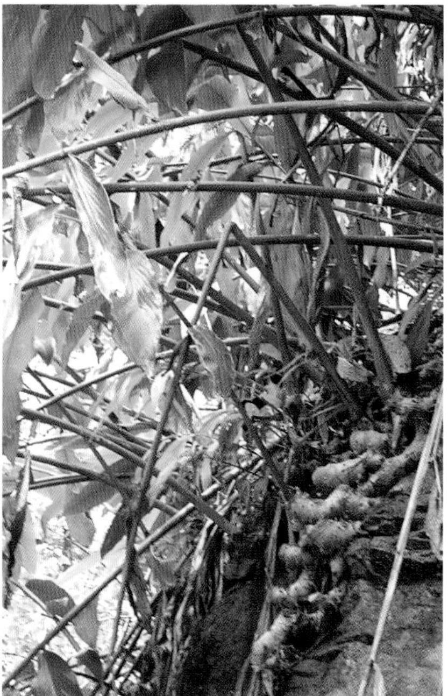

Zingiber officinale Roscoe, formerly *Amomum zingiber* L., *Zingiber blancoi* Massk. • ZING-ee-ber oh-fiss-ih-NAH-lee

Family: Zingiberaceae

Other Names: African ginger, common ginger, ginger root, Jamaica ginger, ardraka (fresh rhizome), shunthi (dried rhizome), jiang, sheng jiang (fresh rhizome), gan jiang (dried rhizome), pao jiang (prepared rhizome), jiang pi (peel)

Parts Used: Rhizome

Distribution: Native to Southeast Asia and cultivated in tropical regions worldwide. It is grown commercially in Africa, China, India, and Jamaica. India is the world's largest producer (Kapoor, 1990).

Selected Constituents: 1% to 4% essential oil, zingiberene, zingiberole, sesquiterpene hydrocarbons (giving the aroma), including zingiberene, arcurcumene, sesquiphellandrene, and bisabolene. Monoterpene aldehydes and alcohols are also present. Gingerols are responsible for the pungent taste of ginger and possibly some of its antiemetic properties, with dehydration products being shogaols (Standard of ASEAN Herbal Medicine, 1993; Bisset, 1994; Yoshikawa, 1993).

O OH

CH_3

$(CH_2)_n$

HO

$n = 3, 4, 5$

OCH_3

Gingerol

Clinical Actions: Carminative, antispasmodic, anti-inflammatory, antiplatelet, diaphoretic

Energetics: Hot, dry

History and Traditional Usage: Ginger is well known across several cultures. It has been used medicinally for more than 2500 years in China and India for conditions such as headache, nausea, rheumatism, and colds. In Traditional Chinese Medicine, ginger is used to warm the body and treat cold extremities, improve a weak and tardy pulse, address a pale complexion, and strengthen the body after blood loss (Chang, 1995).

Other uses described include treatment of patients with dyspepsia, flatulence, colic, vomiting, diarrhea, spasms, and other stomach complaints. Powdered ginger is used for colds and flu, to stimulate the appetite, as a narcotic antagonist (German Commission E Monograph, 1988), and as an anti-inflammatory agent for migraine headache and rheumatic and muscular disorders (Farnsworth, 1995; Srivastava, 1992). Uses described but not supported by clinical data include the treatment of cataracts, toothache, insomnia, baldness, and hemorrhoids, and increased longevity (Farnsworth, 1995; Kapoor, 1990). de Biaracli Levy (1985) recommends powdered ginger mixed with honey for travel sickness; a brew of cloves, peppermint, and ginger for vomiting, a spoonful several times a day; powdered ginger for tapeworm prevention; and ginger root taken internally to repel mosquitoes.

Ethnoveterinary use includes rhizomes for cough and colds, retained placenta, eye disease, bloating, diarrhea, and sprains in poultry, ruminants, and swine. The leaves and rhizomes are used for prevention of mastitis and treatment of wounds, hemorrhagic septicemia, pneumonia, asthma, cough, swelling of nasal mucosa, stomach pain, tympanitis, constipation, dysentery, loss of appetite, lumbar fracture, and stoppage of urination (Williamson, 2002). Gresswell wrote that ginger was often used with other remedies as a tonic and appetite stimulant in horses, and it was given with purgatives to suppress the spasms and "griping" that came with them (Gresswell, 1886). Greig also mentioned its use for rumen impaction in cattle, along with purgatives and nux vomica, and with ginger tincture used for "simple spasmodic colic" in horses (Greig, 1942).

Published Research: Clinical studies support the use of ginger for nausea. Ginger acts directly on the gastrointestinal tract by increasing gastric motility and promoting adsorption of toxins and acids (Mowrey, 1982). In double-blind, randomized studies, the effect of powdered ginger was statistically better than that of placebo in decreasing the incidence of seasickness 4 hours after ingestion (Grontved, 1988). Another investigation compared the effects of seven antiemetic drugs on prevention of seasickness in 1489 subjects and concluded that ginger was as effective as the antiemetic drugs (Schmid, 1994). A systematic review of ginger concluded that ginger was significantly more effective than placebo and equally as effective as metoclopramide for postoperative nausea and vomiting. Of the studies that examined morning sickness and chemotherapy-induced nausea, results collectively favored ginger over placebo (Ernst, 2000).

In a double-blind, randomized, crossover trial, both the degree of nausea and the number of vomiting attacks in pregnancy were significantly reduced with oral powdered ginger (250 mg 4 times daily) (Fischer-Rasmussen, 1991). In a prospective, randomized, double-blind study, significantly fewer cases of postoperative nausea and vomiting were noted in 60 patients given ginger compared with placebo. The effect on postoperative nausea and vomiting was better than that associated with metoclopramide (Bone, 1990). Another double-blind, randomized study concluded that orally administered ginger was ineffective in reducing postoperative nausea and vomiting (Arfeen, 1995).

Anticancer agents such as cisplatin, cyclophosphamide, and methotrexate slow gastric emptying and may cause nausea. In a double-blind study of chemotherapy-induced nausea, 41 patients with leukemia received either ginger or a placebo after administration of compazine. Results showed a significantly greater symptomatic benefit from ginger compared with placebo (Pace, 1987).

Another study investigated the effects of ginger root extract (GRE) on the viability and production of nitric oxide (NO) and prostaglandin E_2 (PGE_2) by sow osteoarthrotic cartilage explants. GRE reduced NO and PGE_2 production by cartilage tissue explants, suggesting an important role for GRE as an antiarthritic agent in osteoarthrosis (Shen, 2003). A different study reported that 113 humans with rheumatic pain and chronic lower back pain, who were injected with 5% to 10% ginger extract into the painful areas, experienced full or partial relief of pain, decreased joint swelling, and improvement in or recovery of joint function (Ghazanfar, 1994). Oral powdered ginger given to patients with rheumatism and musculoskeletal disorders has been reported to provide relief from pain and swelling (Srivastava, 1992).

Antiemetic activity in dogs

Sharma and colleagues induced emesis in healthy mongrel dogs with the use of cisplatin, 3 mg/kg intravenously (iv). Different doses of ethanol and acetone extracts of ginger were tested and compared with granisetron given at 0.5 mg/kg iv. Ginger administration significantly reduced the number of vomiting episodes at doses as low as 25 mg/kg per os. The highest dose tested for both extracts was 200 mg/kg, which led to the fewest vomiting episodes but a shorter latency in minutes to the first episode. The highest doses were most comparable with the antiemetic efficacy of granisetron. Because ginger was ineffective in inhibiting apomorphine-induced emesis (which was mediated through a dopaminergic mechanism), the authors hypothesized that 5-HT_3 receptors may be involved in the activity of ginger (Sharma, 1997).

Antifilarial activity in dogs

Dogs naturally infected with *Dirofilaria immitis* were treated with alcoholic extracts of ginger. Twelve subcutaneous injections of ginger at 100 mg/kg reduced microfilarial concentration in blood by a maximum of 98%. At 55 days after the last injection, 83% reduction in microfilarial concentration was recorded, suggesting partial destruction of adult worms (Datta, 1987).

Tenderization of poultry meat

A study examined the effects of ginger extract on the tenderness of spent hen meat. Spent hen meat chunks were marinated with different concentrations (0%, 1%, 3%, and 5% v/w) of ginger and were evaluated after 24 hours. Ginger treatment increased the pH, moisture, cooking yield, total pigment, water-holding capacity, collagen solubility, protein extractability, muscle fiber diameter, and decreased shear force values. Tenderness scores were higher in samples treated at the postchilled stage. A 3% concentration of ginger was deemed optimum for tenderization (Naveena, 2001).

Indications: Uses supported by clinical data include prophylaxis of nausea and vomiting associated with motion sickness (Reynolds, 1993; Holtmann, 1989); postoperative nausea (Bone, 1990); nausea in pregnancy (Fischer-Rasmussen, 1991); and seasickness (Schmid, 1994). Also, flatulent colic, arthritis, poor peripheral circulation, and fever

Potential Veterinary Indications: Adjunct to nausea control in cancer care and chemotherapy; adjunctive dirofilariasis treatment; osteoarthritis; improving circulation in geriatric or nonambulant animals

Contraindications: Patients taking anticoagulant drugs or those with blood coagulation disorders and those with gallstones (German Commission E Monograph, 1988).

Toxicology and Adverse Effects: *The Botanical Safety Handbook* classifies fresh and dried root separately. Fresh root is rated class 1. Dried root is class 2b, 2d, as patients with gallstones must be treated with caution. Ginger may affect bleeding times and immunologic parameters owing to its ability to inhibit thromboxane synthase and act as a prostacyclin agonist (Backon, 1991). However, a randomized, double-blind study of the effects of dried ginger (2 g daily orally for 14 days) on platelet function showed no difference in bleeding times in patients given ginger or a placebo (Lumb, 1994). Large doses (12-14 g) of ginger may enhance the hypothrombinemic effects of anticoagulant therapy, but the clinical significance of this has yet to be evaluated. Contact dermatitis of the fingertips has been reported in sensitive patients (Seetharam, 1987).

Dosage:

Human:

Dried herb (can be used at the doses below more frequently than noted, in acute conditions).

Motion sickness, adults and children >6 years: 0.5 g, 2-4 times daily

Dyspepsia: 2-4 g/day powdered plant material or extracts (German Commission E Monograph, 1988)

Infusions and decoctions: 5 g per cup of water, with 1 cup of the tea given TID

Tincture (available as 60%-90% ethanol preparations; dose is lower for higher alcohol preparations) 1:2 or 1:3: 0.25-0.75 mL TID, up to 6 times daily for acute conditions

Small Animal:

Dried herb: 15-200 mg/kg, divided daily (optimally, TID)

Infusion: 5 g per cup of water, administered at a rate of ¼-½ cup per 10 kg (20 lb), divided daily (optimally, TID)

Tincture: 1:2-1:3: 0.25-0.5 mL per 10 kg (20 lb), divided daily (optimally, TID) and diluted or combined with other herbs. Higher doses may be appropriate if the herb is used singly and is not combined in a formula.

For nausea associated with travel, 25-50 mg powder per kg divided dose daily, or 0.5 mL per 10 kg (20 lb), 2 to 3 times daily, given at least 30 minutes prior to travel

Historical Veterinary Doses:

Small Animal

Dried herb: 10-20 grains (0.65-1.3 g) (Gresswell, 1887); 0.3-1.3 g (Leeney, 1921); 5-15 grains (0.3-1 g) (Milks, 1948); 10-20 grains (0.65-1.3 g) (Greig, 1942); dogs, 0.3-1 g; cats, 0.1-0.5 g (Hungerford, 1970)

Fresh ginger: 5-15 grains (0.3-1 g) (Winslow, 1908)

Tincture: dog, 0.9-1.2 mL per dose (RCVS, 1920); 5-15 minims (0.3-1 mL) (Milks, 1948); 3-5 minims (0.18-1.3 mL) (Greig, 1942)

Horse

Dried herb: 8-30 g, 5-60 g (Hungerford, 1970); 2 dr-1 oz (8-30 g) (Milks, 1948); 0.5-1 oz (Greig, 1942); fresh ginger: horse: 2 dr-1 oz (8-30 g) (Winslow, 1908)

Tincture: 15-45 mL (RCVS, 1920); 7-42 mL (Leeney, 1921); 0.5-1 oz (Gresswell, 1887); horses, 1-2 oz (Greig, 1942): fluid extract, 2 dr-1 oz (8-30 mL) (Milks, 1948)

Cattle

Dried herb: 5-60 g (Hungerford, 1970); 1-2 oz (Gresswell, 1887); cattle, 1-2 oz (Greig, 1942)

Fresh ginger: 1-4 oz (30-120 g) (Winslow, 1909)

Pig

Dried herb: 1-4 g (Leeney, 1921); 0.5-8 g (Hungerford, 1970); 0.5-1 dr (Gresswell, 1887); 1-2 dr (4-8 g) (Milks, 1948); 0.5-1 oz (Greig, 1942)

Fresh ginger: 1-2 oz (4-8 g) (Winslow, 1908)

Tincture: 2-5 mL (RCVS, 1920)

Sheep

Dried herb: 2-8 g; 0.5-8 g (Hungerford, 1970); 1-2 dr (Gresswell, 1887); 1-2 dr (4-8 g) (Milks, 1948), 1-2 dr (Greig, 1942)

Fresh ginger: 1-2 oz (4-8 g) (Winslow, 1908)

Tincture: 3.5-14 mL (Leeney, 1921)

References

Arfeen Z, Owen H, Plummer JL, Ilsley AH, Sorby-Adams RA, Doecke CJ. A double-blind randomized controlled trial of ginger for the prevention of postoperative nausea and vomiting. Anaesth Intensive Care 1995;23:449-452.

Backon J. Ginger as an antiemetic: possible side effects due to its thromboxane synthetase activity. Anaesthesia 1991;46:705-706.

Bisset NG. *Max Wichtl's Herbal Drugs & Phytopharmaceuticals.* Boca Raton, Fla: CRC Press; 1994.

Bone ME, Wilkinson DJ, Young JR, McNeil J, Charlton S. Ginger root, a new antiemetic. The effect of ginger root on postoperative nausea and vomiting after major gynaecological surgery. Anaesthesia 1990;45:669-671.

Chang CP, Chang JY, Wang FY, Chang JG. The effect of Chinese medicinal herb *Zingiberis rhizoma* extract on cytokine secretion by human peripheral blood mononuclear cells. J Ethnopharmacol 1995;48:13-19.

Datta A, Sukul NC. Antifilarial effect of *Zingiber officinale* on *Dirofilaria immitis.* J Helminthol 1987;61:268-270.

De Bairacli Levy J. *The Complete Herbal Handbook for Farm and Stable.* London: Faber and Faber; 1963.

De Bairacli Levy J. *The Complete Herbal Handbook for the Dog and Cat.* London: Faber and Faber; 1985.

Ernst E, Pittler MH. Efficacy of ginger for nausea and vomiting: a systematic review of randomized clinical trials. Br J Anaesth 2000;84:367-371.

Farnsworth NR, ed. NAPRALERT database. Chicago, Ill: University of Illinois at Chicago; March 15, 1995 production (an online database).

Fischer-Rasmussen W, Kjaer SK, Dahl C, Asping U. Ginger treatment of hyperemesis gravidarum. Eur J Obstet Gynecol Reprod Biol 1991;38:19-24.

German Commission E. Monograph, *Zingiberis rhizoma.* Bundesanzeiger 1988;85:5.

Ghazanfar SA. *Handbook of Arabian Medicinal Plants.* Boca Raton, Fla: CRC Press; 1994.

Greig JR, Boddie GF. *Hoare's Veterinary Material Medica and Therapeutics.* London: Bailliere, Tindall and Cox; 1942.

Gresswell G, Gresswell C, Gresswell A. *The Veterinary Pharmacopeia, Materia Medical and Therapeutics.* London: Bailliere, Tindall and Cox; 1887.

Grontved A, Brask T, Kambskard J, Hentzer E. Ginger root against seasickness. A controlled trial on the open sea. Acta Otolaryngol 1988;105:45-49.

Holtmann S, Clarke AH, Scherer H, Hohn M. The anti–motion sickness mechanism of ginger: a comparative study with placebo and dimenhydrinate. Acta Otolaryngol 1989;108:168-174.

Hungerford T. *Veterinary Physicians Index.* 5th ed. Sydney: Angus & Robertson; 1970.

Kapoor LD. *Handbook of Ayurvedic Medicinal Plants.* Boca Raton, Fla: CRC Press; 1990.

Leeney H. *Home Doctoring for Animals.* 4th ed. London: Macdonald & Martin; 1921.

Lumb AB. Effect of ginger on human platelet function. Thromb Haemost 1994;71:110-111.

Mowrey DB, Clayson DE. Motion sickness, ginger, and psychophysics. Lancet 1982;i:655-657.

Naveena BM, Mendiratta SK. Tenderisation of spent hen meat using ginger extract. Br Poult Sci 2001;42:344-349.

Pace JC. Oral ingestion of encapsulated ginger and reported self-care actions for the relief of chemotherapy associated nausea and vomiting. Diss Abstr Int 1987;47:3297-B.

RCVS (Royal College of Veterinary Surgeons). *Veterinary Counter Practice.* London: Ballantyne Press; 1920.

Reynolds JEF, ed. *Martindale, The Extra Pharmacopoeia.* 30th ed. London: Pharmaceutical Press; 1993:885.

Schmid R, Schick T, Steffen R, Tschopp A, Wilk T. Comparison of seven commonly used agents for prophylaxis of seasickness. J Travel Med 1994;1:203-206.

Sharma SS, Kochupillai V, Gupta SK, Seth SD, Gupta YK. Antiemetic efficacy of ginger *(Zingiber officinale)* against cisplatin-induced emesis in dogs. J Ethnopharmacol 1997;57:93-96.

Shen CL, Hong KJ, Kim SW. Effects of ginger (*Zingiber officinale* Rosc.) on decreasing the production of inflammatory mediators in sow osteoarthrotic cartilage explants. J Med Food 2003;6:323-328.

Srivastava KC, Mustafa T. Ginger *(Zingiber officinale)* in rheumatism and musculoskeletal disorders. Med Hypoth 1992;39:342-348.

Standard of ASEAN Herbal Medicine, vol I. Jakarta: ASEAN Countries; 1993.

Williamson E, ed. *Major Herbs of Ayurveda.* London: Churchill Livingstone; 2002.

Winslow K. *Veterinary Materia Medica and Therapeutics.* New York: William R. Jenkins; 1908.

Yoshikawa M, Hatakeyama S, Chatani N, Nishino Y, Yamahara J. Qualitative and quantitative analysis of bioactive principles in *Zingiberis rhizoma* by means of high performance liquid chromatography and gas liquid chromatography. Yakugaku Zasshi 1993;113:307-315.

Ginkgo

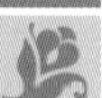

Ginkgo biloba L. • GEEN-ko bi-LOB-uh

Distribution: Native to China, but the fossil record indicates its presence in North America 7 to 24 million years ago. It may exist only in cultivation ("wild" specimens in China may be the result of cultivation by Buddhist monks). The tree has been known to live for 4000 years. It is cultivated worldwide in temperate zones and is very resistant to parasites and other environmental stressors.

Similar Species: None

Other Names: Maidenhair tree, arbol de los escudos. In Traditional Chinese Medicine, the nut is known as bai guo or yin xing.

Family: Ginkgoaceae

Parts Used: In Western herbal medicine, a leaf extract is mainly used. In Traditional Chinese Medicine, the nut or seed is used.

Collection: Green leaves may be collected in late spring and summer and dried.

Selected Constituents: Leaf: terpenoid lactones (ginkgolides A, B, C, etc.), sesquiterpene lactone (bilobalide), flavonoids, tannins, organic acids (e.g., ginkgolic acid), lignans

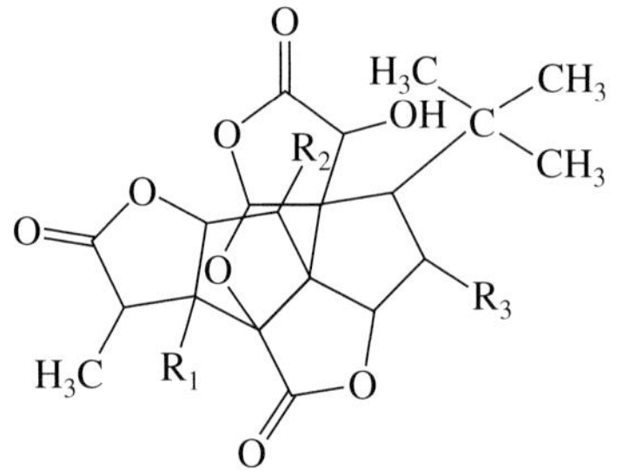

Ginkgolide

Clinical Actions: *Leaf:* anti-inflammatory, cognitive enhancer

Energetics: *Leaf:* bitter, astringent

Seed: seed enters the lung and kidney meridians. It is sweet, bitter, astringent, neutral, and slightly toxic. TCM indications are to expel phlegm, eliminate dampness, and stop discharge. Used for both deficiency and damp heat.

History and Traditional Usage: The leaf was introduced only recently (in 1965) to Western herbal medicine. It is considered an anti-inflammatory and a vasodilator, relaxant, and digestive bitter; the seed (or nut) is used in Traditional Chinese Medicine for bronchitis. The nut has been used in China for at least 700 years and is said to be discussed in the Shen Nong Ben Cao. The nut is considered in Traditional Chinese Medicine as an herb that "stabilizes and binds" and is used for asthma with productive cough, as well as for discharges such as vaginal discharge and urinary incontinence.

Published Research: Ginkgo leaf has no ancient traditional use in Western herbal medicine but may be one of the most well-studied herbs available today. Two standardized extracts (LI 1370 and EGb 761), and an acetone–water extract are the subjects of almost all of the research that has been reported.

Circulatory effects

An extract has been shown to promote peripheral and central blood flow and to protect the brain from oxidative damage. At the same time, the flavonoids stabilize vascular permeability and integrity. The mechanisms at work are not yet well understood but appear to include effects on neurotransmitter receptor changes and uptake, as well as inhibition of nitric oxide and antioxidant effects. The leaf contains ginkgolide B, which demonstrated potent platelet-activating factor (PAF) inhibition in vitro. Only traces of ginkgolide B have been found in ginkgo extract, and it does not inhibit PAF in vivo. Ginkgo appears to be effective in controlling the symptoms of intermittent claudication (Jacoby, 2004).

Effects on cognition

A Cochrane review in 2002 indicated that the results of trials investigating the use of ginkgo for cognitive impairment and dementia are inconsistent but promising. This meta-analysis found benefit for ginkgo in cognition, activities of daily living, mood, and emotional function compared with placebo (Birks, 2002).

Miscellaneous effects

Ginkgo extracts have been shown in laboratory animal studies to inhibit the effects of stress-induced cortisol hypersecretion by reducing secretion of corticosterone and decreasing the number of adrenal peripheral benzodiazepine receptors. Human clinical trials point to benefits for tinnitus and vertigo.

Indications: In humans, evidence-based applications of the leaf include cognitive dysfunction, attention-deficit/hyperactivity disorder (ADHD), headache, vertigo, cerebral trauma, impaired hearing, tinnitus, intermittent claudication, Raynaud's disease, age-related macular degeneration, peripheral arterial occlusive disease, glaucoma, and diabetic retinopathy. It has also been used as a part of protocols to treat asthma, but with poor results. It is used for altitude sickness, but clinical trial evidence tends not to support this use.

Potential Veterinary Indications: Cognitive dysfunction, cardiomyopathy when hypercoagulability is a concern, peripheral circulation disorders, central nervous system ischemia (e.g., from trauma), hypercoagulation disorders, and possibly stress (oxidative, or induced by glucocorticoid excess) from chronic illness. Possibly hyperadrenocorticism or cortisol-induced effects of chronic stress

Contraindications: Bleeding disorders

Toxicology and Adverse Effects: *Leaf:* AHPA class 1. Ginkgo preparations may rarely cause skin reactions (e.g., dermatitis, cheilitis) and mild gastrointestinal problems and, in humans, headache and dizziness. Hyphema and subdural hematoma have been reported in humans who took the leaf for long periods. Ginkgolic acid is slightly toxic and is an allergen; for this reason, some sources suggest using only the standardized extract, which is standardized to the flavonoids and minimizes ginkgolic acid content. Marketers recommend <5ppm ginkgolic acid, but oral ingestion of ginkgolic acid up to 2000ppm has been shown to cause no allergenic reaction. LD_{50} values of the EGb 761 extract were 1100mg/kg iv in rats and mice, 7725mg/kg po in mice, and >10,000mg/kg po in rats.

Seed: no more than 8 to 10 cooked nuts per day is recommended for human adults, and this preparation is not recommended for long-term use (in contrast to the leaf, for which the potential indications usually require 4-6 weeks before benefits may be realized). Seizures have been reported, probably following consumption of the raw nut. Consumption of raw nuts is a common source of adverse effects in Asian children.

Drug Interactions: Except for reports of bleeding when concentrated extracts were taken with aspirin or other anticoagulants, most drug interactions remain theoretical for clinical patients. Several studies in conjunction with aspirin and warfarin show no change in international normalized ratio (INR). In vitro studies show that ginkgo decreases the activity of the enzyme CYP2D6. It may also affect the activity of CYP3A4. Isolated gingkolic acids from gingko inhibit CYP2C19 activity in vitro (Zou, 2002), but a more complete extract in humans appears to induce CYP2C19 (Yin, 2004). Individual case reports have suggested that combination with anticoagulant drugs may increase the chances of coagulopathy and hemorrhage. Ginkgo leaf extract decreased sleep time induced by anesthetics in mice. Ginkgo leaf may enhance the effectiveness of or act additively with cyclosporine, trimipramine, monoamine oxidase (MAO) inhibitors, and hypoglycemic agents. Ginkgo leaf may reduce the cardiotoxicity of doxorubicin, the nephrotoxicity of gentamicin, and the sexual adverse effects of fluoxetine and selective serotonin reuptake inhibitors (SSRIs). Ginkgo nut may have been associated with increased seizure activity—a point for the practitioner to be aware of when using this herb for animals who are being administered anticonvulsants.

Notes of Interest: Ginkgo is considered a living fossil—the tree's morphology has not changed in approximately 200 million years. It is a beautiful ornamental tree whose leaves turn bright gold in the autumn, and it is found on many city streets. Although it takes a long time to mature, this tree is worth planting.

Preparation Notes: The leaf is generally extracted and sold as a standardized extract (standardized to 24% flavone glycosides and 6% triterpene lactones). The nut was eaten in Traditional Chinese Medicine as a food (but sparingly), and safety is enhanced by cooking. The nut can be cooked with konji and ginger, which, in Traditional Chinese Medicine, sedates heat, boosts *Wei Qi,* and builds immunity (Bensky, 1993).

Dosage:

Human:

Dried herb: 3-10gTID

Standardized extract (50:1, with approximately 24% flavonoids, 6% terpene lactones, and less than 5% ginkgolic acids) 30-240mg divided BID or TID

Tincture (usually 50%-75% ethanol): 1:2 or 1:3: 1-5 mL TID, up to 6 times daily for acute conditions

Small Animal:

Dried herb: 25-300 mg/kg, divided daily (optimally, TID)

Standardized extract (50:1 with approximately 24% flavonoids, 6% terpene lactones, and less than 5% ginkgolic acids): 10-50 mg per 10 kg, divided BID or TID

Tincture (usually in 50%-75% ethanol): 1:2-1:3: 0.5-1.0 mL per 10 kg (20 lb), divided daily (optimally, TID) and diluted or combined with other herbs. Higher doses may be appropriate if the herb is used singly and is not combined in a formula.

Selected References

Bensky D, Gamble A. Herbs that expel parasites. In: *Chinese Herbal Medicine: Materia Medica.* Seattle, Wash: Eastland Press Inc.; 1993:441-444.

Birks J, Grimley EV, Van Dongen M. Ginkgo biloba for cognitive impairment and dementia. Cochrane Database Syst Rev 2002;4:CD003120.

Horsch S, Walther C. Ginkgo biloba special extract EGb 761 in the treatmet of peripheral arterial occlusive disease (PAOD)—a review based on randomized controlled studies. Int J Clin Pharmacol Ther 2004;42:63-72.

Jacoby D, Mohler ER 3rd. Drug treatment of intermittent claudication. Drugs 2004;64:1657-1670.

Muller WE, Chatterjee SS. Cognitive and other behavioral effects of EGb 761 in animal models. Pharmacopsychiatry 2003;36(suppl 1):S24–S31.

Ponto LL, Schultz Sk. Ginkgo biloba extract: review of CNS effects. Ann Clin Psychiatry 2003;15:109-119.

Schultz V. Ginkgo extract or cholinesterase inhibitors in patients with dementia: what clinical trials and guidelines fail to consider. Phytomedicine 2003;10(suppl 4):74-79.

Upton R, Graff A. *Ginkgo Leaf; Ginkgo Leaf Dry Extract.* Scotts Valley, Calif: American Herbal Pharmacopeia and Therapeutic Compendium; 2003.

Yin OQ, Tomlinson B, Waye MM, Chow AH, Chow MS. Pharmacogenetics and herb–drug interactions: experience with Ginkgo biloba and omeprazole. Pharmacogenetics 2004;14: 841-850.

Zou L, Harkey MR, Henderson GL. Effects of herbal components on cDNA-expressed cytochrome P450 enzyme catalytic activity, Life Sci 71:1579, 2002.

Goldenrod

Solidago virgaurea L. • so-li-DAY-go virg-AW-ree-uh

Other Names: Solidago, European goldenrod, virgaureae herba, *S. virga aurea* L., verge d'or (French), verge d'oro (Italian), goldruthe, woundwort, Aaron's rod, unestala (Cherokee)

Similar Species: *Solidago odora* (sweet golden rod, fragrant leaved golden rod, sweet scented golden rod, blue mountain tea), *Solidago gigantea,* Aiton (smooth three-ribbed goldenrod), *Solidago canadensis* L. (Canadian goldenrod or early goldenrod)

Distribution: Europe, North America, Northern Africa, parts of Asia

Family: Asteraceae

Parts Used: Flowering tops and leaves

Selected Constituents: Saponins, diterpenes, essential oil, flavonoids (rutin, quercetin, hyperoside, astragalin), 10% catechin tannins

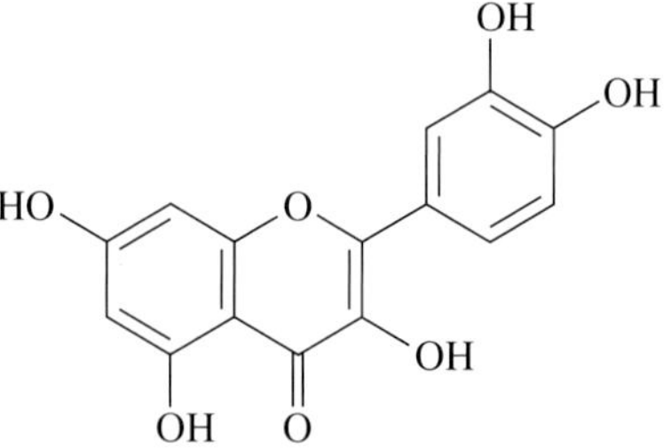

Quercetin

Clinical Action: Gentle diuretic, carminative, diaphoretic, antiseptic

Energetics: Sweet, pungent, warming, drying

History and Traditional Usage: *Solidago californica* was used by a number of North American tribes to treat wounds and as an aid to prevent hair loss. An infusion or decoction of the roots of *S. canadensis* was used for various disorders of children, such as fevers, starting during sleep, and the inability to speak or laugh. *S. canadensis* was also used for flu, fever, diarrhea, and sleeplessness and excessive crying. A decoction of *S. canadensis* and wild tarragon was used as a wash for sores and cuts in horses by the Thompson Indians. *Solidago altissima* was used primarily as a topical treatment for wounds. *Solidago juncea* was used for fever, nausea, jaundice, and diarrhea. *Solidago nemoralis* was used for kidney problems and skin ulcerations. *S. odora* was used by the Cherokee for a variety of disorders, including female obstructions, bloody diarrhea, cough, colds, fevers, sore mouth, nerves, measles, and tuberculosis. Other species of Solidago were used by various North American tribes.

King's describes goldenrod as gently stimulant, carminative, diuretic, and diaphoretic. Other sources describe it as anticatarrhal, anti-inflammatory, antiseptic, mildly antispasmodic, diuretic, diaphoretic, and vulnerary. It is indicated for flatulent colic, amenorrhea, stomach pain, and nausea. The flowers are described as aperient, tonic, astringent, and diuretic and were recommended for gravel, urinary obstruction, renal colic, and ulceration of the bladder. The flowers are a pleasant tasting substitute for tea as well.

Other traditional uses include acute or chronic upper respiratory catarrh, bronchitis, tonsillitis, laryngitis, and possibly influenza.

Published Research: Goldenrod was shown in early studies to promote renal blood flow and increase glomerular filtration rate without causing major electrolyte abnormalities. In a double-blind placebo-controlled study, a diuretic effect was observed in healthy volunteers after a single dose of golden rod tincture (4 mL) (Chodera, 1985). The German Commission E supports the use of goldenrod along with copious fluid intake to treat inflammatory diseases of the lower urinary tract, including urinary calculi; it is also recommended as prophylaxis against urinary calculi (Blumenthal, 1998).

Indications: For flatulence, colicky abdominal pain, nausea, upper respiratory infection or inflammation, urinary tract infection, and other bladder/urethral inflammation. Externally as an anti-inflammatory and antiseptic for wounds
Potential Veterinary Indications: Flatulent colic, cystitis, gastrointestinal spasm, upper respiratory tract inflammation or infection with catarrh. Feline lower urinary tract disease, urolithiasis; topically for hot spots, ulcers
Contraindications: Safety or toxicity in pregnant or lactating patients is unknown. Because copious amounts of water are advised to be taken with goldenrod for urinary conditions, caution is advised in patients with impaired renal or cardiovascular function (Blumenthal, 1998).
Toxicology and Adverse Effects: AHPA class 2d because caution is required with use in renal disease. Allergic reaction and contact dermatitis are common in people who are allergic to plants in the daisy family. Those with sensitivity to other members of the Asteraceae family (such as chamomile—Matricaria recutita—and various species of chrysanthemum) may also be allergic to goldenrod.
Drug Interactions: The mild diuretic effect causes some sources to recommend caution about simultaneous use with diuretics and with drugs such as lithium that are excreted "with water."
Dosage:
Human:
Dried herb: 3-10 g TID, up to 6 times daily for acute conditions
Infusions and decoctions: 5-30 g per cup of water, with 1 cup of the tea given TID, up to 6 times daily acutely
Tincture (usually 40%-45% ethanol): 1:2 or 1:3: 0.5-5 mL TID, up to 6 times daily for acute conditions
Small Animal:
Dried herb: 25-300 mg/kg, divided daily (optimally, TID)
Infusion: 5-30 g per cup of water, administered at a rate of ¼-½ cup per 10 kg (20 lb), divided daily (optimally, TID)
Tincture (usually in 40%-45% ethanol): 1:2-1:3: 0.5-1.5 mL per 10 kg (20 lb), divided daily (optimally, TID) and diluted or combined with other herbs. Higher doses may be appropriate if the herb is used singly and is not combined in a formula.

References

Blumenthal M, ed. *The Complete German Commission E Monographs: Therapeutic Guide to Herbal Medicines.* Austin: American Botanical Council; 1998.

Chodera A, Dabrowska K, Senczuk M, et al. [Diuretic effect of the glycoside from a plant of the *Solidago* L. genus]. Acta Pol Pharm 1985;42:199-204.

Goldenseal

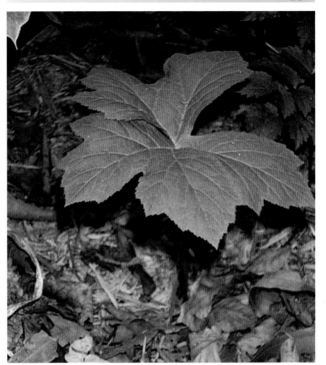

Hydrastis canadensis L. • hy-DRASS-tiss ka-na-DEN-sis
Distribution: North America
Similar Species: Possibly *Hydrastis jeozensis* from Japan
Other Names: Yellow puccoon, yellow root (note that another plant that goes by this name is *Xanthorhiza simplicissima),* goldensiegel, goldsiegel, guldsegl, kanadische gelbwurzel, sigillo d'oro, hydrastis rhizome. Very old names that were being discouraged in the late 1800s but that may persist in rural areas include golden root, Indian dye, Indian paint, Indian turmeric, ground raspberry, jaundice root, Ohio curcuma, orange root, warnera, wild curcuma, wild turmeric, yellow eye, yellow Indian plant, yellow paint root, yellow wort, yellow seal, yellow paint
Family: Ranunculaceae
Parts Used: Rhizome and root; also leaf used in teas
Selected Constituents: Isoquinolone alkaloids (hydrastine); protoberberine alkaloids (berberine, berberastine, canadine), phenolic acids, resin

O, O, N, CH_3, H, H, O, CH_3O, OCH_3, O

Hydrastine

Clinical Action: Digestive bitter, hemostatic, laxative, cholalogue, hepatic

Energetics: Bitter, cold; clears heat and toxins; dries damp. King's American Dispensatory noted that it is valuable in moving blood stasis by stimulating circulation.

History and Traditional Usage: The Cherokee were said to have used goldenseal for cancer, as a wash for local inflammation, for dyspepsia, as a tonic, and as a dye. Other tribes had similar uses for the plant, in addition to using it for earache, diarrhea, gas, biliousness, sore eyes, fever, heart trouble, and pneumonia. A primary indication was for inflammation and ulceration of mucous membranes anywhere in the gastrointestinal tract (e.g., stomatitis, gastric ulcers, anal fissures) and the reproductive tract. Also for liver disorders that may lead to jaundice. To stop bleeding after birth; for nasal catarrh (sinusitis with mucoid dishcarge), hemorrhoids, and vulvovaginitis. Its use for diarrhea is likely related to antimicrobial and antigiardia activity. Used externally for a variety of focal skin infections or inflammation, as well as for eye and ear inflammation.

Titus (1865) recommended goldenseal for farm animals almost exclusively as a tonic and alterative. One of his recipes consisted of 4 oz goldenseal, 2 oz unicorn root, and 1 oz ginger, to be given 1 oz TID. Other variants of goldenseal-containing tonics included poplar bark, capsicum, and table salt. Milks (1949) described its external use as a mucous membrane stimulant that is to be used in chronic catarrhal conditions, and he recommended it orally for genitourinary inflammation. He also recommended it as a bitter stomachic for anorexia and convalescence.

Published Research: When the popularity of this plant is considered, the lack of clinical trials and the preponderance of studies on adverse effects and drug interactions are most surprising. Most of the research that has been conducted on goldenseal actually concentrates on the single alkaloid, berberine, which has positive inotropic, negative chronotropic, antiarrhythmic, and vasodilator properties. Although berberine is a prominent constituent in goldenseal, other components of the plant have powerful activities as well. In vitro studies suggest that the plant's constituents are microbicidal against a number of bacterial pathogens, including Pseudomonas aeruginosa (Scazzocchio, 2001). Berberine and other constituents of goldenseal have individual and additive in vitro antimicrobial activity against oral pathogens, specifically, Streptococcus mutans and Fusobacterium nucleatum (Hwang, 2003). A crude methanol extract of goldenseal root was very active in vitro against Helicobacter pylori, with an MIC_{50} of 12.5 μg/mL. Two of the alkaloids, berberine and beta-hydrastine, were identified as major active constituents (Mahady, 2003).

Goldenseal extracts have vasoactive effects that have yet to be well characterized. The extract relaxes guinea pig trachea in vitro, but individual components of the extract have differing effects in the same model (Abdel-Haq, 2000). Rabbit aorta responds to the total extract differently than to the isolated constituents, with the total extract being more potent in one study (Palmery, 1993; Palmery, 1996). When rabbit detrusor muscle was exposed in vitro to an ethanol extract of goldenseal, relaxation occurred, and the isolated alkaloids did not have such an effect (Bolle, 1997). Rabbit prostate strips were inhibited from contraction with the use of goldenseal extract and berberine (Baldazzi, 1998).

Uterine muscle is also responsive in vitro to goldenseal extract and its various alkaloids in different ways (older studies cited in Brinker, 2004).

Goldenseal has a reputation for being an immune stimulant, but only one study in rats supports this action. Rats given a 1:1 glycerin extract exhibited augmented IgM responses to the test antigen, keyhole limpet hemocyanin (KLH) (Rehman, 1999).

As a bitter digestive tonic, goldenseal may have different effects, depending on the preparation that is used. Brinker (2004) describes studies in which a 54% alcoholic extract enhanced gastric acidity in a person, and a 50% hydroethanolic extract reduced gastric acidity.

To summarize Brinker's findings on the activities of different goldenseal extracts, the glycerine extract has been found to modulate IgM antibody response in rats when the hydroethanolic extracts are antiadrenergic, antiserotonergic, and vasorelaxant in the genitourinary and respiratory tracts. An extract devoid of alkaloids has astringent effects (Brinker, 2004).

Indications: Gastritis, stomatitis, enteritis, giardiasis and other enteric pathogens, colitis, sinusitis. Especially topically for otitis, conjunctivitis, vaginitis, and focal bacterial or fungal skin infections

Potential Veterinary Indications: Gastritis, stomatitis, enteritis, giardiasis and other enteric pathogens, colitis, otitis, conjunctivitis, vaginitis, sinusitis, and focal bacterial or fungal skin infections. The antimicrobial effects are more likely to be a factor with topical use or within the gastrointestinal tract.

Notes of Interest: Goldenseal is highly threatened in the wild. Observers noted in the late 1800s that populations were already declining, and it is still wildcrafted today. Only 34% of marketed goldenseal was derived from cultivated sources in 1999. It is important that goldenseal be obtained from sustainable sources only—buying of wildcrafted plant products should be avoided. For a list of substitutes for various conditions, see Chapter 18, on substitutes for endangered herbs.

Contraindications: Very young animals, hypertension. Modern, more theoretical contraindications include bleeding disorders, cardiovascular disease, hyperbilirubinemia, and jaundice. Safety in pregnancy and lactation not established. One experimental study in diabetic rats suggested that goldenseal may improve signs of diabetes (Swanston-Flatt, 1989), but diabetes is not a recognized contraindication for use of this herb.

Toxicology and Adverse Effects: AHPA class 2b. At high doses, nausea, diarrhea, vomiting, changes in blood pressure. Also reported: anxiety, depression, hallucinations, hyperbilirubinemia, paralysis, and seizures. Topical application may lead to photosensitivity.

Drug Interactions: May interact with drugs metabolized by the CYP 3A4 isozymes, especially in tincture form. Goldenseal inhibits CYP3A4 activity in vitro, but a clinical study in humans examining the effects of goldenseal on a drug metabolized by CYP3A4 (indinavir) showed no effect on disposition of this drug in humans (Sandhu,

2003). In another study in healthy human volunteers, goldenseal strongly inhibited CYP2D6 and CYP3A4/5 as measured by metabolism of drugs other than indinavir (Gurley, 2005).

Most drug interaction research has centered on the single constituent, berberine. This compound has been shown to decrease hepatic damage caused by acetaminophen and to block α-adrenergic activity of phenylephrine, norepinephrine, and caffeine. In addition, berberine may inhibit platelet aggregation, have an additive effect with cardiac glycosides, potentiate the hypotensive action of anesthetics, potentiate the sedative action of central nervous system depressants, and reduce the effects of tetracycline. The whole herb contains other components that may have antiarrhythmic activity and calcium channel blocking activity and that may displace protein-bound drugs.

Dosage:

Human:

Dried herb: 0.125-10 g TID, up to 6 times daily for acute conditions (this is a bitter herb, and the higher doses are not usually required)

Infusions and decoctions: 5-10 g per cup of water, with ¼-1 cup of the tea given TID, up to 6 times daily acutely

Tincture (usually as 45%-60% ethanol): 1:2 or 1:3: 0.5-5 mL TID, up to 6 times daily for acute conditions

Small Animal:

Dried herb: 25-300 mg/kg, divided daily (optimally, TID)

Infusion: 5-10 g per cup of water, administered at a rate of ¼-½ cup per 10 kg (20 lb), divided daily (optimally, TID)

Tincture (usually in 45%-60% ethanol): 1:2-1:3: 0.5-1.0 mL per 10 kg (20 lb), divided daily (optimally, TID) and diluted or combined with other herbs. Higher doses may be appropriate if the herb is used singly and is not combined in a formula.

Large Animal:

Tincture for farm animals (Karreman, 2004): 30-60 mL for horses and cows; 4-15 mL for sheep and goats

Glycerite: 8-30 mL for horses and cows; 4-15 mL for sheep and goats

Fluid extract (1:1): 8-30 mL for horses and cows; 4-8 mL for sheep and goats

Historic Veterinary Doses:

Fluid extract (1:1): horse and cow, 8-30 mL; sheep and swine, 4-8 mL; dog, 0.3-4 mL

Tincture: horse, 30-60 mL; dog, 2-8 mL (Winslow, 1910)

References

Abdel-Haq H, Cometa MF, Palmery M, Leone MG, Silvestrini B, Saso L. Relaxant effects of *Hydrastis canadensis* L. and its major alkaloids on guinea pig isolated trachea. Pharmacol Toxicol 2000;87:218-222.

Baldazzi C, Leone MG, Casini ML, Tita B. Effects of the major alkaloid of *Hydrastis canadensis* L., berberine, on rabbit prostate strips. Phytother Res 1998;12:589-591.

Bolle P, Cometa MF, Palmery M, Tucci P. Further studies of the adrenolytic activity of the major alkaloids from *Hydrastis canadensis* L. on isolated rabbit aorta. Phytother Res 1997;12:S86–S88.

Brinker F. *Complex Herbs, Complete Medicines*. Sandy, Ore: Eclectic Medical Publications; 2004.

Hwang BY, Roberts SK, Chadwick LR, Wu CD, Kinghorn AD. Antimicrobial constituents from goldenseal (the Rhizomes of *Hydrastis canadensis*) against selected oral pathogens. Planta Med 2003;69:623-627.

Gurley BJ, Gardner SF, Hubbard MA, Williams DK, Gentry WB, Khan IA, Shah A. In vivo effects of goldenseal, kava kava, black cohosh, and valerian on human cytochrome P450 1A2, 2D6, 2E1, and 3A4/5 phenotypes. Clin Pharmacol Ther 2005;77:415-426.

Karreman H. *Treating Dairy Cows Naturally: Thoughts and Strategies*. Paradise, Pa: Paradise Publications; 2004.

Mahady GB, Pendland SL, Stoia A, Chadwick LR. In vitro susceptibility of *Helicobacter pylori* to isoquinoline alkaloids from *Sanguinaria canadensis* and *Hydrastis canadensis*. Phytother Res 2003;17:217-221.

Milks HJ. *Practical Veterinary Pharmacology, Materia Medica and Therapeutics*. Chicago, Ill: Alex Eger, Inc.; 1949.

Palmery M. Further studies of the adrenolytic activity of the major alkaloids from *Hydrastis canadensis* L. on isolated rabbit aorta. Phytother Res 1996;10:A47–A49.

Palmery M. Effects of *Hydrastis canadensis* L. and the two major alkaloids berberine and hydrastine on rabbit aorta. Pharmacol Res 1993;27(suppl):73-74.

Rehman J, Dillow JM, Carter SM, Chou J, Le B, Maisel AS. Increased production of antigen-specific immunoglobulins G and M following in vivo treatment with the medicinal plants *Echinacea angustifolia* and *Hydrastis canadensis*. Immunol Lett 1999;68:391-395.

Sandhu RS, Prescilla RP, Simonelli TM, Edwards DJ. Influence of goldenseal root on the pharmacokinetics of indinavir. J Clin Pharmacol 2003;43:1283-1288.

Scazzocchio F, Cometa MF, Tomassini L, Palmery M. Antibacterial activity of *Hydrastis canadensis* extract and its major isolated alkaloids. Planta Med 2001;67:561-564.

Swanston-Flatt SK, Day C, Bailey CJ, Flatt PR. Evaluation of traditional plant treatments for diabetes: studies in streptozotocin diabetic mice. Acta Diabetol Lat 1989;26:51-55.

Titus Nelson N. *The American Eclectic Practice of Medicine, as Applied to the Diseases of Domestic Animals*. New York: Baker and Godwin; 1862. Also available online at: David Winston's Herbal Therapeutics Research homepage: http://www.herbaltherapeutics.net/DomesticAnimalDiseases.pdf.

Winslow K. *Veterinary Materia Medica and Therapeutics*. New York: William R. Jenkins; 1908.

Gotu Kola

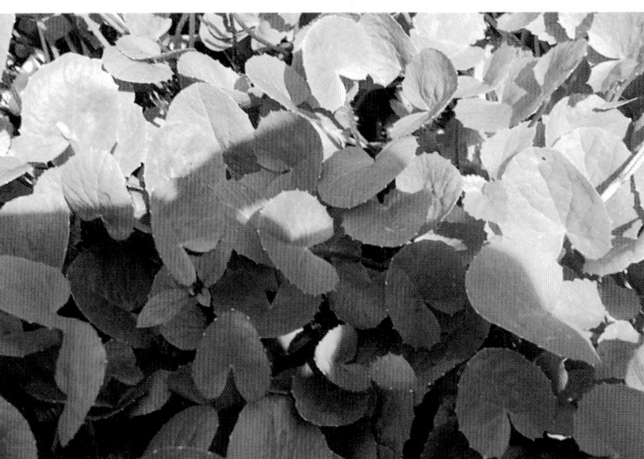

Centella asiatica (L.) Urban, syn. *Hydrocotyle asiatica* L. • sen-TEL-uh a-see-AT-ee-kuh

Distribution: Indigenous to warmer regions of both hemispheres, including Australia, Africa, Cambodia, Central America, China, Indonesia, Pacific Islands, South America, Thailand, Laos, Viet Nam, Madagascar, and southern United States and is especially abundant in the swampy areas of India, Iran, Pakistan, and Sri Lanka

Similar Species: *Centella coriacea, Hydrocotyle lunara,* and *Trisanthus cochinchinensis*

Common Names: Asiatic pennywort, centella, gotu kola, Indian pennywort, luei gong gen, pami, yerba de chavos. This plant is known as "brahmi" in North and West India, and "mandukaparni" in South India. Bacopa *(Bacopa monnieri)* is known as "brahmi" in South India, and as "mandukaparni" in North and West India.

Family: Apiaceae

Parts Used: Aerial parts preferred; however, whole plant, which can include leaves, fruit, seed, and root, is also used.

Selected Constituents: Active constituents: major principles are the triterpenes, asiatic acid and madecassic acid, and their derived triterpene ester glycosides, asiaticoside, and madecassoside.

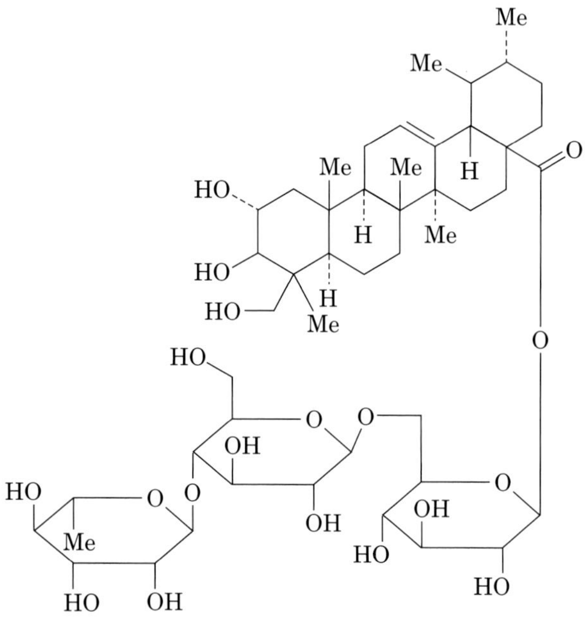

Asiaticoside

Clinical Actions: Adaptogen, connective tissue regenerator, nerve tonic, mild diuretic, alterative

Energetics: Cold, bitter, slightly astringent

History and Traditional Usage: *Centella asiatica* has a long history of traditional medical use, particularly in India and Asia. It was considered useful as a remedy against leprosy in Greek medicine. In Ayurvedic medicine, it was used for chronic eczema and other skin conditions, as well as in scrofula, secondary syphilis, ulcers, and chronic rheumatism. Internally, it was used for skin disorders such as dermatitis, eczema, abscesses, lupus scleroderma, bruises, fractures, snakebites, rheumatic conditions, epilepsy, insanity, and infantile diarrhea, as well as urethritis, bronchitis, asthma, anemia, hematemesis, nephritis, toothache, and furunculosis. Ethnoveterinary uses include the whole plant for jaundice, contagious abortion, foot and mouth disease, colic, and swelling of the respiratory tract (Williamson, 2002).

Published Research: The efficacy of gotu kola in the treatment of wound healing disturbances has been supported by studies on its constituents, the madecassosides and asiaticosides (Brinkhaus, 2000), including delayed-type wound healing (Shukla, 1999a; Maquart, 1999). Gotu kola stimulated collagen synthesis in human fibroblasts (Maquart, 1990), hyaluronic acid, and chondroitin sulphate (Del Vecchio, 1984), activated cells of the germinative layer of the epidermis of porcine skin, and stimulated keratinization (May, 1968). Gotu kola reduces scarring (Widgerow, 2000). The possible mechanism of the effect of asiaticoside on hypertrophic scars is associated with its inhibitory action on fibroblast proliferation and collagen synthesis (Qi, 2000). Madecassol reduces keloid scars and has been shown to have preventive effects on burn scars and postoperative hypertrophic scars. It is as effective as compression bandaging and yields more lasting results than are produced by intralesional cortisone or radiation therapy (Bosse, 1979).

Open wounds in rats treated 3 times daily with formulations (ointment, cream, and gel) of aqueous extract of gotu kola epithelialized faster and the rate of wound contraction was higher when compared with control wounds (Suguna, 1996; Rosen, 1967; Leung, 1980). Healing was improved with the gel formulation when compared with the other two formulations (Sunilkumar, 1998). Scar formation was reduced when asiaticoside was applied during wound healing (Hostettmann, 1995). An extract of gotu kola accelerated the keratinization and transformation of the granular layer into the corneous layer in guinea pig skin (Morisset, 1987). Gotu kola extract administered externally for wound healing in rats accelerated the proliferation of granulation and increased tensile strength. The area of skin necrosis induced by burns was also decreased (Tsumuri, 1973).

Asiaticoside has an accelerating influence on wound healing (particularly in slow-healing wounds) in hospital patients when applied locally as a 1% salve or a 2% powder (Kiesswetter, 1964). Gotu kola extract has been used as a supporting therapy in the treatment of patients with second- and third-degree burns. Topical application expedited the healing of burns (Gravel, 1965). An extract of gotu kola and antiseptic compounds was applied in an open study of patients with soiled wounds or chronic or recurrent atony that was resistant to other forms of treatment (including antibiotic therapy, wound healing agents, debridement, skin flaps, and grafts); 64% of lesions completely healed, and 16% were improved (Morisset, 1987).

Patients with chronically infected ulcers were treated with gotu kola cream (1%); 77% of ulcers completely healed by the end of the treatment period, and 23% did not heal completely but were reduced in size (Kosalwatna, 1988). Extracts of gotu kola exhibited antibacterial activity and antifungal activity (Leungsakul, 1987; Medda, 1995).

The ulcer protective activity of the fresh juice of gotu kola was investigated with induced gastric ulcers in rats. Given orally in doses of 200 and 600 mg/kg twice daily for 5 days, centella showed significant protection against all previous experimental ulcer models, and results were comparable with those elicited by sucralfate (250 mg/kg, po BID ×5 days). At 600 mg/kg, gotu kola juice significantly enhanced gastric mucin secretion and increased mucosal cell glycoproteins. It also reduced cell shedding, indicating improved integrity of the mucosal barrier. Thus, the ulcer protective effect of centella juice may be due to strengthening of mucosal defensive factors (Sairam, 2001).

In vitro, gotu kola extract and purified extracts destroyed cultured cancer cells, retarded the development of solid and ascites tumors, and extended the life span of tumor-bearing mice. Practically no toxic effects were observed in normal human lymphocytes at effective concentrations (Babu, 1995). In lymphoma-bearing mice, 50 mg per kg per day (po) of crude methanol extract of *Centella asiatica* for 14 days significantly increased antioxidant enzymes such as superoxide dismutase, catalase, and glutathione peroxidase and decreased antioxidants such as glutathione and ascorbic acid (Jayashree, 2003).

The total triterpene fraction of gotu kola is active in preventing microangiopathy in people caused by hypertension or diabetes. This extract appears to improve microcirculation and reduce capillary permeability (De Sanctis, 2001; Incandela, 2001; Cesarone, 2001a). One trial also found the extract effective in reducing leg edema from "economy class flight syndrome" (Cesarone, 2001b).

Gotu kola has been used as a cognitive enhancer. An aqueous extract has been shown to decrease markers of oxidative stress and enhance cognitive measures in rat models of human Alzheimer's disease and epilepsy. Doses ranged from 100 to 300 mg/kg (Veerendra, 2002; Veerendra, 2003; Gupta, 2003).

Indications: Treatment of wounds, burns, and ulcerous skin ailments and prevention of keloid and hypertrophic scars. Extracts have been used to treat second- and third-degree burns and topically to accelerate healing, particularly in cases of chronic postsurgical and posttraumatic wounds.

Suggested Veterinary Indications:

Internal Use:

- *Helicobacter pylori* infection with ulceration of the stomach; aspirin/NSAID-induced gastritis
- Lymphoma and possibly other tumors in mice
- Cognitive enhancement

Topically: Wounds, equine granulomatous lesions, acral lick granulomas, posttraumatic degloving injuries, delayed wound healing, feline leprosy ulcers, anal furunculosis

Contraindications: None found.

Toxicology and Adverse Effects: Toxicology studies have shown that even very large doses of asiaticoside are not toxic, and that the toxicity of standardized extract and asiaticoside is very low (Laerum, 1972). Topical sensitization to gotu kola or carriers is possible. It may increase sleeping time when given with phenobarbital.

Notes of Interest: The name hydrocotyle is derived from the Greek "water" and "cup" to describe the habitat, water, and appearance of the cup-shaped leaves.

Dosage:

External Use:

Topically: applied twice daily in a 40% cream

Internal Use:

Human

Dried herb: 3-10 g TID

Infusions and decoctions: 5-30 g per cup of water, with 1 cup of the tea given TID

Tincture (usually 45% ethanol): 1:2 or 1:3: 1-5 mL TID

Small Animal

Dried herb: 25-300 mg/kg, divided daily (optimally, TID)

Infusion and decoction: 5-30 g per cup of water, administered at a rate of ¼-½ cup per 10 kg (20 lb), divided daily (optimally, TID)

Tincture (usually in 25%-40% ethanol): 1:2-1:3: 0.5-1.5 mL per 10 kg (20 lb), divided daily (optimally, TID) and diluted or combined with other herbs. Higher doses may be appropriate if the herb is used singly and is not combined in a formula.

References

Babu TD, Kuttan G, Padikkala J. Cytotoxic and anti-tumour properties of certain taxa of Umbelliferae with special reference to *Centella asiatica* (L.) Urban. J Ethnopharmacol 1995;48:53-57.

Bosse JP, Papillon J, Frenette G, Dansereau J, Cadotte M, Le Lorier J. Clinical study of a new antikeloid agent. Ann Plast Surg 1979;3:13-21.

Brinkhaus B, Lindner M, Schuppan D, Hahn EG. Chemical, pharmacological and clinical profile of the East Asian medical plant *Centella asiatica*. Phytomedicine 2000;7:427-448.

Cesarone MR, Incandela L, De Sanctis MT, Belcaro G, Geroulakos G, Griffin M, Lennox A, Di Renzo AD, Cacchio M, Bucci M. Flight microangiopathy in medium- to long-distance flights: prevention of edema and microcirculation alterations with total triterpenic fraction of *Centella asiatica*. Angiology 2001b;52(suppl 2):S33–S37.

Cesarone MR, Incandela L, De Sanctis MT, Belcaro G, Bavera P, Bucci M, Ippolito E. Evaluation of treatment of diabetic microangiopathy with total triterpenic fraction of *Centella asiatica:* a clinical prospective randomized trial with a microcirculatory model. Angiology 2001a;52(suppl 2):S49–S54.

De Sanctis MT, Belcaro G, Incandela L, Cesarone MR, Griffin M, Ippolito E, Cacchio M. Treatment of edema and increased capillary filtration in venous hypertension with total triterpenic fraction of *Centella asiatica:* a clinical, prospective, placebo-controlled, randomized, dose-ranging trial. Angiology 2001;52(suppl 2):S55–S59.

Del Vecchio A, Senni I, Cossu G, Molinaro M. Effect of *Centella asiatica* on the biosynthetic activity of fibroblasts in culture [Italian]. Farmaco (Prat) 1984;39:355-364.

Gupta YK, Veerendra Kumar MH, Srivastava AK. Effect of *Centella asiatica* on pentylenetetrazole-induced kindling, cognition and oxidative stress in rats. Pharmacol Biochem Behav 2003;74:579-585.

Hostettmann NR, Marston A. *Chemistry and Pharmacology of Natural Products: Saponins.* Cambridge: Cambridge University Press; 1995.

Incandela L, Cesarone MR, Cacchio M, De Sanctis MT, Santavenere C, D'Auro MG, Bucci M, Belcaro G. Total triterpenic fraction of *Centella asiatica* in chronic venous insufficiency and in high-perfusion microangiopathy. Angiology 2001;52(suppl 2):S9–S13.

Jayashree G, Kurup Muraleedhara G, Sudarslal S, Jacob VB. Antioxidant activity of *Centella asiatica* on lymphoma-bearing mice. Fitoterapia 2003;74:431-434.

Kiessetter H. Report on experience in treating wounds with asiaticoside (madecassol). Wien Med Wochenschr 1964;114:124-126.

Kosalwatna S, Shaipanich C, Bhanganada K. The effect of one percent *Centella asiatica* on chronic ulcers. Siriraj Hosp Gaz 1988;40:455-461.

Laerum OD, Iversen OH. Reticuloses and epidermal tumours in hairless mice after topical skin applications of cantharidin and asiaticoside. Cancer Res 1972;32:1463-1469.

Leung AY. *Encyclopaedia of Common Natural Ingredients Used in Food, Drugs and Cosmetics*. New York: John Wiley; 1980.

Leungsakul S. Antipyogenic bacterial activities of extracts from species of medicinal plants. 13th Symposium on Science and Technology of Thailand; October 20-22, 1987; Songkhla, Thailand.

Maquart FX, Bellon G, Gillery P, Wegrowski Y, Borel JP. Stimulation of collagen synthesis in fibroblast cultures by a triterpene extracted from *Centella asiatica*. Connect Tissue Res 1990;24:107-120.

Maquart FX, Chastang F, Simeon A, Birembaut P, Gillery P, Wegrowski Y. Triterpenes from *Centella asiatica* stimulate extracellular matrix accumulation in rat experimental wounds. Eur J Dermatol 1999;9:289-296.

May A. The effect of asiaticoside on pig skin in organ culture. Eur J Pharmacol 1968;4:331-339.

Medda S, Das N, Mahato SB, Mahadevan PR, Basu MK. Glycoside-bearing liposomal delivery systems against macrophage-associated disorders involving *Mycobacterium leprae* and *Mycobacterium tuberculosis*. Indian J Biochem Biophys 1995;32:147-151.

Morisset R, Cote NG. *Evaluation of the Healing Activity of Hydrocotyle Tincture in Treatment of Wounds*. Cothivet: Articles Scientifiques; 1987.

Qi S, Xie J, Li T. Effects of Asiaticoside on hypertrophic scars in a nude mice model. Zhonghua Shao Shang Za Zhi 2000;16:53-56. [Article in Chinese]

Rosen H, Blumenthal A, McCallum J. Effect of asiaticoside on wound healing in the rat. Proc Soc Exp Biol Med 1967;125:279-280.

Sairam K, Rao CV, Goel RK. Effect of *Centella asiatica* Linn on physical and chemical factors induced gastric ulceration and secretion in rats. Indian J Exp Biol 2001;39:137-142.

Shukla A, Rasik AM, Jain GK, Shankar R, Kulshrestha DK, Dhawan BN. In vitro and in vivo wound healing activity of asiaticoside isolated from *Centella asiatica*. J Ethnopharmacol 1999a;65:1-11.

Shukla A, Rasik AM, Dhawan BN. Asiaticoside-induced elevation of antioxidant levels in healing wounds. Phytother Res 1999b;13:50-54.

Suguna L, Sivakumar P, Chandrakasan G. Effects of *Centella asiatica* extract on dermal wound healing in rats. Indian J Exp Biol 1996;34:1208-1211.

Sunilkumar R, Parameshwaraiah S, Shivakumar HG. Evaluation of topical formulations of aqueous extract of *Centella asiatica* on open wounds in rats. Indian J Exp Biol 1998;36:569-572.

Tsumuri KY, Hiramatsu MH, Fugimura H. Effects of madecassol on wound healing. Oyo Yakuri 1973;7:833-843.

Veerendra Kumar MH, Gupta YK. Effect of *Centella asiatica* on cognition and oxidative stress in an intracerebroventricular streptozotocin model of Alzheimer's disease in rats. Clin Exp Pharmacol Physiol 2003;30:336-342.

Veerendra Kumar MH, Gupta YK. Effect of different extracts of *Centella asiatica* on cognition and markers of oxidative stress in rats. J Ethnopharmacol 2002;79:253-260.

Widgerow AD, Chait LA, Stals R, Stals PJ. New innovations in scar management. Aesthet Plast Surg 2000;24:227-234.

Williamson E, ed. *Major Herbs of Ayurveda*. Sydney: Churchill Livingstone; 2002.

Grapes, Grapeseed

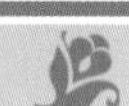

Vitis vinifera L. • VEE-tiss vih-NIFF-er-ah

Family: Vitaceae

Other Names: Grape complex, drue kerne

Parts Used: Seed, fruit skin

Distribution: Cultivated throughout the world

Selected Constituents: Most of the polyphenolic content in grape beverages is derived from the seed and skin of grapes (Prieur, 1994; Souquet, 1996).

Grape skin contains phenolics: hydroxycinnamic acids, flavonols, anthocyanins, and oligomeric proanthocyanidins (OPCs—oligomers of repeating catechin or epicatechin units). Grapeseed contains only a single class of phenolics—a series of OPCs. Grape juice contains the flavonoids quercetin, kaempferol, and myricetin, which are known inhibitors of platelet aggregation in vitro. OPCs were isolated originally by the French scientist Masquelier; he used the term pycnogenol to describe OPCs. Proanthocyanidins (procyanidins) and hydrolyzable tannins are the two major classes of tannins. Procyanidins are oligomers or polymers. These contribute to the color and flavor of red wines. Procyanidins, similar to tannins, characteristically bind and precipitate proteins, including enzymes.

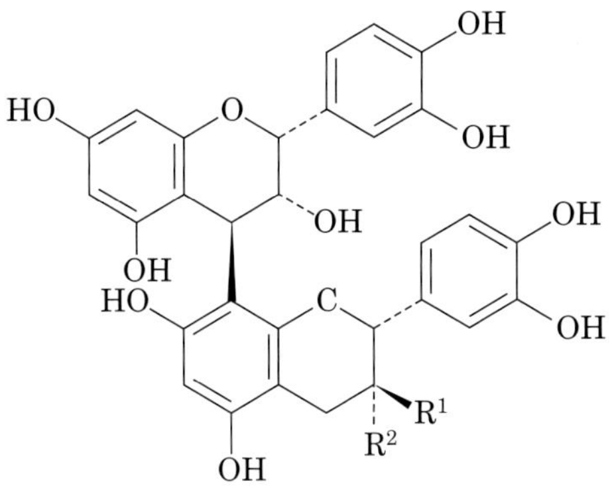

Procyanidin B_1 $R^1{=}OH, R^2{=}H$
Procyanidin B_2 $R^1{=}H, R^2{=}OH$

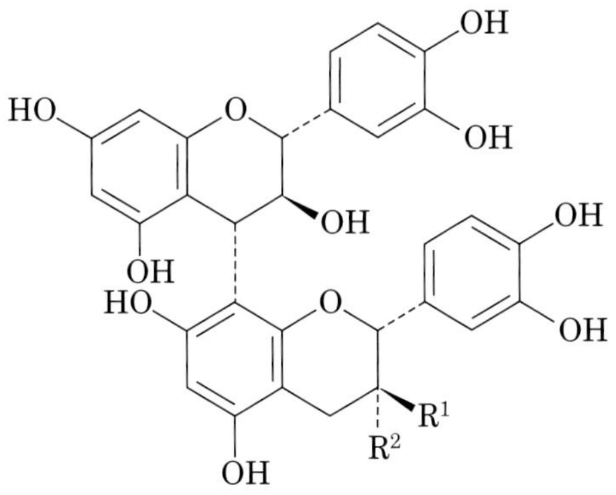

Procyanidin B_3 $R^1{=}OH, R^2{=}H$
Procyanidin B_4 $R^1{=}H, R^2{=}OH$

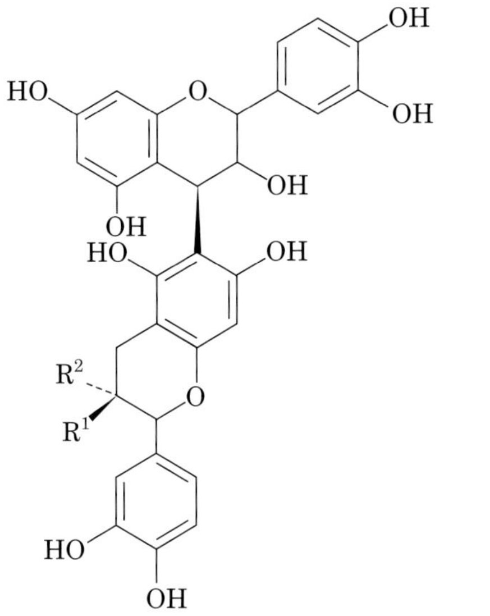

Procyanidin B_5 $R^1{=}H, R^2{=}OH$
Procyanidin B_7 $R^1{=}OH, R^2{=}H$

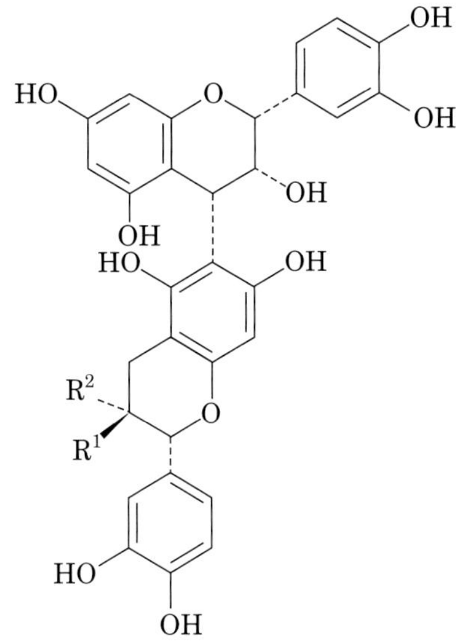

Procyanidin B_6 $R^1{=}OH, R^2{=}H$
Procyanidin B_8 $R^1{=}H, R^2{=}OH$

Structure of the Main Procyanidin Dimers from *V. vinifera*

Clinical Actions: Hemostatic, venotonic, astringent, diuretic, anti-inflammatory

Energetics: Cold, dry

History and Traditional Usage: Use of the common grape dates back to very ancient times. For sustenance, the fruits are eaten fresh or in dried form (raisins), or they are processed to make wine; the leaves are also sometimes eaten. Folk medicine throughout the world makes use of the common grape, as do Traditional Chinese Medicine and the Ayurvedic medical tradition.

For animal use, de Bairacli Levy (1985) indicates anemia; it is also used for internal cleansing and as treatment for mammary tumors. The tendrils and leaves of grape vine and fresh grape juice have been used by the Arabs as an internal and external cure of tumors, for constipation, for debility, for fits (internal cleansing), in the treatment of paralysis, and for faulty pigmentation. Spirit vini rect, or wine, is listed in *Veterinary Counter Practice* (RCVS, 1920).

Published Research: Red wines contain a variety of polyphenolic antioxidants. The total antioxidant activity of some wines investigated was well correlated with phenol content, and polyphenols are, in vitro, significant antioxidants (Lopez-Velez, 2003). OPCs from pine bark and grapeseed demonstrated the strongest free radical scavenging activity when compared with citrus flavinoids and other flavonoids. OPCs from grapeseed were slightly superior to those from pine bark (Schwitters, 1995).

Several epidemiologic studies have found an inverse relationship between the total intake of flavonoids and the incidence of cardiovascular events (Hertog, 1995). Of the numerous food sources of polyphenolics investigated, red wine and other grape products have been shown to inhibit platelet aggregation (and therefore reduce the incidence of atherosclerosis, platelet thrombus formation, and subsequent heart attack) attributed primarily to the polyphenolic compounds in these products (Folts, 1998). However, although several studies have attributed the beneficial effects to a single polyphenolic compound, the beneficial effects observed in the epidemiologic studies mentioned previously might in fact be attributed to synergistic relationships among multiple polyphenolic compounds (Shanmuganayagam, 2002). OPCs reduce cholesterol in rabbits (Wegrowski, 1984).

Extracts of grapeseed and grape skin are effective platelet inhibitors when used individually in dogs and in humans (Demrow, 1995; Osman, 2000; Folts, 1999). A dose of 10 mL of purple grape juice/kg significantly decreased in vivo and ex vivo platelet activity in dogs (Osman, 1998). In the dog, monkey, and human, it has been shown that 5 mL/kg red wine or 5 to 10 mL/kg of purple grape juice inhibited platelet activity and protected against epinephrine activation of platelets (Folts, 2002).

Grapeseed and grape skin together provide a synergistic effect (Shanmuganayagam, 2002). Seven male hound dogs (18.6-27.5 kg) were fed the following treatments for 7 days, with each new treatment starting after a 7-day washout period between treatments: grapeseed (5 mg/kg), grape skin (20 mg/kg), enzyme blend (5 mg/kg), grapeseed (5 mg/kg) + grape skin (20 mg/kg), and grapeseed (5 mg/kg) + grape skin (20 mg/kg) + enzyme blend (2 mg/kg). Feeding grapeseed or grape skin or enzyme blend alone did not affect platelet aggregation, whereas feeding the grape extracts in combination decreased platelet aggregation by 31.9%. When dogs were fed an enzyme blend containing bromelain in addition to both grape extracts, platelet aggregation was decreased by 56.2%. Twenty-four hours later, platelet aggregation was inhibited by 31.5%, suggesting potential residual antiplatelet effects from the final dose. The major finding of this study is that concentrations of grapeseed and grape skin that have little or no effect on platelet activity when used individually elicit a greater antiplatelet effect when used in combination (Shanmuganayagam, 2002).

OPCs increased natural killer cell cytotoxicity, modulated levels of interleukins from immune compromised mice, including those infected with retrovirus (Cheshier, 1996), and demonstrated antimutagenic activity in vitro (Seo, 2001).

Evidence suggests that wine consumption decreases the risk of cancer at several sites, including cancer of the upper digestive tract, lung, and colon, basal cell carcinoma, and non-Hodgkin's lymphoma. The presence of resveratrol, a polyphenol specifically present in red wine, may contribute to these cancer preventive effects. Resveratrol, a phytoalexin found in red wine, inhibits the metabolic activation of carcinogens, has antioxidant and anti-inflammatory properties, decreases cell proliferation, and induces apoptosis (Bianchinin, 2003; Granados-Soto, 2003). It is believed to play a role in the chemoprevention of human cancer. Resveratrol has also been shown to inhibit several leukemia cell lines and the growth of human T-cell lymphotrophic virus-1–infected cell lines, at least in part, by inducing apoptosis mediated by down-regulation in survivin expression (Hayashibara, 2002).

The anticataract activity of a grapeseed extract (GSE) that contains 38.5% procyanidins was investigated in hereditary cataractous rats. Rats were fed a standard diet that contained 0% or 0.213% GSE [0.082% procyanidins in the diet (w/w)] for 27 days. Results suggested that procyanidins and their antioxidative metabolites prevented the progression of cataract formation by their antioxidative action (Yamakoshi, 2002).

Proanthocyanidins (PAs) from grapeseeds have anti-inflammatory effects on experimental inflammation in rats and mice. PA mechanisms of anti-inflammatory action are relevant to oxygen free radical scavenging, antilipid peroxidation, and inhibition of the formation of inflammatory cytokines (Li, 2001). Procyanidins at a dose of 2 mg/kg applied orally to rats 3 times daily for 6 days inhibited carrageenan-induced hind paw edema. Procyanidin stabilized capillary walls and prevented the increase in capillary permeability caused by local cutaneous application of xylene (Zafirov, 1990). OPCs significantly increased the rate of disappearance of postoperative edema (Baruch, 1984).

Semen of different ejaculates collected from breeding rams was mixed and prepared with various antioxidants, including resveratrol, and compared with controls. A significantly higher proportion of motile sperm cells was observed in treated than in control samples. The frequency of acrosomal defects was lower in the treated groups than in the control group. Antioxidants, including resveratrol, may improve the effects of preservation on ram semen (Sarlos, 2002).

Oral administration of bioflavonoid antioxidants (containing grapeseed extract) to cats at risk for oxidative stress may have a beneficial effect on their ability to resist oxidative injury to erythrocytes. Heinz body formation may result from oxidant exposure, as well as from disease processes such as diabetes mellitus, lymphoma, and hyperthyroidism. In an experimental study in which cats were given acetaminophen to induce oxidative injury to red blood cells, administration of 10 mg daily of a commercial grapeseed extract (Proanthozone; Animal Health Options, Golden, Colo) mitigated damage, with no adverse effects (Allison, 2000).

Urinary bladder dysfunction secondary to benign prostatic hyperplasia (BPH) is a major affliction of aging men. A rabbit model of partial outlet obstruction was used to evaluate the ability of a standardized grape suspension to protect the bladder against obstructive bladder dysfunction. Rabbits were divided into 4 groups that were pretreated by oral gavage for 3 weeks with a standardized grape suspension in water or with vehicle; then the bladder was partially ligated, or rabbits were given a sham operation after 3 weeks of treatment. At 3 weeks following surgery, in vivo and in vitro bladder functions were evaluated. The grape suspension significantly reduced the severity of obstructed bladder dysfunction. This is consistent with the hypothesis that ischemia is a major etiologic factor in obstructive dysfunction; treatment with antioxidants and membrane stabilization compounds such as those in the grape suspension may be effective in the treatment of patients with obstructive bladder disease (Argartan, 2004).

Indications: Antioxidant, reduction of edema, venous insufficicncy, diabetic retinopathy, prevention of some cancers, prevention of cardiovascular disease, hypercholesterolemia, stabilization of connective tissue, assistance in the healing of fractures, antiallergic activity, wound healing, and pretreatment for surgery. Impaired circulation, edema, radiation adverse effects, retinal damage, rhinitis, and varicose veins

Potential Veterinary Uses: Feline leukemia viral infection, feline lower urinary tract disease, various ocular disorders, including retinopathy; prevention and treatment of early cataracts and nuclear sclerosis, antioxidant support for geriatric animals or those with cardiovascular disorder, photosensitization and prevention of sunburn in depigmented animals, anti-inflammatory support; prevention of postoperative edema; sports injury edema, systemic mast cell tumor

Contraindications: None described,

Safety and Toxicity: Acute oral toxicity, dermal toxicity, dermal irritation, and eye irritation studies have been conducted on grapeseed extract. The LD_{50} was found to be greater than 5 g/kg when administered once orally via gastric intubation to fasted male and female albino rats. The LD_{50} of grapeseed extract was found to be greater than 2 g/kg when administered once in 24 hours to the clipped intact skin of male and female albino rats. In addition, 2 g/kg was found to be the no-observed-effect level (NOEL) for systemic toxicity under the conditions of the study. In a dermal irritation study, grapeseed extract received a descriptive rating classification of "moderately irritating." Extensive chronic studies were also conducted. Mice were fed 0, 100, 250, or 500 mg grapeseed extgract/kg/day for 6 months, and the effects of exposure on brain, duodenum, heart, kidney, liver, lung, pancreas, and spleen, and on serum chemistry changes in female mice were examined. These acute studies demonstrated that grapeseed extract is safe and that it caused no detrimental effects in vivo under the conditions investigated in this study (Ray, 2001).

The safety of Proanthozone (Animal Health Options, Golden, Colo) was evaluated in four healthy adult cats given 10 mg orally daily for 32 days. No abnormal clinical or laboratory findings attributed to the test compound were seen during, and for 1 week following, the administration period. The supplement was safe when orally administered in healthy cats for 1 month (Burkhard, 1996).

Toxicity was not observed at 60 mg/kg/day for 6 and 12 months in rats and dogs, respectively. OPCs from grapeseed are devoid of toxic, mutagenic, and teratogenic effects.

Renal failure has been associated with the ingestion of grapes and raisins in dogs (Singleton, 2001; Gwaltney-Brant, 2001), but no cause has been identified at the time of this writing.

Preparations: Red wine, resveratrol (a red wine extract), grapeseed extract, grape juice, pycnogenol (a commercial mixture of bioflavonoids), OPC

Dosage:

Human:

Grapeseed extract (Vitis vinifera) standardized to 95% polyphenols: 50 mg daily to 150 to 300 mg per day for specific illnsses

Small Animal:

For dogs, give 1-2 mg per kg of extract daily

Historical Veterinary Doses:

Spirit Vini Rect.: horse, 21-35 mL; pig, 3.5-10.5 mL; dog, 3.5-5.3 mL daily (RCVS, 1920)

References

Agartan CA, Whitbeck C, Sokol R, Chichester P, Levin RM. Protection of urinary bladder function by grape suspension. Phytother Res 2004;18:1013-1018.

Allison RW, Lassen ED, Burhard MJ, Lappin MR. Effect of a bioflavonoid dietary supplement on acetominophen induced oxidative energy to feline erythrocytes. J Am Vet Med Assoc 2000;217:1157-1161.

Baruch J. [Effect of Endotelon in postoperative edema. Results of a double-blind study versus placebo in 32 female patients.] Ann Chir Plast Esthet 1984;29:393-395.

Bianchini F, Vainio H. Wine and resveratrol: mechanisms of cancer prevention? Eur J Cancer Prev 2003;12:417-425.

Burkhard MJ, Meyer DJ, Lappin MR, Christopher MM, Hutchinson JM. The effect of a commercial bioflavonoid in normal cats and cats with acetaminophen induced oxidative erythrocyte injury. Abstract available on the Animal Health Options website: www.animalhealthoptions.com/research.html

Cheshier JE, Ardestani-Kaboudanian S, Liang B, et al. Immunomodulation by pycnogenol in retrovirus-infected or ethanol-fed mice. Life Sci 1996;58:PL87–PL96.

De Bairacli Levy J. *The Complete Herbal Handbook for the Dog and Cat.* London: Faber and Faber; 1985.

Demrow HS, Slane PR, Folts JD. Administration of wine and grape juice inhibits in vivo platelet activity and thrombosis in stenosed canine coronary arteries. Circulation 1995;91:1182-1188.

Folts JD. Antithrombotic potential of grape juice and red wine for preventing heart attacks. Pharm Biol 1998;36:S21–S27.

Folts JD. Potential health benefits from the flavonoids in grape products on vascular disease. Adv Exp Med Biol 2002;505:95-111.

Folts J, Shanmuganayagam D. Commercial mixture of flavonoids, Provex CV(R), inhibits in vivo thrombosis and ex vivo platelet aggregation in dogs and humans (abstract). FASEB J 1999;13:A839.

Granados-Soto V. Pleiotropic effects of resveratrol. Drug News Perspective 2003;16:5.

Gwaltney-Brant S, Holding JK, Donaldson CW, Eubig PA, Khan SA. Renal failure associated with ingestion of grapes or raisins in dogs. J Am Vet Med Assoc 2001;218:1555-1556.

Hayashibara T, Yamada Y, Nakayama S, et al. Resveratrol induces downregulation in survivin expression and apoptosis in HTLV-1–infected cell lines: a prospective agent for adult T cell leukemia chemotherapy. Nutr Cancer 2002;44:193-201,299-307.

Hertog MG, Kromhout D, Aravanis C, et al. Flavonoid intake and long-term risk of coronary heart disease and cancer in the seven countries study. Arch Intern Med 1995;155:381-386.

Li WG, Zhang XY, Wu YJ, Tian X. Anti-inflammatory effect and mechanism of proanthocyanidins from grape seeds. Acta Pharmacol Sin 2001;22:1117-1120.

Lopez-Velez M, Martinez-Martinez F, Del Valle-Ribes C. The study of phenolic compounds as natural antioxidants in wine. Crit Rev Food Sci Nutr 2003;43:233-244.

Osman HE, Maalej N, Shanmuganayagam D, Folts JD. Grape juice but not orange or grapefruit juice inhibits platelet activity in dogs and monkeys. J Nutr 1998;128:2307-2312.

Ray S, Bagchi D, Lim PM, et al. Acute and long-term safety evaluation of a novel IH636 grape seed proanthocyanidin extract. Res Commun Mol Pathol Pharmacol 2001;109:165-197.

RCVS (Royal College of Veterinary Surgeons). *Veterinary Counter Practice.* London: Ballantyne Press; 1920.

Sarlos P, Molnar A, Kokai M, Gabor G, Ratky J. Comparative evaluation of the effect of antioxidants in the conservation of ram semen. Acta Vet Hung 2002;50:235-245.

Schwitters B, Masquelier J. *OPC in Practice.* 2nd ed. Rome: Alfa Omega Editrice; 1995.

Seo K, Jung S, Park M, Song Y, Choung S. Effects of leucocyanidines on activities of metabolizing enzymes and antioxidant enzymes. Biol Pharm Bull 2001;24:592-593.

Shanmuganayagam D, Beahm MR, Osman HE, Krueger CG, Reed JD, Folts JD. Grape seed and grape skin extracts elicit a greater antiplatelet effect when used in combination than when used individually in dogs and humans. J Nutr 2002;132:3592-3598.

Singleton VL. More information on grape or raisin toxicosis. J Am Vet Med Assoc 2001;219:434,436.

Souquet JM, Cheynier V, Brossaud F, Moutounet M. Polymeric proanthocyanidins from grape skins. Phytochemistry 1996;43:509-512.

Wegrowski J, Robert AM, Moczar M. The effect of procyanidolic oligomers on the composition of normal and hypercholesterolemic rabbit aortas. Biochem Pharmacol 1984;33:3491-3497.

Yamakoshi J, Saito M, Kataoka S, Tokutake S. Procyanidin-rich extract from grape seeds prevents cataract formation in hereditary cataractous (ICR/f) rats. J Agric Food Chem 2002;50:4983-4988.

Zafirov D, Bredy-Dobreva G, Litchev V, Papasova M. Antiexudative and capillaritonic effects of procyanidines isolated from grape seeds *(V. vinifera).* Acta Physiol Pharmacol Bulg 1990;16:50-54.

Gravel Root, Joe Pye Weed

Eupatorium purpureum L. • yoo-puh-TOR-ee-um pur-PUR-ee-um

Common Names: Gravelweed, queen of the meadow, purple boneset, sweetscented Joe Pye weed. Note that "gravel root" is also a common name for *Hydrangea arborescens*.

Similar Species: *Eupatorium maculatum*

Family: Asteraceae

Parts Used: Rhizome and root

Distribution: Indigenous to North America

Selected Constituents: Volatile oil, terpenes, flavonoids (euparin, eupatorin), resins (eupatorine, eupurpurin), saponins, silica, pyrrolizidine alkaloids

Clinical Actions: Antilithic, antirheumatic, diuretic

Energetics: Cooling, slightly bitter, drying

History and Traditional Usage: Native Americans used gravel root for difficult urination and kidney problems, for "female problems," to expel afterbirth, as a love potion, and to break fevers, as well as for dyeing. It was used by European settlers for urinary and kidney complaints, as well as for digestive disorders, rheumatism, cough, and prolapse. The plant is named after an American Indian named Joe Pye, who was said to have cured typhus with it. It has been used as a diuretic and stimulant and in dropsy, strangury, gravel, hematuria, gout, rheumatism, and chronic urinary tract disease (Grieve, 1975).

Published Research: An active principle of gravel root has been identified as cistifolium, which is described as an inhibitor of integrin cellular adhesion molecules (ICAMS)—glycoproteins and carbohydrate molecules present on cell surfaces, in particular, leukocytes and platelets. Downregulating ICAMS may prevent the expression of a number of diseases. It has been described as useful for rheumatoid arthritis and may be useful in thrombotic disease, osteoporosis, cancer metastasis, immunological disorders, and parasitic infections (Habtemariam, 1998). Cistifolin showed activity in in vitro and in vivo models of inflammation. Data show that it inhibits monocyte adhesion to fibrinogen in a concentration-dependent manner (Habtemariam, 2001).

Indications: Urinary calculus, cystitis, dysuria, prostatitis, rheumatism, kidney stones or gravel

Potential Veterinary Uses: Urinary tract disorders, including bladder stones

Contraindications: Pregnancy, lactation, hepatic conditions

Toxicology and Adverse Effects: AHPA class 2a, 2b, 2c, 2d. Roots contain pyrrolizidine alkaloids; avoid prolonged use (over 1 month in duration) or use with concurrent liver disease.

Dosage:

Human:

Dried herb: 2-10 g TID

Infusions and decoctions: 5-30 g per cup of water, with 1 cup of the tea given TID

Tincture (usually 40% ethanol): 1:2 or 1:3: 0.5-5 mL TID

Small Animal:

Dried herb: 25-300 mg/kg, divided daily (optimally, TID)

Infusion and decoction: 5-30 g per cup of water, administered at a rate of ¼-½ cup per 10 kg (20 lb), divided daily (optimally, TID)

Tincture (40% ethanol): 1:2-1:3: 0.5-1.5 mL per 10 kg (20 lb), divided daily (optimally, TID) and diluted or combined with other herbs. Higher doses may be appropriate if the herb is used singly and is not combined in a formula.

References

Grieve M. *A Modern Herbal.* London: Jonathan Cape; 1975.

Habtemariam S. Cistifolin, an integrin-dependent cell adhesion blocker from the anti-rheumatic herbal drug, gravel root (rhizome of *Eupatorium purpureum*). Planta Med 1998;64:683-685.

Habtemariam S. Antiinflammatory activity of the antirheumatic herbal drug, gravel root *(Eupatorium purpureum):* further biological activities and constituents. Phytother Res 2001;15:687-690.

Green Tea

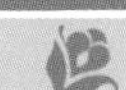

Camellia sinensis (L.) *Kuntze* • kuh-MEE-lee-uh sye-NEN-sis

Family: Theaceae

Parts Used: Young leaves. Green tea is obtained by drying freshly harvested tea leaves, thus causing inactivation of enzymes that initiate the fermentation process. This yields a dry and stable product that contains most of the polyphenols and gives green tea its typical color and taste (Bachrach, 2002). Green tea is rich in polyphenolic compounds, which account for a third of the dry weight of the leaves; the most prominent components are flavonols, commonly known as catechins (Balentine, 1997).

Distribution: Green tea was originally cultivated in China. It is now grown in India, China, Sri Lanka, Japan, Indonesia, Kenya, Turkey, Pakistan, Malawi, and Argentina.

Selected Constituents: Purine alkaloids (caffeine, theobromine, theophylline), triterpene saponins, catechins, caffeic acid derivatives, anorganic ions (fluoride, potassium, aluminum ions), volatile oil. Green tea contains 30% to 40% polyphenols, which are catechins, with potent antioxidant properties and these give green tea its bitter flavor. Green tea contains six primary catechin compounds: catechin, gallaogatechin, epicatechin, epigallocatechin, epicatechin gallate, and apigallocatechin gallate (also known as EGCG). EGCG is considered to be the most active component in green tea.

R = H (EC)
= OH (EGC)

Epicatechin (EC)

R = H (ECg)
= OH (EGCg)

Epigalocatechin (EGC)

Clinical Actions: Stimulant, antioxidant, possible antimutagen

Energetics: Warming, drying

History and Traditional Usage: Archeologic evidence suggests that tea leaves steeped in boiling water were consumed 500,000 years ago. Botanical evidence indicates that India and China were among the first to cultivate tea. In Traditional Chinese and Indian Medicine, green tea has been used as a stimulant, diuretic, and astringent and to improve heart health. Other traditional uses include treating flatulence, regulating body temperature and blood sugar, promoting digestion, and improving mental processes.

Published Research: Tea consumption has been associated with anti-inflammatory, antioxidative, antimutagenic, and anticarcinogenic effects (Benelli, 2002; Weisburger, 2002). Although most experimental studies have focused on EGCG as a major active constituent of green tea, the overall preventive effect of green tea observed in vivo is thought to require the combined actions of several components of tea, rather than a single compound (Williams, 2000). Moreover, green tea extracts are more stable than is pure EGCG because of the presence of other antioxidant constituents in the extract.

Another constituent of green tea is caffeine, which interacts with the polyphenols by improving the antimutagenic activity of regular tea compared with the decaffeinated version (Weisburger, 1998). In vitro, tea with caffeine inhibited the growth of several human cancer cell lines, and tumor prevention in humans and rats was improved by regular green tea consumption (Huang, 1997).

Tea consumption has been shown to afford protection against chemical carcinogen–induced stomach, lung, esophagus, duodenum, pancreas, liver, breast, and colon carcinogenesis in various models. The mechanisms of tea's broad cancer chemopreventive effects are not completely understood. Several theories have been put forward, including inhibition of ultraviolet (UV) and tumor promoter–induced ornithine decarboxylase, cyclooxygenase, and lipoxygenase activities, as well as antioxidant and free radical scavenging activity; enhancement of antioxidant (glutathione peroxidase, catalase, and quinone reductase) and phase II (glutathione-S-transferase) enzyme activities; inhibition of lipid peroxidation; and anti-inflammatory activity (Katiyar, 1997).

Overproduction of nitric oxide contributes to disorders of vascular dysfunction and organ failure during endotoxemia and with diseases such as inflammatory bowel disease, asthma, or lupus nephritis (Pfeilschifter, 2002). Green tea extract in concentrations in the range of the plasma concentration found in humans who drink 6 to 10 cups of green tea per day indirectly dramatically reduces nitric oxide production (Tedeschi, 2004). Because green tea can be consumed over the long term in large quantities without any (currently known) harmful adverse effects, and because epidemiologic data are already available on Chinese and Japanese cohorts (Fujiki, 2002), its possible therapeutic potential in inflammatory disease deserves consideration.

A study investigated the inhibitory effect of the green tea catechin extract, Polyphenon, with epigallocatechin gallate on staphylococcal enterotoxin B in patients with atopic dermatitis. Inhibition of cell activation by catechin was observed in in vivo and in vitro studies, suggesting that catechin may be useful in the treatment of patients with atopic dermatitis (Hisano, 2003).

Another study investigated the body fat–suppressive effects of green tea in rats fed a high-fat diet, to determine whether the effect is associated with β-adrenoceptor activation of thermogenesis in brown adipose tissue. Feeding a high-fat diet that contains a water extract of green tea at 20 g/kg prevented the increase in body fat caused by a high-fat diet without affecting energy intake. The concurrent administration of the β-adrenoceptor antagonist propranolol inhibited the body fat–suppressive effect of green tea extract. It appeared that green tea inhibits body fat deposition, possibly through reduction in digestibility and through increased brown adipose tissue thermogenesis (Choo, 2003).

Green tea polyphenolic compounds have been shown to reduce inflammation in a murine model of inflammatory arthritis, so the effects of these catechins were investigated for chondroprotective effects with the use of bovine and human cartilage cultured with and without agents known to accelerate cartilage matrix breakdown. Catechins were effective at inhibiting proteoglycan and type II collagen breakdown (Adcocks, 2002).

With the use of rodent models of diarrhea, the effects of a hot water extract of black tea *(Camellia sinensis)* on upper gastrointestinal transit and on diarrhea were investigated. Black tea extract was found to possess antidiarrheal activity in all models of diarrhea used. Naloxone significantly inhibited the antidiarrheal activity of the extract and of loperamide, which suggested a role of the opioid system in the antidiarrheal activity of the extract (Besra, 2003).

Two experiments evaluated the effects of protein supplementation of green tea waste on palatability and the performance of lactating cows. It was concluded that green tea waste can be used as a partial replacement for other protein sources with no detrimental effects on the performance of lactating cows (Kondo, 2004).

Antiparasite effects of a hot water infusion and an aqueous acetone extract of green tea *(Camellia sinensis)* on the motility of infective larvae of the sheep nematodes *Teladorsagia circumcincta* and *Trichostrongylus colubriformis* were investigated under in vitro conditions. The infusion and extract doses dependently inactivated the infective larvae, as assessed by the larval migration inhibition (LMI) assay. Fractions that contained epigallocatechin gallate (EGCG) and proanthocyanidin oligomers were most effective (Molan, 2004).

Indications: Prophylaxis against cancer, stimulant, diarrhea, arthritis, atopy

Potential Veterinary Uses: Diarrhea, cancer prevention, adjunctive cancer therapy, atopic dermatitis, topically for "hot spots" and rashes, oral cancers

Contraindications: People with renal disease, thyroid hyperfunction, or anxiety and pregnant or nursing women should be careful of use.

Toxicology and Adverse Effects: Black tea (the fermented form of green tea) has class 2d classification from the AHPA. No health hazards known with proper administration. Hyperacidity, gastric irritation, reduced appetite, obstipation, or diarrhea may result from excessive tea consumption.

Preparation Notes: Black tea (rolled, fermented, dried), green tea (heat treated and rapidly dried and rolled), oolong tea (semifermented). Fermentation (oxidation) changes the color from yellowish green (green tea) to reddish brown (black tea), along with the chemical composition (because of oxidation of polyphenols).

Dosage:

External Use: Plain green tea (the infusion) may be used for excoriations and other minor skin lesions (such as canine hot spots)

Internal Use:

Human

Most Japanese ingest 0.8-1.3 g green tea extract, including 340-540 mg ECCG, in 10 (8 oz) cups daily (Nakachi, 1997).

Infusion: 3 cups of green tea per day (3 g soluble components, or 240 to 320 mg polyphenols)

Standardized extract: 300-400 mg per day of extracts that contain 80% total polyphenols and 55% epigallocatechin

Small Animal

Standardized extract containing 80% polyphenols: 10-20 mg per kg, divided daily

Green tea can be added easily to moist food or given in water, ½-1 cup per 10 kg per day

References

Adcocks C, Collin P, Buttle DJ. Catechins from green tea *(Camellia sinensis)* inhibit bovine and human cartilage proteoglycan and type II collagen degradation in vitro. J Nutr 2002;132:341-346.

Bachrach U, Wang Y-C. Cancer therapy and prevention by green tea: role of ornithine decarboxylase. Amino Acids 2002;22:1-13.

Balentine DA, Wiseman SA, Bouwens LC. The chemistry of tea flavonoids. Crit Rev Food Sci Nutr 1997;37:693-704.

Benelli R, Venè R, Bisacchi D, Garbisa S, Albini A. Anti-invasive effects of green tea polyphenol epigallocatechin-3-gallate (EGCG), a natural inhibitor of metallo and serine proteases. Biol Chem 2002;383:101-105.

Besra SE, Gomes A, Ganguly DK, Vedasiromoni JR. Antidiarrhoeal activity of hot water extract of black tea *(Camellia sinensis)*. Phytother Res 2003;17:380-384.

Choo JJ. Green tea reduces body fat accretion caused by high-fat diet in rats through beta-adrenoceptor activation of thermogenesis in brown adipose tissue. J Nutr Biochem 2003;14:671-676.

Fujiki H, Suganuma M, Imai K, Nakachi K. Green tea: cancer preventive beverage and/or drug. Cancer Lett 2002;188:9-13.

Hisano M, Yamaguchi K, Inoue Y, et al. Inhibitory effect of catechin against the superantigen staphylococcal enterotoxin B (SEB). Arch Dermatol Res 2003;295:183-189.

Huang MT, Xie JG, Wang ZY, et al. Effects of tea, decaffeinated tea, and caffeine on UVB light–induced complete carcinogenesis in SKH-1 mice: demonstration of caffeine as a biologically important constituent of tea. Cancer Res 1997;57: 2623-2629.

Katiyar SK, Mukhtar H. Tea antioxidants in cancer chemoprevention. J Cell Biochem Suppl 1997;27:59-67.

Kondo M, Nakano M, Kaneko A, et al. Ensiled green tea waste as partial replacement for soyabean meal and lucerne hay in lactating cows. Asian-Austral J Anim Sci 2004;17:960-966.

Molan AL, Sivakumaran S, Spencer PA, Meagher LP. Green tea flavan-3-ols and oligomeric proanthocyanidins inhibit the motility of infective larvae of *Teladorsagia circumcincta* and *Trichostrongylus colubriformis* in vitro. Res Vet Sci 2004;77:239-243.

Nakachi K, Imai K, Suga K. Epidemiological evidence for prevention of cancer and cardiovascular disease by drinking green tea. In: Ohigashi H, Osawa T, Terao J, et al, eds. *Food Factors for Cancer Prevention.* Tokyo: Springer; 1997a:105-108.

Pfeilschifter J, Beck KF, Eberhardt W, Huwiler A. Changing gears in the course of glomerulonephritis by shifting superoxide to nitric oxide–dominated chemistry. Kidney Int 2002;61:809-815.

Tedeschi E, Menegazzi M, Yao Y, Suzuki H, Förstermann U, Kleinert H. Green tea inhibits human inducible nitric-oxide synthase expression by down-regulating signal transducer and activator of transcription-1α activation. Mol Pharmacol 2004;65:111-120.

Weisburger JH, Dolan L, Pittman B. Inhibition of PhIP mutagenicity by caffeine, lycopene, daidzein and genistein. Mutat Res 1998;41:125-128.

Weisburger JH. Lifestyle, health and disease prevention: the underlying mechanisms. Eur J Cancer Prev 2002;11(suppl 2):S1–S7.

Williams SN, Shih H, Guenette DK, et al. Comparative studies on the effects of green tea extracts and individual tea catechins on human CYP1A gene expression. Chem Biol Interact 2000;128:211-229.

Guggul 

Commiphora mukul (Hook ex. Stocks) Engl.; Formerly *Balsamodendron mukul* (Hook) • kom-MEE-for-uh MOO kul

Distribution: Arid, rocky regions of central India and Bangladesh

Similar Species: Older descriptions of the source species list *Commiphora roxburghiana* as the source for commercially available guggul (US Dispensatory, 1918), but this species is not presently recognized. Some sources treat guggul and myrrh as botanically synonymous, and others say that guggul is similar to but not as strong as myrrh. *Boswellia serrata* is sometimes referred to as guggul.

Other Names: Guggulu (sanskrit), gugulon, guggal, gum guggul, false myrrh, mukul myrrh tree, common myrrh, bdellium tree. Bdellium (multiple bdelliums were listed in the US Dispensatory) refers to all gums from similar species of trees, but they had different characteristics and uses. Guggul was called *Indian bdellium.*

Family: Burseraceae

Parts Used: Resin. Stem and leaves may also be used.

Collection: Resin is collected in winter after the bark has been cut.

Selected Constituents: Resins known as guggulsterones, volatile oil (containing myrcene and eugenol), lignans, lipids (long-chain tetrols such as eicosan-1,2,3,4-tetrol), and mucilaginous polysaccharides. Guggulipid is a dried ethyl acetate extract of the whole resin.

Guggulsterone-Z

Clinical Actions: Astringent, carminative, diaphoretic, diuretic, emmenagogue, expectorant, alterative, stomachic, sedative

Energetics: Bitter, aromatic, warming

History and Traditional Usage: This herb has been used at least since the days of the New Testament for infected wounds, digestive problems, and bronchitis. Used in traditional Indian medicine for rheumatic complaints, neurologic disorders, skin problems, urinary problems, and obesity. It was also used for women's health and purification rituals. Indians used guggul and/or myrrh to treat animals with rheumatism, cold, and cough.

Published Research: Many trials in people and animals have shown that guggul is effective in lowering blood lipids. The E- and Z-guggulsterones bind two nuclear hormone receptors that regulate cholesterol synthesis (Urizar, 2003) and multiple steroid receptors (Burris 2005). Other mechanisms at work in the lipid-lowering effect may include enhancing excretion and degradation of cholesterol, stimulating thyroid activity, and altering biogenic amines. The most recent controlled trial in people (with TID doses of 1000 mg and 2000 mg of a standardized extract) did not confirm this effect (Szapary, 2003); however, a reanalysis of the data did show that guggul lowered blood glucose and insulin, C-reactive protein levels, and blood pressure.

Older studies have shown an analgesic effect in people taking guggul for arthritis and rheumatism. An uncontrolled trial in people with osteoarthritis of the knee showed that subjects exhibited significant improvement after 1 month of treatment. The dose used was 500 mg TID with food (Singh, 2003). Another uncontrolled trial in India showed that guggul was as effective as tetracycline in controlling nodulocystic acne.

Dixit et al (1980) studied the hypolipidemic effects of a guggul extract in dogs and monkeys. Animals were administered a single dose (25 mg/kg) of guggul powder intravenously, and blood was drawn at 2, 4, 8, 12, 24, and 48 hours after administration. Guggul extract was associated with a peak decrease of 31% in total cholesterol at 4 and 8 hours, and levels were still 11% lower at 48 hours. Triglyceride levels were suppressed by 21% at 24 hours, and they remained 10% lower than preadministration levels at 48 hours. Phospholipid levels were 43% lower at 2 hours, persisted through 8 hours, and remained 10% lower at 48 hours. Lipid levels were more dramatically affected in monkeys than in dogs.

Indications: Hyperlipidemia, hypercholesterolemia, rheumatism, arthritis, acne

Potential Veterinary Indications: Hyperlipidemia, hypercholesterolemia, rheumatic disorders (arthritis, stiff muscles)

Contraindications: Pregnancy. One of the guggulsterones may increase iodine uptake by the thyroid, so this herb should be used with caution in patients with thyroid disorders.

Toxicology and Adverse Effects: AHPA class 2b. Emmenagogue and uterine stimulant. Gastrointestinal distress, nausea, diarrhea. Contact allergy also possible. A single case report suggested that guggul was responsible for the development of rhabdomyolysis in a 55-year-old man who was taking 300 mg TID.

Drug Interactions: Guggulipid oleoresin is similar to that contained in colestipol and cholestryamine, which may account for the finding that administration of guggulipid decreased serum concentrations of diltiazem and propranolol. Guggulsterone binds the pregnane X receptor, which may affect blood levels of coadministered drugs such as cyclophosphamide and acetaminophen.

Notes of Interest: Guggul is used as a calming incense.

Dosage:

Human: Should be used for at least 4 weeks for effects to develop.

Dried resin: 50 mg-10 g TID

Guggulipid: 100-400 mg TID

Guggulsterones (standardized to 2.5%): 6.25-25 mg TID

Tincture (in 80% ethanol): 1:2 or 1:3: 1.5-5 mL TID

Small Animal:

Dried herb: 25-400 mg/kg, divided daily (optimally, TID)

Tincture 1:2-1:3: 0.5-1.5 mL per 10 kg (20 lb), divided daily (optimally, TID) and diluted or combined with other herbs. Higher doses may be appropriate if the herb is used singly and is not combined in a formula.

References

Burris TP, Montrose C, Houck KA, Osborne HE, Bocchinfuso WP, Yaden BC, Cheng CC, Zink RW, Barr RJ, Hepler CD, Krishnan V, Bullock HA, Burris LL, Galvin RJ, Bramlett K, Stayrook KR. The hypolipidemic natural product guggulsterone is a promiscuous steroid receptor ligand. Mol Pharmacol 2005;67:948-954.

Dixit VP, Joshi S, Sinha R, Bharvava SK, Varma M. Hypolipidemic activity of guggul reson *(Commphora mukul)* and garlic (*Allium sativum* Linn) in dogs *(Canis familiaris)* and monkeys (*Presbytis entellus entellus* Dufresne). Biochem Exp Biol 1980;16:421-424.

Singh BB, Mishra LC, Vinjamury SP, Aquilina N, Singh VJ, Shepard N. The effectiveness of *Commiphora mukul* for osteoarthritis of the knee: an outcomes study. Altern Ther Health Med 2003;9:74-79.

Singh RB, Niaz MA, Ghosh S. Hypolipidemic and antioxidant effects of *Commiphora mukul* as an adjunct to dietary therapy in patients with hypercholesterolemia. Cardiovasc Drugs Ther 1994;8:659-664.

Szapary PO, Wolfe ML, Bloedon LT, et al. Guggulipid for the treatment of hypercholesterolemia: a randomized controlled trial. JAMA 2003;290:765-772.

Urizar NL, Moore DD. GUGULIPID: a natural cholesterol-lowering agent. Annu Rev Nutr 2003;23:303-313. Epub 2003 Feb 26.

Gymnema

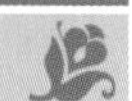

Gymnema sylvestre (Retz) R. Br. ex Schult. • jim-NEE-muh sil-VESS-tree

Other Names: Milkweed, gurmar, merasingi

Family: Asclepiadaceae

Parts Used: Dried leaf, root

Distribution: Native to India and Northern Africa, and grown commercially in Southeast Asia, Australia, Europe, and North America. Gymnema thrives in tropical climates.

Selected Constituents: Two resins, nine gymnemic acids, saponins of the gymnemic acids, and the gymnemagenins; four other saponin triterpenoids, identified as gymnemasin A, B, C, and D4; a peptide that suppresses sweet taste perception; gurmarin; pectin; stigmasterol; quercitol and the amino acid derivatives betaine, choline, and trimethylamine (Kapoor, 1990)

Clinical Actions: Hypoglycemic, pancreatic trophorestorative, astringent; mildly diuretic; reduces sensation of sweetness

Energetics: Slightly cooling

History and Traditional Usage: Gymnema has a long history of medicinal use in India for "honey urine" or diabetes. Its ancient Sanskrit name means "sugar destroyer." It has also been used to treat conditions ranging from malaria and caries prevention to snakebites.

Its ethnoveterinary uses include feeding leaves to cattle as a galactagogue (Williamson, 2002).

Published Research: In animal and human studies, gymnema has been found to reduce hyperglycemia. In induced diabetic rats, gymnema doubled the number of insulin-secreting β cells in the pancreas and returned blood sugars to almost normal (Prakash, 1986; Shanmugasundaram, 1990). Gymnema increased the activity of enzymes responsible for glucose uptake and utilization (Shanmugasundaram, 1983) and inhibited peripheral utilization of glucose by somatotrophin and corticotrophin (Gupta, 1964). Gymnema has also been found to inhibit epinephrine-induced hyperglycemia (Gupta, 1961).

The hypoglycemic effects of extracts from gymnema leaves were investigated in 22 patients with type 2 diabetes who were on conventional oral antihyperglycemic agents. These extracts (400 mg/day) were administered for 18 to 20 months as a supplement to conventional oral drugs. With the extracts, patients showed a significant reduction in blood glucose, glycosylated hemoglobin, and glycosylated plasma proteins, and conventional drug dosage could be decreased. Five patients discontinued conventional drugs and maintained blood glucose homeostasis with the extract alone (Baskaran, 1990).

Antimicrobial activity was also demonstrated with the ethanolic extract of gymnema leaves against *Bacillus pumilis, Bacillus subtilis, Pseudomonas aeruginosa,* and *Staphylococcus aureus,* along with inactivity against *Proteus vulgaris* and *Escherichia coli* (Satdive, 2003).

Indications: Diabetes mellitus (insulin and non–insulin dependent, hypoglycemia, sweet cravings)

Potential Veterinary Indications: Diabetes mellitus. Clinical use suggests that gymnema must be administered for 2 to 3 months for maximum effect.

Contraindications: Gymnema may lower blood sugar levels, so caution is advised when one is also taking prescription drugs that may lower blood sugar levels.

Toxicology and Adverse Effects: A 52-week study of oral repeated dose toxicity of gymnema was conducted in rats. None of the animals studied died during the 52 weeks. No exposure-related changes in body weight, food consumption, hematology, or biochemical examination findings were seen, nor did any histopathologic alterations occur. It was concluded that no toxic effect occurred in rats treated with gymnema at up to 1.00% in the diet for 52 weeks (Ogawa, 2004). Gymnema may alter the ability to taste sweet foods.

Potential Drug Interactions: Some of the effects of gymnema may theoretically be enhanced by antidepressant medications, fenfluramine, salicylates (including aspirin), and tetracyclines. Its actions may be decreased with the use of epinephrine, phenothiazines, and thyroid hormone.

Dosage:

Human:

Standardized extract (to 24% gymnemic acids): 100-200 mg TID with meals

Fluid extract (1:1): 1-3 mL TID with meals

Small Animal:

Dried herb: 50-500 mg/kg, divided daily (optimally, TID)

Fluid extract (1:1): 1.0-2.5 mL per 10 kg (20 lb), divided daily, given with meals

Combinations: Although the herb is available alone, it is more often used in combination with other herbs, including bitter melon, cinnamon, fenugreek, and ginseng, in the treatment of patients with diabetes (Wynn, 2001).

References

Baskaran K, Kizar Ahamath B, Radha Shanmugasunduram K, Shanmugasunduram ER. Antidiabetic effect of a leaf extract from *Gymnema sylvestre* in non–insulin-dependent diabetes mellitus patients. J Ethnopharmacol 1990;30:295-300.

Gupta SS. Inhibitory effect of *Gymnema sylvestre* (Gurmar) on adrenaline induced hyperglycemia in rats. Indian J Med Sci 1961;15:883-887.

Gupta SS, Variyar MC. Experimental studies on pituitary diabetes. IV. Effect of *Gymnema sylvestre* and Cocciniaindica against the hyperglycemia response of somatotropin and corticotrophin hormones. Indian J Med Res 1964;52:200-207.

Kapoor LD. *Handbook of Ayurvedic Medicinal Plants.* Boca Raton, Fla: CRC Press; 1990:200-201.

Ogawa Y, Sekita K, Umemura T, et al. *Gymnema sylvestre* leaf extract: a 52-week dietary toxicity study in Wistar rats [Japanese]. J Food Hyg Soc Jpn 2004;45:8-18.

Prakash AO, Mather S, Mather R. Effect of feeding *Gymnema sylvestre* leaves on blood glucose in berylliumnitrate treated rats. J Ethnopharmacol 1986;18:143-146.

Satdive RK, Abhilash P, Fulzele DP. Antimicrobial activity of *Gymnema sylvestre* leaf extract. Fitoterapia 2003;74:699-701.

Shanmugasundaram ER, Gopinath KL, Radha Shanmugasundaram K, Rajendram VM. Possible regeneration of the islets of Langerhans in streptozotocin-diabetic rats given *Gymnema sylvestre* leaf extracts. J Ethnopharmacol 1990;30:265-279.

Shanmugasundaram KR, Panneerselvam C, Samudram P. Enzyme changes and glucose utilisation in diabetic rabbits: the effect of *Gymnema sylvestre,* R. Br.J Ethnopharmacol 1983;7:205-234.

Williamson E, ed. *Major Herbs of Ayurveda.* Sydney: Churchill Livingstone; 2002.

Wynn S. Diabetes in Veterinary Practice. Altern Med Rev 2001:6(suppl):S17-S23.

Hawthorn

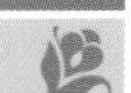

Crataegus laevigata (Poir.) DC *or Crataegus monogyna* Jacq • krah-TEE-gus lee-vih-GAY-tuh, krah-TEE-gus mon-NO-gy-nuh

Distribution: Native to Europe

Similar Species: *Crataegus pentagyna,* Waldst et Kit ex Willd, *Crataegus nigra* Waldst et Kit, *Crataegus azarolus* L. are used in Europe. Species used in Chinese medicine are *Crataegus cuneata* and *Crataegus pinnatifolia.*

Other Names: English hawthorn, whitethorn, may tree, woodland hawthorn. *C. monogyna* is "One seed hawthorn." Shan zha is the pin yin name for the fruit of *Crataegus pinnatifida* Bge.

Family: Rosaceae

Parts Used: Berries, leaves, and flowers have been used in modern research.

Collection: Leaves and flowers, when in bloom. Berries when ripe are used in Traditional Chinese Medicine.

Selected Constituents: Flavonoids (mostly vitexin and vitexin glycosides, rutin, hyperoside; quercetin, and quercetin glycosides), oligomeric proanthocyanidins (OPCs), triterpenoid sapogenins, and biogenic amines (e.g., choline). Leaves contain more vitexin rhamnoside, quercetin, and quercetin glycosides, and less hyperoside.

Clinical Action: Cardiotonic, diuretic, and astringent. The constituent profile of the Western and Asian species and parts is considerably different. Cholesterol-lowering activity has been associated with the Asian species, but no reports of cardioactivity such as the positive inotropic activity associated with Western Crataegus have been documented.

Energetics: Berries are sour, sweet, and slightly warm, and they enter the liver, spleen, and stomach channels. Flower and leaf are slightly sweet, slightly bitter, and astringent.

History and Traditional Usage: The berries, twigs, and root of various *Crataegus* species have been used by Native Americans. The berries were generally used for food and for treatment of patients with diarrhea and stomach disorders; the twigs and root were used for "female disorders," bladder ailments, gastrointestinal problems, and pain. In Traditional Chinese Medicine, the fruit is particularly important for dissolving food stagnation, especially from meat. The action is to nourish heart blood and enhance digestion. It is indicated for abdominal distention, pain, and diarrhea. It is also used for angina, postpartum abdominal pain and masses, congealed blood, and long-term bleeding.

Published Research: Hawthorn extract inhibits Na^+/K^+-ATPase and blocks repolarizing potassium current in ventricular muscle, prolonging the refractory period and resulting in an antiarrhythmic effect. The proanthocyanidins also inhibit angiotensin-converting enzyme activity. The leaf and flower have shown potential for a positive inotropic effect, increased conductivity, decreased excitability, vasodilation of peripheral and coronary arteries, and an antiarrythmic effect. The berry may have mild peripheral vasodilatory and antihypertensive effects. Some studies have documented a mild anxiolytic effect in patients with cardiovascular disease who take the extracts. Controlled trials and large cohort studies in humans have shown that hawthorn increases cardiac maximal workload and decreases symptoms such as dyspnea and fatigue. Hawthorn has also been investigated for the treatment of patients with blood lipid disorders and hypertension, but no clear positive effect has been observed for these disorders (Rigelsky, 2002). Doses used in human trials have ranged from 160 to 900 mg daily.

Pittler et al (2003) conducted a meta-analysis of trials in which hawthorn was used as an adjunct to conventional care in the treatment of humans with chronic heart failure. Eight randomized, double-blind, placebo-controlled studies that enrolled 632 patients with New York Heart Association (NYHA) Class I to III disease were included. Maximal workload, pressure heart rate product, dyspnea, and fatigue were all improved with hawthorn treatment. Adverse effects were temporary and mild and included nausea, dizziness, and cardiac and gastrointestinal problems. The authors concluded that the use of hawthorn extract as adjunctive treatment for patients with chronic heart failure is highly beneficial. In a more recent report to the Heart Failure Society of America (Aaronson, 2004), a study was described that involved 120 patients who were given 450 mg of a proprietary leaf and flower extract (WS 1442, Schwabe, Germany) twice daily. Hawthorn did not provide a benefit in the primary outcome, which was 6-minute walking distance.

Most studies involved the use of proprietary extracts of the leaf and flower, but a single experiment that used hawthorn berries in people with NYHA Class II found that the berry extract improved exercise tolerance to a significantly greater degree than did placebo (Degenring, 2003).

A pilot study in 36 mildly hypertensive people examined the effects of hawthorn, magnesium, and placebo on blood pressure. Systolic and diastolic pressure declined in all groups, including the placebo group (Walker, 2002).

In studies by Roddewig and Hensel (1977), dogs were implanted with heat conduction probes placed in the left ventricular myocardium on a long-term basis. The OPC extract of hawthorn, given orally, led to significant dose-dependent increases in blood flow for up to several hours. When anesthetized cats were given this extract intravenously, myocardial blood flow increased and arterial blood pressure decreased. Taskov (1977) investigated a flavonoid extract in dogs and cats. Intravenous administration of a 2-mg/kg dose led to increased coronary blood flow in dogs, with no change in heart rate or electrocardiogram (ECG) pattern. In cats, increased minute cardiac volume, increased cardiac index, increased left ventricular work, and decreased peripheral resistance occurred with insignificant changes in blood pressure.

Multiple experimental studies used hawthorn in dogs and cats; unfortunately, findings of these studies are published in languages other than English and were unavailable to these authors.

Indications: Congestive heart failure, possibly hyperlipidemia and hypertension (leaf and flower, possibly berry). Also, for poor or slow digestion (berry).

Potential Veterinary Indications: Same as human indications, but especially congestive heart failure, with the possible exception of hypertrophic cardiomyopathy of cats. However, Marsden reports a case of feline hypertrophic cardiomyopathy that resolved on echocardiogram following treatment with hawthorn and a single (individually prescribed) homeopathic remedy (Marsden, personal communication).

Contraindications: Disagreement has been expressed among veterinary herbalists about the use of hawthorn for cats with hypertrophic cardiomyopathy. It would seem that increasing ventricular work would worsen the condition. On the other hand, some herbalists claim that the action is "amphoteric" or normalizing—if the heart works too hard, the antioxidant and antiarrhythmic activities are beneficial in this type of disease as well. Theoretical contraindications have been listed as bleeding disorders (because synthesis of thromboxane A2 is inhibited), chest pain, and low blood pressure.

Herbalists generally do not recommend hawthorn for patients who are sedate, have slow heart beats, or hypotension.

Toxicology and Adverse Effects: AHPA class 1. Intraperitoneal and oral administration of an extract to mice and rats, at a dose of 3 g/kg body weight, did not induce lethal effects. In people, allergic responses have been reported; at large doses, fatigue, sedation, and hypotension are theoretically possible.

Drug Interactions: Studies have shown interactions with cardiac glycosides, theophylline, caffeine, papaverine, sodium nitrate, adenosine, barbiturates, and epinephrine. Interactions may occur with anticoagulants and antihypertensives. Hawthorn flavonoids may affect P-glycoprotein function and have been suspected to cause interactions with digoxin, also a P-glycoprotein substrate. Tankanow (2003) studied the effects of hawthorn on digoxin pharmacokinetic parameters. Eight volunteers were administered digoxin or digoxin plus hawthorn leaf and flower extract (450 mg BID) in a randomized, crossover trial for 10 days during each phase. Hawthorn did not significantly affect the pharmacokinetic parameters for digoxin. Veterinarians should monitor dogs that are being treated with digitalis for a possible potentiating effect of hawthorn, which would allow administration of lower doses of digitalis.

Dosage: Most practitioners believe that the most potent effect is achieved after 6 weeks of therapy.

Human:

Dried herb: 0.1-10 g TID

Standardized extract (4-30 mg of total flavonoids and 30-160 mg of OPC): 150-900 mg daily

Infusions and decoctions: 5-30 g per cup of water, with 1 cup of the tea given TID

Tincture (commonly 25%-45% ethanol; some pharmacies include glycerin to prevent precipitation by tannins) 1:2 or 1:3: 0.25-5 mL TID

Small Animal:

Dried herb: 25-300 mg/kg, divided daily (optimally, TID)

Infusion and decoction: 5-30 g per cup of water, administered at a rate of ¼-½ cup per 10 kg (20 lb), divided daily (optimally, TID)

Tincture (usually in 25%-45% ethanol) 1:2-1:3: 0.5-1.5 mL per 10 kg (20 lb), divided daily (optimally, TID) and diluted or combined with other herbs. Higher doses may be appropriate if the herb is used singly and is not combined in a formula.

References

Aaronson K. HERB-CHF: Hawthorne extract randomized blinded chronic heart failure trial. Presented at: Heart Failure Society of America 8th Annual Scientific Meeting; September 9-15, 2004; Toronto, Ontario, Canada.

Degenring FH, Suter A, Weber M, Saller R. A randomised double blind placebo controlled clinical trial of a standardised extract of fresh Crataegus berries (Crataegisan) in the treatment of patients with congestive heart failure NYHA II. Phytomedicine 2003;10:363-369.

Pittler MH, Schmidt K, Ernst E. Hawthorn extract for treating chronic heart failure: meta-analysis of randomized trials. Am J Med 2003;114:665-674.

Rigelsky JM, Sweet BV. Hawthorn: pharmacology and therapeutic uses. Am J Health Syst Pharm 2002;59:417-422.

Roddewig C, Hensel H. [Reaction of local myocardial blood flow in non-anesthetized dogs and anesthetized cats to the oral and parenteral administration of a Crateagus fraction (oligomere procyanidins).] Arzneimittelforschung 1977;27:1407-1410.

Tankanow R, Tamer HR, Streetman DS, Smith SG, Welton JL, Annesley T, Aaronson KD, Bleske BE. Interaction study between digoxin and a preparation of hawthorn *(Crataegus oxyacantha)*. J Clin Pharmacol 2003;43:637-642.

Taskov M. On the coronary and cardiotonic action of crataemon. Acta Physiol Pharmacol Bulg 1977;3:53-57.

Walker AF, Marakis G, Morris AP, Robinson PA. Promising hypotensive effect of hawthorn extract: a randomized double-blind pilot study of mild, essential hypertension. Phytother Res 2002;16:48-54.

Horehound 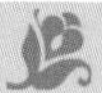

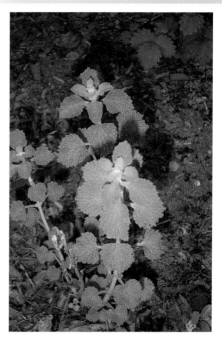

Marrubium vulgare L. • ma-ROO-bee-um vul-GAY-ree

Other Names: White horehound, hoarhound

Family: Lamiaceae

Parts Used: Aerial parts

Selected Constituents: Diterpenoid lactones, including marrubiin, premarrubiin; phenolic acids, flavonoids, essential oil (containing alpha-pinene, sabinene, limonene, camphene, p-cymol, α-terpinolene), sterols, choline, alkaloids

Clinical Action: Expectorant, diuretic, diaphoretic, antispasmodic, bitter tonic, choleretic

Energetics: Bitter, cool

History and Traditional Usage: Various Native American tribes used this plant to flush the kidneys, for breast complaints, and for cough, flu, sore throat, and colds. The Navajo fed the plant to sheep to make the meat bitter. Horehound syrup was used by Eclectics for cough, colds, asthma, chronic catarrh, and other pulmonary affections.

Published Research: Horehound is a folk treatment for diabetes. It was investigated in a double-blind trial in which an infusion was administered to people who were not well controlled under conventional treatment. In this trial, horehound provided significant benefit to diabetic patients (Herrera-Arellano, 2004). Marrubiin, a furane labdane diterpene, has analgesic effects as measured in experimental models of pain in mice (De Jesus, 2000; Meyre-Silva, 2005). Laboratory animal studies have suggested that horehound may have antihypertensive activity (Bardai, 2004; El Bardai, 2001).

Indications: The herb has antispasmodic and bronchial secretagogue activities that account for its traditional use for dry cough. Also used for loss of appetite, nonulcerative dyspepsia, flatulence, and diabetes.

Potential Veterinary Indications: Chronic bronchitis, chronic obstructive pulmonary disease, feline asthma

Contraindications: Use cautiously with hypoglycemics and antihypertensives because the herb exhibits these activities in laboratory animal studies. Safety has not been proved in pregnancy; this herb is a uterine stimulant.
Toxicology and Adverse Effects: AHPA class 2b. High doses may cause arrhythmias and diarrhea, but this is not reported at normal doses.
Drug Interactions: Theoretical concerns exist concerning the concurrent use of antihypertensives and hypoglycemic agents.
Dosage:
Human:
Dried herb: 1-10 g TID (this is a bitter herb, and the higher doses are not usually required)
Infusions: 5-10 g per cup of water, with ¼-1 cup of the tea given TID
Tincture (usually 20%-50% ethanol; some pharmacies include glycerin to prevent precipitation by tannins) 1 : 2 or 1 : 3: 0.25-5 mL TID
Small Animal:
Dried herb: 25-300 mg/kg, divided daily (optimally, TID)
Infusion: 5-10 g per cup of water, administered at a rate of ¼-½ cup per 10 kg (20 lb), divided daily (optimally, TID)
Tincture (usually in 20%-50% ethanol) 1 : 2-1 : 3: 0.5-1.0 mL per 10 kg (20 lb), divided daily (optimally, TID) and diluted or combined with other herbs. Higher doses may be appropriate if the herb is used singly and is not combined in a formula.
Notes of Interest: Henriette Kress' recipe for horehound syrup:
Herbal Syrup:
40 g herb, fresh, chopped up, or 20 g dried, crushed*
9 dL water
450 g sugar

Bring to a boil, leave set on stove for ½ hour, and then strain. Allow set on low heat until you have 2 dL (don't overcook). Add sugar, and dissolve on low heat. Bottle the syrup.

References

Bardai SE, Lyoussi B, Wibo M, Morel N. Comparative study of the antihypertensive activity of *Marrubium vulgare* and of the dihydropyridine calcium antagonist amlodipine in spontaneously hypertensive rat. Clin Exp Hypertens 2004;26:465-474.

De Jesus RA, Cechinel-Filho V, Oliveira AE, Schlemper V. Analysis of the antinociceptive properties of marrubiin isolated from *Marrubium vulgare*. Phytomedicine 2000;7:111-115.

El Bardai S, Lyoussi B, Wibo M, Morel N. Pharmacological evidence of hypotensive activity of *Marrubium vulgare* and *Foeniculum vulgare* in spontaneously hypertensive rat. Clin Exp Hypertens 2001;23:329-343.

Herrera-Arellano A, Aguilar-Santamaria L, Garcia-Hernandez B, Nicasio-Torres P, Tortoriello J. Clinical trial of *Cecropia obtusifolia* and *Marrubium vulgare* leaf extracts on blood glucose and serum lipids in type 2 diabetics. Phytomedicine 2004;11:561-566.

Meyre-Silva C, Yunes RA, Schlemper V, Campos-Buzzi F, Cechinel-Filho V. Analgesic potential of marrubiin derivatives, a bioactive diterpene present in *Marrubium vulgare* (Lamiaceae). Farmaco 2005;60:321-326.

*Herbs for the syrup: 2 parts peppermint, 1 part horehound, ½ part thyme. Heriette Kress's invaluable Web page may be accessed at: http://www.henriettesherbal.com

Horsetail

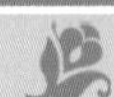

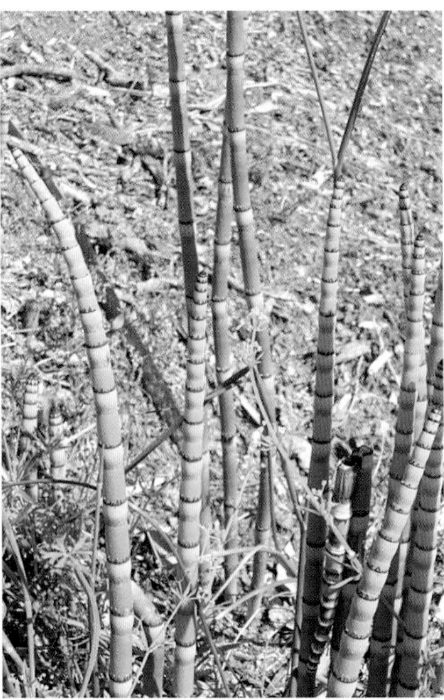

Equisetum arvense L. • ek-wis-SEE-tum ar-VEN-see *or* ar-VEN-say
Common Names: Scouring rush, bottle brush, pewterwort, shavegrass, equisetum, equiseti herba, meadow horsetail
Related Species: *Equisetum myriochaetum, Equisetum bogotense, Equisetum hyemale, Equisetum fluviatile, Equisetum giganteum*
Family: Equisetaceae
Parts Used: Stems arising from a creeping rhizome
Distribution: In waste and moist places throughout Britain, Europe, North America, Australia, and temperate Asia. Prefers nonchalky soil.
Selected Constituents: Horsetail is rich in silicic acid and silicates, providing about 2% to 3% elemental silicon. Sterols include β-sitosterol (60.0%), campesterol (32.9%), isofucosterol (5.9%), alkaloids (nicotine, palustrine), and cholesterol (trace amounts). Flavonoids (luteolin) and saponins (equisetonin) are believed to cause the diuretic effect, and the silicon content is thought to exert connective tissue–strengthening and antiarthritic actions (Weiss, 1988). Some authors have suggested that the element silicon in horsetail is a vital component for bone and cartilage formation (Seaborn, 1993).
Clinical Actions: Antihemorrhagic, anti-inflammatory, diuretic, detoxifying, genitourinary astringent
Energetics: Cold, pungent
History and Traditional Usage: Apparently first recorded by the Roman physician Galen, several cultures have employed horsetail as a remedy for kidney and bladder troubles, arthritis, bleeding ulcers, and tuberculosis.

Horsetail was used topically to stop hemorrhaging from wounds and to promote healing. Other uses included strengthening of hair, nails, and skin; treatment of benign prostatic hyperplasia, gout, menorrhagia, and dysentery; flushing out of stones; and treatment of patients with dyspepsia, dropsy, ulcerations in urinary passages, and kidney affections generally.

"*E. arvense* has been found beneficial in dropsy, gravel, and kidney affections generally, and a drachm of the dried herb, powdered, taken three or four times a day, has proved very effectual in spitting of blood. The ashes of the plant are considered very valuable in acidity of the stomach, dyspepsia, etc., administered in doses of 3 to 10 grains. Besides being useful in kidney and bladder trouble, a strong decoction acts as an emmenagogue; being cooling and astringent, it is of efficacy for hemorrhage, cystic ulceration, and ulcers in the urinary passages. The decoction applied externally will stop the bleeding of wounds and quickly heal them, and will also reduce the swelling of eyelids" (Grieve, 1975). Felter and Remington summarized the effects of horsetail briefly: "Equisetum is diuretic and astringent. It is asserted to greatly relieve irritation due to the presence of gravel and the tenesmic urging to urinate in acute inflammations of the genito-renal tract" (Felter, 1898). Remington (1918) claims that "the diuretic action of *Equisetum* is very feeble."

Published Research: Horsetail has demonstrated anti-inflammatory and analgesic properties in mouse inflammation models (Do Monte, 2004). It contains dicaffeoyl tartaric acids, which have been shown to have vasorelaxant activity in norepinephrine-induced vasocontraction in rat aortas (Sakurai, 2003) and minimal free radical scavenging properties (Myagmar, 2000).

The diuretic activity of *Equisetum* species, including *E. bogotense,* has been evaluated in healthy volunteers (Lemus, 1996) and mice with *E. fluviatile, E. hiemale, E. giganteum,* and *E. myriochaetum,* producing an effect similar to that of hydrochlorothiazide (Perez, 1985). The effects of *E. arvense* on urolithiasis have been studied with the use of female Wistar rats. Variations of the main urolithiasis risk factors (citraturia, calciuria, phosphaturia, pH, and diuresis) were evaluated, and it was concluded that beneficial effects on urolithiasis caused by herb infusion can be attributed to some disinfectant action and, tentatively, to the presence of saponins. Some solvent action with respect to uric stones may occur with the alkalinizing capacity of some herb infusions (Grases, 1994).

Horsetail may provide protection from radiation and may have applications in radiotherapy (Joksic, 2003); it may also provide hepatoprotective effects on induce acute hepatitis (Katikova, 2002). Anecdotal reports suggest that horsetail may be of some use in the treatment of brittle nails (Hamon, 1992).

Indications: Prostatic disease, cystitis with hematuria; posttraumatic and stasis edema; irrigation therapy for bacterial and inflammatory disease of the lower urinary tract and for renal gravel; inflammatory or mild infection of the genitourinary tract (Bradley, 1992). Externally for slowly healing wounds, rheumatic conditions, fractures, sprains.

Potential Veterinary Use: Brittle nails, hooves; urolithiasis; feline lower urinary tract disease (FLUTD)

Contraindications: Cardiac or renal dysfunction (Bradley, 1992)

Toxicology and Adverse Effects: AHPA class 2d (because of contraindications in cardiac or renal disease). Bulls refused hay contaminated (about 12% by mass) by horsetail. Observations seem to imply that cattle recognize the plant by its odor and refuse it if alternative roughage is available, thereby escaping intoxication (Kamphues, 1990).

Horsetail contains significant thiaminase activity. A horse that consumes hay that is contaminated with 20% or more of horsetail plants will show signs of thiamine deficiency in 2 to 5 weeks (Mayer, 1989). Therefore, one should not use unheated or unprocessed horsetail powder orally. Because alcohol, heat, and alkalinity neutralize thiaminase, tinctures, fluid extracts, or preparations of the herb subjected to 100°C temperatures during manufacturing are preferred for medicinal use (Fabre, 1993).

In rats, the effects of dietary field horsetail (*Equisetum arvense* L.) powder were studied. A diet with 4% horsetail caused dermatitis at the neck, head, and back in about 20% to 65% of rats. This dermatitis was reversed when the diet was changed to commercial pellets (Maeda, 1997).

Drug Interactions: Digitalis and its cardiac glycosides might become more toxic because of the loss of potassium that results from the diuretic effect of horsetail; however, the herb is also high in potassium.

Notes of Interest: The Latin name for this herb is derived from the words *equus* (a horse) and *seta* (a bristle), because of the peculiar bristly appearance of the jointed stems of the plants, which has also earned it the popular names of horsetail, bottle-brush, and paddock-pipes. The herb, when finely ground, is excellent for polishing pewter.

Dosage:

External Use:

Compress: 10g in 1L water (German Commission E Monograph, 1988)

Internal Use:

Human

Dried herb: 1-10gTID, up to 6 times daily for acute conditions

Infusions and decoctions: 5-30g per cup of water, with 1 cup of the tea given TID, up to 6 times daily acutely

Tincture (usually 25%-50% ethanol) 1:2 or 1:3: 1-5mLTID, up to 6 times daily for acute conditions

Small Animal

Dried herb: 25-300mg/kg, divided daily (optimally, TID)

Infusion: 5-30g per cup of water, administered at a rate of ¼-½ cup per 10kg (20lb), divided daily (optimally, TID)

Tincture (usually in 25%-50% ethanol) 1:2-1:3: 0.5-1.0mL per 10kg (20lb), divided daily (optimally, TID) and diluted or combined with other herbs. Higher doses may be appropriate if the herb is used singly and is not combined in a formula.

References

Bradley P, ed. *British Herbal Medicine Association British Herbal Compendium,* vol 1. Bournemouth: BHMA; 1992:93.

Do Monte FH, dos Santos JG, Russi M, Bispo Lanziotti VM, Leal LK, de Andrade Cunha GM. Antinociceptive and anti-inflammatory properties of the hydroalcoholic extract of stems from *Equisetum arvense* L. in mice. Pharmacol Res 2004;49: 239-243.

Fabre B, Geay B, Beaufils P. Thiaminase activity in *Equisetum arvense* and its extracts. Plant Med Phytother 1993;26:190-197.

Felter HW, Lloyd JU. *King's American Dispensatory,* 1898. Available online at Henriette's Herbal Homepage at: http://www.henriettesherbal.com/eclectic/kings/index.html.

German Commission E. Monograph, *Zingiberis rhizoma.* Bundesanzeiger 1988;85:5.

Grases F, Melero G, Costa-Bauza A, Prieto R, March JG. Urolithiasis and phytotherapy. Int Urol Nephrol 1994;26:507-511.

Grieve M. *A Modern Herbal.* London: Jonathan Cape; 1931 (Reprint, 1975).

Hamon NW, Awang DVC. Horsetail. Canadian Pharm J 1992; September:399-401.

Joksic G, Stankovic M, Novak A. Antibacterial medicinal plants *Equiseti herba* and *Ononidis radix* modulate micronucleus formation in human lymphocytes in vitro. J Environ Pathol Toxicol Oncol 2003;22:41-48.

Kamphues J. [Refusal of breeding bulls to eat hay contaminated with horsetail *(Equisetum palustre).*] Tierarztl Prax 1990;18:349-351.

Katikova OIu, Kostin IaV, Tishkin VS. [Hepatoprotective effect of plant preparations.] Eksp Klin Farmakol 2002;65:41-43.

Lemus I, Garcia R, Erazo S, Pena R, Parada M, Fuenzalida M. Diuretic activity of an *Equisetum bogotense* tea (Platero herb): evaluation in healthy volunteers. J Ethnopharmacol 1996;54: 55-58.

Maeda H, Miyamoto K, Sano T. Occurrence of dermatitis in rats fed a cholesterol diet containing field horsetail (*Equisetum arvense* L.). J Nutr Sci Vitaminol (Tokyo) 1997;43:553-563.

Meyer P. Thiaminase activities and thiamine content of *Pteridium aquilinum, Equisetum ramosissimum, Malva parviflora, Pennisetum clandestinum* and *Medicago sativa.* Onderstepoort J Vet Res 1989;56:145-146.

Myagmar BE, Aniya Y. Free radical scavenging action of medicinal herbs from Mongolia. Phytomedicine 2000;7:221-229.

Perez Gutierrez RM, Laguna GY, Walkowski A. Diuretic activity of Mexican equisetum. J Ethnopharmacol 1985;14:269-272.

Remington JP, Wood HC. *The Dispensatory of the United States of America* (1918). Available at: www.henriettesherbal.com. Accessed June 2005.

Sakurai N, Iizuka T, Nakayama S, Funayama H, Noguchi M, Nagai M. [Vasorelaxant activity of caffeic acid derivatives from *Cichorium intybus* and *Equisetum arvense.*] Yakugaku Zasshi 2003;123:593-598.

Seaborn CD, Nielsen FH. Silicon: a nutritional beneficence for bones, brains and blood vessels? Nutr Today 1993;28:13-18.

Weiss RF. *Herbal Medicine.* Gothenburg, Sweden: Ab Arcanum; 1988:238-239.

Juniper

Juniperus communis L. • jew-NIP-er-us KOM-yoo-nis

Common Names: Juniper berries, juniperi fructus

Family: Cupressaceae

Distribution: Native to Europe, Asia, and the United States. It often occurs in groups (hence, the species name, *communis*) as an undergrowth in mixed open forests, or in heaths and moorelands.

Related Species: *Juniperus oxycedrus, Juniperus phoenicea, Juniperus virginiana*

Parts Used: The medicinal portions of the plant are referred to as berries, but they are actually dark blue-black scales from the cones of the tree. In contrast to other pine cones, juniper cones are fleshy and soft.

Selected Constituents: The volatile oils, up to 2% of the pulp, particularly terpinen-4-ol, may cause an increase in urine volume (Tyler, 1994). Flavonoids, resin, tannins, bitter principles, and sugar up to 30%.

Clinical Actions: Diuretic, antiseptic, carminative, stomachic, antirheumatic

Energetics: Warm, pungent, dry

History and Traditional Usage: Juniper has been used as a flavoring agent in gin, and has been used in the manufacture of soap and perfume, among other things. Juniper has been used to treat patients with arthritis, gout, warts and skin growths, cancer, dyspepsia, and various urinary tract and kidney diseases (Duke, 1985). It has also been used as a diuretic and for dropsy.

Oil of juniper has been used as a diuretic, stomachic, and carminative for indigestion and flatulence, and for diseases of the kidney and bladder. According to Grieve (1975), the oil mixed with lard was also used in veterinary practice as an application to exposed wounds; it prevents irritation from flies, and the "fruit" is readily eaten by most animals, especially sheep; it is said to prevent and cure dropsy in the latter (Grieve, 1975). Milks (1949) stated that juniper was not frequently used, except as a diuretic and as a stimulating expectorant in chronic respiratory disease.

Published Research: According to some sources, juniper increases urine volume without loss of electrolytes such as potassium (Blumenthal, 2000). The infusion and the essential oil of juniper berries (*Juniperus communis* L.) were tested for a diuresis response in rats, which was compared with the effect of vasopressin (antidiuretic hormone). During a 3-day experiment, diuresis was stimulated after the second and third applications of test solutions. Among tested preparations, a 10% infusion exerted the most considerable diuretic activity; the cumulative urine volume was 44% above the control value. Results suggest that the diuretic activity of juniper berries cannot be attributed only to the essential oil but is also related to hydrophilic constituents (Stanic, 1998).

The essential oil from ripe and unripe berries and from leaves of *Juniperus* species has been tested against a wide variety of bacteria and fungi with nonsignificant inhibitory effects (Angioni, 2003; Filipowicz, 2003; Shin, 2003). *J. communis* was found to have inhibitory activity on prostaglandin biosynthesis and platelet-activating factor (PAF)-induced exocytosis in vitro (Tunon, 1995).

Juniperus communis may have use as a surgical implant. The wood is dense, durable, and strong and has naturally impregnated essential oils that display antiseptic properties. One study (Gross, 2003) investigated the toxicity of the oil, the effects of sterilization on the mechanical properties of the wood, and bone attachment potential. Femoral implants were shaped from the wood and implanted into rabbits. They demonstrated good acceptance by the body up to a period of 3 years with bone apposition, abutment into pores, and growth into drilled cavities observed.

The hypoglycemic activity of juniper "berries" *(Juniperus communis)* in induced diabetic rats was investigated. Juniper decoction decreased glucose levels in normoglycemic rats at doses of 250 mg/kg and 125 mg/kg in streptozotocin-diabetic rats. In the latter group, treatment for 24 days resulted in a reduction both in blood glucose levels and in the mortality index; treatment also prevented loss of body weight (Sanchez, 1994).

Juniper berry oil is rich in 5,11,14-eicosatrienoic acid—a polyunsaturated fatty acid similar to one found in fish oil, yet less prone to peroxidation. Because dietary fish oil treatment has been shown to effectively reduce reperfusion injury, the effects of juniper berry oil were compared with those of fish oil in the diet of rats. Both juniper berry oil and fish oil treatment improved rates of bile flow. Juniper berry oil reduced cell death in the liver by 75% and blunted increases in intracellular calcium and release of prostaglandin E_2 by cultured Kupffer cells stimulated by endotoxin. This study suggested that feeding a diet with juniper berry oil reduces reperfusion injury by inhibiting activation of Kupffer cells, thus reducing vasoactive eicosanoid release and improving hepatic microcirculation in livers undergoing oxidant stress (Jones, 1998).

An ethanolic extract of *Juniperus communis* showed 60% to 70% anti-implantation activity in female rats, which affected fertility (Prakash, 1985). Sheep have been treated for psoroptic mange with *J. communis* extract (Srivastava, 1969).

Indications: Acute and chronic cystitis, flatulent colic, rheumatism, topically for rheumatic pain in joints and muscles

Potential Veterinary Indications: Cystitis, flatulent colic, diabetes, fertility control in mice, topically for wounds

Contraindications: Pregnancy

Toxicology and Adverse Effects: AHPA class 2b, 2d. Not for use in inflammatory kidney disease and should not be used longer than 4 to 6 weeks.

It is often claimed that juniper exerts nephrotoxic effects, and that the essential oil works as a diuretic by irritating the kidneys; however, nephrotoxic effects are related to extremely high doses of the essential oil not used in human medicine, or to confusion in observations concerning turpentine oil. All available literature from 1844 to 1994 has been reviewed, and the conclusion is that juniper berry herbal medicine can be used safely (Schilcher, 1994).

The nephrotoxicity of juniper oil was evaluated in male Sprague-Dawley rats after oral administration. Terpinene-4-ol, a compound with postulated aquaretic activity that can be found in essential juniper oil up to an amount of 10 mg%, was also tested at a dosage of 400 mg/kg. Neither of the tested substances induced change in function or morphology in the kidneys at tested doses, and both were revealed to be nontoxic (Schilcher, 1997).

Acute studies of animals show little dermal toxicity from the oil or tar. Oils derived from *J. communis, J. virginiana,* and *J. oxycedrus* tar were not skin irritants in animals. Oil from *J. virginiana* was not a sensitizer, and oil from *J. communis* was not phototoxic in animal tests. *J. communis* extract affected fertility and was abortifacient in studies that used albino rats. Clinical tests showed no evidence of irritation or sensitization with any of the tested oils; however, some evidence of sensitization to the tar was noted. These data were not considered sufficient to justify assessment of the safety of these ingredients (Unknown, 2001).

J. communis dry needles contain high levels of isocupressic acid, which has been identified as the abortifacient in cattle (Gardner, 1998; Wu, 2002).

Dosage:

Human:

Dried herb: 1-5 g TID

Essential oil: maximum adult, 3 drops 3 times daily

Infusions and decoctions: 5-10 g per cup of water, with 1 cup of the tea given TID

Tincture (usually 45%-80% ethanol; higher alcohol preparations may require lower dose rates) 1:2 or 1:3: 1-2 mL TID

Small Animal:

Dried herb: 25-200 mg/kg, divided daily (optimally, TID)

Infusion: 5-30 g per cup of water, administered at a rate of ¼-½ cup per 10 kg (20 lb), divided daily (optimally, TID)

Tincture (usually 45%-80% ethanol; higher alcohol preparations may require lower dose rates) 1:2-1:3: 0.5-1.0 mL per 10 kg (20 lb), divided daily (optimally, TID) and diluted or combined with other herbs

Historical Veterinary Doses:

Dog

Juniper berries: 15-60 grains (approximately 1-4 g) (Milks, 1949)

Juniper oil: 0.1-0.2 mL (RCVS, 1920)

Large Animal

Juniper berry: horse, 30-60 g or 1-2 oz (Milks, 1949) per day; pig, 7-15 g (RCVS, 1920)

Juniper oil: horse, 1-7 mL; pig, 0.25-0.9 mL (RCVS, 1920)

References

Angioni A, Barra A, Russo MT, Coroneo V, Dessi S, Cabras P. Chemical composition of the essential oils of *Juniperus* from ripe and unripe berries and leaves and their antimicrobial activity. J Agric Food Chem 2003;51:3073-3078.

Blumenthal M, Goldberg A, Brinckman J. *Herbal Medicine: Expanded Commission E Monographs.* Newton, Mass: Integrative Medicine Communications; 2000:218-220.

Duke JA. *CRC Handbook of Medicinal Herbs.* Boca Raton, Fla: CRC Press; 1985:256.

Filipowicz N, Kaminski M, Kurlenda J, Asztemborska M, Ochocka JR. Antibacterial and antifungal activity of juniper berry oil and its selected components. Phytother Res 2003;17:227-231.

Gardner DR, Panter KE, James LF, Stegelmeier BL. Abortifacient effects of lodgepole pine *(Pinus contorta)* and common juniper *(Juniperus communis)* on cattle. Vet Hum Toxicol 1998;40:260-263.

Grieve M. *A Modern Herbal.* London: Jonathan Cape; 1931 (Reprint, 1975).

Gross KA, Ezerietis E. Juniper wood as a possible implant material. J Biomed Mater Res 2003;64A:672-683.

Jones SM, Zhong Z, Enomoto N, Schemmer P, Thurman RG. Dietary juniper berry oil minimizes hepatic reperfusion injury in the rat. Hepatology 1998;28:1042-1050.

Milks HJ. *Practical Veterinary Pharmacology, Materia Medica and Therapeutics.* Chicago, Ill: Alex Eger, Inc.; 1949.

Prakash AO, Saxena V, Shukla S, et al. Anti-implantation activity of some indigenous plants in rats. Acta Eur Fertil 1985;16:441-448.

RCVS (Royal College of Veterinary Surgeons). *Veterinary Counter Practice.* London: Ballantyne Press; 1920.

Sanchez de Medina F, Gamez MJ, Jimenez I, Jimenez J, Osuna JI, Zarzuelo A. Hypoglycemic activity of juniper "berries." Planta Med 1994;60:197-200.

Schilcher H, Heil B. Nephrotoxicity of juniper berry preparations: a critical review of the literature from 1844-1993. Zeitschrift fur Phytotherapie 1994;15:203-213.

Schilcher H, Leuschner F. [The potential nephrotoxic effects of essential juniper oil.] Arzneimittelforschung 1997;47:855-858.

Shin S. Anti-*Aspergillus* activities of plant essential oils and their combination effects with ketoconazole or amphotericin B. Arch Pharm Res 2003;26:389-393.

Srivastava SC, Sisodia CS. Treatment of psoroptic mange in sheep with *Juniperus communis* (hipush) extract. Indian Vet J 1969; 46:826-828.

Stanic G, Samarzija I, Blazevic N. Time dependent diuretic response in rats treated with juniper berry preparations. Phytother Res 1998;12:494-497.

Tunon H, Olavsdotter C, Bohlin L. Evaluation of anti-inflammatory activity of some Swedish medicinal plants: inhibition of prostaglandin biosynthesis and PAF-induced exocytosis. J Ethnopharmacol 1995;48:61-76.

Tyler VE. *Herbs of Choice: The Therapeutic Use of Phytomedicinals.* Binghamton, NY: Pharmaceutical Products Press; 1994:76-77.

Unknown. Final report on the safety assessment of *Juniperus communis* extract, *Juniperus oxycedrus* extract, *Juniperus oxycedrus* tar, *Juniperus phoenicea* extract, and *Juniperus virginiana* extract. Int J Toxicol 2001;20(suppl 2):41-56.

Wu LS, Chen JC, Sheu SY, et al. Isocupressic acid blocks progesterone production from bovine luteal cells. Am J Chin Med 2002;30:533-541.

Kava

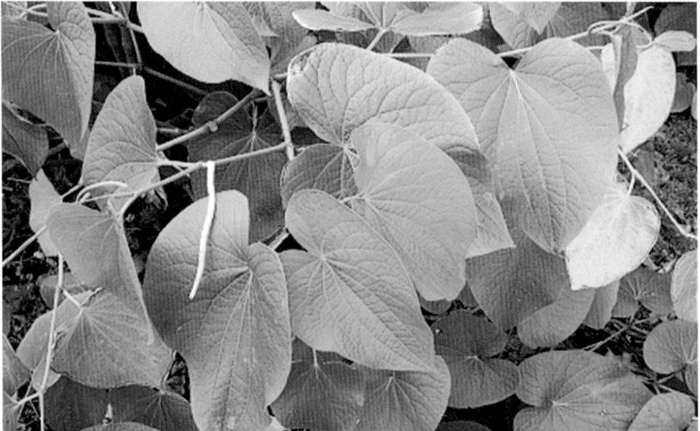

Piper methysticum G. Forst. • PIP-er *or* PYE-per Me-THIS-tik-um

Other Names: Kava kava, awa, kava pepper, yangona

Family: Piperaceae

Parts Used: Dried rhizome

Distribution: Kava is indigenous to and has been cultivated for longer than 3000 years in the Pacific Islands, from Hawaii to Papua New Guinea, with the exceptions of New Caledonia, New Zealand, and most of the Solomon Islands (Singh, 1992). It thrives in tropical to subtropical climates.

Selected Constituents: The major constituents are kava lactones, also known as kava pyrones. The major lactones are kawain (1.8%), methysticin (1.2%), dihydromethysticin (0.5%), demethoxyyangonin (1.0%), yangonin (1.0%), and dihydrokawain (1.0%). At least 13 other lactones, 2 chalcones, and a number of free aromatic acids are known (Farnsworth, 1998; Singh, 1992; Bruneton, 1995).

OCH$_3$ O O

Kavain

OCH$_3$ O O O O

Methysticin

OCH$_3$ O O H$_3$CO

Yangonin

Clinical Actions: Anesthetizing (to mucous membranes), anxiolytic, sedative, antispasmodic, antimicrobial

Energetics: Pungent, neutral, dry

History and Traditional Usage: Kava has been and still is used as a ceremonial intoxicating drink. Uses described in pharmacopoeias and in traditional systems of medicine include the following: to induce relaxation, reduce weight, treat fungal infections, and treat patients with asthma, common cold, cystitis, gonorrhea, headache, menstrual irregularities, urinary infection, and warts (Singh, 1992). *King's American Dispensatory* lists the specific indications as "neuralgia, particularly of the trifacial nerve; toothache; earache; ocular pain; reflex neuralgia; anorexia; dizziness and despondency; gonorrhea; chronic catarrhal inflammation; vesical irritation; painful micturition; dysuria."

Published Research: For centuries, kava has been used by Pacific Islanders for its tranquilizing and sedative effects. Human clinical trials suggest that kava is safe and effective for the treatment of patients with anxiety. Kava extract produced statistically significant dose-dependent anxiolytic-like behavioral changes and a profound decrease in locomotor activity in mice. Sedation was not mediated through the benzodiazepine-binding site on the GABA (gamma-aminobutyric acid) (A) receptor complex (Garrett, 2003).

A placebo-controlled, double-blind outpatient trial investigated the dosage range and efficacy of a kava special extract in patients with nonpsychotic anxiety. A total of 50 patients were treated with 3 × 50 mg/day over 4 weeks followed by a 2-week safety observation phase. Kava was well tolerated with no drug-related adverse events or withdrawal symptoms. It was found that 150 mg/day is an effective and safe treatment for nonpsychotic anxiety syndromes (Geier, 2004). An 8-week, randomized, reference-controlled, double-blind, multicenter clinical trial investigated kava kava in generalized anxiety disorder. It was concluded that kava kava is well tolerated and is as effective as buspirone and opipramol in the acute treatment of patients with generalized anxiety disorder (Boerner, 2003).

The effectiveness and safety of kava extract for treating patients with anxiety were assessed in a major review of the literature that included all publications that described randomized, double-blind, placebo-controlled trials of kava extract for anxiety. Eleven trials with 645 participants met the inclusion criteria. A meta-analysis of six studies suggested a significant reduction in anxiety in patients receiving kava extract compared with placebo. Adverse events were mild, transient, and infrequent. It was concluded that compared with placebo, kava extract is an effective symptomatic treatment option for anxiety and is relatively safe for short-term use (Pittler, 2003).

A hydroalcoholic extract of kava inhibited the growth in vitro of *Aspergillus fumigatus, Aspergillus niger, Penicillium digitatum, Rhizopus nigricans, Trichophyton mentagrophytes, Candida albicans,* and *Saccharomyces pastorianus* (Guerin, 1984). However, an aqueous extract did not inhibit the growth in vitro of *Trichophyton rubrum, Microsporum canis,* or *Epidermophyton floccosum* (Locher, 1995).

Indications: Anxiety, insomnia, nervous tension, cystitis

Potential Veterinary Indications:

- Alleviation of anxiety due to fireworks, thunderstorms, stress, separation, and other causes.
- Interstitial cystitis and other lower urinary tract disorders in cats
- Feline inappropriate elimination
- Topically, a teaspoon of kava powder can be mixed with 1 tbsp calendula ointment and applied to painful wounds and lick granulomas (Basko, 2004)
- Muscle relaxant

Contraindications: During pregnancy and lactation and in patients with endogenous depression or liver disease. The effectiveness of centrally acting drugs such as alcohol, barbiturates, and other psychopharmacologic agents may be potentiated (Blumenthal, 1998).

Toxicology and Adverse Effects: AHPA class 2b, 2c, 2d. *The Botanical Safety Handbook* warns that the recommended dose should not be exceeded. Concerns have been expressed in the literature regarding the potential hepatotoxcity of kava because a number of cases of adverse events associated with kava have been reported. As of June 2005, 80 cases of toxicity had been reported worldwide (primarily from German products), and none have been reported in communities where kava use is traditional, even among heavy kava drinkers. Upon analysis, a causal relationship was associated in four cases. Considering that some 250 million daily doses of ethanolic kava extract have been ingested over the past 10 years, this is a very low incidence (Schmidt, 2001). However, the herb should not be used in cases of acute or chronic hepatic disease, or when hepatotoxic drugs are administered concurrently.

One study analyzed 29 novel cases of hepatitis concurrent with kava ingestion. Hepatic necrosis or cholestatic hepatitis was noted with both alcohol and acetone extracts of kava. Nine patients developed fulminant liver failure, and three died. In others, complete recovery occurred after withdrawal of kava. The report noted the potential hepatotoxicity of Kava (Stickel, 2003). In a surveillance study of 4049 patients who were given a standardized kava extract that contained 70% Kava pyrones (150 mg extract, equivalent to 105 mg kava pyrones) orally daily for 7 weeks, adverse reactions were reported in 61 patients (1.5%). Major reactions included gastrointestinal complaints and allergic skin reactions. In a study of 3029 patients given 30% kava pyrones (800 mg extract, equivalent to 240 mg kava pyrones) orally daily for 4 weeks, adverse reactions were reported in 2.3% of patients. Nine cases of allergic reactions, 31 cases of gastrointestinal complaints, 22 cases of headache or dizziness, and 11 cases of other undefined problems were reported (Blaschek, 1998).

Anke (2004) and Bauer (2003) reviewed hepatotoxicity reports to date, noting that some reports were duplicates, and that many patients were co-ingesting hepatotoxic drugs or alcohol. Kavalactones have been regarded as the "toxic principles"; however, Anke writes that pipermethystin is a more likely candidate. These authors also note that in a case report, patients were deficient in the P450 enzyme, CYP2D6, and that complex interactions between co-ingested drugs and genetic polymorphisms in the P450 systems may be at work.

Heavy long-term consumption of kava is associated with a pellagroid dermopathy (Ruze, 1990). Long-term administration may cause transient, yellow discoloration of the skin and nails, which is reversible with discontinuation. One study in an Australian aboriginal community found that chronic abuse of kava led to malnutrition and weight loss, increased levels of γ-glutamyltransferase, decreased levels of plasma protein, and reduced platelet volume and lymphocyte numbers (Mathews, 1988). Kava should not be taken for longer than 3 months without medical advice (Blumenthal, 1998).

Dosage:

External Use: Kava can be used topically in the form of a liniment and a transdermal lotion for muscle pain

Internal Use:

Human

Dried herb: 1.7-3.4 g per day, equivalent to 60-120 mg kavapyrones (Blumenthal, 2000); 6-12 g/day (Mills, 2005); 1-10 g TID (Yarnell)

Standardized extract: equivalent to 60-210 mg Kava pyrones/lactones, divided daily (Mills, 2005)

Tincture (commonly 60% ethanol) 1:2 or 1:3: 1-4 mL TID (Mills, 2005)

Small Animal

Dried herb: 25-300 mg/kg, divided daily (optimally, TID)

Tincture (60% ethanol): 1:2-1:3: 0.5-1.5 mL per 10 kg (20 lb), divided daily (optimally, TID) and diluted or combined with other herbs. Higher doses may be appropriate if the herb is used singly and is not combined in a formula.

Large Animal

Dried herb: horses, 1-2 tbsp; horses suffering from tying-up syndrome can be given 1 tbsp 4 times a day (Basko, 2004)

References

Anke J, Ramzan I. Kava hepatotoxicity: are we any closer to the truth? Planta Med 2004;70:193-196.

Bauer R, Kopp B, Nahrstedt A. Relevant hepatotoxic effects of kava still need to be proven: a statement of the Society for Medicine Plant Research. Planta Med 2003;69:971-972.

Blaschek W, ed. *Hagers Handbuch der pharmazeutischen Praxis. Folgeband 2: Drogen A-K.* 5th ed. Berlin: Springer-Verlag; 1998.

Blumenthal M, Goldberg A, Brinckmann J, eds. *The Complete German Commission E Monographs.* Austin, Tex: American Botanical Council; 2000.

Boerner RJ, Sommer H, Berger W, Kuhn U, Schmidt U, Mannel M. Kava-kava extract LI 150 is as effective as opipramol and buspirone in generalised anxiety disorder—an 8-week randomized, double-blind multi-centre clinical trial in 129 out-patients. Phytomedicine 2003;10(suppl):38-49.

Bruneton J. *Pharmacognosy, Phytochemistry, Medicinal Plants.* Paris: Lavoisier; 1995.

Farnsworth NR, ed. NAPRALERT database. Chicago, Ill: University of Illinois at Chicago; February 9, 1998 production.

Garrett KM, Basmadjian G, Khan IA, Schaneberg BT, Seale TW. Extracts of kava *(Piper methysticum)* induce acute anxiolytic-like behavioral changes in mice. Psychopharmacology (Berl) 2003;170:33-41.

Geier FP, Konstantinowicz T. Kava treatment in patients with anxiety. Phytother Res 2004;18:297-300.

Guérin JC, Réveillère HP. Activité antifongique d'extraits végétaux à usage thérapeutique. I. Étude de 41 extraits sur 9 souches fongiques. Ann Pharmaceut Franç 1984;42:553-559.

Holm E, Staedt U, Heep J, et al. Untersuchungen zum Wirkungsprofil von D,L-Kavain. Zerebrale Angriffsorte und Schlaf-Wach-Rhythmus im Tierexperiment. Arzneimittelforschung 1991;41:673-683.

Jamieson DD, Duffield PH, Cheng D, Duffield AM. Comparison of the central nervous system activity of the aqueous and lipid extract of kava *(Piper methysticum).* Arch Int Pharmacodyn Thér 1989;301:66-80.

Locher CP, Burch MT, Mower HF, et al. Anti-microbial activity and anti-complement activity of extracts obtained from selected Hawaiian medicinal plants. J Ethnopharmacol 1995; 49:23-32.

Mathews JD, Riley MD, Fejo L, et al. Effects of the heavy usage of kava on physical health: summary of a pilot survey in an Aboriginal community. Med J Aust 1988;148:548-555.

Mills S, Bone K. *The Essential Guide to Herbal Safety.* St. Louis, Mo: Elsevier; 2005.

Pittler MH, Ernst E. Kava extract for treating anxiety [Review]. Cochrane Database Syst Rev 2003;1:CD003383.

Ruze P. Kava-induced dermopathy: a niacin deficiency? Lancet (Brit ed) 1990;335:8703,1442-1445.

Schmidt J. Analysis of kava side effects. Reports concerning the liver. [Lindenmaier M, Brinckmann J, translators.] Unpublished report. Silver Springs, Md: American Herbal Products Association; 2001.

Seitz U, Schule A, Gleitz J. [3H]-monoamine uptake inhibition properties of kava pyrones. Planta Med 1997;63:548-549.

Singh YN. Kava: an overview. J Ethnopharmacol 1992;37: 13-45.

Stickel F, Baumuller HM, Seitz K, et al. Hepatitis induced by Kava *(Piper methysticum rhizoma).* J Hepatol 2003;39:62-67.

Lavender

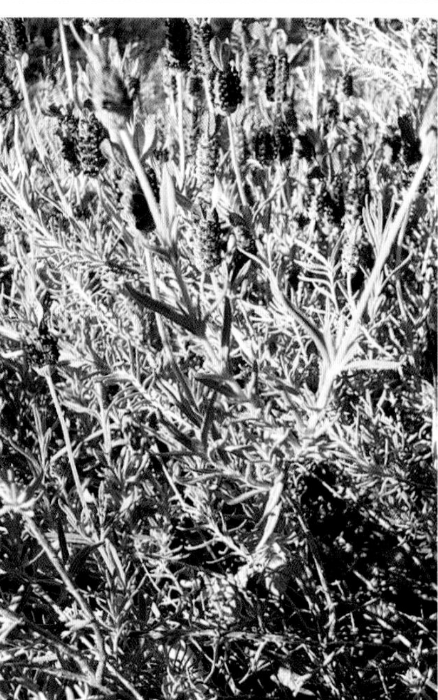

Lavandula angustifolia Mill. syn. *Lavandula officinalis* Chaix., *Lavandula spica* L., *Lavandula vera* DC. • lav-AN-dew-lah an-gus-tee-FOH-lee-uh

Family: Lamiaceae

Parts Used: Flowers. Essential oil from fresh flowers

Distribution: Lavender is indigenous to the Mediterranean and is cultivated in many parts of the world.

Selected Constituents: The essential oil contains linalyl acetate, linalool, camphor, β-ocimene, and 1,8-cineol. The herb also contains tannins.

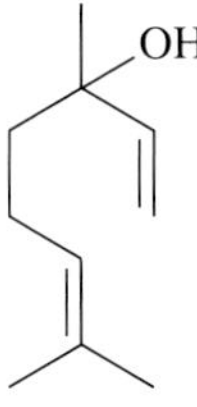

Linalool

Clinical Actions: Spasmolytic, carminative, antidepressant, antirheumatic, local anesthetic, mild diuretic
Energetics: Hot, dry
History and Traditional Usage: Lavender has been used as an antispasmodic, carminative, diuretic, and general tonic. Extracts have been used to treat patients with conditions ranging from acne to migraines (Leung, 1980). It has been thought to increase bile flow output and flow into the intestine (Weiss, 1988) and has been used as an antidiabetic agent (Gamez, 1987). Lavender is usually administered as an infusion, decoction, or oil and is taken internally or applied topically for relief of neuralgia. Lavender oil and extracts are used as pharmaceutical fragrances and in cosmetics.

Lavender oil was also used in veterinary practice; according to Grieve (1975), it is effective in killing lice and other parasites. Its germicidal properties are pronounced. It was considered a useful vermifuge in France (Grieve, 1975). The Eclectics used official preparations of the plant as a carminative and as a stimulant, which contrasts with the present theory that lavender is calming. They also made use of it as a local anesthetic.

de Bairacli Levy (1985) recommends a douche of lavender infusion for metritis in dogs. She claimed that it was eaten eagerly by sheep and goats and it gives a sweet flavor to milk and cheese, and also that it prevents the rapid souring of milk. It has been used in the treatment of patients with vomiting, faintness, sunstroke, headache, and paralysis, and as a douche for female ailments and a lotion for foul mouth and loose teeth. A dose of 2 handfuls of the herb to 1½ pints of water, with 1 cup given 3 times daily, was recommended, or it was used externally (de Bairacli Levy, 1963).
Published Research: In a study that explored plant-derived essential oils that possess an "anticonflict effect" in mice, lavender essential oil increased the response rate during the alarm period in a manner similar to the anxiolytic diazepam (an anticonflict effect), but buspirone did not (Umezu, 2000).

Local anesthetic activity of the essential oil of lavender was investigated. The essential oil reduced the electrically evoked contractions of rat phrenic hemidiaphragm in vitro and in vivo; in a rabbit conjunctival reflex test, treatment with a solution of essential oil of lavender confirmed the local anesthetic activity observed in vitro (Ghelardini, 1999).

A hydroalcoholic extract, a polyphenolic fraction, and essential oil of lavender leaves were investigated for their analgesic effects and anti-inflammatory activity in mice. All extracts tested suppressed some aspects of pain responses in the experimental animals (Hajhashemi, 2003).

The diuretic activity of an infusion of lavender was studied in rats and was compared with that of acetazolamide. The aqueous extract of lavender accelerated elimination of fluid. At the peak of diuretic response, urinary osmolarity was significantly less than that of controls, and sodium excretion was moderate compared with acetazolamide. The stability of aldosterone and the absence of correlation with plasma sodium concentrations, coupled with observed clearance of free water, showed that increased diuresis was of tubular origin. Analysis of hexane extracts in the infusion and in urine indicated that four or five constituents may be involved in the diuretic effect (Elhajili, 2001).

Lavender essential oil and some of its main constituents—linalool, linalyl acetate, and camphor—were tested in vitro for their bioactivities against the *Psoroptes cuniculi* mite of the rabbit. Essential oil and linalool were found to have powerful miticidal activities (Perrucci, 1994).
Indications: Internal: mood disturbances such as restlessness or insomnia, functional abdominal complaints, colic, depression associated with digestive dysfunction, headache. External oil: treatment of patients with functional circulatory disorders, rheumatic pain
Potential Veterinary Indications:
Topical Use: Mites, mild anesthetic and topical anti-inflammatory for skin, douche
Internal Use: Anxiety, restlessness, colic associated with anxiety
Contraindications: Conservative sources list pregnancy as a contraindication; however, *The Botanical Safety Handbook* does not.
Toxicology and Adverse Effects: AHPA class 1. Nausea, vomiting, headache, and chills are sometimes reported after lavender is inhaled or absorbed through the skin. These effects, as well as constipation, appetite loss, confusion, and drowsiness, have been reported after large doses of lavender or perillyl alcohol have been given. The essential oil of lavender may be toxic if taken by mouth. Lavender may cause skin rash and sun sensitivity. Drowsiness is rarely reported with lavender aromatherapy. Some patients with cancer have experienced low blood cell counts (neutropenia) after using high doses of perillyl alcohol.
Drug Interactions: Lavender may increase drowsiness caused by benzodiazepines, barbiturates, narcotics, alcohol, and valerian. In theory, oral use of lavender may increase the risk of bleeding when used with anticoagulants or antiplatelet drugs, and may add to the cholesterol-lowering effects of other drugs and herbs. Lavender may have additive effects when used with certain antidepressants.
Dosage:
External Use:
Aromatherapy: 2-4 drops lavender oil to 2-3 cups boiling water; inhale the steam once per day
Bath: 6 drops lavender oil or ¼-½ cup dried lavender flowers added to bath water
Massage: Add 1-4 drops lavender to a base oil
Internal Use:
Human
Dried herb: 0.5-10 g TID
Infusion: 5-30 g per cup of water, with 1 cup of the tea given TID
Tincture (commonly 70% ethanol) 1:2 or 1:3: 1-5 mL TID
Small Animal
Dried herb: 25-200 mg/kg, divided daily (optimally, TID)
Infusion: 5-30 g per cup of water, administered at a rate of ¼-½ cup per 10 kg (20 lb), divided daily (optimally, TID)

Tincture (70% ethanol) 1:2-1:3: 0.5-1.0 mL per 10 kg (20 lb), divided daily (optimally, TID) and diluted or combined with other herbs. Higher doses may be appropriate if the herb is used singly and is not combined in a formula.

References

De Bairacli Levy J. *The Complete Herbal Handbook for Farm and Stable.* London: Faber and Faber; 1963.

De Bairacli Levy J. *The Complete Herbal Handbook for the Dog and Cat.* London: Faber and Faber; 1985.

Elhajili M, Baddouri K, Elkabbaj S, Meiouat F, Settaf A. Diuretic activity of the infusion of flowers from *Lavandula officinalis* [French]. Reprod Nutr Dev 2001;41:393-399.

Gamez MJ, Jimenez J, Risco S, Zarzuelo A. Hypoglycemic activity in various species of the genus *Lavandula.* Part 1: *Lavandula stoechas* L. and *Lavandula multifida* L. Pharmazie 1987;42:706-707.

Ghelardini C, Galeotti N, Salvatore G, Mazzanti G. Local anaesthetic activity of the essential oil of *Lavandula angustifolia.* Planta Med 1999;65:700-703.

Grieve M. *A Modern Herbal.* London: Jonathan Cape; 1931 (Reprint, 1975).

Hajhashemi V, Ghannadi A, Sharif B. Anti-inflammatory and analgesic properties of the leaf extracts and essential oil of *Lavandula angustifolia* Mill. J Ethnopharmacol 2003;89:67-71.

Leung AY. *Encyclopedia of Common Natural Ingredients Used in Food, Drugs and Cosmetics.* New York: John Wiley and Sons; 1980.

Perrucci S. Acaricidal agents of natural origin against *Psoroptes cuniculi.* Parassitologia 1994;36:269-271.

Umezu T. Behavioral effects of plant-derived essential oils in the Geller type conflict test in mice. Jpn J Pharmacol 2000;83:150-153.

Weiss RF. *Herbal Medicine.* Stuttgart: Hippokrates Verlag; 1988.

Lemon Balm

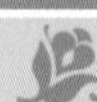

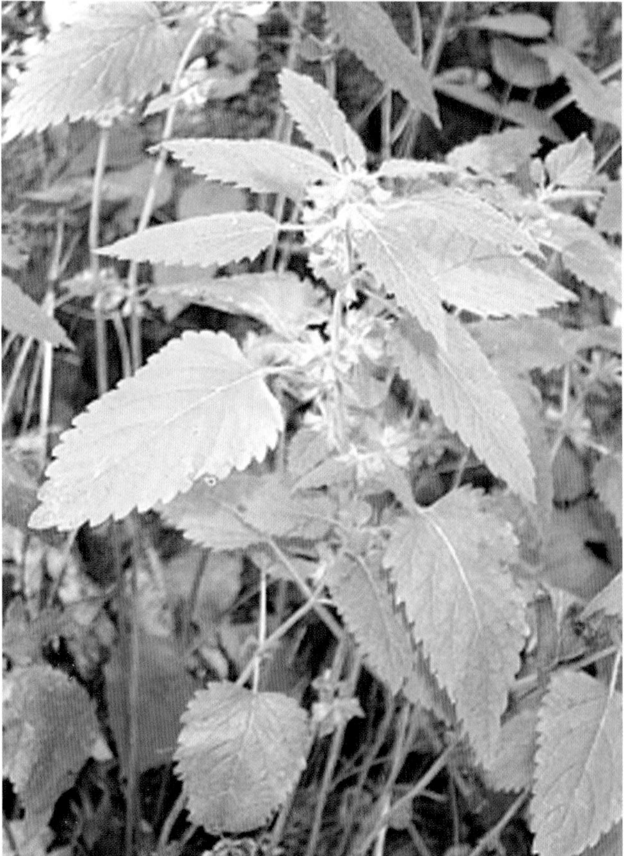

Melissa officinalis L. • mel-ISS-uh oh-fiss-ih-NAH-liss

Other Names: Balm, Melissa, Melissa balm, bee balm, honeyplant, sweet balm, *Folium melissae* being the dried leaves

Family: Lamiaceae

Parts Used: (Dried) leaves picked at or just prior to flowering

Distribution: Indigenous to Western Asia and the Eastern Mediterranean region. Cultivated in Central, Eastern, and Western Europe and America

Selected Constituents: The major characteristic constituents are the hydroxycinnamic acids—rosmarinic (<6%), p-coumaric, caffeic, and chlorogenic acids. Essential oil (1%-2%) composed of >40% monoterpenes and >35% sesquiterpenes. The most significant terpenoid components are citral (a mixture of the isomers neral and geranial), citronellal, geraniol, nerol, linalool, farnesyl acetate, humulene (α-caryophyllene), β-caryophyllene, and eremophilene. Others components include flavonoids, tannins, bitter, resin, and acidic triterpenes (e.g., ursolic and oleanolic acids) (Bisset, 1994; Bruneton, 1995: Blumenthal, 1998).

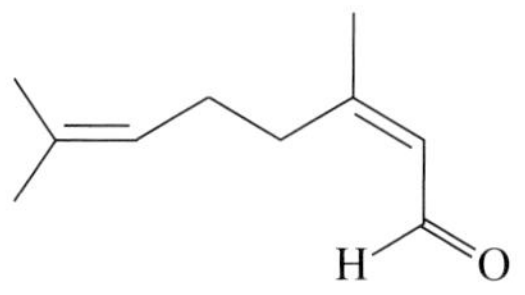

H O

Citral

History and Traditional Usage: Lemon balm is traditionally taken orally as a carminative for gastrointestinal disorders and as a sedative for treatment of patients with nervous disturbances of sleep (British Herbal Pharmacopoeia, 1996; Blumenthal, 1998). Other traditional uses include treatment of those with amenorrhea, asthma, bee stings, cough, dizziness, dysmenorrhea, migraine headache, tachycardia, toothache, tracheobronchitis, and urinary incontinence (Farnsworth, 1998).

Old European herbals documented lemon balm as having memory-improving properties. It is interesting to note that cholinergic activities have now been identified in lemon balm extracts (Perry, 1998).

In Italy, folk use of lemon balm included use to promote milk production in cows about to calve or after calving (Viegi, 2003).

Published Research: An open multicenter study of 115 patients with herpes simplex infection of the skin and transitional mucosa showed that topical 1% aqueous extract of lemon balm in a cream base reduced the healing time of herpetic lesions from 10 to 14 days to 6 to 8 days. A randomized, double-blind, placebo-controlled study of 116 patients with herpes simplex infection showed significant reduction in the size of herpetic lesions within 5 days when patients were treated with the same cream ($P = .01$) as compared with placebo treatment (Vogt, 1991; Wölbling, 1994).

Antimicrobial activity of lemon balm essential oil was tested against 13 bacterial strains and 6 fungi. The most effective antibacterial activity was seen with *Shigella sonei;* significant antifungal activity was exhibited on *Trichophyton* species (Mimica-Dukic, 2004).

The efficacy and safety of lemon balm extract in 42 patients with mild to moderate Alzheimer's disease were examined in a 4-month, parallel-group, placebo-controlled trial. A 1:1 extract in 45% alcohol was dosed at 60 drops daily. This study showed that lemon balm extract produced a significantly better outcome in terms of cognitive function than occurred with placebo, and agitation was more common in the placebo group ($P = .03$). It was concluded that lemon balm extract is of value in Alzheimer's disease, and that it mitigates agitation (Akhondzadeh, 2003).

The cognitive and mood effects of single doses of dried lemon balm leaf were assessed in a randomized, placebo-controlled, double-blind, balanced crossover study. A total of 20 healthy young participants received single doses of 600, 1000, and 1600 mg of encapsulated dried leaf, or a matching placebo, at 7-day intervals. No cholinesterase inhibitory properties were detected. The most notable effects were improved memory and increased "calmness" at all postdose points for the highest (1600 mg) dose. Results suggested that high doses of lemon balm can improve cognitive performance and mood in the treatment of patients with Alzheimer's disease (Kennedy, 2003).

The value of aromatherapy with essential oil of lemon balm for agitation in people with severe dementia was investigated in a placebo-controlled trial. In all, 72 people with clinically significant agitation with severe dementia were randomly assigned to aromatherapy with *Melissa* essential oil (n = 36) or placebo (sunflower oil) (n = 36). No significant adverse effects were observed. It was noted that 60% of the active treatment group and 14% of the placebo-treated group experienced a 30% reduction in agitation. Quality of life indices also improved to a greater extent in people given essential balm oil (Ballard, 2003).

Indications: Flatulence, depression, dementia, Alzheimer's disease, herpes simplex infection (topically), sleep disorders, tenseness, irritability

Potential Veterinary Indications: Cognitive dysfunction, depression; anxiety related to cognitive dysfunction; herpesviral infection, topically for ringworm

Contraindications: None found.

Toxicology and Adverse Effects: AHPA class 1. None known.

Preparation Notes: Should be dried at >35° to preserve the volatile oil. Rapid drying is essential. It should be stored in a tightly closed container and protected from light and should not be stored in plastic containers (Bisset, 1994).

Dosage:

External Use:

Topical cream containing 1% concentrated aqueous extract (70:1): 2-3 times per day for a maximum of 14 days

Tincture: 1:2-1:3 tincture may also be used topically for human herpes lesions (Yarnell, 2005)

Internal Use:

Human

Dried herb: 2-10 g TID

Infusions and decoctions: 5-30 g per cup of water, with 1 cup of the tea given TID

Tincture (usually 45% ethanol) 1:2 or 1:3: 1-5 mL TID

Glycerite (80% glycerin): 1:5: 4.5-6 mL QID

Small Animal

Dried herb: 25-300 mg/kg, divided daily (optimally, TID)

Infusion: 5-30 g per cup of water, administered at a rate of ¼-½ cup per 10 kg (20 lb), divided daily (optimally, TID)

Tincture (usually 45% ethanol) 1:2-1:3: 0.5-1.5 mL per 10 kg (20 lb), divided daily (optimally, TID) and diluted or combined with other herbs. Higher doses may be appropriate if the herb is used singly and is not combined in a formula.

References

Akhondzadeh S, Noroozian M, Mohammadi M, Ohadinia S, Jamshidi AH, Khani M. *Melissa officinalis* extract in the treatment of patients with mild to moderate Alzheimer's disease: a double blind, randomised, placebo controlled trial. J Neurol Neurosurg Psychiatry 2003;74:863-866.

Ballard CG, O'Brien J, Reichelt K, et al. Aromatherapy as a safe and effective treatment for the management of agitation in severe dementia: the results of a double-blind, placebo-controlled trial with *Melissa*. J Clin Psychiatry 2003;64:732.

Bisset NG. *Herbal Drugs and Phytopharmaceuticals*. Boca Raton, Fla: CRC Press; 1994.

Blumenthal M, Busse WR, Goldberg A, eds. *The Complete German Commission E Monographs*. Austin, Tex: American Botanical Council; 1998.

Bombik E, Bombik T, Saba L. The effect of herb extracts on the level of selected microelements in blood serum of calves [Polish]. Instytut Zootechniki Biuletyn Informacyjny 2002a; 40:279-285.

Bombik T, Saba L. The effect of an herb extract on the level of selected macroelements in blood serum of calves [Polish]. Roczniki Naukowe Zootechniki 2002b;1:155-165.

Bombik T, Bombik A, Saba L. Effects of an herb extract on the level of selected biochemical indicators in the blood of calves [Polish]. Medycyna Weterynaryjna 2002c;58:464-466.

British Herbal Pharmacopoeia. London: British Herbal Medicine Association; 1996.

Bruneton J. *Pharmacognosy, Phytochemistry, Medicinal Plants*. Paris: Lavoisier; 1995.

Farnsworth NR, ed. NAPRALERT database. Chicago, Ill: University of Illinois at Chicago; February 9, 1998 production (an online database available through the University of Illinois).

Kennedy DO, Wake G, Savelev S, et al. Modulation of mood and cognitive performance following acute administration of single doses of *Melissa officinalis* (Lemon balm) with human CNS nicotinic and muscarinic receptor-binding properties. Neuropsychopharmacology 2003;28:1871-1881.

Konig B, Dustmann JH. The caffeoylics as a new family of natural compounds. Naturwissenschaften 1985;72:659-661.

Kucera LS, Herrmann EC. Antiviral substances in plants of the mint family (Labiatae). II. Tannin of *Melissa officinalis*. Proc Soc Exp Biol Med 1967;124:865-869.

Mimica-Dukic N, Bozin B, Sokovic M, Simin N. Antimicrobial and antioxidant activities of *Melissa officinalis* L. (Lamiaceae) essential oil. J Agric Food Chem 2004;52:2485-2489.

Perry EK, Pickering AT, Wang WW, Houghton P, Perry NS. Medicinal plants and Alzheimer's disease: integrating ethnobotanical and contemporary scientific evidence [Review]. J Altern Complement Med 1998;4:419-428.

Van den Berghe DA, Vlichink AJ, Van Hoof I. Present status and prospects of plant products as antiviral agents. In: Vlietinck AJ, Dommisse RA, eds. *Advances in Medicinal Plant Research*. Stuttgart: Wissenschaftliche Verlagsgesellschaft; 1985: 47-99.

Viegi L, Pieroni A, Guarrera PM, Vangelisti R. A review of plants used in folk veterinary medicine in Italy as a basis for a databank. J Ethnopharmacol 2003;89:221-244.

Vogt HJ, Tausch I, Wolbling RH, et al. Melissenextrakt bei Herpes simplex. Allgemeinarzt 1991;13:832-841.

Wölbling RH, Leonhardt K. Local therapy of herpes simplex with dried extract from *Melissa officinalis*. Phytomedicine 1994;1:25-31.

Yarnell E, Abascal K. Herbs for treating herpes simplex infections. Altern Complement Ther 2005;11:83-88.

Licorice

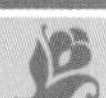

Glycyrrhiza glabra L. syn. *Glycyrrhiza glandulifera* Waltst and Kit. • gly-ky-RY-zuh *or* glis-uh-RY-zuh GLAY-bruh *or* GLAB-ruh

Other Names: *Radix glycyrrhizae*, yashtimadhu, guang guo gan caop, gan cao, Russian licorice, Spanish licorice, Turkish licorice

Family: Fabaceae

Parts Used: Dried roots and rhizomes

Distribution: Native to Central and Southwestern Asia and the Mediterranean. Licorice is cultivated in Africa, Southern Europe, and India.

Selected Constituents: The major constituents are triterpene saponins, including glycyrrhizin (glycyrrhizic acid, glycyrrhizinic acid) (2%-9%); minor components occur in proportions that vary depending on the species and geographic location (Sagara, 1986; Okada, 1981). Glycyrrhizin occurs as a mixture of potassium and calcium salts (Bradley, 1992).

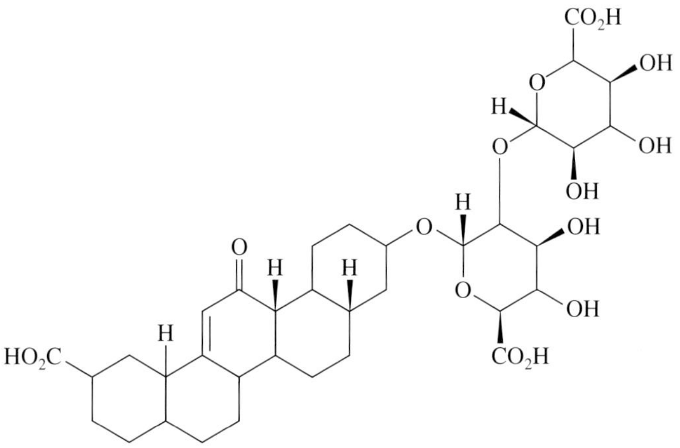

Glycyrrhizin

Clinical Actions: Anti-inflammatory, adaptogen, antiviral (topically), antispasmodic, laxative, estrogenic, taste improver, antiulcerogenic, expectorant

Energetics: Sweet, neutral

History and Traditional Usage: Licorice has a long history of medicinal use since ancient Egyptian, Greek, and Roman times and since the Former Han era (the 2nd-3rd century BC) in ancient China. In Traditional Chinese Medicine today, licorice is still one of the most frequently used herbs. The oldest specimen of licorice from China in the 8th century still exists in the Imperial Storehouse in Japan (Shibata, 2000).

Traditional uses include the following: as a demulcent in the treatment of sore throats and as an expectorant in the treatment of cough and bronchial catarrh; for prophylaxis and treatment of gastric and duodenal ulcers and dyspepsia; as an anti-inflammatory agent in the treatment of allergic reactions (Hikino, 1985), rheumatism, and arthritis; to prevent liver toxicity; and to treat tuberculosis and adrenocorticoid insufficiency

(Bradley, 1992). It is also used as a laxative, emmenagogue, contraceptive, galactagogue, antiasthmatic drug, and antiviral agent, and in the treatment of dental caries, kidney stones, heart disease (Farnsworth, 1995), consumption, epilepsy, loss of appetite, appendicitis, dizziness, tetanus, diphtheria, snakebite, and hemorrhoids (Chin, 1992).

In India, licorice has been extensively used in veterinary medicine for similar purposes to those in humans, for example, for cough, as an expectorant, and as a wound-healing agent in ruminants (Williamson, 2002). It was recommended by Gervase Markham, an authority on husbandry and farriery in the early part of the 17th century for the treatment of certain horse ailments (Grieve, 1975). It is recommended by de Bairacli Levy (1963) as a treatment for cough, inflamed throat, pneumonia, pleurisy, catarrhal conditions, chronic constipation, female infertility, and mild worms in young animals, and colic pain. She makes mention that a poultice of chewed leaves can be used on sores on the backs of horses. For coughing in dogs, "one should make a strong infusion of licorice root, using 1 tablespoon of the root or a 1-oz piece of solid juice; 1 pint of cold water should be added; then the mixture should be boiled, and 1 teaspoon of honey added to each tablespoon of the licorice brew; 2 tablespoons should be given before meals" (de Bairacli Levy, 1985). Winslow (1909) noted that licorice is demulcent and slightly laxative but emphasized its use in making medication balls because the sweet taste covered other tastes so well.

Published Research: Licorice has been used to treat patients with gastrointestinal ulceration. Peptic ulcers have been treated with a glycyrrhetinic acid (GA) extract and a glycyrrhizin (GL) preparation has been used clinically as an antiallergic and an antihepatitis agent. However, GL and GA may induce edema, hypertension, and hypokalemia in patients treated with high doses and with long-term administration. This induced pseudoaldosteronism is due to the 11-hydroxy-steroid dehydrogenase inhibitory activity of GL and GA, which reduce alanine transaminase and aspartate transaminase in serum. To exclude the potential for adverse effects and to enhance therapeutic activities, chemical modification of GL and GA has been performed. Deoxoglycyrrhetol (DG; deglycyrrhizinated licorice [DGL]) also has anti-inflammatory, antiallergic, and antiulcer activities in animal experiments. Immunomodulating effects of GL, GA, and DG have been demonstrated (Shibata, 2000).

The mechanism of antiulcer activity involves acceleration of mucin excretion through increased synthesis of glycoprotein and prolonged life of the epithelial cells and antipepsin activity (Dehpour, 1995); it may protect the stomach against its own peptic secretions (Yamamoto, 1992). Oral deglycyrrhizinated licorice (380 mg 3 times daily) given to 169 patients with chronic duodenal ulcers was as effective as antacid or cimetidine treatment (Kassir, 1985).

Topical licorice extract was evaluated in atopic dermatitis. An extract was standardized; formulations (1% and 2%) were studied in a double-blind clinical trial and were compared with a base gel over 2 weeks (30 patients in each group). Quantities of glycyrrhizinic acid were 20.3% in the extract and 19.6% in the topical preparation. The 2% licorice topical gel was more effective than a 1% gel in reducing the scores for erythema, edema, and itching over 2 weeks (Saeedi, 2003).

The vulnerary effect of licorice extract on open skin wounds in rabbits was investigated. Creams containing 5%, 10%, and 15% (w/w) extract in eucerin base were applied 2 times daily. Phenytoin cream 1% was used as standard control. Results confirmed that licorice cream with 10% extract performed better than phenytoin cream (Arzi, 2003).

One study investigated whether hypertensive patients were more sensitive to licorice-induced inhibition of 11 β-hydroxysteroid dehydrogenase (11 β-HSD) than were normotensive subjects, and whether the response varies according to sex. Healthy volunteers and patients with essential hypertension consumed 100 g of licorice daily for 4 weeks, which corresponded to 150 mg glycyrrhetinic acid. The mean rise in systolic blood pressure (BP) after 4 weeks was 3.5 mm Hg ($P < .06$) in normotensive and 15.3 mm Hg ($P = .003$) in hypertensive subjects ($P = .004$). The mean rise in diastolic BP was 3.6 mm Hg ($P = .01$) in normotensive and 9.3 mm Hg ($P < .001$) in hypertensive subjects ($P = .03$). Licorice induced more pronounced clinical symptoms in women than in men ($P = .0008$), although the difference in BP was not significant. It was concluded that patients with essential hypertension were more sensitive to the inhibition of 11 β-HSD by licorice than were subjects with normal blood pressure (Sigurjonsdottir, 2003).

Licorice may suppress coughing. A 50% methanol extract (100 mg/kg po) led to a greater than 60% reduction in the number of capsaicin-induced coughs, whereas neither the water-eluted nor the 100% ethanol–eluted fractions of water extract of licorice had antitussive effects. Licorice root contains an antitussive compound, liquilitin apioside, the effects of which may depend on peripheral and central mechanisms (Kamei, 2003).

Glycyrrhetinic acid increases mineralocorticoid activity; a case report describes the use of licorice in a 4-year-old dog with Addison's disease. Licorice was added to the diet to reduce persistent hyperkalemia despite conventional veterinary treatment (Jarrett, 2005).

Indications: Cough, asthma, bronchitis, gastric ulceration, Addison's disease; to augment steroid treatment; topically for eczema

Potential Veterinary Indications: To flavor formulas; for atopic dermatitis and Addison's disease; to augment corticosteroid use; to treat those with gastric ulcers, bronchitis, and cough

Contraindications: Licorice is contraindicated in patients with hypertension, cholestatic disorders, or cirrhosis of the liver, hypokalemia, or chronic renal insufficiency, and during pregnancy (German Commission, 1985; Bradley, 1992). Because it increases potassium loss, licorice should not be administered for prolonged use with thiazide and loop diuretics or cardiac glycosides (German Commission, 1985).

Toxicology and Adverse Effects: AHPA class 2b, 2d. Not for prolonged use or in high doses unless given under the supervision of a qualified professional.

Prolonged use of large doses (>50 g/day) of the drug for extended periods (>6 wk) may increase water accumulation. Sodium excretion is reduced and potassium excretion is increased. Blood pressure may rise. Prolonged use can lead to pseudoaldosteronism (Bradley, 1992; Stewart, 1987). In rare cases, myoglobinuria and myopathy may occur (Caradonna, 1992).

It is believed that licorice derivatives may cause retinal or occipital vasospasm, giving rise to transient monocular or binocular visual loss/aberrations. Of five patients who reported recent ingestion of a licorice candy (¼-2 lb), two had documented visual loss (Dobbins, 2000). In the United States, licorice candy is most often flavored with anise—not licorice.

Notes of Interest: Dioscorides left one of the earliest records of the ancient Greek name for this plant, Glykrrhiza (Greek *glukos,* sweet, and *riza,* a root). The plant is often found under the name *Liquiritia officinalis.* The Latin name *Liquiritia,* whence is derived the English name Liquorice (Lycorys in the 13th century), is a corruption of Glycyrrhiza, as is shown in the transitional form, Gliquiricia. The Italian Regolizia, the German Lacrisse or Lakriz, the Welsh Lacris, and the French Reglisse have the same origin (Grieve, 1975).

Dosage:

Human: Licorice should not be used for longer than 4-6 weeks without medical advice, and should not be used at doses that provide more than 100 mg glycyrrhizin per day for longer than 2 weeks without regular blood pressure monitoring

Dried herb: 5-15 g total daily, corresponding to not more than 250 mg daily of glycyrrhizin. Doses of other preparations should be calculated accordingly

DGL powder or tablets: 800-1600 mg chewed 15 min before meals (must be chewed, as capsules are ineffective)

Tincture (usually 30%-35% ethanol) 1:2 or 1:3: 1-5 mL TID

DGL (deglycyrrhizinated licorice): 1.2-4.8 mL per day

Small Animal:

Dried herb: 25-300 mg/kg, divided daily (optimally, TID)

Infusion: 5-30 g per cup of water, administered at a rate of ¼-½ cup per 10 kg (20 lb), divided daily (optimally, TID)

Tincture (usually in 30%-35% ethanol) 1:2-1:3: 0.5-1.0 mL per 10 kg (20 lb), divided daily (optimally, TID) and diluted or combined with other herbs. Higher doses may be appropriate if the herb is used singly and is not combined in a formula.

Historical Veterinary Doses:

Dried herb:

Horse: 15-45 g (RCVS, 1920); 30-60 g (Hungerford, 1970)
Pig: 2-6 g (RCVS, 1920); 4-12 g (Hungerford, 1970)
Cattle: 30-60 g (Hungerford, 1970)
Dog: 1-4 g (RCVS, 1920); 1.3-4 g (Hungerford, 1970)

References

Arzi A, Hemmati AA, Amin M. Stimulation of wound healing by licorice in rabbits. Saudi Pharmaceut J 2003;11:57-60.

Bradley PR, ed. *British Herbal Compendium,* vol 1. Bournemouth: British Herbal Medicine Association; 1992:145-148.

Caradonna P, Gentiloni N, Servidei S, Perrone GA, Greco AV, Russo MA. Acute myopathy associated with chronic licorice ingestion: reversible loss of myoadenylate deaminase activity. Ultrastruct Pathol 1992;16:529-535.

Chin WY, Keng H. *An Illustrated Dictionary of Chinese Medicinal Herbs.* Singapore: CRCS Publications; 1992.

De Bairacli Levy J. *The Complete Herbal Handbook for Farm and Stable.* London: Faber and Faber; 1963.

De Bairacli Levy J. *The Complete Herbal Handbook for the Dog and Cat.* London: Faber and Faber; 1985.

Dehpour AR, Zolfaghari ME, Samadian T, et al. Antiulcer activities of licorice and its derivatives in experimental gastric lesion induced by ibuprofen in rats. Int J Pharmaceut 1995;119:133-138.

Dobbins KR, Saul RF. Transient visual loss after licorice ingestion. J Neuro-ophthalmol 2000;20:38-41.

Farnsworth NR, ed. NAPRALERT database. Chicago, Ill: University of Illinois at Chicago; March 15, 1995 production (an online database of subjects). BMJ 1977;1:488-490.

German Commission E. Monograph: *Liquiritiae radix.* Bundesanzeiger 1985;90:15.

Grieve M. *A Modern Herbal.* London: Jonathan Cape; 1931 (Reprint, 1975).

Hikino H. Recent research on Oriental medicinal plants. In: Wagner H, Hikino H, Farnsworth NR, eds. *Economic and Medicinal Plant Research,* vol 1. London: Academic Press; 1985:53.

Hungerford T. *Veterinary Physicians Index.* 5th ed. Sydney: Angus & Robertson; 1970.

Jarrett RH, Norman EJ, Squires RA. Liquorice and canine Addison's disease. N Z Vet J 2005;53:214.

Kamei J, Nakamura R, Ichiki H, Kubo M. Antitussive principles of *Glycyrrhizae radix,* a main component of the Kampo preparations Bakumondo-to (Mai-men-dong-tang). Eur J Pharmacol 2003;469:159-163.

Kassir ZA. Endoscopic controlled trial of four drug regimens in the treatment of chronic duodenal ulceration. Irish Med J 1985;78:153-156.

Okada K, Tanaka J, Miyashita A, et al. High-speed liquid chromatographic analysis of constituents in licorice root. I. Determination of glycyrrhizin. Yakugaku Zasshi 1981;101:822-828.

RCVS (Royal College of Veterinary Surgeons). *Veterinary Counter Practice.* London: Ballantyne Press; 1920.

Saeedi M, Morteza-Semnani K, Ghoreishi MR. The treatment of atopic dermatitis with licorice gel. J Dermatol Treat 2003;14:153-157.

Sagara K. Determination of glycyrrhizin in pharmaceutical preparations by ion pair high-performance liquid chromatography. Shoyakugaku Zasshi 1986;40:77-83.

Shibata S. A drug over the millennia: pharmacognosy, chemistry, and pharmacology of licorice [Review]. Yakugaku Zasshi 2000;120:849-862.

Sigurjonsdottir HA, Manhem K, Axelson M, et al. Subjects with essential hypertension are more sensitive to the inhibition of 11 beta-HSD by licorice. J Hum Hypertens 2003;17:125-131.

Stewart PM, et al. Mineralocorticoid activity of licorice: 11-β hydroxysteroid dehydrogenase deficiency comes of age. Lancet 1987;ii:821-824.

Williamson E, ed. *Major Herbs of Ayurveda.* Sydney: Churchill Livingstone; 2002.

Winslow K. *Veterinary Materia Medica and Therapeutics.* New York: William R. Jenkins; 1908.

Yamamoto K, Kakegawa H, Ueda H, et al. Gastric cytoprotective anti-ulcerogenic actions of hydroxychalcones in rats. Planta Med 1992;58:389-393.

Lobelia

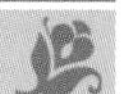

Lobelia inflata L. • low-BEE-lee-uh in-FLAT-uh *or* in-FLAY-tuh

Distribution: Eastern North America

Other Names: Indian tobacco, puke weed, asthma weed, indianascher tabak, tabac indien

Family: Campanulaceae

Parts Used: Aerial parts

Collection: Collect in late summer/fall when the seed capsule is inflated.

Selected Constituents: Piperidine alkaloids (lobeline, isolobinine, etc), resin, volatile oil

Lobeline

Nicotine

Acetylcholine

Clinical Action: Respiratory stimulant, antispasmodic, sedative expectorant, emetic, central nervous system depressant

Energetics: Pungent, bitter, neutral; moves *Qi*

History and Traditional Usage: Native Americans used the root and herb topically for sores and ulcers, and to relieve body pain. It was chewed or taken internally as an emetic, for cough and asthma, for headache, and to "break the smoking habit." The Eclectics used lobelia for spasmodic bronchitis, asthma, and spasms in other systems as well—colic and epilepsy are two examples. It has also been used topically for insect bites, bruises, sprains, and muscle spasms. Lobelia has been used as an aid to stop smoking because lobeline is somewhat chemically similar to nicotine, but adverse effects are unpleasant.

Milks (1949) suggested that lobelia may be useful for heaves in horses; it was combined with belladonna for those cases. It is not mentioned in the Eclectic veterinary text by Titus (1865).

Published Research: Lobeline is a nicotinic receptor antagonist; it has been found to inhibit dopamine uptake and promote dopamine release (Dwoskin, 2002). It crosses the blood–brain and placental barriers and enhances gastrointestinal tone and mobility. Lobelia stimulates the respiratory center (Bradley, 1992).

Indications: Chronic obstructive pulmonary disease (COPD), asthma, and as an aid to stop smoking

Potential Veterinary Indications: Chronic bronchitis, asthma, pneumonia

Contraindications: Pregnancy, lactation, nausea, dyspnea, hypotension

Toxicology and Adverse Effects: AHPA class 2b, 2d. Causes immediate vomiting at doses slightly higher than a therapeutic dose (which may naturally limit toxicity).

This is a strong herb that should not be used by untrained pet owners; however, the toxicity of the herb has been greatly exaggerated. Bergner (2001) claims that part of the reason for this is that lobelia was a symbol of the conflict between regular medicine and the new sects that sprang up in the early 19th century that opposed regular medicine. The medical literature has repeatedly cited "many cases" of fatal poisoning by lobelia, but primary references cannot be found. The only cases that can be confirmed are one involving Samuel Thomson, who was acquitted by the jury in the case, and one in London, in which the practitioner was convicted of practicing without a license. Other cases (all in London) were probably due to the natural course of the epidemic cholera, and the practitioners were acquitted. No human cases of fatality due to lobelia have been reported in the subsequent two centuries. Bergner quotes William Cook, who described Yale professor William Tully's experiments on cats, dogs, and rabbits. Despite administration of large doses by enema, none of the experimental animals was killed.

Adverse effects described in the medical literature include nausea, vomiting, tachycardia, bradycardia, dizziness, dyspnea, hypotension, diaphoresis, respiratory depression, and seizures, although according to Bergner (2004), toxicology references generally fail to include Lobelia; because high doses lead to vomiting, adverse effects are rare.

Drug Interactions: None reported.

Dosage:

Human: (see Chapter 12 in which Poppenga notes that toxicity has been associated with a dose of 50 mg dried herbs, or 1 mL of tincture.)

Dried herb: 12.5-200 mg up to TID

Infusions and decoctions: 0.05-0.6 g in water TID *or* $\frac{1}{4}$-$\frac{1}{2}$ tsp dried herb in 1 cup water; administer $\frac{1}{4}$-1 cup up to TID

Tincture (usually 40%-60% ethanol; some pharmacies include vinegar to better extract alkaloids) 1:2 or 1:3: 0.25-1 mL TID

Small Animal:

Dried herb: 1-5 mg/kg up to TID (do NOT increase an individual dose above 5 mg/kg unless one's individual experience with a particular lobelia product suggests that this is safe)

Tincture (usually 40%-60% ethanol; some pharmacies include vinegar to better extract alkaloids) 1:2-1:3: 0.1-1.0 mL divided daily (optimally, TID) and diluted or combined with other herbs

Large Animal (Karreman, 2004):

Tincture: horse, 30-60 mL

Tincture: cattle, 30-60 mL

Tincture: sheep and goats, 4-15 mL

Historical Veterinary Doses:

Small Animals:

Dogs

Fluid extract: 0.03-1.3 mL

Tincture: 0.2-2 mL (Milks, 1949)

Horses

Fluid extract: 4-30 mL

Tincture: 30-60 mL (Milks, 1949)

Notes of Interest: This is the first herb championed by Samuel Thomson that led to extensive investigation of herbal medicine in the United States; he and the movements he inspired rebelled against "regular medicine of the early 1800s."

Selected References

Bergner P. Lobelia: is lobelia toxic? Medical Herbalirm 2001; 10:15-17,20-25. Available online at: http://medherb.com/Materia_Medica/Lobelia_-_Is_lobelia_toxic_.htm. Accessed April 30, 2006.

Bradley PR, ed. *British Herbal Compendium.* Bournemouth: British Herbal Medicine Association, Scientific Committee; 1992:158-159.

Dwoskin LP, Crooks PA. A novel mechanism of action and potential use for lobeline as a treatment for psychostimulant abuse. Biochem Pharmacol 2002;63:89-98.

Karreman H. *Treating Dairy Cows Naturally: Thoughts and Strategies.* Paradise, Pa: Paradise Publications; 2004.

Milks HJ. *Practical Veterinary Pharmacology, Materia Medica and Therapeutics.* Chicago, Ill: Alex Eger, Inc.; 1949.

Yarnell E. *Clinical Botanical Medicine.* Larchmont, NY: Mary Ann Liebert, Inc.; 2003.

Maitake

Grifola frondosa (Dicks ex. Fr.) S.F. Gray; formerly, *Polyporus frondosus* • Grif-O-luh fron-DO-suh

Similar Species: None found.

Other Names: Hen of the woods, dancing mushroom, mushikusa, king of mushrooms, cloud mushrooms

Family: Polyporaceae

Parts Used: Fruiting bodies

Selected Constituents: B-glucans, lipids, sterols

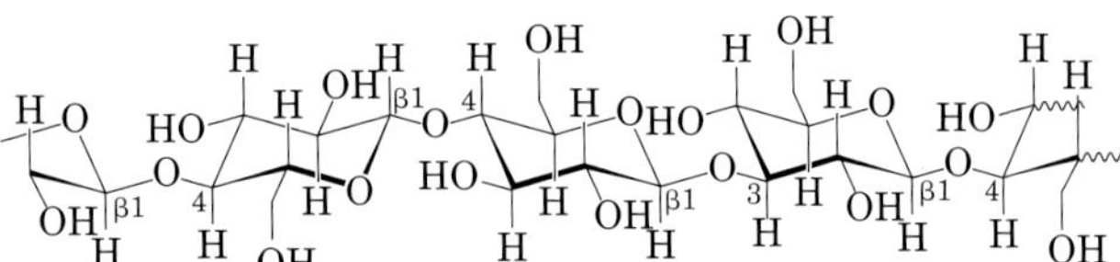

Beta-glucan with β1 ⟶ 4 and β1 ⟶ 3 linkages

Clinical Action: Immunomodulant, antibacterial, antitumor

Energetics: Sweet

History and Traditional Usage: English (and subsequently, American) culinary culture has been described as "mycophobic," which contrasts with virtually the rest of the world. This fungus has no traditional use in Western Herbal Medicine, but it has been the subject of recent scientific investigation. In Japan, the mushroom was used as a tonic.

Published Research: A well-publicized but uncontrolled case series in human patients with cancer reported percentages of people who had tumor regression or symptom improvement when taking the MD fraction, which contains β-1,6 glucan with β-1,3 branched chains. Those patients with liver cancer, breast cancer, and lung cancer had better outcomes than those with leukemia, stomach cancer, and brain cancer. Because the latter group of cancers are generally more aggressive under most circumstances anyway, these results are not easily interpretable. In vitro trials have shown enhanced bone marrow colony formation and decreased doxorubicin toxicity, which lead to cell death and growth inhibition in canine cancer cell lines (Konno, 2004). Maitake may enhance immune function by activating macrophages and T cells. Laboratory animal and human studies show that maitake D-fraction enhances natural killer (NK) cell activity; it also enhances Th-1 dominant immune responses in tumor-bearing mice (Adachi 1987; Kodama, 2005; Kodama, 2003; Harada, 2003; Kodama, 2002a; Lin, 2001).

Animal studies have indicated that maitake extract has hypoglycemic activity (Talpur, 2002; Horio, 2001) and may lower blood lipids (Kubo, 1997).

Indications: Cancer, immune suppression, hypertension, hyperlipidemia, diabetes

Potential Veterinary Indications: Immune suppression related to chronic disease, cancer, hyperlipidemia, diabetes

Notes of Interest: Maitake mushroom is used for food.

Contraindications: None reported.

Toxicology and Adverse Effects: AHPA class 1. None reported.

Drug Interactions: Animal studies showed that maitake increased insulin levels and decreased blood glucose levels, suggesting that the herb may have an additive effect in diabetic patients who are administered hypoglycemic agents.

Dosage:

Human:

Dried herb: 5-30 g TID

D-Fraction: Doses vary widely, from 5.5-70 mg TID

Tincture (usually 30% ethanol) 1:2 or 1:3: 5-15 mL TID

Small Animal:

Dried herb: 200-500 mg/kg to 1 g/kg, divided daily

Tincture (usually 30% ethanol) 1:2-1:3: 2.0-5.0 mL per 10 kg (20 lb), divided daily, and diluted or combined with other herbs

Selected References

Adachi K, Nanba H, Kuroda H. Potentiation of host-mediated antitumor activity in mice by beta glucan obtained from *Grifola frondosa* (maitake). Chem Pharm Bull 1987;35:262-270.

Harada N, Kodama N, Nanba H. Relationship between dendritic cells and the D-fraction–induced Th-1 dominant response in BALB/c tumor-bearing mice. Cancer Lett 2003;192:181-187.

Horio H, Ohtsuru M. Maitake *(Grifola frondosa)* improve glucose tolerance of experimental diabetic rats. J Nutr Sci Vitaminol 2001;47:57-63.

Kodama N, Asakawa A, Inui A, Masuda Y, Nanba H. Enhancement of cytotoxicity of NK cells by D-fraction, a polysaccharide from *Grifola frondosa.* Oncol Rep 2005;13:497-502.

Kodama N, Harada N, Nanba H. A polysaccharide, extract from *Grifola frondosa,* induces Th-1 dominant responses in carcinoma-bearing BALB/c mice. Jpn J Pharmacol 2002a;90:357-360.

Kodama N, Komuta K, Nanba H. Effect of maitake *(Grifola frondosa)* D-fraction on the activation of NK cells in cancer patients. J Med Food 2003;6:371-377.

Kodama N, Komuta K, Sakai N, Nanba H. Effects of D-fraction, a polysaccharide from *Grifola frondosa,* on tumor growth involve activation of NK cells. Biol Pharm Bull 2002b;25:1647-1650.

Konno S. Potential growth inhibitory effect of maitake D-fraction on canine cancer cells. Vet Ther 2004;5:263-271.

Konno S, Tortorelis DG, Fullerton SA, Samadi AA, Hettiarachchi J, Tazaki H. A possible hypoglycaemic effect of maitake mushroom on type 2 diabetic patients. Diabet Med 2001; 18:1010.

Kubo K, Nanba H. Anti-hyperliposis effect of maitake fruit body *(Grifola frondosa).* Biol Pharm Bull 1997;20:781-785.

Lin H, She YH, Cassileth BR, Sirotnak F, Cunningham Rundles S. Maitake beta-glucan MD-fraction enhances bone marrow colony formation and reduces doxorubicin toxicity in vitro. Int Immunopharmacol 2004;4:91-99.

Matsui K, Kodama N, Nanba H. Effects of maitake *(Grifola frondosa)* D-fraction on the carcinoma angiogenesis. Cancer Lett 2001;172:193-198.

Talpur N, Echard B, Dadgar A, Aggarwal S, Zhuang C, Bagchi D, Preuss HG. Effects of Maitake mushroom fractions on blood pressure of Zucker fatty rats. Res Commun Mol Pathol Pharmacol 2002;112:68-82.

Marshmallow

Althaea officinalis L. • AL-thay-uh *or* AL-thee-uh oh-fiss-ih-NAH-liss

Other Names: Schloss tea, guimauve tea, malve, guimauve, malvavisco, malvavisce, gul-khairu, k'uei, *Althaeae radix*

Family: Malvaceae

Distribution: Native to Europe and Asia

Similar Species: *Althaea taurinensis, Althaea rosea, Malva sylvestris, Malva rotundifolia,* and *Malva vulgaris* are stated by *King's* as equivalent in action.

Parts Used: Root from 2-year plants, in early spring or autumn. The fleshy part is used and woody parts discarded. The leaf is sometimes used.

Selected Constituents:
Root: 5%-35% mucilage; asparagines, tannins
Leaf: mucilage, flavonoids, phenolic acids

Clinical Action: Nutritive, demulcent, vulnerary, diuretic

Energetics: Sweet, bitter, cool

Traditional Usage: *King's* states that the decoction is advantageous for nearly every kidney and bladder problem; it lists "diseases of the mucous tissues" that affect most systems, which include hoarseness, respiratory problems, cystitis, urethritis, and diarrhea. It has also been used as a poultice for local inflammatory disorders such as wounds, cellulitis, tumors, and burns. The German Commission E recommends marshmallow root for irritation of the oral and pharyngeal mucosa and associated dry cough, and for mild inflammation of the gastric mucosa.

Published Research: Nosal'ova (1992) compared the antitussive capacity of marshmallow extract and its isolated polysaccharide with the nonnarcotic drugs prenoxdiazine and dropropizine. Unanesthetized cats were stimulated to cough through mechanical irritation of laryngopharyngeal and tracheobronchial mucus achieved with the use of a nylon fiber (diameter, 0.35 mm). The number of cough efforts was measured on the basis of changes in tracheal pressure. The polysaccharide dosed at 50 mg/kg body weight PO inhibited the cough as well as it was inhibited by 1000 mg/kg body weight po of Althaea syrup. The complex extract was less effective than the polysaccharide.

Indications: Digestive complaints, especially gastroenteritis, gastric ulcer, colitis, diarrhea, urinary tract inflammation (cystitis, nephritis, urethritis), stomatitis, laryngitis, and bronchitis. Topically for ruptured abscesses, ulcers, and open wounds

Potential Veterinary Indications: Digestive complaints, especially gastroenteritis, gastric ulcer, colitis, diarrhea, urinary tract inflammation (cystitis, nephritis, urethritis), stomatitis, laryngitis, bronchitis, and other chronic coughs. Topically for ruptured abscesses, ulcers, and open wounds

Contraindications: None reported.

Toxicity and Adverse Effects: AHPA class 1. None reported.

Drug Interactions: The mucilage may theoretically reduce absorption of drugs, glucose, and other soluble molecules from the gut, although the same could be said of many foodstuffs.

Preparations: Decocting destroys mucilage. Cold infusion is best for mucilages.

Dosage:

Human:

Dried root or leaf: 5-10 g TID (usually supplied as the cold infusion), up to 6 times daily for acute conditions

Syrup: ¼-1 tsp as needed for cough

Infusions and decoctions: 5-30 g per cup of water, with 1 cup of the tea given TID, up to 6 times daily acutely

Tincture (usually 25%-30% ethanol, but this is not the optimal form for supplying this herb) 1:2 or 1:3: 1-5 mL TID, up to 6 times daily for acute conditions

Small Animal:
Dried herb: 25-300 mg/kg, divided daily (optimally, TID)
Infusion: 5-30 g per cup of water, administered at a rate of ¼-½ cup per 10 kg (20 lb), divided daily (optimally, TID)
Tincture (usually in 25%-30% ethanol or glycetract) 1:2-1:3: 0.5-1.5 mL per 10 kg (20 lb), divided daily (optimally, TID) and diluted or combined with other herbs. Higher doses may be appropriate if the herb is used singly and is not combined in a formula.

Selected Reference

Nosal'ova G, Strapkova A, Kardosova A, Capek P, Zathurecky L, Bukovska E. [Antitussive action of extracts and polysaccharides of marsh mallow (*Althaea officinalis* L., var. robusta).] Pharmazie 1992;47:224-226.

Meadowsweet

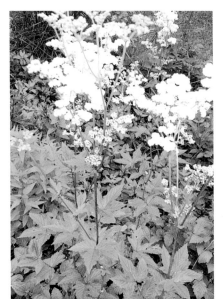

Filipendula ulmaria (L.) Maxim • fil-ih-PEN-dyoo-luh ul-MAR-ee-uh

Other Names: Queen of the meadow, lady of the meadow, *Spiraea ulmaria, Spiraea herba, Philipendula ulmaria*

Family: Rosaceae

Parts Used: The flowers and flowering tops are primarily used in herbal preparations, although historical references are made to use of the root.

Distribution: Meadowsweet is found in Northern and Southern Europe, North America, and Northern Asia.

Selected Constituents: Flavonoids: spiraeoside (quercetin 4′-glucoside), quercetin, hyperoside, rutin, avicularin, and kaempferol derivatives. Tannins. Phenolic glycosides: spiraein, monotropitin (gaultherin), spireine, 6-xylosylglucosides of salicylaldehyde, and methyl salicylate. Essential oil: salicylaldehyde (75%), phenylethyl alcohol, benzyl alcohol, anisaldehyde, methyl salicylate, ethylsalicylate, and methoxybenzaldehyde. Polyphenolics: mainly hydrolysable tannides (10%-15%) and rugosin-D

Other: chalcones, phenylcarboxylic acids, coumarin (trace), ascorbic acid (trace). Although meadowsweet flowers are high in flavonoids, the primary constituents are salicylates, including salicin, salicylaldehyde, and methyl salicylate (Newall, 1996). In the digestive tract, these compounds are oxidized into salicylic acid.

Clinical Actions: Antacid, antiulcerogenic, anti-inflammatory, astringent, mild urinary antiseptic

Energetics: Dry, cool

History and Traditional Usage: Meadowsweet has a history of use in conditions associated with the gastrointestinal tract, particularly for diarrhea, and especially in disorders of children. It was also used to treat patients with rheumatic complaints of the joints and muscles (Bruneton, 1995). Meadowsweet is well indicated for diarrhea and provides soothing and astringent effects. It is considered a corrector and alterative to the stomach. The salicyin content probably provides some diaphoretic action and may give a mild anti-inflammatory effect. Nicholas Culpeper, a 17th century English pharmacist, mentioned the use of meadowsweet to help break fever and to promote sweating during a cold or flu. Herbal references indicate its uses as a diuretic and as an antacid to treat stomach complaints, including heartburn.

De Bairacli Levy (1963) mentions its use by gypsies as a spring tonic for animals and explains that it is eaten by goats and sheep and is used to treat people with fever, blood disorders, diarrhea, and dropsy. She recommends a strong infusion of meadowsweet to control hemorrhage from deep wounds, with leaves and flowers administered externally and internally. In addition, she recommends that meadowsweet be used internally for eczema, and internally and externally for heat rash, scurf, and heat spots (de Bairacli Levy, 1985).

Published Research: The antiulcerogenic properties of *Filipendula ulmaria* have been investigated. An infusion of dried leaves, stems, and flowers (1:10) was tested on mice with carrageenan-induced inflammation. Although a 60% rate of ulcer occurrence was noted in the control group, no ulcers were identified for all concentrations of Meadowsweet tested (0.35, 1.25, 5.0, 10.0 mL/kg) (Gorbacheva, 2002). A decoction (1:10, 1:20) from flowers of *Filipendula ulmaria* was found to reduce the ulcerogenic action of ligation of the pylorus and to reduce the formation of lesions of the glandular part of the stomach after injection of reserpine to rats and mice or phenylbutazone to rats. The decoction prevented acetylsalicylic acid–induced lesions of the stomach in rats. It promoted healing of chronic ulcers of the rat stomach induced by injection of 70% ethanol. The decoction did not protect rats from the ulcerogenic action of cinchophen, but it increased the bronchosphastic and ulcerogenic properties of histamine in guinea pigs (Barnaulov, 1980). Alcohol and water extracts of meadowsweet flowers showed preventive action against the evolution of experimental erosion and stomach ulcers in mice.

A clinical trial of 500 middle-aged men found that *Filipendula ulmaria* reduced the risk of angina (Filipendula alone) and myocardial infarction (Filipendula with Cratageus) (Kielczynski, 1998).

A total of 48 women with cervical dysplasia were treated with topical application of *Filipendula ulmaria* flowers (ointment) to the cervix. Positive responses were recorded in 32 patients (67%), including complete regression in 25 cases (52%). No recurrence was observed in 10 completely cured patients after 12 months (Peresun'ko, 1993).

The anticoagulant activities of flower and seed extracts of *Filipendula ulmaria* were assessed on the basis of recalcification time in plasma from healthy rats after addition of thrombin. It was concluded that both flower and seed extracts of *Filipendula ulmaria* have significant anticoagulant effects (Lyapina, 1993).

Extracts of roots, herb, and flowers of *Filipendula ulmaria* were investigated for in vitro immunomodulatory properties. The ethyl acetate extracts of roots and flowers, all methanol extracts, and the aqueous root extract exhibited strong inhibition toward the classical pathway of complement (Halkes, 1997).

Indications: Acid reflux, gastric ulcer, indigestion, diarrhea, rheumatic conditions, urinary disorders, cervical dysplasia, and repair of the vagina and cervix topically

Potential Veterinary Indications: Gastric ulceration and prevention of ulceration in horses, gastrointestinal inflammation, gastritis, colitis

Contraindications: Salicylate sensitivity. The salicylate content has been estimated to be approximately 388 μg/mL of a 1 : 2 fluid extract. The normal human diet provides a daily intake of 10 to 200 mg salicylates; recommendations for a low salicylate diet require approximately 1.5 to 2 mg daily. A daily dose of 3 mL of meadowsweet is equivalent to approximately 1.16 mg salicylates (Burgoyne, 1995). Published aspirin doses to be administered to cats range up to 25 mg/kg daily of acetylsalicylic acid, but the toxic dose of salicylic acid in cats is not well known. See Chapter 12 for more information on salicylate toxicity.

Toxicology and Adverse Effects: AHPA class 1. In a Bearded Collie with acute weakness, hematemesis, melena, painful abdomen, and pale mucous membranes, a hematocrit of 13% and panhypoproteinemia were found that had been caused by severe gastrointestinal bleeding. Despite intensive investigations, no systemic or local cause could be identified. After repeated client interrogation, it was found that the dog had been receiving a food supplement formulated for horses. This supplement contained a shell extract plus willow *(Salicaceae)* and meadowsweet. The ingestion of this supplement was considered a possible cause of gastrointestinal bleeding (Rohner, 2004).

Potential Drug Interactions: Meadowsweet flowers may potentiate anticoagulant drugs, although this has not been reported.

Notes of Interest: Aspirin is named after the plant used by Bayer as the source of salicylic acid. "A" stood for acetyl chloride, and "spir" was from *Spirea ulmaria*. This is the former botanical name for meadowsweet.

Dosage:

Human:

Dried herb: 1-10 g TID, or more often as needed

Infusions and decoctions: 5-30 g per cup of water, with 1 cup of the tea given TID, up to 6 times daily acutely (Bradley, 1992; Yarnell, 2003)

Tincture (commonly 25% ethanol; some pharmacies include glycerin to prevent precipitation by tannins) 1:2 or 1:3: 1-5 mL TID, up to 6 times daily for acute conditions

Small Animal:

Dried herb: 25-300 mg/kg, divided daily (optimally, TID)

Infusion: 5-30 g per cup of water, administered at a rate of ¼-½ cup per 10 kg (20 lb), divided daily (optimally, TID)

Tincture (commonly 25% ethanol; some pharmacies include glycerin to prevent precipitation by tannins) 1:2-1:3: 0.5-1.5 mL per 10 kg (20 lb), divided daily (optimally, TID) and diluted or combined with other herbs. Higher doses may be appropriate if the herb is used singly and is not combined in a formula.

References

Barnaulov OD, Denisenko PP. Anti-ulcer action of a decoction of the flowers of the dropwort, *Filipendula ulmaria* (L.) Maxim. Farmakol Toksikol 1980;43:700-705.

Bradley PR, ed. *British Herbal Compendium*. Bournemouth: British Herbal Medicine Association, Scientific Committee; 1992:158-159.

Bruneton J. *Pharmacognosy, Phytochemistry, Medicinal Plants*. Paris: Lavoisier; 1995.

Burgoyne B. Salicylates in herbs. Mod Phytother 1995;1:3-6.

De Bairacli Levy J. *The Complete Herbal Handbook for Farm and Stable*. London: Faber and Faber; 1963.

De Bairacli Levy J. *The Complete Herbal Handbook for the Dog and Cat*. London: Faber and Faber; 1985.

Halkes SB, Beukelman CJ, Kroes BH. *In vitro* immunomodulatory activity of *Filipendula ulmaria*. Phytother Res 1998;11:518-520.

Kielczynski W. Clinical outcome of herbal prevention of vascular disease in 500 middle aged males. Proceedings of NHAA International Conference; 1998; Sydney, Australia.

Lyapina LA, Koval'chuk GA. A comparative study of the effects of *Fillipendula ulmaria* flower and seed extracts on hemostasis. Biol Bull Russian Acad Sci 1993;20:505-507.

Newall CA, Anderson LA, Phillipson JD. *Herbal Medicines: A Guide for Health-Care Professionals*. London: The Pharmaceutical Press; 1996:191-192.

Peresun'ko AP, Bespalov VG, Limarenko AI, et al. Clinico-experimental study of using plant preparations from the flowers of *Filipendula ulmaria* (L.): maxim for the treatment of precancerous changes and prevention of uterine cervical cancer. Vopr Onkol 1993;39:291-295.

Rohner MM, Glaus TM, Reusch CE. Life threatening intestinal bleeding in a Bearded Collie associated with a food supplement for horses [German]. Schweiz Arch Tierheilkd 2004;146:479-482.

Yarnell E. *Clinical Botanical Medicine*. Larchmont, NY: Mary Ann Liebert, Inc.; 2003.

Milk Thistle

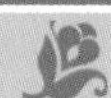

Silybum marianum L. Gaertn. • SIGH-lee-bum mar-ee-AH-num

Distribution: Southern and Western Europe; naturalized to South America and North America

Similar Species: *Silybum eburneum* is an inferior species with which *S. marianum* can cross-pollinate. Many thistle species may have similar uses.
Common Names: Holy thistle, marian thistle, our lady's thistle, Mary thistle, St. Mary's thistle, wild artichoke, mariendistel (Germany), Chardon-Marie (French). Milk thistle should not be confused with blessed thistle, *Cnicus benedictus*. Former botanical name was *Carduus marianus*. Legalon (Madaus, Cologne, Germany) and Thisilyn (Nature's Way, Springville, Utah, United States) are the two most studied products. In Chinese medicine, milk thistle is known as *shui fei ji*.
Family: Asteraceae
Parts Used: Seed collected in late summer. (In Europe, the leaves were historically used similarly to spinach; once the spines had been removed, the fruit was eaten like an artichoke.)
Selected Constituents: Silymarin is a flavonoid complex made up of three parts: silibinin, silidianin, and silichristine. Silibinin is thought most active and is probably responsible for the benefits attributed to silymarin. Also contains sterols, fixed oil, flavonoids (apigenin, quercetin, kaempferol), lignans, biogenic amines (tyramine, betaine), and mucilage

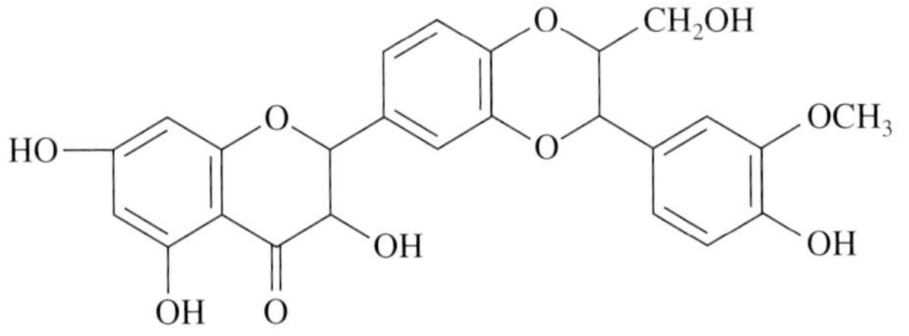

HO OH O OH CH_2OH OCH_3 OH

Silibinin

Clinical Action: Hepatoprotective, demulcent, cholagogue, galactagogue, antioxidant
Energetics: Bitter, warm; has been described in contradicting ways. Holmes (1997) states that it is drying, and Kenner (2001) claims that it is a yin tonic.
History and Traditional Usage: This plant has been used since ancient times, and it was mentioned in many of the great Herbals of the 16th and 17th centuries. Gerard recommended it for liver disease (melancholy). No record can be found of its use in North America by native people, although the plant was brought to the West by European settlers. It was not introduced into Eclectic practice until 1898. Specific indications in Eclectic use were as follows: "splenic, hepatic and renal congestion, face sallow, appetite, capricious; nervous irritability; despondency; physical debility; pain in either hypochondriac; pelvic tension and weight; congestion of the parts supplied by the coeliac axis; and non-malarial splenic hypertrophy."
Published Research: Silymarin is thought to have the following effects (Flora, 1998):

- Acts as an antioxidant
- Inhibits lipid peroxidation in hepatocyte plasma membranes, thereby protecting against many toxins
- Protects against genomic injury through suppression of lipoxygenase, hydrogen peroxide, and superoxide
- Increases hepatocyte protein synthesis via stimulation of RNA polymerase
- Suppresses nuclear factor (NF)-kappaB
- Chelates iron and decreases glutathione destruction in iron overload conditions
- Stabilizes mast cells
- Slows calcium metabolism
- Decreases activity of tumor promoters

A total of 20% to 40% of an oral dose is found in bile, and 3% to 8% is excreted in the urine. Silybin levels peak in bile at between 2 and 9 hours post ingestion, and excretion in the bile continues for 24 hours. Extensive enterohepatic circulation is suspected. Absorption is said to be enhanced if silymarin is administered with phosphatidylcholine (Flora, 1998).

Liver disorders

Controlled clinical trials in various hepatic disorders, including toxin- and drug-induced hepatitis, alcoholic liver disease, viral hepatitis, and cirrhosis, suggest that milk thistle decreases aminotransferase activity and improves various clinical parameters on a less consistent basis. In an evidence report/technology assessment paper prepared by the US Department of Health and Human Services, a literature review revealed the following:

Of 16 prospective placebo-controlled trials, study design was found to be of variable quality, and interpretation overall was difficult. However, results revealed that four of six studies on alcoholic liver disease showed significant improvement in at least one measure of liver function. Three of three studies on viral hepatitis showed improvement in clinical disease, and two of three showed improvement in histology. In two of two studies on cirrhosis (alcoholic and nonalcoholic), administration of milk thistle was associated with improvement. Of three trials that evaluated milk thistle in the treatment or prevention of damage due to hepatotoxic drugs, results were mixed (Agency for Healthcare Research and Quality, 2000).

Milk thistle and silymarin have been submitted to later critical reviews in the treatment of patients with hepatitis B and C. These compounds do not appear to influence viral infection; however, they may attenuate damage caused by infection (Mayer, 2005; Rambaldi, 2005).

Kidney diseases

Silybin reduces oxidative damage to kidney cells in vitro (Sanhueza, 1992). In rats, silibinin prevented cisplatin-induced nephrotoxicity (Gaedeke, 1996; Bokemeyer, 1996), but it did not prevent cyclosporine-induced glomerular damage, except for lipid peroxidation (Zima, 1998).

Blood lipids

Animal studies have suggested that silymarin can help control blood lipid levels (Skottova, 2004; Skottova, 2003), possibly by modulating absorption of cholesterol (Sobolova, 2005). Humans given silymarin in an open clinical trial did not display significant changes in blood lipid profiles (Somogyi, 1989). Fifteen patients who underwent cholecystectomy received placebo or silymarin (420 mg daily for 1 month). Silymarin administration led to a significant decrease in biliary cholesterol concentration. The authors suggest that silymarin decreases hepatic cholesterol synthesis (Nassuato, 1991).

Pancreatic disorders

Experimental damage of the pancreas in rats can be ameliorated with the use of silymarin (Soto, 1998). Silibyn protects the pancreas from cyclosporine toxicity. In rats given cyclosporin A, or cyclosprin A plus silymarin, silibinin mitigated changes in amylase secretion, but the combination of cyclosporine and silibinin had an additive effect on inhibiting insulin secretion (von Schonfeld, 1997). In a human clinical trial, 60 alcoholics with hepatic cirrhosis and insulin-dependent diabetes were treated with silymarin (200 mg TID) or placebo. Silymarin administration resulted in significant decreases in fasting glucose, glycosuria, and insulin needs over 6 months (Velussi, 1997; Velussi, 1993).

Cancer

Silibinin and silymarin have been investigated in animal studies as cancer preventive agents. In prostate cancer cells, for example, these compounds alter cell cycle progression, inhibit cell survival signaling and mitogenic signaling, synergize the effects of doxorubicin, inhibit secretion of proangiogenic factors, inhibit growth, and enhance apoptosis. Silibinin also inhibits growth of implanted prostate tumor cells in nude mice (Singh, 2004). Silibinin may improve repair of mouse skin DNA damaged by UV radiation (Singh, 2005); silymarin, applied topically, inhibits chemical carcinogenesis in mice (Katiyar, 2005).

Veterinary trials

In two trials of dogs given hepatotoxic chemicals, silymarin or silibinin improved biochemical and histologic measures of hepatotoxicity, and survival was improved.

In the first trial, beagles were given 85 mg/kg *Amanita phalloides* lyophilizate orally. In addition to a control group, 4 groups of 6 to 10 dogs were given the following:

- Prednisolone, 30 mg/kg IV at 5 and 24 hours
- Cytochrome C, 50 mg/kg IV at 5 and 24 hours
- Penicillin G, 1000 mg/kg IV at 5 hours
- Silymarin, 50 mg/kg IV at 5 hours and 30 mg/kg IV at 24 hours

Blood was sampled at 5, 24, 48, 96, and 192 hours. Results of this study showed that all liver enzymes of dogs that received milk thistle remained nearly normal throughout the testing period, whereas those of control dogs increased precipitously (Floersheim, 1978).

Vogel (1984) administered 85 mg/kg of amanita lysate to beagles, then treated half of them with silibinin (78 mg/kg IV at 5 and 24 hours). In the control group, 4 of 12 dogs died, and histopathology showed severe liver necrosis. None died in the silibinin-treated group, and liver histopathology was nearly normal.

In one trial of postparturient cattle given milk thistle seeds, milk production was increased and ketonuria reduced, as compared with controls. Tedesco (2004a, 2004b) found that 10 g of silymarin (the extract) daily protected postparturient cows from a loss in body condition and improved lactation performance. No silymarin residues were found in milk or colostrum. The same group examined liver histology and biochemistry of periparturient cows and found that silymarin had no observable effect on fat accumulation or biochemical parameters of liver disease.

Tedesco (2004c) also examined the effect of a silymarin–phospholipid/phytocome complex administered to 14-day-old broiler chicks to determine whether it provided protection against aflatoxin B1. A total of three groups of chicks were administered diet alone, diet plus 0.8 mg/kg of feed of the aflatoxin B1, or diet plus aflatoxin plus 600 mg/kg of the silymarin phytosome. The silymarin complex resulted in lower alanine aminotransferase (ALT) levels and better weight gain than were noted in birds given aflatoxin but no silymarin. Birds receiving aflatoxin and silymarin had body weight gain and ALT levels equivalent to those of birds given no aflatoxin.

Giardia and interactions with metronidazole

Chon (2005) investigated the efficacy of silymarin for the treatment of giardiasis, measured with use of the giardia antigen test. Dogs that tested positive for giardia were treated orally for 2 weeks with silymarin (3.5 mg/kg QD), metronidazole (50 mg/kg QD), metronidazole and silymarin at the same doses, or nothing. Seven days into the trial, no significant difference in infection levels was observed between the silymarin and metronidazole and metronidazole alone groups, but by the 10th day, the combination group showed significantly less infection than did the group given metronidazole alone. By the end of 2 weeks, the metronidazole and the metronidazole + silymarin groups tested negative for giardia; the silymarin and placebo groups remained positive. It is interesting to note that dogs treated with silymarin in addition to metronidazole did not experience weight loss, and liver measurements were similar to those seen in the metronidazole alone group.

Indications: Used for a variety of liver diseases, but especially as protection against toxic ingestion such as occurs in alcoholism; for hypercholesterolemia and varicose veins. It is used by some herbalists to increase lactation.

Potential Veterinary Indications: Hepatitis, cholangiohepatitis, toxic injury to liver (especially aflatoxicosis), hepatic lipidosis; adjunct for giardia treatment or during metronidazole administration to decrease adverse effects; for protection of the pancreas during pancreatitis or protection from drug damage; hyperlipidemia; to increase lactation and protect dairy cows from ketonemia

Contraindications: No known contraindications have been reported. Milk Thistle has been recommended for problems associated with the gallbladder during pregnancy, and so it is likely to be safe even for pregnant and lactating animals. Patients allergic to members of the daisy family may be sensitive to milk thistle.

Toxicology and Adverse Effects: AHPA class 1. Milk thistle is relatively nontoxic, and the seeds, plant, and root have been used as food. In one study, mice tolerated a dose of 20 g/kg. The most common adverse reactions were allergy, urticaria, and gastrointestinal distress. The European Agency for Evaluation of Medicinal Products, Committee for Veterinary Medicinal Products, has determined that milk thistle is safe in food-producing animals when used as the homeopathic mother tincture (an alcohol tincture of 1 part dried seed and 2 parts alcohol) and in all homeopathic dilutions. This author (SW) has noted at least 2 cases in which milk thistle administration (prescribed for elevated liver enzymes) led to increased ALT in dogs; when the herb was discontinued, ALT returned to the former level. This occurs in only a small minority of treated cases in this practice, however, and has thus far been attributed to a hypersensitivity reaction.

Potential Drug Interactions: Milk thistle reduces the activity of CYP3A4 and other liver enzymes in vitro, but clinical trials did not demonstrate any effect on anti–human immunodeficiency virus (HIV) drugs (Brinker, 1998). A clinical trial in healthy volunteers suggests that the effect is minimal and perhaps not clinically significant (Gurley, 2004). Silymarin has been reported to stimulate activity of the p-glycoprotein drug transporter (Zhou, 2004).

Milk thistle may reduce insulin requirements in some patients with diabetes. Silymarin has been shown to protect against organ toxicity induced by cisplatin, acetaminophen, butyrophenones, halothane, phenothiazines, tacrine, and vincristine.

Preparation Notes: Flavonolignans are not very water soluble, so dried seeds or liquid extracts must be alcohol based. Even so, Brinker notes that water extracts have been used traditionally; this suggests that other components in the herb may be beneficial as well.

Notes of Interest: The characteristic spiked leaves display white veins, which were said to carry the breast milk of the Virgin Mary. Dioscorides made mention of the leaf, and Gerard (1596) had this to say of it: "My opinion is that this is the best remedy that grows against all melancholy (bile-liver) diseases." Culpeper also made use of Milk Thistle.

Dosage: Milk thistle is usually supplied as a solid extract, standardized to 70% to 80% silymarin. Milk thistle should be used for at least 8 weeks before results such as improvement in biochemistry are expected.

Human:

Dried herb: 1-10 g TID

Standardized extract (standardized to 70% silymarin): 140-200 mg TID; reduce to 90 mg TID after 6 weeks

Infusions and decoctions: Not recommended

Fluid extract (1:1) (usually 60%-80% ethanol): 10-15 mL per day

Glycetract (1:1): 5-9 mL per day, divided

Small Animal:

Dried herb: 50-100 mg/kg, divided daily (optimally, TID) if extracted and dried; triple or quadruple dose for unprocessed herb

Dry standardized extract (70% silymarin): 10-15 mg/kg, divided daily

Fluid extract (1:1) (usually 60%-80% ethanol): 1.0-2.0 mL per 10 kg (20 lb), divided daily and diluted or combined with other herbs

Glycetract (1:1): 1.0-2.0 mL per 10 kg (20 lb), divided daily and diluted or combined with other herbs

Cattle:

Dried herb: 10 g daily

References

Agency for Healthcare Research and Quality. *Milk Thistle: Effects on Liver Disease and Cirrhosis and Clinical Adverse Effects.* Summary, Evidence Report/Technology Assessment: Number 21, September 2000. Available at: http://www.ahrq.gov/clinic/epcsums/milktsum. Accessed May 2, 2006.

Bokemeyer C, Fels LM, Dunn T, et al. Silibinin protects against cisplatin-induced nephrotoxicity without compromising cisplatin or ifosfamide antitumour activity. Br J Cancer 1996;74:2036-2041.

Brinker F, ed. *Herb Contraindications and Drug Interactions.* 2nd ed. Sandy, Ore: Eclectic Medical Publications; 1998:74-75.

Chon SK, Kim NS. Evaluation of silymarin in the treatment on asymptomatic *Giardia* infections in dogs. Parasitol Res 2005;97:445-451.

Floersheim GL, Eberhard M, Tschumi P, Duckert F. Effects of penicillin and silymarin on liver enzymes and blood clotting factors in dogs given a boiled preparation of *Amanita phalloides.* Toxicol Appl Pharmacol 1978;46:455-462.

Flora K, Hahn M, Rosen H, Benner K. Milk thistle *(Silybum marianum)* for the therapy of liver disease. Am J Gastroenterol 1998;93:139-143.

Gaedeke J, Fels LM, Bokemeyer C, Mengs U, Stolte H, Lentzen H. Cisplatin nephrotoxicity and protection by silibinin. Nephrol Dial Transplant 1996;11:55-62.

Gurley BJ, Gardner SF, Hubbard MA, Williams DK, Gentry WB, Carrier J, Khan IA, Edwards DJ, Shah A. In vivo assessment of botanical supplementation on human cytochrome P450 phenotypes: *Citrus aurantium, Echinacea purpurea,* milk thistle, and saw palmetto. Clin Pharmacol Ther 2004;76:428-440.

Holmes P. *The Energetics of Western Herbs.* Boulder, Colo: Snow Lotus Press; 1997.

Katiyar SK. Silymarin and skin cancer prevention: anti-inflammatory, antioxidant and immunomodulatory effects. Int J Oncol 2005;26:169-176.

Kenner D, Requena Y. *Botanical Medicine.* Brookline, Mass: Paradigm Publications; 2001.

Mayer KE, Myers RP, Lee SS. Silymarin treatment of viral hepatitis: a systematic review. J Viral Hep 2005;12:559-567.

Nassuato G, Iemmolo RM, Strazzabosco M, Lirussi F, Deana R, Francesconi MA, Muraca M, Passera D, Fragasso A, Orlando R, Comos G, Okolicsanyi L. Effect of Silibinin on biliary lipid composition experimental and clinical study. J Hepatol 1991; 12:290-295.

Paulova J, Dvorak M, Kolouch F, Vanova L, Janeckova L. [Verification of the hepatoprotective and therapeutic effect of silymarin in experimental liver injury with tetrachloromethane in dogs.] Vet Med (Praha) 1990;35:629-635.

Rambaldi A, Jacobs BP, Iaquinto G, Gluud C. Milk thistle for alcoholic and/or hepatitis B or C liver diseases—a systematic cochrane hepato-biliary group review with meta-analyses of randomized clinical trials. Am J Gastroenterol 2005;100:2583-2591.

Sanhueza J, Valdes J, Campos R, Garrido A, Valenzuela A. Changes in the xanthine dehydrogenase/xanthine oxidase ratio in the rat kidney subjected to ischemia-reperfusion stress: preventive effect of some flavonoids. Res Commun Chem Pathol Pharmacol 1992;78:211-218.

Singh RP, Agarwal R. Prostate cancer prevention by silibinin. Curr Cancer Drug Targets 2004;4:1-11.

Singh RP, Agarwal R. Mechanisms and preclinical efficacy of silibinin in preventing skin cancer. Eur J Cancer 2005;41:1969-1979.

Skottova N, Kazdova L, Oliyarnyk O, Vecera R, Sobolova L, Ulrichova J. Phenolics-rich extracts from *Silybum marianum* and *Prunella vulgaris* reduce a high-sucrose diet induced oxidative stress in hereditary hypertriglyceridemic rats. Pharmacol Res 2004;50:123-130.

Skottova N, Vecera R, Urbanek K, Vana P, Walterova D, Cvak L. Effects of polyphenolic fraction of silymarin on lipoprotein profile in rats fed cholesterol-rich diets. Pharmacol Res 2003;47:17-26.

Sobolova L, Skottova N, Vecera R, Urbanek K. Effect of silymarin and its polyphenolic fraction on cholesterol absorption in rats. Pharmacol Res 2006;53:104-112. Epub 2005 Nov 4.

Somogyi A, Ecsedi GG, Blazovics A, Miskolczi K, Gergely P, Feher J. Short term treatment of type II hyperlipoproteinaemia with silymarin. Acta Med Hung 1989;46:289-295.

Soto CP, Perez BL, Favari LP, Reyes JL. Prevention of alloxan-induced diabetes mellitus in the rat by silymarin. Compar Pharmacol Toxicol 1998;119:125-129.

Tedesco D, Tava A, Galletti S, et al. Effects of silymarin, a natural hepatoprotector, in periparturient dairy cows. J Dairy Sci 2004a;87:2239-2247.

Tedesco D, Domeneghini C, Sciannimanico D, Tameni M, Steidler S, Galletti S. Silymarin, a possible hepatoprotector in dairy cows: biochemical and histological observations. J Vet Med 2004b;A51:85-89.

Tedesco D, Steidler S, Galletti S, Tameni M, Sonzogni O, Ravarotto L. Efficacy of silymarin-phospholipid complex in reducing the toxicity of aflatoxin B1 in broiler chicks. Poult Sci 2004c;83:1839-1843.

Velussi M, Cernigoi AM, De Monte A, Dapas F, Caffau C, Zilli M. Long-term (12 months) treatment with an anti-oxidant drug (silymarin) is effective on hyperinsulinemia, exogenous insulin need and malondialdehyde levels in cirrhotic diabetic patients. J Hepatol 1997;26:871-879.

Velussi M, Cernigoi AM, Viezzoli L, Dapas F, Caffau C, Zilli M. Silymarin reduces hyperinsulinemia, malondialdehyde levels, and daily insulin needs in cirrhotic diabetic patients. Curr Ther Res 1993;53:533-545.

Vogel G, Tuchweber B, Trost W, Mengs U. Protection by silibinin against *Amanita phalloides* intoxication in beagles. Toxicol Appl Pharmacol 1984;73:355-362.

Vojtisek B, Hronova B, Hamrik J, Jankova B. [Milk thistle (*Silybum marianum*, L., Gaertn.) in the feed of ketotic cows.] [Article in Czech] Vet Med (Praha) 1991;36:321-330.

von Schonfeld J, Weisbrod B, Muller MK. Silibinin, a plant extract with antioxidant and membrane stabilizing properties, protects exocrine pancreas from cyclosporin A toxicity. Cell Mol Life Sci 1997;53:917-920.

Zhou S, Lim LY, Chowbay B. Herbal modulation of P-glycoprotein. Drug Metab Rev 2004;36:57-104.

Zima T, Kamenikova L, Janebova M, Buchar E, Crkovska T, Tesar V. The effect of silibinin on experimental cyclosporine nephrotoxicity. Renal Failure 1998;20:471-479.

Mullein

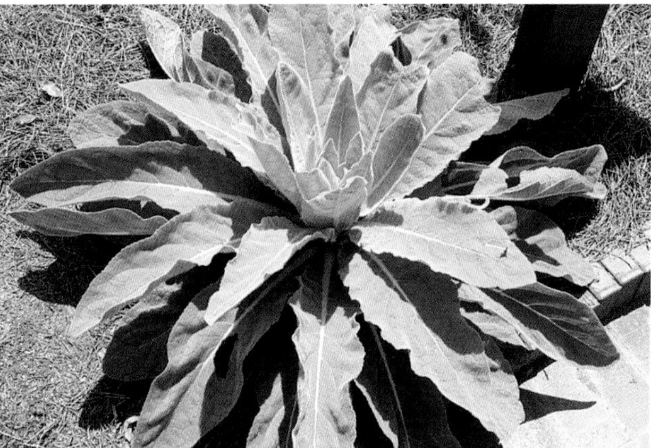

Verbascum thapsus L. • ver-BASK-um THAP-sus

Other Names: Aaron's rod, *Verbascum schraderi*

Family: Scrophulariaceae

Parts Used: Leaves, flowers, and tops

Distribution: Mullein is indigenous to Europe, India, Asia, Egypt, North Africa, and Ethiopia. It is a weed that is now widely established across temperate North America.

Selected Constituents: Polysaccharides, including verbascose, heptaose, and octaose. Flavonoids, including 3′-methylquercitin, hesperidin, and verbascoside. Saponins, including verbasterol. Volatile oil.

Clinical Actions: Demulcent, emollient, expectorant, mild sedative, mild diuretic

Energetics: Cool, slightly astringent and bitter

History and Traditional Usage: The demulcent, expectorant, and astringent properties of the leaves and flowers have been used for thousands of years. Mullein tea is given to treat patients with influenza, catarrh, bronchitis, and tracheitis and is thought to be effective because of the mucilage content, which coats and soothes irritated mucous membranes, and the mild expectorant action of saponins. In folk medicine, mullein tea was used as a diuretic and antirheumatic and for treating those with wounds, gout, piles, cramps, convulsions, skin conditions, and ear problems. Mullein was given to patients with tuberculosis in Europe, the United Kingdom, and the United States in the 19th century. According to Blumenthal and others (2000), naturopathic physicians and medical herbalists prescribe mullein for chronic otitis media and eczema of the ear. The German Commission E recognizes mullein flowers for treating catarrh, and clinical studies have shown antiviral action against fowl plague virus, influenza A and B, and herpes simplex virus (Blumenthal, 2000). The soft, padded leaves can also be used as natural bandages or insoles for sore-footed hitchhikers.

According to Grieve (1975), the origins of the name mullein include *Moleyn* in Anglo-Saxon and *Malen* in Old French, derived from the Latin *malandrium* (i.e., the malanders, or leprosy).

The term "malandre" also applied to diseases of cattle and to lung disease among the rest, and the plant was used as a remedy; thus, it acquired its names of "mullein" and "Bullock's lungwort." It is mentioned in Coles, in 1657, in *Adam in Eden,* that "Husbandmen of Kent do give it their cattle against the cough of the lungs.

Mullein is "famed for its powers in pulmonary ailments, being much used in lung ailments in cattle, one of its names being cow lungwort. The powdered roots are used to fatten poultry" (de Bairacli Levy, 1963). It is used for treatment of cough, pneumonia, pleurisy, bronchitis, tuberculosis, asthma, diarrhea, and internal bleedings of the lungs and bowels, and externally for neuralgia, pains, and cramps.

Published Research: Antibacterial activity (especially the water extract) was observed in vitro with *Klebsiella pneumonia, Staphylococcus aureus, Staphylococcus epidermidis,* and *Escherichia coli* (Turker, 2002). Mullein was shown in vitro to inhibit viral infectivity against pseudorabies virus strain RC/79 (herpes suis virus) (Zanon, 1999) and herpes virus type 1 (McCutheon, 1995).

Indications: Bronchitis with hard cough, respiratory catarrh, tracheitis, gastrointestinal conditions requiring demulcency—ulcers, diarrhea

Potential Veterinary Indications: Contagious bronchitis; bronchitis; diarrhea; topically for inflamed mucosa

Contraindications: None known.

Toxicology and Adverse Effects: AHPA class 1. Flowers are approved in the United States as a flavoring for alcoholic beverages. No adverse effects have been reported; however, the leaf hairs (trichomes) of Mullein species can cause skin irritation in susceptible persons. The leaves contain rotenone and coumarins (Foster, 1990).

Notes of Interest: The down on the leaves and stem makes excellent tinder when dry, readily igniting on the slightest spark; it was, before the introduction of cotton, used for lamp wicks, hence its older names Candlewick Plant, Hag's, Our Lady's Candle, and Torches (Grieve, 1975).

Dosage:

Human:

Dried herb: 1-10gTID, up to 6 times daily for acute conditions

Infusions and decoctions: 5-30g per cup of water, with 1 cup of the tea given TID, up to 6 times daily acutely

Tincture (usually 25%-35% ethanol) 1:2 or 1:3: 1.5-5mL TID, up to 6 times daily for acute conditions

Small Animal:

Dried herb: 50-300mg/kg, divided daily (optimally, TID)

Infusion: 5-30g per cup of water, administered at a rate of ¼-½ cup per 10kg (20lb), divided daily (optimally, TID)

Tincture (usually in 25%-35% ethanol) 1:2-1:3: 1.0-1.5mL per 10kg (20lb), divided daily (optimally, TID) and diluted or combined with other herbs. Higher doses may be appropriate if the herb is used singly and is not combined in a formula.

References

Blumenthal M, Goldberg A, Brinckmann J. *Herbal Medicine: Expanded Commission E Monographs.* Newton, Mass: American Botanical Council, Integrative Medicine Communications; 2000:270-272.

Coles W. *The Art of Simpling: An Introduction to the Knowledge and Gathering of Plants.* St Catharine's, Ontario: Kessinger Publishing; 1968.

De Bairacli Levy J. *The Complete Herbal Handbook for Farm and Stable.* London: Faber and Faber; 1963.

Foster S, Duke JA. *Eastern/Central Medicinal Plants (Peterson Field Guide).* New York: Houghton Mifflin; 1990.

Grieve M. *A Modern Herbal.* London: Jonathan Cape; 1931 (Reprint, 1975).

McCutcheon AR, Roberts TE, Gibbons E, et al. Antiviral screening of British Columbian medicinal plants. J Ethnopharmacol 1995;49:101-110.

Turker AU, Camper ND. Biological activity of common mullein, a medicinal plant. J Ethnopharmacol 2002;82:117-125.

Zanon SM, Ceriatti FS, Rovera M, Sabini LJ, Ramos BA. Search for antiviral activity of certain medicinal plants from Cordoba, Argentina. Rev Latinoam Microbiol 1999;41:59-62.

Myrrh 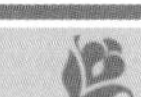

Commiphora myrrha (Nees) Engl., formerly, *Commiphora molmol* Engl. • kom-MEE-for-uh MIR-uh

Distribution: Somalia, Ethiopia, Kenya, Iran, India, Arabia

Similar Species: *Commiphora guidotti, Commiphora abyssinica, Commiphora gileadensis, Commiphora Africana, Commiphora erythraea, Commiphora madagascariense, Commiphora schimperi*

Other Names: Myrrhe, mirra, mur, mulmul, mukula, heerabole, mo yao shu, mo yao

Family: Burseraceae

Parts Used: Resin that exudes from the bark

Collection: Natural exudation product. Lower-quality product is said to result if the bark of a shrub is intentionally damaged.

Selected Constituents: Triterpenoids, sesquiterpenes, essential oil (limonene, dipentene, elemene, lindestrene, boubonene), resins (commiphoric acids, heerabomyrrols, burseracin), gum (contains proteoglycans)

History and Traditional Usage: Long used in Chinese, Tibetan, and Unani traditions. Expectorant, emmenagogue, vermifuge, stimulant, antimicrobial, vulnerary. Used for gonorrhea, laryngitis, bronchitis, asthma, stomatitis, gum disease, aphthous ulcers, chronic gastritis, and muscle pain. Powder used topically for wounds and chronic ulcers.

Milks (1949) reported that myrrh is an emmenagogue, a stimulant to mucous membranes, and a stimulating expectorant. It was combined with iron or aloes as an emmenagogue (an unusual recommendation in an old veterinary textbook, presumably referring to human uses or to stimulation of estrus cycles in general). As a stimulant to mucous membranes, the tincture was diluted and used as a wash for stomatitis.

Energetics: Aromatic, bitter, warm

Published Research: A proprietary brand of myrrh known as Mirazid (Pharco Pharmaceuticals, Alexandria, Egypt) has been investigated extensively for its parasite control activity. Clinical trials in humans suggest that it may be effective for controlling schistosomiasis (Abo-Madyan, 2004a), but a trial from another laboratory found that it had no effect (Barakat, 2005). In a field study, the product was found effective in the treatment of human liver flukes (Abo-Madyan, 2004b). In sheep, a dose of 3600 mg daily (on an empty stomach) for 4 days yielded 100% cure for *Moniezia expansa* infection (Haridy, 2004). A dose of 900 to 1200 mg of the same preparation resulted in 100% clearance of *Fasciola hepatica* (Haridy, 2003). Sheep infected with *Dicrocoelium dendriticum* were completely cleared of the parasite after they were given 600 mg daily (on an empty stomach) for 4 days (Al-Mathal, 2004).

Indications: Gum disease, mouth ulcers, liver flukes, schistosomiasis; topically for skin lesions

Potential Veterinary Indications: Stomatitis, gingivitis, topically for skin lesions, possibly rheumatism. In large animals especially, may be considered for fascioliasis and gastrointestinal parasites

Notes of Interest: One of the oldest known remedies, it is believed to be one of the precious gifts offered by the Magi to the infant Jesus.

Contraindications: Pregnancy, uterine bleeding

Toxicology and Adverse Effects: AHPA class 2b, 2d. Contact dermatitis has been reported, and *The Botanical Safety Handbook* suggests that kidney irritation and diarrhea can occur at human doses greater than 2 to 4 g (McGuffin, 1997). It is considered GRAS (generally recognized as safe) by the US Food and Drug Administration (FDA) as a food and beverage flavoring.

Drug Interactions: None reported.

Dosage:

External Use: Tinctures can be diluted in water for a mouthwash

Internal Use:

Human

Dried herb: 1-10 g TID

Infusions and decoctions not used in infusion form because they are not water soluble, although the finely powdered gum can be suspended if necessary

Tincture (usually 80%-90% ethanol) 1:5: 1-5 mL TID

Small Animal

Dried herb: 10-20 mg/kg, divided daily (optimally, TID)

Tincture (usually 80%-90% ethanol) 1:5: 0.5 mL per 10 kg (20 lb), divided daily (optimally, TID) and diluted or combined with other herbs. Higher doses may be appropriate if the herb is used singly and is not combined in a formula.

Large Animal

Tincture (Karreman, 2004): Cows and horses, 8-15 mL; sheep and goats, 4-8 mL

Historical Veterinary Doses: *Dog:* dried herb, 5-30 grains (0.3-2 g); tincture, 0.5-2 dr (2-4 mL) (Winslow, 1909)

Horse and cow: dried herb, 2-4 dr (3.5-7 g); tincture, 1-2 oz (Winslow, 1909)

Sheep and swine: dried herb, 3-6 dr (5-10 g); tincture, 3-6 dr (12-24 mL) (Winslow, 1909)

Selected References

Abo-Madyan AA, Morsy TA, Motawea SM. Efficacy of Myrrh in the treatment of schistosomiasis (haematobium and mansoni) in Ezbet El-Bakly, Tamyia Center, El-Fayoum Governorate, Egypt. J Egypt Soc Parasitol 2004a;34:423-446.

Abo-Madyan AA, Morsy TA, Motawea SM, Morsy AT. Clinical trial of Mirazid in treatment of human fascioliasis, Ezbet El-Bakly (Tamyia Center) Al-Fayoum Governorate. J Egypt Soc Parasitol 2004b;34:807-818.

Al-Mathal EM, Fouad MA. Myrrh *(Commiphora molmol)* in treatment of human and sheep *Dicrocoeliasis dendriticum* in Saudi Arabia. J Egypt Soc Parasitol 2004;34:713-720.

Barakat R, Elmorshedy H, Fenwick A. Efficacy of myrrh in the treatment of human *Schistosomiasis mansoni.* Am J Trop Med Hyg 2005;73:365-367.

Haridy FM, Dawoud HA, Morsy TA. Efficacy of *Commiphora molmol* (Mirazid) against sheep naturally infected with *Monieziasis expansa* in Al-Santa Center, Gharbia Governorate, Egypt. J Egypt Soc Parasitol 2004;34:775-782.

Haridy FM, El Garhy MF, Morsy TA. Efficacy of Mirazid *(Commiphora molmol)* against fascioliasis in Egyptian sheep. J Egypt Soc Parasitol 2003;33:917-924.

Karreman H. *Treating Dairy Cows Naturally: Thoughts and Strategies.* Paradise, Pa: Paradise Publications; 2004.

McGuffin M, Hobbs C, Upton R, Goldberg A. *Botanical Safety Handbook.* Boca Raton, Fla: CRC Press; 1997.

Milks HJ. *Practical Veterinary Pharmacology, Materia Medica and Therapeutics.* Chicago, Ill: Alex Eger, Inc.; 1949.

Winslow K. *Veterinary Materia Medica and Therapeutics.* New York: William R. Jenkins; 1908.

Neem 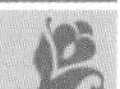

Azadirachta indica A. Juss. (also, *Melia azadirachta* L.) • ay-zad-ih-RAK-tuh IN-dih-kuh *or* in-DEE-kuh

Distribution: Native to India, Sri Lanka, and Burma, but now grown in many tropical areas

Similar Species: *Azadirachta siamensis* (or *A. azadirachta* var. siamensis) and *Azadirachta excelsa*

Common Names: Sanskrit: nimba, *Sarva Roga Nirvani* (curer of all ailments), margosa, margousier, nimbaum, neembaum, nem, bead tree, pride of China, nim, holy tree, indiar, lilac tree

Family: Meliaceae

Parts Used: Root bark, bark, and seed (or nut) are most commonly used, but also fruit, leaves, juice, nut oil, and flowers.

Selected Constituents: Limonoid triterpenes (including azadirachtin, salannin, nimbin, gedunin), flavonoids, tannins, fixed oil

Azadirachtin

Clinical Action: Antibacterial, antifungal, bitter tonic, insecticidal (antifeedant), anthelmintic, antimalarial, astringent, antifertility, vulnerary
Energetics: Bitter, astringent, pungent, cold. In Ayurvedic medicine, it balances kapha and pitta.
History and Traditional Usage: Neem twigs have traditionally been used in India for cleaning teeth and are used for treatment of patients with infection and chronic disease of all types. Neem was and is especially valued for external conditions like wounds, ulcers, eczema, ringworm, vulvovaginitis, and leprosy, for which leaf preparations are applied topically. It is taken orally for the treatment of those with malaria, fever, and intestinal worms. It is also used for external parasites in people (lice) and animals. Neem seed oil is most commonly used externally as a stimulant (for rheumatism and some skin problems), and the leaf and bark are usually taken internally. The bark, leaves, and seeds are used for a large number of conditions in farm animals. A full listing given by Williamson (2002) is found in Box 24-1.
Published Research: Constituents of neem leaf have been shown to have antimalarial, antifungal, antibacterial, antiviral, antioxidant, anticarcinogenic, immunemodulatory, anti-inflammatory, antihyperglycemic, and antiulcer activities (Subapriya, 2005).

Ectoparasite infestations

Neem has antifeedant, antifecundity, sterilization, and growth effects on insects (Mulla, 1999). It has proved effective against a number of insect parasites of crops.

Various parts of neem tree and its constituents have demonstrated repellent or larvicidal activity against biting midges (Blackwell, 2004), and mosquitoes (Wandscheer, 2004; Batra, 1998; Mishra, 1995; Su, 1999). It has variable benefit with parasites of cattle, showing efficacy against ixodid ticks but not against myaisis. In sheep treated for *Bovicola ovis,* neem spray was apparently as effective as cypermethrin (Heath, 1995). Psoroptic mites in sheep appeared susceptible to neem (O'Brien, 1999).

A single trial examined the benefits of neem, alone and in combination with other insecticides, in controlling fleas in dogs and cats. A total of 36 racing Greyhounds were naturally infested with *Ctenocephalides felis* and 9 caged cats were inoculated twice with fleas. Animals were treated with a combination of neem and N,N-diethyl-m-toluamide (DEET). All concentrations of neem used on these dogs reduced flea numbers by 94% to 100% for the first 12 hours, but as time went on, only neem extract adjusted to 2400 ppm (the highest concentration) inhibited flea populations (by manual count) by 53% to 96% for 19 days. Lower concentrations had some inhibiting effect but were not 100% effective. In cats administered the combination of DEET and neem, flea populations fell progressively until 100% reduction was achieved at days 2 to 6. DEET alone did not significantly reduce flea numbers. Investigators noted that even though higher concentrations of neem were effective, they were not as cost effective as were combinations with DEET and D-limonene. They also noted that azadirachtin is light and oxidation sensitive and is probably better protected when applied with an oil base (Guerrini, 1998).

BOX 24-1

Ethnoveterinary Uses of Neem in India

Poultry
Diarrhea
Wounds
Ticks
Lice

Ruminants
Abscesses
Castration sites
Bleeding
Udder infections
Fever
Footrot
Lice ticks
Insect repellent
Stomatitis
Glossitis
Escherichia coli bacillosis
Hepatic swelling
Jaundice
Bloody dysentery
Intestinal wounds
Constipation
Indigestion
Respiratory disorders
Throat disorders
Asthma
Pleuropneumonia
Mucous membrane irritation anywhere in the respiratory tract
Ringworm
Alopecia
Eczema
Urticaria
Scabies
Ticks
Lice
Metritis
Orchitis
Tetanus
Anuria
Nephritis
Mastitis
Otitis
Rinderpest
Rheumatism

Animal feed

The seed has been investigated as feed for poultry, with good results noted in chickens but toxicity reported in quail. White Leghorns fed 100 g/kg of neem kernel meal showed no adverse effects, but at higher concentrations, weight gain, shell quality, fertility, and some blood parameters were adversely effected (Gowda, 1998). Broiler chicks fed 135 or 300 g/kg of alkali-treated neem kernel cake exhibited similar growth and feed efficiency as chicks fed standard diets (Nagalakshmi, 1996). Investigators concluded that neem may have a sparing effect on other protein sources used by humans in developing countries. On the other hand, when Japanese quail were fed neem seed at 0, 50, 75, or 100 g/kg, long-term effects included lower feed efficiency, fatty infiltration of the liver, and degeneration of the kidneys (Elangovan, 2000).

Immune effects

Sadekar (1998) administered powdered neem leaves to a flock of broiler chickens that had survived an outbreak of infectious bursal disease (IBD). A dose of 2 g/kg appeared to enhance antibody titers against Newcastle's disease antigen.

Gastrointestinal parasites

Dawo (2001) examined more than 50 goats divided into seven treatment groups. Subjects were divided into a control (no treatment) group, a group that received albendazole, and five groups that were given dried neem leaf—one each at 0.5, 1, 2, 5, and 10 g/kg. Neem leaves reduced fecal egg counts by only 16.99%, but albendazole reduced counts by 94.82%. Further, at 21 days, goats administered neem leaves had lower packed cell volume (PCV) values.

Dried neem leaves were mixed with feed and were fed to sheep for 3 months while fecal egg counts, worm burden, hematocrit, and weight gain were monitored (Costa, 2006). Sheep were divided into 4 groups that received 100 mg neem/kg of food, 200 mg/kg, closantel, or nothing. At these doses, neem had no anthelmintic effect in sheep.

Ulcer healing

In rats and dogs, nimbidin alone enhanced healing of ulcers induced with acetic acid (Pillai, 1984). A case series in humans with gastroduodenal and esophageal ulcers found that a dried, aqueous extract of neem bark reduced gastric acid secretion and may have enhanced healing of ulcers (Bandyopadhyay, 2004). The dose administered was 30 to 60 mg BID.

Dental care

Pai (2004) compared the antiplaque effects of a dental gel that contained 25 mg/g of neem leaf extract with those of a chlorhexidine dentrifice and a control. Semiquantitative methods were used to determine that neem use was associated with a significant ($P < .05$) reduction in plaque index and bacterial count.

Contraception

An extract of neem appears effective as a spermicidal contraceptive in humans, primates, and rabbits (Garg, 1998; Khillare, 2003; Talwar, 1997).

Diabetes

Laboratory animal studies suggest that neem may improve glucose control. In stressed and normoglycemic dogs, a 50% w/v aqueous leaf extract given at 0.15 mg/kg intravenously led to a significant decrease in blood glucose levels (Shukla, 1973).

Indications: Some external parasites and skin infections as a topical treatment, possibly as a dentrifice

Potential Veterinary Indications: External parasiticide, wound healing, skin and dental infections, possibly diabetes

Contraindications: Pregnancy, lactation, and possibly hypoglycemia

Toxicology and Adverse Effects: Not rated in *The Botanical Safety Handbook*. High doses can lead to nausea, vomiting, and diarrhea. The LD_{50} (dose that kills 50% of a sample) of a 50% ethanolic extract of stem bark was >1000 mg/kg. Experimental studies have shown lung, liver, and kidney toxicity when animals are fed high doses of neem products. Long-term oral use has been reported to result in anemia, weakness, loss of appetite, and weight loss. High-dose toxic effects (probably of the oil) have been listed as convulsions, respiratory distress, stupor, coma, death, metabolic acidosis, and seizures (Herr, 2002). Neem oil has produced vomiting, diarrhea, drowsiness, acidosis, and encephalopathy in humans. In calves, administration of the oil led to reduced hemoglobin content and growth suppression (Biswas, 2000).

Drug Interactions: May have additive effects with insulin and oral glycemics. Less than 15 mg/kg of a 50% aqueous extract resulted in reduced blood glucose levels in dogs.

Dosage:

External Use:

Neem oil: add 25 mL of oil to 400 mL of shampoo for topical use

Dried neem leaf: add 1 cup leaf to 1 L of water, and bring to low simmer for 5 min; cool and use as topical spray

Internal Use:

Human

Dried leaf: 0.25-2 g TID

Infusion: 2.5-20 mL

Oil: 0.05-1 mL total daily dose (Williamson, 2002)

Tincture (usually 50%-80% ethanol; higher alcohol preparations are more potent): 1.5-3.5 mL divided daily

Small Animal

Dried leaf: 25-50 mg/kg, divided daily

Infusion: 5 g per cup of water, administered at a rate of ¼-½ cup per 10 kg (20 lb), divided daily (optimally, TID)

Tincture (usually 50%-80% ethanol; higher alcohol preparations are more potent) 1:2: 0.25-0.5 mL per 10 kg (20 lb), divided daily and diluted or combined with other herbs

Selected References

Bandyopadhyay U, Biswas K, Sengupta A, et al. Clinical studies on the effect of Neem *(Azadirachta indica)* bark extract on gastric secretion and gastroduodenal ulcer. Life Sci 2004;75: 2867-2878.

Batra CP, Mittal PK, Adak T, Sharma VP. Efficacy of neem oil-water emulsion against mosquito immatures. Indian J Malariol 1998;35:15-21.

Biswas K, Chattopadhyay I, Banerjee RK, Bandyopadhyay U. Biological activities and medicinal properties of neem *(Azadirachta indica)*. Curr Sci 2000;82:1336-1345. Available on the Web at: http://www.ias.ac.in/currsci/jun102002/1336.pdf. Accessed May 4, 2006.

Blackwell A, Evans KA, Strang RH, Cole M. Toward development of neem-based repellents against the Scottish Highland biting midge *Culicoides impunctatus*. Med Vet Entomol 2004;18:449-452.

Costa CT, Bevilaqua CM, Maciel MV, Camurca-Vasconcelos AL, Morais SM, Monteiro MV, Farias VM, da Silva MV, Souza MM. Anthelmintic activity of *Azadirachta indica* A. Juss against sheep gastrointestinal nematodes. Vet Parasitol 2006;137:306-310.

Dawo F, Asseye Z, Tibbo M. Comparative evaluation of crude preparation of *Azadirachta indica* leaf and albendazole in naturally infected goats with internal parasites. Bull Anim Health Prod Afr 2001;49:140-144.

Elangovan AV, Verma SV, Sastry VR, Singh SD. Laying performance of Japanese quail fed graded levels of neem *(Azadirachta indica)* kernel meal incorporated diets. J Sci Food Agric 2000; 88:113-120.

Garg S, Talwar GP, Upadhyay SN. Immunocontraceptive activity guided fractionation and characterization of active constituents of neem *(Azadirachta indica)* seed extracts. J Ethnopharmacol 1998;60:235-246.

Gowda SK, Verma SV, Elangovan AV, Singh SD. Neem *(Azadirachta indica)* kernel meal in the diet of White Leghorn layers. Br Poult Sci 1998;39:648-652.

Guerrini VH, Kriticos CM. Effects of azadirachtin on *Ctenocephalides felis* in the dog and the cat. Vet Parasitol 1998; 74:289-297.

Heath AC, Lampkin N, Jowett JH. Evaluation of nonconventional treatments for control of the biting louse *(Bovicola ovis)* on sheep. Med Vet Entomol 1995;9:407-412.

Herr SM. In: Ernst E, Young VSL, eds. *Herb–Drug Interaction Handbook*. 2nd ed. Nassau, NY: Church Street Books; 2002.

Khillare B, Shrivastav TG. Spermicidal activity of *Azadirachta indica* (neem) leaf extract. Contraception 2003;68:225-229.

Mishra AK, Singh N, Sharma VP. Use of neem oil as a mosquito repellent in tribal villages of Mandla district, Madhya Pradesh. Indian J Malariol 1995;32:99-103.

Mulla MS, Su T. Activity and biological effects of neem products against arthropods of medical and veterinary importance. J Am Mosq Control Assoc 1999;15:133-152.

Nagalakshmi D, Sastry VR, Agrawal DK, Katiyar RC, Verma SV. Performance of broiler chicks fed on alkali-treated neem *(Azadirachta indica)* kernel cake as a protein supplement. Br Poult Sci 1996;37:809-818.

O'Brien DJ. Treatment of psoroptic mange with reference to epidemiology and history. Vet Parasitol 1999;83:177-185.

Pai MR, Acharya LD, Udupa N. Evaluation of antiplaque activity of *Azadirachta indica* leaf extract gel—a 6-week clinical study. J Ethnopharmacol 2004;90:99-103.

Pillai NR, Santhakumari G. Effects of nimbidin on acute and chronic gastroduodenal ulcer models in experimental animals. Planta Med 1984;50:143.

Sadekar RD, Kolte AY, Barmase BS, Desai VF. Immunopotentiating effects of *Azadirachta indica* (Neem) dry leaves powder in broilers, naturally infected with IBD virus. Indian J Exp Biol 1998;36:1151-1153.

Shukla R, Singh S, Bhandari CR. Preliminary clinical trials on antidiabetic actions of *Azadirachta indica*. Med Surg 1973; 13:11.

Su T, Mulla MS. Effects of neem products containing azadirachtin on blood feeding, fecundity, and survivorship of *Culex tarsalis* and *Culex quinquefasciatus* (Diptera: Culicidae). J Vector Ecol 1999;24:202-215.

Subapriya R, Nagini S. Medicinal properties of neem leaves: a review. Curr Med Chem Anticancer Agents 2005;5:149-146.

Talwar GP, Raghuvanshi P, Misra R, Mukherjee S, Shah S. Plant immunomodulators for termination of unwanted pregnancy and for contraception and reproductive health. Immunol Cell Biol 1997;75:190-192.

Wandscheer CB, Duque JE, da Silva MA, Fukuyama Y, Wohlke JL, Adelmann J, Fontana JD. Larvicidal action of ethanolic extracts from fruit endocarps of *Melia azedarach* and *Azadirachta indica* against the dengue mosquito *Aedes aegypti*. Toxicon 2004;44:829-835.

Williamson E, ed. *Major Herbs of Ayurveda*. London: Churchill Livingstone; 2002.

Winslow K. *Veterinary Materia Medica and Therapeutics*. New York: William R. Jenkins; 1908.

Nettle

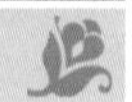

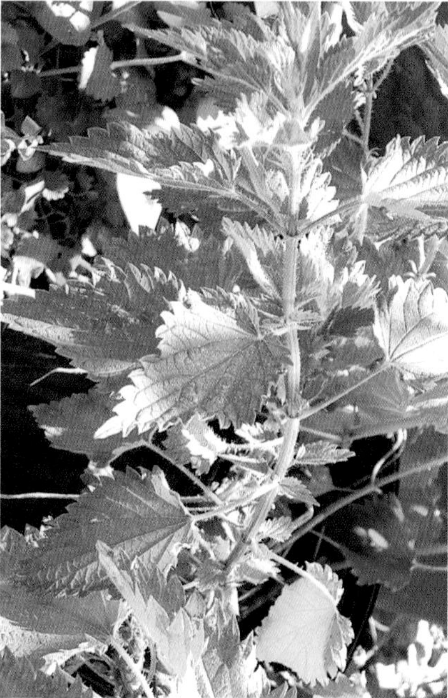

Urtica dioica L. sp. Dioica • UR-ti-kuh dy-oh-EE-kuh

Similar Species: *Urtica urens*, others

Common Names: Nettles, stinging nettle, dwarf nettle, urtica

Family: Urticaceae

Parts Used:

Leaf: For inflammatory disease

Root: For prostatic disease

Seed: For renal disease

Selected Constituents: Flavonoids, acetylcholine, phenolic acids, coumarin, sterols. As a nutritive tonic, this herb is particularly high in calcium, chromium, magnesium, zinc, cobalt, manganese, phosphorus, potassium, protein, riboflavin, selenium, silicon, thiamine, vitamin A, and vitamin C. The seed contains glycerol, linoleic acid, linolenic acid, oleic acid, and palmitic acid.

Clinical Action: Anti-inflammatory, diuretic, nutritive, hemostatic, antidiarrheal. Root is used for prostatic disease, particularly for benign prostatic hypertrophy (BPH) in men. The seed may be a kidney trophorestorative.

Energetics: Sweet, cool

Published Research: Nettle contains a lectin that binds N-acetylglucosamine on cell surfaces and is known to be a major histocompatibility complex (MHC) I and MHC II superantigen. A phenolic extract inhibits proinflammatory cytokine production via cyclooxygenase, including LTB4; a whole plant extract, IDS23, partially inhibits lipoxygenase-derived inflammatory products and inhibits NF-kappaB activation.

Allergies

In a double-blind, randomized trial comparing freeze-dried nettle (600 mg) with placebo given at onset of symptoms to 69 human patients with allergic rhinitis, nettle was rated higher than placebo on symptom assessments (Mittman, 1990).

Prostatic hypertrophy

Wilt (2000) conducted a systematic review of phytotherapy for BPH in 18 trials involving 2939 men. Saw palmetto *(Serenoa repens)* was more effective than other plant therapies, including nettle root. Studies that involved nettle were, however, inadequate for investigators to fully judge its efficacy. A subsequent randomized, double-blind, placebo-controlled trial found that ingestion of a dry extract of the root led to significant improvement in international prostate symptom scores, but no differences in maximum urinary flow rate or residual urine volume were observed. Fewer adverse events were reported in the treatment group as well (Schneider, 2004).

Renal disease

Nettle seed was first suggested for the treatment of patients with renal disease by herbalist David Winston. A paper reported two cases of humans with persistently elevated serum creatinine that required them to undergo long-term dialysis (Treasure, 2003). A hydroethanolic (1:5) tincture of Nettle seed (5 mL TID) led to reductions in serum creatinine in both patients. In one patient, discontinuation of Nettle seed was associated with a subsequent rise in creatinine; when the herb was started again, creatinine fell once more.

Osteoarthritis

Randall (1999) surveyed 18 patients with arthritis to determine whether nettle had been helpful in the treatment of their arthritis. Almost all associated nettle with improvement or cure, and the only reported adverse effect was a transient urticarial rash. The same group (Randall, 2000) then conducted a randomized, controlled, double-blind, crossover study in 27 patients with thumb or index finger base arthritis. Nettle leaf was applied topically to sting the area, once daily for 1 week. After 5 weeks of washout, placebo (white nettle, *Lamium album*) was applied similarly. Active nettle provided significantly better pain control than was produced by placebo, according to visual analogue scale and disability questionnaires.

Indications: *Leaf:* chronic diarrhea, kidney disease, cystitis, eczema, warts, suppression of bleeding, osteoarthritis, allergic rhinitis. *Root:* prostatitis, benign prostatic hypertrophy. *Seed:* chronic renal disease

Potential Veterinary Indications: *Leaf:* chronic diarrhea, cystitis, osteoarthritis allergic rhinitis. Topically as a hemostatic for hot spots. *Root:* prostate cancer, prostatitis, benign prostatic hypertrophy. *Seed:* chronic renal disease

Contraindications: Cautious authors have suggested that diabetes, congestive heart failure, kidney disease, edema, pregnancy, and lactation are contraindications for this herb (Herr, 2002). The authors do not agree and believe this to be a very safe herb in practice.

Adverse Effects: AHPA class 1. The European Medicines Agency saw fit to establish *no* maximum intake on nettle herb for animals. Overindulgence in the herb can result in transient urticaria. The most obvious adverse effect is contact dermatitis that is caused by touching the fresh plant. Massive exposure has been reported to cause trembling, salivation, dyspnea, vomiting, pain, and weakness in hunting dogs (atropine and rapid-acting corticosteroids are said to provide effective treatment). More recent reports claim that these effects were due to misidentification of the culprit plant, which was believed by these latter authors to be *Urtica chamaedryoides,* or possibly, a "nettle" of another genus, such as *Cnidoscolus, Jatropha,* or *Solanum.* Another possibility is that these effects were caused by inhalation of pollen or another factor elaborated by the plant (Edom, 2002).

Dosage:

External Use:

Fresh plant juice

Internal Use:

Human

Dried leaf, root, or seed: 1-10 g TID, up to 6 times daily for acute conditions

Concentrated root extract (5:1 to 10:1): 300-400 mg TID

Infusions and decoctions: 5-30 g per cup of water, with 1 cup of the tea given TID, up to 6 times daily acutely

Tincture (usually 30%-35% ethanol) 1:2 or 1:3: 1-5 mL TID, up to 6 times daily for acute conditions

Small Animal

Dried herb: 50-600 mg/kg, divided daily (optimally, TID)

Infusion: 5-30 g per cup of water, administered at a rate of ¼-½ cup per 10 kg (20 lb), divided daily (optimally, TID)

Tincture (usually in 30%-35% ethanol) 1:2-1:3: 1.0-3.0 mL per 10 kg (20 lb), divided daily (optimally, TID) and diluted or combined with other herbs. Higher doses may be appropriate if the herb is used singly and is not combined in a formula.

Notes of Interest: Handled with gloves, nettle leaf can be sauteed in butter and is tastier than spinach. The exact agent responsible for the sting of nettle is unknown; however, nettle hairs and whole plant extract have been found to contain high levels of leukotrienes and histamine, and so resemble insect venoms and cutaneous mast cells with regard to their mediators (Bone, 2003). When the "sting" is initiated, acetylcholine, histamine, and serotonin are released, in addition to a fourth, unidentified substance thought to be an enzyme.

Selected References

Bone K. *A Clinical Guide to Blending Liquid Herbs.* Sydney: Churchill Livingstone; 2003.

Edom G. The uncertainty of the toxic effect of stings from the Urtica nettle on hunting dogs. Vet Hum Toxicol 2002;44:42-44.

Herr SM. In: Ernst E, Young VSL, eds. *Herb–Drug Interaction Handbook*. 2nd ed. Nassau, NY: Church Street Books; 2002.

Mittman P. Randomized, double-blind study of freeze-dried *Urtica dioica* in the treatment of allergic rhinitis. Planta Med 1990;56:44-47.

Randall C, Meethan K, Randall H, Dobbs F. Nettle sting of *Urtica dioica* for joint pain—an exploratory study of this complementary therapy. Complement Ther Med 1999;7:126-131.

Randall C, Randall H, Dobbs F, Hutton C, Sanders H. Randomized controlled trial of nettle sting for treatment of base-of-thumb pain. J R Soc Med 2000;93:305-309.

Schneider T, Rubben H. Stinging nettle root extract (Bazoton-uno) in long term treatment of benign prostatic syndrome (BPS). Results of a randomized, double-blind, placebo controlled multicenter study after 12 months. Urologe A 2004;43:302-306.

Treasure J. Urtica semen reduces serum creatinine levels. J Am Herb Guild 2003;4:22-25.

Wilt TJ, Ishani A, Rutks I, MacDonald R. Phytotherapy for benign prostatic hyperplasia. Public Health Nutr 2000;3:459-472.

Noni

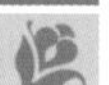

Morinda citrifolia L. • Moh-RIN-duh sit-tru-FOH-lee-uh

Distribution: Southeast Asia, Polynesian Islands; found in open coastal regions, often along lava flows

Similar Species: *Morinda officinalis* (Ba Ji Tian), *Morinda lucida*

Common Names: Indian mulberry, nono or nonu, cheese fruit, nhau, hog apple

Family: Rubiaceae

Parts Used: Roots, stems, bark, leaves, flowers, fruit

Selected Constituents: Terpenoids, alkaloids, anthraquinones (damnacanthal, morindone, rubiadin, rubiadin-1-methyl ether, anthraquinone glycoside), β-sitosterol, flavone glycosides, linoleic acid, caprylic acid, proxeronine. Proxeronine is the most touted constituent in noni. It is converted to the patented alkaloid, xeronine. One investigator claims that a unique enzyme called proxeroninase is responsible for this conversion, and that xeronine is capable of altering the structure of a wide variety of proteins in the body, making it a normal metabolic coregulator. Xeronine has proved very difficult to isolate, and attention has recently been focused on the anthraquinone, damnacanthal.

Damnacanthal

History and Traditional Usage: Said to have been in use by Polynesian Islanders for 2000 years, the noni plant has multiple traditional uses, and all parts of the plant can be used. The root was used to produce yellow or red dyes. The fruit was eaten for food in Polynesia, Southeast Asia, India, and Australia (likely only in times of starvation—it is disgusting and when ripened, ferments immediately). Medicinally, it is used as an emmenagogue and for broken bones (likely with the leaves externally as a poultice), lacerations, bruises, sores, wounds (also probably externally), infectious disease, breast cancer, and eye problems. By the 1930s, Hawaiians used the plant mixed with ginger, coconut milk, and sugar cane juice for tuberculosis, intestinal worms, and sexually transmitted diseases, and as a blood purifier. Only the fruit extract and a juice made with the fruit are sold commercially at this time.

Published Research: In vitro studies suggest that noni suppresses growth or replication of numerous bacterial species, human immunodeficiency virus (HIV), and, to a lesser extent, *Mycobacterium tuberculosis;* it paralyzes the human roundworm. Noni juice appears to have cyclooxygenase (COX)-1 and COX-2 inhibitory activity in vitro. Two animal studies show that noni root has central analgesic properties. Noni root showed hypotensive activity in anesthetized dogs.

The fruit juice may have immunomudulatory activity; it increased thymus weight in mice and may enhance TH-1–type immunologic responses. Researchers have speculated that enhancement of immune function may account for some of the antitumor activity noted in other studies.

Noni juice suppressed carcinogen-induced DNA damage in two laboratory animal studies. In a randomized, double-blind, placebo-controlled trial, human cigarette smokers were found to produce lower plasma superoxide anion and lipid peroxidation activity when given noni juice as compared with placebo (Wang, 2002). Most in vitro and laboratory animal studies center on activity against tumor promotion and growth (Furusawa, 2003; Hornick, 2003). In a small clinical trial in humans, noni juice improved mental functioning and high-frequency hearing (Lanford, 2004). In summary, noni has clear antioxidant activity and contains anthraquinones with antitumor capacity; quality clinical trials undertaken to investigate its use in the treatment of patients with osteoarthritis, pain, and cancer are lacking.

Indications: Primarily an antioxidant; may have immune modulating activity. Arthritis and cancer are currently the primary indications. Although the fruit is most often used, the root may be more effective for pain control and hypertension.

Suggested Veterinary Indications: Conditions that benefit from antioxidant activity such as cancer and arthritis. Pain control (the root); immune support. The high sugar content of the commercially available sweetened fruit juice should be taken into account for overweight patients, and as understanding is enhanced about the possible promotional role of carbohydrates in the growth and metastasis of cancer.

Contraindications: Hyperkalemia and conditions that may predispose to it—a single case report of a man in chronic renal failure suggested that noni juice had high levels of potassium (56.3 mEq/L, similar to that in orange juice and tomato juice) that led to the development of hyperkalemia in those on a low-potassium diet (Mueller, 2000).

Toxicology and Adverse Effects: Laboratory studies showed that up to 8 mL/kg of the juice and the concentrated equivalent of 80 mL/kg of the juice were nontoxic in laboratory animals. Constipation is said to be a common adverse effect of ingestion of the fruit juice. Hepatotoxicity following noni juice ingestion has been reported (Stadlbauer, 2005). One case was described of a man who had evidence 10 months previously of paracetamol toxicity and had taken a Chinese herbal formula for 9 days before admission, along with 1.5 L of noni juice during the previous 3 weeks. The other was of a woman who had taken noni juice (2 L, apparently a cumulative dose) alone and had milder clinical symptoms. If reported doses are indeed cumulative, this is a low dose of the juice, and in one of these cases, the assignment of cause to noni juice is suspect. A final case involved a man who was taking no other medication, and whose liver enzymes normalized when noni ingestion was discontinued (Millonig, 2005).

Drug Interactions: None known, but some have suggested that laboratory animal studies showing hypoglycemic activity warrant caution in patients with diabetes who use hypoglycemic drugs.

Dosage:

Human:

Noni juice: ¼-2 oz of the sweetened fruit juice BID on an empty stomach for prevention and long-term use. Pharmacokinetic studies suggest that acute dosing should occur at least every 4 hours

Small Animal:

Noni juice: 2-6 mL per kg, divided doses

Large Animal:

Noni juice: 100 mL per 100 kg, divided doses

Notes of Interest: Almost all supportive research has been done by companies that produce the product; others have pointed to claims about the broad activity of xeronine as flawed.

References

Furusawa E, Hirazumi A, Story S, Jensen J. Antitumour potential of a polysaccharide-rich substance from the fruit juice of *Morinda citrifolia* (noni) on sarcoma: 180 ascites tumours in mice. Phytother Res 2003;17:1158-1164.

Hornick CA, Myers A, Sadowski-Krowicka H, Anthony CT, Woltering EA. Inhibition of angiogenic initiation and disruption of newly established human vascular networks by juice from *Morinda citrifolia* (noni). Angiogenesis 2003;6:143-149.

Langford J, Doughty A, Wang M, Clayton L, Babich M. Effects of *Morinda citrifolia* on quality of life and auditory function in postmenopausal women. J Altern Complement Med 2004; 10:737-739.

Li RW, Myers SP, Leach DN, Lin GD, Leach G. A cross cultural study: anti-inflammatory activity of Australian and Chinese plants. J Ethnopharmacol 2003;85:25-32.

Millonig G, Stadlmann S, Vogel W. Herbal hepatotoxicity: acute hepatitis caused by a Noni preparation *(Morinda citrifolia)*. Eur J Gastroenterol Hepatol 2005;17:445-447.

Mueller BA, Scott MK, Sowinski KM, Prag KA. Noni juice *(Morinda citrifolia)*: hidden potential for hyperkalemia? Am J Kidney Dis 2000;35:310-312.

Stadlbauer V, Fickert P, Lackner C, Schmerlaib J, Krisper P, Trauner M, Stauber RE. Hepatotoxicity of Noni juice: report of two cases. World J Gastroenterol 2005;11:4758-4760.

Wang MY, West BJ, Jensen CJ, et al. *Morinda citrifolia* (Noni): a literature review and recent advances in Noni research. Acta Pharmacol Sin 2002;23:1127-1141.

Oats

Avena sativa L. • av-VEE-nuh sa-TEE-vuh

Other Names: Oats, groats

Family: Poaceae

Parts Used: The above-ground parts (fresh or dried), the seeds (grain), and the dried, threshed leaf and stem. Immature Oat seeds are known as "milky oats." Some herbalists believe that only the milky oats are effective clinically.

Distribution: The cultivated oat, *Avena sativa,* is a major human and animal food that is grown in many countries. Wild Oats are considered weeds.

Selected Constituents: Oat grass greens contain the following: aconitic acid, apigenin, avenarin, caffeic acid, calcium, carbohydrates, carotene, β-carotene, chlorine, chlorophyll A and B, chromium, cobalt, copper, rhamnosides, glucosides, fat, fiber, fructose, glutamic acid, glutaric acid, guanine, hypoxanthine, iodine, iron, isoleucine, leucine, lignin, luteolin, lysine, magnesium, malic acid, manganese, methionine, niacin, oxalic acid, pantothenic acid, pentosans, phosphorus, potassium, proline, protein, pyridoxine, riboflavin, selenium, silicon, silicon oxide, β-sitosterol, sodium, spermidine, spermine, sugars, sulfur, tartaric acid, thiamine, threonine, the antioxidant tricin, tryptophan, uronic acids, valine, vanillin, and zinc

Clinical Actions: General tonic, nervine tonic, stimulant, antidepressant

Energetics: Warm, sweet

History and Traditional Usage: Oats have been used as food and medicine since antiquity. Paleobotanists suggest that this ancient cereal grass was cultivated as early as 2000 BC. Traditionally, tinctures and extracts of oat straw and immature seed are used in Europe as a nervous system restorative, to assist convalescence, and to strengthen a weakened constitution; recently, European herbal practitioners have recommended oat straw extract for treating patients with multiple sclerosis. It is also used to treat shingles, herpes zoster, herpes simplex, and neurasthenia. The Commission E has approved oat straw for external use in treating those with inflammatory and seborrheic skin disease, especially conditions involving itching, similar to the use of colloidal oatmeal preparations (Blumenthal, 2000).

Oats are made into gruel and are used for nervine, stimulant, and antispasmodic properties. Grieve (1975) describes the preparation as "boiling 1 oz Oatmeal or groats in 3 pints water until reduced to 1 quart, then straining it; sugar, lemons, wine, or raisins may be added as flavoring". Gruel is a mild, nutritious remedy that can be used in inflammatory cases and fever; after parturition, and employed in poisoning from acid substances. It has also been used as a demulcent enema and an emollient poultice. Grieve (1975) says that in horses, it was said to cause excitement. Modern herbalists believe that only milky oats (preferably fresh or extracted fresh) are active as a nervine, and oat straw is used only as a nutritive mineral source.

In dogs, oats have been used for convalescence, teeth problems, thinness, and growth abnormalities like hip dysplasia (de Bairacli Levy, 1985). In *A Practical Treatise on the Veterinary Art,* Briddon (1846) formulated a poultice for general purposes, but especially for wounds of the stifle joint in horses. This comprised the dregs of ale and sufficient oatmeal to form a stiff paste; it could be mollified with hog's lard.

Published Research: One study compared the efficacy of two products—one containing liquid paraffin with 5% colloidal Oatmeal, and the other liquid paraffin alone—for the treatment of patients with pruritus caused by post-burn injuries. A total of 35 patients with acute burns were monitored in an assessor-blinded clinical trial. Patients were asked to rate their discomfort from itch and pain twice daily and to monitor their antihistamine use. Results showed that the group who used the product with colloidal oatmeal reported significantly less itch and requested significantly less antihistamine than did those who used the oil that contained liquid paraffin alone (Matheson, 2001).

β-Glucan, extracted from oats, has immune modulatory effects and was studied in immune suppressed mice infected with *Eimeria vermiformis.* Fecal oocyst shedding was reduced in the β-glucan–treated groups compared with control groups. Control groups showed more severe clinical signs of disease and 50% mortality; minimal clinical signs and no mortality were recorded in the β-glucan–treated groups. Total immunoglobulins of β-glucan–treated groups were higher than those in nontreated groups, and interferon-γ– and interleukin-4–secreting cells were noted in the spleen and mesenteric lymph nodes of β-glucan–treated groups only (Yun, 1997).

Indications: Malnutrition, immune support, depression, insomnia, exhaustion, convalescence

Potential Veterinary Indications: Convalescence; topically for pruritus

Contraindications: None known.

Toxicology and Adverse Effects: AHPA class 1. None known.

Potential Drug Interactions: None described.

Dosage:

External Use:

For external use against skin irritation and itching: 100g of milky oats (seed heads) for 1 full bath, or equivalent preparations

Internal Use:

Human

Oat is a common food that is used, for example, in porridge, granola, and oatcakes

Dried herb: 1-10gTID, up to 6 times daily for acute conditions

Infusions and decoctions: 5-30g per cup of water, with 1 cup of the tea given TID, up to 6 times daily acutely

Tincture (usually 25%-40% ethanol, or 75%-80% glycerin) 1:2 or 1:3: 1-8mLTID, up to 6 times daily for acute conditions

Small Animal

Oats can be fed to large and small animals as a gruel

Infusion: 5-30g per cup of water, administered at a rate of ½-4 cups, divided daily (optimally, TID)

Tincture (usually 25%-40% ethanol, or 75%-80% glycerin) 1:2-1:3: 0.5-1.5mL per 10kg (20lb), divided daily (optimally, TID) and diluted or combined with other herbs. Higher doses may be appropriate if the herb is used singly and is not combined in a formula.

References

Blumenthal M, Goldberg A, Brinckmann J. *Herbal Medicine: Expanded Commission E Monographs.* Newtown, Mass: American Botanical Council, Integrative Medicine Communications; 2000:281-282.

Briddon J. *A Practical Treatise on the Veterinary Art.* London: Simpkin, Marshall and Co; 1846:105.

De Bairacli Levy J. *The Complete Herbal Handbook for the Dog and Cat.* London: Faber and Faber; 1985.

Grieve M. *A Modern Herbal.* London: Jonathan Cape; 1931 (Reprint, 1975).

Matheson JD, Clayton J, Muller MJ. The reduction of itch during burn wound healing. J Burn Care Rehabil 2001;22:76-81; discussion 75.

Yun CH, Estrada A, Van Kessel A, Gajadhar AA, Redmond MJ, Laarveld B. Beta-(1- > 3, 1- > 4) oat glucan enhances resistance to *Eimeria vermiformis* infection in immunosuppressed mice. Int J Parasitol 1997;27:329-337.

Oregon Grape

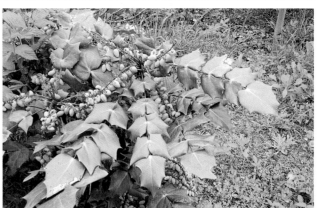

Mahonia aquifolium (Pursh) Nutt., also known as *Berberis aquifolium* Pursh • Ma-HO-nee-uh a-kwee-FOH-lee-um

Other Names: Mountain grape, holy grape, creeping barberry

Similar Species: Indian barberry *(Berberis aristala)*

Family: Berberidaceae

Parts Used: Root

Distribution: Grows wild throughout Europe and North and South America

Selected Constituents: Alkaloids berbamine, berberine, canadine, corypalmine, mahonine, oxyacanthine. Quaternary alkaloids palmatine and jatrorrhizine. Aporphine alkaloids, corytuberine, magnoflorine, isothebaine, and isocorydine. Bisbenzylisoquinoline alkaloids, armoline, baluchistine, obamegine, aquifoline. Resin and tannin

Clinical Actions: Cholagogue, mild laxative, liver tonic, bitter tonic, alterative, antiemetic, anticatarrhal

Energetics: Bitter and cooling

History and Traditional Usage: Native Americans used *Berberis aquifolium* root tea to treat patients with recurrent fever and dysentery, to tone, and to stop rectal hemorrhage. It is believed to stimulate bile and kidney secretions and to improve digestion. The root's antibacterial properties explain its successful use in treating those with skin and internal infection. Extracts were used as a blood cleanser to treat acne, nausea, eczema, psoriasis, and cold sores. The decoction acts as a digestive and liver tonic to improve appetite and relieve rheumatic inflammation. The alkaloids make it an effective antiseptic and treatment for diarrhea. Berberine has been shown to possess fungicidal and antibacterial activities, as well as activity against protozoa.

Currently, predominant clinical uses of berberine include bacterial diarrhea, intestinal parasite infection, and ocular trachoma infection (Anonymous, 2000).

Published Research: Berberine has antimutagenic activity (Cernakova, 2002b) and antitumor effects (Bone, 2000).

Antimicrobial activity

Berberine, from *Berberis aquifolium,* has demonstrated antibacterial (Cernakova, 2002a) and antifungal activity (Vollekova, 2001, 2003) against a variety of organisms, including resistant strains of *Pseudomonas aeruginosa* and *Escherichia coli.*

Antitussive activity

A glucuronoxylan isolated from stems of *Berberis aquifolium* was tested for antitussive activity on mechanically induced coughing in cats. It exhibited a much greater effect in comparison with drugs used in clinical practice to treat those with cough (Kardosova, 2002).

Dermatologic activity

Berberis aquifolium has been used to treat patients with psoriasis (Wiesenauer, 1996; Gieler, 1995). Products of lipoxygenase metabolism are known to play a role in the pathogenesis of psoriasis, and alkaloids in *Berberis* inhibit lipid peroxide substrate accumulation by direct reaction with peroxide or by scavenging of lipid-derived radicals (Bezakova, 1996).

Indications: Externally for acne, psoriasis, vulvovaginitis. Internally as a digestive bitter; for hepatitis, enteritis, inflammatory skin disorders, and possibly infections such as urinary tract infection

Potential Veterinary Indications: Chronic skin disease; giardia, enteritis; possibly other types of infection such as urinary tract infection and topically for skin and ear infections

Contraindications: Berberine and other alkaloids can stimulate the uterus and should not be used during pregnancy.

Toxicology and Adverse Effects: AHPA class 2b. At recommended dosages, berberine is considered to be nontoxic. If taken in large quantities, it has been reported to cause acute and even fatal poisoning. Injections may produce hyperpigmentation.

Dosage:

External Use:

Topically as a cream (containing 10% tincture) or decoction of stem bark or root: 1.5-3 g per day, divided

Internal Use:

Human

Dried herb: 1-10 g TID

Infusions and decoctions: 5 g per cup of water, with ½-1 cup of the tea given TID, up to 6 times daily acutely

Tincture (usually 25%-50% ethanol) 1:2 or 1:3: 1-5 mL TID

Small Animal

Dried herb: 25-300 mg/kg, divided daily (optimally, TID)

Infusion: 5 g per cup of water, administered at a rate of ¼-½ cup per 10 kg (20 lb), divided daily (optimally, TID)

Tincture (usually in 25%-50% ethanol) 1:2-1:3: 0.5-1.5 mL per 10 kg (20 lb), divided daily (optimally, TID) and diluted or combined with other herbs. Higher doses may be appropriate if the herb is used singly and is not combined in a formula.

References

Anonymous. Berberine. Altern Med Rev 2000;5:175-177.

Bezakova L, Misik V, Malekova L, Svajdlenka E, Kostalova D. Lipoxygenase inhibition and antioxidant properties of bisbenzylisoqunoline alkaloids isolated from *Mahonia aquifolium.* Pharmazie 1996;51:758-761.

Bone K, Mills S. *Principles and Practice of Phytotherapy.* Sydney: Churchill Livingstone; 2000.

Cernakova M, Kost'alova D. Antimicrobial activity of berberine—a constituent of *Mahonia aquifolium.* Folia Microbiol 2002a; 47:375-378.

Cernakova M, Kost'alova D, Kettmann V, Plodova M, Toth J, Drimal J. Potential antimutagenic activity of berberine, a constituent of *Mahonia aquifolium.* BMC Complement Altern Med 2002b;2:2.

Gieler U, Weth A, von der Heger M. *Mahonia aquifolium*—a new type of topical treatment for psoriasis. J Dermatol Treat 1995; 6:31-34.

Kardosova A, Malovkova A, Patoprsty V, Nosal'ova G, Matakova T. Structural characterization and antitussive activity of a glucuronoxylan from *Mahonia aquifolium* (Pursh) Nutt. Carbohydrate Polymers 2002;47:27-33.

Vollekova A, Kost'alova D, Kettmann V, Toth J. Antifungal activity of *Mahonia aquifolium* extract and its major protoberberine alkaloids. Phytother Res 2003;17:834-837.

Vollekova A, Kost'alova D, Sochorova R. Isoquinoline alkaloids from *Mahonia aquifolium* stem bark are active against *Malassezia* spp. Folia Microbiol 2001;46:107-111.

Wiesenauer M, Ludtke R. *Mahonia aquifolium* in patients with psoriasis vulgaris—an intraindividual study. Phytomedicine 1996;3:231-235.

Panax Ginseng

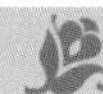

Panax ginseng C.A. Mey. • PAN-aks JIN-sing

Other Common Names: Radix ginseng, Korean ginseng, red ginseng, Chinese ginseng, ren shen

Family: Araliaceae

Parts Used: Main root

Distribution: Mountain regions of China, Korea, Japan, and Eastern Siberia

Selected Constituents: The major chemical constituents are the triterpene saponins dammarane and ginsenosides (derived from oleanolic acid) (Shibata, 1985; Bruneton, 1989; Cui, 1995). The dammarane saponins are derivatives of protopanaxadiol or protopanaxatriol.

Clinical Actions: Adaptogenic, stimulant, tonic, thymolepic, hypoglycemic, immune stimulant, hepatoprotective, cardioprotective, antiarrhythmic; increases adrenocorticotrophic hormone (ACTH)

Energetics: Sweet, slightly bitter, slightly warming

History and Traditional Usage: Used traditionally as a tonic, particularly for geriatrics, as a prophylactic and restorative agent for enhancement of mental and physical capacities; in cases of weakness, exhaustion, tiredness, and loss of concentration; during convalescence (Hallstrom, 1982; D'Angelo, 1986; Pieralisi, 1991; Forgo, 1985). Ginseng has been used in the treatment of patients with diabetes and impotence and in the prevention of hepatotoxicity and gastrointestinal disorders such as gastritis and ulcers (Bruneton, 1989).

Other uses include treatment of those with liver disease, cough, fever, tuberculosis, rheumatism, vomiting during pregnancy, hypothermia, dyspnea, and nervous disorders (Bruneton, 1989).

Published Research

Physical performance

Ginseng has an adaptogenic effect that produces a nonspecific increase in defenses against exogenous stress factors and noxious chemicals; it promotes overall improvement in physical and mental performance (Wagner, 1994; Phillipson, 1984). A randomized, double-blind, crossover study of the effects of ginseng on circulatory, respiratory, and metabolic functions during maximal exercise in 50 men showed that ginseng increased the work capacity of participants by improving oxygen utilization (Pieralisi, 1991). A placebo-controlled, crossover study determined the effects of ginseng on the physical fitness of 43 male triathletes. Participants received 200 mg ginseng twice daily for 2 consecutive 10-week training periods. No significant changes were observed during the first 10 weeks, but ginseng prevented the loss of physical fitness during the second 10-week period (Van Schepdael, 1993). Placebo-controlled, double-blind trials have demonstrated significant athletic improvement in the ginseng group as compared with the placebo group (Forgo, 1983). Similar results were reported in athletes in whom the differences lasted for 3 weeks after the last ginseng dose (Forgo, 1985).

Ginseng (1200 mg) effects were assessed in a placebo-controlled, double-blind crossover study of fatigued night nurses and were compared with those of placebo and with effects on nurses engaged in daytime work. Ginseng restored ratings on tests of mood, competence, and general performance; study investigators concluded that Ginseng had antifatigue activity (Hallstrom, 1982).

Seven healthy men were subjected to treadmill tests before and after administration of a ginseng extract (2 g TID) for 8 weeks. In addition, blood was analyzed for serum malondialdehyde, catalase, and superoxide dismutase levels as a measure of oxidant stress. At the end of the trial, subjects exhibited significantly increased exercise capacity, and ginseng extract attenuated markers of oxidant stress (Kim, 2005).

Respiratory function

Pulmonary function tests were monitored in 92 humans with moderate to severe chronic obstructive pulmonary disease (COPD). Patients took a placebo or 100 mg BID of a ginseng extract in this randomized, placebo-controlled trial. Function tests were studied every 2 weeks for 3 months, and all parameters were found to be improved above baseline compared with placebo (Gross, 2002). No adverse effects were observed.

Immune function

In a placebo-controlled, double-blind study of immune modulatory actions of ginseng, a total of 60 healthy volunteers were divided into three groups of 20 each; volunteers were given placebo or 100 mg of aqueous ginseng extract, or 100 mg of a standardized ginseng extract, every 12 hours for 8 weeks. Blood samples compared with those of the placebo group revealed an increase in chemotaxis of polymorphonuclear leukocytes, phagocytic index, and total numbers of T3 and T4 lymphocytes after 4 and 8 weeks of ginseng therapy. The group given the standardized extract also showed increased T4:T8 ratio of natural killer cells activity. It was concluded that ginseng extract stimulated the immune system in humans, and that the standardized extract was more effective than the aqueous extract (Scaglione, 1990).

Administration of 5.4 g daily of *Panax ginseng* to HIV-1–infected patients slowed progression of the disease; this did not occur in patients who took no ginseng. Patients were not being treated with antiretroviral drugs. Ginseng slowed the loss of CD4 lymphocytes associated with progression of the disease, and it slowed the increase in CD8-associated markers. It was determined that HLA subtype (which is associated with prognosis) was not involved in this change in progression (Sung, 2005).

Cognitive function

Rat studies have shown that administration of ginseng improved specific learning and memory tasks (Nishijo, 2004). A double-blind, placebo-controlled clinical study assessed the effects of standardized ginseng (100 mg twice daily for 12 weeks) on psychomotor performance in 16 healthy humans and showed a positive effect on attention, processing, integrated sensory motor function, and auditory reaction time. Ginseng was superior to placebo in improving certain psychomotor functions in healthy subjects (D'Angelo, 1986). In a double-blind, counterbalanced, placebo-controlled study, 200 mg of *Panax ginseng* extract was given to 28 young adult humans, and cognitive and mood effects were assessed. Ingestion of this herb led to improved task performance and enhanced speed of memory task performance (Kennedy, 2004).

Reay (2005) examined whether the cognitive enhancement activity of ginseng extract (200 mg and 400 mg) in healthy people was related to its hypoglycemic effects.

In a placebo-controlled, double-blind, crossover trial, 30 humans completed cognition tests before and after administration of ginseng or placebo. Blood glucose was also measured before and after treatment. Both doses of ginseng led to significant reductions in blood glucose, and the 200-mg dose significantly improved some mental function test results. The authors suggest that ginseng can improve "mental performance and subjective feeling of mental fatigue during sustained mental activity," and that this may be associated with the blood glucose changes related to ginseng ingestion.

Diabetes

Oral ginseng (200 mg daily for 8 weeks) given to 36 non–insulin-dependent patients elevated mood, improved physical performance, reduced fasting blood glucose and serum procollagen concentrations, and lowered glycated hemoglobin levels (Sontaneimi, 1995). A randomized, single-blind, placebo-controlled trial of healthy people in whom hyperglycemia was induced showed variable effects of *Panax ginseng* on blood glucose. The authors note that different concentrations of ginsenosides or simply differences in batch may have been responsible for the inconsistent results (Sievenpiper, 2003).

Hypolipidemic effects

Kim (2003) investigated the effects on lipid metabolism of people when 6 g ginseng extract was ingested daily. Results suggested that after 8 weeks of administration, ginseng may decrease cholesterol, triglycerides, low-density lipoprotein, and plasma malondialdehyde. Ginseng also increased superoxide dismutase and catalase activities, and the authors suggest that an antioxidant mechanism may be involved.

Erectile dysfunction

A double-blind, placebo-controlled, crossover trial in 45 men with erectile dysfunction suggested that administration of ginseng (900 mg TID) improved function scores (Hong, 2002).

Veterinary Trials

Immune function: pigs and cows

Cows with subclinical mastitis caused by *Staphylococcus aureus* were injected subcutaneously with ginseng extract at 8 mg/kg per day for 6 days, or with saline as a control. The numbers of *S. aureus*–infected quarters and milk SCCs (somatic cell counts) decreased in ginseng-treated cows. Phagocytosis and oxidative burst activity were significantly increased 1 week after initiation of ginseng treatment. The number of monocytes in ginseng cows was significantly higher 1 week post treatment, and the number of lymphocytes was significantly higher at 2 and 3 weeks than was the preinfusion number. These findings indicated that ginseng can activate innate immunity and accelerate recovery from mastitis (Hu, 2001).

Adjuvant effects of a crude ginseng extract and purified ginsenoside R(b1) were evaluated in dairy cattle that had been immunized with ovalbumin (OVA) or an *S. aureus* bacterin (used for prevention of bovine mastitis). In all, 36 lactating cows were randomly divided into six groups. Cows were inoculated twice intramuscularly at 2-week intervals with saline solution, OVA in saline, or OVA in combination with 4, 16, or 64 mg ginseng, or aluminium hydroxide adjuvant. The antibody response in serum was significantly higher in animals immunized with OVA and ginseng than in those immunized with OVA alone. A significant increase in milk antibody titers was noted 2 weeks after the second immunization with OVA and 4 mg ginseng. Addition of R(b1) resulted in significantly higher antibody production and lymphocyte proliferation than occurred in the control group. Ginseng induced significantly higher lymphocyte proliferation. It was concluded that both ginseng and R(b1) were safe adjuvants, and that R(b1) had the strongest adjuvant effects (Hu, 2003).

In pigs, the adjuvant effect of ginseng was demonstrated by vaccinating them against porcine parvovirus (PPV) and *Erysipelothrix rhusiopathiae* infections with the use of commercially available vaccines. It was found that the addition of 2 mg ginseng per vaccine dose significantly potentiated the antibody titer response to both vaccines without altering their safety. Aluminium hydroxide–adjuvanted vaccines favored the production of IgG1 antibodies. Vaccines supplemented with ginseng favored IgG2. The study concluded that ginseng used as an adjuvant provides a safe and inexpensive alternative for improving the potency of aluminium hydroxide–adjuvanted vaccines (Rivera, 2003).

Miscellaneous trials

In White Leghorn poultry, females were fed for 4 weeks a corn-based diet (control) or an experimental diet with 0.25% ginseng or petroleum ether (PESF), methyl alcohol (MESF), or water (WASF) extract. Each ginseng treatment lowered serum total cholesterol level (67%-83% of control) and serum low-density lipoprotein cholesterol level (53%-81% of control). PESF treatment was the most effective suppressor of each, and WASF had significant impact. PESF effected a change in the ratio of low- to high-density lipoprotein cholesterol from 1.46 (control) to 0.88. In companion studies, broiler females were fed 0.28% ginseng root powder or fractions. Results confirmed those recorded earlier. Ginsenosides are considered to be the active agents for suppression of cholesterogenesis and lipogenesis (Qureshi, 1983).

In dogs, a study investigated the effects of ginseng on liver morphologic change and function. Fifteen adult dogs were divided into three groups: control (40% hepatectomy, untreated), a 250 group (40% hepatectomy, 250 mg/kg of ginseng PO), and a 500 group (40% hepatectomy, 500 mg/kg of ginseng PO). Liver regeneration rates were higher in treated groups than in controls. Blood values returned to normal ranges except for leukocyte counts for 3 days postoperatively. Aspartate aminotransferase (AST) and alanine aminotransferase (ALT) in treated groups were significantly decreased compared with control values. Degenerative cells and connective tissue were significantly decreased with ginseng. It was concluded that ginseng accelerates liver regeneration and ameliorates liver injury in dogs (Kwon, 2003).

Indications: To aid with short-term stress, recovery from disease or surgery; to minimize adverse effects of chemotherapy, cardiac arrhythmia; to improve resistance to infection, low sperm count, erectile dysfunction, chronic inflammation; for long-term use in geriatric patients and those with diabetes, asthma, cancer, depression, and cognitive disorders

Potential Veterinary Indications: Improving immune function; adjuvant for vaccination; mastitis treatment in cattle; diabetes mellitus; liver disease in dogs; tonic for convalescing animals or those with chronic debilitating disease; performance animals; fertility improvement in male animals

Contraindications: Ginseng should be avoided in hypertension, although a trial using a related species—*Panax quinquefolius* (American ginseng)—in hypertensive people for 12 weeks found no adverse effect on blood pressure after administration of the herb (Stavro, 2006).

Toxicology and Adverse Effects: AHPA class 2d. See contraindication provided earlier. One case of ginseng-associated cerebral arteritis was reported in a patient who consumed a high dose of an ethanol extract of ginseng root (6g) (Ryu, 1995). Two cases of mydriasis and disturbance in accommodation and dizziness have been reported after large doses (3-9g) (Lou, 1989). Estrogenic-like adverse effects have been reported in women. Seven cases of mastalgia (Palmer, 1978; Koriech, 1978) and one of vaginal bleeding in a postmenopausal woman were reported. Increased libido in premenopausal women has been reported (Punnonen, 1980). However, clinical studies have demonstrated that standardized ginseng extract does not cause a change in male or female hormonal status (Buchi, 1984; Reinhold, 1990).

Potential Drug Interactions: Ginseng intake may slightly reduce blood glucose levels (Kwan, 1994; Sotaneimi, 1995). Two instances of interaction have been reported between ginseng and phenelzine, a monoamine oxidase inhibitor (Jones, 1987; Shader, 1985). The clinical significance of this has not been evaluated.

Preparation Notes: Red ginseng is *Panax ginseng* that has been steamed before drying.

Dosage:

Human:

Dried herb: 1-10g TID

5:1 dried extract: 200mg daily

Infusions and decoctions: 5-30g per cup of water, with 1 cup of the tea given TID

Tincture (usually 60%-70% ethanol) 1:2 or 1:3: 1-5mL TID

Small Animal:

Dried herb: 25-300mg/kg, divided daily (optimally, TID)

Decoction: 5-30g per cup of water, administered at a rate of ¼-½ cup per 10kg (20lb), divided daily (optimally, TID)

Tincture (usually 60%-70% ethanol) 1:2-1:3: 0.5-1.5mL per 10kg (20lb), divided daily (optimally, TID) and diluted or combined with other herbs. Higher doses may be appropriate if the herb is used singly and is not combined in a formula.

References

Bradley PR, ed. *British Herbal Compendium*, vol 1. Guildford, UK: British Herbal Medicine Association; 1992:115-118.

Bruneton J. *Pharmacognosy, Phytochemistry, Medicinal Plants*. Paris: Lavoisier; 1995.

Buchi K, Jenny E. On the interference of the standardized ginseng extract G115 and pure ginsenosides with agonists of the progesterone receptor of the human myometrium. Phytopharmacy 1984:1-6.

Cui JF. Identification and quantification of ginsenosides in various commercial ginseng preparations. Eur J Pharmaceut Sci 1995;3:77-85.

D'Angelo L, Grimaldi R, Caravaggie M, et al. Double-blind, placebo-controlled clinical study on the effect of a standardized ginseng extract on psychomotor performance in healthy volunteers. J Ethnopharmacol 1986;16:15-22.

Forgo I. Effect of drugs on physical performance and hormone system of sportsmen. Münchener Medizinische Wochenschrift 1983;125:822-824.

Forgo I, Schimert G. The duration of effect of the standardized ginseng extract in healthy competitive athletes. Notabene Med 1985;15:636-640.

Gross D, Shenkman Z, Bleiberg B, Dayan M, Gittelson M, Efrat R. Ginseng improves pulmonary functions and exercise capacity in patients with COPD. Monaldi Arch Chest Dis 2002; 57:242-246.

Hallstrom C, Fulder S, Carruthers M. Effect of ginseng on the performance of nurses on night duty. Compar Med East West 1982;6:277-282.

Hong B, Ji YH, Hong JH, Nam KY, Ahn TY. A double-blind crossover study evaluating the efficacy of Korean red ginseng in patients with erectile dysfunction: a preliminary report. J Urol 2002;168:2070-2073.

Hu S, Concha C, Johanisson A, Meglia G, Walker KP. Effect of subcutaneous injection of ginseng on cows with subclinical *Staphylococcus aureus* mastitis. J Vet Med B Infect Dis Vet Public Health 2001;48:519-528.

Hu S, Concha C, Lin F, Persson Waller K. Adjuvant effect of ginseng extracts on the immune responses to immunisation against *Staphylococcus aureus* in dairy cattle. Vet Immunol Immunopathol 2003;91:29-37.

Jones BD, Runikis AM. Interaction of ginseng with phenelzine. J Clin Psychopharmacol 1987;7:201-202.

Kennedy DO, Haskell CF, Wesnes KA, Scholey AB. Improved cognitive performance in human volunteers following administration of guarana *(Paullinia cupana)* extract: comparison and interaction with *Panax ginseng*. Pharmacol Biochem Behav 2004;79:401-411.

Kim SH, Park KS. Effects of *Panax ginseng* extract on lipid metabolism in humans. Pharmacol Res 2003;48:511-513.

Kim SH, Park KS, Chang MJ, Sung JH. Effects of *Panax ginseng* extract on exercise-induced oxidative stress. J Sports Med Phys Fitness 2005;45:178-182.

Koriech OM. Ginseng and mastalgia. BMJ 1978;297:1556.

Kwan HJ, Wan JK. Clinical study of treatment of diabetes with powder of the steamed insam (ginseng) produced in Kaesong, Korea. Tech Info 1994;6:33-35.

Kwon YS, Jang KH, Jang IH. The effects of Korean red ginseng *(Ginseng radix rubra)* on liver regeneration after partial hepatectomy in dogs. J Vet Sci 2003;4:83-92.

Lou BY, Li CF, Li PY, Ruan JP. Eye symptoms due to ginseng poisoning. Yan Ke Xue Bao 1989;5:96-97.

Morris AC, Jacobs I, Kligerman TM. No ergogenic effect of ginseng extract after ingestion. Med Sci Sports Exerc 1994;26:S6.

Nishijo H, Uwano T, Zhong YM, Ono T. Proof of the mysterious efficacy of ginseng: basic and clinical trials: effects of red ginseng on learning and memory deficits in an animal model of amnesia. J Pharmacol Sci 2004;95:145-152.

Owen RT. Ginseng: a pharmacological profile. Drugs Today 1981;17:343-351.

Palmer BV, Montgomery AC, Monteiro JC. Ginseng and mastalgia. BMJ 1978;279:1284.

Phillipson JD, Anderson LA. Ginseng-quality, safety and efficacy? Pharmaceut J 1984;232:161-165.
Pieralisi G, Ripari P, Vecchiet L. Effects of a standardized ginseng extract combined with dimethylaminoethanol bitartrate, vitamins, minerals, and trace elements on physical performance during exercise. Clin Ther 1991;13:373-382.
Punnonen R, Lukola A. Oestrogen-like effect of ginseng. BMJ 1980;281:1110.
Qureshi AA, Abuirmelah N, Din ZZ, Ahmad Y, Burger WC, Elson CE. Suppression of cholesterogenesis and reduction of LDL cholesterol by dietary ginseng and its fractions in chicken liver. Atherosclerosis 1983;48:81-94.
Reay JL, Kennedy DO, Scholey AB. Single doses of *Panax ginseng* (G115) reduce blood glucose levels and improve cognitive performance during sustained mental activity. J Psychopharmacol 2005;19:357-365.
Reinhold E. Der Einsatz von Ginseng in der Gynäkologie. Natur Ganzheits Medizin 1990;4:131-134.
Rivera E, Daggfeldt A, Hu S. Ginseng extract in aluminium hydroxide adjuvanted vaccines improves the antibody response of pigs to porcine parvovirus and *Erysipelothrix rhusiopathiae*. Vet Immunol Immunopathol 2003;91:19-27.
Ryu SJ, Chien YY. Ginseng-associated cerebral arteritis. Neurology 1995;45:829-830.
Scaglione F, Ferrara F, Dugnani S, Falchi M, Santoro G, Fraschini F. Immunomodulatory effects of two extracts of *Panax ginseng*. Drugs Exp Clin Res 1990;26:537-542.
Shader RI, Greenblatt DJ. Phenelzine and the dream machine—ramblings and reflections. J Clin Psychopharmacol 1985;5:67.
Shibata S, Tanaka O, Shoji J, et al. Chemistry and pharmacology of *Panax*. In: Wagner H, Farnsworth NR, Hikino H, eds. *Economic and Medicinal Plants Research,* vol 1. London: Academic Press; 1985.
Sievenpiper JL, Arnason JT, Leiter LA, Vuksan V. Null and opposing effects of Asian ginseng (*Panax ginseng* C.A. Meyer) on acute glycemia: results of two acute dose escalation studies. J Am Coll Nutr 2003;22:524-532.
Sotaniemi EA, Haapakoski E, Rautio A. Ginseng therapy in non–insulin-dependent diabetic patients. Diabetes Care 1995; 18:1373-1375.
Stavro PM, Woo M, Leiter LA, Heim TF, Sievenpiper JL, Vuksan V. Long-term intake of North American ginseng has no effect on 24-hour blood pressure and renal function. Hypertension 2006;47:791-796. Epub 2006 Mar 6.
Sung H, Kang SM, Lee MS, Kim TG, Cho YK. Korean red ginseng slows depletion of CD4 T cells in human immunodeficiency virus type 1–infected patients. Clin Diagn Lab Immunol 2005;12:497-501.
Van Schepdael P. Les effets du ginseng G115 sur la capacité physique de sportifs d'endurance. Acta Ther 1993;19:337-347.
Wagner H, Norr H, Winterhoff H. Plant adaptogens. Phytomedicine 1994;1:63-76.

Parsley

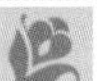

Petroselinum crispum (Mill.) Nyman ex. A.W. Hill • pet-roh-sel-EE-num KRISP-um

Family: Apiaceae

Distribution: A native of Mediterranean countries, it is now naturalized around the world.

Parts Used: The herb, root, and fruit (which looks like a seed), but mainly the root for therapeutic purposes

Selected Constituents: Apiol, essential oil *(Parsley camphor),* myristicin mainly in the seed and root. Bergapten, a furanocoumarin, flavonoids (apiin, luteolin, apigenin glycosides), fatty oil (in seeds), vitamin C, provitamin A, iron, calcium, phosphorus, manganese. Tannins, sterols, triterpenes, cumarines, imperatorin

Apiol

Bergapten

Clinical Actions: Antispasmodic, diuretic, expectorant, antirheumatic, antimicrobial, carminative

Energetics: Sweet, bland, warm

History and Traditional Usage: Parsley is used traditionally as a carminative (similar to fennel and dill, which also contain apiol) for reducing flatulence and colic. In Germany, it has been used for the treatment of patients with anorexia to stimulate appetite. Parsley also has a tradition of use in constipation and is used as a traditional remedy to decrease blood sugar in diabetes and dropsy (edema). Galen said, "It provoketh the urine mightily." In France, it was used to treat those with kidney stones. Parsley has a long tradition of use in anemia and iron deficiency disorders; it is high in vitamin C and iron, and the vitamin C component improves the bioavailability of iron. Parsley has also been used as a remedy for rheumatism and gout.

Grieves (1975) writes, "Hares and rabbits will come from a great distance to seek for it, so that it is scarcely possible to preserve it in gardens to which they have access. Sheep are also fond of it, and it is said to be a sovereign remedy that preserves them from footrot, provided it is given to them in sufficient quantities." "The foliage is well liked by sheep and goats. It improves their milk yield and keeps them free from foot ills. It is used for the treatment of all disorders of the kidneys and bladder, gravel, stone, congestion, cystitis, jaundice, obesity, dropsy, worms, rheumatism, sciatica, neuritis, arthritis, and swellings of the joints" (De Bairacli-Levy, 1963). The root is used for constipation, obstruction of the intestine, and fever, the seed for colic and fever (de Bairacli Levy, 1963). de Bairacli (1985) states that parsley alone has cured even severe cases of rheumatism and arthritis, and it can be used to improve eye health. Steamed parsley roots can be fed following gastroenteritis and can be used for anemia and bad breath.

Published Research: Parsley leaf (ethanolic extract) was tested for its ability to inhibit gastric secretion and to protect the gastric mucosa against induced physical and chemical injury in vivo. In doses of 1 and 2 g/kg body weight, it had significant antiulcerogenic activity. Acute toxicity tests showed a large margin of safety for the extract (Al-Howiriny, 2003).

A mechanism of action for laxative effects has been investigated. In the rat colon, an aqueous extract of parsley seeds significantly reduced net water absorption from the colon, as compared with controls. Results suggest that parsley acts by inhibiting sodium and consequently water absorption through inhibition of the Na^+/K^+ pump, stimulating the Na-K-Cl transporter, and increasing electrolyte and water secretion (Kreydiyyeh, 2001). The same mechanism of action leads to a reduction in Na^+ and K^+ reabsorption and a diuretic action. This was demonstrated in a study in which rats were offered an aqueous parsley seed extract to drink. Rats eliminated a significantly larger volume of urine daily compared with when they drank water alone. This effect was apparent in the presence of amiloride and furosemide and in the absence of sodium—but not in the absence of potassium. Reduced reabsorption led to an osmotic water flow into the lumen and diuresis (Kreydiyyeh, 2002).

In one study, parsley extract was given to male rats with diabetes. The numbers of secretory granules and cells in islets and other morphologic changes were not different from those of the control diabetic group; however, blood glucose levels were reduced compared with the diabetic group. It was suggested that parsley can provide blood glucose homeostasis but cannot regenerate B cells of the endocrine pancreas (Yanardag, 2003).

Parsley leaves (methanolic extract) showed potent estrogenic activity, similar to that of isoflavone glycosides from soybeans. The methanolic extracts of parsley, apiin, and apigenin restored uterine weight in ovariectomized mice when orally administered for 7 consecutive days. These compounds were shown to have proliferative activity in an estrogen-sensitive breast cancer cell line (Yoshikawa, 2000).

Antioxidant activity has been demonstrated in vitro (Fejes, 1998) and in rats (Hempel, 1999). The antioxidative properties of parsley have also been demonstrated in a randomized crossover trial in 14 human subjects. The urinary excretion of flavones and biomarkers for oxidative stress were measured. Erythrocyte glutathione reductase and superoxide dismutase activities increased during intervention with parsley ($P < .005$) as compared with levels in the basic diet (Nielsen, 1999).

Indications: Colic, flatulence, dysuria, cystitis, dysmenorrhea, myalgia

Potential Veterinary Uses: Mild colic and flatulence; cystitis, dysuria, and urinary calculi; incontinence in females; diabetes

Contraindications: Inflammatory kidney disease, pregnancy

Toxicology and Adverse Effects: AHPA class 2b, 2d, because of the contraindications listed earlier. In isolation, apiol (a chemical extracted from the seed) is toxic in large doses, causing irritation to mucous membranes, liver damage, cardiac arrhythmia, and central paralysis; it is an abortifacient. Parsley, however, has no reputation at all for toxicity in humans. Phytophotodermatitis has been described in pigs exposed to parsley (Griffiths, 2000).

Drug Interactions: The effect of parsley on mice (pretreated with parsley juice) was investigated in terms of the hypnotic action of pentobarbital and the analgesic action of paracetamol and aminopyrine—drugs that rely on the cytochrome P450 superfamily for their metabolism. In mice pretreated with parsley juice, the action of pentobarbital was prolonged compared with its effects in controls. Parsley increased and prolonged the analgesic action of aminopyrine and paracetamol. Parsley juice caused a significant decrease in cytochrome P450 in the liver compared with control values (Jakovljevic, 2002).

Dosage:

Human:

Fresh leaves: A handful a day

Dried herb: 1-10 g TID, up to 6 times daily for acute conditions

Infusions: 5-30 g per cup of water, with 1 cup of the tea given TID, up to 6 times daily acutely

Tincture (usually 45% ethanol) 1:2 or 1:3: 1-5 mL TID, up to 6 times daily for acute conditions

Small Animal:

Fresh Parsley leaves (minced): 1 teaspoon per 5 kg of body weight in food

Dried herb: 25-500 mg/kg, divided daily (optimally, TID)

Infusion: 5-30 g per cup of water, administered at a rate of ¼-½ cup per 10 kg (20 lb), divided daily (optimally, TID)

Tincture (usually 45% ethanol) 1:2-1:3: 0.5-2.5 mL per 10 kg (20 lb), divided daily (optimally, TID) and diluted or combined with other herbs. Higher doses may be appropriate if the herb is used singly and is not combined in a formula

References

Al-Howiriny T, Al-Sohaibani M, El-Tahir K, Rafatullah S. Prevention of experimentally-induced gastric ulcers in rats by an ethanolic extract of "Parsley" *Petroselinum crispum.* Am J Chin Med 2003;31:699-711.

De Bairacli Levy J. *The Complete Herbal Handbook for Farm and Stable.* London: Faber and Faber; 1963.

De Bairacli Levy J. *The Complete Herbal Handbook for the Dog and Cat.* London: Faber and Faber; 1985.

Fejes S, Kery A, Blazovics A, et al. [Investigation of the in vitro antioxidant effect of *Petroselinum crispum.*] Acta Pharm Hung 1998;68:150-156.

Griffiths IB, Douglas RG. Phytophotodermatitis in pigs exposed to parsley *(Petroselinum crispum).* Vet Rec 2000;146:73-74.

Hempel J, Pforte H, Raab B, Engst W, Bohm H, Jacobasch G. Flavonols and flavones of parsley cell suspension culture change the antioxidative capacity of plasma in rats. Nahrung 1999;43:201-204.

Jakovljevic V, Raskovic A, Popovic M, Sabo J. The effect of celery and parsley juices on pharmacodynamic activity of drugs involving cytochrome P450 in their metabolism. Eur J Drug Metab Pharmacokinet 2002;27:153-156.

Kreydiyyeh SI, Usta J. Diuretic effect and mechanism of action of parsley. J Ethnopharmacol 2002;79:353-357.

Kreydiyyeh SI, Usta J, Kaouk I, Al-Sadi R. The mechanism underlying the laxative properties of parsley extract. Phytomedicine 2001;8:382-388.

Nielsen SE, Young JF, Daneshvar B, et al. Effect of parsley *(Petroselinum crispum)* intake on urinary apigenin excretion, blood antioxidant enzymes and biomarkers for oxidative stress in human subjects. Br J Nutr 1999;81:447-455.

Yanardag R, Bolkent S, Tabakoglu-Oguz A, Ozsoy-Sacan O. Effects of *Petroselinum crispum* extract on pancreatic B cells and blood glucose of streptozotocin-induced diabetic rats. Biol Pharm Bull 2003;26:1206-1210.

Yoshikawa M, Uemura T, Shimoda H, Kishi A, Kawahara Y, Matsuda H. Medicinal foodstuffs. XVIII. Phytoestrogens from the aerial part of *Petroselinum crispum* Mill. (Parsley) and structures of 6″-acetylapiin and a new monoterpene glycoside, petroside. Chem Pharm Bull (Tokyo) 2000;48:1039-1044.

Passionflower

Passiflora incarnata L., other species also used; *Passiflora edulis, Passiflora caerulea* • pass-iff-FLOR-uh in-kar-NAH-tuh

Other Names: Passionvine, maypop, apricot vine, wild passionflower, passiflore, fleur de la passion, fleischfarben passionsblume, pasiflora

Family: Passifloraceae

Parts Used: Aerial parts. The yellow pulp from the berry is edible.

Distribution: Passionflower is indigenous from Southeast United States to Argentina and Brazil. It is cultivated in other parts of the world as a garden plant.

Selected Constituents: Flavonoids (up to 2.5%): in particular, C-glycosyl-flavones, including, among others, isovitexin-2″-o-glucoside, schaftoside, isoschaftoside, isoorientin, isoorientin-2″-o-flucoside, vicenin-2, and lucenin-2; cyanogenic glycosides: gynocardine (<0.1%); volatile oil: trace

Clinical Actions: Antispasmodic, antitussive, anxiolytic, sedative, hypnotic, anodyne

Energetics: Cool, bitter

History and Traditional Usage: Evidence suggests prehistoric use of passionflower fruit by natives of North America and evidence of cultivation when Europeans arrived. Seeds found at archaeologic sites are several thousand years old. It has been used internally for hysteria, general nervous agitation, insomnia, and nervous gastrointestinal complaints. The herb is used externally for hemorrhoids and as a bath additive for nervous agitation. It was approved by the German Commission E for nervous restlessness and insomnia (Blumenthal, 1997).

Published Research: Passionflower has been used for the treatment of patients with central nervous system (CNS) disorders. The methanol leaf extract of *P. incarnata* was evaluated for various CNS effects in mice (200 mg/kg). It exhibited significant sedative, anticonvulsant, and CNS-depressant activities at this dose, as well as analgesic and anti-inflammatory activities against induced pain and induced edema, respectively, in mice (Kamaldeep, 2003). The methanol extracts of leaves, stems, flowers, and whole plant displayed anxiolytic effects at 100, 125, 200, and 300 mg/kg, respectively. Roots were practically devoid of anxiolytic effects (Dhawan, 2001). *Passiflora edulis* and *P. alata* extracts have also shown anxiolytic activity in rat studies at doses of 200 to 800 mg/kg of body weight (Reginatto, 2006). An extract of *P. edulis* rind (at 10 mg/kg and 50 mg/kg of body weight) has also been shown to control systolic blood pressure in spontaneously hypertensive rats (Ichimura, 2006).

The efficacy of oxazepam was compared with that of passionflower in a double-blind, randomized trial of 36 humans with generalized anxiety disorder. Patients were allocated in a random fashion for a 4-week trial: 18 to the passionflower extract at 45 drops/day plus placebo tablet group, and 18 to oxazepam 30 mg/day plus placebo drops. Both were effective in the treatment of those with generalized anxiety disorder, with no significant difference noted between the 2 protocols. Oxazepam provided a more rapid onset of action but a significantly greater number of adverse effects related to impaired job performance. Results suggest that passionflower is an effective treatment for the management of generalized anxiety disorder and is associated with a low incidence of impaired job performance (Akhondzadeh, 2001a).

Passionflower was shown effective as an aid in opiate withdrawal in a double-blind, randomized trial in which opiate addicts experienced improved mental symptoms when the herb was added to an established clonidine protocol (Akhondzadeh, 2001b).

P. incarnata significantly inhibited inflammation in rodent models (Borrelli, 1996) and demonstrated anti-asthma effects against induced bronchospasm in guinea pigs with a 7-day treatment regimen at a 100-mg/kg dose (Dhawan, 2003a). Passionflower leaves (100 and 200 mg/kg po) exhibited significant antitussive activity in sulfur dioxide–induced cough in mice; cough inhibition (39.4% and 65.0%, respectively) was comparable with that of codeine phosphate (10 and 20 mg/kg po, respectively) (Dhawan, 2002).

The aphrodisiac properties of the methanol extract of passionflower leaves were evaluated in mice through observation of mounting behavior. Methanol extract exhibited significant aphrodisiac behavior in male mice at all doses (i.e., 75, 100, and 150 mg/kg). Among these, the highest level of activity was observed with the 100-mg/kg dose when mountings were calculated about 95 minutes after administration of the test extracts (Dhawan, 2003b).

Indications: Anxiety, neuralgia, epilepsy

Potential Veterinary Indications: Anxiety, nervousness; adjunct for treatment of stress due to travel or transportation; seizures

Contraindications: None found.

Toxicology and Adverse Effects: AHPA class 1. No adverse effects are expected at normal dosage; however, a 34-year-old woman developed severe nausea, vomiting, drowsiness, prolonged QT interval, and ventricular tachycardia following ingestion of Passionflower at therapeutic doses (Fisher, 2000).

Potential Drug Interactions: Theoretically, passionflower may have additive effects with anxiolytics and CNS depressants.

Dosage:

Human:

Dried herb: 1-10 g TID; for insomnia, double the dose 30 min before bedtime

Infusions: 5-30 g per cup of water, with 1 cup of the tea given TID, up to 6 times daily acutely

Tincture (usually 35% ethanol) 1:2 or 1:3: 1-5 mL TID, up to 6 times daily for acute conditions

Small Animal:

Dried herb: 25-300 mg/kg, divided daily (optimally, TID)

Infusion: 5-30 g per cup of water, administered at a rate of ¼-½ cup per 10 kg (20 lb), divided daily (optimally, TID)

Tincture (usually 35% ethanol) 1:2-1:3: 0.5-1.5 mL per 10 kg (20 lb), divided daily (optimally, TID) and diluted or combined with other herbs. Higher doses may be appropriate if the herb is used singly and is not combined in a formula.

References

Akhondzadeh S, Naghavi HR, Vazirian M, Shayeganpour A, Rashidi H, Khani M. Passionflower in the treatment of generalized anxiety: a pilot double-blind randomized controlled trial with oxazepam. J Clin Pharm Ther 2001a; 26:363-367.

Akhondzadeh S, Kashani L, Mobaseri M, Hosseini SH, Nikzad S, Khani M. Passionflower in the treatment of opiate withdrawal: a double-blind randomized controlled trial. J Clin Pharm Ther 2001b;26:369-373.

Blumenthal M, ed. (Klein S, trans.) *German Commission E Therapeutic Monographs on Medicinal Herbs for Human Use.* Austin, Tex: American Botanical Council; 1997.

Borrelli F, Pinto L, Izzo AA, et al. Anti-inflammatory activity of *Passiflora incarnata* L. in rats. Phytother Res 1996;10(suppl): S104–S106.

Dhawan K, Kumar S, Sharma A. Anxiolytic activity of aerial and underground parts of *Passiflora incarnata.* Fitoterapia 2001; 72:922-926.

Dhawan K, Sharma A. Antitussive activity of the methanol extract of *Passiflora incarnata* leaves. Fitoterapia 2002;73:397-399.

Dhawan K, Kumar S, Sharma A. Antiasthmatic activity of the methanol extract of leaves of *Passiflora incarnata.* Phytother Res 2003a;17:821-822.

Dhawan K, Kumar S, Sharma A. Aphrodisiac activity of methanol extract of leaves of *Passiflora incarnata* Linn in mice. Phytother Res 2003b;17:401-403.

Fisher AA, Purcell P, Le Couteur DG. Toxicity of *Passiflora incarnata* L. J Toxicol Clin Toxicol 2000;38:63-66.

Ichimura T, Yamanaka A, Ichiba T, Toyokawa T, Kamada Y, Tamamura T, Maruyama S. Antihypertensive effect of an extract of *Passiflora edulis* rind in spontaneously hypertensive rats. Biosci Biotechnol Biochem 2006;70:718-721.

Kamaldeep D, Suresh K, Anupam S. Evaluation of central nervous system effects of *Passiflora incarnata* in experimental animals. Pharmaceut Biol 2003;41:87-91.

Reginatto FH, De-Paris F, Petry RD, Quevedo J, Ortega GG, Gosmann G, Schenkel EP. Evaluation of anxiolytic activity of spray dried powders of two South Brazilian Passiflora species. Phytother Res 2006;20:348-351.

Pau D'Arco

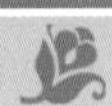

Tabebuia impetiginosa (Mart. ex D.C.) Standl. • TAB-eb-u-ee-ah im-pet-eye-gin-OH-suh

Tabebuia avellanedae Lorentz. ex Griseb. • TAB-eb-u-ee-ah avay-AN-eday

Tabebuia heptaphylla (Vell.) Toledo.

Distribution: Central and South America

Similar Species: *Herbs of Commerce* states that *T. impetiginosa, T. avellanedae,* and *T. heptaphylla* are synonyms. *Tabebuia rosea* (an endangered species)

Other Names: Lapacho, taheebo, ipe roxo, ipes. *T. heptaphylla* is also known as lapacho Colorado and lapacho morado.

Family: Bignoniaceae

Parts Used: Inner bark

Selected Constituents: Naphthoquinones (lapachone, lapachol), anthraquinones, and furanonaphthoquinones are the main active constituents and are not consistently present in commercial products. Also, phenolic acids, tannins, coumarins, flavonoids, saponins

Lapachol

Clinical Action: Antibacterial, antifungal, immune modulator, astringent, anti-inflammatory

Energetics: Sour, bitter, cold

History and Traditional Usage: In the 1960s, a Brazillian news magazine reported "miracle cures" of leukemia and cancer following treatment with pau d'arco tea, and the plant is very popular for the treatment of patients with cancer. Used by South Americans for rheumatism, bronchitis, gastrointestinal disorders, and fever; topically for eczema, fungal infection, and skin cancer

Published Research: Lapachol and an anthraquinone constituent of *T. impetiginosa* bark were evaluated in a bacterial sensitivity system against human intestinal bacteria. Anthraquinone-2-carboxylic acid strongly inhibited *Clostridium paraputrificum,* but this compound and lapachol were only weakly active against *C. perfringens* and *Escherichia coli.* No activity was noted against *Bifidobacterium* and *Lactobacillus* species (Park, 2005). Pereira (2006) tested beta-lapachone, 3-hydroxy-beta-N-lapachone, and alpha-lapachone against methicillin-resistant *Staphylococcus aureus, Streptococcus epidermidis,* and *Streptococcus haemolyticus* strains. These compounds had some antibacterial activity and were found to be safe when applied to rabbit skin. The authors suggested that these compounds could be used topically for serious skin infections, including infection by methicillin-resistant *S. aureus.* A *T. avellanedae* extract had some antifungal activity (Portillo, 2001).

The pau d'arco constituent lapachol has demonstrated some antitumor activity in rodent studies (deSanatan, 1968; Rau, 1968), which might account for the popularity of pau d'arco; however, a clinical trial was stopped prematurely because of adverse events associated with treatment. No studies involving use of the whole plant have been conducted. A recent study showed that lapachol has potential for preventing metastasis (Balassiano, 2005); however, lapachol was not detected in the aqueous extract (Steinert, 1996). Antinociceptive and antiedematogenic effects of *T. avellanedae* inner bark aqueous extract were demonstrated in mice; acute toxicity was low. These results may validate the plant's popular use as an analgesic and anti-inflammatory agent (deMiranda, 2001).

Indications: Gastroenteritis, upper respiratory infection and allergy, cystitis/urethritis, fever. Used topically for skin inflammation and infection and wounds

Potential Veterinary Indications: Topically and perhaps systemically for infection (fungal, bacterial, yeast) of the gastrointestinal, respiratory, and urinary tracts.

Contraindications: Possibly bleeding disorders and pregnancy

Toxicology and Adverse Effects: Skin and upper respiratory irritations have occurred on exposure to the powdered herb. Possibly, nausea, vomiting, and increased bleeding

Drug Interactions: Lapachol antagonizes vitamin K and may interact with anticoagulants.

Dosage:

Human:

Dried herb: 1-10 g TID

Decoctions: 5-30 g per cup of water, with 1 cup of the tea given TID

Tincture (generally 45%-50% ethanol; some pharmacies include glycerin to prevent precipitation by tannins) 1:2 or 1:3: 1-5 mL TID

Small Animal:

Dried herb: 25-300 mg/kg, divided daily (optimally, TID)

Decoction: 5-30 g per cup of water, administered at a rate of ¼-½ cup per 10 kg (20 lb), divided daily (optimally, TID)

Tincture (usually 45%-50% ethanol; some pharmacies include glycerin to prevent precipitation by tannins) 1:2-1:3: 0.5-1.5 mL per 10 kg (20 lb), divided daily (optimally, TID) and diluted or combined with other herbs. Higher doses may be appropriate if the herb is used singly and is not combined in a formula.

Selected References

Balassiano IT, De Paulo SA, Henriques Silva N, et al. Demonstration of the lapachol as a potential drug for reducing cancer metastasis. Oncol Rep 2005;13:329-333.

de Almeida ER, da Silva Filho AA, dos Santos ER, Lopes CA. Antiinflammatory action of lapachol. J Ethnopharmacol 1990; 29:239-241.

de Miranda FG, Vilar JC, Alves IA, Cavalcanti SC, Antoniolli AR. Antinociceptive and antiedematogenic properties and acute toxicity of *Tabebuia avellanedae* Lor. ex Griseb. inner bark aqueous extract. BMC Pharmacol 2001;1:6. Epub 2001 Sep 13.

de Santana CF, de Lima O, d'Albuquerque IL, Lacerda AL, Martins DG. [Antitumoral and toxicological properties of extracts of bark and various wood components of Pau d'arco *(Tabebuia avellanedae)*.] Rev Inst Antibiot (Recife) 1968;8:89-94.

Park BS, Kim JR, Lee SE, Kim KS, Takeoka GR, Ahn YJ, Kim JH. Selective growth-inhibiting effects of compounds identified in *Tabebuia impetiginosa* inner bark on human intestinal bacteria. J Agric Food Chem 2005;53:1152-1157.

Pereira EM, Machado TB, Leal IC, Jesus DM, Damaso CR, Pinto AV, Giambiagi-deMarval M, Kuster RM, Santos KR. *Tabebuia avellanedae* naphthoquinones: activity against methicillin-resistant staphylococcal strains, cytotoxic activity and in vivo dermal irritability analysis. Ann Clin Microbiol Antimicrob 2006;5:5.

Portillo A, Vila R, Freixa B, Adzet T, Canigueral S. Antifungal activity of Paraguayan plants used in traditional medicine. J Ethnopharmacol 2001;76:93-98.

Rimpler M. High-performance liquid chromatographic separation of some naturally occurring naphthoquinones and anthraquinones. J Chromatogr A 1996;723:206-209.

Steinert J, Khalaf H, Rau KV, McBride TJ, Oleson JJ. Recognition and evaluation of lapachol as an anti-tumor agent. Cancer Res 1968;28:1952-1954.

Peppermint

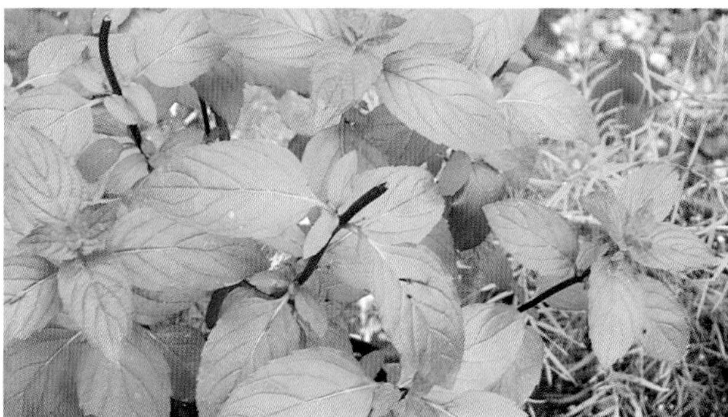

Mentha x piperita L. • MEN-thuh pip-er-EE-tuh

Distribution: Most is currently grown in the United States, but this plant does not occur in nature. It is a sterile triple hybrid between *Mentha aquatica* and *Mentha spicata* (which is itself a hybrid of *Mentha suaveolens* and *Mentha longifolia).*

Similar Species: *M. spicata* (spearmint), *M. arvensis* (field mint)

Other Names: Folia *Menthae piperitae,* bo he, mionnt, menta, pfefferminze, minze, podina, hakka, pepaminto, pereminde, pudina, nana, eqama, *Menthe poivrée,* sentebon, Fefermints, and many others

Part Used: Leaves

Family: Lamiaceae

Selected Constituents: Essential oil (includes menthol, menthone, and others; sometimes pulegone and carvone); tannins, triterpenes, flavonoids, coumarins, biogenic amines

H CH_3 HO H_3C CH_3

Menthol

Clinical Action: Carminative, antispasmodic, choleretic, aromatic, diaphoretic, antiemetic, nervine, antiseptic, analgesic

Energetics: Bitter, pungent, cool. In Traditional Chinese Medicine, disperses wind heat, benefits the throat, and clears the eyes; enters stomach, liver, and lung meridians; moves stagnant Liver *Qi* and vents rashes

History and Traditional Usage: Native American tribes used this plant for gastrointestinal problems; to relieve colic pain; for headaches, food, flavoring, fevers, and colds; and as a vermifuge. The Eclectics viewed peppermint as having stimulant, antispasmodic, carminative, stomachic, antiseptic, and weak anodyne properties. Indications for use included flatulence, painful gastrointestinal spasms (colic), nausea, vomiting, and a variety of digestive disorders. It was also recommended for headaches and, when nebulized, for bronchitis and pneumonia. Traditional herbalists claim that peppermint inhibits mucous secretion and that it has antianxiety and tension-relieving properties; in women, it may relieve menstrual pain. It is used as well for ulcerative colitis, Crohn's disease, fever, colds, and influenza, and as an inhalant for nasal catarrh. It may relieve itching when used topically. In Traditional Chinese Medicine, peppermint disperses wind heat, mostly from the head and eyes, and promotes eruption (and resolution) of rashes. It is used for headache, inflammation of the eyes, upper respiratory infection, sore throat, and mouth ulcers. Also helps suppress rebellious *Qi* that causes vomiting.

Milks (1949) mentioned peppermint briefly as a valuable veterinary carminative for colic and flatulence and for external use as an antiseptic.

Published Research: Peppermint constituents are absorbed from the gastrointestinal tract, glucuronidated in the liver, and excreted in urine and bile. Menthol feels cooling to the skin and mucosa because it stimulates cold receptors (Hensel, 1951). It has topical analgesic activity because it blocks skin and mucosal nociceptors (Green, 1992). Peppermint and menthol may have calcium channel blocking activity in smooth muscle (Grigoleit, 2005a). Peppermint appears to reduce intestinal spasm (Grigoleit, 2005c), and, in animal studies, peppermint oil has been shown to decrease the gut contractile response to histamine, serotonin, acetylcholine, and substance P (Hills, 1991).

Grigoleit (2005b) reviewed 15 clinical trials on peppermint oil in the treatment of irritable bowel syndrome, along with a paper on abdominal pain in children. In all, 15 clinical trials enrolled a total of 651 patients and lasted from 2 weeks to 6 months. Twelve trials were randomized, double blinded, and placebo controlled, and 2 were open-label studies. Peppermint oil was compared with psychotherapy and anticholinergic smooth muscle relaxants. In three trials that compared peppermint oil with smooth muscle relaxants, no difference was observed between treatment groups. Thirteen trials included enteric-coated peppermint oil capsules, and three trials did not describe the form of peppermint used. Eight of 12 placebo-controlled trials showed a positive effect for peppermint over placebo. Adverse events were mild and included heartburn, anal "burning," and peppermint taste. Reviewers concluded that a dose of 180 to 200 mg of peppermint oil given TID for 2 to 4 weeks is likely efficacious. Peppermint oil may also be effective for the treatment of recurrent abdominal pain in children (Weydert, 2003).

Peppermint has been advocated for the treatment of nausea. One placebo-controlled study examined the effect of peppermint oil in patients undergoing gynecologic surgery and found that peppermint was effective (Tate, 1997). A different group investigated the use of peppermint oil administered in the form of aromatherapy for postsurgical patients who complained of nausea. A total of 33 patients rated the severity of nausea on a visual analogue scale and were then randomly assigned to treatment with peppermint oil, isopropyl alcohol, and saline on gauze sponges, to be breathed in with deep, controlled breaths. Peppermint treatment did not result in improvements beyond those seen with placebo treatment (Anderson, 2004).

Peppermint oil was shown to suppress gastric spasm in people during upper gastrointestinal endoscopy (Hiki, 2003). Peppermint oil was added to barium for use in barium enema, and the effect on colonic muscle spasm was investigated in 141 human patients. A highly significant benefit was found with the use of peppermint oil for this procedure, compared with the use of conventional barium (Sparks, 1995).

Topical peppermint has proved effective in treatment of headache in human subjects in randomized, placebo-controlled, double-blind, crossover studies (Gobel, 1994; Gobel, 1996).

Peppermint is often recommended for the treatment of cough. Menthol is thought to have an anesthetic action on the throat, to suppress cough, and to lower surfactant surface tension (Zanker, 1980). In animal models in which coughing is induced, menthol dose dependently suppresses cough (Laude, 1994). In humans, induced coughing is also suppressed by menthol inhalation (Morice, 1994). Human asthmatic patients who nebulized menthol twice daily did not experience improvements in some respiratory measures, but they had fewer wheezing episodes and used fewer bronchodilators (Tamaoki, 1995).

In dogs and guinea pigs—but not cats—menthol stimulated reflex inhibition of respiration (Sant'Ambrogio, 1992; Davies, 1987). In dogs and cats, vaporized menthol stimulated respiratory tract cold receptors (Sant'Ambrogio, 1991; Schafer, 1986). Inhalation of menthol has the same inhibitory effect on respiration in humans (De Cort, 1993; Javorka, 1980).

Peppermint is believed to act as a nasal decongestant. Menthol applied topically to the nasal mucosa leads to congestion (Fox, 1982). Human study participants report a subjective increase in airflow after menthol is inhaled (Ahijevych, 2004; Naito, 1991; Eccles, 1990a; Eccles, 1990b). The reason for the sensation of increased airflow is not the peppermint smell, but the stimulation of cold receptors innervated by the trigeminal nerve (Eccles, 1983; Eccles, 1988a; Eccles, 1988b).

Peppermint given to laying hens gave an aromatic flavor to their eggs (Richter, 2002).

Indications: Gastroenteritis, vomiting, flatulence, fever, bronchitis, upper respiratory tract infection, nasal congestion, asthma, headache, inflammatory bowel disease, Crohn's disease
Potential Veterinary Indications: Gastroenteritis, flatulence, nausea and vomiting, colic, upper respiratory congestion, bronchitis
Contraindications: Bile duct obstruction, gallbladder inflammation, severe liver damage, gastrointestinal reflux. Traditional herbalists warn nursing mothers not to take peppermint because it may decrease lactation. In Traditional Chinese Medicine, contraindications include exterior deficiency and yin deficiency with heat signs.

The European Agency for the Evaluation of Medicinal Products, Veterinary Medicines Evaluation Unit, assessed *Mentha piperita* for potential problems in food animal medicine. No special precautions were advised.
Toxicology and Adverse Effects: AHPA class 1. Peppermint is generally recognized as safe (GRAS) by the US Food and Drug Administration (FDA). Allergic reaction is possible, as is irritation, if undiluted oil is placed on mucous membranes. Inhalation of the oil can cause apnea and laryngoconstriction, and young children and animals are thought particularly susceptible. In one study of dogs, doses of 25 to 125 mg/kg given for 5 weeks caused no ill effects. As with most aromatic essential oils, caution is advised for use in the cat, although the herb itself may be used.
Drug Interactions: None reported. Non–enteric-coated preparations may cause mild nausea and gastritis. Some sources suggest that these forms should be considered for patients on H2 blockers because enteric-coated forms may not be broken down. May interact with drugs metabolized through the CYP3A4, CYP1A2, and CYP2E enzyme systems
Preparation Notes: Essential oil of peppermint and tannins are extracted by hot infusion (tea); the essential oil is better extracted in alcohol.
Dosage:
External Use:
Volatile oil topically (headache, arthralgia): dilute 50% and apply 3-5 drops to temples or joint (more for larger joints)
Internal Use:
Human
Dried herb: 1-10 g TID, up to 6 times daily for acute conditions
Enteric coated capsules: 1-2 caps TID of those delivering 0.2 mL menthol/cap
Essential oil: 1-3 drops TID
Infusions: 5-30 g per cup of water, with 1 cup of the tea given TID, up to 6 times daily acutely
Tincture (usually 45% ethanol) 1:2 or 1:3: 0.5-5 mL TID, up to 6 times daily for acute conditions
Small Animal
Dried herb: 25-300 mg/kg, divided daily (optimally, TID)
Enteric-coated capsules containing essential oil: 0.1 mL per 10 kg
Essential oil: 1 drop—added to a 25-mL (1-oz) bottle of herbal formula
Infusion: 5-30 g per cup of water, administered at a rate of ¼-½ cup per 10 kg (20 lb), divided daily (optimally, TID)
Tincture (usually 45% ethanol) 1:2-1:3: 0.5-1.0 mL per 10 kg (20 lb), divided daily (optimally, TID) and diluted or combined with other herbs. Higher doses may be appropriate if the herb is used singly and is not combined in a formula.
Historic Veterinary Doses:
Peppermint oil for farm animals: 1-2 mL for horses and cows; 0.3-0.6 mL for sheep and goats (Milks, 1949)
Combinations: Tiger balm is a traditional balm that is used as a topical analgesic, particularly for headaches, insect bites, and sore muscles in people. If this balm is used on dogs or cats, they should be prevented from licking it. Following is one of several recipes for a similar homemade balm (found on Henriette's Herbal Homepage at: http://www.henriettesherbal.com/faqs/medi-4-4-balm.html)
Tigerbalm Oil:
- Peppermint oil, 25 mL
- Camphor oil, 15 mL
- Wintergreen oil, 20 mL
- Lavender oil, 15 mL
- Eucalyptus oil, 15 mL
- Jojoba oil, 10 mL

The oil can be made into an ointment by adding melted beeswax to the warmed oil; Vaseline may be substituted if necessary.

Selected References

Ahijevych K, Garrett BE. Menthol pharmacology and its potential impact on cigarette smoking behavior. Nicotine Tobacco Res 2004;6(suppl 1):S17–S28.
Anderson LA, Gross JB. Aromatherapy with peppermint, isopropyl alcohol, or placebo is equally effective in relieving postoperative nausea. J Perianesth Nurs 2004;19:29-35.
Davies AM, Eccles R. Electromyographic responses of a nasal muscle to stimulation of the nasal vestibule in the cat. J Physiol (Lond) 1987;391:25-38.
De Cort S, et al. Cardiorespiratory effects of inhalation of L-menthol in healthy humans. J Physiol 1993;473:47.
Eccles R, Jones AS. The effect of menthol on nasal resistance to air flow. J Laryngol Otol 1983;97:705-709.
Eccles R, Griffiths DH, Newton CG, Tolley NS. The effects of menthol isomers on nasal sensation of airflow. Clin Otolaryngol Allied Sci 1988a;13:25-29.
Eccles R, et al. The effects of D and L isomers of menthol upon nasal sensation of airflow. J Laryngol Otol 1988b;102:506-508.
Eccles R, Jawad MS, Morris S. The effects of oral administration of (−)-menthol on nasal resistance to airflow and nasal sensation of airflow in subjects suffering from nasal congestion associated with the common cold. J Pharm Pharmacol 1990a; 42:652-654.
Eccles R, Morris S, Jawad MS. The effects of menthol on reaction time and nasal sensation of airflow in subjects suffering from the common cold. Clin Otolaryngol 1990b;15:39-42.
Fox N. Effect of camphor, eucalyptol and menthol on the vascular state of the mucous membrane. Arch Otolaryngol Head Neck Surg 1927;6:112-122.
Freise J, Kohler S. [Peppermint oil–caraway oil fixed combination in non-ulcer dyspepsia—comparison of the effects of enteric preparations.] Pharmazie 1999;54:210-215.
Gobel H, Fresenius J, Heinze A, Dworschak M, Soyka D. [Effectiveness of *Oleum menthae piperitae* and paracetamol in therapy of headache of the tension type.] Nervenarzt 1996;67:672-681.

Gobel H, Schmidt G, Soyka D. Effect of peppermint and eucalyptus oil preparations on neurophysiological and experimental algesimetric headache parameters. Cephalalgia 1994;14: 228-234; discussion, 182.

Green BG. The sensory effects of l-menthol on human skin. Somatosensory Motor Res 1992;9:235-244.

Grigoleit HG, Grigoleit P. Pharmacology and preclinical pharmacokinetics of peppermint oil. Phytomedicine 2005a;12: 612-616.

Grigoleit HG, Grigoleit P. Peppermint oil in irritable bowel syndrome. Phytomedicine 2005b;12:601-606.

Grigoleit HG, Grigoleit P. Gastrointestinal clinical pharmacology of peppermint oil. Phytomedicine 2005c;12:607-611.

Hensel H, Zotterman Y. The effects of menthol and thermoreceptors. Acta Physiol Scand 1951;24:27-34.

Hiki N, Kurosaka H, Tatsutomi Y, Shimoyama S, Tsuji E, Kojima J, Shimizu N, Ono H, Hirooka T, Noguchi C, Mafune K, Kaminishi M. Peppermint oil reduces gastric spasm during upper endoscopy: a randomized, double-blind, double-dummy controlled trial. Gastrointest Endosc 2003;57:475-482.

Hills JM, Aaronson PI. The mechanism of action of peppermint oil on gastrointestinal smooth muscle. Gastroenterology 1991;101:55-65.

Javorka K, Tomori Z, Zavarska L. Protective and defensive airway reflexes in premature infants. Physiol Bohemoslov 1980;29:29-35.

Laude EA, Morice AH, Grattan TJ. The antitussive effects of menthol, camphor and cineole in conscious guinea-pigs. Pulm Pharmacol 1994;7:179-184.

Milks HJ. *Practical Veterinary Pharmacology, Materia Medica and Therapeutics*. Chicago, Ill: Alex Eger, Inc.; 1949.

Morice AH, Marshall AE, Higgins KS, Grattna TJ. Effect of inhaled menthol on citric acid induced cough in normal subjects. Thorax 1994;49:1024-1026.

Naito K, Ohoka E, Kato R, Kondo Y, Iwata S. The effect of L-menthol stimulation of the major palatine nerve on nasal patency. Auris Nasus Larynx 1991;18:221-226.

Richter T, Braun P, Fehlhaber K. [Influence of spiced feed additives on taste of hen's eggs.] Berl Munch Tierarztl Wochenschr 2002;115:200-202.

Sant'Ambrogio FB, Anderson JW, Sant'Ambrogio G. Menthol in the upper airway depresses ventilation in newborn dogs. Respir Physiol 1992;89:299-307.

Sant'Ambrogio FB, Anderson JW, Sant'Ambrogio G. Effect of l-menthol on laryngeal receptors. J Appl Physiol 1991;70:788-793.

Schafer K, Braun HA, Isenberg C. Effect of menthol on cold receptor activity: analysis of receptor processes. J Gen Physiol 1986;88:757-776.

Sparks MJ, O'Sullivan P, Herrington AA, Morcos SK. Does peppermint oil relieve spasm during barium enema? Br J Radiol 1995;68:841-843.

Tate S. Peppermint oil: a treatment for postoperative nausea. J Adv Nurs 1997;26:543-549.

Weydert JA, Ball TM, Davis MF. Systematic review of treatments for recurrent abdominal pain. Pediatrics 2003;111:e1-e11.

Zanker KS, Tolle W, Blumel G, Probst J. Evaluation of surfactant-like effects of commonly used remedies for colds. Respiration 1980;39:150-157.

Plantain

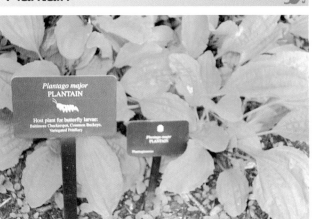

Plantago major L. • plan-TA-go MAY-jor

Distribution: Asia, Europe, naturalized to the New World and Australia

Similar Species: *Plantago lanceolata* L. (English plantain, ribgrass, ribwort, narrow leaf plantain, spitzwegerich, llantén menor), *Plantago media* (hoary plantain)

Other Names: Broad leaf plantain, greater plantain, white man's foot, che qian cao, waybroad, waybread, wegerich, platano, piantaggine

Family: Plantaginaceae

Parts Used: Leaf

Selected Constituents: Iridoids (e.g., aucubin, catalpol), mucilage, phenolic acids, flavonoids (apigenin, scutellarin, baicalein, nepetin, plantagoside), tannins, saponin, coumarins. The seeds contain some mucilage, but not as much as the seeds of *Plantago ovata, Plantago psyllium,* and other sources of the fiber laxative known as psyllium.

Aucubin

Clinical Action: Anti-inflammatory, astringent, emollient, demulcent, vulnerary

Energetics: Sweet, cold; clears heat; drains dampness

History and Traditional Usage: North American natives used plantain for gastrointestinal and gynecologic disorders, but especially for skin problems, as a poultice. It was used for upper respiratory inflammation (dry cough, sore throat, bronchitis, allergic rhinitis, etc.), mild gastroenteritis, and cystitis, similar to other plants that contain mucilage and tannins. Topically, this herb is well known for use in skin ulcers, rashes, insect bites, cuts, wounds, and poison ivy. The young leaves can be cooked and eaten.

Published Research: Experimental studies suggest that plantain has spasmolytic, vulnerary, weak antibacterial, anti-inflammatory, and immune modulatory activity (Wegener, 1999; Samuelsen, 2000).

Clinical trials published in Bulgaria suggest that plantain may be effective for the treatment of patients with chronic bronchitis (Koichev, 1983). Matev (1982) studied 25 humans with chronic bronchitis for their response to plantain treatment over 1 month. The authors concluded that 80% of subjects improved in subjective and some objective measures.

An old study examining the effect of plantain in a base of petroleum jelly found that it may have been beneficial for people with impetigo and ecthyma (Aliev, 1950).

Indications: Topically, as a poultice, for skin wounds, rashes, insect bites, etc. For upper respiratory inflammation, chronic bronchitis, mild gastroenteritis

Suggested Veterinary Indications: Topically, as a poultice, for skin wounds, rashes, insect bites, etc. For upper respiratory inflammation, chronic bronchitis, mild gastroenteritis

Notes of Interest: This plant can be found in most parts of the world and is the favorite of herbalists as a fresh, at-hand treatment for patients with wounds, insect bites, poison ivy, cough, and diarrhea. Suppliers have, in the past, misidentified the plant and accidentally sold *Digitalis* leaves instead, resulting in bradycardia and emergency department visits.

Contraindications: None reported.

Toxicology and Adverse Effects: AHPA class 1. Rare allergic reactions

Drug Interactions: May decrease drug levels of carbamazepine and lithium, although this has not been reported.

Dosage:

External Use:

Fresh juice may be pressed from the leaves for topical use

Internal Use:

Human

Dried herb: 1-10 g TID

Infusions: 5-30 g per cup of water, with 1 cup of the tea given TID

Tincture (usually 30%-40% ethanol) 1:2 or 1:3: 2-6 mL TID

Small Animal

Dried herb: 50-500 mg/kg, divided daily (optimally, TID)

Infusion: 5-30 g per cup of water, administered at a rate of ¼-½ cup per 10 kg (20 lb), divided daily (optimally, TID)

Tincture (usually 30%-40% ethanol) 1:2-1:3: 1.0-3.0 mL per 10 kg (20 lb), divided daily (optimally, TID) and diluted or combined with other herbs

Selected References

Aliev RK. A wound healing preparation from the leaves of the large plantain (Plantago major L.). *Am J Pharm* 1950;122:24-26.

Koichev A. Complex evaluation of the therapeutic effect of a preparation from *Plantago major* in chronic bronchitis. Probl Vatr Med 1983;11:61-69.

Matev M, Angelova I, Koichev A, Leseva M, Stefanov G. Clinical trial of a *Plantago major* preparation in the treatment of chronic bronchitis. Vutr Boles 1982;21:133-137.

Samuelsen AB. The traditional uses, chemical constituents and biological activities of *Plantago major* L. A review. J Ethnopharmacol 2000;71:1-21.

Wegener T, Kraft K. Plantain (*Plantago lanceolata* L.): anti-inflammatory action in upper respiratory tract infections. Wien Med Wochenschr 1999;149:211-216.

Pleurisy Root

Asclepias tuberosa L. • ass-KLE-pee-us tew-ber-OH-suh

Distribution: North America

Other Names: Butterfly Weed, Orange Milkweed, Asclepiade Tubereuse, Knollige Schwalbenwurz

Family: Asclepiadaceae

Parts Used: Rhizome

Selected Constituents: Cardenolides, flavonoids, choline sugars

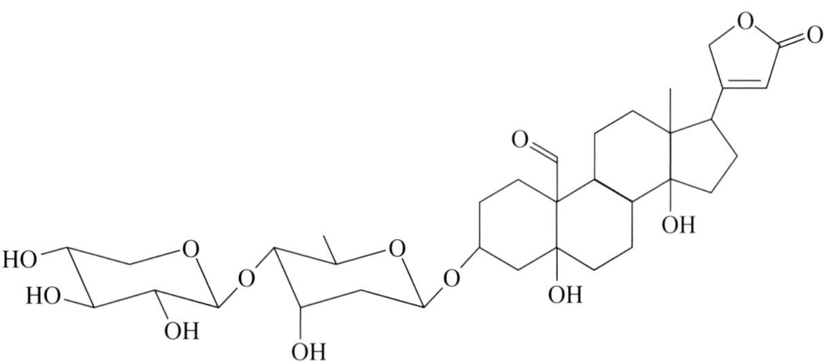

Cardenolide diglycoside 2, a cardiac glycoside of pleurisy root

Clinical Action: Diaphoretic, diuretic, laxative, tonic, carminative, expectorant
Energetics: Bitter, pungent
History and Traditional Usage: The Cherokees used Asclepias as an expectorant, for heart trouble, as a laxative, for diarrhea, and as an analgesic for breast, stomach, and intestinal pain. Other tribes had similar uses, in addition to employing the root for dermatologic problems and as a ceremonial medicine. *King's American Dispensatory* praises pleurisy root as one of the best available diaphoretics because it stimulates perspiration that is more like natural skin secretions, including "solid" matter. Scudder's specific indication was as follows:

"Pulse strong, vibratile . . . the urine is scanty; . . . vascular excitement is marked in the parts supplied by the bronchial arterioles; inflammation of serous tissues; gastrointestinal. Catarrhal troubles due to recent colds."
Published Research: No relevant clinical trials found.
Indications: Pleurisy, flu, bronchitis, pneumonia, and other respiratory conditions
Potential Veterinary Indications: Respiratory disorders, especially bronchitis and pneumonia, rhinitis
Contraindications: Pregnancy
Toxicology and Adverse Effects: AHPA class 2b, 2d. May cause nausea and vomiting. Contains cardiac glycosides and may interact with pharmaceutical cardiac glycosides.
Drug Interactions: Cardiac glycosides may lead to additive effects when used with digoxin or other cardiac glycosides.
Dosage:
Human:
Dried herb: 1-5 g TID
Decoctions: 5 g per cup of water, with 1 cup of the tea given TID
Tincture (usually 45%-60% ethanol) 1:2 or 1:3: 1-2.5 mL TID
Small Animal:
Dried herb: 25-50 mg/kg, divided daily (optimally, TID)
Decoctions: 5 g per cup of water, administered at a rate of ¼-½ cup per 10 kg (20 lb), divided daily (optimally, TID)
Tincture (usually 45%-60% ethanol) 1:2-1:3: 0.5-1.0 mL per 10 kg (20 lb), divided daily (optimally, TID) and diluted or combined with other herbs

Poke Root 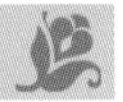

Phytolacca americana L., previously *Phytolacca decandra* L. • fy-toh-LAK-uh am-er-ih-KAH-nuh *or* am-er-ih-KAY-nuh
Distribution: North America; also, the Mediterranean
Similar Species: *Phytolacca dodecandra* (from Africa), *Phytolacca acinosa* (from East Asia), *Phytolacca esculenta*
Other Names: Pokeweed, poke root, pigeonberry, inkberry, Virginian poke, garget, garget-weed, scoke, scokeweed, coacum, coakum, cocum, mechoacan, cancer-root, jalap cancer-root, red nightshade, American nightshade, redweed, and scoke jalap. A plant known as Indian poke was actually *Veratrum viride*. In Europe, gewöhnlicheker mesbeere, herbe de la laque, fitolacca
Family: Phytolaccaceae
Parts Used: Root, sometimes berries, and rarely leaves. The root is collected in the spring as the first sprouts appear (preferably), or in the fall after the plant has died. All parts of the plant are considered toxic.
Selected Constituents: Triterpene saponins (phytolaccosides), lignans, lectins (pokeweed mitogen is one), genins, histamine, starches, γ-aminobutyric acid (GABA)
Clinical Action: Alterative, lymphatic, antirheumatic, anticatarrhal, emetic, purgative, and anti-inflammatory
Energetics: Sweet, pungent; transforms phlegm
History and Traditional Usage: North American natives used the root and berry for arthritis and rheumatism, and as a blood purifier. They used it topically for sores, sore breasts, and glandular swellings. It was popular for rheumatism, breast inflammation, lumps, breast cancer, and scrofula (lymphadenopathy). A remedy for rheumatism was made with the berries steeped in gin. *King's* states that the herb kills scabies mites and is useful for other skin conditions in which scaly, vesicular, or pustular eruptions are noted, especially with lymphatic enlargement. It was recommended to be used both locally and systemically for skin problems. It was also used to treat patients with diseases of the mouth and throat, especially stomatitis, tracheitis, pharyngitis, and faucitis. For mastitis, it was also used topically and orally. It is to be considered for all hard swellings of glands—lymphatic, salivary, breast, testicular, and so forth. *King's* claims that it has cured lymphoma. One source (Bartram, 1995) suggests that persistent internal and external treatment may be effective for lipoma.

Nelson (1865) recommended that a seton of Poke root should be placed between the jaws and in the breast for the treatment of glanders in horses. This was to be followed by an application of tar up the nose daily.
Published Research: No clinical studies have been found. A glycosidase, pokeweed antiviral protein (PAP), inactivates ribosomes and has antiviral activity against many plant and animal viruses. Pokeweed mitogen is a common laboratory reagent for stimulating proliferation of B and T lymphocytes. Uckun (1999) studied the effects of pokeweed antiviral protein on human immunodeficiency virus (HIV)-infected chimpanzees and humans. The protein suppressed viral load in chimpanzees and was well tolerated at a dose of 20 μg/kg daily after 2 months. Infected humans received a single dose of 100 μg/kg, and plasma half-life was approximately 12 hours.

Birds are frequently seen eating poke berries. Toxicity of these berries was examined in turkeys. At 5% and 10% of the diet, changes in growth rate, ataxia, inability to walk, ascites, and enlargements or deformities of the hock joints were noted. Mortality rate was up to 43% with 10% poke berries in the diet (Barnett, 1975).

Species of *Phytolacca* are molluscicidal and may slow the growth of *Schistosoma* parasites, making this plant the subject of study in areas with endemic schistosomiasis.
Indications: This herb is not in common use, but traditional indications for rheumatism, breast inflammation and lumps, and lymphadenopathy guide modern herbalists.
Potential Veterinary Indications: Stomatitis, rheumatic disorders, lymphadenopathy, lymphoma, mammary

cancer, and possibly other tumors, and inflammatory skin disorders (topically and orally) such as scabies, atopic dermatitis, ringworm, and pemphigus

Contraindications: Pregnancy, lactation, gastrointestinal irritation (due to saponin content). Lymphocytic leukemia has also been listed as a contraindication (Mills, 2004) because of its mitogenic activity in vitro, but given that lymphoma and lymphadenopathy are traditional indications for the herb and that other herbs have mitogenic activity with no similar contraindications, this should be considered theoretical.

Toxicology and Adverse Effects: AHPA class 3. A total of ½ oz of berries or root is considered fatal. Intake of 10 berries is said to be fatal for infants. The root is an irritant to skin and mucous membranes. Toxic doses cause nausea, persistent vomiting and diarrhea, drowsiness, hypotension, tachycardia or bradycardia, tremors, tetanic convulsions, respiratory paralysis, and death. Heart block has been reported in family members who ate the raw or cooked leaves. Treatment of patients with poisoning should include emesis, gastric lavage, activated charcoal, and supportive care. Poisoned patients have exhibited elevated globulin levels (probably caused by pokeweed mitogens).

Drug Interactions: None found; concurrent use with immunosuppressive drugs should be avoided.

Notes of Interest: Although the plant is considered toxic, the young shoots and leaves, known as poke sallat or poke salad, are a traditional green in the southeastern part of the United States. The young leaf is safe for ingestion only when subjected to multiple boiling water baths. *King's* states that severe purging has occurred when people ate pigeons that had partaken of poke berries. Poke root is one of the ingredients in the Hoxsey formula.

Dosage:

Human: This is a toxic herb that should be used only by experienced herbalists. It is frequently used in homeopathic potency for different indications—3× is common.

Dried herb: 1-2 g TID; more conservative sources state 15-60 mg, divided daily

Decoction: 2-5 g per cup of water, with ⅒-½ cup of the tea given TID

Tincture (usually 45% ethanol) 1:2-1:3: 0.05-1 mL TID (1:10 tinctures are much more commonly available and are safer than 1:2)

Small Animal:

Dried herb: 5 mg/kg

Tincture (45% ethanol) 1:5: 0.1 mL per 10 kg (20 lb), divided daily (optimally, TID) and diluted or combined with other herbs

Historic Veterinary Doses: Fluid extract for farm animals (Karreman, 2004): 4-8 mL for horses and cows; 1.3-3 mL for sheep and goats

Selected References

Barnett BD. Toxicity of pokeberries (fruit of *Phytolacca americana* large) for turkey poults. Poult Sci 1975;54:1215-1217.

Bartram T. *Bartram's Encyclopedia of Herbal Medicine.* New York: Marlowe and Company; 1995.

Karreman H. *Treating Dairy Cows Naturally: Thoughts and Strategies.* Paradise, Pa: Paradise Publications; 2004.

Mills S, Bone K. *The Essential Guide to Herbal Safety.* St. Louis: Mosby; 2004.

Titus NN. *The American Eclectic Practice of Medicine, As Applied to the Diseases of Domestic Animals.* New York: Baker and Godwin; 1862. Also available online at David Winston's Herbal Therapeutics Research homepage at: http://www.herbaltherapeutics.net/DomesticAnimalDiseases.pdf.

Uckun FM, Bellomy K, O'Neill K, Messinger Y, Johnson T, Chen CL. Toxicity, biological activity, and pharmacokinetics of TXU (anti-CD7)-pokeweed antiviral protein in chimpanzees and adult patients infected with human immunodeficiency virus. J Pharmacol Exp Ther 1999;291:1301-1307.

Potentilla

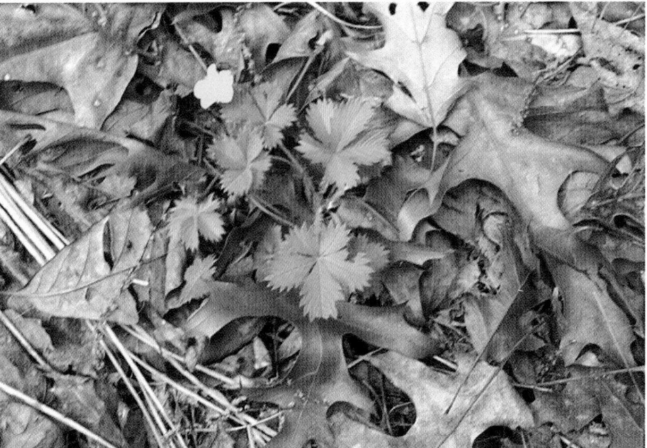

Potentilla reptans L. = *Potentilla tormentilla* Stokes • poh-ten-TILL-uh REP-tanz

Other Names: Cinquefoil, creeping cinquefoil, European five-finger, five leaf grass tormentil, biscuits, earthbank, ewe daisy, flesh and blood, septfoil, shepherd's knot

Similar Species: *Potentilla erecta* (L.) Räusch; also known as cinquefoil, tormentil, and erect cinquefoil

Family: Rosaceae

Distribution: Commonly found throughout North America, Europe, Caucasus, and West Siberia.

Parts Used: Root

Selected Constituents: Roots containing tannins (up to 20%), phlobaphene ("tormentil red"), the triterpene alcohol tormentol, a glycoside (tormentillin), starch, sugars, and a bitter compound (chinovic acid)

Clinical Actions: Astringent, tonic, hemostatic, anti-inflammatory, vulnerary, antiseptic

Energetics: Drying, astringing

History and Traditional Usage: The Latin word *tormentilla* stems from tormentum, "pain"; the herb has traditionally been used to relieve stomach pain and toothache. The root was traditionally used to reduce bowel inflammation associated with diarrhea and for mild painful menstruation and sore throat and ulcerated throat, and also as a douche in leukorrhea. The fluid extract acts as a styptic to cuts, wounds, and so forth. A strong decoction is recommended as a wash for piles and inflamed eyes. "If a piece of lint be soaked in the decoction and kept applied to warts, they will disappear" (Grieve, 1975).

De Bairacli Levy (1963) recommended tormentil for gastritis, dysentery, colic, diarrhea, bowel hemorrhage, sour stomach and intestines, and cramps, and externally for wounds, bleeding ulcers, sores, and warts.

Published Research: Potentilla has demonstrated cyclooxygenase-inhibiting activity (Tunon, 1995).

In a randomized, double-blind, placebo-controlled trial, 40 children ranging in age from 3 months to 7 years with rotavirus diarrhea were treated with tormentil root extract or placebo. All patients received 3 drops of tormentil root extract or placebo per year of life, 3 times daily, until diarrhea resolved, or for a maximum of 5 days. The duration of diarrhea in the tormentil root extract treatment group was 2 to 3 days shorter than in the control group. Eight of 20 (40%) children in the treatment group were free of diarrhea 48 hours after admission to the hospital, compared with 1 of 20 (5%) in the control group. It was concluded that the administration of tormentil root extract shortened the duration of rotavirus diarrhea and decreased the requirement for rehydration (Subbotina, 2003).

Indications: Astringent; diarrhea (especially rotavirus diarrhea), dysentery; intestinal hemorrhage; externally for wounds with delayed healing, for sores and ulcers

Potential Veterinary Indications: Diarrhea, hemorrhagic enteritis, dysentery, wound healing

Contraindications: None found.

Toxicology and Adverse Effects: AHPA class 1

Dosage:

Human:

Dried herb: 1-10gTID, up to 6 times daily for acute conditions

Decoctions: 5-30g per cup of water, with 1 cup of the tea given TID, up to 6 times daily acutely

Tincture 1:2 or 1:3: 1-5mLTID, up to 6 times daily for acute conditions

Small Animal:

Dried herb: 25-300mg/kg, divided daily (optimally, TID)

Decoction: 5-30g per cup of water, administered at a rate of 1/4-1/2 cup per 10kg (20lb), divided daily (optimally, TID)

Tincture 1:2-1:3: 0.5-1.5mL per 10kg (20lb), divided daily (optimally, TID) and diluted or combined with other herbs. Higher doses may be appropriate if the herb is used singly and is not combined in a formula.

References

De Bairacli Levy J. *The Complete Herbal Handbook for Farm and Stable*. London: Faber and Faber; 1963.

De Bairacli Levy J. *The Complete Herbal Handbook for the Dog and Cat*. London: Faber and Faber; 1985.

Grieve M. *A Modern Herbal*. London: Jonathan Cape; 1931 (Reprint, 1975).

Subbotina MD, Timchenko VN, Vorobyov MM, Konunova YS, Aleksandrovih YS, Shushunov S. Effect of oral administration of tormentil root extract *(Potentilla tormentilla)* on rotavirus diarrhea in children: a randomized, double blind, controlled trial. Pediatr Infect Dis J 2003;22:706-711.

Tunon H, Olavsdotter C, Bohlin L. Evaluation of anti-inflammatory activity of some Swedish medicinal plants: inhibition of prostaglandin biosynthesis and PAF-induced exocytosis. J Ethnopharmacol 1995;48:61-76.

Prickly Ash

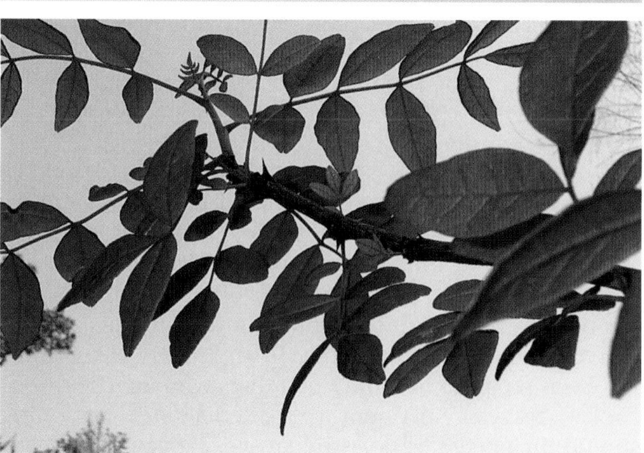

Zanthoxylum americanum Mill., formerly *Xanthoxylum fraxineum* • Zan-THOX-uh-lum am-er-ih-KAH-num

Zanthoxylum clava-herculis L. = *Xanthoxylum macrophyllum* Nutt (Southern Prickly Ash) • Zan-THOX-uh-lum KLAV-uh HER-kew-lis

Distribution: The Northern species is found from southern Canada throughout northern, central, and western United States. The Southern species is found in central and southern United States.

Similar Species: *Zanthoxylum xanthoxyloides* (African species used for rheumatism), *Zanthoxylum bungeanum* (Chinese species used for cold patterns causing abdominal pain), *Zanthoxylum capense* (African species used for colic)

Other Names: Toothache bark, Hercules' club, zahnwehgelbholz, clavalier, *Clava erculea*

Family: Rutaceae

Parts Used: Bark, sometimes berries

Selected Constituents: Amides (herclavin and others), lignans, and benzophenathridine alkaloids (chelerythrine, nitidine and others). *Z. americanum* contains coumarins.

Clinical Action: Counterirritant, topical anodyne, anti-inflammatory, antirheumatic, bitter tonic, diaphoretic, circulatory stimulant

Energetics: Pungent, warm, bitter

History and Traditional Usage: Native North Americans used the bark topically for toothaches and skin problems, and orally for colds, pain, rheumatism, cramps, heart and kidney troubles, bronchitis, and sore throat. The Cree applied the infusion to dog noses to improve scent capacity. The Pawnee used the fruit as a diuretic for horses.

Used topically and orally for rheumatism. Applied as a paste to painful teeth. Used orally for impaired circulation, hepatic congestion, mild diarrhea and gas, ascites, cystitis, and upper respiratory infection. Well known for stimulating peripheral circulation. *Cook's Physiomedical Dispensatory* considered prickly ash more warming than ginger and less so than capsicum.

Published Research: *Z. clava-herculis* was found to be highly microbicidal against methicillin-resistant *Staphylococcus* in vitro. Bowen et al (1996) examined the neuromuscular effects of various extracts of *Z. clava-herculis* in rats, rabbits, and a dog. Specific extracts appeared to exert action on neuromuscular transmission through blockade of postjunctional end plate receptors or enhanced release of neurotransmitters.
Indications: Rheumatism, leg cramps and other peripheral circulatory disorders, Raynaud's syndrome, leg ulcers
Suggested Veterinary Indications: Rheumatism, circulatory disorders
Contraindications: Pregnancy, lactation, gastric ulcer
Toxicology and Adverse Effects: AHPA class 2b. Nausea is possible in clinical patients.

Cattle have been reported to exhibit signs of toxicity after eating unspecified amounts of bark stripped from prickly ash trees (Bowen, 1996). Signs of toxicity included apparent blindness, high stepping gait, and inability to drink and to swallow. The authors prepared two extremely concentrated extracts for testing in vitro (on diaphragmatic muscle) and in vivo. The first extract preparation resulted in an unspecified volume of extract, beginning with 50 g of powdered bark. The second extract was started with 1 kg of dried powdered bark; an unspecified volume of extract resulted. These extracts were reconstituted to 10 mg/mL in methanol. When a 9.1-kg anesthetized dog was administered 2 mg and 4 mg of this extract intravenously, muscular contraction was partially inhibited. An intravenous dose of 10 mg led to a sharp decrease in blood pressure that did not resolve during the course of the experiment. The authors also instilled the extract into the eyes of rabbits and detected no topical anesthetic effect (Bowen, 1996).
Drug Interactions: None reported.
Dosage:
Human:
Dried herb: 0.25-2 g TID
Decoctions: 5-10 g per cup of water, ¼-1 cup TID
Tincture (usually 45%-70% ethanol) 1:2 or 1:3: 0.125-2 mL TID
Small Animal:
Dried herb: 25-200 mg/kg, divided daily (optimally, TID)
Decoction: 5-10 g per cup of water, administered at a rate of ¼-½ cup per 10 kg (20 lb), divided daily (optimally, TID)
Tincture (usually in 45%-70% ethanol; some pharmacies include glycerin to prevent precipitation by tannins) 1:2-1:3: 0.5-1.0 mL per 10 kg (20 lb), divided daily (optimally, TID) and diluted or combined with other herbs. Higher doses may be appropriate if the herb is used singly and it is not combined in a formula.
Historic Veterinary Doses: Fluid extract in farm animals: 15-60 mL in horses and cows; 4-12 mL in sheep and goats

Selected Reference

Bowen JM, Cole RJ, Bedell D, Schabdach D. Neuromuscular effects of toxins isolated from southern prickly ash *(Zanthoxylum clava-herculis)* bark. Am J Vet Res 1996;57:1239-1244.

Rehmannia

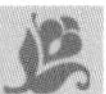

Rehmannia glutinosa Libosch. Ex Fisch and Mey = *Rehmannia glutinosa* Steud. • re-MAN-nee-uh gloo-tin-OH-suh
Distribution: East Asia
Similar Species: None identified that are used medicinally.
Common Names: Chinese foxglove, di huang, sheng di huang (raw root of rehmannia), shu di huang (cured root of rehmannia), shojio (Japanese), saengjihwang (Korean)
Family: Scrophulariaceae
Parts Used: Root
Selected Constituents: Bitter constituents (iridoids, including ajugol, rehmanniosides), phenylethanoid glycosides (verbascoside, echinacoside), sugars, sterols, etc.
Clinical Action: Antioxidant, aperient, bitter tonic, anti-inflammatory, antipyretic, antibacterial, diuretic, hepatoprotectant
Energetics:

- Sheng Di Huang—sweet, slightly bitter, cold (uncured/raw)
- Shu Di Huang—sweet, slightly warm (cured/cooked)

Enters kidney, heart, and liver meridians.
History and Traditional Usage: This herb was used primarily in Oriental medicine, and its traditional usage must be described in the language of that system. Rehmannia clears heat, cools blood, nourishes *Yin,* generates fluids, and cools upward blazing of Heart Fire. It is used for treatment in all warm-febrile diseases in which heat pathogens cause high fever, thirst, and a very red tongue. Also used for hemorrhage caused by heat entering the Blood level. For *Yin* deficiency with Heat signs and for injury to bodily fluids. Signs include continuous low-grade fever, dry mouth, constipation, and throat pain. For mouth and tongue sores, irritability, insomnia, skin rash, afternoon or low-grade fever, and malar flush. An important indication is "thirsting and wasting" disorder (often characteristic of diabetes mellitus and chronic renal failure). Contraindicated in Spleen deficiency with Dampness and *Yang* deficiency. Also contraindicated in pregnancy with blood deficiency or Spleen or Stomach deficiency.

In Western terms, Sheng Di Huang is indicated in the treatment of fever, bleeding, rash, and diabetes mellitus. Shu Di Huang is used to regulate menstrual disorders caused by blood deficiency, to enhance production of blood, and to treat patients with anemia, dizziness, weakness, tinnitus, amenorrhea, and metrorrhagia.
Published Research: In laboratory animal studies, administration of the root seemed to reverse adrenal hormone production and morphologic changes associated with long-term steroid administration.

Kidney disease

In a study in which acute renal failure was induced in rats in an ischemia-reperfusion model, rehmannia root extract improved creatinine clearance, urine sodium excretion, and urine osmolality. In addition, administration of rehmannia influenced expression of certain renal electrolyte and fluid transport channels (Kang, 2005). In a diabetic nephropathy rat model, rehmannia extract reduced increases in BUN and glucose, as well as histopathologic changes in kidneys (Yokozawa, 2004).

In a Chinese case series, a combination of astragalus and rehmannia may have improved the clinical status of people with chronic nephritis, with significant improvement observed for 91% of the treatment group compared with 67% of the control group (Su, 1993). The classical formula liu wei di huang enhanced renal blood flow and reduced hypertension in rats (Li, 1974).

Diabetes

Rats rendered hyperglycemic through various means were administered rehmannia extract and experienced lower blood glucose levels (Zhang, 2004a). The authors found that an extract high in stachyose was most effective (Zhang, 2004b).

Atopic dermatitis

In humans and dogs, formulas that contain rehmannia reduce pruritus and other signs of atopic dermatitis. The human formula contained 10 herbs, including rehmannia, and was called zemaphyte. The veterinary formula consisted of three herbs: *Rehmannia glutinosa,* white peony *(Paeonia lactiflora),* and licorice *(Glycyrrhiza glabra).* Investigators at the University of Minnesota studied 50 atopic dogs in a randomized, double-blind, placebo-controlled trial (Nagle, 2001). Dogs were given the formula just described or a placebo that contained dextrose and food coloring; they were assessed by veterinarians and owners. In all, 37.5% of the herb group improved, compared with 13% of the placebo group, but this was not a statistically significant difference. Deterioration of the itch score was significantly worse in the placebo group at the final visit, and more dropouts were reported in the placebo group because of worsening of clinical signs. No significant differences were observed in surface damage, seborrhea, coat condition, or general demeanor.

Indications: Fever, anemia, rash, diabetes, dehydration, constipation, hepatitis, fatigue, and eczema. Chinese studies suggest that rehmannia alone may be useful for rheumatoid arthritis, asthma, urticaria, and chronic nephritis.

Potential Veterinary Indications: Atopic dermatitis and other dry inflammatory skin diseases, kidney disease, diabetes mellitus

Contraindications: None described, except energetic (see Indications, earlier)

Toxicology and Adverse Effects: AHPA class 2d. Contraindicated with diarrhea and indigestion. Safe—generally used over the long term, usually in formulas. Diarrhea was described in a small number of subjects in Chinese studies.

Drug Interactions: None reported.

Dosage:

Human:

Dried herb: 1-10 g TID

Decoctions: 5-30 g per cup of water, with 1 cup of the tea given TID

Tincture (usually 25%-35% ethanol) 1:2 or 1:3: 1.5-5 mL TID

Small Animal:

Dried herb: 50-400 mg/kg, divided daily (optimally, TID)

Decoction: 5-30 g per cup of water, administered at a rate of ¼-½ cup per 10 kg (20 lb), divided daily (optimally, TID)

Tincture (usually 25%-35% ethanol) 1:2-1:3: 1.0-2.0 mL per 10 kg (20 lb), divided daily (optimally, TID) and diluted or combined with other herbs. Higher doses may be appropriate if the herb is used singly and is not combined in a formula.

References

Kang DG, Sohn EJ, Moon MK, Lee YM, Lee HS. Rehmannia glutinose ameliorates renal function in the ischemia/reperfusion-induced acute renal failure rats. Biol Pharm Bull 2005;28:1662-1667.

Li CP. *Chinese Herbal Medicine.* Washington, DC: US Department of Health, Education, and Welfare, Public Health Service, National Institutes of Health; 1974:21-23. DHEW Publication No. (NIH)76-732.

Nagle TM, Torres SM, Horne KL, Brover R, Stevens MT. A randomized, double-blind, placebo-controlled trial to investigate the efficacy and safety of a Chinese herbal product (P07P) for the treatment of canine atopic dermatitis. Vet Dermatol 2001;12:265-274.

Su ZZ, He YY, Chen G [Clinical and experimental study on effects of man-shen-ling oral liquid in the treatment of 100 cases of chronic nephritis.] Zhongguo Zhong Xi Yi Jie He Za Zhi 1993;13:269-272, 259-260.

Yokozawa T, Kim HY, Yamabe N. Amelioration of diabetic nephropathy by dried Rehmanniae Radix (Di Huang) extract. Am J Chin Med 2004;32:829-839.

Zhang R, Zhou J, Jia Z, Zhang Y, Gu G. Hypoglycemic effect of *Rehmannia glutinosa* oligosaccharide in hyperglycemic and alloxan-induced diabetic rats and its mechanism. J Ethnopharmacol 2004a;90:39-43.

Zhang RX, Jia ZP, Kong LY, Ma HP, Ren J, Li MX, Ge X. Stachyose extract from *Rehmannia glutinosa* Libosch. to lower plasma glucose in normal and diabetic rats by oral administration. Pharmazie 2004b;59:552-556.

Sage

Salvia officinalis L. • SAL-vee-uh oh-fiss-ih-NAH-liss

Other Names: Sage, garden sage, red sage, dalmatian sage, broad leaved sage, sawge, salbeiblätter, edelsalbei, gartensalbei, *Feuilles de sauge officinale, Feuilles de sauge commune*

Family: Lamiaceae

Similar Species: *S. officinalis* is native to the Mediterranean and was brought to North America as a garden plant; many subvarieties are now available for culinary use. *Salvia triloba* may have similar properties.

Parts Used: Leaves

Selected Constituents: Essential oil, which contains thujone, pinene, and other volatile constituents, as well as diterpene bitters, flavonoids (salvigenin, genkwanin, etc.), phenolic acids, and salviatannin (a catechin)

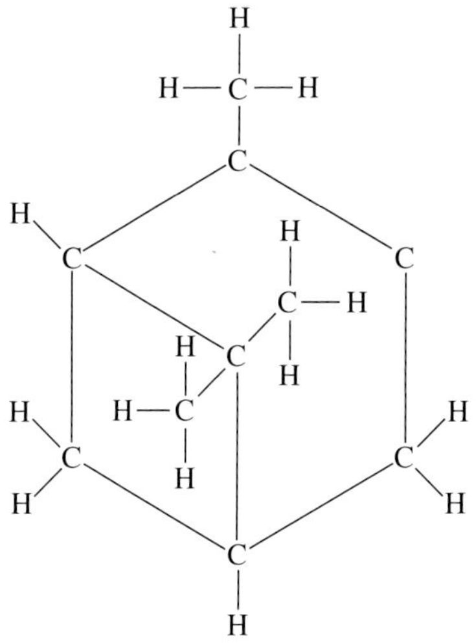

α-pinene

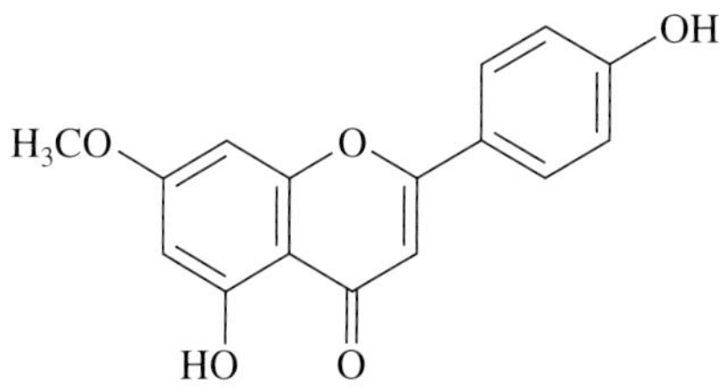

Genkwanin

Clinical Action: Carminative, antispasmodic, anti-inflammatory, antimicrobial

Energetics: Aromatic, pungent, slightly bitter

History and Traditional Usage: Native North American tribes used leaves of *Salvia apiana* (white sage) for colds and cough, as an analgesic, for epilepsy and miscellaneous other disorders, and for flavorings. From *King's:* "Sage is feebly tonic, astringent, expectorant, and diaphoretic, and has properties common to aromatics." It was used as a diaphoretic in fever, as a carminative in some cases of flatulence, as a gargle for sore and inflamed throat, as an anthelmintic, and as an anaphrodisiac (to suppress sexual desire). A specific indication was to enhance circulation.

Titus (1865) mentioned a sage tea drench as a remedy for colic in horses. He recommended that it should be strong tea and should (incidentally) contain 1 oz paregoric for every quart of tea.

Published Research: Hubbert (2006) investigated the efficacy of a *Salvia officinalis* extract spray in the treatment of people with acute viral pharyngitis. With the use of a visual analogue scale, 286 people rated their throat pain after application of salvia spray or placebo in this randomized, double-blind trial. Various concentrations of the extract were investigated, and the 15% salvia spray was found to be significantly more effective than placebo in reducing throat pain. Minor adverse effects were observed, including a dry throat or mild burning.

A placebo-controlled, parallel-group trial in 42 patients with Alzheimer's disease showed that *S. officinalis* improved cognition (Akhondzadeh, 2003). Drugs that inhibit the degradation of acetylcholine in synapses are effective in reducing the destruction of neurons in this disease. Sage has cholinergic binding capacity in vitro (Akhondzadeh, 2003).

The essential oil of another species, *S. lavandulaefolia* (Spanish sage), has been tested in two controlled trials. It improved memory in 24 healthy young humans in a double-blind, placebo-controlled, crossover trial (Tildesley, 2003). Subjects in a second trial reported that they felt more calm, contented, and alert (Tildesley, 2005).

Water extracts of *Salvia officinalis* demonstrated hepatoprotective effects against azathioprine-induced hepatotoxicity in rats (Amin, 2005).

Indications: Pharyngitis, gingivitis, stomatitis; topically for wounds; gastrointestinal disorders such as flatulence, diarrhea, enteritis. May improve memory. Suppresses sweating and lactation

Potential Veterinary Indications: Stomatitis, gingivitis, flatulence, diarrhea, cognitive dysfunction, adjunct to azathioprine treatment

Contraindications: Pregnancy, may induce uterine contractions; lactation, unless drying off is desired

Toxicology and Adverse Effects: AHPA class 2b, 2d. Large doses or prolonged use may lead to tachycardia, hot flashes, seizures, and dizziness. Approved by the US Food and Drug Administration (FDA) as GRAS (generally recognized as safe) for flavoring. Sage leaf contains thujone, which may be neurotoxic with long-term use of very high doses.

Drug Interactions: None described.

Dosage:

Human:

Dried herb: 1-10 g TID

Essential oil: 1-3 drops TID

Infusion: 5-30 g per cup of water, with 1 cup of the tea given TID

Tincture (usually 40%-60% ethanol) 1:2 or 1:3: 0.25-5 mL TID

Small Animal:

Dried herb: 25-200 mg/kg, divided daily (optimally, TID)

Infusion: 5-30 g per cup of water, administered at a rate of ¼-½ cup per 10 kg (20 lb), divided daily (optimally, TID)

Tincture (usually 40%-60% ethanol) 1:2-1:3: 0.5-1.0 mL per 10 kg (20 lb), divided daily (optimally, TID) and diluted or combined with other herbs. Higher doses may be appropriate if the herb is used singly and is not combined in a formula.

Notes of Interest: Smudging is used by Native Americans for purification of people or spaces. Smudge sticks (used more by non-Natives) are tight bundles of herbs—usually sage, but others such as wormwood, lavender, and rosemary may be used—that may be stored in drawers or closets, or burned. (Note: The common Western sagebush is actually *Artemisia tridentata.*) Smudge sticks are usually burned during rituals for clearing. One procedure for making smudge sticks is described in *The Herbalist's Garden* (de la Tour, 2001).

References

Akhondzadeh S, Noroozian M, Mohammadi M, Ohadinia S, Jamshidi AH, Khani M. *Salvia officinalis* extract in the treatment of patients with mild to moderate Alzheimer's disease: a double blind, randomized and placebo-controlled trial. J Clin Pharm Ther 2003;28:53-59.

Amin A, Hamza AA. Hepatoprotective effects of Hibiscus, Rosmarinus and Salvia on azathioprine-induced toxicity in rats. Life Sci 2005;77:266-278. Epub 2005 Feb 17.

de la Tour S, de la Tour R. *The Herbalist's Garden.* Pownal, Vt: Storey Books; 2001.

Hubbert M, Sievers H, Lehnfeld R, Kehrl W. Efficacy and tolerability of a spray with *Salvia officinalis* in the treatment of acute pharyngitis—a randomised, double-blind, placebo-controlled study with adaptive design and interim analysis. Eur J Med Res 2006;11:20-26.

Tildesley NT, Kennedy DO, Perry EK, Ballard CG, Wesnes KA, Scholey AB. Positive modulation of mood and cognitive performance following administration of acute doses of *Salvia lavandulaefolia* essential oil to healthy young volunteers. Physiol Behav 2005;83:699-709.

Tildesley NT, Kennedy DO, Perry EK, et al. *Salvia lavandulaefolia* (Spanish sage) enhances memory in healthy young volunteers. Pharmacol Biochem Behav 2003;75:669-674.

Titus NN. *The American Eclectic Practice of Medicine, as Applied to the Diseases of Domestic Animals.* New York: Baker and Godwin; 1862. Also available online at the David Winston's Herbal Therapeutics Research homepage: http://www.herbaltherapeutics.net/DomesticAnimalDiseases.pdf

Sarsaparilla

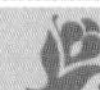

Smilax aristolochiaefolia Mille. (previously *Smilax medica* Schltdl. and Cham., or *Smilax ornata* Lem), *Smilax febrifuga, Smilax regelii* (previously *Smilax officinalis* Kunth or *Smilax utilis* Hemsl.) • SMIL-aks ah-rist-o-lo-kee-uh FOL-ee-uh

Distribution: *Smilax* species are distributed worldwide.

Similar Species: *Smilax china, Smilax febrifuga, Smilax cordifolia, Smilax tonduzii, Smilax glauca*

Other Names: Gray sarsaparilla, Mexican sarsaparilla, Santa Cruz sarsaparilla *(S. aristolochiofolia),* Ecuadorian sarsaparilla *(S. febrifuga),* Jamaican sarsaparilla, Honduran sarsaparilla, brown sarsaparilla *(S. regelii).* Also, sarsaparille, salsepareille, zarzaparrilla, salsapariglia, maghrabi, ashbah, salasá. Species local to southeastern United States are commonly called catbriar and greenbriar.

Family: Smilacaceae

Parts Used: Rhizome. The rhizome can be dug at any time because the plant is evergreen. It is difficult to follow the underground stems to the rhizome; subsequently, it is difficult to dig it out!

Selected Constituents: Steroid saponins (1%-3%)—various species contain sapogenin, smilagenin, diosgenin; flavonoids, phytosterols (beta-sitosterol, epsilon sitosterol), organic acids, starch, and resin.

Sarsaspogenin

Clinical Action: Alterative, antirheumatic, diaphoretic, diuretic

Energetics: Pungent, sweet; transforms phlegm.

History and Traditional Usage: Native North Americans used various *Smilax* species for rheumatism and kidney and stomach trouble, as a tonic, and topically for sores and scratches; the root was also used to make breads. *Smilax lancaefolia* is a South and Central American species used by indigenous peoples as a blood tonic and for fatigue, anemia, rheumatism, and skin conditions. The Eclectics used the plants as alteratives for various chronic skin disorders such as psoriasis, as well as for other chronic problems such as rheumatoid arthritis, rheumatism, hepatic disorders, and syphilis.

Published Research: Laboratory animal studies on *Smilax glabra* (Chinese sarsaparilla) suggest that an aqueous extract is capable of modulating inflammation in adjuvant-induced arthritis (Jiang, 2003). The aqueous extract of *S. china* L. demonstrated significant antinociceptive and anti-inflammatory effects compared with controls in rats; it works in part by inhibiting cyclooxygenase (COX)-2 activity and COX expression (Shu, 2005).

Sitosterol in *Smilax* species may reduce cholesterol absorption from the gastrointestinal tract (Fernandez, 2005). Sarsaparilla root extract (2.4 g/day) reduced serum urea in patients with nephritis and healthy patients, possibly because of increased excretion of urea. Symptoms of uremia were alleviated (Rittman, 1930).

Indications: Psoriasis, inflammatory skin disorders, rheumatism, hypercholesterolemia, possibly kidney disorders

Suggested Veterinary Indications: Atopic dermatitis and other chronic inflammatory skin disorders, rheumatism, hypercholesterolemia

Contraindications: None described, although higher than recommended doses are to be avoided in pregnancy.

Toxicology and Adverse Effects: AHPA class 1. Generally recognized as safe (GRAS) for flavoring alcoholic beverages and root beer. Adverse reactions are rare but are reported by the German Commission E to include gastrointestinal irritation, occupational asthma, skin irritation, and temporary kidney impairment; *The Botanical Safety Handbook* notes that this is unsubstantiated.

Drug Interactions: This herb may promote absorption of bismuth and cardiac glycosides. It may also enhance excretion of hypnotics, but none of these interactions has been demonstrated.

Dosage: The action of this herb is slow, and it is often used for weeks to months before clinical effects are expected.

Human:

Dried herb: 1-10 g TID

Decoctions: 5-30 g per cup of water, with 1 cup of the tea given TID

Tincture (ethanol percentage ranges from 20%-60%; doses are significantly higher for low-alcohol preparations) 1:2 or 1:3: 1-5 mL TID

Small Animal:

Dried herb: 25-300 mg/kg, divided daily (optimally, TID)

Decoction: 5-30 g per cup of water, administered at a rate of ¼-½ cup per 10 kg (20 lb), divided daily (optimally, TID)

Tincture (usually 20%-60% ethanol, doses are significantly higher for low-alcohol preparations) 1:2-1:3: 0.5-1.5 mL per 10 kg (20 lb), divided daily (optimally, TID) and diluted or combined with other herbs. Higher doses may be appropriate if the herb is used singly and is not combined in a formula

Historical Veterinary Doses:

Farm Animals (Karreman, 2004)*:*

Fluid extract (1:1): (30-60 mL for horses and cows; 4-8 mL for sheep and goats)

References

Fernandez ML, Vega-Lopez S. Efficacy and safety of sitosterol in the management of blood cholesterol levels. Cardiovasc Drug Rev 2005;23:57-70.

Jiang J, Xu Q. Immunomodulatory activity of the aqueous extract from rhizome of *Smilax glabra* in the later phase of adjuvant-induced arthritis in rats. J Ethnopharmacol 2003; 85:53-59.

Karreman H. *Treating Dairy Cows Naturally: Thoughts and Strategies.* Paradise, Pa: Paradise Publications; 2004.

Rittman R, Schneider F. Klin Wochschr 1930;9:401-408, cited in Bone K. *Clinical Guide to Blending Liquid Herbs.* Sydney: Churchill Livingstone; 2003.

Shu XS, Gao ZH, Yang XL. Anti-inflammatory and antinociceptive activities of *Smilax china* L. aqueous extract. J Ethnopharmacol 2006;103:327-332. Epub 2006 Jan 18.

Saw Palmetto

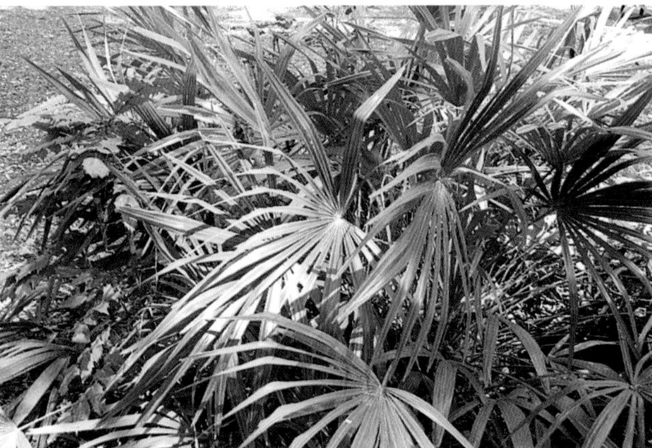

Serenoa repens (W. Bartram) Small (syn. *Serenoa serrulata* [Michx.] G. Nichols., *Sabal serrulata* [Michx] Nutt ex Schult and Schult.f.) • se-REN-oh-uh REE-penz

Common Names: Sabal fructus, sabal, sabal palm

Distribution: Indigenous to southeastern North America

Family: Arecaceae

Parts Used: Dried ripe fruit; semimature or immature fruits are typically harvested.

Selected Constituents: The berries contain fatty oil with fatty acids, esters, phytosterols, and polysaccharides.

The main constituents include carbohydrates (inverted sugar, mannitol, high-molecular-weight polysaccharides with galactose, arabinose, uronic acid), fixed oils (free fatty acids and their glycerides), steroids, flavonoids, resin, pigment, tannin, and volatile oil (Newall, 1996). The fruits and seeds are rich in triacylglycerol-containing oil (50% of the fatty acids contain 14 or fewer carbons) (Bruneton, 1995).

Clinical Actions: Urinary antiseptic, diuretic, antihyperprostatic, endocrine agent

Energetics: Warm, pungent, sweet

History and Traditional Usage: The Southern Cherokee tribes used saw palmetto berry as a food only. The medicinal value of saw palmetto berry has been reported since the 1800s, and it has been recommended for various prostatic conditions. It was an official drug that was listed in two editions of the *US Pharmacopoeia* from 1906 to 1916, and in the *National Formulary* from 1926 to 1950 (Boyle, 1991). *King's American Dispensatory* says of Saw Palmetto,

> ". . . It is said to enlarge wasted organs, as the breasts, ovaries, and testicles, while the paradoxical claim is also made that it reduces hypertrophy of the prostate . . . it has been lauded as the 'old man's friend,' giving relief from the many annoyances commonly attributed to enlarged prostate. May its results not be due to its control over urethral irritation, and thereby reducing swollen conditions not in reality amounting to hypertrophy? Besides this, it increases the tonus of the bladder, allowing a better contraction and more perfect expulsion of the contents of that viscus. Thus, it overcomes the tenesmic pain so dreaded by the sufferer" (Felter, 1898).

In Europe, phytotherapeutic agents have long been used in the treatment of patients with benign prostatic hyperplasia (BPH). French researchers in the 1960s began to examine the chemical composition of the saw palmetto berry. A breakthrough was the development of the proprietary lipophilic (fat-soluble portion) extract of saw palmetto berries (Permixon; Pierre Fabre, France). Rich in fatty acids and sterols, lipophilic (also called liposterolic) extracts of saw palmetto berries are currently approved by the French and German governments for the treatment of patients with BPH (Brown, 1996; Tyler, 1993).

Published Research: Saw palmetto has been reported to contain diuretic, urinary antiseptic, endocrinologic, and anabolic properties (Newall, 1996). The liposterolic extract has been subject to many open and double-blind clinical trials; however, the galenical forms of saw palmetto such as extracts and tinctures should not be discounted.

Spasmolytic effects of a lipid extract from saw palmetto fruits were demonstrated in vitro in rat uterus (Gutierrez, 1996) and may be partially due to interference with intracellular calcium mobilization or to activity on ion exchange pumps.

Anti-inflammatory effects were investigated. Ethanol extract of saw palmetto (5.0 g/kg) inhibited edema in rats (Hiermann, 1989); a carbon dioxide extract of the fruit inhibited cyclooxygenase and 5-lipoxygenase in vitro. These inhibitory effects may explain the in vivo anti-inflammatory and antiedema activities of the lipophilic saw palmetto extract (Breu, 1992).

A polysaccharide fraction of saw palmetto isolated from the fruit and given intraperitoneally to mice (10 mg/kg) showed significant immunostimulating activity (Wagner, 2002). An increased rate of phagocytosis by human polymorphonuclear leukocytes was observed in cells treated with the extract (Wagner, 2002).

Prostatic disease

A systematic review of the literature assessed the effects of *Serenoa repens* in the treatment of patients with BPH. A total of 3369 men from 24 randomized trials that lasted 4 to 48 weeks were evaluated. *Serenoa repens* was superior to placebo in urinary symptom scores, clinical symptoms, and flow measures. Evidence shows that saw palmetto provided mild to moderate improvement in urinary symptoms and flow measures, comparable with finasteride, but caused fewer adverse events (Wilt, 2006). A more recent randomized, double-blind, placebo-controlled trial found no effects when saw palmetto was used for 1 year in 225 men with moderate to severe symptoms of BPH (Bent, 2006).

Two review articles (Koch, 1994; Niederprum, 1994) explored the 5α-reductase–inhibiting properties of the free fatty acids in saw palmetto berry. This action is critical to the herb's activity with respect to BPH. The pathogenesis of BPH is linked to the accumulation of dihydrotestosterone (DHT), the active form of testosterone (T), in prostatic tissue. 5α-Reductase is involved in the conversion of free testosterone to 5α-dihydrotestosterone (DHT), which is 5 times more potent than testosterone. Inhibitors of 5α-reductase (such as the drug finasteride) block this conversion and have been found to reduce the size of the prostate, leading to an increase in peak urinary flow rate and a reduction in symptoms (Farmer, 1997). The fruit of saw palmetto has been shown in vitro to inhibit the 5α-reductase and aromatase enzymes that are significant in the development of BPH (Koch, 1994), perhaps accounting for its action. This action was confirmed in vivo in growing pigs. Kinetic parameters of porcine 5α-reductase in the presence of *Serenoa repens* extracts revealed uncompetitive, noncompetitive, and mixed types of inhibition. Results showed the inhibitory action of *S. repens* on prostatic porcine microsomal 5α-reductase activity (Palin, 1998).

Effects on canine prostatic hyperplasia

A total of 20 mature male dogs with BPH were assigned to one of three comparable groups and were treated with 500 mg saw palmetto po TID or 100 mg TID, or they were given no treatment. Prostatic volume, prostatic weight, prostatic histologic characteristics, radiographic and ultrasonographic assessments of prostatic size, complete blood count (CBC) results, serum biochemical analyses, urinalysis, serum testosterone concentration, and semen characteristics were determined before and after 91 days of treatment, by investigators who were blinded to the treatment groups. Although no adverse effects were observed, no positive effect could be discerned in either saw palmetto treatment group (Barsanti, 2000). One criticism of this study is that the dogs were free of clinical signs from the outset, and saw palmetto may have effects other than on prostate size (such as on urethral function and urine flow parameters).

Indications: Commission E approved the internal use of saw palmetto berry for urination problems in BPH stages I and II. May also be used for testicular atrophy

Potential Veterinary Uses: Potential therapy in prostate disorders such as prostatitis and BPH; interstitial cystitis in cats; spasmolytic effect for pain of dysuria

Contraindications: None known

Toxicology and Adverse Effects: AHPA class 1. In humans, rare cases of gastritis. In acute toxicity studies conducted on the mouse, rat, and dog over 13 to 26 weeks, the LD_{50} could not be determined. With intraperitoneal injection at a dose of 1080 mg/kg, the rat exhibited signs of depression, dyspnea, and greasy fur; however, the rat and the dog given oral doses of 50 g/kg and 10 g/kg, respectively, exhibited no clinical signs. The authors concluded that the LD_{50} should be considered higher than these doses (Bombardelli, 1997).

Potential Drug Interactions: None known. Theoretical concerns exist regarding concurrent use of drugs with sex hormone–like effects.

Dosage:

Human:

Dried herb: 3-10 g TID

Liposterolic extract standardized to 85%-95% fatty acids and sterols: 320 mg once per day

Tincture (usually 45%-80% ethanol) 1:2 or 1:3: 1-5 mL TID

Small Animal:

Dried herb: 25-400 mg/kg, divided daily (optimally, TID)

Tincture (usually 45%-80% ethanol) 1:2-1:3: 0.5-2.0 mL per 10 kg (20 lb), divided daily (optimally, TID) and diluted or combined with other herbs. Higher doses may be appropriate if the herb is used singly and is not combined in a formula.

References

Barsanti JA, Finco DR, Mahaffey MM, et al. Effects of an extract of *Serenoa repens* on dogs with hyperplasia of the prostate gland. Am J Vet Res 2000;61:880-885.

Bent S, Kane C, Shinohara K, Neuhaus J, Hudes ES, Goldberg H, Avins AL. Saw palmetto for benign prostatic hyperplasia. N Engl J Med 2006;354:557-566.

Bombardelli E, Marrazzoni M. Unpublished research conducted at the University of Pavia, 1997. Provided by Indena Corp, Milan, Italy.

Bone K. Saw palmetto—a critical review, part 2. MediHerb Professional Review 1998;61:1-4.
Boyle W. *Official Herbs: Botanical Substances in the United States Pharmacopoeias 1820-1990.* East Palestine, Ohio: Buckeye Naturopathic Press; 1991.
Breu W, Hagenlocher M, Redl K, Tittel G, Stadler F, Wagner H. Anti-inflammatory activity of sabal fruit extracts prepared with supercritical carbon dioxide: in vitro antagonists of cyclooxygenase and 5-lipoxygenase metabolism. Arzneimittelforschung 1992;42:547-551.
Brown DJ. *Herbal Prescriptions for Better Health.* Rocklin, Calif: Prima Publishing; 1996:167-172.
Bruneton J. *Pharmacognosy, Phytochemistry, Medicinal Plants.* Paris: Lavoisier Publishing; 1995.
Farmer A, Noble J. Drug treatment for benign prostatic hyperplasia. BMJ 1997;314:1215-1216.
Felter HW, Lloyd JU. *King's American Dispensatory,* vols 1, 2. Portland, Ore: Eclectic Medical Publications [reprint of 1898 original]; 1985:1750-1752.
Gutierrez M, Hidalgo A, Cantabrana B. Spasmolytic activity of a lipidic extract from *Sabal serrulata* fruits: further study of the mechanisms underlying this activity. Planta Med 1996;62:507-511.
Hiermann A. [The contents of sabal fruits and testing of their anti-inflammatory effect.] Arch Pharm (Weinheim) 1989;322:111-114.
Koch E, Biber A. Pharmacological effects of Sabal and Urtica extracts as a basis for a rational medication of benign prostatic hyperplasia. Urologe 1994;34:3-8.
Newall CA, Anderson LA, Phillipson JD. *Herbal Medicines: A Guide for Health-Care Professionals.* London: The Pharmaceutical Press; 1996.
Niederprum HJ, Schweikert HU, Zonker KS. Testosterone 5-α-reductase inhibition by free fatty acids from *Sabal serrulata* fruits. Phytomedicine 1994;1:127-133.
Palin MF, Faguy M, LeHoux JG, Pelletier G. Inhibitory effects of *Serenoa repens* on the kinetic of pig prostatic microsomal 5alpha-reductase activity. Endocrine 1998;9:65-69.
Tyler VE. *The Honest Herbal.* 3rd ed. New York: Pharmaceutical Products Press; 1993:285-287.
Wagner H, Proksch A, Riess-Maurer I, et al. *Serenoa repens* for benign prostatic hyperplasia. Cochrane Database Syst Rev 2002;3:CD001423.
Wilt T, Ishani A, Mac Donald R. *Serenoa repens* for benign prostatic hyperplasia. Cochrane Database Syst Rev 2006;2.

Schisandra

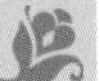

Schisandra chinensis (Turcz.) Baill. • shiz-AN-druh chi-NEN-sis

Other Names: Schisandra, Schizandra, Chinese magnolia vine, wu wei zi

Family: Schisandraceae

Parts Used: Fruit and seed

Distribution: Indigenous to China. Schisandra is a member of the magnolia family, with many variants growing in the United States, Korea, Japan, and Russia.

Selected Constituents: Gomisins (dibenzocyclooctane lignans), schisandrins (dibenzocyclooctane lignans)

Gomisin A

Gomisin G

Clinical Actions: Hepatoprotective, adaptogenic, antitussive, nervine tonic, antioxidant; enhances phase I/II detoxification

Energetics: Warm, sweet, sour

History and Traditional Usage: Schisandra has a long history of use in China, where it has been used to support the kidneys and lungs and as a sedative. It was valued for its ability to promote a youthful appearance and as a sexual tonic. In Russia, it has been used as an adaptogen to enhance the body's ability to fight disease and stress due to various causes. It has also been used traditionally for coughing and wheezing, spontaneous sweating, chronic diarrhea, and insomnia. Schisandra has been reported to enhance human endurance and mental and physical performance and to improve the sensitivity of sight, hearing, and touch.

Published Research: In mature rabbits, schisandra increased RNA, glycogen, and enzymes in the kidneys and gonads, returning these values to those of 3-month-old rabbits. It also increased the numbers of reproductive cells in males and females (Peng, 1989). Oral administration of schisandra tincture improved the working capacity of mice (Azizov, 1998).

In a randomized, double-blind, crossover study, 18 healthy horses were given a single dose of schisandra concentrate (equivalent to about 50g dried berries, containing 1.2% schisandrins) or placebo 30 minutes before exercising. For race horses, the exercise consisted of an 8-minute race over 5.6km. Show-jump horses were taken over a 700-m obstacle course with 12 jumps. Treatment with schisandra reduced heart rate and respiratory frequency, increased plasma glucose, and decreased lactate levels in both exercise groups, although the effects were more marked in the race horse group. Schisandra-treated show-jump horses completed the circuit in a shorter time than did controls (Hancke, 1994).

In an earlier study involving thoroughbred horses, a single dose of extract equivalent to 192 g schisandra fruit produced similar results to those described in the previous study. The race horses ran on average 1.8 seconds faster over 800 m (Ahumada, 1989). It was hypothesized that schisandra may cause a lower rate of lactate synthesis by muscle tissue under anaerobic conditions; it may also stimulate lactate clearance by the liver. Significant reductions in serum levels of glutamic pyruvic transaminase (GPT), glutamic oxaloacetic transaminase (GOT), and creatine kinase were observed in poorly performing horses at days 7 and 14 after oral administration of standardized schisandra extract ($P < .01\text{-}.05$) compared with baseline values. Horses selected for the trial had persistently high enzyme levels. Horses treated with placebo did not experience significant reductions in any enzyme (Hancke, 1996).

Research has focused on the potential for gomisins contained in schisandra to support and enhance liver health (Maeda, 1985; Kubo, 1992). Studies indicate that they may be effective in protecting the liver from toxins, and they may stimulate liver repair (Shiota, 1996; Ohtaki, 1996). Related studies have suggested that schisandra lignoids may aid in the treatment of patients with certain types of hepatitis. In a controlled trial in patients with chronic viral hepatitis, 68% of the people who received schisandra extract (60-100 mg, corresponding to 1.5 g fruit) showed normalized serum GPT levels after 4 weeks compared with 44% of patients treated on average for 8 weeks with a liver extract and vitamin E control. After withdrawal of treatment, GPT remained at normal levels. Improvement in other liver function parameters was less pronounced. Schisandra was also effective in relieving symptoms of sleeplessness, fatigue, abdominal tension, and diarrhea. Four patients who were given schisandra developed mild and transient nausea, headache, and stomach upset (Hikino, 1984).

Nitric oxide (NO) may be a marker for the level of adaptation to heavy exercise. In athletes, the effect of schisandra on the concentration of nitric oxide in saliva was investigated in a randomized, double-blind, placebo-controlled study. Schisandra extract (182.2 mg, standardized to contain 6.2 mg schisandrins) or placebo was administered daily for 8 days. Schisandra significantly increased the basal level of salivary NO compared with placebo ($P < .05$). It was suggested that schisandra induced an increase in physical performance by stimulating NO production (Panossian, 1999).

Effects of schisandra on the growth and immunization of male chicks were investigated. It was added to the basal diet at 1% levels; the control was the basal diet supplemented with 50 mg/kg bacitracin zinc (BZ). Body weights were recorded at 1, 21, and 42 days after hatching. The birds were vaccinated against Newcastle's disease (ND) at 21 days of age and at 49 days of age. Serum antibody titers of the schisandra group were significantly increased in contrast to controls on day 21 or 28 after the first vaccine, which suggested that schisandra could augment antibody formulation. Compared with controls, antibody titers in the Schisandra group were higher after the second vaccination (Ma, 2003).

Indications: Acute or chronic liver disease, including hepatitis, chemical liver damage, and poor liver function; to improve mental, physical, and sensory performance and resistance to the effects of stress; for nervous system disorders

Potential Veterinary Indications: Acute or chronic liver disease, including hepatitis, chemical liver damage, and poor liver function; for improving sports performance; as adjunct to vaccination; to improve fertility

Contraindications: In Traditional Chinese Medicine, schisandra is contraindicated in the early stages of cough or rash and with excessive heat patterns (Bensky, 1986). Schisandra is used during late pregnancy to promote childbirth. This would imply caution for its use in early pregnancy, although no adverse effects have been documented.

Toxicology and Adverse Effects: AHPA class 1. Rare occurrences of appetite suppression, stomach upset, and urticaria have been reported. Oral LD_{50} values include >21 g/kg (Schisandra extract, standardized to 2% schisandrins) in rats (Burgos, 1999). No toxicity was observed in pigs after oral intake of schisandra extract (2% schisandrins) for 90 days at daily doses of 0.07 to 0.72 g/kg. No embryotoxic effects were observed in rats or mice after oral dosages of 0.1 to 0.5 g/kg (Hanke, 1999).

Potential Drug Interactions: Although no interactions have been documented, the potential for drug–herb interactions with corticosteroid medications, reserpine, and drugs metabolized by the cytochrome P450 pathway has been suggested. Because schisandra enhances phase I/II metabolism, it might promote the clearance of several drugs, and caution should be exercised with those drugs that have a narrow therapeutic window, such as digoxin, coumarin, and anticonvulsants. Use of Schisandra should be discontinued about 1 week before surgery is performed.

Dosage:

Human:

Dried herb: 1-10 g TID

Infusions: 5-30 g per cup of water, with 1 cup of the tea given TID

Tincture (usually 45%-60% ethanol; some pharmacies include glycerin to prevent precipitation by tannins) 1:2 or 1:3: 1-5 mL TID

Small Animal:

Dried herb: 50-400 mg/kg, divided daily (optimally, TID)

Infusion: 5-30 g per cup of water, administered at a rate of ¼-½ cup per 10 kg (20 lb), divided daily (optimally, TID)

Tincture (usually 45%-60% ethanol; some pharmacies include glycerin to prevent precipitation by tannins) 1:2-1:3: 1.0-2.0 mL per 10 kg (20 lb), divided daily (optimally, TID) and diluted or combined with other herbs. Higher doses may be appropriate if the herb is used singly and is not combined in a formula.

References

Ahumada F, Hermosilla J, Hola R, et al. Studies on the effect of *Schizandra chinensis* extract on horses submitted to exercise and maximum effort. Phytother Res 1989;3:175-179.

Azizov AP, Seifulla RD. [The effect of elton, leveton, fitoton and adapton on the work capacity of experimental animals.] Eksperimentalnaia I Klinicheskaia Farmakologiia 1998;61:61-63.

Bensky D, Gamble A. *Chinese Herbal Medicine Materia Medica.* Seattle: Eastland Press; 1986:541-543.

Burgos RA, Hancke JL. Toxicological studies on *S. chinensis.* Fitoterapia 1999;70:451-471.

Hancke J, Burgos R, Caceres D, et al. Reduction of serum hepatic transaminases and CPK in sport horses with poor performance treated with a standardized *Schizandra chinensis* fruit extract. Phytomedicine 1996;3:237-240.

Hancke J, Burgos R, Wikman G, et al. *Schisandra chinensis,* a potential phytodrug for recovery of sport horses. Fitoterapia 1994;65:113-118.

Hikino H, Kiso Y, Taguchi H, et al. Antihepatotoxic actions of lignoids from *Schizandra chinensis* fruits. Planta Med 1984;50:213-218.

Kubo S, Ohkura Y, Mizoguchi Y, et al. Effect of gomisin A (TJN-101) on liver regeneration. Planta Med 1992;58:489-492.

Ma DY, Shan AS, Li QD, et al. Effects of Chinese medicinal herb on growth and immunization of laying chicks. J Northeast Agric Univ (English ed) 2003;10:121-125.

Maeda S, Takeda S, Miyamoto Y, Aburada M, Harada M. Effects of gomisin A on liver functions in hepatotoxic chemical–treated rats. Jpn J Pharmacol 1985;38:347-353.

Ohtaki Y, Hida T, Hiramatsu K, et al. Deoxycholic acid as an endogenous risk factor for hepatocarcinogenesis and effects of gomisin A, a lignan component of Schizandra fruits. Anticancer Res 1996;16:751-755.

Panossian AG, Oganessian AS, Ambartsumian M, et al. Effects of heavy physical exercise and adaptogens on nitric oxide content in human saliva. Phytomedicine 1999;6:17-26.

Peng GR, Xu ZQ, Zeng XG, et al. Effects of *Schisandra chinensis* on the contents of DNA, glycogen and enzymes in kidneys and gonads of rabbits. Shanghai J Tradit Chin Med 1989;2:43-45. Cited in Abstracts of Chinese Medicine 1989;3:157.

Shiota G, Yamada S, Kawasaki H. Rapid induction of hepatocyte growth factor mRNA after administration of gomisin A, a lignan component of Shizandra fruits. Res Commun Mol Pathol Pharmacol 1996;94:141-146.

Sheep Sorrel

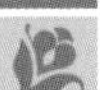

Rumex acetosella L. • ROO-meks a-see-TOE-sell-uh *or* a-kee-TOE-sell-uh

Other Names: Sour weed, field sorrel, sorrel, red weed, sour dock, sour grass, dog-eared sorrel

Family: Polygonaceae

Parts Used: Leaves, fresh and dried

Distribution: Sheep sorrel grows in pastures and dry gravelly places in most parts of the world, except the tropics; it has also been found in Arctic and Alpine regions.

Selected Constituents: Aerial parts contain rutin 0.53%, flavone glycosides (hyperoside or quercitin-3d-galactoside) 0.05%, and hyperin (12 mg/100 g), as well as vitamins C, A, B complex, D, E, K, P, and U. Also included are calcium, phosphorus, magnesium, potassium, silicon, iron, sulphur, copper, iodine, manganese, and zinc. Carotenoids, chlorophyll, organic acids (malic, oxalic, tannic, tartaric, and citric) and phytoestrogens, anthraquinones, emodin, aloe emodin, chrysophanol, rhein, and physcion are other ingredients.

Clinical Actions: Anti-inflammatory, antioxidant, laxative, diuretic

Energetics: Drying, cooling

History and Traditional Usage: Indigenous peoples of Canada and the United States have used this plant as food and medicine. The tea was also used traditionally as a diuretic and to treat patients with fever, inflammation, and scurvy (Turner, 1991). Sheep sorrel contains phytoestrogens similar to the isoflavone phytoestrogens common to red clover, licorice, and soy—all legumes known for their health restorative properties. The herb also contains several anthraquinones that are antioxidants and radical scavengers (Duke, 1985). The seeds were used occasionally for diarrhea. Southeastern folk herbalist Tommy Bass claimed that the plant was used for sore throat and topically for cancer (Crellin, 1997). Sheep sorrel is related to the tangy salad green, French sorrel, and it can be used similarly.

The plant is much enjoyed by grazing animals and is used for blood ailments, fever, and kidney ailments and externally for skin irritations (de Bairacli Levy, 1963).

Published Research: No published trials have evaluated the efficacy of sheep sorrel for any proposed claims. It is one of four components of Essiac, a proprietary tea that has been reported to demonstrate anticancer activity in vitro, although its effects in vivo remain a matter of debate. A recent study indicated that Essiac tea possesses antioxidant and DNA-protective activity—properties that are common to natural anticancer agents (Leonard, 2006).

Indications: Scurvy, vascular disorders; possibly as an alterative because of its diuretic and aperient qualities

Potential Veterinary Indications: Possibly antioxidant and alterative for chronic disorders

Contraindications: Sheep Sorrel and other plants of the Polygonaceae family contain oxalates in their fresh and cooked leaves and are contraindicated in cases of oxalate urolithiasis.

Toxicology and Adverse Effects: Sorrel leaves contain enough oxalates and anthraquinone to cause poisoning and possibly death if eaten in excessive amounts. Ruminants have been reported to be poisoned by consuming sheep sorrel *(Rumex acetosella)* in addition to other plants that are recognized poisons; these include autumn crocus *(Colchicum autumnale),* cowbane *(Cicuta virosa),* Bracken fern *(Pteridium aquilinum),* and St. John's wort *(Hypericum perforatum).* Animals died after they consumed this combination of plant intoxications (Schrader, 2001). Sheep sorrel is also a common allergen for which canines with atopic dermatitis are tested.

Drug Interactions: In large dosages, the anthraquinone-type laxative compounds may enhance the action of other laxatives and should not be taken.

Notes of Interest: *Acetosella* means vinegar salts. Sheep sorrel was considered the most active herb in Essiac for stimulating cellular regeneration, detoxification, and cleansing, according to reports by Rene Caisse, the nurse behind the famous Essiac formula that has been promoted for cancer treatment. No scientific evidence has been published to suggest that the Essiac formula has clinical efficacy; however, anecdotal evidence exists, and popularity among clients is considerable.

Dosage: This herb can be used as an occasional fresh food addition to the diet, unless high-oxalate foods are contraindicated.

Human:

Dried herb: 1-10 g TID

Infusions: 5-30 g per cup of water, with 1 cup of the tea given TID

Tincture 1:2 or 1:3: 1-5 mL TID

Small Animal:

Dried herb: 25-500 mg/kg, divided daily (optimally, TID)

Infusion: 5-30 g per cup of water, administered at a rate of ¼-½ cup per 10 kg (20 lb), divided daily (optimally, TID)

Tincture 1:2-1:3: 0.5-2.5 mL per 10 kg (20 lb), divided daily (optimally, TID) and diluted or combined with other herbs. Higher doses may be appropriate if the herb is used singly and is not combined in a formula.

References

Crellin J, Philpott J. *Reference Guide to Medicinal Plants: Herbal Medicine Past and Present.* Durham, NC: Duke University Press; 1997.

De Bairacli Levy J. *The Complete Herbal Handbook for Farm and Stable.* London: Faber and Faber; 1963.

Duke JA. *Rumex crispus* L. In: *Handbook of Medicinal Herbs.* Boca Raton, Fla: CRC Press; 1985:414-415.

Leonard SS, Keil D, Mehlman T, et al. Essiac tea: scavenging of reactive oxygen species and effects on DNA damage. J Ethnopharmacol 2006;103:288-296. Epub 2005 Oct 13.

Schrader A, Schulz O, Volker H, Puls H. [Recent plant poisoning in ruminants of northern and eastern Germany. Communication from the practice for the practice.] Berl Munch Tierarztl Wochenschr 2001;114:218-221.

Turner N, Kuhnlein H. Traditional plant foods of Canadian indigenous peoples. Nutrition, botany and use. In: *Food and Nutrition in History and Anthropology,* vol 8. Philadelphia, Pa: Gordon & Breach Science Publishers; 1991:222.

Shiitake

Lentinula edodes (Berk.) Singer • Len-TIN-ew-luh ee-DOE-deez

Other Names: Shitake, black mushroom, hua gu, fragrant mushroom

Family: Tricholomataceae

Parts Used: Fruiting body

Distribution: China, Japan, and throughout Asia. Commercially grown worldwide

Selected Constituents: Polysaccharide (lentinan), purine alkaloid (eritadenin), proteins, fatty acids, and vitamins D, B_2, and B_{12}. The proteins contain all essential amino acids, commonly occurring nonessential amino acids, and amides. The fatty acids are largely unsaturated, and shiitakes are rich in vitamins and minerals. Commercial preparations employ the powdered mycelium of the mushroom before the cap and stem grow; this is called lentinan edodes mycelium extract (LEM). LEM is also rich in polysaccharides and lignans. The most thoroughly investigated bioactive molecule isolated from shiitake is the pure β(1-3)-D-glucan lentinan. Crude mushrooms are also used in the manufacture of extracts.

Clinical Actions: Immune modulating, nutritive

Energetics: Neutral, sweet

History and Traditional Usage: Shiitake has had a long reputation as an elixir of life because of its high nutritional content (Crisan, 1978). The therapeutic importance of *L. edodes* has been known since the Ming dynasty (1368-1644). Wu Ri, a famous physician from the Chinese Ming Dynasty (AD 1368-1644), wrote extensively about this mushroom, noting its ability to increase energy, cure colds, and eliminate worms (Ito, 1978).

The Chinese have always regarded the mushroom as having special properties. Mushrooms are regarded as "spirit medicine" because they are believed to nourish the shen, or spirit. Shiitake is particularly thought to replenish *Qi* and support the spleen and stomach channels.

In Japan, lentinan is used as a popular anticancer drug and has been studied in numerous clinical trials, although none of these studies was placebo controlled or double blind (Ooi, 2000).

Published Research: In vitro and in vivo studies show that shiitake has an inhibitory effect on dental plaque. A significantly improved score was observed in rats infected with *Streptococcus mutans* and fed a cariogenic diet containing 0.25% shiitake extract compared with controls fed the cariogenic diet without shiitake extract (Shouji, 2000).

Perhaps one of the most interesting aspects of shiitake is that it is used as an alternative to antibiotics for use in animals that are used for food. Preparations of *Lentinus edodes* and a polysaccharide extract were investigated in vitro with the use of microflora from chicken ceca. The mushroom showed potential for improving microbial activity and composition in chicken ceca (Guo, 2003). This was also confirmed in vivo.

One trial compared the effects of polysaccharide extracts of *Lentinula edodes, Tremella fuciformis* (a different mushroom), and *Astragalus membranaceus* on growth performance and gastrointestinal tract organ weight in broiler chickens with an antibiotic treatment group (20 mg/kg, virginiamycin) and in nonsupplemented birds. No significant differences were discerned between the extract-supplemented groups and the antibiotic groups. Birds fed with shiitake showed greater body weight gain and lower feed conversion ratios than did those fed *Tremella* and *Astragalus* extracts. The optimal concentration for enhancing growth efficiency was 2 g/kg (Guo, 2004a).

Researchers also investigated the effects of polysaccharide extracts from *Lentinula edodes* on the cellular and humoral immune responses of *Eimeria tenella*–infected chickens. A total of 150 broiler chicks were infected with *E. tenella* and were fed the extract from 8 to 14 days of age at a dose of 1 g/kg of the diet. A significantly higher production of specific immunoglobulin (Ig)A, IgM (at days 14 and 21 post infection), and IgG (at day 21 post infection) was detected in the *Eimeria*-infected groups fed the extract than in the control group. Cecal antibody production showed a similar trend to that seen with serum antibodies (Guo, 2004b).

Another experiment was conducted to study the potential prebiotic effects of mushroom and herb polysaccharide extracts, *Lentinus edodes* extract (LenE), *Tremella fuciformis* extract, and *Astragalus membranaceus* root extract on chicken growth and the cecal microbial ecosystem, as compared with the antibiotic apramycin (APR). Extracts significantly stimulated growth of chickens infected with avian *Mycoplasma gallisepticum* and increased the number of potentially beneficial bacteria (bifidobacteria and lactobacilli), but they reduced the number of potentially harmful bacteria (*Bacteroides* spp and *Escherichia coli*). LenE was associated with the greatest quantity of cecal bifidobacteria and lactobacilli. With each increase in LenE dose, birds tended to have greater body weight gain and higher total aerobe and anaerobe counts. The numbers of predominant cecal bacteria—in particular, *E. coli,* bifidobacteria, and lactobacilli—were significantly increased with increases in the LenE dose. It was suggested that these specific mushroom and herb polysaccharide extracts are potential modifiers of intestinal microbial populations in diseased chickens (Guo, 2004c).

Alternatives to growth-promoting antibiotics in pig nutrition include nondigestible oligosaccharides or polysaccharides. Lentinan or dried *L. edodes* mycelium was added to the diet of piglets. Four groups of five newly weaned piglets received one of four diets: a control diet, a diet supplemented with 50 mg/kg of avilamycin, a diet supplemented with 0.1% of lentinan, or a diet supplemented with 5% of dried *L. edodes* mycelium powder. The diet that contained 5% dried *L. edodes* produced lower viable counts of total bacteria, *E. coli,* streptococci, and lactic acid bacteria. Luminal and mucosal effects corresponded with this finding. Acetate and butyrate concentrations in the distal jejunum were doubled—an obvious advantage when their trophic effects on enterocytes and colonocytes are considered (van Nevel, 2003).

Lentinan from *L. edodes* has also shown anticancer activity. Mice treated with a carcinogen, N-butyl-N'butanolnitrosoamine, received 5% dried, powdered Shiitake in the diet, or a control diet. One hundred percent of the control group developed urinary bladder carcinoma (10/10); the incidence was reduced to 52.9% in the experimental group (9/17) (Kurashige, 1997).

Lentinan is in clinical use (i.e., 0.5-1.0 mg lentinan/day, iv), especially in Japan and China, for adjuvant tumor therapy; clinical studies have been conducted in Asia (Lindequist, 2005). In a study of patients with advanced colorectal cancer, median survival times were 200 days in the lentinan-treated group (2 mg/week, 23 patients) and 94 days in the control group (Taguchi, 1982). In patients with stomach cancer, colon cancer, and other carcinomas, application of parenteral lentinan with chemotherapy led to prolongation of survival time, restoration of immunologic parameters, and improvements in quality of life compared with patients who were given chemotherapy alone (Hazama, 1995). In a randomized multicentric study of 89 patients with stomach cancer, median survival time in the group treated with chemotherapy and lentinan (2 mg/week, IV) was 189 days, compared with the control group (with only chemotherapy) time of 109 days (Ochiai, 1992). Supplementation of a shiitake polysaccharide extract was investigated in 62 men with prostate cancer. The open-label study monitored PSA (prostate-specific antigen) over 6 months. Results suggested that Shiitake extract was not effective in the treatment of patients with prostate cancer (deVere, 2002).

Lentinan has been tested in the treatment of patients with human immunodeficiency virus. Gordon (1998) enrolled people with HIV to be treated with lentinan (2, 5, or 10 mg of lentinan) or placebo IV. Investigators noted trends toward improvement in the CD4 count or in neutrophil activity, although these did not reach statistical significance. Adverse effects, including anaphylactoid reaction, were notable when lentinan was administered rapidly, but when it was administered intravenously over 30 minutes, it was better tolerated.

Indications: Chemotherapy support, hepatitis, human immunodeficiency virus (HIV) support

Potential Veterinary Indications: To enhance growth efficiency in food animals; immune support; adjunct to chemotherapy

Contraindications: None found.

Toxicology and Adverse Effects: AHPA class 1. Shiitake has an excellent record of safety but has been known to induce diarrhea and abdominal bloating when used in high dosages. One patient was found to have occupational allergic contact dermatitis to shiitake mushroom (Curnow, 2003). Rash, abdominal discomfort, and eosinophilia led to withdrawal of 17 of 49 patients involved in a trial to examine the possibility that shiitake may lower blood cholesterol. Subjects ingested 4 g of dried powdered herb daily (Levy, 1998). Chronic hypersensitivity pneumonitis (HP) caused by shiitake mushroom spores was diagnosed (Suzuki, 2001; Moore, 2005).

Dosage:

Human:

Dried herb: 5-30 g TID

LEM (lentinan edodes mycelium extract): intake is 1-3 g 2 to 3 times per day until the condition improves

Infusions: 5-30 g per cup of water, with 1 cup of the tea given TID

Tincture (usually 30% ethanol) 1:2 or 1:3: 1-5 mL TID

Small Animal:

Dried (and soaked) or fresh mushroom: 2-4 chopped mushrooms per 10 kg (20 lb) in food daily

Dried herb: 50-400 mg/kg, divided daily (optimally, TID)

Infusion: 5-30 g per cup of water, administered at a rate of ¼-½ cup per 10 kg (20 lb), divided daily (optimally, TID)

Tincture (usually 30% ethanol) 1:2-1:3: 1.0-2.0 mL per 10 kg (20 lb), divided daily (optimally, TID) and diluted or combined with other herbs. Higher doses may be appropriate if the herb is used singly and is not combined in a formula.

References

Crisan EV, Sands A. Nutritional value. In: Chang ST; Hayes WA, eds. *The Biology and Cultivation of Edible Mushrooms*. London: Academic Press; 1978:137-165.

Curnow P, Tam M. Contact dermatitis to Shiitake mushroom. Austral J Dermatol 2003;44:155-157.

deVere White RW, Hackman RM, Soares SE, Beckett LA, Sun B. Effects of a mushroom mycelium extract on the treatment of prostate cancer. Urology 2002;60:640-644.

Gordon M, Bihari B, Goosby E, Gorter R, Greco M, Guralnik M, Mimura T, Rudinicki V, Wong R, Kaneko Y. A placebo-controlled trial of the immune modulator, lentinan, in HIV-positive patients: a phase I/II trial. J Med 1998;29:305-330.

Guo FC, Kwakkel RP, Williams BA, et al. Effects of mushroom and herb polysaccharides, as alternatives for an antibiotic, on growth performance of broilers. Br Poult Sci 2004a;45:684-694.

Guo FC, Kwakkel RP, Williams BA, Parmentier HK, Li WK, Yang ZQ, Verstegen MW Effects of mushroom and herb polysaccharides on cellular and humoral immune responses of *Eimeria tenella*–infected chickens. Poult Sci 2004b;83:1124-1132.

Guo FC, Williams BA, Kwakkel RP, Li HS, Li XP, Luo JY, Li WK, Verstegen MW. Effects of mushroom and herb polysaccharides, as alternatives for an antibiotic, on the cecal microbial ecosystem in broiler chickens. Poult Sci 2004c;83:175-182.

Guo FC, Williams BA, Kwakkel RP, Verstegen MW. In vitro fermentation characteristics of two mushroom species, an herb, and their polysaccharide fractions, using chicken cecal contents as inoculum. Poult Sci 2003;82:1608-1615.

Hazama S, Oka M, Yoshino S, Iizuka N, Wadamori K, et al. Clinical effects and immunological analysis of intraabdominal and intrapleural injection of lentinan for malignant ascites and pleural effusion of gastric carcinoma. *Cancer Chemother* 1995;22:1595-1597.

Ito T. Cultivation of *Lentinus edodes*. In: Chang ST; Hayes WA, eds. *The Biology and Cultivation of Edible Mushrooms*. London: Academic Press; 1978:461-473.

Kurashige S, Akuzawa Y, Endo F. Effects of *Lentinus edodes, Grifola frondosa* and *Pleurotus ostreatus* administration on cancer outbreak and activities of macrophages and lymphocytes in mice treated with carcinogen, N-butyl-N'butanolnitrosoamine. Immunopharmacol Immunotoxicol 1997;19: 175-183.

Levy AM, Kita H, Phillips SF, Schkade PA, Dyer PD, Gleich GJ, Dubravec VA. Eosinophilia and gastrointestinal symptoms after ingestion of shiitake mushrooms. J Allergy Clin Immunol 1998;101:613-620.

Lindequist U, Niedermeyer THJ, Jülich WD. The pharmacological potential of mushrooms. eCAM 2005;2:285-299. Available at: http://ecam.oxfordjournals.org/cgi/content/full/2/3/285. Accessed November 2005.

Moore JE, Convery RP, Millar BC, Rao JR, Elborn JS. Hypersensitivity pneumonitis associated with mushroom worker's lung: an update on the clinical significance of the importation of exotic mushroom varieties. Int Arch Allergy Immunol 2005; 136:98-102.

Ochiai T, Isono K, Suzuki T, Koide Y, Gunji Y, Nagata M, et al. Effect of immunotherapy with lentinan on patients' survival and immunological parameters in patients with cancer. Int J Immunother 1992;8:161-169.

Ooi VEC, Liu F. Immunomodulation and anti-cancer activity of polysaccharide-protein complexes. Curr Med Chem 2000;7: 715-729.

Shouji N, Takada K, Fukushima K, Hirasawa M. Anticaries effect of a component from shiitake (an edible mushroom). Caries Res 2000;34:94-98.

Suzuki K, Tanaka H, Sugawara H, et al. Chronic hypersensitivity pneumonitis induced by Shiitake mushroom spores associated with lung cancer. Intern Med 2001;40:1132-1135.

Taguchi T, Furue H, Kimura T, Kondoh T, Hattori T, Itoh I, et al. Life-span prolongation effect of lentinan on patients with advanced or recurrent colorectal cancer. *Int J Immunopharmacol* 1982;4:271.

van Nevel CJ, Decuypere JA, Dierick N, Molly K. The influence of Lentinus edodes (Shiitake mushroom) preparations on bacteriological and morphological aspects of the small intestine in piglets. Arch Tierernahr 2003;57:399-412.

Skullcap

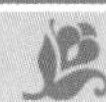

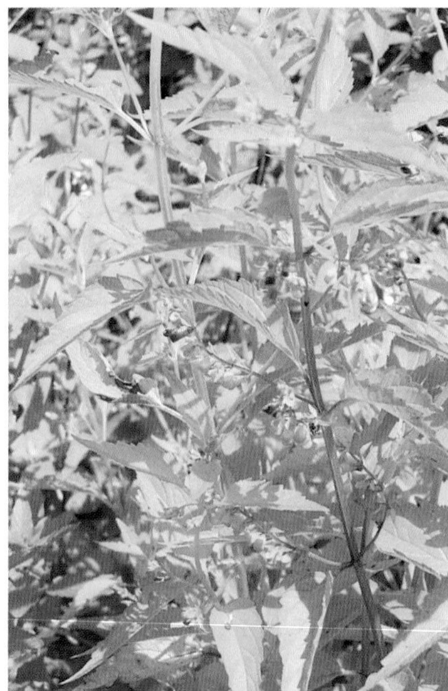

Scutellaria lateriflora L. • skew-teh-LARE-ee-uh la-ter-uh-FLOR-uh

Other Names: Hoodwort, helmut flower, scullcap, blue skullcap

Family: Lamiaceae

Parts Used: Aerial parts

Distribution: Skullcap is a perennial herb that is native to North America and is also found in Asia and Europe.

Selected Constituents: Skullcap contains flavonoids (apigenin, hispidulin, luteolin), scutellarein, scutellarin (bitter glycoside), iridoids (catalpol) and volatile oils (limonene, terpineol [monoterpenes], δ-cadinene, caryophyllene, trans-β-farnesene, and β-humulene [sesquiterpenes]); other constituents include lignin, resin, and tannin.

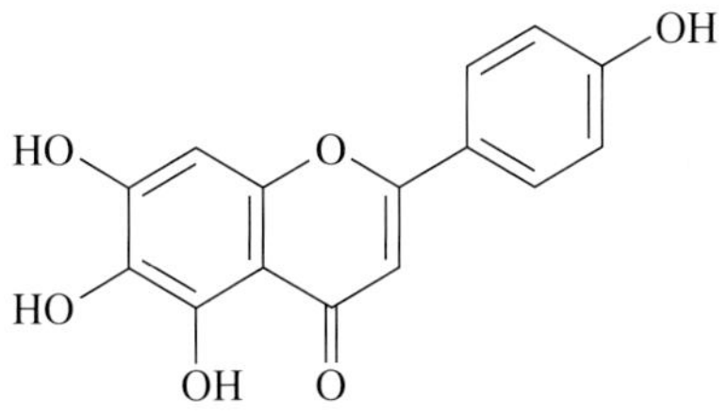

HO, HO, OH, O, O, OH

Scutellarein

Clinical Actions: Anticonvulsant, sedative, nervine, anti-inflammatory, antispasmodic, astringent, febrifuge, tonic
Energetics: Bitter, cool
History and Traditional Usage: Traditionally, skullcap has been used as a mild sedative (BHMA, 1996) and in the management of headache (Grieve, 1971). In folk medicine, it has been used to treat patients with epilepsy, chorea, hysteria, nervousness, and grand mal seizures. Skullcap has been used by Native Americans for generations, generally to treat female problems and nervous disorders.

de Bairacli Levy (1963, 1985) suggested that skullcap should be used for treatment of all patients with nervous complaints, including meningitis, fits, nervous spasm, distemper, gastroenteritis, lack of appetite, sterility, and rabies. (Note: The authors do not recommend treating any animal with rabies!)

Published Research: A double-blind, placebo-controlled study of healthy subjects demonstrated the anxiolytic effects of skullcap. Nineteen healthy people 20 to 70 years of age were supplied with separate and coded packets of four different herbal preparations (2 placebo capsules; 350-mg capsule organically grown, freeze-dried skullcap; 100-mg capsule organic, freeze-dried skullcap extract; and 2 capsules with each containing 100 mg organic, freeze-dried skullcap extract). Of the three variables (energy, cognition, and anxiety), the effect on anxiety was the most pronounced, and results were superior to those of placebo and to baseline measurements (Wolfson, 2003).

Male rats were given a single systemic injection of lithium (3 mEq/kg) and pilocarpine (30 g/kg) to induce status epilepticus. One week later, they were administered one of three herbal treatments through the water supply for 30 days; a fourth group was administered colloidal minerals and diluted food grade hydrogen peroxide in water; a fifth group of rats received only tap water as a control. Spontaneous seizures were recorded for each rat during the treatment period and during an additional 30 days, when only tap water was given. Rats given *Scutellaria lateriflora* experienced no seizures during treatment, compared with controls, which exhibited seizure activity. However, when herbal treatment was discontinued, the rats in this group and controls displayed comparable numbers of spontaneous seizures (Peredery, 2004).

The anxiolytic effects of oral *S. laterifolia* were investigated in rats through observation of behavior. Significant increases in the number of entries into the center of an "open-field arena," the number of unprotected head dips, the number of entries, and the length of time spent on the open arms of a maze test were seen, indicating reduced anxiety. Baicalin and baicalein are known to bind to the benzodiazepine site of GABA-A (gamma-aminobutyric acid) (Awad, 2003).

Indications: Epilepsy, nervous tension, insomnia, chorea
Potential Veterinary Indications: Anxiety, epilepsy, nervousness
Contraindications: None found.
Toxicology and Adverse Effects: AHPA class 1. Excessive use or overdose may cause giddiness, stupor, confusion, and seizures. Hepatotoxic reactions have been reported after ingestion of some preparations that reportedly contain skullcap. Adulteration of skullcap herb by germander has been documented in cases of hepatitis (Larrey, 1992). Germander is a known hepatotoxin.
Potential Drug Interactions: May theoretically interact with other central nervous system depressants.
Preparation Notes: Some herbalists have stated that this herb loses potency when dried; tinctures of fresh plant may be preferred.
Dosage:
Human: Last dose may be taken 30 min before bedtime and may be doubled for insomnia
Dried herb: 1-10 g TID
Infusions and decoctions: 5-30 g per cup of water, with 1 cup of the tea given TID
Tincture (usually 40% ethanol) 1:2 or 1:3: 1-5 mL TID, up to 6 times daily for acute conditions
Glycerite (80% glycerin) 1:5: 4-5 mL TID
Small Animal:
Dried herb: 25-400 mg/kg, divided daily (optimally, TID)
Infusion: 5-30 g per cup of water, administered at a rate of ¼-½ cup per 10 kg (20 lb), divided daily (optimally, TID)
Tincture (usually 40% ethanol) 1:2-1:3: 0.5-2.0 mL per 10 kg (20 lb), divided daily (optimally, TID) and diluted or combined with other herbs. Higher doses may be appropriate if the herb is used singly and is not combined in a formula.

References

Awad R, Arnason JT, Trudeau V, et al. Phytochemical and biological analysis of skullcap (*Scutellaria lateriflora* L.): a medicinal plant with anxiolytic properties. Phytomedicine 2003;10:640-649.

British Herbal Medicine Association (BHMA). *British Herbal Pharmacopoeia (BHP).* Exeter (UK): BHMA; 1996.

De Bairacli Levy J. *The Complete Herbal Handbook for Farm and Stable.* London: Faber and Faber; 1963.

De Bairacli Levy J. *The Complete Herbal Handbook for the Dog and Cat.* London: Faber and Faber; 1985.

Grieve M. *A Modern Herbal,* vol 1, 2. New York, NY: Dover Publications; 1971.

Larrey D, Vial T, Pauwels A, et al. Hepatitis after germander *(Teucrium chamaedrys)* administration: another instance of herbal medicine toxicity. Am Call Phys 1992;117:129-213.

Peredery O, Persinger MA. Herbal treatment following post-seizure induction in rat by lithium pilocarpine: *Scutellaria lateriflora* (Skullcap), *Gelsemium sempervirens* (Gelsemium) and *Datura stramonium* (Jimson Weed) may prevent development of spontaneous seizures. Phytother Res 2004;18:700-705.

Wolfson P, Hoffmann DL. An investigation into the efficacy of *Scutellaria lateriflora* in healthy volunteers. Altern Ther Health Med 2003;9:74-78.

Slippery Elm

Ulmus rubra Muhl. = *Ulmus fulva* Michx. • UL-mus REW-bruh

Distribution: Eastern Canada and the United States

Similar Species: Other species *(Ulmus glabra, Ulmus laevis, Ulmus carpinifolius)* have been used for similar purposes. Dioscorides described a species in the 1st century AD.

Other Names: Red elm, Indian elm, sweet elm, ulme, orme, olmo, rotulme

Family: Ulmaceae

Parts Used: Inner bark, which should be collected in the spring or fall

Selected Constituents: Mucilage (a mixture of polyuronides that consists of sugar and uronic acid units that form a hydrocolloid in the gut), tannins, phytosterols

Clinical Action: Demulcent, emollient, antitussive, astringent, nutritive, laxative

Energetics: Sweet, neutral

History and Traditional Usage: The inner bark and, rarely, the leaves were used by Native Americans for food, in the treatment of gastrointestinal troubles, topically for wounds and skin problems, and for sore throat and eye problems. The powder has been cooked and used for convalescing patients and weak babies. It has been used for upper respiratory tract irritation—sore throat, tracheitis, bronchitis, and dry cough; and inflammation of the gastrointestinal tract, including gastritis, gastric ulcer, colitis, and irritable bowel. It has been used topically (as a poultice) for skin inflammation, burns, and wounds; as an eyewash for styes; and as a mouthwash for patients with stomatitis. Also used for cystitis, urethritis, and other inflammatory disorders of the urinary tract.

Published Research: No relevant trials found.

Indications: Inflammatory bowel disease, diarrhea, irritable bowel syndrome, and gastrointestinal disease that is fiber responsive; dry ticklish cough; and topically for slow-healing wounds and anal fissures

Potential Veterinary Indications: Fiber-responsive gastrointestinal problems such as inflammatory bowel disease, diarrhea, constipation, and colitis; for dry cough, perianal fistulas, and anal gland abscesses; feline lower urinary tract disease; topically for burns; and as a sweetener and demulcent

Notes of Interest: Although slippery elm is not an endangered plant, United Plant Savers considers it at risk because it is not in cultivation, because it has been affected by Dutch Elm disease, and because sales of the bark have increased in recent years. Possible substitutes include psyllium, marshmallow, and fenugreek.

Contraindications: Known allergy.

Toxicology and Adverse Effects: AHPA class 1. Allergic reactions (including contact dermatitis and urticaria) possible.

Drug Interactions: As with any soluble fiber, absorption of drugs from the gut may be altered if they are administered simultaneously.

Preparation Notes: The fiber is best extracted in cold water.

Dosage:

Dried: 5-10 g TID (usually supplied as the cold infusion), up to 6 times daily for acute conditions

Infusion of powder: 5-30 g per cup of water, with 1 cup of the tea given TID, up to 6 times daily acutely

Tincture (usually 25%-30% ethanol 1:2 or 1:3: 1-5 mL TID, up to 6 times daily for acute conditions

Small Animal:

Dried herb: 50-400 mg/kg, divided daily (optimally, TID) added to moist food

Infusion of powder: 5 g per cup of cold water, administered at a rate of ¼-½ cup per 10 kg (20 lb), divided daily (optimally, TID)

Tincture (in 25%-30% ethanol) 1:2-1:3: 1.0-2.0 mL per 10 kg (20 lb), divided daily (optimally, TID) and diluted or combined with other herbs. Higher doses may be appropriate if the herb is used singly and is not combined in a formula.

St. John's Wort

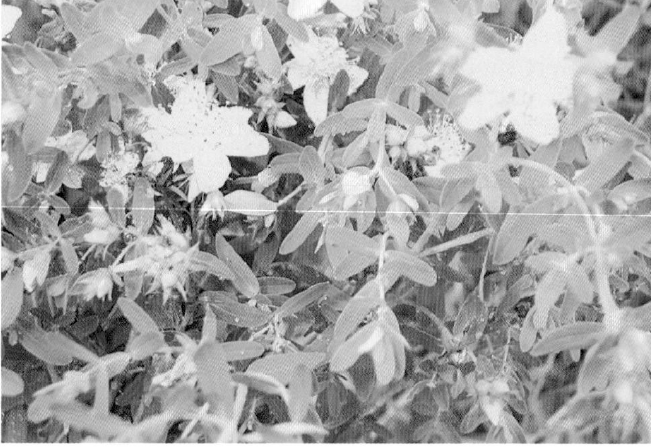

Hypericum perforatum L. • hy PER ee kum per for Ay tum

Other Names: Herba hyperici, millepertuis perforé, echtes Johanniskraut, tüpfel-Johanniskraut, iperico, erba di San Giovanni

Family: Clusiaceae

Parts Used: Dried flowering tops or aerial parts

Distribution: Indigenous to Northern Africa, South Africa, South America, Asia, Australia, Europe, and New Zealand. Naturalized in the United States (Bisset, 1994).

Selected Constituents: Major characteristic constituents include 0.05% to 0.30% naphthodianthrones (hypericin, pseudohypericin, hyperforin, adhyperforin—the latter two compounds are classified as phloroglucinols); 2% to 4% flavonoids (hyperoside, quercitrin, isoquercitrin, rutin); and 7% to 15% catechin tannins (Bisset, 1994; Nahrstedt, 1997).

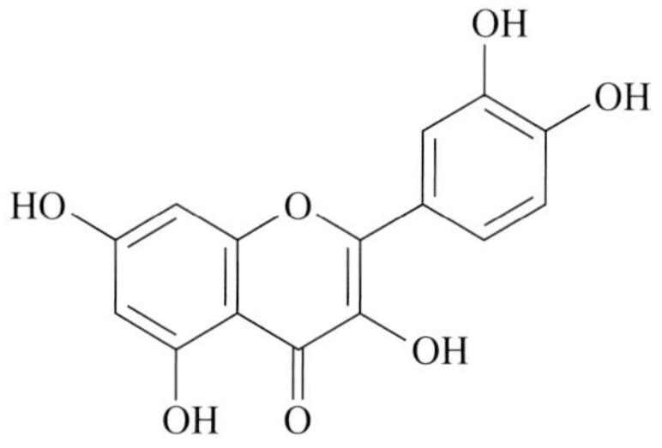

Quercetin

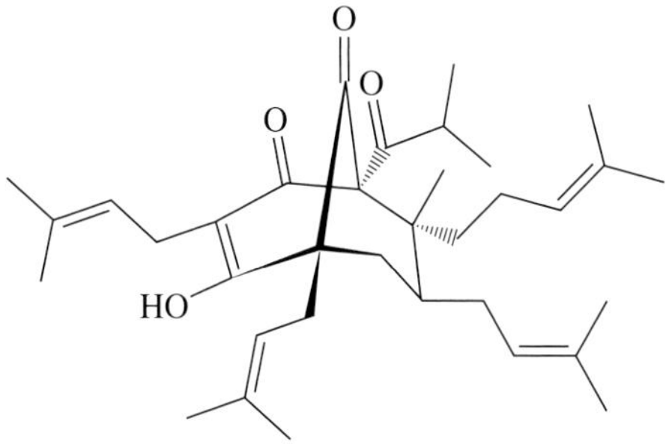

Hyperforin

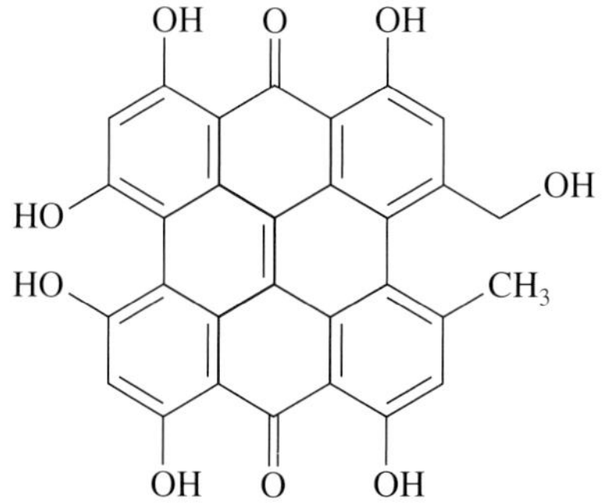

Pseudohypericin

Clinical Actions: Nervine tonic, antidepressant, vulnerary, anti-inflammatory, antiviral

Energetics: Bitter, cool

History and Traditional Usage: Uses reported in pharmacopoeias and in traditional systems of medicine: externally for the treatment of minor cuts, burns, and skin ulcers (Bombardelli, 1995; Blumenthal, 1998). Topical use for viral infection (Ivan, 1979). Aromatic, astringent, expectorant, and nervine. Used in pulmonary and bladder inflammation; hemoptysis; for worms, diarrhea, hysteria, nervous depression, neuralgia, migraine headaches, sciatica, ulcers, hemorrhage; for jaundice, biliary disorders, diabetes, hemorrhoids; as a diuretic, emmenagogue, and antimalarial agent (Farnsworth, 1998; Bombardelli, 1995; Grieves, 1975). For bedwetting children and externally for hard tumors, caked breasts, and ecchymosis (Grieves, 1975).

de Bairacli Levy (1985, 1963) suggests St. John's wort for jaundice, tail injuries (applied as a salve), and sickness in farm animals; for coughs, inflammation of the chest and lungs, rheumatism, jaundice, lymphoma, dropsy, earache, worms, and inflammation; externally for wounds, eruptions, ulcers, swellings, and skin inflammation.

Published Research: A meta-analysis published in 2005 that included 37 randomized, double-blind, controlled trials found significant positive response to St. John's wort for mild to moderate depression (Linde, 2005). Trials involved various proprietary extracts of *Hypericum perforatum;* 26 comparisons were made with placebo and 14 with synthetic standard antidepressants. St. John's wort extracts were more effective than placebo in patients with mild to moderate depression, and less so in those with major depression. No difference was noted between the clinical effects of St. John's wort and those of conventional antidepressants. Adverse effects were less commonly observed with St. John's wort than with conventional antidepressants. The authors suggest that inconsistency observed in these results may be attributed to pharmaceutical differences in the various extracts tested. Schulz (2006) reviewed 38 trials, which comprised a total of 34,804 patients, for the safety of St. John's wort. Adverse events were mild and transient in almost all cases; the major consideration for use of St. John's wort involves potential interaction with other drugs. The adverse event rate and dropout rate for St. John's wort are at least 10-fold lower than those reported for synthetic antidepressants.

Current thinking suggests that hyperforin is one of the more active constituents of St. John's wort. In vitro, hyperforin leads to nonselective inhibition of uptake of many neurotransmitters, as well as interaction with dopamine and opioid receptors. However, hyperforin levels in the brain do not mirror the concentrations that cause these changes. Hypericum extract is theorized to indirectly activate sigma receptors (Mennini, 2004). Other constituents that may be at work (Butterweck, 2003; Simmen, 2001) include amentoflavone (inhibits binding at 5-HT[1D], 5-HT [2C], D3 dopamine receptors, delta opiate receptors, and benzodiazepine receptors in vitro); I3,II8-biapigenin (inhibits in vitro binding at the estrogen-alpha receptor and the benzodiazepine receptor); other flavonoids that inhibit dopamine hydroxylase activity in vitro; hyperin (decreases malondialdehyde and nitric oxide in animal models); and pseudohypericin (inhibits activation of NMDA receptors in vitro). St. John's wort caused significant increases in salivary cortisol and plasma growth hormone in human volunteers and rats; however, it decreased plasma prolactin versus placebo. In animal studies, acute treatment with St. John's wort, hyperforin, and hypericin caused significant increases in plasma corticosterone (Franklin, 2001).

The efficacy of St. John's wort for obsessive-compulsive disorder was investigated. Twelve humans with a diagnosis of obsessive-compulsive disorder for at least 12 months were evaluated. Treatment involved 450 mg of 0.3% hypericin given twice daily for 12 weeks, and participants were monitored weekly and monthly. A significant change from baseline to endpoint occurred at 1 week and continued to increase throughout the trial. By the end of the trial, 5 of 12 patients were rated much or very much improved, 6 were minimally improved, and 1 exhibited no change. The most common adverse effects reported were diarrhea and restless sleep (Taylor, 2000).

Hyperforin may inhibit the growth of some tumor cells according to in vitro studies. The antiproliferative effects of serotonin-reuptake inhibitors and serotonin antagonists have been demonstrated in prostate tumors. One paper reported a significant reduction in tumor growth and numbers of metastases, suggesting that St. John's wort may be useful in the treatment of patients with prostate cancer (Martarelli, 2004).

Indications: Seasonal affective disorder, mild to moderate depression, menopausal depression, fibrositis, obsessive-compulsive disorder, anxiety and irritability, nervous fatigue, neuralgia; topically for wounds

Potential Veterinary Indications: Peripheral neuropathy, mild depression (e.g., associated with pain), anxiety, obsessive-compulsive disorder

Contraindications: None found.

Toxicology and Adverse Effects: AHPA class 2d (see "Potential Drug Interactions" later). Ultraviolet or prolonged exposure to sunlight should be avoided because photosensitization may occur in light-sensitive individuals (Blumenthal, 1998). St. John's wort has low toxicity; mice given 2 g/kg/day for up to 1 year showed no signs of toxic change (Okpanyi, 1990). Two case histories and a review of existing literature showed that it may cause serotonin syndrome in sensitive patients and may be associated with hair loss (Parker, 2001).

Awasi sheep given chopped St. John's wort at 0, 4, 8, 12, and 16 mg/kg in feed for 14 days were monitored for signs of poisoning. Blood samples were collected at 0, 7, and 14 days after the start of dosing. Clinical signs included restlessness, photophobia, tachycardia, polypnea, congested mucous membranes, diarrhea, and hyperthermia. Skin lesions involved redness of exposed parts of the tail and legs, edema of the eyelids, and swelling and secretions from the ears. After 1 week, signs worsened and included salivation, alopecia of the face and head, keratoconjunctivitis, severe congestion of the mucous membranes, loss of eyelashes, corneal opacity, and blindness. Hemoglobin, red cell count, packed cell volume, total protein, glucose, triglycerides, and serum alkaline phosphatase activity were all decreased. Blood urea nitrogen, sodium, potassium, and total and direct bilirubin values, as well as aspartate aminotransferase, alanine aminotransferase, lactate dehydrogenase, and γ-glutamyltransferase activities, were all increased (Kako, 1993).

The roles of shade, fleece length, and wool type in the protection of sheep from *Hypericum perforatum* poisoning (3 mg hypericin/kg body weight) were investigated. After treatment, hypericin poisoning was evident in 26.5% of woolled sheep that were exposed to sunlight, but in none of those that were fully shaded. Among recently shorn sheep, 94% showed hypericin poisoning when exposed to sunlight. It was concluded that Merinos with at least 14 weeks' wool growth are not poisoned by a single oral dose of 3 mg hypericin/kg. Because hypericin persists in the circulation for several days, this safe dose is reduced in the face of continuous daily ingestion. Sheep with access to substantial areas of shade may ingest much greater amounts of hypericin safely. Wool removal clearly increases the risk of poisoning. The ability of ruminant livestock to graze St. John's wort safely is probably better predicted by the level of skin protection against incident sunlight than by differences in hypericin metabolism and excretion capacity (Bourke, 2003).

Potential Drug Interactions: Several herb–drug interactions have been well documented for St. John's wort. A systematic review of potential St. John's wort–drug interactions was undertaken to examine trial quality and the results of these trials (Mills, 2004). Twenty-two trials of pharmacokinetics were located, 5 of which involved clinical patients, and 12 of which involved healthy volunteers. Three of 19 trials found no important drug–herb interactions; 17 noted a decrease in the systemic availability of conventional drugs.

Pharmacokinetic interactions may be the result of drug-metabolizing enzymes (P450) or drug-transporting proteins (P-glycoprotein). Clinical risk is determined by the therapeutic range of the conventional drug. Schulz (2006) has suggested that clinical interactions are relatively rare, and that they might be expected with "antidepressants, with coumarin-type anticoagulants, the immunosuppressants cyclosporine and tacrolimus, protease and reverse transcriptase inhibitors used in anti-HIV treatment, or with specific antineoplastic agents."

St. John's wort may potentiate the effects of monoamine oxidase (MAO) inhibitors. Coadministration of theophylline and St. John's wort lowered the serum level of theophylline in a patient who had been previously stabilized, requiring an increase in theophylline dose (Nebel, 1999). St. John's wort and digoxin taken together reduced serum digoxin concentrations after 10 days of treatment (Johne, 1999). Decreases in serum cyclosporine, warfarin, and phenprocoumon concentrations were seen in patients after they had additionally taken St. John's wort (Ernst, 1999). Concomitant use of St. John's wort in five patients who had been stabilized on serotonin reuptake inhibitors resulted in symptoms of central serotonin excess (Lantz, 1999). Significant drug interaction has been noted between St. John's wort and indinavir (Piscitelli, 2000).

Notes of Interest: Many ancient superstitions arose regarding this herb. Its name *Hypericum* is derived from the Greek and means "over an apparition,"—a reference to the belief that the herb was so obnoxious to evil spirits that a whiff of it would cause them to fly.

Dosage:

External Use: Oil or ointment is used for burns and minor wounds. The tincture is also used topically by some herbalists to treat human herpes lesions.

Internal Use:

Human

Dried herb: 1-10 g TID

Standardized tinctures or fluid extracts up to a daily dose of 900 mg extract (equivalent to 0.2-2.7 mg total hypericin) (Woelk, 1994). A move is growing to standardize to 2%-3% hyperforin and hypericins (0.3%)

Infusion: 5-30 g per cup of water, with 1 cup of the tea given TID, up to 6 times daily acutely

Tincture (usually 45%-60% ethanol) 1:2 or 1:3: 0.5-5 mL TID

Small Animal

Dried herb: 25-300 mg/kg, divided daily (optimally, TID)

Infusion: 5-30 g per cup of water, administered at a rate of ¼-½ cup per 10 kg (20 lb), divided daily (optimally, TID)

Tincture (usually 45%-60% ethanol) 1:2-1:3: 0.5-1.5 mL per 10 kg (20 lb), divided daily (optimally, TID) and diluted or combined with other herbs

References

Bisset NG. *Herbal Drugs and Phytopharmaceuticals.* Boca Raton, Fla: CRC Press; 1994.

Blumenthal M, et al, eds. *The Complete German Commission E Monographs.* Austin, Tex: American Botanical Council; 1998.

Bombardelli E, Morazzoni P. *Hypericum perforatum.* Fitoterapia 1995;66:43-68.

Bourke CA. The effect of shade, shearing and wool type in the protection of Merino sheep from *Hypericum perforatum* (St John's wort) poisoning. Aust Vet J 2003;81:494-498.

Butterweck V. Mechanism of action of St John's wort in depression: what is known? CNS Drugs 2003;17:539-562.

De Bairacli Levy J. *The Complete Herbal Handbook for Farm and Stable.* London: Faber and Faber; 1963.

De Bairacli Levy J. *The Complete Herbal Handbook for the Dog and Cat.* London: Faber and Faber; 1985.

Ernst E. Second thoughts about safety of St John's wort. Lancet 1999;354:2014-2016.

Farnsworth NR, ed. NAPRALERT database. Chicago, Ill: University of Illinois at Chicago; February 9, 1998 production.

Franklin M, Cowen PJ. Researching the antidepressant actions of *Hypericum perforatum* (St. John's wort) in animals and man. Pharmacopsychiatry 2001;34(suppl 1):S29-S37.

Grieve M. *A Modern Herbal* (1931). London: Jonathan Cape; Reprint 1975.

Ivan H. Preliminary investigations on the application of *Hypericum perforatum* in herpes therapy. Gyogyszereszet 1979; 23:217-218.

Johne A, Brockmöller J, Bauer S, Maurer A, et al. Interaction of St John's wort extract with digoxin. Eur J Clin Pharmacol 1999;6:80.

Kako MDN, Al-Sultan II, Saleem AN. Studies of sheep experimentally poisoned with *Hypericum perforatum.* Vet Human Toxicol 1993;35:298-300.

Lantz MS, Buchalter E, Giambanco V. St John's wort and antidepressant drug interactions in the elderly. J Geriatr Psychiatry Neurol 1999;12:7-10.

Linde K, Mulrow CD, Berner M, Egger M. St John's wort for depression. Cochrane Database Syst Rev 2005;2:CD000448.

Martarelli D, Martarelli B, Pediconi D, Nabissi MI, Perfumi M, Pompei P. *Hypericum perforatum* methanolic extract inhibits growth of human prostatic carcinoma cell line orthotopically implanted in nude mice. Cancer Lett 2004;210:27-33.

Mennini T, Gobbi M. The antidepressant mechanism of *Hypericum perforatum.* Life Sci 2004;75:1021-1027.

Mills E, Montori VM, Wu P, Gallicano K, Clarke M, Guyatt G. Interaction of St John's wort with conventional drugs: systematic review of clinical trials. BMJ 2004;329:27-30.

Nahrstedt A, Butterweck V. Biologically active and other chemical constituents of the herb of *Hypericum perforatum* L. Pharmacopsychiatry 1997;30:129-134.

Nebel A, Schneider BJ, Baker RK, Kroll DJ. Potential metabolic interaction between St John's wort and theophylline. Ann Pharmacother 1999;33:502.

Okpanyi SN, et al. Genotoxizität eines standardisierten Hypericum Extrakts. Arzneimittelforschung 1990;40:851-855.

Parker V. Adverse reactions to St John's Wort. Can J Psychiatry 2001;46:77-79.

Piscitelli SC, Burstein AH, Chaitt D, Alfaro RM, Falloon J. Indinavir concentrations and St John's wort. Lancet 2000; 355:547-548.

Schulz V. Safety of St. John's Wort extract compared to synthetic antidepressants. Phytomedicine 2006;13:199-204.

Simmen U, Higelin J, Berger-Buter K, et al. Neurochemical studies with St. John's wort in vitro. Pharmacopsychiatry 2001; 34(suppl 1):S137-S142.

Taylor LH, Kobak KA. An open-label trial of St. John's Wort *(Hypericum perforatum)* in obsessive-compulsive disorder. J Clin Psychiatry 2000;61:575-578.

Woelk H, Burkard G, Grunwald J. Benefits and risks of the Hypericum extract LI 160: drug monitoring study with 3250 patients. J Geriatr Psychiatry Neurol 1994;7(suppl 1):S34-S38.

Sweet Wormwood

Artemisia annua L. • art-em-MIZ-ee-uh ANN-yew-uh

Distribution: China, Korea, Japan, Vietnam, and Russia; widely naturalized in the United States

Similar Species: Many species of *Artemisia* are used as medicine worldwide.

Common Names: Sweet Annie, qing hao, annual wormwood

Family: Asteraceae

Parts Used: Aerial parts

Collection: Leaves collected in summer before blooming.

Constituents: Sesquiterpene lactones (such as artemisinin, arteannuin B), volatile oil (with abrotamine, β-bourbonene), flavonoids, vitamin A

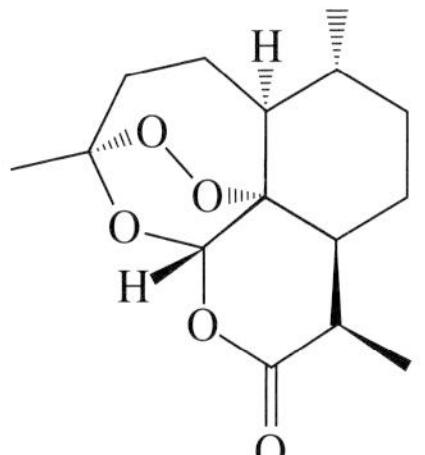

Artemisinin

Clinical Action: Antimalarial, antipyretic, possibly antineoplastic

Energetics: Bitter and cold; enters the kidney, liver, and gallbladder meridians

History and Traditional Usage: This herb was first mentioned by name in 168 bc. In Traditional Chinese Medicine, qing hao clears summer heat, clears fevers from deficiency, cools the blood, and stops bleeding. Used for summer heat with low fever, headache, dizziness, and stifling sensation in the chest. Especially used for fevers that are unremitting or that occur at night. For morning coolness caused by heat in the blood. Used for malaria to relieve the alternating fever and chills.

Published Research: Early Chinese research indicated that qing hao is effective against some fungal skin disease and leptospirosis. It is plasmodicidal, even against multiresistant strains of the malarial agent, *Plasmodium falciparum* (Young, 2004; Sriram, 2004)

Researchers believe that artemisinin reacts with free intracellular iron through the endoperoxide bridge in the molecule. Cancer cells and malarial parasites both contain high levels of iron. When the artemisinin reacts, free radicals result; these induce cell death (Zhang, 1992). Artemisinin and artemether are as effective as conventional antimalarial drugs, with variable efficacy and adverse effect profiles (WHO, 1998).

Numerous in vitro studies have indicated that artemisinin has antineoplastic activity. In a canine study, dihydroartemisinin was applied to the oral mucosa of dogs that had been challenged with the canine oral papillomavirus. Dihydroartemisinin inhibited virus-induced tumor formation but did not prevent papillomavirus replication. These findings suggest that some artemisinin derivatives may be useful for the topical treatment of epithelial papillomavirus lesions (Disbrow, 2005).

Artemisinin, when applied to cultured cells infected with *Neospora caninum,* inhibited intracellular tachyzoite multiplication. Extracts of the whole plant have been examined in the treatment of chicks with coccidian infection. Artemisinin reduces oocyst output when fed at levels of 8.5 and 17 ppm in the diet. Investigators suggested that artemisinin works by inducing oxidative stress (Allen, 1997, 1998). Artemisinin and, less consistently, the whole plant suppress lesions caused by *Eimeria tenella* (Kim, 2002).

Most published research focuses on the single extract, artemisinin. Different plant harvests contain variable levels of artemisinin—even none at all.

Indications: Possibly certain cancers. Malara: "Artemisinin derivatives presently show no cross-resistance with known antimalarials and as such are important for treating severe malaria in areas of multidrug resistance; however, they require long treatment courses and, when used alone, recrudescence may occur" (WHO, 1998).

Potential Veterinary Indications: Certain cancers (as an adjunct to effective conventional care); some blood and gastrointestinal parasites, oral and genital papillomas

Contraindications: None known.

Toxicology and Adverse Effects: AHPA class 2b. Central nervous system depression and seizures were observed in dogs given 40 to 80 mg/kg of artemether (a synthetic derivative of artemisinin) intramuscularly. Dogs given up to 600 mg/kg orally demonstrated no adverse effects (Classen, 1995).

Potential Drug Interactions: Artemisinin induces CYP3A4 within 7 to 10 days (Giao, 2001). This difficulty has been approached clinically by administration of each dose with 4 to 8 oz grapefruit juice and by the use of pulsed therapy (10 days on, 5 days off). Artemisinin may also induce CYP2C19 (Svennson, 1998). No drug interactions have been described at the time of this writing, however.

Dosage:

Human: The traditional human dose for the whole herb used in Chinese medicine is 20 to 40 g taken daily, in decoction

Dried herb: 1-10 g TID

Artemisinin: 400-500 mg TID

Infusion: 5-15 g per cup of water, with 1 cup of the tea given TID

Tincture 1:2 or 1:3: 1-5 mL TID

Small Animal:

Dried herb: 25-500 mg/kg, divided daily (optimally, TID)

Artemisinin: 2-4 mg/kg daily, divided dose

Infusion: 5-15 g per cup of water, administered at a rate of ¼-½ cup per 10 kg (20 lb), divided daily (optimally, TID)

Tincture 1:2-1:3: 0.5-2.5 mL per 10 kg (20 lb), divided daily (optimally, TID) and diluted or combined with other herbs

References

Allen PC, Danforth HD, Augustine PC. Dietary modulation of avian coccidiosis. Int J Parasitol 1998;28:1131-1140.

Allen PC, Lydon J, Danforth HD. Effects of components of *Artemisia annua* on coccidian infections in chickens. Poult Sci 1997;76:1156-1163.

Bone K. Artemisia annua: herbal use vs isolated active. Townsend Letter for Doctors and Patients, April 2005. Available at: http://www.tldp.com/. Accessed July 2005.

Classen W, Altmann B, Gretener P, Souppart C, Skelton-Stroud P, Krinke G. Differential effects of orally versus parenterally administered qinghaosu derivative artemether in dogs. Exp Toxicol Pathol 1999;51:507-516.

Disbrow G, Baege AC, Kierpiec KA, et al. Dihydroartemisinin is cytotoxic to papillomavirus-expressing epithelial cells *in vitro* and *in vivo*. *Cancer Res* 2005;65:10854-10861.

Giao PT, de Vries PJ. Pharmacokinetic interactions of antimalarial agents. Clin Pharmacokinet 2001;40:343-373.

Jung M, Lee K, Kim H, Park M. Recent advances in artemisinin and its derivatives as antimalarial and antitumor agents. Curr Med Chem 2004;11:1265-1284.

Kim JT, Park JY, Seo HS, et al. In vitro antiprotozoal effects of artemisinin on *Neospora caninum*. Vet Parasitol 2002;103:53-63.

Sriram D, Rao VS, Chandrasekhara KV, Yogeeswari P. Progress in the research of artemisinin and its analogues as antimalarials: an update. Nat Prod Res 2004;18:503-527.

Svensson US, Ashton M, Trinh NH, Bertilsson L, Dinh XH, Nguyen VH, Nguyen TN, Nguyen DS, Lykkesfeldt J, Le DC. Artemisinin induces omeprazole metabolism in human beings? Clin Pharmacol Ther 1998;64:160-167.

World Health Organization Malaria Fact Sheet, 1998. Available at: http://www.who.int/malaria/docs/artrep.htm. Accessed May 12, 2006.

Zhang F, Gosser DK. Hemin-catalyzed decomposition of artemisinin (qinghaosu). Biochem Pharmacol 1992;43:1805-1809.

Tea Tree Oil

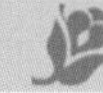

Melaleuca alternifolia (Maiden and Betche) Cheel. • me-luh-LOO-kuh al-tern-ee-FOH-lee-uh

Other Names: "Tea tree" may refer to many different species within the *Melaleuca* and *Leptospermum* genera.

Family: Myrtaceae
Parts Used: Volatile oil extract of the leaves of *Melaleuca alternifolia*
Distribution: Native to Australia and parts of New Zealand
Selected Constituents: Major compounds include terpenes γ-terpinene, p-cymene, 1,8-cineol, and 1-terpinen-4-ol.

gamma-Terpinene

P-cymene

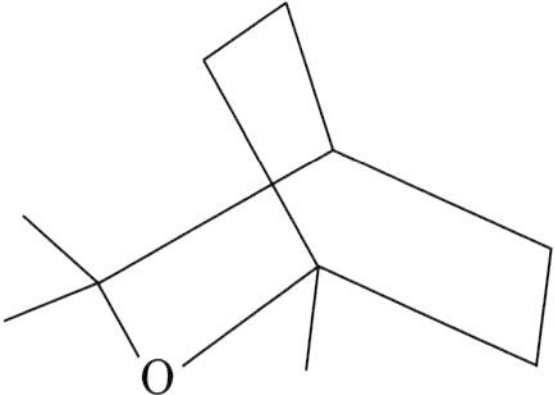

1,8-cineole

Clinical Actions: Antimicrobial
Energetics: Pungent, cooling (leaf)
History and Traditional Usage: The leaves of many *Melaeuca* species were used traditionally by Australian indigenous people. Leaves were crushed or made into tea and used to treat patients with cough, colds, and skin infection. The herb came to be known as tea tree in the late 1700s, when James Cook gave the tea to his men to prevent scurvy. Tea tree oil has been used topically to treat those with skin, joint, and muscle conditions, including acne, athlete's foot, boils and burns, insect bites, lice, scabies, body and foot odor, vaginal infection, sinus congestion, hemorrhoids, ringworm, mouth and throat infections, herpes, warts, sprains, rheumatism, and sore muscles.
Published Research: Studies that began in the 1920s revealed the oil's antibacterial and antiseptic properties; it has proved effective as an antifungal and germicide.

Tea tree has been investigated for its effects on oral microorganisms and pathogens. In one trial that compared 5-week treatments with oral rinses containing 0.2% tea tree oil, garlic, or chlorhexidine in 30 people, tea tree showed intermediate tolerability, but efficacy was not as great as with chlorhexidine or garlic (Groppo, 2002). Two prospective, single-center, open-label studies evaluated the capacity for tea tree oil to affect fluconazole-resistant oral candidiasis (thrush) in patients with HIV (Vazquez, 2002; Jandourek, 1998). Treatments were reasonably effective. Because animals cannot be instructed to avoid swallowing the oil, toxicity limits its usefulness for oral infection in small animals.

The efficacy of tea tree cream (10%) was investigated in patients with methicillin-resistant *Staphylococcus aureus* (MRSA). In all, 224 patients were treated with tea tree 10% cream and 5% body wash, or mupirocin 2% nasal ointment; clinical results were approximately equivalent (46% clearance with tea tree regimen vs. 56% clearance with mupirocin treatment). Tea tree treatment was more effective than chlorhexidine or silver sulfadiazine in clearing superficial skin lesions and sites, but less effective at clearing nasal carriage, than mupirocin. Tea tree preparations were safe and well tolerated (Dryden, 2004).

Antifungal activity has also been demonstrated in a randomized, controlled, double-blind study of 158 patients with a dermatophyte infection (*Tinea Pedis*). Patients received placebo or 25% or 50% tea tree oil solution applied twice daily to affected areas, for 4 weeks; they were examined after 2 and 4 weeks. Mycologic cure was assessed by culture of skin scrapings taken at baseline and after 4 weeks. The cure rate was 64% in the 50% tea tree oil group, compared with the placebo group (31%) (Satchell, 2002). An earlier study that used a 10% tea tree cream or placebo in the treatment of tinea pedis found this concentration ineffective (Tong, 1992).

Investigators have studied the anti-inflammatory effects of tea tree oil in vitro (Finlay-Jones, 2001). In a human clinical trial, 27 volunteers and subjects were injected intradermally (study and control) with histamine diphosphate. Topical liquid paraffin had no significant effect on histamine-induced wheal, and mean wheal volume significantly decreased with tea tree oil (Koh, 2002).

Bassett (1990) compared a 5% tea tree oil gel with 5% benzoyl peroxide for the treatment of 124 patients with mild to moderate acne. These treatments were both effective, and although tea tree was slower to act, those receiving this treatment had fewer adverse effects than did those treated with benzoyl peroxide.

The yeast *Malassezia pachydermatis* is frequently involved in skin diseases such as seborrhoeic dermatitis, especially in dogs and cats. The in vitro activity of tea tree oil was confirmed against several strains of *Malassezia pachydermatis*. All tested strains showed remarkably high susceptibility to tea tree oil (Weseler, 2002).

A commercial preparation, Bogaskin (Bogar, AG Zurich), a 10% emulsion of the oil in a water-based cream, was administered twice daily to 53 canine dermatology patients for 4 weeks in an open, multicenter trial. Dogs treated during the previous 2 weeks with antibiotics, anti-inflammatory agents, or other herbal therapy were excluded from the trial. Significant improvements were noted in pruritus, erythema, pustules, oozing, crusts, erosions, alopecia, hyperkeratosis, and scaling (Fitzi, 2002). The same group tested a 10% tea tree cream in dogs with focal dermatitis, manifested as pruritic skin lesions, skin fold pyoderma, and other conditions that were associated with positive fungal or bacterial testing. A total of 57 dogs seen by 7 different practitioners were randomly assigned to practitioner-blinded treatment with a commercial skin cream or with tea tree cream twice daily for 10 days. Application of tea tree cream led to significantly better clinical improvement. A single adverse event was reported in the tea tree group; investigators suspected that this was unrelated to treatment (Reichling, 2004).

Indications: Bacterial infection; fungal infection; inflammatory skin lesions

Potential Veterinary Indications: Fungal, yeast, and bacterial skin infection; inflammatory skin lesions

Contraindications: Known allergy.

Toxicology and Adverse Effects: Tea tree oil should not be ingested and should not be used over long periods.

The LD_{50} value of tea tree oil in rats is 1 to 2 g/kg—a dose that is considered mildly toxic (Tisserand, 1995).

The essential oil of *Melaleuca alternifolia* was investigated for skin irritation by means of an occlusive patch test given to 28 human subjects for 21 days. In all, 3 of 28 subjects were withdrawn because of severe allergic (not irritant) response to tea tree oil (Southwell, 1997).

About 30 mL tea tree oil was applied to a raw eczematous skin lesion on a 10-year-old dog. The dog became unconscious 20 minutes later and was later treated by a veterinarian. Two days after this occurred, the dog was seizing, semicomatose, and dehydrated and had putrid diarrhea. After other possible causes were ruled out and further unsuccessful treatment was administered, the dog was euthanized (Thornton, 1990).

Two cats were treated with tea tree oil spray (strength unknown) for flea prevention. One cat with unbroken skin was normal; the other had several small, moist areas of dermatitis. The latter cat presented to a veterinarian in a collapsed state 2 hours after receiving treatment. Intensive treatment was provided, and the cat initially improved, but its condition deteriorated and the cat died after 12 hours (Norris, 1990). Three purebred cats were poisoned with tea tree oil (Bischoff, 1998).

A rescued baby spectacled flying fox was treated all over with tea tree oil to kill flies on its body. The flying fox was presented to a veterinarian with dehydration, severe depression, and bloody diarrhea. It was assumed that the tea tree oil had been absorbed through the delicate wing membrane and was ingested during fastidious cleaning. The oral mucosa was ulcerated, and clinical signs revealed ulceration throughout the entire gastrointestinal tract. The flying fox recovered after undergoing intensive therapy (Olsson, 1993).

Preparation Notes: For a 1% solution, suspend 5 mL tea tree oil with 500 mL or just over 2 cups distilled water. This solution may be used as a disinfecting wash and room spray, after it is well shaken.

For an antiseptic wash, 30 to 40 drops essential oil should be added to 1 cup distilled, sterile, or filtered water, or to an infusion of tea tree leaves.

Dosage: *Ointments and creams:* 1%-10% tea tree oil in animals; human studies on fungal onychomycosis suggest that 50% creams are effective and safe in that species; many use 100% tea tree oil on toenails or on very thick skin on the feet.

References

Bassett IB, Pannowitz DL, Barnetson RS. A comparative study of tea-tree oil versus benzoylperoxide in the treatment of acne. Med J Aust 1990;153:455-458.

Bischoff K, Guale F. Australian tea tree *(Melaleuca alternifolia)* oil poisoning in three purebred cats. J Vet Diagn Invest 1998;10:208-210.

Dryden MS, Dailly S, Crouch M. A randomized, controlled trial of tea tree topical preparations versus a standard topical regimen for the clearance of MRSA colonization. J Hosp Infect 2004;56:283-286.

Finlay-Jones J, Hart P, Riley T, Carson C. Anti-inflammatory activity of tea tree oil. RIRDC Publication No. 01/10, 2001. Available at: http://www.rirdc.gov.au/reports/TTO/01-10.pdf

Fitzi J, Furst-Jucker J, Wegener T, Saller R, Reichling J. Phytotherapy of chronic dermatitis and pruritis of dogs with a topical preparation containing tea tree oil (Bogaskin®). Schweiz Arch Tierheilk 2002;144:223-231.

Groppo FC, Ramacciato JC, Simoes RP, Florio FM, Sartoratto A. Antimicrobial activity of garlic, tea tree oil, and chlorhexidine against oral microorganisms. Int Dent J 2002;52:433-437.

Jandourek A, Vaishampayan JK, Vazquez JA. Efficacy of melaleuca oral solution for the treatment of fluconazole refractory oral candidiasis in AIDS patients. AIDS 1998;12:1033-1037.

Koh KJ, Pearce AL, Marshman G, Finlay-Jones JJ, Hart PH. Tea tree oil reduces histamine-induced skin inflammation. Br J Dermatol 2002;147:1212-1217.

Norris J. Tea tree oil poisoning in a cat. Control and Therapy Series, Postgraduate Foundation in Veterinary Science of the University of Sydney, December 1990.

Olsson A. Tea tree oil poisoning: flying foxes. Control and Therapy Series, Postgraduate Foundation in Veterinary Science of the University of Sydney, December 1993.

Satchell AC, Saurajen A, Bell C, Bametson RS. Treatment of interdigital tinea pedis with 25% and 50% tea tree oil solution: a randomized, placebo-controlled, blinded study. Australas J Dermatol 2002;43:175-178.

Southwell IA, Freeman S, Rubel D. Skin irritancy of tea tree oil. J Essential Oil Res 1997;9:47-52.

Thornton M. Tea tree oil poisoning: possible case. Control and Therapy Series, Postgraduate Foundation in Veterinary Science of the University of Sydney, April 1990.

Tisserand R, Balacs T. *Essential Oil Safety: A Guide for Health Care Professionals.* Edinburgh: Churchill Livingstone; 1995.

Tong MM, Altman PM, Barnetson RS. Tea tree oil in the treatment of tinea pedis. Australas J Dermatol 1992;33:145-149.

Vazquez JA, Zawawi AA. Efficacy of alcohol-based and alcohol-free melaleuca oral solution for the treatment of fluconazole-refractory oropharyngeal candidiasis in patients with AIDS. HIV Clin Trials 2002;3:379-385.

Weseler A, Geiss HK, Saller R, Reichling J. Antifungal effect of Australian tea tree oil on *Malassezia pachydermatis* isolated from canines suffering from cutaneous skin disease. Schweiz Arch Tierheilkd 2002;144:215-221.

Thuja

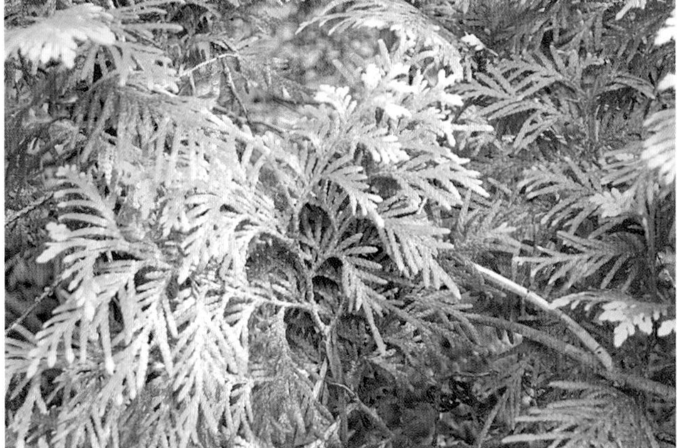

Thuja occidentalis L. • THOO-yuh ock-sih-den-TAY-liss

Other Names: Eastern white cedar, Northern white cedar, Eastern arborvitae, arborvitae, arbor vitae, American arborvitae, swamp-cedar, hackmatack, abendländischer lebensbaum, amerikanischer lebensbaum, heckenthuja, lebensbaum, livsträ, thuya d'occident, tuja, livsträd, zerav zapadni

Family: Cupressaceae (Cypress)

Parts Used: Leaves and twigs

Distribution: Eastern white cedar is native to Northeastern North America from Nova Scotia and Quebec to Manitoba, Minnesota, Ohio, New York, and Northern New England. It is most often associated with cool, moist, nutrient-rich sites, particularly on organic soils near streams or other drainageways, or on calcareous mineral soils.

Selected Constituents: Volatile oil, flavonoids, mucilage, astringent. Bitter principle: pinipicrin, tannic acids, and thujin, thujigenin, and thujetin. The essential oil consists of 65% thujone. High-molecular-weight glycoproteins and polysaccharides are the focus of recent research (Chang, 2000).

Thujone

Clinical Actions: Expectorant, immune enhancing, antiviral, astringent, diuretic, depurative, antifungal

Energetics: Cool, dry

History and Traditional Usage: The name Arborvitae, or "tree of life," dates from the 16th century when the French explorer Jacques Cartier learned from Native Americans how to use the tree's foliage to treat scurvy and a variety of ailments. The branches were used in steam baths for colds and fever, as poultices for swelling and skin problems, and as decoctions for pneumonia, colic in babies, cystitis, and rheumatism; for periparturient conditions; and for a variety of other diseases. Eastern white cedar is valued for its soft, rot-resistant, easily worked wood, which can be made into canoe ribs, toboggans, shingles, and fence posts.

The decoction has been used with intermittent fever, rheumatism, dropsy, cough, and scurvy, and as an emmenagogue. An ointment of the leaves was used in rheumatism. Injection of the tincture was thought to cure venereal warts (Grieve, 1975).

Milks treated thuja oil as unproven and listed its reported uses as removing excrescences from skin and mucous membranes, retarding growth of malignant cells, removing warts and papillomas, and healing mucocutaneous fissures. The oil, when given internally, was said to act as an antiseptic expectorant (Milks, 1949).

Published Research: Although many preclinical investigations are documented in the literature, no data on clinical trials in which thuja was used as a single herbal substance were available at this writing.

Water-soluble polysaccharides from thuja increase T-lymphocyte counts. When mice were injected with a thuja extract, activity of tumor necrosis factor-α, interleukin-6, and interleukin-1 was increased. Antibody responses in mice are stimulated in Peyer's patches after oral administration of the extract (Naser, 2005).

One study in mice was designed to investigate the theory that thuja may be effective in the treatment of patients with male pattern baldness (androgenetic alopecia). Thuja seed extract inhibited 5α-reductase activity (although not as well as finasteride). When it was applied topically to rats, sebum secretion and sebaceous gland size decreased. Alopecia was less pronounced in a rat alopecia model when treatment consisted of topical thuja, compared with vehicle alone (Park, 2003).

Indications: Bronchitis with cardiac weakness, warts (oral and topical use), cystitis, rheumatism, psoriasis, sinusitis

Potential Veterinary Indications: Topically for warts and possibly other skin conditions; potentially for chronic otitis externa; orally for sinusitis and upper respiratory tract infection

Contraindications: Thuja has abortifacient and emmenagogue properties—not for use during pregnancy or lactation.

Toxicology and Adverse Effects: AHPA class 2b, 2d. Not for long-term use or at doses exceeding manufacturer recommendations. Symptoms, in people, of intoxication from the fresh thuja plant include gastroenteritis followed by absorption disorders, headache, nervous agitation, and chronic convulsions, as well as symptoms of liver and renal toxicity that may extend to arrhythmia and myocardial bleeding (Frohne, 1997). Excessive oral intake of thuja extracts induced severe metabolic disturbances. Intoxication was accompanied by irritant effects on the gastrointestinal tract, uterus, liver and kidney. Infants who ingested leaves and twigs of fresh plant showed mild gastrointestinal disorders and vomiting (EMEA, 1999). These reactions can be explained by the high contents of thujone in the fresh plant.

As with any plant that is high in essential oils, caution should be observed at any dose considered for use in the cat.

Notes of Interest: The name thuja is a Latinized form of a Greek word, meaning "to fumigate," or *thuo* ("to sacrifice"), for the fragrant wood was burned by the ancients during sacrifice rituals. The tree was described as "arbor vita" by Clusius, who saw it in the royal garden of Fontainebleau after it had been imported from Canada. It was introduced into Britain in about 1566 (Grieve, 1975).

Dosage:

Human:

Tincture (usually 60%-80% ethanol; some pharmacies include glycerin to prevent precipitation by tannins) 1:2 or 1:3: 0.5-1 mLTID, up to 6 times daily for acute conditions

Small Animal:

Tincture (usually 60%-80% ethanol; some pharmacies include glycerin to prevent precipitation by tannins) 1:2-1:3: 0.5 mL per 10 kg (20 lb), divided daily (optimally, TID) and diluted or combined with other herbs

Historical Veterinary Dose: Topical (Milks, 1949): 10% ointment or oil, or applied undiluted

References

Chang LC, Song LL, Park EJ, et al. Bioactive constituents of *Thuja occidentalis*. J Nat Prod 2000;63:1235-1238.

EMEA Committee for Veterinary Medicinal Products—*Thuja occidentalis*. EMEA—The European Agency for the Evaluation of Medicinal Products Summary Report 1999.

Frohne D. Giftpflanzen: Cupressaceae. Stuttgart: Wissenschaftliche Verlagsgesellschaft mbH; 1997:153-156.

Grieve M. *A Modern Herbal* (1931). London: Jonathan Cape; Reprint 1975.

Milks HJ. *Practical Veterinary Pharmacology, Materia Medica and Therapeutics*. Chicago, Ill: Alex Eger, Inc.; 1949.

Naser B, Bodinet C, Tegtmeier M, Lindequist U. *Thuja occidentalis* (Arbor vitae): a review of its pharmaceutical, pharmacological and clinical properties. Evid Based Complement Alternat Med 2005;2:69-78. Epub 2005 Feb 9.

Park WS, Lee CH, Lee BG, Chang IS. The extract of *Thujae occidentalis* semen inhibited 5alpha-reductase and androchronogenetic alopecia of B6CBAF1/j hybrid mouse. J Dermatol Sci 2003;31:91-98.

Tribulus

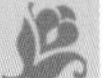

Tribulus terrestris L. • TRY-bew-lus ter-RES-triss

Other Names: Gokshura, chota gokhru, small caltrops, puncture vine, "cow-scratcher"

Family: Zygophyllaceae

Parts Used: Fruit, root, leaf

Distribution: Throughout India, China, and Vietnam and in parts of Europe and South Africa on wasteland

Selected Constituents: Steroidal saponins (Xu, 2001), including protodioscin and protogracilin, and phytosterols such as β-sitosterol. Tribulus leaf standardized extract (TLSE) is a product obtained from the aerial parts of *Tribulus terrestris,* which contains mainly saponins of the furostanol type (not less than 45%, calculated as protodioscin) and was developed in Bulgaria from Mediterranean varieties of tribulus. Tribestan is a standardized tribulus leaf extract that contains not less than 45% steroidal saponins. It is about 30 to 40 times more concentrated than tribulus leaf. The methanol extract of the *Tribulus cistoides* leaf was found to contain nine steroid saponins, among them the cardioactive cistocardin (Achenbach, 1994).

R = Glucose: Rhamnose (1:2)

Protodioscin

Clinical Actions: Antispasmodic, fertility enhancer, antihypertensive, diuretic, antilithic

Energetics: Sweet, cold

History and Traditional Usage: The fruit of tribulus is used in Traditional Chinese Medicine for pruritus, insufficient milk production, and sore eyes. In Ayurveda, the fruit is used for urinary tract problems and for male and female reproductive tract disorders. In Bulgaria, the leaves have gained a reputation among body builders and athletes as an herbal equivalent to anabolic steroids, despite the lack of scientific support. However, Bulgarian research has focused on the potential of tribulus as a reproductive tonic for impotence, infertility in both sexes, and menopausal symptoms. tribulus has been commonly used in folk medicine as a diuretic, and in Turkey, it has been used to treat patients with colic pain, hypertension, and hypercholesterolemia (Arcasoy, 1998).

Ethnoveterinary usage includes bloody dysentery, urinary disorders in ruminants, and rheumatism (Williamson, 2002).

Published Research: To validate the claim of *T. terrestris* as an aphrodisiac, the sexual behavior of rats and intracavernous pressure measurements were investigated. Weight gain, increased intracavernous pressure, and improvement in sexual behavior were observed, and authors believed that these were possibly due to the androgen-enhancement property of protodioscin (PTN). The dose used was 2.5 to 10 mg/kg/day (Gauthaman, 2003). In male rats, tribulus showed considerable stimulation of sperm production. Also, sperm cells were more viable, which suggests improved fertility (Zarkova, 1984).

In another study, it was observed that PTN produced a moderate increase in testosterone, dihydrotestosterone, and dehydroepiandrosterone sulfate levels in primates given intravenous tribulus extract at doses of 7.5, 15, and 30 mg/kg body weight. It also improved libido, sexual activity, and intracavernous pressure in rats after oral administration for 8 weeks (at doses of 2.5, 5, and 10 mg/kg body weight) and had a proerectile effect on the corpus cavernosum smooth muscle of rabbits (orally for 8 weeks at doses of 2.5, 5, and 10 mg/kg body weight) (Adaiken, 2001).

Neychev (2005) treated 21 healthy young men with 2 different doses of tribulus extract (10 mg/kg or 20 mg/kg, divided TID) or placebo for 4 weeks. Serum testosterone, androstenedione, and luteinizing hormone levels were tested before treatment and at intervals up to 24 days after starting supplementation. No changes in hormone levels were detected in any group treated, and all results remained within the normal range.

The stimulating effect of a proprietary tribulus extract (Tribestan) on rams that were intended for breeding, as well as on rams that exhibited sexual impotence and deteriorating semen qualities, was studied. Treatment led to extension of the duration of sexual activity and improved semen production over the service period. Results of therapy with rams with reduced libido showed that the animals could recover by the seventh or eighth day with no essential morphologic changes in the structure of testes and epididymides. Treatment was associated with increased testosterone levels, and the sexual activity of rams affected with coital impotence was normalized (Dimitrov, 1987). Tribestan (250 mg/day) increased testosterone levels and accelerated sexual development in rams and male lambs, respectively (Georgiev, 1988). Libido and sexual reflexes were restored in 71% of boars with long-term sexual impotence (70 mg/kg/day) (Zarkova, 1981).

The effects of tribulus on body composition and exercise performance in resistance-trained human males were also investigated. Fifteen men were randomly assigned to placebo or tribulus (3.21 mg/kg body weight daily). Body weight, body composition, maximal strength, dietary intake, and mood states were monitored before and after 8 weeks of periodized resistance training and supplementation. No changes were noted in body weight, percentage fat, total body water, dietary intake, or mood state in either group. Supplementation with tribulus did not enhance body composition or exercise performance in resistance-trained men in this study (Antonio, 2000).

It has been suggested that *T. terrestris* L. or its saponin mixture may be useful in the treatment of some patients with smooth muscle spasms or colic pain. A saponin extract of dried and powdered *T. terrestris* caused a significant decrease in peristaltic movement of isolated sheep ureter and rabbit jejunum preparations in a dose-dependent manner (Arcasoy, 1998).

T. terrestris has hypotensive effects in rats. In hypertensive rats treated with a single daily dose of 10 mg/kg of lyophilized aqueous extract of tribulus fruit orally for 4 weeks, systolic blood pressure (SBP) was significantly decreased compared with that of hypertensive rats that were not so treated. Angiotensin-converting enzyme (ACE) activity in all tissues of tribulus-fed hypertensive rats was significantly lower than that in control hypertensive rats; this was more pronounced in the kidney. Results suggested a negative correlation between consumption of tribulus and ACE activity in serum and various tissues of rats (Sharifi, 2003).

In a human clinical trial, treatment with the saponin fraction of *T. terrestris* in 406 patients with coronary heart disease resulted in remission in 82.3% of cases. The saponin fraction was claimed to dilate the coronary artery and improve coronary circulation. The authors suggest that tribulus was safe and would be effective in the treatment of patients with angina pectoris (Wang, 1990).

The decoction of tribulus may inhibit gluconeogenesis and influence glycometabolism in normal mice. This decoction may also reduce plasma triglyceride and cholesterol levels (Li, 2001).

An ethanolic extract of the fruits of *T. terrestris* demonstrated significant dose-dependent protection against (glass bead implantation–induced) uroliths in rats by preventing deposition of calculogenic material around a glass bead; it also protected against leukocytosis and elevation in serum urea levels (Anand, 1994). In rats, an oral dose (5 g/kg) of aqueous extract of *T. terrestris* elicited positive diuresis, which was slightly greater than that of furo-semide. Urinary Na(+), K(+), and Cl(+) concentrations also increased. In addition to this diuretic activity, *T. terrestris* evoked contractile activity in guinea pig ileum. The diuretic and contractile effects of *T. terrestris* may indicate that it has the potential to propel urinary stones (Al-Ali, 2003).

T. terrestris was found to be a rich source of calcium and iron (Duhan, 1992).

Indications: Infertility, decreased libido

Potential Veterinary Indications: Improving reproductive performance

Contraindications: None found.

Toxicology and Adverse Effects: Tribulus is a ground weed with sharp spines. It causes photosensitization and liver damage in sheep that consume too much. Tribulus toxicity has been reported in Australia (Bourke, 1992), the United States (McDonough, 1994), South Africa (Wilkins, 1996), and Argentina (Tapia, 1994). However, no toxicity in humans has been reported when tribulus is used as an herbal medicine.

The LD_{50} of a saponin extract was 813 mg/kg (mice, intraperitoneal) (Arcasoy, 1998). Photosensitization and cholangiohepatopathy have been noted in sheep grazing *T. terrestris* (Tapia, 1994). Two β-carboline indolamines (harmane and norharmane) isolated from plant material of *T. terrestris* have been implicated as causing central nervous system effects in sheep that have grazed on *Tribulus* over a period of months. Researchers proposed that harmane and norharmane accumulate in tryptamine-associated neurones of the central nervous system and gradually interact irreversibly with a specific neuronal gene DNA sequence (Bourke, 1992).

Large amounts of tribulus are required for toxicity to occur.

Dosage:

Human:

Dried herb: 0.25-5 g TID

Standardized extract (standardized to 100 mg of furostanol saponins (calculated as protodioscin per tablet): 1 tablet TID-QID. Higher doses may be necessary in some cases, especially for male impotence

Infusions and decoctions: 5-10 g per cup of water, with ¼-1 cup of the tea given TID

Tincture (usually 45%-60% ethanol; higher alcohol preparations may require lower dose rates; some pharmacies include glycerin to prevent precipitation by tannins) 1:2 or 1:3: 1-2.5 mL TID

Small Animal:

Dried herb: 25-300 mg/kg, divided daily (optimally, TID)

Infusion and decoction: 5-10 g per cup of water, administered at a rate of ¼-½ cup per 10 kg (20 lb), divided daily (optimally, TID)

Tincture 2:1 (not 1:2): 1.5-2.5 mL per 10 kg (20 lb), divided daily and diluted or combined with other herbs

Large Animal:

Suggested from literature with Tribestan or Tribulus leaf standardized extract (TLSE): sheep, rams, and lambs: 250 mg/day

Boars: 70 mg/kg/day

References

Achenbach H, Hubner H, Brandt W, Reiter M. Cardioactive steroid saponins and other constituents from the aerial parts of *Tribulus cistoides*. Phytochemistry 1994;35:1527-1543.

Adaikan PG, Gauthaman K, Prasad RNV. History of herbal medicines with an insight on the pharmacological properties of *Tribulus terrestris*. The Aging Male 2001;4:163-169.

Al-Ali M, Wahbi S, Twaij H, Al-Badr A. *Tribulus terrestris:* preliminary study of its diuretic and contractile effects and comparison with *Zea mays*. J Ethnopharmacol 2003;85:257-260.

Anand R, Patnaik G, Kulshreshtha D. Activity of certain fractions of *Tribulus terrestris* fruits against experimentally induced urolithiasis in rats. Indian J Exp Biol 1994;32:548-552.

Antonio J, Uelmen J, Rodriguez R, Earnest C. The effects of *Tribulus terrestris* on body composition and exercise performance in resistance-trained males. Int J Sport Nutr Exerc Metab 2000;10:208-215.

Arcasoy HB, Erenmemisoglu A, Tekol Y, Kurucu S, Kartal M. Effect of *Tribulus terrestris* L. saponin mixture on some smooth muscle preparations: a preliminary study. Boll Chim Farm 1998;137:473-475.

Bourke CA, Stevens GR, Carrigan MJ. Locomotor effects in sheep of alkaloids identified in Australian *Tribulus terrestris*. Aust Vet J 1992;69:163-165.

Dimitrov M, Georgiev P, Vitanov S. [Use of Tribestan on rams with sexual disorders.] Vet Med Nauki 1987;24:102-110.

Duhan A, Chauhan BM, Punia D. Nutritional value of some non-conventional plant foods of India. Plant Foods Hum Nutr 1992;42:193-200.

Gauthaman K, Ganesan AP, Prasad RN. Sexual effects of puncturevine *(Tribulus terrestris)* extract (protodioscin): an evaluation using a rat model. J Altern Complement Med 2003;9:257-265.

Georgiev P, Dimitrov M, Vitanov S. The effect of the preparation Tribestan on the plasma concentration of testosterone and spermatogenesis of lambs and rams. Vet Sib 1988;3:20-22.

Li M, Qu W, Chu S, Wang H, Tian C, Tu M. [Effect of the decoction of *Tribulus terrestris* on mice gluconeogenesis.] Zhong Yao Cai 2001;24:586-588.

McDonough SP, Woodbury AH, Galey FD, Wilson DW, East N, Bracken E. Hepatogenous photosensitization of sheep in California associated with ingestion of *Tribulus terrestris* (puncture vine). J Vet Diagn Invest 1994;6:392-395.

Neychev VK, Mitev VI. The aphrodisiac herb *Tribulus terrestris* does not influence the androgen production in young men. J Ethnopharmacol 2005;101:319-323.

Sharifi AM, Darabi R, Akbarloo N. Study of antihypertensive mechanism of *Tribulus terrestris* in 2K1C hypertensive rats: role of tissue ACE activity. Life Sci 2003;73:2963-2971.

Tapia MO, Giordano MA, Gueper HG. An outbreak of hepatogenous photosensitization in sheep grazing *Tribulus terrestris* in Argentina. Vet Hum Toxicol 1994;36:311-313.

Wang B, Ma L, Liu T. 406 cases of angina pectoris in coronary heart disease treated with saponin of *Tribulus terrestris*. Chung Hsi I Chieh Ho Tsa Chih 1990;10:85-87.

Wilkins AL, Miles CO, De Kock WT, Erasmus GL, Basson AT, Kellerman TS. Photosensitivity in South Africa. IX. Structure elucidation of a beta-glucosidase-treated saponin from *Tribulus terrestris,* and the identification of saponin chemotypes of South African *T. terrestris*. Onderstepoort J Vet Res 1996;63:327-334.

Williamson E, ed. *Major Herbs of Ayurveda*. Sydney: Churchill Livingstone; 2002.

Xu YJ, Xie SX, Zhao HF, Han D, Xu TH, Xu DM. [Studies on the chemical constituents from *Tribulus terrestris*.] Yao Xue Xue Bao 2001;36:750-753.

Zarkova S. Steroid saponins of *Tribulus terrestis* L. having a stimulant effect on the sexual functions. Rev Port Ciencias Vet 1984;79:117-126.

Zarkova S. *Tribestan: Experimental and Clinical Investigations*. Sofia Bulgaria: Chemical Pharmaceutical Research Institute; 1981.

Turmeric

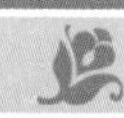

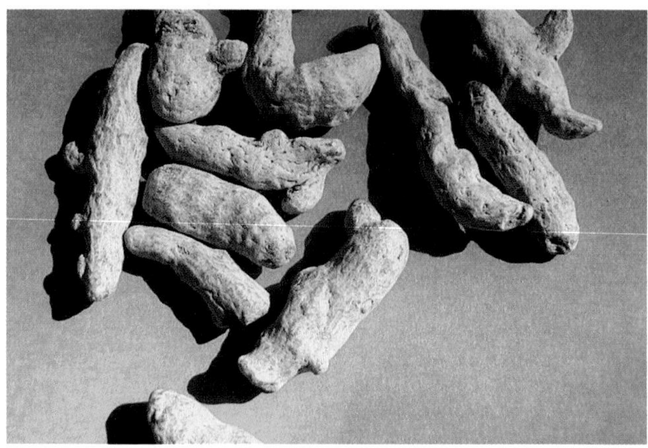

Curcuma longa L. syn. *Curcuma domestica* Valeton (dried rhizomes of *Curcuma wenyujin, Curcuma kwangsiensis,* and *Curcuma phaeocaulis* are also official sources of turmeric in China) (Pharmacopoeia of the People's Republic of China, 1992). • KER-koo-muh LONG-uh

Other Names: Haridra, haldi, Indian saffron, yellow ginger, jiang huang (rhizome), yu jin (root tuber)

Family: Zingiberaceae

Parts Used: Dried rhizome, tuber

Distribution: Cambodia, China, India, Indonesia, Lao People's Democratic Republic, Madagascar, Malaysia, the Philippines, and Vietnam. It is extensively cultivated in China, India, Indonesia, Africa, and Thailand, and throughout the tropics.

Selected Constituents: Volatile oil (6%) composed of monoterpenes and sesquiterpenes, including zingiberene, curcumene, and α- and β-turmerone. The coloring principles (5%) are curcuminoids, 50% to 60% of which are a mixture of curcumin, monodesmethoxycurcumin, and bisdesmethoxycurcumin (Bruneton, 1995).

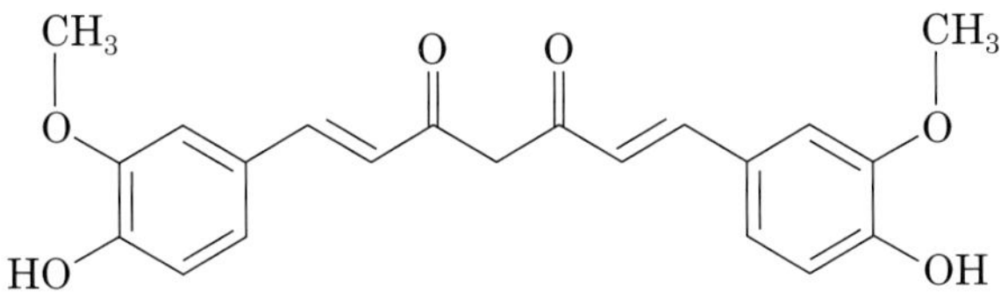

Curcumin

Clinical Actions: Anti-inflammatory, antioxidant, antiplatelet, cholagogue, hepatoprotective, anticancer, cholesterol reducing
Energetics: Warm, pungent, drying
History and Traditional Usage: Turmeric has been used to treat patients with peptic ulcer and pain and inflammation due to rheumatoid arthritis (Medicinal Plants in Viet Nam, 1990), as well as those with amenorrhea, dysmenorrhea, diarrhea, epilepsy, pain, and skin disease (Chang, 1986). Other uses include asthma, boils, bruises, cough, dizziness, epilepsy, hemorrhage, insect bites, jaundice, ringworm, urinary calculi, and slow lactation (Chang, 1986; Medicinal Plants in Viet Nam, 1990) and as a general tonic, blood purifier, and anti-inflammatory.

Ethnoveterinary uses include external application for abscesses, ulcers, ticks, castration wounds, bleeding, eye disorders, and fungal disease. It is also used to treat animal patients with diarrhea and rheumatism; for worms in poultry; for constipation, udder infection, swollen teats, and sprains; for cough and colds in ruminants and poultry; and for jaundice and swinepox. The rhizome is used for gastrointestinal tract disorders, glossitis, *Escherichia coli* bacillosis, threadworm, irregular growth of teeth, loss of appetite, and colic. Respiratory disease, asthma, pneumonia, swelling of the throat, tonsillitis, leeches in the nostrils, and renal disease are other uses. Other indications include lumbar and compound fractures, hemorrhagic septicemia, rinderpest, hematuria, anthrax, and baldness (Williamson, 2002).
Published Research: Turmeric may benefit patients with arthritis. A short-term, double-blind, crossover study of 18 patients with rheumatoid arthritis showed that patients who were given curcumin (1200 mg/day) or phenylbutazone (30 mg/day) had significant improvement in morning stiffness, walking time, and joint swelling (Deodhar, 1980). In another study, the effectiveness of curcumin and phenylbutazone for postoperative inflammation was investigated in a double-blind study. Both resulted in a better anti-inflammatory response than was produced by placebo (Satoskar, 1986), but the degree of inflammation varied greatly among patients.

A randomized, double-blind, placebo-controlled, parallel-group clinical trial of P54FP (an extract of Indian and Javanese turmeric, *Curcuma domestica,* and *Curcuma xanthorrhiza,* respectively) as a treatment for patients with osteoarthritis of the canine elbow or hip was conducted to assess its efficacy and safety. A total of 61 dogs with osteoarthritis were recruited through general practices and then were randomly allocated to receive P54FP or a placebo (orally twice daily for 8 weeks). They were reexamined after 4, 6, and 8 weeks of treatment. No differences were noted between 25 P54FP-treated dogs and 29 placebo-treated dogs when the affected limb was evaluated. Investigators' assessment showed a statistically significant treatment effect of P54FP, but owners' assessment failed to show statistical significance. No adverse effects were recorded, but 2 dogs given P54FP and 4 dogs given placebo were withdrawn because their condition deteriorated (Innes, 2003).

In atherosclerosis and related cardiovascular disease, free radical–induced blood lipid peroxidation and peroxidized low-density lipoprotein cholesterol (LDL) play a central role in the pathogenesis of disease. One study showed that daily oral administration of turmeric significantly decreased LDL and apo B and increased high-density lipoprotein cholesterol (HDL) and apo A of healthy subjects; this herb may be useful as a complement to standard treatments for patients with atherosclerosis (Ramirez-Bosca, 2000).

In 32 patients with chronic anterior uveitis (CAU), curcumin was administered orally at a dose of 375 mg 3 times a day for 12 weeks. A total of 18 patients received curcumin alone, and 14 patients were given curcumin with antitubercular treatment (tuberculosis is the most common cause of anterior uveitis in India). Patients in both groups showed improvement after 2 weeks. All patients who received curcumin alone improved, whereas the group given antitubercular therapy along with curcumin had a response rate of 86%. Follow-up for the next 3 years indicated recurrence rates of 55% in the group receiving curcumin alone and 36% in the group given combination therapy. Comparable numbers of patients in each group lost their vision during the follow-up period because of complications, but no other adverse effects were reported. The efficacy of curcumin and incidences of recurrence after treatment are comparable with those associated with corticosteroid therapy (Lal, 1999).

In broiler chickens, the effect of turmeric as a feed additive on performance was investigated. Turmeric was included in the diet at 0.25%, 0.5%, and 1.0%. Birds fed turmeric had greater body weight gain at 0.5% followed by 0.25% and 1% compared with controls. Similarly, feed conversion of birds receiving 0.5% turmeric was best as compared with controls. Protein percentages of breast and thigh muscles of birds in different groups were nearly the same. The lowest fat percentage was recorded in carcasses at 1.0% turmeric, followed by 0.5%, control, and 0.25%. Higher levels of turmeric inclusion (0.5% and 1.0%) increased erythrocytic and total leukocytic counts. Turmeric did not induce any abnormal flavor, color, or smell. Results indicate that turmeric as a feed additive at the level of 0.5% can enhance the overall performance of broiler chickens (Al-Sultan, 2003).

Dogs envenomated with nonlethal doses of *Bothrops alternatus* snake venom received standard antivenom therapy, intramuscular injections of flunixin meglumine, or topical treatment with aqueous Turmeric extract for a comparison of efficacy. No significant difference was noted in the efficacy of antivenom and turmeric in terms of local effects, but flunixin treatment had lower efficacy. Serum levels of antivenom reached their maximum 2 to 4 hours after administration and were not detected after day 5 (Jacome, 2002).

Turmeric extracts have a hepatoprotective effect in laboratory animal studies; they protect the liver against inflammation caused by galactosamine, lipopolysaccharide, diethylnitrosamine, and carbon tetrachloride, and they improve the clearing function of the liver when it has been damaged (Chuang, 2000; Lukita-Atmadja, 2002; Deshpande, 2003). Doses administered to mice by gavage ranged from 40 mg/kg of curcuminoids to 600 mg/kg curcumin to 5% turmeric extract in the diet.

Curcumin has shown antiangiogenic effects and proapoptotic activities against Ehrlich ascites tumor cells. It has also been found to be cytotoxic in vitro to melanoma cells resistant to doxorubicin, and in vivo studies show that curcumin may serve as a tool against melanoma (Odot, 2004). Curcumin is known to inhibit the growth of ovarian cancer cells (Zheng, 2004). Curcumin has been found to induce apoptosis in lung cancer cell lines (Radhakrishna, 2004). Studies suggest that the chemopreventive action of curcumin may be due to its ability to induce apoptosis and arrest the cell cycle.

Indications: Turmeric is used principally for the treatment of patients with acid, flatulent, or atonic dyspepsia (German Commission E, 1985). It is also used to prevent cardiovascular disease and cancer; arthritis, asthma, and eczema, and to improve the function of the gastrointestinal tract and liver; anterior uveitis is associated with tuberculosis.

Potential Veterinary Indications: Adjunct cancer treatment; arthritis, hepatitis. Improvement in broiler chicken performance; topically for viper envenomation

Contraindications: Obstruction of the biliary tract. Hypersensitivity to turmeric

Herb–Drug Interactions: Turmeric should not be used for patients with gastrointestinal ulceration or hyperacidity, according to *The Botanical Safety Handbook;* however, it may protect against the development of ulcers. Supporting studies show that gastrointestinal ulceration occurred only when mice were administered 50,000 ppm (50 g/kg of diet) of turmeric oil, which was estimated to deliver 7700 to 9300 mg/kg body weight after 2 years (National Toxicology Program, 1993). Clinical trials in animals (Rafatullah, 1990) and a case series in people (Prucksunand, 2001) suggest that turmeric may enhance gastric ulcer healing; at the very least, it may not inhibit healing.

Toxicology and Adverse Effects: AHPA class 2b, 2d. One study evaluated the oral acute and 28-day feeding toxicity of turmeric powder in rats. The acute oral LD_{50} of turmeric powder was greater than 5000 mg/kg. No toxic effects were found through evaluation of clinical signs, body weight, feed consumption and efficiency, hematology, and autopsy in the turmeric- and curcumin-treated groups. No acute oral toxicity was observed, and the higher daily intake (1000 mg/kg) of turmeric for 28 days resulted in no significant toxic effects in rats (Liao, 2003).

Allergic dermatitis from turmeric has been reported. Reactions to patch testing occurred in persons regularly exposed to the substance and in those in whom dermatitis of the fingertips had already been diagnosed. Persons who were not previously exposed to the drug had few allergic reactions (Seetharam, 1987).

Potential Drug Interactions: Caution is advised with antiplatelet or anticoagulation medication.

Dosage:

Human:

Dried herb: 1-10 g TID, up to 6 times daily for acute conditions; 1.5-3.0 g daily (European Pharmacopoeia, 1997)

Curcumin: 400-600 mg TID, up to 6 times per day acutely

Decoctions: 5-30 g per cup of water, with 1 cup of the tea given TID, up to 6 times daily acutely

Tincture (usually 45%-60% ethanol) 1:2 or 1:3: 2-5 mL TID, up to 6 times daily for acute conditions

Small Animal:

Curcumin: canine, 50-250 mg TID; feline, 50-100 mg QD (Silver, 1997)

Dried herb: 50-600 mg/kg, divided daily (optimally, TID) (to maximum palatability tolerance)

Decoction: 5-30 g per cup of water, administered at a rate of ¼-½ cup per 10 kg (20 lb), divided daily (optimally, TID)

Tincture (usually in 45%-60% ethanol) 1:2-1:3: 1.0-3.0 mL per 10 kg (20 lb), divided daily (optimally, TID) and diluted or combined with other herbs. Higher doses may be appropriate if the herb is used singly and is not combined in a formula

Horses:

Curcumin: 1200-2400 mg daily

References

Al-Sultan SI. The effect of *Curcuma longa* (turmeric) on overall performance of broiler chickens. Int J Poult Sci 2003;2:351-353.

Bruneton J. *Pharmacognosy, Phytochemistry, Medicinal Plants.* Paris: Lavoisier; 1995.

Chang HM, But PPH, eds. *Pharmacology and Applications of Chinese Materia Medica,* vol 1. Singapore: World Scientific Publishing; 1986.

Chuang SE, Cheng AL, Lin JK, Kuo ML. Inhibition by curcumin of diethylnitrosamine-induced hepatic hyperplasia, inflammation, cellular gene products and cell-cycle–related proteins in rats. Food Chem Toxicol 2000;38:991-995.

Deodhar SD, Sethi R, Srimal RC. Preliminary study on antirheumatic activity of curcumin (diferuloyl methane). Indian J Med Res 1980;71:632-634.

Deshpande UR, Joseph LJ, Samuel AM. Hepatobiliary clearance of labelled mebrofenin in normal and D-galactosamine HCl–induced hepatitis rats and the protective effect of turmeric extract. Indian J Physiol Pharmacol 2003;47:332-336.

European Pharmacopoeia. 3rd ed. Strasbourg: Council of Europe; 1997.

German Commission E. Monograph: *Curcumae longae* rhizoma. Bundesanzeiger 1985;223:30.

Innes JF, Fuller CJ, Grover ER, Kelly AL, Burn JF. Randomised, double-blind, placebo-controlled parallel group study of P54FP for the treatment of dogs with osteoarthritis. Vet Rec 2003;152:457-460.

Jacome D, Melo MM, Santos MM, Heneine LG. Kinetics of venom and antivenom serum and clinical parameters and treatment efficacy in *Bothrops alternatus* envenomed dogs. Vet Hum Toxicol 2002;44:334-338.

Lal B, Kapoor AK, Asthana OP, et al. Efficacy of curcumin in the management of chronic anterior uveitis. Phytother Res 1999;13:318-322.

Liao JW, Tsai SJ, Wang SC, et al. Safety evaluation of turmeric (*Curcuma longa* L.) powder via oral gavage for 28 days in rats [Chinese]. Plant Protect Bull 2003;45:237-255.

Lukita-Atmadja W, Ito Y, Baker GL, McCuskey RS. Effect of curcuminoids as anti-inflammatory agents on the hepatic microvascular response to endotoxin. Shock 2002;17:399-403.

National Toxicology Program. *NTP Toxicology and Carcinogenesis Studies of Turmeric Oleoresin (CAS No. 8024-37-1) (Major Component 79%-85% Curcumin, CAS No. 458-37-7) in F344/N Rats and B6C3F1 Mice (Feed Studies).* Research Triangle Park, NC: National Toxicology Program; 1993:1-275.

Odot J, Albert P, Carlier A, Tarpin M, Devy J, Madoulet C. In vitro and in vivo anti-tumoral effect of curcumin against melanoma cells. Int J Cancer 2004;111:381-387.

Pharmacopoeia of the People's Republic of China (English ed). Guangzhou: Guangdong Science and Technology Press; 1992.

Prucksunand C, Indrasukhsri B, Leethochawalit M, Hungspreugs K. Phase II clinical trial on effect of the long turmeric (*Curcuma longa* Linn) on healing of peptic ulcer. Southeast Asian J Trop Med Public Health 2001;32:208-215.

Radhakrishna Pillai G, Srivastava AS, Hassanein TI, Chauhan DP, Carrier E. Induction of apoptosis in human lung cancer cells by curcumin. Cancer Lett 2004;208:163-170.

Rafatullah S, Tariq M, Al-Yahya MA, Mossa JS, Ageel AM. Evaluation of turmeric *(Curcuma longa)* for gastric and duodenal antiulcer activity in rats. J Ethnopharmacol 1990;29:25-34.

Ramirez-Bosca A, Soler A, Carrión MA, et al. An hydroalcoholic extract of *Curcuma longa* lowers the apo B/apo A ratio: implications for atherogenesis prevention. Mechanisms Ageing Development 2000;119:41-47.

Satoskar RR, Shah Shenoy SG. Evaluation of antiinflammatory property of curcumin (diferuloyl methane) in patient with postoperative inflammation. Int J Clin Pharmacol Ther Toxicol 1986;24:651-654.

Seetharam KA, Pasricha JS. Condiments and contact dermatitis of the finger-tips. Indian J Dermatol Venereol Leprol 1987;53:325-328.

Silver RJ. Ayurvedic veterinary medicine. In: Schoen AM, Wynn SG, eds. *Complementary and Alternative Veterinary Medicine.* St Louis, Mo: Mosby, Inc.; 1997:463-464.

Williamson E, ed. *Major Herbs of Ayurveda.* Sydney: Churchill Livingstone; 2002.

World Health Organization. *Medicinal Plants in Viet Nam.* Manila: WHO Regional Publications, Western Pacific Series, No. 3; 1990.

Zheng L, Tong Q, Wu C. Growth-inhibitory effects of curcumin on ovary cancer cells and its mechanisms. J Huazhong Univ Sci Technolog Med Sci 2004;24:55-58.

Uva Ursi

Arctostaphylos uva ursi (L.) Spreng. • ark-toh-STAF-ih-los OO-va UR-see

Common Names: Bearberry, kinnickinick, mountain cranberry, uva ursi, uvae ursi folium

Family: Ericaceae

Parts Used: Leaves

Distribution: Indigenous to Europe, the United Kingdom, Asia, Northern America, and Canada

Selected Constituents: The glycoside arbutin, the main active constituent in uva ursi, accounts for up to 10% of the plant by weight. Hydroquinone derived from arbutin and methylarbutin is a powerful antibacterial agent that is thought to be responsible for the ability of uva ursi to treat urinary tract infection (Matsuda, 1992a). Polyphenols consist of tannins (6%-40%), including gallotannins, ellagic acid, catechin, and anthocyanidins (with astringent and antioxidant properties); phenolic gallic, p-coumaric, and syringic acids; flavanoids—mainly glycosides of quercetin, hyperoside, and myricetin; and the triterpenes ursolic acid, amyrin, montropein, and allantoin.

HO

OH

O

O

OH

HO OH

Arbutin

Clinical Actions: Urinary antiseptic, astringent

Energetics: Cold

History and Traditional Usage: Uva ursi use was recorded as early as the 13th century by the Welsh Physicians of Myddfai. It was listed in the London Pharmacopoeia for the first time in 1788 (Grieve, 1975).

It is a traditional herb of American Indians, who used the leaves for ceremonial smoking. Uses by Eclectic physicians included chronic irritation of the bladder, enuresis, excessive mucus and bloody discharges in the urine, chronic diarrhea, dysentery, menorrhagia, leukorrhea, diabetes, and strangury.

Howard Milks (1949) described the herb as a urinary antiseptic recommended for the same uses as buchu, but he considered it inferior to buchu. He noted that it renders the urine dark green.

Published Research: The antibacterial effects of uva ursi are due to hydroquinone esters such as arbutin, as well as to free hydroquinone; the activity of arbutin was directly correlated with the β-glucosidase activity of bacteria (this enzyme converts arbutin to hydroquinone) (Jahodar, 1985). Arbutin metabolites are excreted in human urine variably, ranging from approximately 5% of the administered dose for one metabolite to 75% over 24 hours (Schindler, 2002; Quintus, 2005).

Uva ursi extracts have shown a broad spectrum of antimicrobial activity in vitro against *Escherichia coli, Proteus vulgaris, Enterobacter aerogenes, Streptococcus faecalis, Staphylococcus aureus, Salmonella typhi,* and *Candida albicans* (Holopainen, 1988). One study on the use of uva ursi extract in the course of acute bacterial pyelonephritis in rats showed that at a dose of 25 mg/kg, uva ursi extract had marked antibacterial and nephroprotective effects (Nikolaev, 1996).

One of the probable and potentially important mechanisms of action for bearberry is its ability to influence the surface characteristics of microbial cells, thereby affecting their ability to adhere to host cells. This is thought to be important in the development of gram-negative infections. One of the characteristics that uva ursi influences is the surface hydrophobicity of microbial cells. In one study, the hydrophobicity of 155 *E. coli* strains was determined. Among the strains isolated from fecal samples of calves and pigs with diarrhea, some 40.0% to 60.0% of *E. coli* strains were aggregative. Decoctions of uva ursi leaves significantly increased the hydrophobicity of both microbial species; however, bactericidal action was relatively low (Turi, 1997).

A methanolic extract of uva ursi enhanced the inhibitory effects of dexamethasone on allergic and inflammatory models (Matsuda, 1992b). It is suggested that the suppressive effects of uva ursi against immune-mediated inflammation are due to arbutin. Arbutin enhanced the inhibitory action of prednisolone on induced contact dermatitis, allergic hypersensitivity, and adjuvant-induced arthritis, and it synergized prednisolone or dexamethasone anti-inflammatory activity (Matsuda, 1990). Topical application of uva ursi might increase the anti-inflammatory effects of other steroid-like compounds such as plant-derived saponins (Matsuda, 1992b).

Uva ursi may have use as an adjunct treatment for patients with diabetes. Arbutin reduced postprandial blood glucose elevation following glucose ingestion by mice; blood glucose reductions of between 40% and 52% were observed (Takii, 1997). Bearberry reduced hyperphagia, weight loss, and polydipsia in an induced model of diabetes in mice. However, no effect on insulin or glucose concentration was observed (Swanston-Flatt, 1989).

Bearberry extract may assist in the treatment of patients with hyperpigmentary disorders, in that arbutin inhibits melanin synthesis in vitro by inhibiting tyronase activity (Matsuda, 1992a). Melanogenesis in brown-haired guinea pigs was reduced by 80% through topical application of arbutin (Nishimura, 1995).

Indications: Urinary tract infection and bacterial prostatitis (as a general urinary antiseptic); potentially for diabetes; perhaps as adjuvant treatment for those with inflammatory conditions

Potential Veterinary Uses: Urinary tract infection, perhaps diabetes

Contraindications: Pregnancy, kidney disease, inflammatory digestive conditions. Not for use in urinary tract infection when urine is acidic.

Toxicology and Adverse Effects: AHPA class 2b, 2d. Not for use longer than 2 weeks at a time. Hydroquinone is toxic in high doses—oral LD_{50} in rats is 320 mg/kg, and it is 400 mg/kg in mice, 550 mg/kg in guinea pigs, 70 mg/kg in cats, and 200 mg/kg in dogs (ESCOP, 1997). Maculopathy due to long-term ingestion for 3 years has been reported (Wang, 2004).

Potential Drug Interactions: Urinary acidifiers inhibit the conversion of arbutin to active hydroquinone, making uva ursi less effective. No other clinical interactions have been described. One constituent (coraligin) restored beta lactam activity against methicillin-resistant *Staphylococcus aureus* in vitro. May potentiate anti-inflammatory actions of steroids.

Notes of Interest: The generic name, derived from the Greek, and the Latin specific name, uva ursi, mean the same thing: the bear's grape. The name may have been given to the plant because of the notion that bears eat the fruit with relish, or it may derive from its very rough, unpleasant flavor, which may have been considered fit only for bears (pithy but not unpleasant).

The tannin in the leaves is so abundant that they have been used in Sweden and Russia for tanning leather.

Dosage: Herb should be used for no longer than 1 month.

Human:

Dried herb: 1-10 g TID, up to 6 times daily for acute conditions

Infusions: 5-30 g per cup of water, with 1 cup of the tea given TID, up to 6 times daily acutely

Tincture (usually 45% ethanol; some pharmacies include glycerin to prevent precipitation by tannins) 1:2 or 1:3: 1.5-5 mL TID, up to 6 times daily for acute conditions

Small Animal:

Dried herb: 50-400 mg/kg, divided daily (optimally, TID)

Infusion: 5-30 g per cup of water, administered at a rate of ¼-½ cup per 10 kg (20 lb), divided daily (optimally, TID)

Tincture (usually 45% ethanol; some pharmacies include glycerin to prevent precipitation by tannins) 1:2-1:3: 1.0-2.0 mL per 10 kg (20 lb), divided daily (optimally, TID) and diluted or combined with other herbs. Higher doses may be appropriate if the herb is used singly and is not combined in a formula.

Historic Veterinary Doses:

Dogs: fluid extract (1:1): 2-8 mL per dose (Milks, 1949)

Horses: fluid extract (1:1): 15-60 mL per dose (Milks, 1949)

References

ESCOP *Monographs on the Medical Uses of Plants*. European Scientific Cooperative on Phytotherapy, Exeter UK 1997

Grieve M. *A Modern Herbal*. London: Jonathan Cape; 1931 (Reprint 1975).

Jahodar L, Jilek P, Paktova M, Dvorakova V. [Antimicrobial effect of arbutin and an extract of the leaves of *Arctostaphylos uva-ursi* in vitro.] Cesk Farm 1985;34:174-178.

Matsuda H, Nakamura S, Shiomoto H, Tanaka T, Kubo M. [Pharmacological studies on leaf of *Arctostaphylos uva-ursi* (L.) Spreng. IV. Effect of 50% methanolic extract from *Arctostaphylos uva-ursi* (L.) Spreng. (bearberry leaf) on melanin synthesis.] Yakugaku Zasshi 1992a;112:276-282.

Matsuda H, Nakamura S, Tanaka T, Kubo M. [Pharmacological studies on leaf of *Arctostaphylos uva-ursi* (L.) Spreng. V. Effect of water extract from *Arctostaphylos uva-ursi* (L.) Spreng. (bearberry leaf) on the antiallergic and antiinflammatory activities of dexamethasone ointment.] Yakugaku Zasshi 1992b;112:673-677.

Matsuda H, Nakata H, Tanaka T, Kubo M. [Pharmacological study on *Arctostaphylos uva-ursi* (L.) Spreng. II. Combined effects of arbutin and prednisolone or dexamethazone on immuno-inflammation.] Yakugaku Zasshi 1990;110:68-76.

Matsuda H, Tanaka T, Kubo M. [Pharmacological studies on leaf of *Arctostaphylos uva-ursi* (L.) Spreng. III. Combined effect of arbutin and indomethacin on immuno-inflammation.] Yakugaku Zasshi 1991;111:253-258.

Milks HJ. *Practical Veterinary Pharmacology, Materia Medica and Therapeutics*. Chicago, Ill: Alex Eger, Inc.; 1949.

Nikolaev SM, Shantanova LN, Mondodoev A, et al. Pharmacological activity of the dry extract from the leaves of *Arc-*

tostaphylos uva-ursi L. in experimental nephropyelitis. Rastitel'nye Resursy 1996;32:118-123.
Nishimura T, Kometani T, Okada S, Ueno N, Yamamoto T. [Inhibitory effects of hydroquinone-alpha-glucoside on melanin synthesis.] Yakugaku Zasshi 1995;115:626-632.
Quintus J, Kovar KA, Link P, Hamacher H. Urinary excretion of arbutin metabolites after oral administration of bearberry leaf extracts. Planta Med 2005;71:147-152.
Schindler G, Patzak U, Brinkhaus B, et al. Urinary excretion and metabolism of arbutin after oral administration of *Arctostaphylos uvae ursi* extract as film-coated tablets and aqueous solution in healthy humans. J Clin Pharmacol 2002;42:920-927.
Swanston-Flatt SK, Day C, Bailey CJ, Flatt PR. Evaluation of traditional plant treatments for diabetes: studies in streptozotocin diabetic mice. Acta Diabetol Lat 1989;26:51-55.
Takii H, Matsumoto K, Kometani T, Okada S, Fushiki T. Lowering effect of phenolic glycosides on the rise in postprandial glucose in mice. Biosci Biotechnol Biochem 1997;61:1531-1535.
Turi M, Turi E, Koljalg S, Mikelsaar M. Influence of aqueous extracts of medicinal plants on surface hydrophobicity of *Escherichia coli* strains of different origin. APMIS 1997;105:956-962.
Wang L, Del Priore LV. Bull's-eye maculopathy secondary to herbal toxicity from uva ursi. Am J Ophthalmol 2004;137:1135-1137.

Valerian

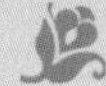

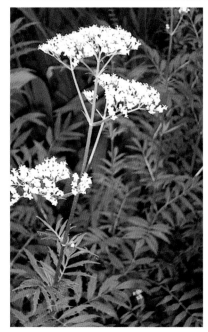

Valeriana officinalis L. • va-ler-ee-AH-nuh oh-fiss-ih-NAH-liss

Distribution: Europe, Northern Asia

Similar Species: *Valeriana dioica* (Linn.) (Marsh Valerian) may be a common inferior substitute. *Valeriana milkanii* (Syme) and *Valeriana sambucifolia* (Mikan) are two common English species used in the 20th century in trade. *Valeriana celtica* (Saliunca) was used in the East in ancient times for aromatic baths. *Valeriana sitchensis* is an American species considered in older Russian research to be a very potent species. *Valeriana edulis* and *Valeriana wallichi* (Indian Valerian) from China and India are used in Mexico, and *Valeriana chinensis* var. Batalin has been used for longer than 1000 years in China; *Valeriana fauriei* is used in China and Japan today. *Valeriana capensis* is used in Africa for epilepsy and nervous disorders.

Common Names: Setwall, setewale, great wild valerian, all-heal, amantilla, capon's tail, phu (galen or dioscorides), baldrianwurzel (German)

Family: Valerianaceae

Parts Used: Root. The odor makes valerian root easy to distinguish from pretenders.

Selected Constituents: Volatile oil (contains α- and β-pinene, borneol, etc.); sesquiterpenes (valerenic acid, valeranone, etc.); baldrinols and phenolic acids. The dried root contains γ-aminobutyric acid (GABA), but the alcoholic extract does not.

Valepotriate

Clinical Action: Sedative, hypnotic, antispasmodic, anticonvulsant, stimulant tonic

Energetics: Warm, pungent; some consider valerian to be a *Qi* mover with particular influence on the cardiovascular system.

History and Traditional Usage: Used since the Middle Ages for promoting sleep, relieving anxiety, suppressing maniacal and aggressive behavior, and controlling seizures. The Blackfoot tribe of North America administered decoctions of the root of *V. dioica* to horses for colic and distemper; both *V. dioica* and *V. sitchensis* were used externally for sores and wounds in horses (note anecdote relayed in Chapter 21 about a horse that colicked when given valerian, however). Various *Valeriana* species were used by Native Americans for diarrhea and stomach troubles, for seizures in babies, as a mild sedative, topically for wounds, and as flavor for smoking mixtures and incense. The Eclectics used valerian for nervous irritability and weakness, nervous headache, and epilepsy. The specific indication was as follows: "A cerebral stimulant. [Indicated for] hysteria, chorea, hemicrania; all with mental depression and despondency; cerebral anemia; mild spasmodic movements." The apparently paradoxical effects (e.g., cerebral stimulant, hypnotic) are resolved in this description of indications for this herb from *King's:*

"The cases requiring it are those evidencing enfeebled cerebral circulation; there is despondency and marked mental depression, often amounting to hypochondria. In properly selected cases, it relieves irritability and pain, and favors rest and sleep."

Milks (1949) stated that valerian is carminative and slightly stimulates the heart and vasomotor and respiratory centers. He explained that the antispasmodic and antihysteric actions in humans were probably not applicable to veterinary patients, in that the herb acted by stimulating the "highest centers which exert psychic control." He noted that although valerian had been recommended for chorea in dogs, it was not very effective.

Published Research: Valepotriates, valeric acid, and volatile oils interact with GABA. Valepotriates dissipate in days to weeks and are not contained in most commercial preparations. Aqueous extracts of valerian root contain significant amounts of GABA, although the oral bioavailability of this neurotransmitter in the context of valerian root is not known. Valerenic acid acts directly on the amygdaloid body in the brain and inhibits the breakdown of GABA, which leads to sedation (Houghton, 1999). Valerian extract and valerenic acid appear to modulate GABA receptor function as well (Yuan, 2004). Valepotriate activities are not as well understood, but they seem to act as prodrugs that are converted to homobaldrinol, a chemical that has been shown to reduce spontaneous motility in mice. The lignan, hydroxypinoresinol, binds benzodiazepine receptors (Houghton, 1999). Recent studies have shown that dichloromethane and petroleum ether extracts of valerian bind the 5-HT(5a) receptor, which is notably found in the suprachiasmatic nucleus of the brain, the area implicated in the sleep–wake cycle (Dietz, 2005).

Insomnia

In an Internet-based, randomized, double-blind, placebo-controlled trial, 391 participants with both anxiety and insomnia were asked whether taking kava, valerian, or the combination of both improved their sleep. Neither herb performed better than placebo in this trial (Jacobs, 2005). In a different trial, a series of 42 n-of-1 placebo-controlled trials showed that valerian was no better than placebo at improving sleep (Coxeter, 2003). Older trials were generally more positive.

A double-blind, placebo-controlled trial compared valerian (a 400-mg aqueous extract) with placebo. A total of 128 volunteers were studied for changes in sleep latency, sleep quality, sleepiness on awakening, night awakening, and dream recall. Valerian was significantly more effective than placebo in improving sleep latency and sleep quality (Leathwood, 1982). The same group conducted a double-blind trial, in which 8 people were given 450 mg or 900 mg of a valerian extract, or placebo. Again, ingestion of valerian was associated with better sleep (Leathwood, 1985). Other studies have had positive results (Donath, 2000; Balderer,1985); doses ranged from 450 to 900 mg. Valerian increased the number of alpha waves as measured by electroencephalogram and reduced anxiety, which appeared to be a main contributor to its benefit for insomnia (Poyares, 2002). In a trial in which oxazepam and valerian (600 mg/day of a proprietary extract) were compared for the treatment of patients with insomnia, valerian showed efficacy equal to that of oxazepam (Dorn, 2000).

Despite these promising results, a comprehensive review of valerian for insomnia concluded that results were inconsistent, and that valerian should be studied further for its use in insomnia (Stevinson, 2000).

If valerian is used for the treatment of those with insomnia, the onset of action occurs generally 2 to 3 weeks after supplementation is begun (Wheatley, 2005).

Stress

In laboratory stress tests, humans given valerian showed decreased heart rate and blood pressure (Cropley, 2002). In all, 70 hospitalized patients with various psychosomatic diagnoses were given Valmane (a valepotriate extract) at 150 to 300 mg daily. Tachycardia, hypertension, sweating, restless legs, and other conditions were positively affected by treatment (Boeters, 1969). In a different study, adults underwent laboratory social stress tests in a double-blind trial. Valerian was effective in reducing symptoms of anxiety in these subjects (Kohnen, 1988). In a randomized, double-blind study of 80 people with various anxiety syndromes, 270 mg daily of a standardized valerian extract was as effective and well tolerated as clobazam, according to standardized anxiety questionnaires (Sousa, 1992).

Cats given 10 mg/kg valerian extract by gastric lavage showed significant decreases in restless, fearful, and aggressive behaviors (von Eickstedt, 1969).

Cardiovascular disorders

Valerian has shown coronary vasodilating and antiarrhythmic activity in laboratory rabbits and mice (Petkov, 1979). In cats, intravenous valerian extract significantly increased coronary blood flow while temporarily reducing heart rate and blood pressure (Zhang, 1982).

Indications: Anxiety, nervous tension, insomnia, uterine cramps

Potential Veterinary Indications: Anxiety, insomnia, and possibly as an adjunct for the treatment of patients with epilepsy. May be useful in cats with hypertrophic cardiomyopathy

Contraindications: Some theoretical concern has been expressed that valerian may worsen the symptoms of schizophrenia or bipolar disorder in humans.

Toxicology and Adverse Effects: AHPA class 1. Some authors report paradoxical excitement or overstimulation after valerian is used. Tachycardia is also a common adverse effect in some people, as is a hung-over feeling the day after use. Overdose may cause nausea and stupor; in humans, headache and blurred vision have been reported. Rare allergic contact dermatitis has been documented. Valerian is considered a very safe herb and is generally recognized as safe (GRAS) by the U.S. Food and Drug Administration (FDA); it has been approved for use in food. Safety for long-term use has not been established.

Drug Interactions: Valerian may interact with barbiturates and other central nervous system depressants. It may also enhance the effects of benzodiazepines. Anecdotal reports have described valerian use that resulted in positive drug tests for reserpine in horses.

Notes of Interest: Mrs. Grieve (1975) has this to say about valerian and animals:

> "Valerian has an effect on the nervous system of many animals, especially cats, which seem to be thrown into a kind of intoxication by its scent. It is scarcely possible to keep a plant of valerian in a garden after the leaves or root has been bruised or disturbed in any way, for cats are at once attracted and roll on the unfortunate plant. It is equally attractive to rats and is often used by rat-catchers to bait their traps. It has been suggested that the famous Pied Piper of Hamelin owed his irresistible power over rats to the fact that he secreted Valerian roots about his person."

Dosage:

Human: For insomnia, take the last dose 30 min before you go to bed, doubling the amount. Valerian does not usually work immediately; consistent use over 3 to 4 weeks is required.

Dried herb: 1-10 g TID

Decoctions: 5-30 g per cup of water, with 1 cup of the tea given TID, up to 6 times daily acutely

Tincture (usually 45%-55%) 1:2 or 1:3: 1-5 mL TID

Small Animal:

Dried herb: 25-300 mg/kg, divided daily

Decoction: 5-30 g per cup of water, administered at a rate of ¼-½ cup per 10 kg (20 lb), divided daily

Tincture (usually 45%-55% ethanol) 1:2-1:3: 0.5-1.5 mL per 10 kg (20 lb), divided daily and diluted or combined with other herbs. Higher doses may be appropriate if the herb is used singly and is not combined in a formula

Large Animal (Karreman, 2004)*:*

Horses: fluid extract, 30-60 mL; oil, 2-4 mL

Farm animals: fluid extract: cow, 30-60 mL; sheep and goat, 4-8 mL ; oil cow, 2-4 mL; sheep and goat, 0.6-1.3 mL

Historical Veterinary Doses:

Horse and Cow

Dried herb: 1-2 oz (Milks, 1949)

Dog

Dried herb: 1-7.5 g

Tincture: 7-15 mL (Milks, 1949)

References

Balderer G, Borbely AA. Effect of valerian on human sleep. Psychopharmacology [Berl] 1985;87:406-409.

Boeters U. Treatment of control disorders of the autonomic nervous system with valepotriate (Valmane). Munch Med Wochenschr 1969;111:1873-1876.

Cropley M, Cave Z, Ellis J, Middleton RW. Effect of kava and valerian on human physiological and psychological responses to mental stress assessed under laboratory conditions. Phytother Res 2002;16:23-27.

Dietz BM, Mahady GB, Pauli GF, Farnsworth NR. Valerian extract and valerenic acid are partial agonists of the 5-HT5a receptor in vitro. Brain Res Mol Brain Res 2005;138:191-197.

Donath F, Quispe S, Diefenbach K, Maurer A, Fietze I, Roots I. Critical evaluation of the effect of valerian extract on sleep structure and sleep quality. Pharmacopsychiatry 2000;33:47-53.

Dorn M. [Efficacy and tolerability of Baldrian versus oxazepam in non-organic and non-psychiatric insomniacs: a randomised, double-blind, clinical, comparative study.] [Article in German] Forsch Komplementarmed Klass Naturheilkd 2000;7:79-84.

Grieve M. *A Modern Herbal*. London: Jonathan Cape; 1931 (Reprint, 1975).

Houghton PJ. The scientific basis for the reputed activity of Valerian. J Pharm Pharmacol 1999;51:505-512.

Jacobs BP, Bent S, Tice JA, Blackwell T, Cummings SR. An Internet-based randomized, placebo-controlled trial of kava and valerian for anxiety and insomnia. Medicine (Baltimore) 2005;84:197-207.

Karreman H. *Treating Dairy Cows Naturally: Thoughts and Strategies*. Paradise, Pa: Paradise Publications; 2004.

Kohnen R, Oswald WD. The effects of valerian, propranolol, and their combination on activation, performance, and mood of healthy volunteers under social stress conditions. Pharmacopsychiatry 1988;21:447-448.

Leathwood PD, Chauffard F, Heck E, Munoz-Box R. Aqueous extract of valerian root (*Valeriana officinalis* L.) improves sleep quality in man. Pharmacol Biochem Behav 1982;17:65-71.

Leathwood PD, Chauffard F. Aqueous extract of valerian reduces latency to fall asleep in man. Planta Med 1985;2:144-148.

Milks HJ. *Practical Veterinary Pharmacology, Materia Medica and Therapeutics*. Chicago, Ill: Alex Eger, Inc.; 1949.

Petkov V. Plants and hypotensive, antiatheromatous and coronarodilatating action. Am J Chin Med 1979;7:197-236.

Poyares DR, Guilleminault C, Ohayon MM, Tufik S. Can valerian improve the sleep of insomniacs after benzodiazepine withdrawal? Prog Neuropsychopharmacol Biol Psychiatry 2002;26:539-545.

Sousa MPD, Pacheco P, Roldao V. Double-blind comparative study of the efficacy and safety of Valdispert vs clobazapam. KaliChemie Medical Research and Information, 1992. In Blumenthal M, Hall T, Goldberg A, Kunz T, Dinda K, Brinkman J, et al, eds. The ABC Clinical Guide to Herbs. Austin, TX, The American Botanical Counal, 2003.

Stevinson C, Ernst E. Valerian for insomnia: a systematic review of randomized clinical trials. Sleep Med 2000;1:91-99.

von Eickstedt KW. Modification of the alcohol effect by valepotriate. Arzneimittelforschung 1969;19:995-997.

Wheatley D. Kava and valerian in the treatment of stress-induced insomnia. Phytother Res 2001;15:549-551.

Wheatley D. Medicinal plants for insomnia: a review of their pharmacology, efficacy and tolerability. J Psychopharmacol 2005;19:414-421.

Yuan CS, Mehendale S, Xiao Y, Aung HH, Xie JT, Ang-Lee MK. The gamma-aminobutyric acidergic effects of valerian and valerenic acid on rat brainstem neuronal activity. Anesth Analg 2004;98:353-358, table of contents.

Zhang BH, Meng HP, Wang T, et al. Effects of *Valeriana officinalis* L. extract on cardiovascular system. Yao Hsueh Hsueh Pao 1982;17:382-384.

Varuna

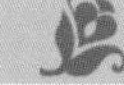

Crataeva nurvala Buch.-Ham. syn. *Crateva nurvala* Buch.-Ham. • *kray TA vuh ner VAH luh*

Common Names: Varuna, Three-Leaved Caper

Family: Capparidaceae

Parts Used: Stem and root bark and leaves

Distribution: Throughout India and cultivated worldwide.

Selected Constituents: Varuna contains lupeol (a triterpene), the most active principle, which has antiurolithic properties and reverses biochemical and histopathologic changes caused by calculosis (Anand, 1990); it also contains glucosinolates, triterpenoid saponins, sterols (including β-sitosterol), and flavonoids (e.g., catechin).

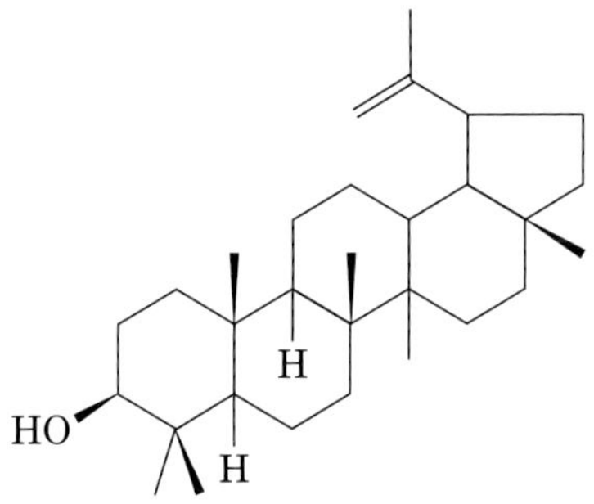

Clinical Actions: Anti-inflammatory, antilithic, bladder tonic, urinary antiseptic
Energetics: Cooling
History and Traditional Usage: Crataevus was a Greek botanist from whom the name of crataeva is derived. The plant was known to ancient physicians, who used it as a blood purifier and for maintenance of homeostasis. Ayurvedic medicine texts dating back to 1100 AD record the use of varuna in urinary tract disorders; Varuna is the name of the God of Water in the Hindu religion.

It is used in the treatment of patients with urinary tract infection, calculi, and crystalluria and is valued as a bitter, astringent, demulcent, laxative, rubifacient, tonic, liver stimulant, and vesicant; it is also used for malaria and tumors.

Ethnoveterinary usage includes the treatment of animals with renal lithiasis, swelling of the liver, and diarrhea (Williamson, 2002).

Published Research: In human studies, 50 mL of decoction given twice daily for 3 months significantly improved incontinence, pain, and retention in patients with prostatic hypertrophy with hypotonic bladder (Deshpande, 1982). After 4 weeks of treatment, 68% of patients had achieved symptomatic relief from chronic urinary tract infection; 17% were devoid of microorganisms and white cells (Deshpande, 1982).

Water extract of the stem bark increased tone in guinea pig, dog, and human skeletal and smooth muscle (intestine and ureter) in vitro (Das, 1974); after oral treatment with varuna was provided for 40 days, a significant increase in bladder tone was observed in dogs (Deshpande, 1982).

The role of lupeol in calcium oxalate experimental rat urolithiasis was studied. Lupeol administration (25 mg/kg body weight/day) significantly reduced oxalate excretion by kidneys. It also decreased levels of damage marker enzymes in urine, which may indicate a reduction in tubular damage. Such effects may be beneficial in minimizing the deposition of stone-forming constituents in the kidney (Malini, 1995). Administration of lupeol and its structural analogue betulin to hyperoxaluric rats minimized tubular damage and reduced markers of crystal deposition in the kidneys, and lupeol was found to be more effective than betulin (Vidya, 2000).

In rats, lupeol produced a dose-dependent (10-50 mg/kg po) (up to 95%) reduction in weight of the formed urolith (protective effect). In preformed stones after 16 weeks of lupeol at 10 to 50 mg/kg po, a weight reduction of 15% to 55% was observed in stones, but no size reduction was detected. Very small stones had disappeared, suggesting their dissolution or subsequent flushing. Biochemical and urinary abnormalities were markedly normalized (Anand, 1994). Stem bark decoction was used in patients with calcium oxalate stones. After 12 weeks, pain and dysuria were significantly reduced, as was the size of stones (Singh, 1991).

In an experimental model in rats, Crataeva significantly inhibited bladder stone formation. Bladders of treated animals showed less edema, ulceration, and cellular infiltration when compared with controls (Deshpande, 1982). Among 46 patients with calcium oxalate stone who used 50 mL decoction twice daily for between 1 and 47 weeks, 28 passed the stone and 18 experienced symptomatic relief. These outcomes were thought to be due to the tonic contractile action of the drug on smooth muscle (Deshpande, 1982).

In rats, crude extract given at 100 mg/kg PO significantly reduced stone formation (81%) (Prabhakar, 1997). In an earlier study, crataeva decoction prevented the expected elevation of the oxalate-synthesizing liver enzyme, glycolate oxidase, produced by feeding of glycollic acid; it was thought that crataeva had a regulatory action on endogenous oxalate synthesis. On the other hand, protein-bound carbohydrates were increased in the renal tissues during calculosis, but these changes were not reversed with crataeva. Increased deposition of stone-forming constituents in the kidneys of calculogenic rats was lowered with decoction administration. Increased urinary excretion of the crystalline constituents, along with lowered magnesium excretion found in stone-forming rats, was partially reversed by decoction treatment (Varalakshmi, 1990).

A pharmacologic study showed that crataeva influenced small intestinal sodium and potassium adenosine triphosphatase (ATPase), which may in turn influence transport of minerals (Varalakshmi, 1991).

Lupeol is an effective antioxidant (Baskar, 1996). The effects of lupeol and lupeol linoleate on the development of complement in adjuvant arthritis in rats were studied and compared with those of indomethacin as a model for rheumatoid arthritis in people. Results suggest that the anti-inflammatory activity of the triterpenes may be due to their anticomplementary activity (Geetha, 1999a). Lupeol and lupeol linoleate were administered orally (50 mg/kg) for 8 days to arthritic rats, after the 11th day of adjuvant injection. Lupeol linoleate was more effective than lupeol, possibly because it caused stabilization of the lysosomal membrane of cells (Geetha, 1999b).

Indications: Chronic urinary tract infection; prevention of kidney and bladder stones; benign prostatic hyperplasia; hypotonic and atonic bladder; incontinence; adjunct treatment for urinary calculi (calcium oxalate)

Potential Veterinary Uses: Calcium oxalate and possibly other uroliths; urinary tract infection; atonic and hypotonic bladder; incontinence
Contraindications: None found.
Toxicology and Adverse Effects: The LD_{50} of a 50% ethanolic extract of stem bark was found to be greater than 1000 mg/kg administered intraperitoneally to adult rats.
Dosage:
Human:
Dried herb: 4.5-8 g TID
Traditional decoction: 1 part powdered stem bark boiled in 16 parts water and evaporated until ¼ remains
Tincture (generally 25% ethanol) 1:2: 6-14 mL, divided daily
Small Animal:
Dried herb: 50-400 mg/kg, divided daily (optimally, TID)
Tincture (generally 25% ethanol) 1:2: 1.0-3.0 mL per 10 kg (20 lb), divided daily and diluted or combined with other herbs

References

Anand R, Patnaik G, Jain P, et al. Antiurolithic activity of *Crataeva nurvala* in Albino rats. Indian J Pharmacol 1990; 222:23-24.
Anand R, Patnaik G, Kulshreshtha D, et al. Antiurolithiatic activity of lupeol, the active constituent isolated from *Crataeva nurvala*. Phytother Res 1994;8:417-421.
Baskar R. Effect of lupeol isolated from *Crataeva nurvala* stem bark against free radical induced toxicity in experimental urolithiasis. Fitoterapia 1996;67:121-125.
Das P. Antiinflammatory and antiarthritic activity of Varuna. J Res Indian Med 1974;9:49.
Deshpande P, Sahu M, Kumar P. *Crataeva nurvala* Hook and Forst (Varun): the Ayurvedic drug of choice in urinary disorders. Indian J Med Res 1982;76(suppl):46-53.
Geetha T, Varalakshmi P. Anticomplement activity of triterpenes from *Crataeva nurvala* stem bark in adjuvant arthritis in rats. Gen Pharmacol 1999a;32:495-497.
Geetha T, Varalakshmi P. Effect of lupeol and lupeol linoleate on lysosomal enzymes and collagen in adjuvant-induced arthritis in rats. Mol Cell Biochem 1999b;201:83-87.
Malini MM, Baskar R, Varalakshmi P. Effect of lupeol, a pentacyclic triterpene, on urinary enzymes in hyperoxaluric rats. Jpn J Med Sci Biol 1995;48:211-220.
Prabhakar Y, Kumar S. *Crataeva nurvala:* an Ayurvedic remedy for urological disorders. Br J Phytother 1997;4:103-109.
Singh R. Evaluation of antilithic properties of varun *(Crataeva nurvala):* an indigenous drug. J Res Indian Med 1991;10:35-39.
Varalakshmi P, Latha E, Shamila Y, Jayanthi S. Effect of *Crataeva nurvala* on the biochemistry of the small intestinal tract of normal and stone-forming rats. J Ethnopharmacol 1991;31:67-73.
Varalakshmi P, Shamila Y, Latha E. Effect of *Crataeva nurvala* in experimental urolithiasis. J Ethnopharmacol 1990;28:313-321.
Vidya L, Varalakshmi P. Control of urinary risk factors of stones by betulin and lupeol in experimental hyperoxaluria. Fitoterapia 2000;71:535-543.
Williamson E, ed. *Major Herbs of Ayurveda*. Sydney: Churchill Livingstone; 2002.

Wild Cherry

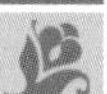

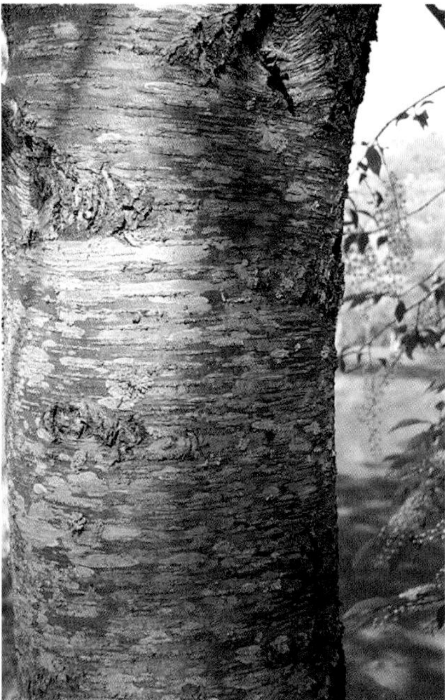

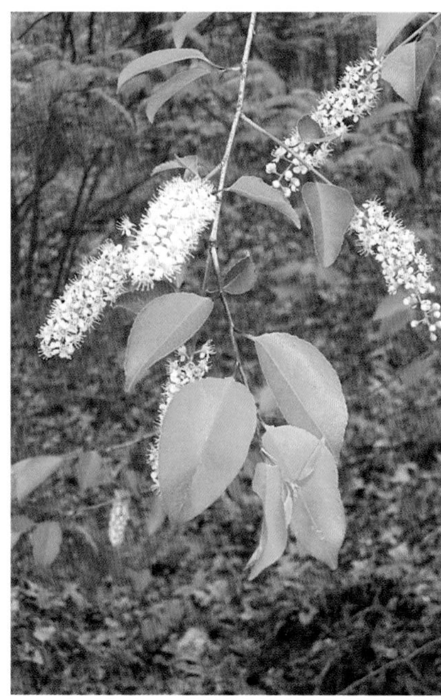

Prunus serotina Ehrh., formerly *Prunus virginiana* • PROO-nus se-roh-TEE-nuh
Distribution: Native to North America
Other Names: Black cherry, wild black cherry, Virginia prune, sauerkirsch, griottier, cerezo, ciliegio, ying tao
Family: Rosaceae
Parts Used: Inner bark
Collection: Bark harvested in the spring contains more tannins, and bark collected in the autumn is higher in starch and prussic acid. Fall-harvested bark is viewed as more desirable.
Selected Constituents: Cyanogenic glycosides (prunasin), tannins, flavonoids, sugars, coumarins (scopoletin)

Prunasin

Clinical Action: Antitussive, antispasmodic, mildly astringent

Energetics: Astringent, bitter, aromatic

History and Traditional Usage: Native Americans used the bark and roots for diarrhea, fever, "female problems," and pain; topically for skin problems and cough. The berries were used for food. Used as a cough suppressant for bronchitis, whooping cough, pneumonia, and asthma to relieve the cough—usually as part of a formula to address other aspects of these conditions. Also used topically as an eyewash for keratitis. *King's* claimed that it is best for chronic problems. It can also be used for fever and inflammatory problems, sore throat, gastrointestinal problems, and diarrhea.

Published Research: Clinical research on this herb appears to be lacking.

Indications: Persistent, irritating cough

Potential Veterinary Indications: Chronic bronchitis, asthma (should be combined with an expectorant herb)

Contraindications: Pregnancy and lactation

Toxicology and Adverse Effects: AHPA class 2d. Not for long-term use. Enzymatic hydrolysis of prunasin yields prussic acid (hydrogen cyanide) and benzaldehyde. The agent has been classified as GRAS (generally recognized as safe) and is used as a flavoring for syrups; however, it is dangerous in large doses or when taken for a long period. Cases of livestock poisoning after animals have eaten from low or fallen branches have been well recognized.

Drug Interactions: May affect the metabolism of drugs processed through the CYP3A4 P450 isozymes, although clinical interactions have not been reported.

Dosage: Some authors state that cold infusion is the preferred form; it best extracts the cyanogenic glycosides

Human:

Dried herb: 0.25-10 g TID, up to 6 times daily for acute conditions

Decoctions: 5-30 g per cup of water, with 1 cup of the tea given TID, up to 6 times daily acutely

Tincture (usually 40%-50% ethanol) 1:2 or 1:3: 0.25-5 mL TID, up to 6 times daily for acute conditions

Small Animal:

Dried herb: 25-300 mg/kg, divided daily (optimally, TID)

Decoction: 5-30 g per cup of water, administered at a rate of ½-4 cups, divided daily (optimally, TID)

Tincture (usually 40%-50% ethanol) 1:2-1:3: 0.5-2.0 mL per 10 kg (20 lb), divided daily (optimally, TID) and diluted or combined with other herbs

Historic Veterinary Doses:

Fluid extract (1:1): horse, ½-1 oz; dog, 1-7 mL (Bunn, circa 1920)

Syrup: dog, 2-7 mL (Bunn, circa 1920)

Reference

Bunn, JF. veterinary school lectures, undated (approximately 1920, Concord, NC).

Wild Yam

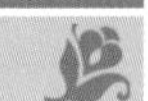

Dioscorea villosa L. • di-oh-SKOR-ee-uh vil-OH-suh

Distribution: North and Central America

Similar Species: *Dioscorea batatas* or *Dioscorea opposita* is Shan Yao used in Chinese medicine.

Other Names: Colic root, China root, North American wild yam, rheumatism root, igname sauvage, racines de colique, zottige yamswurzel, dioscorea, Atlantic yam

Family: Dioscoreaceae

Parts Used: Rhizome

Selected Constituents: Steroidal saponins (diosgenin glycosides, including dioscin), polysaccharides, alkaloid (dioscorin), tannins

Diosgenin

History and Traditional Usage: Native North Americans used the root as food and for pain relief during childbirth. Antispasmodic, anti-inflammatory, cholagogue. Used to relieve pain from spasm in the gastrointestinal tract, gallbladder, and uterus; also used for rheumatism. For nausea, colic (gallbladder, hepatic, gastric, or intestinal), ovarian and uterine spasm. Commonly used today by women for a supposed progesterone-like effect (for menopausal symptoms and birth control) because marketers claim that it contains dehydroepiandrosterone (DHEA) or progesterone; this is inaccurate. (Anecdotes that support a progesterone-like effect may be associated with products that are spiked with synthetic progesterone.)

Energetics: Bitter, mildly pungent, and sour; moves *Qi*

Published Research: Evidence from in vitro trials from the 1920s supports the presence of antirheumatic, antispasmodic properties (Brinker 1996). Wild yam (80 mg/kg) reduced intestinal inflammation and normalized bile secretion in an experimental model (Yamada, 1997).

Diosgenin can be converted in vitro to a number of hormonal agents (e.g., progesterone, dihydroepiandrosterone). Although it has been suggested that this conversion may occur in vivo, existing objective evidence does not support this claim (Arahiniknam, 1996; Dollbaum, 1996).

A trial in menopausal women that compared a wild yam cream with placebo showed that the cream was ineffective in relieving symptoms of menopause (Komesaroff, 2001). By contrast, postmenopausal women were instructed to replace their staple food (which was usually rice) with white yam (*Dioscorea alata,* 390 g daily for 30 days) or sweet potato (240 g daily). Significant increases in serum concentrations of estrone and sex hormone binding globulin, as well as near significant increases in estradiol, were noted in the group that ate yams. Urinary estrogen metabolites decreased and serum androgen increased. Plasma cholesterol decreased slightly, but significantly. Only serum estrone, estradiol, and sex hormone binding globulin were measured in the control group; these levels did not change (Wu, 2005).

Many laboratory animal studies suggest that wild yam beneficially modulates blood lipids. Diosgenin alone was effective in some studies in increasing biliary cholesterol output (Ulloa, 1985; Nervi, 1984). Diosgenin may block intestinal reuptake of intraluminal cholesterol (Zagoya, 1971). Hypercholesterolemic animal models showed decreasing cholesterol absorption, increasing hepatic cholesterol synthensis, and increasing biliary cholesterol secretion when diosgenin was added to the diet (Nervi, 1988; Cayen, 1979; Uchida, 1984). Dioscorea treatment was associated with a decrease in serum triglycerides, but no change in serum cholesterol was seen in humans with ischemic heart disease (Zakharov, 1977). Seven elderly volunteers were given doses of wild yam pills; no increases in serum DHEA were noted. However, lower serum triglycerides and higher HDL were seen (Araghiniknam, 1996).

Other species of *Dioscorea* have shown hypoglycemic, hypocholesterolemic, and antirheumatic activity in animal and human trials.

Indications: Irritable bowel, biliary colic, intestinal colic, flatulent colic, dysmenorrheal symptoms, menstrual pain, hyperlipidemia

Potential Veterinary Indications: Tenesmus and painful colitis, inflammatory bowel disease, flatulent colic, abdominal spasms, hyperlipidemia

Notes of Interest: Mexican wild yam has been and is still used commercially as a source for partial synthesis of pharmaceutical steroids and contraceptives, although total synthesis (via cell culture systems) is increasingly used. No evidence suggests that steroidal saponins contained in the herb are converted to steroids in vivo. Relatives of this plant provide the edible yam, but they are members of the sweet potato family (Convolvulaceae).

Contraindications: Use with caution in pregnancy and lactation. The most conservative sources list gallbladder and hepatic disease as contraindications, in direct contrast to some traditional uses.

Toxicology and Adverse Effects: AHPA class 1. Overdose of the tincture may lead to nausea, vomiting, diarrhea, and headache.

Drug Interactions: Animal studies have suggested that wild yam, in combination with clofibrate, synergistically lowers low-density lipoprotein (beyond the effects of clofibrate alone) (Cayen, 1978).

Dosage:

Human:

Dried herb: 0.5-10 g TID

Decoctions: 5-30 g per cup of water, with 1 cup of the tea given TID

Tincture (usually 40%-60% ethanol) 1:2 or 1:3: 1-5 mL TID, up to 6 times daily for acute conditions

Small Animals:

Dried herb: 25-300 mg/kg, divided daily (optimally, TID)

Decoction: 5-30 g per cup of water, administered at a rate of ¼-½ cup per 10 kg (20 lb), divided daily (optimally, TID)

Tincture (usually 40%-60% ethanol) 1:2-1:3: 0.5-1.5 mL per 10 kg (20 lb), divided daily (optimally, TID) and diluted or combined with other herbs. Higher doses may be appropriate if the herb is used singly and is not combined in a formula.

Horses:

Fluid extract (1:1): 8-24 mL ((Karreman, 2004)

Farm Animals:

Fluid extract (1:1): horses and cows, 8-24 mL; sheep and goats, 2-4 mL (Karreman, 2004)

Combinations: Should be used with carminatives such as ginger and fennel for gastrointestinal spasm and gas.

References

Araghiniknam M, Chung S, Nelson-White T et al. Antioxidant activity of disocorea and dehydroepiandrosterone (DHEA) in older humans. Life Sci 1996;59:147-157.

Boon H, Smith M. *Botanical Pharmacy.* Kingston: Quarry Press; 1999.

Brinker FA. A comparative view of eclectic female regulators. J Naturopathic Med 1996;7:11-26.

Cayen MN, Dvornik D. Combined effects of clofibrate and diosgenin on cholesterol metabolism in rats. Atherosclerosis 1978; 29:317-328.

Cayen MN, Dvornik D. Effects of diosgenin on lipid metabolism in rats. J Lipid Res 1979;20:162-174.

Dollbaum C. Lab analyses of salivary DHEA and progesterone following ingestion of yam-containing products. Townsend Letter for Doctors and Patients 1996;Aug/Sept:101.

Karreman H. *Treating Dairy Cows Naturally: Thoughts and Strategies.* Paradise, Pa: Paradise Publications; 2004.

Komesaroff PA, Black CV, Cable V, Sudhir K. Effects of wild yam extract on menopausal symptoms, lipids and sex hormones in healthy menopausal women. Climacteric 2001;4: 144-150.

Nervi F, Bronfman M, Allalon W, Depiereux E, Pozo RD. Regulation of biliary cholesterol secretion in the rat: role of hepatic cholesterol esterification. J Clin Invest 1984;74:2226-2237.

Nervi F, Marinovic I, Rigotti A, Ulloa N. Regulation of biliary cholesterol secretion: functional relationship between the canalicular and sinusoidal cholesterol secretory pathways in the rat. J Clin Invest 1988;82:1818-1825.

Uchida K, Takase H, Nomura Y, Takeda Ki, Takeuchi N, Ishikawa Y. Effects of diosgenin and B-sitosterol on bile acids. J Lipid Res 1984;25:236-245.

Ulloa N, Nervi F. Mechanism and kinetic characteristics of the uncoupling by plant steroids of biliary cholesterol from bile salt output. Botanika et Biophysica Acta 1985;837:181-189.

Wu WH, Liu LY, Chung CJ, Jou HJ, Wang TA. Estrogenic effect of yam ingestion in healthy postmenopausal women. J Am Coll Nutr 2005;24:235-243.

Yamada T, Hoshino M, Hawakawa T, et al. Dietary diosgenin attenuates subacute intestinal inflammation associated with indomethacin in rats. Am J Physiol 1997;273(2 Pt 1):G355-G364.

Zagoya JCD, Laguna J, Guzman-Garcia J. Studies on the regulation of cholesterol metabolism by the use of the structural analogue, diosgenin. Biochem Pharmacol 1971;20:3471-3480.

Zakharov VN. Hypolipemic effect of diosponine in ischemic heart disease depending on the type of hyperlipoproteinemia. Kardiologiia 1977;17:136-137.

Willow Bark 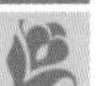

Salix alba L. • SAL-iks *or* SAY-liks AL-buh

Common Names: White willow bark, willow, salix cortex, bail liu, bai liu gen (root), bai liu ye (leaf)

Similar Species: The name *white willow* caught on among herbalists, even though it was not a preferred source of the bark. Several other species are preferred. Many *Salix* species (e.g., crack willow *[S. fragilis]*, purple willow *[S. purpurea]*, and *S. daphnoides*) are used interchangeably with white willow. *Salix acrophylla* is used in India for fever. *Salix alba* is among the poorest sources of salicin among *Salix* species.

Family: Salicaceae

Parts Used: Bark (inner bark); outer bark can be very corky. Originally, bark of branches—not trunk bark—was used. The bark is stripped from branches of 2- to 5-year-old trees in the spring.

Distribution: *Salix alba* is native to much of Europe. It is also found in North Africa and Asia, and it thrives in damp areas such as river banks.

Selected Constituents: *Salix* contains phenolic glycosides, including salicin, salicortin, salireposide, picein, and triandrin. Salicylates calculated as salicin vary between species (e.g., 0.5% in *S. alba,* 1%-10% in *S. fragilis,* 3%-9% in *S. purpurea*). Up to 20% of *Salix* bark consists of tannins; *Salix* also contains catechins and flavonoids.

Salicin **Acetylsalicylic acid**

Clinical Actions: Anti-inflammatory, antirheumatic, antipyretic, antiseptic, analgesic, astringent

Energetics: Cold, dry

History and Traditional Usage: Salicylate-containing plants have been used since antiquity. The Assyrians and the Egyptians were aware of the analgesic effects of a decoction of willow leaves for joint pain. Hippocrates recommended chewing willow leaves for analgesia in childbirth. In 1827, salicin was extracted from meadowsweet (*Filipendula ulmaria,* formerly *Spiraea ulmaria*), and French chemists discovered how to convert salicin into salicylic acid. Salicylic acid, however, was too irritating on the stomach to be taken orally. Charles Gerhardt was the first to synthesize acetylsalicylic acid, or aspirin, but Felix Hoffman from Bayer in Germany reportedly tested the rediscovered agent on himself and on his father (Levesque, 2000). Bayer began marketing acetylsalicylic acid in 1899 under the trade name *aspirin.* Bayer named the drug after the German word (spirsäure) for salicylic acid, which had first been isolated from meadowsweet (spirea). Spirea (meadowsweet) was never a commercial source for the drug; acetylsalicylic acid was synthesized because Hoffman developed that process for Bayer.

Willow bark has a long history of folk use for relief of headache. It has been used to treat patients with many different kinds of pain, including rheumatic pain, back pain, toothache, headache, and menstrual cramps. It is also used to relieve sore throat, fever, and headache associated with upper respiratory tract infection and influenza (Friend, 1974). It has been approved by the U.S. Food and Drug Administration (FDA) as a topical treatment for warts and calluses, bunions, corns, and acne. Salicylic acid is a strong antiseptic because of its carboxylated phenol base. The European Scientific Cooperative on Phytotherapy (ESCOP) has approved willow bark extract to treat patients with fever, pain, and mild rheumatic complaints (Anon, 1997)

Cattle and horses eat the young shoots and foliage, and the bark has been used for fever, debility, enteritis, colic, pleurisy, rheumatism, rickets, and cramps (de Bairacli Levy, 1963). The herb does not have prominence in the authors' historic books, but salicin and salicylic acid, once synthesized in the 19th century, began to appear in 20th century veterinary *Materia Medica* texts.

Published Research: Willow bark extract has anti-inflammatory activities that are comparable with those of acetylsalicylic acid (ASA), and it shows antinociceptive and antipyretic action. A daily dose of 1572 mg willow bark extract of a proprietary preparation (Assalix; standardized to 15.2% salicin, i.e., 240 mg salicin per day) produced no adverse effects, in contrast to ASA, on the stomach mucosa. In two open studies, with active treatments as controls, Willow Bark extract exhibited advantages against routinely prescribed nonsteroidal antirheumatic drugs; it also displayed similar efficacy to the cyclooxygenase (COX)-2 inhibitor refecoxib (Marz, 2002). The proprietary willow bark extract (Assalix; Bionorica, Neumarkt, Germany) is a selective inhibitor of COX-2–mediated prostaglandin E_2 release. It inhibits the release of cytokines to a greater or lesser degree—possibly enough to have a preventive effect on cartilage destruction (Chrubasik, 2001; Goldring, 1999).

A very early study showed that an extract (1 : 1) of fresh willow bark (1 tsp diluted in half a glass of water three times daily after meals) for the treatment of patients with chronic rheumatic disease was a strong antirheumatic, antineuralgic, and antipyretic, with no undesirable adverse effects. The dose was increased to 2 to 3 teaspoons three times daily in cases of acute illness or fever (Mayer, 1949).

In patients with osteoarthritis, a double-blind, placebo-controlled study on the efficacy of a standardized willow bark extract showed that a daily dose of 1572 mg of the aforementioned Assalix was significantly superior to placebo. Patients had osteoarthritis of the hip and knee or chronic low back pain. The study concluded that the willow bark extract showed a moderate analgesic effect in osteoarthritis and was well tolerated (Schmid, 2001b).

In another randomized, placebo-controlled, blinded trial, the effectiveness of willow bark extract for the treatment of low back pain was investigated. Patients were randomly assigned to receive an oral willow bark extract with 120 mg (low dose) or 240 mg (high dose) of salicin, or placebo, with tramadol as the sole rescue medication, in a 4-week blinded trial. In the last week of treatment, the numbers of pain-free patients were highest in the group receiving high-dose extract, next highest in the group receiving low-dose extract, and significantly lower in the placebo group. Response in the high-dose group was evident after only 1 week of treatment. Willow Bark extract may be a useful and safe treatment for those with low back pain (Chrubasik, 2000).

The analgesic effects of a standardized willow bark extract (240 mg salicin/day) in patients with osteoarthritis of the knee or hip were investigated in a randomized, double-blind, placebo-controlled clinical trial. The analgesic effect was reportedly comparable with the effect of tenoxicam (20 mg/day) and approximately 40% lower than the effect of diclofenac (150 mg/day) (Schmid, 1998).

The effects of salicin, saligenin (an aglycone of salicin), and salicylic acid (an active metabolite of salicin) were compared in pharmacokinetic and pharmacologic studies in rats. Salicylic acid appeared rapidly in the plasma after sodium salicylate and saligenin were administered, but not after salicin was given. Salicin did not induce gastric lesions at a dose of 5 mmol/kg, but sodium salicylate and saligenin induced severe gastric lesions dose dependently. This study suggests that salicin is a prodrug that is gradually transported to the lower part of the intestine, is hydrolyzed to saligenin by intestinal bacteria, is converted to salicylic acid after absorption, and provides antipyretic effects without causing gastric ulceration (Akao, 2002).

Willow bark extract also shows antithrombocyte activity, but the activity is clearly weak (Marz, 2002). In a placebo-controlled study, acetylsalicylate (100 mg) had a significant inhibitory effect on platelet aggregation compared with willow extract and placebo. Daily consumption of willow extract with 240 mg salicin per day affects platelet aggregation to a far lesser extent than does intake of acetylsalicylate (Krivoy, 2001); therefore willow should not be used as a substitute for aspirin in a preventive thrombolytic protocol against stroke and heart attack. On the other hand, salicin preparations from crude willow bark do not present a hemorrhagic risk and may be clinically advantageous for the treatment of pain some patients.

Indications: Rheumatoid arthritis, ankylosing spondylitis, respiratory catarrh

Potential Veterinary Indications: Anti-inflammatory; antipyretic; osteoarthritis, ankylosing spondylitis, myositis

Contraindications: Salicylate sensitivity

Toxicology and Adverse Events: AHPA class 1. Safety has been described in cats: Assuming that willow bark *(Salix alba)* contains 0.5% to 1% salicins and that a 1:2 extract contains 500 mg willow in 1 mL, 1% is 5000 μg or 5 mg. A 1-mL dose would provide 5 mg salicin or 10% of the normal dose of aspirin (50 mg) in cats; thus, the risk of reaching toxic levels with normal doses in cats is very low (Fougere, 2003).

In brushtail possums, salicin was administered orally by incorporation in food for 6 days at three dose levels (0.05%, 0.5%, and 1.5% wet weight). Salicyl alcohol glucuronide accounted for 56% to 64% of urinary metabolites, salicyluric acid 15% to 26%, and salicin 10% to 18%; smaller amounts of free (2%-4%) and conjugated (0%-6%) salicylic acid were included. Hydrolysis of dietary salicin enabled reconjugation of its aglycone, salicyl alcohol, with a more polar sugar, glucuronic acid, thus enhancing its renal excretion and resulting in little net loss of substrates for conjugation and a low measurable metabolic cost of excretion (McLean, 2001).

In humans and rats, willow is considered to be a safe herb. It is possible that signs of toxicity associated with salicylates may occur with willow consumption. However, given the large amount of willow bark that must be consumed to equal the salicylate content of one aspirin, this is an unlikely possibility. Salicin has been documented to cause skin rash. Safety during pregnancy, lactation, or childhood has not been established.

Nephropathy has been associated with *Salix* ingestion in six okapis *(Okapia johnstoni)* (relatives of the giraffe). Although the cause and pathogenesis are unclear, primary damage of the renal tubular epithelium appears to be the most likely cause, and toxicity from ingested plant material, possibly willow, is possible (Haenichen, 2001).

Potential Drug Interactions: Nonsteroidal anti-inflammatory drugs (NSAIDs), particularly aspirin, have the potential to interact with herbal supplements that are known to possess antiplatelet activity (Abebe, 2002). Note that the activity of salicin is very low.

Notes of Interest: Of importance when the use of willow bark preparations is considered is the decision of whether to use anti-inflammatory agents at all in patients with fever. Inflammation is a homeostatic response to pathogens and tissue injury. Inhibiting such processes may do more harm than good and may be associated with some degree of cellular and organ system toxicity. The use of anti-inflammatory agents should therefore be carefully considered, restricted to a limited time, and followed by more appropriate therapies to address the underlying cause of inflammation.

Dosage: Improvement from willow bark treatment is usually observable within 1 to 4 weeks and is sometimes preceded by a transient worsening of symptoms that is followed by a significant decrease in discomfort, swelling, and inflammation. In some cases, improvement is seen within the first few days of initiation of therapy (Schmid, 1998).

Human:

Dried herb: 1-10 g TID

Dry standardized extract: tablets 500 mg TID (with 240 mg salicin)

Decoctions: 5-30 g per cup of water, with 1 cup of the tea given TID

Tincture (usually 35% ethanol; some pharmacies include glycerin to prevent precipitation by tannins) 1:2-1:3: 1-5 mL TID

Small Animal:

Dry standardized (to salicins) extract: 10 mg per day (cats)
Dried herb: 25-500 mg/kg, divided daily (optimally, TID)
Tincture (usually in 35% ethanol) 1:2-1:3: 0.5-2.5 mL per 10 kg (20 lb), divided daily (optimally, TID) and diluted or combined with other herbs. Higher doses may be appropriate if the herb is used singly and is not combined in a formula.

References

Abebe W. Herbal medication: potential for adverse interactions with analgesic drugs. J Clin Pharm Ther 2002;27:391-401.

Akao T, Yoshino T, Kobashi K, Hattori M. Evaluation of salicin as an antipyretic prodrug that does not cause gastric injury. Planta Med 2002;68:714-718.

Anonymous. *Monographs on the Medicinal Uses of Plants*. Exeter: European Scientific Cooperative on Phytotherapy; 1997.

Chrubasik S, Eisenberg E, Balan E, Weinberger T, Luzzati R, Conradt C. Treatment of low back pain exacerbations with willow bark extract: a randomized double-blind study. Am J Med 2000;109:9-14.

Chrubasik S, Künzel O, Model A, Conradt C , Black A. Treatment of low back pain with an herbal or synthetic anti-rheumatic: a randomized controlled study: Willow bark extract for low back pain. Rheumatology 2001;40:1388-1393.

de Bairacli Levy J. *Herbal Handbook for Farm and Stable*. London: Faber and Faber; 1963.

Fougere B. Salicylate safety and cats. In: *Proceedings of the Veterinary Business Management Association Symposium;* September 19-20, 2003; Durham, North Carolina.

Friend D. Aspirin: the unique drug. Arch Surg 1974;108:765-769.

Goldring MB. The role of cytokines as inflammatory mediators in osteoarthritis: lessons from animal models. Connect Tissue Res 1999;40:1-11.

Haenichen T, Wisser J, Wanke R. Chronic tubulointerstitial nephropathy in six okapis *(Okapia johnstoni)*. J Zoo Wildlife Med 2001;32:459-464.

Krivoy N, Pavlotzky E, Chrubasik S, Eisenberg E, Brook G. Effect of *Salicis cortex* extract on human platelet aggregation. Planta Med 2001;67:209-212.

Levesque H, Lafont O. [Aspirin throughout the ages: a historical review.] Rev Med Interne 2000;21(suppl 1):8s-17s.

Marz RW, Kemper F. Willow bark extract—effects and effectiveness: status of current knowledge regarding pharmacology, toxicology and clinical aspects. Wien Med Wochenschr 2002; 152:354-359.

Mayer R, Mayer M. Mayer R, Mayer M. Biological salicyl therapy with cortex salicus [Weidenrinde]. Pharmazie 1949;4:77-81.

McLean S, Pass GJ, Foley WJ, Brandon S, Davies NW. Does excretion of secondary metabolites always involve a measurable metabolic cost? Fate of plant antifeedant salicin in common brushtail possum, *Trichosurus vulpecula*. J Chem Ecol 2001;27: 1077-1089.

Schmid B, Kotter I, Heide L. Pharmacokinetics of salicin after oral administration of a standardised willow bark extract. Eur J Clin Pharmacol 2001a;57:387-391.

Schmid B, Ludtke R, Selbmann HK, et al. Efficacy and tolerability of a standardized willow bark extract in patients with osteoarthritis: randomized placebo-controlled, double blind clinical trial. Phytother Res 2001b;15:344-350.

Schmid BM. Handling of Cox and gonarthroses with a dry extract of *Salix purpurea x daphnoides* [dissertation]. Tubingen, 1998.

Witch Hazel

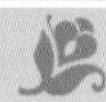

Hamamelis virginiana L. • ham-uh-MEE-lis *or* ham-uh-MAY-lis vir-jin-ee-AN-uh

Other Names: Spotted alder, winterbloom, snapping hazelnut

Family: Hamamelidaceae

Parts Used: Dried or fresh leaves or dried bark

Distribution: Indigenous to the Atlantic coast of North America (Bisset, 1994)

Selected Constituents: Major constituents of the dried leaf and bark are tannins (up to 10%) (Bisset, 1994; Bruneton, 1995). Leaf tannins are a mixture of gallic acid (10%), hydrolyzable hamamelitannin (1.5%), and condensed proanthocyanidins. Bark tannins are similar qualitatively but have a much higher hamamelitannin level—up to 65% of a hydroalcoholic extract (Bruneton, 1995). Essential oil and flavonoids are also present (Bisset, 1994).

Clinical Actions: Astringent, hemostatic, venotonic, anti-inflammatory

Energetics: Cold

History and Traditional Usage: It is used topically as a hemostat (Reynolds, 1996). For the treatment of colitis, diarrhea, dysentery, dysmenorrhea, eye inflammation, hematuria, kidney pain, and neuralgia; as a poultice for swellings, nosebleeds, and excessive menstruation. Also as a tonic (Farnsworth, 1998; Newall, 1996). It has been used for controlling internal and external hemorrhage; for hemorrhoids, bruises, and inflammatory swellings; also for diarrhea, dysentery, and mucous discharges. North American Indians used it as a poultice for painful swellings and tumors. It has been used for ophthalmia, menorrhagia, stomach and bowel complaints, and hemoptysis (Grieve, 1975).

In animals, it has been recommended for use in uterine, vaginal, and udder inflammation, as well as for torn udders that result in milk leakage, sore eyes, inflamed ears, wounds, sores, bruises, and ulcers in farm animals; internally, it was used for ulcerated and burned tissues from poisonings (de Bairacli Levy, 1963). It can be used for umbilical cords of the newborn and anal glands, for cleaning ears, and for treating patients with metritis and tail injuries (de Bairacli Levy, 1985). Veterinary *Materia Medica* texts make it clear that witch hazel has little systemic effect, but it is valued for its local effects, whether applied to skin lesions or directly onto the mucosa of the gastrointestinal or urinary tract. Winslow (1908) recommended it as an astringent and styptic for oozing wounds and to reduce the swelling and pain of bruises and sores. It was also recommended for anal irritation.

Published Research: In a randomized clinical trial involving 266 patients undergoing episiotomy, the efficacy of three analgesic treatments, including a cream containing witch hazel, a reference cream containing 1% hydrocortisone, and a local anesthetic and ice packs, was investigated to determine their effects on pain, bruising, and edematous swelling. The efficacy of all three analgesic treatments was found to be equal (Moore, 1989).

One study evaluated the antibacterial activity of six plants, including witch hazel leaves. The methanol extract of witch hazel showed inhibiting activity against many of the species tested. Results suggested that alcohol extracts of witch hazel could be used for topical periodontal prophylaxis (Iauk, 2003). Another study evaluated the antimicrobial activity of a distillate of witch hazel and urea formulated as a topical dermatologic preparation in 15 healthy volunteers. Significant antimicrobial activity for a product containing witch hazel distillate (90%) and urea (5%) was demonstrated (Gloor, 2002).

Another ointment prepared with witch hazel bark was assessed for efficacy and safety in a randomized, double-blind, placebo-controlled study for the treatment of patients with *Herpes labialis* infection. Thirty-four patients were treated within 48 hours of symptom recurrence; treatment lasted for 8 days. By the time therapy had ceased, the size of the inflamed area was significantly reduced in patients treated with witch hazel ointment as compared with placebo (Baumgaertner, 1998).

The phenolic constituents of witch hazel are responsible for its astringent activity (Vennat, 1992). Application of witch hazel preparations to the skin and mucosa in low concentrations sealed cell membranes and reduced capillary permeability (Steinegger, 1992). Higher concentrations precipitated proteins and thickened colloidal tissue, forming a thin membrane in the wound region (Laux, 1993). Alcohol extracts of witch hazel had strong astringent action, with the bark extract being slightly superior to the leaf extract (Grascza, 1987).

A randomized, double-blind, placebo-controlled trial compared the efficacy of three creams that contained witch hazel distillate, 0.5% hydrocortisone, or a drug-free vehicle for the symptomatic treatment of 72 patients with moderately severe atopic eczema. All treatments reduced the incidences of itching, scaling, and erythema after 1 week of treatment. The cream that contained witch hazel was no more effective than that containing placebo (Korting, 1995).

A randomized, double-blind comparison study assessed the efficacy of ointments that contain a standardized extract of witch hazel or bufexamac in the treatment of 22 patients with bilateral, moderately severe endogenous eczema (neurodermatitis). Patients were treated three times daily for an average of 17 days. Both treatments reduced the severity of symptoms such as desquamation of the skin, redness, itching, and lichenification, with desquamation showing the highest reduction; their efficacy was found to be the same (Swoboda, 1991). Later, in a pilot study of 37 patients with endogenous eczema (neurodermatitis), a cream witch hazel leaf extract was applied twice daily for 2 weeks. Following treatment, considerable improvement in symptoms such as inflammation and itching was noted in 24 patients (Wokalek, 1993).

A randomized, double-blind trial compared the efficacy of rectal ointments containing witch hazel, bismuth subgallate, or a local anesthetic in the treatment of 90 patients with acute, stage 1 hemorrhoidal symptoms. The local anesthetic was present in two control ointments, which also contained policresulen or fluocinolone acetonide. After 21 days, all four ointments were deemed equally effective in improving pruritus, bleeding, burning sensation, and pain (Knoch, 1992).

Indications: Topical application for minor skin lesions, bruises, sprains, local inflammation of the skin and mucous membranes, hemorrhoids, and varicose veins (Blumenthal, 1998; ESCOP Monographs, 1997). Diarrhea, colitis

Potential Veterinary Indications: Colitis, anal furunculosis, local inflammation of the skin and mucous membranes, ear cleaning, episiotomy, stomatitis

Contraindications: None found.

Toxicology and Adverse Effects: AHPA class 1. *The Botanical Safety Handbook* notes that the tannins in witch hazel may cause gastritis in susceptible individuals. Allergic contact dermatitis may occur in sensitive individuals (Bruynzeel, 1992; Granlund, 1994).

Preparation: The fluid extract of witch hazel leaves and bark was made by maceration and percolation with alcohol, glycerin, and water. It should be noted that "witch hazel water" is made of the bark that is macerated in water and distilled, with alcohol added to the distillate. Witch hazel water does not contain tannins, which are thought to be essential for the astringent and possibly anti-inflammatory effects.

Dosage:

External Use: Steam distillates are commonly available but are not thought to contain tannins. Herbalists do not recommend this form.

Decoction: 5-10 g to 250 mL water for poultices and wound irrigation

Rectal suppositories: 1-3 times daily, with the quantity of a preparation corresponding to 0.1-1.0 g crude drug

Infusion: undiluted or diluted 1:3 with water

Other preparations: several times daily, corresponding to 0.1-1.0 g drug in preparations (Blumenthal, 1998)

Internal Use: Rarely used internally

Human

Tincture 1:2-1:3: 1-2 mL TID, up to 6 times daily for acute conditions

Small Animal

Not used internally

Historical Veterinary Doses:

Horses: Hamamelis liquid extract, 30-60 mL per dose (RCVS, 1920)

Cows: 30-60 mL per dose (Winslow, 1908)

Pigs: Hamamelis liquid extract, 3.5-7 mL per dose (RCVS, 1920)

Dogs: Hamamelis liquid extract, 1.7-3.5 mL daily (RCVS, 1920); dogs, 2-8 mL (Winslow, 1908)

References

Baumgärtner M. A Hamamelis-Spezialextrakt zur lokalen Behandlung des Herpes labialis. Zs Allg Med 1998;74:158-161.

Bisset NG. *Herbal Drugs and Phytopharmaceuticals.* Boca Raton, Fla: CRC Press; 1994.

Blumenthal M, Goldberg A, Brinckman J, eds. *The Complete German Commission E Monographs.* Austin, Tex: American Botanical Council; 1998.

Bruneton J. *Pharmacognosy, Phytochemistry, Medicinal Plants.* Paris: Lavoisier; 1995.
Bruynzeel DP, van Ketel WG, Young E, van Joost T, Smeenk G. Contact sensitization by alternative topical medicaments containing plant extracts. Contact Dermatitis 1992;27:278-279.
De Bairacli Levy J. *The Complete Herbal Handbook for Farm and Stable.* London: Faber and Faber; 1963.
De Bairacli Levy J. *The Complete Herbal Handbook for the Dog and Cat.* London: Faber and Faber; 1985.
ESCOP Monographs on the Medicinal Uses of Plant Drugs. Fascicule 5. Devon: European Scientific Cooperative on Phytotherapy; 1997.
Farnsworth NR, ed. NAPRALERT database. Chicago, Ill: University of Illinois at Chicago; February 9, 1998 production.
Gloor M, Reichling J, Wasik B, Holzgang HE. Antiseptic effect of a topical dermatological formulation that contains Hamamelis distillate and urea. Forschende Komplementarmedizin und Klassische Naturheilkunde 2002;9:153-159.
Granlund H. Contact allergy to witch hazel. Contact Dermatitis 1994;31:195.
Grascza L. Adstringierende Wirkung von Phytopharmaka. Deutsche Apotheker Zeitung 1987;44:2256-2258.
Grieve M. *A Modern Herbal.* London: Jonathan Cape; 1931 (Reprint 1975).
Iauk L, Lo Bue AM, Milazzo I, Rapisarda A, Blandino G. Antibacterial activity of medicinal plant extracts against periodontopathic bacteria. Phytother Res 2003;17:599-604.
Knoch HG, Klug W, Hubner WD et al. Ointment treatment of 1st degree hemorrhoids: comparison of the effectiveness of a phytogenic preparation with two new ointments containing synthetic drugs. Fortschr Med 1992;110:135-138. [German]
Korting HC, Schafer-Korting M, Hart H, et al. Comparative efficacy of Hamamelis distillate and hydrocortisone cream in atopic eczema. Eur J Clin Pharmacol 1995;48:461-465.
Laux P, Oschmann R. Die Zaubernuss—*Hamamelis virginiana* L. Zeitschrift für Phytotherapie. 1993;14:155-166.
Moore W, James DK. A random trial of three topical analgesic agents in the treatment of episiotomy pain following instrumental vaginal delivery. J Obstet Gynaecol 1989;10:35-39.
Newall CA, Anderson LA, Phillipson JD. *Herbal Medicines: A Guide for Healthcare Professionals.* London: The Pharmaceutical Press; 1996.
RCVS (Royal College of Veterinary Surgeons). *Veterinary Counter Practice.* London: Ballantyne Press; 1920.
Reynolds JEF, Prasad AB. *Martindale, The Extra Pharmacopoeia.* 30th ed. London: The Pharmaceutical Press; 1996.
Steinegger E, Hansel R. *Pharmakognosie.* Berlin: Springer; 1992.
Swoboda M, Meurer J. Therapie von Neurodermitis mit Hamamelis virginiana Extrakt in Salbenform. Zeitschrift für Phytotherapie 1991;12:114-117.
Vennat B, Gross D, Pourrat A, et al. *Hamamelis virginiana:* identification and assay of proanthocyanidins, phenolic acids and flavonoids in leaf extracts. Pharmaceut Acta Helvet 1992;67:11-14.
Winslow K. *Veterinary Materia Medica and Therapeutics.* New York: William R. Jenkins; 1908.
Wokalek H. Zur Bedeutung epidermaler Lipide und des Arachidonsäurestoffwechsels bei feuilles d'hamamelis. Journal de Pharmacie de Belgique 1993;27:498-506.

Yellow Dock

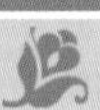

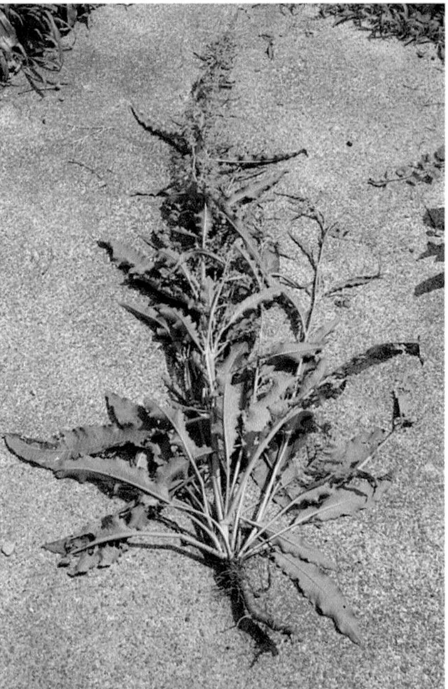

Rumex crispus L. • ROO-meks KRISP-us

Other Names: Curled dock, curly dock, narrow-leafed dock

Family: Polygonaceae

Parts Used: Root

Distribution: Native to Europe originally. Now a very common free-growing plant in many parts of the world.

Selected Constituents: Anthraquinone glycosides, including rhein and chrysophanol. Tannins, resin, volatile oil, oxalic acid, calcium oxalate, and vitamins A, B_1, B_2, B_3, and C

Clinical Actions: Alterative, cholagogue, purgative

Energetics: Cold, dry

History and Traditional Usage: Yellow dock has been used traditionally as an alterative for debility caused by cancer and necrosis. The root has laxative, alterative, and mildly tonic action and is used in "bilious complaints, rheumatism, and diphtheria"; it is used in the treatment of patients with blood diseases from jaundice to scurvy and with chronic skin disease. The anthraquinones have a gentle cathartic action on the bowel (Grieve, 1975). The Eclectics considered the root an alterative and an astringent. *Cook's Physiomedical Dispensatory* (1869) describes its indications and actions most succinctly as follows:

> "The greater portion of its power is expended upon the skin; but the gall-ducts, small intestines, and kidneys feel its impressions to a fair extent. Though not cathartic, it is fairly laxative; and exerts a desirable tonic and diluent influence upon the entire hepatic and alvine structures. It moderately resembles rhubarb, in the same botanical family. The chief use made of it is in scrofulous affections of the skin, scrofulous ulcers, and scrofulous forms of diarrhea; for all which it is of superior efficacy. . . . In nearly all forms of dry, scaly, and pustular skin disease, it has a deserved reputation,

both as an inward and an outward remedy; in itch and eczema . . ."

Published Research: Little published research exists despite the fact that it is a popular herbal medicine. The antioxidant activities, radical-scavenging activities, and antimicrobial activities of various extracts of the leaves and seeds of yellow dock were studied. The antioxidant activities increased with increasing amount of extracts (50-150 μg). Water extracts of both leaves and seeds showed antioxidant activity. The ether extracts of both leaves and seeds and the ethanol extract of leaves showed antimicrobial activities. None of the water extracts showed antimicrobial activity (Yildirim, 2001). It should be noted that these studies did not explore the root, which is the part that has been and is used medicinally.
Indications: Skin disease, chronic skin disease, jaundice, constipation
Potential Veterinary Indications: Chronic skin disease; constipation
Contraindications: Should not be used in high doses for prolonged periods. One should start at a low dose and increase to the point of normal motion. Griping may be due to free anthraquinones. Habituation may occur, and long-term use can lead to potassium loss. Calcium oxalate urolithiasis
Toxicology and Adverse Effects: AHPA class 2d because of oxalate content (see Contraindications, earlier) and anthraquinone content

Ten of 100 mature ewes exhibited acute oxalate poisoning within 40 hours after being penned on a small plot that contained patches of yellow dock, in which they ate aerial portions of the plant—which are not the subject of this monograph. Clinical signs included excess salivation, tremor, ataxia, and recumbency. Affected ewes were hypocalcemic and azotemic. Gross post mortem lesions in two ewes revealed perirenal edema and renal tubular degeneration. Oxalate poisoning was confirmed by histologic findings. Samples of yellow dock contained 6.6% to 11.1% oxalic acid, dry weight basis (Panciera, 1990).

A case of fatal poisoning due to ingestion of yellow dock (aerial parts) has been described. The patient, a 53-year-old man, presented with gastrointestinal symptoms, severe hypocalcemia, metabolic acidosis, and acute hepatic insufficiency (Reig, 1990).
Dosage:
Human:
Dried herb: 1-10 g TID (this is a bitter herb and the higher doses are not usually required)
Decoctions: 5-10 g per cup of water, with ½-1 cup of the tea given TID
Tincture (usually 25%-40% ethanol; some pharmacies include glycerin to prevent precipitation by tannins) 1:2-1:3: 0.5-3 mL TID
Small Animal:
Dried herb: 25-200 mg/kg, divided daily (optimally, TID)
Decoction: 5-10 g per cup of water, administered at a rate of ¼-½ cup per 10 kg (20 lb), divided daily (optimally, TID)
Tincture (usually 25%-40% ethanol) 1:2-1:3: 0.5-1.0 mL per 10 kg (20 lb), divided daily (optimally, TID) and diluted or combined with other herbs. Higher doses may be appropriate if the herb is used singly and is not combined in a formula.

References

Grieve M. *A Modern Herbal.* London: Jonathan Cape; 1931 (Reprint, 1975).
Panciera RJ, Martin T, Burrows GE, Taylor DS, Rice LE. Acute oxalate poisoning attributable to ingestion of curly dock *(Rumex crispus)* in sheep. J Am Vet Med Assoc 1990;196:1981-1984.
Reig R, Sanz P, Blanche C, Fontarnau R, Dominguez A, Corbella J. Fatal poisoning by *Rumex crispus* (curled dock): pathological findings and application of scanning electron microscopy. Vet Hum Toxicol 1990;32:468-470.
Yildirim A, Mavi A, Kara AA. Determination of antioxidant and antimicrobial activities of *Rumex crispus* L. extracts. J Agric Food Chem 2001;49:4083-4089.

Yerba Santa

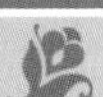

Eriodictyon californicum (Hook. Et Arn), Torr. = *Eriodictyon glutinosum* Benth. • Eh-err-o-DIK-tee-on kal-ih-FOR-nik-um
Other Names: California yerba santa, woolly yerba santa
Family: Hydrophyllaceae
Parts Used: Leaf
Selected Constituents: Flavonoids, volatile oil, tannins, catechins (eriodictyol), organic acids, resin

Eriodictyol

Clinical Action: Anti-inflammatory, antimicrobial, expectorant, carminative, diuretic
Energetics: Sweet, warm, pungent; transforms phlegm
History and Traditional Usage: Colds, cough, asthma, and other pulmonary disorders; stomachache; as a steam or bath for rheumatism; as an analgesic poultice for headache; a "blood purifier"; eyewash. Used by Coahuilla people as a poultice for sores on animals. *King's American Dispensatory* describes its use in "chronic mucous affections of the respiratory tract," chronic bladder catarrh, and catarrhal gastritis, but it is not very enthusiastic about its efficacy. The specific indication is as follows:

> "Chronic asthma with cough, profuse expectoration, thickening of the bronchial mucous membrane, loss of a petite, impaired digestion, emaciation" . . . "Cough, with abundant and easy expectoration."

Milks (1949) claimed that the leaves destroy bitter tastes but theorized that they would render alkaloids insoluble because of the tannic acid content. He also

warned that in many cases, the bitter taste had to be tasted for the herb to be effective.
Published Research: No relevant clinical trials found
Indications: Suppresses bitter taste and is used to mask the taste of bitter herbs in formulas. Used for bronchitis, asthma, cystitis, and rheumatism.
Potential Veterinary Indications: Upper and lower respiratory disorders requiring expectoration. As a flavor enhancer for herbal formulas
Contraindications: None reported.
Toxicology and Adverse Effects: AHPA class 1. None reported.
Dosage:
Human:
Dried herb: 1-10 g TID
Infusions: 5-30 g per cup of water, with 1 cup of the tea given TID
Tincture (usually high in ethanol) 1:2-1:3: 1-5 mL TID
Small Animal:
Dried herb: 25-500 mg/kg, divided daily (optimally, TID)
Infusion: 5-30 g per cup of water, administered at a rate of ¼-½ cup per 10 kg (20 lb), divided daily (optimally, TID)
Tincture 1:2-1:3: 0.5-2.5 mL per 10 kg (20 lb), divided daily (optimally, TID) and diluted or combined with other herbs. Higher doses may be appropriate if the herb is used singly and is not combined in a formula.
Historic Veterinary Doses (Karreman, 2004): Fluid extract (1:1): horses and cows, 15-60 mL; sheep and goat, 2-8 mL

References

Karreman H. *Treating Dairy Cows Naturally: Thoughts and Strategies.* Paradise, Pa: Paradise Publications; 2004.
Milks HJ. *Practical Veterinary Pharmacology, Materia Medica and Therapeutics.* Chicago, Ill: Alex Eger, Inc.; 1949.

Yucca

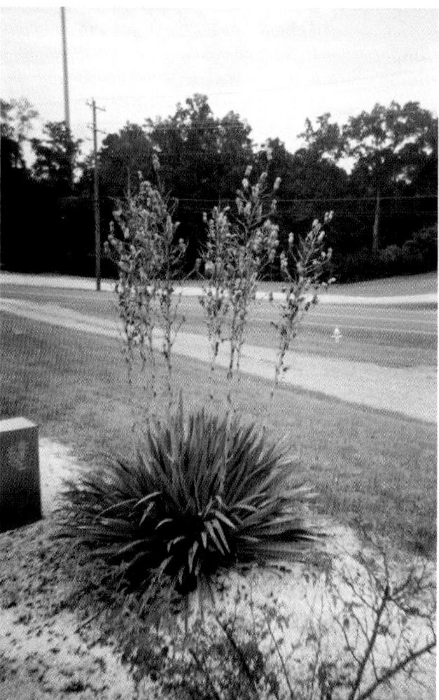

Yucca schidigera Roezl ex Ortgies • YUK-uh shi-di-GER-uh

Distribution: Southwestern United States to Northern Mexico; has spread to Eastern United States
Similar Species: *Yucca filamentosa, Yucca aloifolia* L., *Yucca filamentosa* L., *Yucca glauca* Nutt
Common Names: Mojave yucca, Spanish dagger, amole, Spanish bayonet, soapweed, soapwell, Adam's needle
Family: Liliaceae
Parts Used: Stalk, root, leaves
Selected Constituents: Steroidal saponins (including tigenin, smilagenin)
Clinical Action: Anti-inflammatory, antirheumatic, alterative, laxative
Energetics: Sweet, bland, cool
History and Traditional Usage: Poultices or baths for skin sores and other diseases. For inflammation of all sorts, including joint inflammation and bleeding. Other uses include arthritis, rheumatism, gout, urethritis, and prostatitis. Native Americans washed their hair with yucca to fight dandruff and hair loss. The plant was used more often as food and a source of string, or to make baskets or other usefulness, than for medicine. Root poultices were used for sprains, wounds, and ulcers; they were also applied to saddle sores on horses. The Lakota burned the root and believed the fumes allowed horses to be caught and haltered easily. Currently popular as a veterinary treatment for arthritis.
Published Research: In a preliminary trial, yucca has shown some benefit in the treatment of people with arthritis. The dose used was 1 g TID (Bingham, 1975).

In heifers given up to 6 g daily of *Yucca schidigera,* rumen propionate levels increased (Hristov, 1999). The authors concluded that this change was probably due to a selective inhibitory effect of yucca on rumen microbial species. Wilson (1998) found that in multiparous Holstein cows given 9 g of yucca daily, no effect on ruminal pH or ammonia was noted, and that milk yields were not benefited by supplementation.

Two different groups have studied the effects of yucca supplementation to canine and feline diets in reducing the odor of flatus (Giffard, 2001; Lowe, 1997a; Lowe, 1997b). Yucca appears to change the volatile components in the colon and specifically reduces hydrogen sulfide production. Lowe (1997b) also found that in cats, administration of yucca was correlated with a significant rise in serum urea nitrogen. Colina (2001) found that the addition of *Yucca schidigera* extract to the diet of nursery pigs reduced ammonia concentrations in the nursery room. In contrast to the study in cats, blood urea nitrogen levels were not increased.

Yucca was investigated in lambs for antigiardial activity and was found ineffective at controlling infection at doses of 10 g per lamb daily (McAllister, 2001).
Indications: Rheumatism, urethritis, prostatitis; as a poultice for wounds or sores
Potential Veterinary Indications: To reduce fecal odor. Some use it for osteoarthritis.
Contraindications: None reported.
Toxicology and Adverse Effects: AHPA class 1. Saponins may have a laxative effect when Yucca is taken in high doses. Some concern has been raised regarding the potential for saponins to be absorbed and cause intravascular

hemolysis, but this is a theoretical concern. Yucca is approved for use in foods as a foaming agent (particularly in root beer). Some people experience nausea, probably because of the saponin content, and should take the herb with food.

Drug Interactions: None reported.

Notes of Interest: The leaf fibers were used by Native Americans for cord, cloth, baskets, and sandals. Raw flowers were eaten in salads or were boiled as vegetables. The immature pods were roasted and peeled before eating. Dried seed pods are ground into flour and are used in the cooking of South and Central America. The roots have been used for soap.

Dosage:

Human:

Dried herb: 1 g TID

Tincture 1:2-1:3: 2-3 mL TID

Small Animal:

Dried herb: 25-200 mg/kg, divided daily (optimally, TID); cats: ¼ tsp daily (Tilford, 1999)

Tincture 1:2-1:3: 0.5-1.0 mL per 10 kg (20 lb), divided daily (optimally, TID) and diluted or combined with other herbs

References

Bingham R, Bellew BA, Bellew JG. Yucca plant saponin in the management of arthritis. J Appl Nutr 1975;27:45-50.

Colina JJ, Lewis AJ, Miller PS, Fischer RL. Dietary manipulation to reduce aerial ammonia concentrations in nursery pig facilities. J Anim Sci 2001;79:3096-3103.

Giffard CJ, Collins SB, Stoodley NC, Butterwick RF, Batt RM. Administration of charcoal, *Yucca schidigera,* and zinc acetate to reduce malodorous flatulence in dogs. J Am Vet Med Assoc 2001;218:892-896.

Hristov AN, McAllister TA, Van Herk FH, Cheng KJ, Newbold CJ, Cheeke PR. Effect of *Yucca schidigera* on ruminal fermentation and nutrient digestion in heifers. J Anim Sci 1999;77:2554-2563.

Lowe JA, Kershaw SJ. The ameliorating effect of *Yucca schidigera* extract on canine and feline faecal aroma. Res Vet Sci 1997a;63:61-66.

Lowe JA, Kershaw SJ, Taylor AJ, Linforth RS. The effect of *Yucca schidigera* extract on canine and feline faecal volatiles occurring concurrently with faecal aroma amelioration. Res Vet Sci 1997b;63:67-71.

McAllister TA, Annett CB, Cockwill CL, Olson ME, Wang Y, Cheeke PR. Studies on the use of *Yucca schidigera* to control giardiosis. Vet Parasitol 2001;97:85-99.

Tilford MW, Tilford G. *All You Ever Wanted to Know about Herbs for Pets*. Irvine, Calif: Bow Tie Press; 1999.

Wilson RC, Overton TR, Clark JH. Effects of *Yucca shidigera* extract and soluble protein on performance of cows and concentrations of urea nitrogen in plasma and milk. J Dairy Sci 1998;81:1022-1027.

Zizyphus, Chinese Date

Ziziphus jujuba Mill • ZIZ-ih-fuss JOO-joo-buh

Other Names: *Ziziphus jujuba* Mill is jujube = da zao (the fruit), Chinese date, Chinese jujube, jujube date. *Ziziphus jujube* Mill var. *spinosa* (Bunge) Hu ex H.E. Chow is a different herb—it is the seed of this plant, known as sour Chinese date, wild Chinese jujube, mountain jujube, suan dzao ren, suan zao or suan zao ren

Family: Rhamnaceae

Parts Used: Seed

Distribution: Zizyphus is indigenous to China and commonly grows on the mountains on the outskirts of Beijing. It also grows in India, Malaysia, Afghanistan, and Japan.

Selected Constituents: Saponins, including jujubosides (Tang, 1992), which are considered to be the active constituents. Also, fixed oil and volatile oil. Nutrients include vitamins A, B_2, and C and the minerals calcium, phosphorus, and iron. The triterpenoid glycoside ziziphin suppresses the sweet taste sensation.

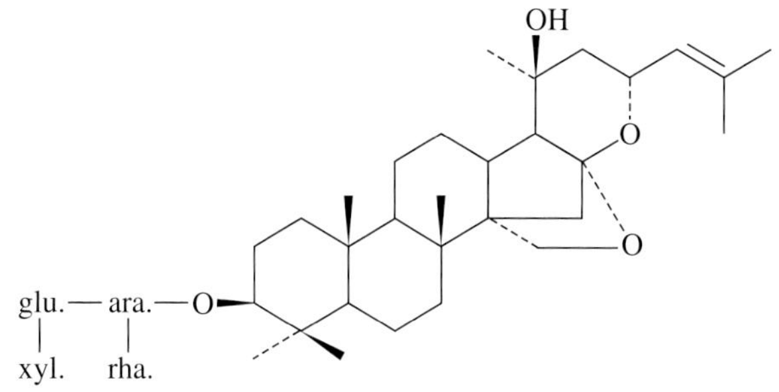

OH O O glu.— ara.—O xyl. rha.

Jujuboside

Clinical Actions: Sedative, hypnotic, hypotensive, anticonvulsant, antihydrotic, digestive tonic, nutritive, relaxant, stomachic

Energetics: Sour, neutral, sweet, mild

History and Traditional Usage: Zizyphus use is recorded as far back as the fifth century AD, for insomnia, palpitations, neurasthenia, forgetfulness, and nightmares (Leung, 1996). Zizyphus is also noted for abnormal sweating, including nightsweats, especially when accompanied by feelings of anxiety and irritability (Trickey, 1998). In Traditional Chinese Medicine, it acts on the liver and heart channels; it nourishes the heart and calms the nerves and is therefore used in insomnia and restless sleep. Zizyphus tonifies the spleen and benefits the stomach and is therefore used for weakness and shortness of breath. It nourishes the nutritive *Qi* and calms the spirit and is thus indicated for irritability, emotional debility, and convulsions. Zizyphus also moderates and harmonizes the characteristics of harsh herbs in a formulation (Bensky, 1986).

Published Research: In all, 50 Korean traditional plants were screened for effects on choline acetyltransferase and attenuation of scopolamine-induced amnesia. The methanolic extracts of Zizyphus, and especially oleamide, showed the highest activatory effect on choline acetyltransferase in vitro (Heo, 2003).

Jujuboside A is a main constituent extracted from the seed of *Ziziphus jujuba,* which is widely used in traditional medicine for the treatment of patients with insomnia and anxiety. A study examined the effects of jujuboside A on the glutamate-mediated excitatory signal pathway in the hippocampus. Results suggested that Jujuboside A has inhibitory effects on glutamate-mediated excitatory signal pathways in the hippocampus and probably acts through its anticalmodulin action (Zhang, 2003).

Antisteroidogenic activity has been shown in adult female mice treated with the ethyl acetate extract of *Ziziphus jujuba* bark. Changes in estrus cycle, body weight, weight of ovaries, steroidogenic enzymes, and substrates were assessed. It arrested the normal estrus cycle in the mice at diestrus stage and significantly reduced the weight of ovaries. Significant inhibition of δ(5)-3beta-hydroxysteroid dehydrogenase and glucose-6-phosphate dehydrogenase—two key enzymes in ovarian steroidogenesis—was also observed. Hematologic profiles and biochemical estimations were unaltered. Normal estrus cycle and ovarian steroidogenesis were restored after withdrawal of treatment, and antifertility activities were found to be reversible (Gupta, 2004).

Indications: For nervous depletion, anxiety, insomnia, excess sweating and palpitations, exhaustion, irritability, hypertension

Potential Veterinary Indications: Anxiety and restlessness, insomnia; cognitive dysfunction; reducing fertility in mice; hyperthyroidism (as an adjunct)

Contraindications: Zizyphus is contraindicated in conditions of excess dampness such as symptoms of epigastric distention and bloating. Caution should be used in cases of diarrhea. Zizyphus may have synergistic effects with a range of sedatives and hypnotics (Chang, 1987).

Toxicology and Adverse Effects: AHPA class 1. Very low toxicity if used orally. At 50 g/kg by decoction, it did not produce any toxicity in mice (Chang, 1987).

Dosage:

Human:

Dried herb: 1-10 g TID

Tincture 1:2 or 1:3: 1-5 mL TID

Small Animal:

Dried herb: 50-500 mg/kg, divided daily (optimally, TID)

Tincture 1:2-1:3: 1.0-3.0 mL per 10 kg (20 lb), divided daily (optimally, TID) and diluted or combined with other herbs

References

Bensky D, Gamble A. *Chinese Herbal Medicine Materia Medica.* Seattle, Wash: Eastland Press; 1986:580-581.

Chang HM, But PP. *Pharmacology and Applications of Chinese Materia Medica,* vol 2. Singapore: World Scientific; 1987.

Gupta M, Mazumder UK, Vamsi ML, Sivakumar T, Kindar CC. Anti-steroidogenic activity of the two Indian medicinal plants in mice. J Ethnopharmacol 2004;90:21-25.

Heo HJ, Park YJ, Suh YM, et al. Effects of oleamide on choline acetyltransferase and cognitive activities. Biosci Biotechnol Biochem 2003;67:1284-1291.

Leung A, Foster S. *Encyclopaedia of Common Natural Ingredients Used in Food, Drugs and Cosmetics.* New York: John Wiley; 1996:475-476.

Tang W, Eisenbrand G. *Chinese Drugs of Plant Origin.* Berlin: Springer Verlag; 1992.

Trickey R. *Women, Hormones & the Menstrual Cycle: Herbal and Medical Solutions from Adolescence to Menopause.* St. Leonards, NSW, Australia: Allen & Unwin; 1998:364.

Zhang M, Ning G, Shou C, Lu Y, Hong D, Zheng X. Inhibitory effect of jujuboside A on glutamate-mediated excitatory signal pathway in hippocampus. Planta Med 2003;69:692-695.

Weights and Measures Conversions*

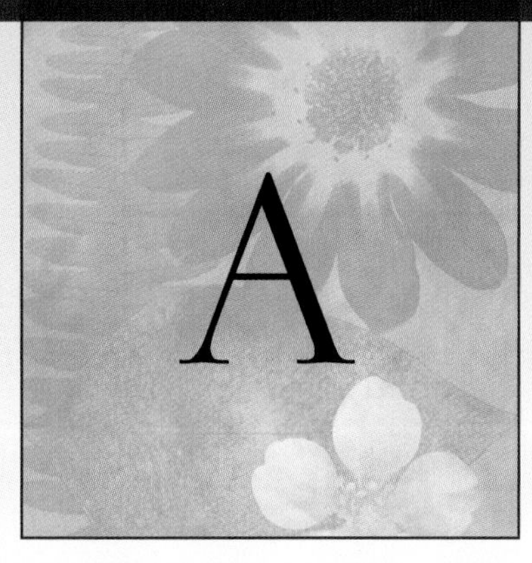

APPENDIX

Dry Weights

Measure	Symbol	Avoirdupois (this system is still common in the United States)	Troy	Apothecary
Pound	lb, lb avdp, or #	16 ounces 7000 grains 0.454 kilogram	1 lb t 12 ounces 240 pennyweight 5760 grains 0.373 kilogram	1 lb ap 12 ounces 5760 grains 0.373 kilogram
Ounce	℥ oz or oz avdp	16 drams 437.5 grains 0.0625 pound 28.350 grams	1 oz t 20 pennyweight 480 grains 0.083 pound 31.103 grams	1 oz ap 8 drams 480 grains 0.083 pound 31.103 grams
Dram	ʒ dr or dr avdp	27.344 grains 0.0625 ounce 1.772 grams		1 dr ap 3 scruples 60 grains 3.888 grams
Scruple	℈			1 s ap 20 grains 0.333 dram 1.296 grams
Grain	gr	0.037 dram 0.002286 ounce 0.0648 gram	0.042 pennyweight 0.002083 ounce 0.0648 gram	1 gr 0.05 scruple 0.002083 ounce 0.0166 dram 0.0648 gram
Pennyweight	dwt, pwt		24 grains 0.05 ounce 1.555 grams	
Kilogram	kg	2.2046 pounds		
Gram	g	0.035 ounce		
Milligram	mg	0.015 grain		
Microgram	µg	0.000015 grain		

* Merriam Webster online. An excellent online converter can be found at: http://www.people.virginia.edu/~rmf8a/convert.html. (accessed February 15, 2005).

Liquid Measures

Measure	Symbol	US Liquid	US Dry	British Imperial Liquid and Dry
Gallon	gal	4 quarts (231 cubic inches) 3.785 liters		4 quarts (277.420 cubic inches) 4.546 liters
Quart	qt	2 pints (57.75 cubic inches) 0.946 liter	2 pints (67.201 cubic inches) 1.101 liters	2 pints (69.355 cubic inches) 1.136 liters
Pint	pt	4 gills (28.875 cubic inches) 473.176 milliliters	1/2 quart (33.600 cubic inches) 0.551 liter	4 gills (34.678 cubic inches) 568.26 milliliters
Bushel	bu		4 pecks (2150.42 cubic inches) 35.239 liters	4 pecks (2219.36 cubic inches) 36.369 liters
Peck	pk		8 quarts (537.605 cubic inches) 8.810 liters	2 gallons (554.84 cubic inches) 9.092 liters
Gill	gi	4 fluid ounces (7.219 cubic inches) 118.294 milliliters		5 fluid ounces (8.669 cubic inches) 142.066 milliliters
Fluid ounce	fl oz	8 fluid drams (1.805) cubic inches) 29.573 milliliters		8 fluid drams (1.7339 cubic inches) 28.412 milliliters
Fluid dram	fl dr	60 minims (0.226 cubic inch) 3.697 milliliters		60 minims (0.216734 cubic inch) 3.5516 milliliters
Minim	♏	1 min cubic inch) 0.061610 milliliter	1/60 fluid dram (0.003760	1/60 fluid dram (0.003612 cubic inch) 0.059194 milliliter
Liter	L	61.02 cubic inches 1.057 quarts	0.908 quart	
Milliliter	mL	0.061 cubic inch	0.27 fluid dram	
Microliter	μL	0.000061 cubic inch	0.00027 fluid dram	

OTHER CONVERSIONS

ppm = mg/kg
1000 μg = 1 mg
1000 mg = 1 g

OTHER OLD WEIGHTS (Christopher, 1976)

1 teaspoon—1/2 dessertspoon, 1 dram, 60 grains, 4–5 mL, 3 scruples
1 dessertspoon—2 drams, 1/4 fluid oz, 120 grains, 8 mL, 6 scruples, 1/2 tablespoon, 1/8–1/10 teacup
1 tablespoon—4 drams
1 wineglass—2 oz
1 cup—8 oz

Capsules*

2 "0" sized capsules hold 3/4 teaspoon of dried herb, or about 1000 mg of dried herb.
2 "00" sized capsules will hold 1 teaspoon or 1300 mg of dried herb. They will also hold 60 drops or 1 teaspoonful of tincture.
2 "000" sized capsules hold approximately 1 1/3 teaspoon or 1600 mg of dried herb.
1 oz. of dried herb will make approx. 60 "0" sized capsules and 30 "00" sized capsules.

*The weights held by any specific capsule size will vary depending on the density of the herb

Suppliers

APPENDIX

U.S. SUPPLIERS

Veterinary Products Only

Jing Tang Herbal Company
9791 NW 160th Street
Reddick, FL 32686
Phone: 352-591-3165
Fax: 352-591-0988

Hilton Herbs, Ltd.
US Distributor
Chamisa Ridge
3212a Richard's Lane
Santa Fe, NM 87505
Phone: 1-800-743-3188
Fax: 1-505-438-4811
www.chamisaridge.com

Equilite, Inc.
437 Kulp Road
Pottstown, PA 19465
Toll Free: 1-800-942-LITE (5483)
Direct: 610-326-6480
Fax: 610-326-6481
http://www.equilite.com/

Animals' Apawthecary
P.O. Box 212
Conner, MT 59827
Phone: 406-821-4090

Buck Mountain Botanicals
HC 30
Miles City, Montana 59301
Phone: 406-232-1185
Fax: 406-232-4491
www.buckmountainbotanicals.com

Healing Herbs for Pets
4292-99 Fourth Avenue
Ottawa, Ontario
Canada K1S 5B3
Phone: 613-230-9966
Fax: 613-230-0750
wwilmot@petherbs.com

Suppliers of Combination Nutraceutical/ Herb Formulas

Vetri-Science Laboratories
20 New England Drive-C 1504
Essex Junction, VT 05453-1504
Phone: 800-882-9993

Rx Vitamins for Pets
200 Myrtle Boulevard
Larchmont, NY 10538
Phone: 800-792-2222
Fax: 914-834-1804
www.rxvitamins.com

Genesis/Resources Ltd.
4093 Oceanside Boulevard, Suite B
Oceanside, CA 92056
Phone: 1-760-631-6225
Fax: 1-760-631-6227
Toll-Free: 1-877-P-E-T-S-4-L-I-F-E

Thorne Research, Inc.
25820 Highway 2 West
P.O. Box 25
Dover, ID 83825
Phone: 800-228-1966
www.thorne.com

Natural Animal Feeds
Telephone: 813-920-7613
Fax: 813-920-1642
http://www.naf-usa.com

Suppliers of Human Herbal Products

Chinese herbs

Health Concerns
8001 Capwell Drive
Oakland, CA 94621
Phone: 800-233-9355

Lotus Herbs
1124 N. Hacienda Boulevard
La Puente, CA 91744

Phone: 626-916-1070
Fax: 626-917-7763

Brion Corporation
9200 Jeronimo Road
Irvine, CA 92718
Phone: 800-333-4372

Institute of Traditional Medicine
2017 S.E. Hawthorne
Portland, OR 97214
Phone: 503-233-4907

MayWay Trading Company
1338 Cypress Street
Oakland, CA 94607
Phone: 510-208-3113

Nuherbs Co.
3820 Penniman Avenue
Oakland, CA 94519
Phone: 800-233-4307
Chinese herb combos

Golden Flower Chinese Herbs
P.O. Box 781
Placitas, NM 87043
Phone: 800-729-8509

Ayurvedic Medicine

Ayush Herbs, Inc.
2115 112th N.E.
Bellevue, WA 98006
Phone: 206-637-1400
Fax: 206-451-2670
ayurveda@ayush.com

Western Herbal Medicine

Herbalist and Alchemist
P.O. Box 553
Broadway, NJ 08808-0553
Phone: 908-689-9020
Toll-Free: 800-611-8235
Fax: 908-689-9071
www.herbalist-alchemist.com

Herb Pharm
P.O. Box 116
Williams, OR 97544
Phone: 800-348-4372
Fax: 541-846-6112

Wise Woman Herbals
P.O. Box 279
Creswell, OR 97426
Phone: 541-895-5172
Fax: 541-895-5174
http://www.wisewomanherbals.com/

Gaia Herbs
108 Island Ford Road
Brevard, NC 28712
Phone: 800-831-7780

Murdock Pharmaceuticals, Inc.
1400 Mountain Springs Park
Springville, UT 84663
Phone: 800-962-8873

Eclectic Institute, Inc.
14385 S.E. Lusted Road
Sandy, OR 97055
Phone: 800-332-4372

Essential Wholesale
8850 S.E. Herbert Court
Clackamas, OR 97015
Phone: 503-722-7557
Fax: 503-296-5631
http://www.essentialwholesale.com/
Unscented creams, shampoos, and cosmetic ingredients for use in formulating topical formulas

AUSTRALIAN SUPPLIERS

Veterinary Herbs

The Natural Vet Company
Drummoyne, Sydney, N.S.W.
Australia
Phone: 02-97198462
www.naturalvetcompany.com

Western Herbs

Mediherb
MediHerb Pty Ltd.
P.O. Box 713
Warwick QLD 4370
Australia
Toll-Free: 1-800-639-122
www.mediherb.com.au
Medical grade herbal medicines, excellent technical support

Phytomedicine

P.O. Box 1995
Dee Why N.S.W. 2099
Phone: 02-9939-1380
Toll-free: 1-800-822-922
www.phytomedicine.com.au
Medical grade herbal medicines

Chinese Herbs

Sun Ten
P.O. Box 830
Hamilton, Queensland 4007
Phone: 07-3260-3300
Phone (country and interstate): 1-800-777-648
Chinese herbs—singles and formulas

Acuneeds Australia
622 Camberwell Road
Camberwell, VIC 3124

Australia
www.acuneeds.com.au
Toll-Free: 1-800-678-789
Phone: 03-9889-4100
Variety of Chinese herbal products

Helio Supply Company
Chippendale Sydney N.S.W.
Australia
Phone: 02 9698-5555
Variety of Chinese herbal products

Other Supplies

Plasdene
6 Sheridan Close
Milperra N.S.W. 2214
Phone: 02-9773-8666
Toll-Free: 1-800-252-709
Glass dispensing bottles

UNITED KINGDOM SUPPLIERS

Natural Animal Feeds (NAF) and Nutrilabs
Wonastow Road Industrial Estate West
Monmouth
NP25 5JA
United Kingdom
Tel : 0800 373106 (Freephone)
Fax: 01600 710701
http://www.naf-uk.com/

Dorwest Herbs Ltd.
Shipton Gorge
Bridport Dorset
United Kingdom
DT6 4LP
Phone: +44-0-870-733-7272
Fax: +44-0-870-733-7929
info@dorwest.com

Wendals Herbs
Phone: +44-01945-780880
Fax: +44-01945-780044
United States & Canada
Toll-Free: 1-800-981-0320
Republic of Ireland
0503 75006
http://www.wendals.com/

Dodson and Horrell
Dodson & Horrell Ltd.
Ringstead
Northamptonshire
NN14 4BX
United Kingdom
Phone: +44-0-1832-737300
Fax: +44-0-1832-737303
http://www.dodsonandhorrell.com

Hilton Herbs
Downclose Farm
North Perrott
Crewkerne
Somerset
England
TA18 7SH
Phone: +44-1460-270700
Fax: +44-1460-270702
http://www.hiltonherbs.com

Global Herbs Ltd.
Tamarisk House
12 Kingsham Ave.
Chichester
W. Sussex PO19 2AN
United Kingdom
Tel: 01243 773363
Fax 01243 788775
http://www.globalherbs.co.uk/

CANADIAN SUPPLIERS

The Natural Path Herb Company
8215-102 Street
Edmonton AB Canada
T6E4A5
fax: 780-438-0465
ph: 780-436-3040
email:naturvet@telusplanet.net
www.nphc.ca

Seroyal International Inc.
44 East Beaver Creek Road, Suite 17
Richmond Hill ON l4B 1G8
Phone: 905-764-6355
Fax: 905-764-6357
Supplements

T.C. Unicorn
Toronto
Phone: 1-800-567-1668
Herbs

Eastern Current Distributing Ltd.
#200A 3540 West 41st Avenue
Vancouver, BC V6N 3E6
Toll-Free: 1-800-667-6866
Phone: 604-263-5042
Fax: 604-263-8781
www.acupuncturetcm.com
Herbs, AP needles, and other supplies

Nutra Med
3168 Drinkwater Road
Duncan, BC
Phone: 250-746-9397
Fax: 250-746-3966
Supplements

Lucid Distributors, Inc.
Animal Health Products
Unit B 9444 190th Street
Surrey, BC
V4N 3S2

Phone: 604-882-9918
Fax: 604-882-9443
Supplements

NutriScience
51 Beverly Hills Drive
Toronto, Ontario M3L 1A2
Phone: 416-240-1234
Toll-Free: 1-800-661-2434
Fax: 419-249-0341
Supplements

Training in Herbal Medicine

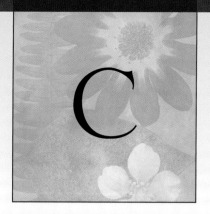

APPENDIX

VETERINARY HERBAL MEDICINE

U.S. Courses in Veterinary Herbal Medicine

Integrative Veterinary Herbalism
Tufts University School of Veterinary Medicine
200 Westboro Road
North Grafton, MA 01536
Phone: 508-839-5302
http://www.tufts.edu/vet/continedu/vetCEinfo@tufts.edu
Offered episodically through the Continuing Education Program

International College of Veterinary Herbal Medicine
http://www.vetherbalmedicine.com *Basic to advanced online education*

Chi Institute
9708 West Highway 318
Reddick, FL 32686
Phone: 1-800-891-1986, 352-591-5385
Fax: 352-591-2854
www.tcvm.com
admin@tcvm.com
In-depth course on Chinese veterinary herbal medicine

Healing Oasis Wellness Center
2555 Wisconsin Street
Sturtevant, WI 53177
Phone: 262-884-9549
Fax: 262-886-6460
www.thehealingoasis.com
In-depth course on Chinese and Western veterinary herbal medicine

International Veterinary Acupuncture Society
P.O. Box 271395
Fort Collins, CO 80527-1395
Phone: 970-266-0666
Fax: 970-266-0777
Ivasoffice@aol.com
www.ivas.org
In-depth course on Chinese veterinary herbal medicine

New Mexico Chinese Herbal Veterinary Medicine Course
1925 Juan Tabo N.E., Suite E
Albuquerque, NM 87112
Phone: 505-450-4325
Fax: 505-332-4775
In-depth course on Chinese veterinary herbal medicine

Veterinary Botanical Medicine Association
Jasmine C. Lyon, Executive Director
1785 Poplar Dr.
Kennesaw, GA 30144
http://www.vbma.org
Various online courses, annual Veterinary Herbal Medicine Symposium

Veterinary Information Network
www.vin.com
Offers introductory and intermediate courses online from time to time

UK Courses in Veterinary Herbal Medicine

Introduction to Veterinary Herbal Medicine
Course coordinator: Jimmy Symmonds, MRCVS
Phone: +44-0-1869-349955
courses@healthybeast.com
www.healthybeast.com

Canadian Courses in Veterinary Herbal Medicine

Academy of Veterinary Acupuncturists of Canada
C.P. 73
Beaconsfield
Québec, Canada
H9W 5T6
Phone: 514-697-0295
office@avac.ca

Australian Courses in Veterinary Herbal Medicine

Introduction and Intermediate Veterinary Herbal Medicine (Western)
Course coordinator: Barbara Fougere
www.naturalvet.com.au
courses@naturalvet.com.au

Courses in Traditional Chinese Herbal Veterinary Medicine

Course coordinator: Barbara Fougere
Contact: courses@naturalvet.com.au

HUMAN HERBAL MEDICINE

Selection of U.S. Courses

Herbal Therapeutics
Principle Instructor: David Winston, AHG
School of Botanical Medicine
P.O. Box 553
Broadway, NJ 08808
classes@herbaltherapeutics.net

Botanologos
Principal Instructor: Patricia Kyritsi Howell
P.O. Box W
Mountain City, GA 30562
Phone: 706-746-5485
info@botanologos.com
http://www.botanologos.com/

Planet Herbs Home Study Course
Principal Instructors: Michael and Lesley Tierra
East West School of Herbology
P.O. Box 275
Ben Lomond, CA 95005
Phone: 800-717-5010
herbcourse@planetherbs.com

Tai Sophia Institute for the Healing Arts
Principal Instructor: Simon Mills
7750 Montpelier Road
Laurel, MD 20723
Phone: 410-888-9048
Fax: 301-725-1674
Toll-Free: 800-735-2968
http://www.tai.edu/

Southwest School of Botanical Medicine
Principal Instructor: Michael Moore
P.O. Box 4565
Bisbee, AZ 85603
Phone: 520-432-5855
http://www.swsbm.com/homepage/

Foundations in Herbal Medicine
Principal Instructor: Tierona Low Dog, MD, AHG
P.O. Box 4544
Albuquerque, NM 87196
Phone: 888-857-1976
Fax: 505-266-2160
Fihm1@aol.com
http://www.fihm.com

Selection of European Courses

The Scottish School of Herbal Medicine
Unit 20, Alexander Stephen House
91 Holmfauld Road
Glasgow G51 3BA
Phone: 0141-445-2500
sshm@herbalmedicine.org.uk
www.herbalmedicine.org.uk

Middlesex University
Queens Way
Enfield
EN3 4SA
Phone: 0208-411-5161
enadmissions@mdx.ac.uk
www.mdx.ac.uk

University of Westminster
115 New Cavendish Street
London
W1M 6UW
Phone: 0207-911-5000
http://www.wmin.ac.uk/sih/page-45

The University of Central Lancashire
Preston
PR2 2HE
Phone: 44/0-1772-201-201
www.uclan.ac.uk/parttime/section1/19.htm

Napier University
Faculty of Health and Life Sciences
School of Community Health
Canaan Lane Campus
74 Canaan Lane
Edinburgh EH9 2TB
Phone: 0131-455-5653 or 5315 (course tutors)
www.napier.ac.uk

University of Lincoln
Brayford Pool
Lincoln
LN6 7TS
Phone: +44-0-1522-882000
www.lincoln.ac.uk

Selection of Australian Courses

The National Herbalists Association of Australia (NHAA) is the peak herbal medicine body in Australia. It does not accredit training institutions—only individual courses. Its professional process ensures that full membership in the NHAA is granted only when a person has successfully completed the required course content. See www.nhaa.org.au to ensure that any course undertaken is accredited.
Australasian College of Natural Therapies
P.O. Box K1356
Haymarket N.S.W. 1240
Australia
Phone: 02-9218-8888
Toll-Free: 1-800-46-2268

For postgraduate courses
The Australian College of Phytotherapy Pty, Ltd.
P.O. Box 661
Warwick
Queensland 4370
Australia
Phone: +61-7-4661-9653
www.herbaleducation.com.au

Herbal Terminology

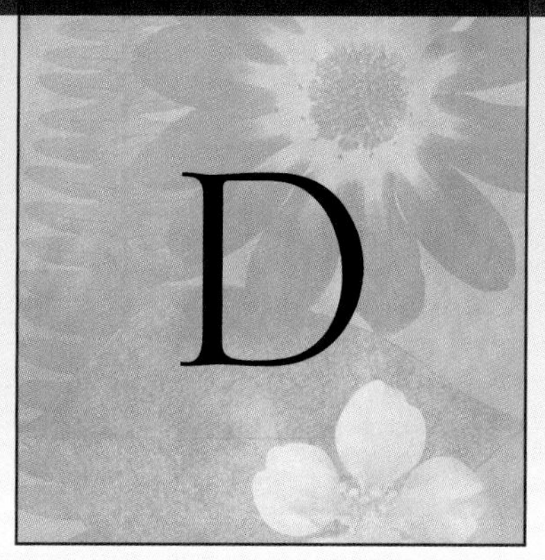

APPENDIX

These traditional categorizations of herbs are based on their clinical actions.

Adaptogen A plant adaptogen is a "smooth" pro-stressor that reduces reactivity of host defense systems and decreases damaging effects of various stressors caused by increased basal levels of mediators involved in the stress-response (Panossian, 1999). Adaptogens allow easy adaptation of the entire body to the environment or illness; they achieve this by enhancing homeostatic mechanisms. Adaptogens act on nervous, endocrine, or immune function via the hypothalamic-pituitary-adrenal axis. Some think the term is synonymous with "tonic"; however, tonics may act simply as nutritional supplements, or they may have direct immune-modulating effects. The term was originally coined by Soviet researchers, who defined an adaptogen as a substance that (1) increases nonspecific responses to stress, (2) is mild, without strong adverse effects, and (3) can be taken for extended periods, similar to a food.

Alterative A traditional term for an herb that "cleanses and purifies" the blood by gradually modulating tissue metabolism; it restores absorptive and excretory functions and most have mild diuretic or laxative properties. An alterative herb may change the course of a chronic condition by improving overall physiological functioning of the patient. Some equate "alterative" with "depurative."

Amphoteric A substance that normalizes organ or system dysfunction. If deficient, the herb stimulates activity; if excessive, the herb may normalize or even blunt activity. It has opposite physiologic action (e.g., it lowers and elevates blood pressure). This bidirectional modulation of physiology occurs because of the multitude of constituents in the herb; the body takes what it needs and "knows what to do."

Analgesic Relieves pain when administered orally

Anodyne Relieves pain via topical application

Anitcatarrhal Diminishes secretions, inflammation, and congestion of all mucous membranes

Antiphlogistic Relieves and counters inflammation

Antispasmodic Relieves muscle spasms

Aperient Mild laxative; gentle and nonirritating purgative causing slight increase in peristalsis

Aromatic Herbs with strong odor that stimulate the digestive system

Asthenia Lack or loss of strength; debility; any weakness, but especially one originating in muscular or cerebellar disease

Asthenic Weak; pertaining to asthenia; body constitution characterized by a narrow, shallow thorax, a long thoracic cavity, and a short abdominal cavity

Astringent Contracts and firms tissues and organs; decreases secretions and discharges. Binds proteins, glycoproteins, and carbohydrates (mucin) in the body and on microorganisms

Balsam A soothing and healing agent

Bitter An agent that increases tone and activity of gastric mucosa, improves the appetite, and stimulates gastric juices. The term covers a number of different types of phytochemicals. Bitters that are prescribed for gastrointestinal problems are meant to be tasted to stimulate secretion of saliva and stomach acids; this may limit their traditional use in animals.

Calmative Nourishes the entire body and nervous system

Carminative Promotes proper intestinal function, relieves indigestion, abdominal distention, and flatulence

Cathartic Strong laxative that causes rapid evacuation of the colon

Cholagogue Cholagogues stimulate release and flow of bile formed in the liver; generally a property of bitters, but produced by other plant constituents as well.

Choleretic Choleretics stimulate bile production by hepatocytes and most have effective cholagogue properties as well.

Counterirritant External application to relieve more deep-seated pain through hyperemia or local irritation

Decoction Herb extracted by boiling (used for hard parts of plants like seeds, roots, and bark)

Demulcent Soothes, protects, and restores mucous membranes; relieves irritation of inflamed or abraded surfaces, usually through mucilage content

Depurative "Blood purifying"; aids in the removal of metabolites, mineral, drugs, and so forth from the body via the gastrointestinal tract, urine, skin, or lungs
Diaphoretic Promotes perspiration via dilation of vessels in the skin
Diathesis Constitutional predisposition to certain disease conditions
Diuretic Increases the flow of urine
Emmenagogue Promotes and normalizes menstrual flow
Emollient Softening, soothing, and/or protecting
Escharotic An herbal paste (sometimes caustic or corrosive) that is capable of producing an eschar (or scab) that is most often used for the removal of warts and tumors
Expectorant Promotes and dispels mucus from lungs and bronchi
Febrifuge Assists the body to reduce fever
Fluid extract Plant extract 1:1 (i.e., 1 mL of liquid equals 1 gram of herb)
Galactagogue Promotes lactation
Galenical Standard medicinal preparation (as an extract or tincture) that contains usually one or more active constituents of a plant; made by a process that leaves the inert and other undesirable constituents of the plant undissolved
Glycetract Herb extracted in glycerine or alternatively extracted in alcohol, then the alcohol is removed and replaced with glycerine as a preservative.
Hemostatic Stops the flow of blood
Hypnotic Powerful relaxant and sedative that promotes drowsiness
Infusion Herbal extract prepared with warm or cold water as a tea (without boiling); used for soft parts of the plant like leaves, flower, or green parts
Liniment Soothing, liquid preparation for rubbing on the skin
Mucilaginous Contains mucins (complex carbohydrates) that are demulcent, emollient, and soothing
Narcotic Central nervous system depressant; relieves pain and promotes sleep
Nervine Herbs that tone, nourish, and strengthen the central nervous system; some stimulate, and some are relaxing or sedative
Neurocirculatory asthenia Psychosomatic disorder characterized by mental and physical fatigue, dyspnea, giddiness, precordial pain, and palpitation, especially on exertion
Nutritive Nourishes the body or affects metabolic processes; increases weight by providing supplies for tissue building; supplies vitamins, minerals, trace elements, amino acids, and/or fats
Oxymel Medicinal vinegar with added honey
Oxytocic Accelerates or facilitates childbirth
Parturient Stimulates uterine contractions that induce and assist labor
Pectoral Having an effect on diseases of the chest
Phytotherapy Using plants as medicine; a term used mainly in Europe, the UK, and Australia; a term that refers to both scientific and traditional herbal medicine
Protective Lessens damage from environmental influences, including what is taken into the body
Purgative Watery evacuation of the colon
Relaxant Eases tension and pain in the body and organs; nonsedating
Restorative Restores normal function of the body, organ, or system
Rubefacient Externally applied; reddens the skin by causing capillary dilation
Scrofula An obsolete term frequently seen in historical texts; refers to a variety of tuberculous adenitis. This is thought to consist of secondary involvement of cervical lymph nodes as a result of localized hematogenous spread from a pulmonary lesion. Most common in childhood.
Sedative Calms or tranquilizes by lowering functional activity
Sialagogue Promotes the flow of saliva
Stomachic Promotes normal physiologic function of the stomach
Styptic External application stops blood flow by constricting blood vessels
Succus Plant juice
Sudorific Promotes perspiration; stronger effect than diaphoretic
Tonic Slowly restores and strengthens the tone of the body, organ, or system; it stimulates nutrition and enhances or normalizes physiologic function
Troche Lozenge for slow dissolution in the mouth; commonly used for demulcent herbs
Trophorestorative Herb that restores function and morphology of a specific organ or tissue
Vermicide Kills intestinal worms
Vermifuge Dispels intestinal worms
Vesicant Causes blistering
Vital Force Energy that makes body, tissue, or cells grow, develop and restore enthalpy
Vulnerary Aids in wound and skin healing; usually applied externally

Client Handout: Hints on Administering Herbs to Animals*

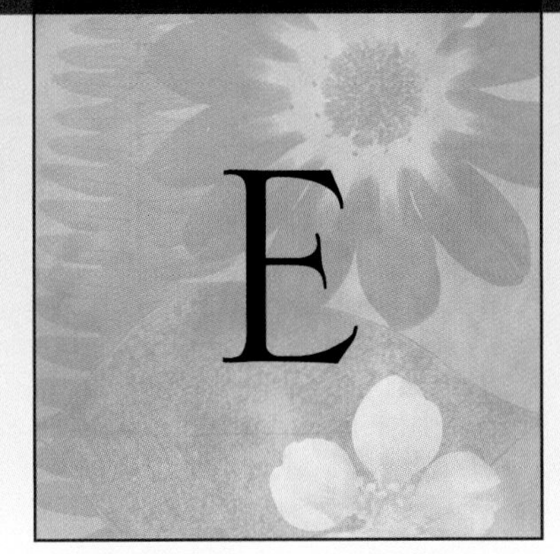

APPENDIX

Compiled by members of the Veterinary Botanical Medicine Association

Herbs can be beneficial to animals when medications are not working or are resulting in adverse effects, or when the practitioner or owner would prefer to try the natural medicine approach first. Administration of these herbs can be challenging at times. Here are a few suggestions on how to make their administration easier for both you and your animal companion. Sometimes, the effect of the herb varies according to the patient's actual ability to taste it, but in most cases, we have the option of trying to trick pets into taking herbs by disguising the taste in an "herb delivery system."

(Please consult your veterinary herbalist for information on the best quality herbs, the correct doses, and the best ways of giving them to your animals. Giving the wrong herbs or giving the correct herbs at incorrect doses can seriously damage your animal's health. This is especially important if your animal is taking other medication as well. Drug–herb interactions are real. Talk to your veterinary herbalist about this.)

MEDICATING DOGS AND CATS

Dogs and cats can be given powdered herbs, powder herb extracts, and liquid herb extracts in their meals. If your pet's appetite is poor because of illness or learned preferences, you may need to disguise the taste further by using especially strong-smelling foods, like tuna, sardines, or braunschweiger. For some pets, baby food or canned cat food is such a novelty that they will take the herbs mixed into these foods. Some pharmacies and veterinary manufacturers make flavored "tab wraps" for dogs and cats; these are especially designed to hide small tablets. Other tasty treats to hide the herbs include cream cheese, jelly, peanut or other nut butters, ground meat or liver, and fruit. Applesauce is particularly recommended by some herbalists. Flavored gravies for pets can also be used to dilute the herbs and mask the taste. If your pet's appetite is suppressed because of illness, do not mix medicines in regular meals—administer the herbs separately in a different food treat.

Powdered herbs may be mixed into small "pills" of butter, then frozen to increase firmness. You can blend them with anchovy paste, organic peanut butter, jelly, jam, sandwich pastes, or other thick tasty foods. It may be easier in some cases to administer the powdered or liquid herbs by mixing them into a liquid that is to be gently and slowly administered by syringe. Vehicles that have been recommended include meat or poultry broth, clam juice, flavored syrups (one veterinary product is VAL Syrup™, (Fort Dodge Animal Health, Overland, KS), and fruit juice.

You can take advantage of your cat's fastidiousness by mixing the herb in a hairball gel (such as VetBasis [petroleum free] (Pet Living, Inc, Bloomington, MN) or Laxatone™ (Evsco Pharmaceuticals, Buena, NJ) vegemite or anchovy paste, and smearing it on his or her paws—only very sick cats will let that insult go unchallenged! Some herbalists make traditional teas using meat broth instead of plain water, then frozen in ice cube trays to preserve until the day of use.

Liquid herbal extracts are often not accepted in any form by some animals. In this case, you can use a dropper to put the extract into a capsule, close it, and administer it to the animal in that form quickly. *Always* dilute liquid extracts (preferably with something sweet-tasting) if giving directly into the mouth.

If herb capsules must be administered, they often "go down" more easily if one end is covered in butter. Be sure to administer water or broth afterward to ensure that the capsule passes quickly from the esophagus to the stomach.

RABBITS AND BIRDS

Rabbits can be medicated by grinding herbs into their pellets with a coffee grinder. Mix dried herbs with good quality honey. Strawberry jam is effective in disguising the taste before administration to exotic species. Birds, especially parrots, seem to accept liquid extracts when dropped onto a cracker.

Your veterinary herbalist may also recommend other routes of administration, such as by enema. This is especially appropriate for vomiting animals.

If your pet has food allergies or any other illness, check the herb delivery system with your veterinarian before using it.

MEDICATING HORSES AND FARM ANIMALS

Horses and ruminant farm animals are herbivores—natural grazers, used to eating many different plant materials. They usually accept herbs mixed in their grain and pellet rations. If that doesn't work, applesauce, molasses, or frozen concentrated fruit juices can be effective vehicles.

FINAL CAUTIONS

Some animals will not tolerate herbs in any form, and we must accept that in some cases, insisting on the continued administration of these medications may affect their quality of life. If your pet won't accept herbs, discuss this with your veterinary herbalist.

Index

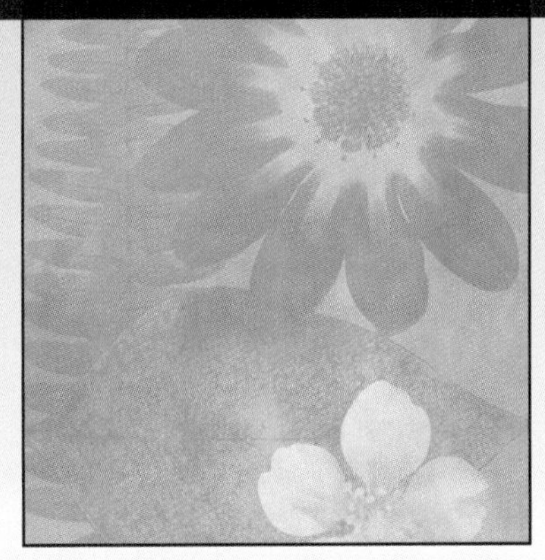

Page numbers followed by f indicate figures; t, tables; b, boxes

E

G

H

N

Q

R

T